Lippincott's

Nursing Procedures

FIFTH EDITION

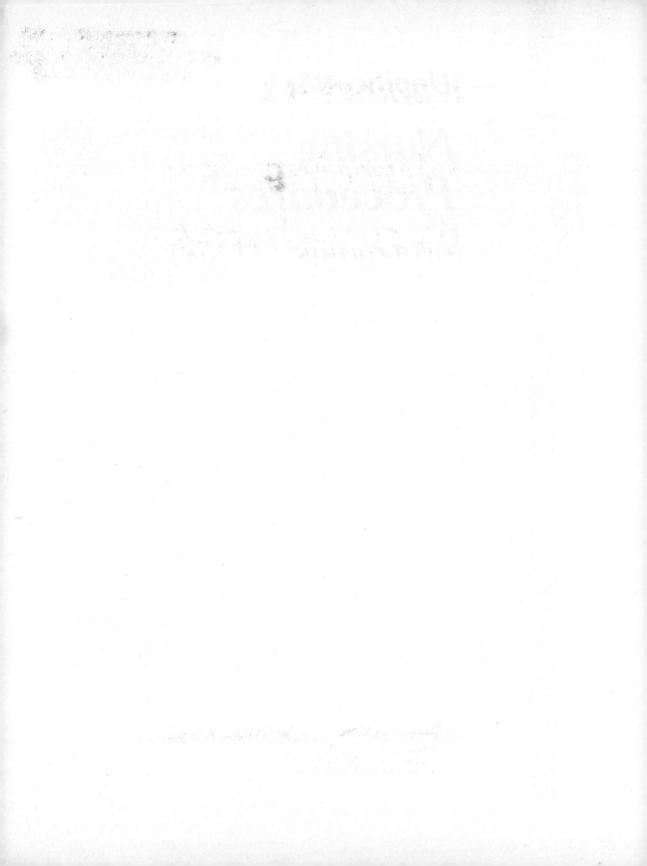

[redacted]

Lippincott's

Nursing Procedures

FIFTH EDITION

Wolters Kluwer Health | Lippincott Williams & Wilkins

Philadelphia • Baltimore • New York • London
Buenos Aires • Hong Kong • Sydney • Tokyo

Staff

Executive Publisher
Judith A. Schilling McCann, RN, MSN

Editorial Director
H. Nancy Holmes

Clinical Director
Joan M. Robinson, RN, MSN

Art Director
Elaine Kasmer

Clinical Project Manager
Jennifer Meyering, RN, BSN, MS, CCRN

Editor
Jennifer P. Kowalak

Copy Editors
Kimberly Bilotta (supervisor), Carol Brown, Scotti Cohn, Heather Ditch, Jeannine Fielding, Amy Furman, Linda Hager, Elizabeth Mooney, Dona Perkins, Pamela Wingrod

Designers
Linda J. Franklin, Susan Hopkins Rodzewich, Joseph John Clark, Larry Didona (cover design)

Digital Composition Services
Diane Paluba (manager), Joyce Rossi Biletz, Donna S. Morris

Associate Manufacturing Manager
Beth J. Welsh

Editorial Assistants
Karen J. Kirk, Jeri O'Shea, Linda K. Ruhf

Indexer
Barbara Hodgson

Acknowledgment
Photographs of the bariatric bed, page 95, and the Vollman Prone Positioner, pages 598 and 599, courtesy of Hill-Rom, Inc., Batesville, Ind.

LNP5010508

Library of Congress Cataloging-in-Publication Data

Lippincott's nursing procedures.—5th ed.
p. ; cm.
Rev. ed. of: Nursing procedures. 4th ed. c2004.
Includes bibliographical references and index.
1. Nursing. I. Lippincott Williams & Wilkins. II. Nursing procedures. III. Title: Nursing procedures.
[DNLM: 1. Nursing Care. WY 100 L765 2009]
RT41.N886 2009
610.73—dc22
ISBN-13: 978-0-7817-8689-8 (alk. paper)
ISBN-10: 0-7817-8689-4 (alk. paper) 2008000920

Contents

Advisory board

Contributors and consultants

Deborah H. Allen, RN, MSN, FNP, APRN,BC, AOCNP
Preston Robert Tisch Brain Tumor Center at Duke & Tug McGraw Quality of Life Research Center at Duke University
Durham, N.C.

Susan E. Antczak, RN, OCN
Clinical Instructor, CNA program
Staff Nurse, per diem pool
Fox Chase Cancer Center
Philadelphia

Rosemary Ashby, ARNP-C, BSN, MS, CGRN
Nurse Practitioner, Gastroenterology & Hepatology
James A. Haley Veteran's Hospital
Tampa, Fla.

Leslie A. Atkins, RN, PhD
Staff Nurse Intensive Care Unit
Norman (Okla.) Regional Hospital

Rita Bates, RN, MSN
Assistant Professor
University of Arkansas
Fort Smith

M. Brucene Bechtel, RN, MSN, CNS
CNS Psychiatry
Gaston Memorial Hospital—CaroMont Health
Gastonia, N.C.

Debbie Berry, RN, MSN, CPHQ
Internal Consultant, Resource Management
MedStar Health
Lutherville, Md.

Cheryl L. Brady, RN, MSN
Assistant Professor
Kent State University
Salem, Ohio

Denise Brehmer, RN, MSN
Visiting Lecturer
Indiana University, Kokomo

Tamara Capik, RN, BSN, CCRN
Registered Nurse—SICU
St. Joseph Hospital—Ministry Health Care
Marshfield, Wis.

Kathy Cochran, RN, MSN
Division Chair Health Technologies
Director and Instructor of Practical Nursing
Coosa Valley Technical College
Rome, Ga.

Cathy Conner, RN, ADN
Practical Nursing Instructor
Concorde Career College
Jacksonville, Fla.

Wendy Tagan Conroy, FNP,BC, MSN
Family Nurse Practitioner
Connecticut Valley Hospital
Middletown

Kim Cooper, RN, MSN
Nursing Department Chair
Ivy Tech Community College
Terre Haute, Ind.

Claire Cottrell, RN, MSN
Nursing Instructor
Mississippi Gulf Coast Community College
Perkinston

Lillian Craig, RN, MSN, FNP-C
Adjunct Faculty
Oklahoma Panhandle State University
Goodwell

Sherry Currie, RN, MN
Lead Instructor
Butler Community College
El Dorado, Kans.

Michelle Deligencia, RN, MSN, CNOR
Clinical Consultant
San Diego

Louise Diehl-Oplinger, RN, MSN, APRN-BC, CCRN, NP-C
Nurse Practitioner, Practice Owner
Lehigh Valley Wellness Center
Phillipsburg, N.J.

Jennifer E. DiMedio, CRNP, MSN, FNP
Family Nurse Practitioner
University of Pennsylvania—West Chester

Laurie Donaghy, RN, CEN
Staff Nurse
Frankford Hospital
Philadelphia

David Dunham, RN, MS, CRNI
Assistant Professor of Nursing
Hawaii Pacific University
Kaneohe

Shelba Durston, RN, MSN, CCRN
Nursing Instructor
San Joaquin Delta College
Stockton, Calif.

Anna Easter, APRN,BC, PhD, ACNP, CNS
Advanced Practice Nurse
Central Arkansas Veterans Health Systems
Little Rock

Patricia Eisenbraun, RN, ADN, ONC
Research Coordinator — Cardiovascular Area
North Central Heart Institute
Sioux Falls, S. Dak.

Judith Faust, RN, MSN
Assistant Professor
Ivy Tech Community College
Lafayette, Ind.

Emilie M. Fedorov, RN, MSN, CS, CNRN
Neuroscience/Surgical Intensive Care Unit Director
St. Mary's Hospital
Madison, Wis.

Cynthia L. Frozena, RN, MSN, OCN
Medical Writer
Enzymatic Therapy
Green Bay, Wis.

Vivian Gamblian, RN, MSN
Nursing Faculty
Baylor University, Louise Herrington School of Nursing
Dallas

Stephen Gilliam, RN, PhD, APRN-BC
Assistant Professor
Medical College of Georgia, School of Nursing
Athens

Margaret M. Gingrich, RN, MSN
Professor
Harrisburg (Pa.) Area Community College

Catherine Grant, CRNP, MSN
Instructor
Carlow University
Pittsburgh

Kim Graves, RN, MSN
Critical Care Nurse
Jewish Hospital
Cincinnati

Sandy Hamilton, RN, BSN, MEd, CRNI
Independent Contractor
Usana Health Sciences
Las Vegas

Allen Hanberg, RN, MSN
Assistant Professor of Nursing
Weber State University
Ogden, Utah

Donna Headrick, RN, MSN, FNP
Instructor
Taft (Calif.) Community College
Family Nurse Practitioner
Advanced Cosmetic Dermatology
Bakersfield, Calif.

Joy L. Herzog, RN
Director of Nursing Services
Golden Living Center of Doylestown (Pa.)

Nichole Lea Howe, RN, BSN
Charge Nurse — Women's Life Center
Newman Regional Health
Instructor — Maternal Child Nursing
Flint Hills Technical Center
Emporia, Kans.

Timothy L. Hudson, RN, MS, MEd, CCRN, FACHE
Evening/Night Nursing Supervisor
Martin Army Hospital
Ft. Benning, Ga.

Angela R. Irvin, RN, MSN, ARNP, NP-C
Assistant Professor of Nursing
Western Kentucky University
Bowling Green

Pamela L. Isbell, RN, MSN, CEN
Staff Nurse
Orlando (Fla.) Regional Medical Center

Fiona Johnson, RN, MSN, CCRN
Clinical Education Specialist/MedSurg Residency Coordinator
Memorial Health University Medical Center
Savannah, Ga.

Karla Jones, RN, MSN
Associate Professor
School of Nursing
University of Alaska
Anchorage

Christine Kennedy, RN, MSN
Staff Nurse — Specialty Clinics Area
Veterans Administration Connecticut Healthcare System
Adjunct Nursing Faculty
Excelsior College
West Haven

Laura Kierol-Andrews, RN, PhD, ACNP, APRN
Acute Care Nurse Practitioner
Manager of Medical Rapid Response Team
Department of Critical Care Medicine
The Hospital of Central Connecticut
New Britain General Campus

Susan M. Kilroy, RN, MS
Clinical Nurse Specialist
Massachusetts General Hospital
Boston

Carol T. Lemay, RN, ADN
Consultant
Brattleboro, Vt.

Grace G. Lewis, RN, MS, BC
Assistant Professor of Nursing
Georgia Baptist College of Nursing of Mercer University
Atlanta

Pamela Y. Mahon, RN, PhD, CNAA
Professor of Nursing
CUNY/Kingsborough
Brooklyn, N.Y.

Patricia J. McBride, RN, MSN, CIC
Infection Control Manager
Bryn Mawr (Pa.) Hospital

Nancy L. Miller, RNC, MSN, CCM
Nursing Professor
Keiser University
Ft. Lauderdale, Fla.

Nicolette C. Mininni, RN, MEd, CCRN
Advanced Practice Nurse, Critical Care
University of Pittsburgh Medical Center Shadyside

Pamela Moody, CRNP, MSN, PhD
Nurse Administrator Public Health—Area 3
Alabama Department of Public Health
Tuscaloosa

Jill Morsbach, RNC, MSN
Staff Nurse
St. Joseph Medical Center
Kansas City, Mo.
Nurse Entrepreneur
Nursing Station
Overland Park, Kans.

Beverly J. Murphy, RN, BSN, MS, APN, CRNA
Certified Registered Nurse Anesthetist
Anesthesia Associates of Northeast Illinois
Tinley Park
Adjunct Faculty
University of St. Francis
Joliet, Ill.

William J. Pawlyshyn, RN, BSN, MS, MN, APRN,BC, MDiv
Nurse Practitioner
Mid & Upper Cape Community Health Center
Hyannis, Mass.

Noel C. Piano, RN, MS
Instructor/Coordinator
Lafayette School of Practical Nursing
Williamsburg, Va.
Adjunct Faculty
Thomas Nelson Community College
Hampton, Va.

Susan Markel Poole, CRNI, BSN, MS, CNSN
Senior Director
Option Care
Buffalo Grove, Ill.

Monica Narvaez Ramirez, RN, MSN
Nursing Instructor
University of the Incarnate Word School of Nursing & Health Professions
San Antonio, Tex.

Jacqueline Regennitter, ADN, ANCC
Staff Nurse
Loring Care Center
Sac City, Iowa

Charles W. Reick, MS, RRT
Specialist, Respiratory Care
Greater Baltimore Medical Center
Towson, Md.

Lauren R. Roach, LPN, HCS-D
Nurse Support Coordinator
Good Samaritan Home Care Services, LLC
Vincennes, Ind.

Tracy A. Robinson, RN, BSN, CWOCN
Home Health Care
MacNeal Hospital
Berwyn, Ill.

Catherine Shields, RN, BSN
Nurse Educator
Ocean County Vocational School
Toms River, N.J.

Concha Carrillo Sitter, FNP-BC, MS, APN, CGRN
Gastroenterology Nurse Practitioner
Sterling (Ill.) Rock Falls Clinic

Angela Starkweather, CCRN, MSN, PhD, ACNP-C
Assistant Professor
Washington State University Intercollegiate College of Nursing
Spokane

Kimberly Such-Smith, RN, BSN, LNC
CEO, Nurse Case Manager, Nurse Supervisor, Legal Nurse Consultant
Nursing Analysis & Review, LLC
Byron, Minn.

Allison J. Terry, RN, MSN, PhD
Director, Center for Nursing
Alabama Board of Nursing
Montgomery

Janelle Wahlman, RN, MS, ACNM
Certified Nurse Midwife
Faculty
Midwifery Institute of Philadelphia University

Mary E. Walker, RN, MSN, CCRN, CCNS
Clinical Instructor, Department of Chronic Nursing Care
University of Texas Health Science Center at San Antonio

Marsha Wamsley, RN, MSN
Associate Professor
Sinclair Community College
Dayton, Ohio

Kate Willcutts, RD, MS, CNSD
Assistant Clinical Nutrition Manager/Assistant Professor
University of Virginia Hospital
Charlottesville

Kelly Witter, RN, MSN
Director
Great Oaks School of Practical Nursing
Cincinnati

Evelyn Yeaw, RN, PhD
Professor
University of Rhode Island College of Nursing
Kingston

Hollace Yowler, RN, MSN
Associate Professor
Ivy Tech Community College
Madison, Ind.

Dawn M. Zwick, RN, MSN, CRNP
Lecturer
Kent (Ohio) State University
Nurse Practitioner
Cleveland Clinic Foundation

Foreword

I commend you on your decision to include *Lippincott's Nursing Procedures*, Fifth Edition, among your clinical references. The health care market demands nurses who are clinically competent and able to provide optimum care, and that requires a clinical reference to assist us in meeting our patients' needs. Experienced practitioners, new graduates, and nursing students alike will discover the latest edition of this valuable reference to be an essential resource for providing safe, appropriate care in everyday practice.

Lippincott's Nursing Procedures, Fifth Edition, presents a wide scope of conceptual and practical clinical information. It discusses several hundred clinical procedures in step-by-step detail and includes full-color illustrations that depict correct technique for performance. Its reader-friendly features enable the student nurse to acquire knowledge of nursing skills and procedures and their rationales, allow a new graduate to gain confidence in performing those skills and procedures in the clinical setting, and assist the experienced practitioner to maintain competency.

New subject matter in this edition runs the gamut of nursing practice from basic to more advanced: sexual assault examination, communicating with difficult patients, basic sterile technique, immunization guidelines, patient-controlled analgesia, use of bariatric beds, hearing aid care, intake and output assessment, iontophoresis, medication error reduction, epicardial pacing wire removal, arterial and venous sheath removal, laryngeal mask airways, tracheostomy and ventilator speaking valves, continuous positive airway pressure, chest tube removal, peripheral nerve stimulation, amnioinfusion, vacuum extraction, intra-abdominal pressure monitoring, and tocolytic therapy.

Initial chapters detail fundamental procedures and skills, such as basic physical assessment techniques, infection control, specimen collection, application of restraints, and venipuncture. Successive chapters feature comprehensive body systems assessment along with common nursing activities such as the treatment, management, and evaluation of care rendered to patients with typical modifications of function. In addition to chapters detailing psychiatric care, maternal-neonatal, and pediatric care is the incorporation of geriatric care procedures and clinical alerts into all appropriate chapters for a more comprehensive understanding of care needs in this patient population. Of particular note is the focus on advance directives that helps you understand the different forms of legal direction patients may give for their treatment choice decisions. A focus on documentation will remind you of the importance of entries in the medical record as well as enable you to include essential facts about a patient's condition. Throughout the text, the graphic icons *Nursing alert* and *Equipment* highlight information critical to operating clinical equipment and rendering care safely.

As regulatory agencies continue to focus on patient safety, *Lippincott's Nursing Procedures,* Fifth Edition, will help you acquire knowledge and proficiency in critical thinking and skill performance when providing patient care. Whether you're a student, new graduate, or experienced practitioner, you'll find this an indispensable theoretical and clinical reference for providing nursing care in a variety of health care settings.

Christine Greenidge, APRN,BC, MSN, DHA
Director of Nursing Professional Practice
Interim Clinical Director of Nursing, Medicine Care Center
Montefiore Medical Center
Bronx, N.Y.

1 ■ Fundamental Procedures

INTRODUCTION

Patients come to hospitals and other health care facilities because they need skilled clinical observation and treatment. According to the American Hospital Association, about 37 million people undergo hospitalization each year, and for most, it's a trying experience. After all, hospitalization challenges the patient's sense of privacy and control of his life. He must relinquish at least part of his normal routine. He must rely on you and your coworkers to meet his fundamental needs. Depending on the complexity of his health problem, he and his family may also require teaching, counseling, coordination of services, development of community support systems, and help in coping with health-related changes in his life.

In many facilities, staff nurses, primary nurses, clinical nurse specialists, and nurse practitioners deliver these vital services. This chapter serves as a starting point to help you understand and perform many of these tasks confidently and effectively. It thoroughly covers all the fundamentals: admission, transfer, and discharge procedures; assessment (including a section on writing a nursing care plan); ensuring patient safety and mobility (including proper use of restraints and assistive devices); practicing correct body mechanics and patient transfer techniques; and using special orthopedic beds. The chapter also includes a comprehensive review of personal hygiene and comfort measures, nutrition, elimination, surgical care, spiritual care, and postmortem care.

Before turning to these nursing care specifics, however, review the broader aims of your care such as helping the patient cope with restricted mobility; giving him a comfortable, stimulating environment; making sure his stay is free from hazards; promoting an uneventful recovery; and helping him return to his normal life.

Dealing with restricted mobility

Whenever a patient's condition impairs or prevents mobility, your nursing goals include promoting his independence by motivating him; helping him set goals, to prevent injury and the complications of immobility; teaching him needed skills; and fostering a positive body image, especially if he faces long-term or permanent immobility.

Promoting a comfortable environment

By manipulating physical factors in the patient's environment—temperature, humidity, lighting—you can affect his comfort, condition and, at times, his response to treatment. For example, a room temperature of 68° to 72° F (20° to 22.2° C) and a relative humidity of 30% to 60%, although comfortable for most patients, may be too cold for elderly patients. Also, proper artificial or natural lighting helps duplicate the day-night cycle.

Providing sensory stimulation

Sensory stimulation (such as therapeutic touch) contributes to patient well-being. Although the amount and type of required stimulation varies with each patient, you can prevent sensory overload or deprivation by accurately assessing his needs. When evaluating stimuli in the patient's environment, remember that illness is a stressor that may intensify the patient's responses, especially to noise and odors.

Promoting safety

Besides weakening the patient, illness and any accompanying treatment may impair his judgment and contribute to accidents. Be alert to hazards in the patient's environment, and teach him and his family to recognize and correct them. When caring for a patient with restricted mobility, you must help him as he's moved, lifted, and transported. By using proper body mechanics and appropriate assistive devices, you can prevent injury, fatigue, and discomfort for the patient and yourself.

Preventing complications

For the bedridden patient, immobility poses special hazards such as pressure on bony prominences; venous, pulmonary, and urinary stasis; and disuse of muscles and joints. These can lead to such complications as pressure ulcers, thrombi, phlebitis, pneumonia, urinary calculi, and contractures. To prevent complications, be sure to use correct positioning, meticulous skin care, assistive devices, and regular turning and range-of-motion exercises.

Promoting rehabilitation

The first step toward rehabilitation typically is progressive ambulation, which should begin as soon as possible—if necessary, using such assistive devices as a cane, crutches, or a walker. Effective rehabilitation may also require you to teach positioning, transfer, and mobilization techniques to the patient and his family. Give him and his family the opportunity to demonstrate the skill or technique so that problems may be corrected. Demonstrating a technique—such as transferring from a bed to a wheelchair—during hospitalization helps the patient and his family to understand it. Allowing them to practice it under your supervision gives them the confidence to perform it at home. Encourage them to provide positive reinforcement to motivate the patient to work toward his goals.

ADMISSION, TRANSFER, AND DISCHARGE PROCEDURES

ADMISSION

Admission to the nursing unit prepares the patient for his stay in the health care facility. Whether the admission is scheduled or follows emergency treatment, effective admission procedures should accomplish the following goals: confirm the patient's identity using two patient identifiers according to your facility's policy, and assess his clinical status, make him as comfortable as possible, introduce him to his roommates and the staff, orient him to the environment and routine, and provide supplies and special equipment needed for daily care.

Nurses should be directly involved in the admission process—assigning a patient to a room, making sure that the necessary diagnostic tests are completed, and providing for continuity of care when the patient is admitted. Admitting personnel should confer with the nursing staff to make sure that the patient's room assignment is based on the patient's condition, health care needs, and personal preferences. Consideration of these factors during the admission process reduces the patient's anxiety and promotes cooperation, contributing to the patient's recovery.

The initial contact with the patient sets the foundation for your relationship. Be prepared to give the patient and his family, if present, your undivided attention during the admission process. Taking the time to listen to and assess your patient fulfills his physiologic and safety needs and establishes a therapeutic relationship. When orienting the patient and his family to the facility's routine, remember to mention that two or more nurses may care for the patient (depending on shift requirements) during his hospitalization.

The Joint Commission requires that each patient have an admission assessment performed by a registered nurse. During this assessment, the nurse must prioritize the patient's needs, and she should always be conscious of the patient's levels of fatigue and comfort. The admission process can be exhausting, especially when the patient is delayed in the admitting office for a room assignment. When the patient is experiencing physical or psychological problems, the nurse should decide whether any portion of the admission assessment can be postponed.

It's also important to maintain the patient's privacy while obtaining his health history. According to the Patient Care Partnership, the patient has the right to expect this. Examination, consultation, and treatment should be conducted in a way that protects the patient's privacy.

Admission routines that are efficient and show appropriate concern for the patient can ease his anxiety and promote cooperation and receptivity to treatment, thus contributing to his recovery. Conversely, admission routines that the patient perceives as careless or excessively impersonal can heighten anxiety, reduce cooperation, impair his response to treatment, and perhaps aggravate symptoms.

Equipment

Gown ▪ personal property form ▪ valuables envelope ▪ admission form ▪ nursing assessment form ▪ thermometer ▪ emesis basin ▪ bedpan or urinal ▪ bath basin ▪ water pitcher, cup, and tray ▪ urine specimen container, if needed.

An admission pack usually contains soap, comb, toothbrush, toothpaste, mouthwash, water pitcher, cup, tray, lotion, facial tissues, and thermometer. *Because the patient's pack is included in his bill,* he can take it home with him. *An admission pack helps prevent cross-contamination and increases nursing efficiency.*

Preparation of equipment

Obtain a gown and an admission pack.

Position the bed as the patient's condition requires. If the patient is ambulatory, place the bed in the low position; if he's arriving on a stretcher, place the bed in the high position. Fold down the top linens.

Prepare any emergency or special equipment, such as oxygen or suction, as needed.

Implementation

- Adjust the room lights, temperature, and ventilation.
- Make sure all equipment is in working order before the patient's admission.

Admitting the adult patient

- Speak slowly and clearly, greet the patient by his proper name, and introduce yourself and any staff present.
- Confirm the patient's identity using two patient identifiers according to your facility's policy. Verify the name and its spelling with the patient. Notify the admission office of any corrections.
- Quickly review the admission form and the practitioner's orders. Note the reason for admission, any restrictions on activity or diet, and any orders for diagnostic tests requiring specimen collection.

Using patient care reminders

When placed at the head of the patient's bed, care reminders call attention to the patient's special needs and help ensure consistent care by communicating these needs to the hospital staff, the patient's family, and other visitors.

You can use a specially designed card or a plain piece of paper to post important information about the patient, such as:

- allergies
- dietary restrictions
- fluid restrictions
- specimen collection
- patient deaf or hearing-impaired in right ear
- foreign-language speaker.

You can also use care reminders to post special instructions, such as:

- complete bed rest
- no blood pressure on right arm
- turn every 1 hour
- nothing by mouth
- infection control or isolation procedures.

Never violate the patient's privacy by posting his diagnosis, details about surgery, or any information he might find embarrassing

- Escort the patient to his room and, if he isn't in great distress, introduce him to his roommate. Then wash your hands, and help him change into a gown or pajamas; if the patient is sharing a room, provide privacy. Itemize all valuables, clothing, and prostheses on the nursing assessment form or in your notes if your facility doesn't use such a form. Encourage the patient to store valuables or money in the safe or, preferably, to send them home along with any medications he may have brought with him. Show the ambulatory patient where the bathroom and closets are located.
- Take and record the patient's vital signs, and collect specimens if ordered. Measure his height and weight if possible. If he can't stand, use a chair or bed scale and ask him his height. *Knowing the patient's height and weight is important for planning treatment and diet and for calculating medication and anesthetic dosages.*
- Show the patient how to use the equipment in his room. Be sure to include the call system, bed controls, TV controls, telephone, and lights.
- Explain the routine at your health care facility. Mention when to expect meals, vital sign checks, and medications. Review visiting hours and any restrictions.
- Take a complete patient history. Include all previous hospitalizations, illnesses, and surgeries; current drug therapy; and food or drug allergies. Ask the patient to tell you why he came to the facility. Record the answers (in the patient's own words) as the chief complaint. Follow up with a physical assessment, emphasizing complaints. Record any wounds, marks, bruises, or discoloration on the nursing assessment form.
- After assessing the patient, inform him of any tests that have been ordered and when they're scheduled. Describe what he should expect.
- Before leaving the patient's room, make sure he's comfortable and safe. Adjust his bed, and place the call bell and other equipment (such as water pitcher and cup, emesis basin, and facial tissues) within easy reach.
- Post patient care reminders (concerning such topics as allergies or special needs) at the patient's bedside *to notify coworkers.* (See *Using patient care reminders.*)

Admitting the pediatric patient

- Your initial goal will be to establish a friendly, trusting relationship with the child and his parents *to help relieve fears and anxiety, which can hinder treatment.* Remember that a child under age 3 may fear separation from his parents; an older child may worry about what will happen to him.
- Speak directly to the child, and allow him to answer questions before obtaining more information from his parents.
- While orienting the parents and child to the unit, describe the layout of the room and bathroom, and tell them the location of the playroom, television room, and snack room, if available.
- Teach the child how to call the nurse. Stress that she'll always be available to take care of his needs, such as helping him to the bathroom.
- Explain the facility's rooming-in and visiting policies *so the parents can take every opportunity to be with their child.*
- Inquire about the child's usual routine *so that favorite foods, bedtime rituals, toileting, and adequate rest can be incorporated into the routine.*
- Encourage the parents to bring some of their child's favorite toys, blankets, or other items *to make the child feel more at home amid unfamiliar surroundings.*

Special considerations

- If the patient doesn't speak English and isn't accompanied by a bilingual family member, contact the appropriate resource (usually the social services department) to secure an interpreter.

■ Keep in mind that the patient admitted to the emergency department requires special procedures. (See *Managing emergency admissions.*)
■ If the patient brings medications from home, take an inventory and record this information on the nursing assessment form. Instruct the patient not to take any medication unless authorized by the practitioner. Send authorized medications to the pharmacy for identification and relabeling. Send other medications home with a responsible family member, or store them in the designated area outside the patient's room until he's discharged. *The use of unauthorized medication may interfere with treatment or cause an overdose.*
■ Find out the patient's normal routine, and ask him if he would like to make any adjustments to the facility regimen; for example, he may prefer to shower at night instead of in the morning. *By accommodating the patient with such adjustments whenever possible, you can ease his anxiety and help him feel more in control of his potentially threatening situation.*

Documentation

After leaving the patient's room, complete the nursing assessment form or your notes, as required. The completed form should include the patient's vital signs, height, weight, allergies, and drug and health history; a list of his belongings and those sent home with family members; the results of your physical assessment (see "Physical assessment," page 32); and a record of specimens collected for laboratory tests. Also document any patient teaching you performed.

SELECTED REFERENCES

Bickely, L. *Bates' Guide to Physical Examination and Health History Taking*, 9th ed. Philadelphia: Lippincott Williams & Wilkins, 2007.

Gallagher, A., and Lynch, D. "Multidisciplinary Meetings in Medical Admission Units," *Nursing Times* 100(44):34-36, November 2004.

The Joint Commission. "Standards: Frequently Asked Questions: Hospital," 2006. Available at *www.jointcommission.org/Standards/FAQs/*.

TRANSFER

Patient transfer—either within your facility or to another one—requires thorough preparation and careful documentation. Preparation includes an explanation of the transfer to the patient and his family, discussion of the patient's condition and care plan with the staff at the receiving unit or facility, and arrangements for transportation if necessary. Documentation of the patient's condition before and during transfer and adequate communication between nursing staffs ensure continuity of nursing care and provide legal protection for the transferring facility and its staff.

Managing emergency admissions

For the patient admitted through the emergency department (ED), immediate treatment takes priority over routine admission procedures. After ED treatment, the patient arrives on the nursing unit with a temporary identification bracelet, a practitioner's order sheet, and a record of treatment. Read this record and talk to the nurse who cared for the patient in the ED *to ensure continuity of care and to gain insight into the patient's condition and behavior.*

Next, record any ongoing treatment, such as an I.V. infusion, in your notes. Take and record the patient's vital signs, and follow the practitioner's orders for treatment. If the patient is conscious and not in great distress, explain any treatment orders to him. If family members accompany the patient, ask them to wait in the lounge while you assess the patient and begin treatment. Permit them to visit the patient after he's settled in his room. When the patient's condition allows, proceed with routine admission procedures.

Equipment

Admission inventory of belongings ■ patient's chart, medication record, and nursing Kardex ■ medications ■ bag or suitcase ■ wheelchair or stretcher, as necessary ■ transfer order form.

Implementation

■ Obtain a transfer order.
■ Explain the transfer to the patient and his family. If the patient is anxious about the transfer or his condition precludes patient teaching, be sure to explain the reason for the transfer to his family members, especially if the transfer is the result of a serious change in the patient's condition. Assess his physical condition *to determine the means of transfer,* such as a wheelchair or a stretcher.
■ Using the admissions inventory of belongings as a checklist, collect the patient's property. Be sure to check the entire room, including the closet, bedside stand, overbed table, and bathroom. If the patient is being transferred to another facility, don't forget valuables or personal medications that have been stored.

- Gather the patient's medications from the cart and the refrigerator. If the patient is being transferred to another unit, send the medications to the receiving unit; if he's being transferred to another facility, return them to the pharmacy.
- Notify the business office and other appropriate departments of the transfer.
- Have a staff person notify the dietary department, the pharmacy, and the facility telephone operator about the transfer (if within the facility).
- Contact the nursing staff on the receiving unit about the patient's condition and drug regimen, and review the patient's nursing care plan with them *to ensure continuity of care.*

Transfer within the facility

- If the patient is being transferred from or to an intensive care unit, your facility may require new care orders from the patient's practitioner. If so, review the new orders with the nursing staff at the receiving unit.
- Send the patient's chart, laboratory request slips, Kardex, special equipment, and other required materials to the receiving unit.
- Use a wheelchair to transport the ambulatory patient to the newly assigned room unless it's on the same unit as his present one, in which case he may be allowed to walk. Use a stretcher to transport the bedridden patient.
- Introduce the patient to the nursing staff at the receiving unit. Then take the patient to his room and, depending on his condition, place him in the bed or seat him in a chair. Introduce him to his new roommate, if appropriate, and tell him about any unfamiliar equipment such as the call bell.

Transfer to an extended-care facility

- Make sure the patient's practitioner has written the transfer order on his chart and has completed the special transfer form. This form should include the patient's diagnosis, care summary, drug regimen, and special care instructions, such as diet and physical therapy.
- Complete the nursing summary, including the patient's assessment, progress, required nursing treatments, and special needs, *to ensure continuity of care.*
- Keep one copy of the transfer form and the nursing summary with the patient's chart, and forward the other copies to the receiving facility. However, don't send the patient's medications, Kardex, or chart. A transcript of the chart may be requested by the receiving facility.

Transfer to an acute-care facility

- Make sure the practitioner has written the transfer order on the patient's chart and has completed the transfer form as discussed above. Then complete the nursing summary.
- Depending on the practitioner's instructions, send one copy of the transfer form and nursing summary and photocopies of pertinent excerpts from the patient's chart—such as laboratory test and X-ray results, patient history and physical progress notes, and records of vital signs—to the receiving facility with the patient. Alternatively, following your facility's policy, substitute a written summary of the patient's condition and facility history for the excerpts from the patient's chart. Make sure this information is complete. If the Kardex isn't considered part of the patient's record in your facility, be sure to document all pertinent information for the receiving institution—by photocopying the nurse's notes if necessary. *This information legally protects the transferring facility and its staff and completes the patient's chart.*

Special considerations

- If the patient requires an ambulance to take him to another facility, arrange transportation with the social services department. Ensure that the necessary equipment is assembled to provide care during transport.
- Be especially careful that all documentation is complete when the patient is being transferred to another facility. *A communications breakdown can hurt the patient's chances for recovery.*
- If the patient is being transferred to a different facility, make sure none of these patient care measures have been omitted: suctioning of airway, administering prescribed medications, changing soiled dressing, bathing an incontinent patient, and emptying drainage collection devices.

Documentation

Record the time and date of transfer, the patient's condition before and during transfer, the name of the receiving unit or facility, and the means of transportation. Include any equipment accompanying the patient, such as I.V. lines and pumps, surgical drains, and oxygen therapy. Note the name and title of the person you gave the report to; also include the names of staff or family members accompanying the patient.

SELECTED REFERENCES

Cortes, C.A., et al. "The Transition of Elderly Patients between Hospitals and Nursing Homes. Improving Nurse-to-nurse Communication," *Journal of Gerotonlogical Nursing* 30(6):10-5, June 2004.

Crolty, M., et al. "Transitional Care Facility for Elderly People in Hospital Awaiting a Long Term Care Bed: Randomised Controlled Trial," *British Medical Journal* 331(7525):1110, November 2005.

Emergency Medical Treatment and Labor Act. Available at *www.medlaw.com/regs.htm.*

Holen, K.A. "Post-Hospital Transition to a Skilled Nursing Facility—Compliance, Competence, and Communication," *Journal of Gerontological Nursing* 32(9):5-9, September 2006.

Holleran, R., and Rhoades, C. "What Important Step Must be Considered before Transferring a Patient from One Facility to Another?" *Critical Care Nurse* 25(1):58-59, February 2005.

The Joint Commission. *Comprehensive Accreditation Manual for Hospitals: The Official Handbook.* PC.15.10-PC.15.30. 2007. Available at *www.jointcommission.org/PatientSafety/NationalPatientSafetyGoals/08_cah_npsgs.htm.*

The Joint Commission. "2008 National Patient Safety Goals: Improve the Effectiveness of Communication Among Caregivers." Available at *www.jointcommission.org/PatientSafety/NationalPatientSafetyGoals/08_cah_npsgs.htm.*

The Joint Commission. "2008 National Patient Safety Goals: Accurately and Completely Reconcile Medications Across the Continuum of Care." Available at *www.jointcommission.org/PatientSafety/NationalPatientSafetyGoals/08_cah_npsgs.htm.*

Joyce, C., et al. "Transfer Admission Discharge Teams Keep Things Moving," *Nursing Management* 36(11):36, 38-39, November 2005.

Strahan, E.H., and Brown, R.J. "A Qualitative Study of the Experiences of Patients Following Transfer from Intensive Care," *Intensive and Critical Care Nursing* 21(3):160-71, June 2005.

Watson, D. "Planning to Ensure the Safe Transfer of Hospital Patients," *Nursing Times* 102(9):21-22, February-March 2006.

DISCHARGE

Although discharge from a health care facility is usually considered routine, effective discharge requires careful planning and continuing assessment of the patient's needs during his hospitalization. Ideally, discharge planning begins shortly after admission. Discharge planning aims to teach the patient and his family about his illness and its effect on his lifestyle, to provide instructions for home care, to communicate dietary or activity instructions, and to explain the purpose, adverse effects, and scheduling of drug treatment. It can also include arranging for transportation, follow-up care if necessary, and coordination of outpatient or home health care services.

Equipment

Wheelchair, unless the patient leaves by ambulance ■ patient's chart ■ patient instruction sheet ■ discharge summary sheet ■ plastic bag or patient's suitcase for personal belongings.

> **Dealing with a discharge against medical advice**
>
> Although a patient can choose to leave a health care facility against medical advice (AMA) at any time, the law requires clear evidence that he's mentally competent to make such a choice. In most health care facilities, an AMA form serves as a legal document to protect you, the practitioners, and the facility if problems arise from a patient's unapproved discharge.
>
> The AMA form should clearly document that the patient knows he's leaving AMA, that he has been advised of the risks of leaving and understands them, and that he knows he can come back.
>
> If a patient refuses to sign the AMA form, document this refusal on the form and enter it in his chart. Use the patient's own words to describe his refusal.
>
> Provide routine discharge care. Even though your patient is leaving AMA, his rights to discharge planning and care are the same as those for a patient who's signed out with medical advice. So, if the patient agrees, arrange follow-up care, and offer other routine health care measures.

Implementation

■ Confirm the patient's identity using two patient identifiers according to your facility's policy.

■ Inform the patient's family of the time and date of discharge as soon as it's known. If the patient's family can't arrange transportation, notify the social services department. (Always confirm arranged transportation on the day of discharge.)

■ Obtain a written discharge order from the practitioner. If the patient discharges himself against medical advice, obtain the appropriate form. (See *Dealing with a discharge against medical advice.*)

■ If the patient requires home medical care, confirm arrangements with the appropriate facility department or community agency.

■ On the day of discharge, review the patient's discharge care plan (initiated on admission and modified during his hospitalization) with the patient and his family. List prescribed drugs on the patient instruction sheet along with the dosage, prescribed time schedule, and adverse reactions that he should report to the practitioner. Ensure that the drug schedule is consistent with the patient's lifestyle *to prevent*

HOME CARE

Discharge teaching goals

Your discharge teaching should aim to ensure that the patient:
- understands his illness
- complies with his drug therapy
- carefully follows his diet
- manages his activity level
- understands his treatments
- recognizes his need for rest
- knows about possible complications
- knows when to seek follow-up care.

Remember that your discharge teaching must include the patient's family or other caregivers *to ensure that the patient receives proper home care.*

improper administration and to promote patient compliance. (See *Discharge teaching goals.*)

- Review procedures the patient or his family will perform at home. If necessary, demonstrate these procedures, provide written instructions, and check performance with a return demonstration.
- List dietary and activity instructions, if applicable, on the patient instruction sheet, and review the reasons for them. If the practitioner orders bed rest, make sure the patient's family can provide daily care and will obtain necessary equipment.
- Check with the practitioner about the patient's next office appointment; if the practitioner hasn't yet done so, inform the patient of the date, time, and location. If scheduling is your responsibility, make an appointment with the practitioner, outpatient clinic, physical therapy, X-ray department, or other health services, as needed. If the patient can't arrange transportation, notify the social services department.
- Retrieve the patient's valuables from the facility's safe, and review each item with him. Then obtain the patient's signature *to verify receipt of his valuables.*
- Obtain from the pharmacy any drugs the patient brought with him. Return these to the patient if drug therapy is unchanged. If giving a new prescription, provide an explanation of the dosage, schedule, and adverse effects.
- If appropriate, take and record the patient's vital signs on the discharge summary form. Notify the practitioner if any signs are abnormal such as an elevated temperature. *If necessary, the practitioner may alter the patient's discharge plan.*
- Help the patient get dressed if necessary.
- Collect the patient's personal belongings from his room, compare them with the admission inventory of belongings, and help place them in his suitcase or a plastic bag.
- After checking the room for misplaced belongings, help the patient into the wheelchair, and escort him to the exit; if the patient is leaving by ambulance, help him onto the litter.
- After the patient has left the area, strip the bed linens and notify the housekeeping staff that the room is ready for terminal cleaning.

Special considerations

- Whenever possible, involve the patient's family in discharge planning *so they can better understand and perform patient care procedures.*
- Before the patient is discharged, perform a physical assessment. If you detect abnormal signs or the patient develops new symptoms, notify the practitioner and delay discharge until he has seen the patient.

Documentation

Although your facility's policy determines the extent and form of discharge documentation, you'll usually record the time and date of discharge, family members or caregivers present for teaching, details of instructions given to the patient, including medications, activity and diet, treatments and the use of medical equipment, signs and symptoms to report to the practitioner, and the date, time, and location of follow-up appointments.

SELECTED REFERENCES

The Joint Commission. "2008 National Patient Safety Goals, Goal 8: Accurately and Completely Reconcile Medications Across the Continuum of Care." Available at *www.jointcommission.org/PatientSafety/NationalPatientSafetyGoals/08_cah_npsgs.htm.*

The Joint Commission. "Standards, Rationales, Elements of Performance Scoring," *PC* 15(10):202, 2005.

Macleod, A. "The Nursing Role in Preventing Delay in Patient Discharge," *Nursing Standards* 21(1):43-48, September 2006.

Maramba, P.J., et al. "Discharge Planning Process: Applying a Model for Evidence-Based Practice," *Journal of Nursing Care Quality* 19(2):123-29, April-June 2004.

Sands, J.R. "Transforming the Traditional Discharge Planning Manual," *Case Manager* 17(6):TCM 66-68, November-December 2006.

ADVANCE DIRECTIVES

The Patient Self-Determination Act requires health care facilities to provide information about the patient's right to choose and refuse treatment. An advance directive is a legal document used as a guideline for providing life-sustaining medical care to a patient with an advanced disease or disability who can no longer indicate his own wishes. Advance directives include living wills and durable powers of attorney for health care.

All patients should be encouraged to have an advance directive as part of any admission, before any routine medical treatment, or at their primary practitioner's office on annual physical examinations. All adults, regardless of their current health status, should make their preferences about medical treatment known before any serious injury or unplanned illness. The advance directive should be discussed with the practitioner, family, and health care proxy.

If a person is terminally ill or in a persistent vegetative state or coma, a living will instructs health care providers about the patient's preferences about life-sustaining treatment. In making a living will, a legally competent patient states which procedures he does or doesn't want carried out, such as intubation and mechanical ventilation, feeding tubes, artificial nutrition and hydration, antibiotics, dialysis, and cardiopulmonary resuscitation. The living will goes into effect when a person can no longer communicate his choices on medical care. (See *The living will,* page 10.)

In the durable power of attorney for health care (also called health care surrogate or proxy), the patient designates another person to make decisions about medical care if the patient can't make his own decisions. (See *Durable power of attorney for health care,* page 11.)

Equipment

Advance directive forms ■ medical record ■ optional as required by the state: witness or notary public.

Implementation

- Confirm the patient's identity using two patient identifiers according to your facility's policy.
- Ask the patient if he has an advance directive as required by the Patient Self-Determination Act.
- If the patient has an advance directive, review it with him and confirm that it still reflects his current wishes.
- Place the advance directive in the medical record *so that it's easily accessible to all health care providers.*
- Notify the practitioner that the patient has an advance directive *so that it can be used to guide care.*
- Determine whether the durable power of attorney for health care has a copy of the advance directive.
- Encourage the patient to discuss his advance directive with his family and durable power of attorney *so they understand the patient's wishes and can ask questions while the patient is competent and can explain his decisions.*
- If the patient doesn't have an advance directive, provide him with verbal and written information *so that he can make an informed decision about developing one.*
- Answer the patient's questions about advance directives, or have a social worker or patient representative discuss advance directives with him *to provide accurate information.*
- Assist in the assessment of the patient's level of competency *to assure he can make decisions.* This may include the patient's ability to understand information, consider the alternatives, evaluate the alternatives in relation to his own situation, make a decision, and communicate his choice. According to your facility's policy, the patient's capacity for making decisions may be determined by a practitioner.

Special considerations

- If family members express opposition to the advance directive, notify the patient's practitioner, the nursing supervisor, and the risk manager. Encourage family members to discuss their feelings with the patient and these individuals. A consult to the facility ethics committee may be made, as indicated.
- The patient may revoke his advance directive at any time. For example, the patient may revoke his directive if he changes his mind about his previous decision or if his condition mandates that he revise his directive. The patient can revoke an advance directive either orally or in writing.

Documentation

Document the presence of an advance directive, and that the practitioner was notified of its presence. Include the name of the practitioner and the time of notification. Include the name, address, and telephone number of the durable power of attorney for health care. If the patient's wishes differ from those of his practitioner or family, note the discrepancies.

If the patient doesn't have an advance directive, document that he was given written information concerning his rights under state law to make decisions regarding health care. If the patient refuses information on an advance directive, document this refusal using the patient's own words, in quotes, if possible. Record any conversations with the patient regarding his decision making. Document that proof of competency was obtained.

SELECTED REFERENCES

Dobbins, E.H. "Helping Your Patient to a 'Good Death'," *Nursing* 35(2):43-45, February 2005.

The living will

The living will is an advance care document that specifies a person's wishes with regard to medical care, should he become terminally ill, incompetent, or unable to communicate. The will is commonly used in combination with the patient's durable power of attorney.

All states and the District of Columbia have living will laws that outline the documentation requirements for living wills. The sample document below is from Ohio.

Living will

If my attending doctor and one other doctor who examines me determine, to a reasonable degree of medical certainty and in accordance with reasonable medical standards, that I am in a terminal condition or in a permanently unconscious state, and if my attending doctor determines that at that time I no longer am able to make informed decisions regarding the administration of life-sustaining treatment, and that, to a reasonable degree of medical certainty and in accordance with reasonable medical standards, there is no reasonable possibility that I will regain the capacity to make informed decisions regarding the administration of life-sustaining treatment, then I direct my attending doctor to withhold or withdraw medical procedures, treatment, interventions, or other measures that serve principally to prolong the process of my dying, rather than diminish my pain or discomfort.

I have used the term "terminal condition" in this declaration to mean an irreversible, incurable, and untreatable condition caused by disease, illness, or injury from which, to a reasonable degree of medical certainty as determined in accordance with reasonable medical standards of my attending doctor and one other doctor who has examined me, both of the following apply:

1. There can be no recovery.
2. Death is likely to occur within a relatively short time if life-sustaining treatment is not administered.

I have used the term "permanently unconscious state" in this declaration to mean a state of permanent unconsciousness that, to a reasonable degree of medical certainty, is determined in accordance with reasonable medical standards by my attending doctor and one other doctor who has examined me, as characterized by both of the following:

1. I am irreversibly unaware of myself and my environment.
2. There is a total loss of cerebral cortical functioning, resulting in my having no capacity to experience pain or suffering.

Nutrition & Hydration

I hereby authorize my attending doctor to withhold or withdraw nutrition and hydration from me when I am in a permanent unconscious state if my attending doctor and at least one other doctor who has examined me determine, to a reasonable degree of medical certainty and in accordance with reasonable medical standards, that nutrition or hydration will not or no longer will serve to provide comfort to me or alleviate my pain.

[Sign here for withdrawal of nutrition or hydration] ____________________

I hereby designate [Print name of person to decide] as the person who I wish my attending doctor to notify at any time that life-sustaining treatment is to be withdrawn or withheld pursuant to this Declaration.

____________________ ____________________
[Sign your name here] [Today's date]

Witness by: ____________________

____________________ ____________________
[First witness signs here] [Second witness signs here]

[Living will person's name] voluntarily signed or directed another individual to sign this Living Will in the presence of the following who each attests that the Declarant appears to be of sound mind and not under or subject to duress, fraud, or undue influence.

Durable power of attorney for health care

The sample document below is an example of a durable power of attorney, which allows a competent patient to delegate to another person the authority to consent to or refuse health care treatment. *This helps the patient ensure that his wishes will be carried out should he become incompetent.*

Each state with a durable power of attorney for health care law has specific requirements for executing the document. The sample form below is from Nebraska.

Power of Attorney for Health Care

I appoint ____________________

whose address is ____________________

and whose telephone number is ____________________

as my attorney in fact for health care. ____________________

I appoint ____________________

whose address is ____________________

and whose telephone number is ____________________

as my successor attorney in fact for health care. ____________________

I authorize my attorney in fact appointed by this document to make health care decisions for me when I am determined to be incapable of making my own health care decisions. I have read the warning which accompanies this document and understand the consequences of executing a power of attorney for health care.

I direct that my attorney in fact comply with the following instructions or limitations (optional):

I direct that my attorney in fact comply with the following instructions on life-sustaining treatment (optional):

I direct that my attorney in fact comply with the following instructions on artificially administered nutrition and hydration (optional):

I have read this power of attorney for health care. I understand that it allows another person to make life and death decisions for me if I am incapable of making such decisions. I also understand that I can revoke this power of attorney for health care at any time by notifying my attorney in fact, my physician, or the facility in which I am a patient or resident. I also understand that I can require in this power of attorney for health care that the fact of my incapacity in the future be confirmed by a second physician.

____________________ ____________________

[Signature of person making designation] [Date]

Griffie, J., et al. "Acknowledging the 'Elephant': Communication in Palliative Care," *American Journal of Nursing* 104(1):48-57, January 2004.

Gross, A.G. "End-of-Life Care Obstacles and Facilitators in the Critical Care Units of a Community Hospital," *Journal of Hospice and Palliative Care* 8(2):92-102, March-April 2006.

The Joint Commission. *Comprehensive Accreditation Manual for Hospitals: The Official Handbook.* Standard RI2.10-RI.2.200. 2007.

Lynn-McHale Wiegand, D.J., and Carlson, K.K., eds. *AACN Procedure Manual for Critical Care,* 5th ed. Philadelphia: W.B. Saunders Co., 2005.

Scanlon, C. "Ethical Concerns in End-of-Life Care," *AJN* 103(1):48-55, January 2003.

Scherer, Y., et al. "Advance Directives and End-of-Life Decision Making: Survey of Critical Care Nurses' Knowledge, Attitude, and Experience," *Critical Care Nurse* 26(4):30-40, August 2006.

ASSESSMENT

TEMPERATURE

Body temperature represents the balance between heat produced by metabolism, muscular activity, and other factors and heat lost through the skin, lungs, and body wastes. A stable temperature pattern promotes proper function of cells, tissues, and organs; a change in this pattern usually signals the onset of illness.

Temperature can be measured with an electronic, or a chemical-dot thermometer. A special electronic thermometer, called a *tympanic thermometer*, can be used to obtain a temperature reading from the ear canal. Oral temperature in adults normally ranges from 97° to 99.5° F (36.1° to 37.5° C); rectal temperature, the most accurate reading, is usually 1° F (0.6° C) higher; axillary temperature, the least accurate, reads 1° to 2° F (0.6° to 1.1° C) lower; and tympanic temperature reads 0.5° to 1° (0.3° to 0.6° C) higher.

Temperature normally fluctuates with rest and activity. Lowest readings typically occur between 4 and 5 a.m.; the highest readings occur between 4 and 8 p.m. Other factors also influence temperature, including gender, age, emotional conditions, and environment. Keep the following principles in mind. Females normally have higher temperatures than males, especially during ovulation. Normal temperature is highest in neonates and lowest in elderly persons. Heightened emotions raise temperature; depressed emotions lower it. A hot external environment can raise temperature; a cold environment lowers it.

Equipment

Thermometer (electronic, chemical-dot, or tympanic) ■ water-soluble lubricant or petroleum jelly (for rectal temperature) ■ gloves (for rectal temperature) ■ facial tissue ■ disposable thermometer sheath or probe cover ■ alcohol pad.

Preparation of equipment

Obtain a thermometer from the nurses' station or central supply department. If you use an electronic thermometer, make sure it has been recharged. (See *Types of thermometers.*)

Implementation

- Confirm the patient's identity using two patient identifiers according to your facility's policy.
- Explain the procedure to the patient, and wash your hands. If the patient has had hot or cold liquids, chewed gum, or smoked, wait 15 minutes before taking an oral temperature.
- To use a disposable sheath, disinfect the thermometer with an alcohol pad. Insert it into the disposable sheath opening; then twist to tear the seal at the dotted line. Pull it apart.

Using an electronic thermometer

- Insert the probe into a disposable probe cover. If taking a rectal temperature, lubricate the probe cover *to reduce friction and ease insertion.* Leave the probe in place until the maximum temperature appears on the digital display.

Using a chemical-dot thermometer

- Remove the thermometer from its protective dispenser case by grasping the handle end with your thumb and forefinger, moving the handle up and down to break the seal, and pulling the handle straight out. Keep the thermometer sealed until use.

Using a tympanic thermometer

- Make sure the lens under the probe is clean and shiny. Attach a disposable probe cover.
- Examine the patient's ears. They should be free from cerumen *to obtain an accurate reading.* If the patient has any visible lesions or drainage, don't perform a tympanic temperature.
- Stabilize the patient's head; then gently pull the ear straight back (for children up to age 1) or up and back (for children age 1 and older to adults).
- Insert the thermometer until the entire ear canal is sealed. The thermometer should be inserted toward the tympanic membrane in the same way that an otoscope is inserted. Then press the activation button and hold it for 1 second. The temperature will appear on the display.

PEDIATRIC ALERT *For infants younger than age 3 months, take three readings, and use the highest.*

EQUIPMENT

Types of thermometers

You can take an oral, rectal, or axillary temperature with such instruments as a chemical-dot device, an electronic digital thermometer, or a tympanic thermometer.

You'll usually use the oral route for adults who are awake, alert, oriented, and cooperative. For infants, young children, and confused or unconscious patients, you may need to take the temperature rectally. The tympanic route may be used on many patients.

Chemical-dot thermometer

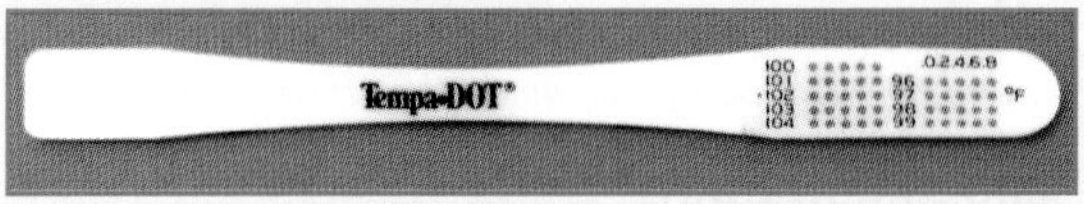

Individual electronic digital thermometer

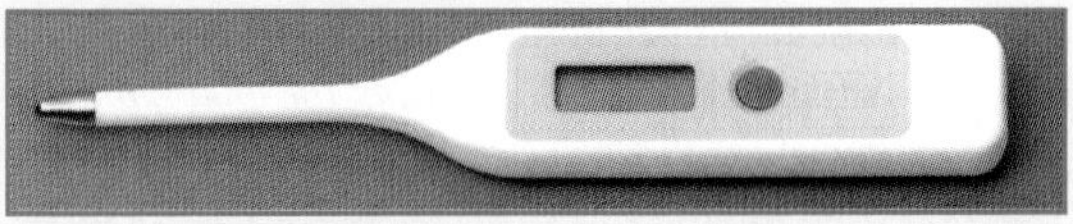

Institutional electronic digital thermometer

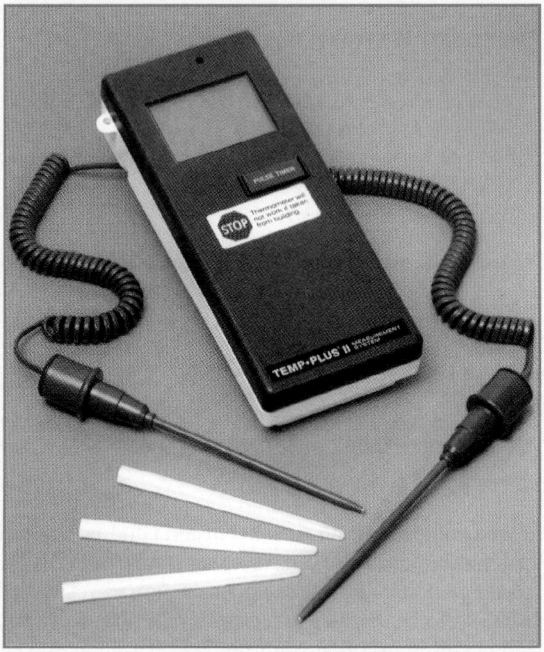

Typanic thermometer

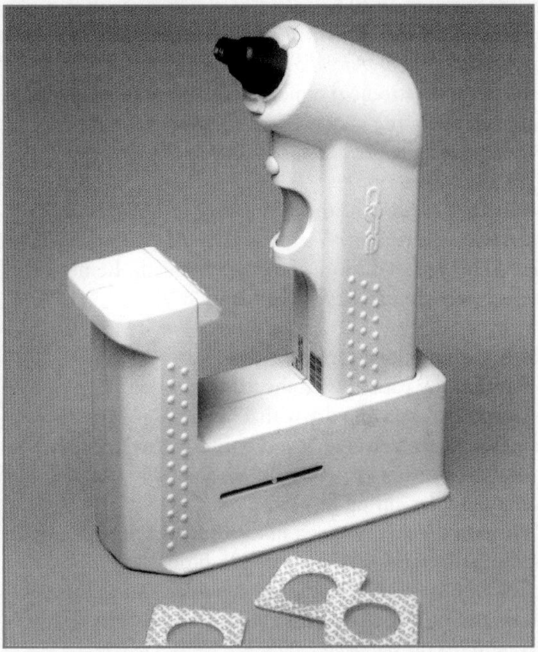

Taking an oral temperature

- Position the tip of the thermometer under the patient's tongue, as far back as possible on either side of the frenulum linguae. *Placing the tip in this area promotes contact with superficial blood vessels and contributes to an accurate reading.*
- Instruct the patient to close his lips but to avoid biting down with his teeth.
- Leave a chemical-dot thermometer in place for 45 seconds *to register temperature;* for an electronic thermometer, wait until the maximum temperature is displayed.
- For an electronic thermometer, note the temperature; then remove and discard the probe cover. For the chemical-dot thermometer, read the temperature as the last dye dot that has changed color, or fired; then discard the thermometer and its dispenser case.

Taking a rectal temperature

- Position the patient on his side with his top leg flexed, and drape him to provide privacy. Then fold back the bed linens to expose the anus.
- Squeeze the lubricant onto a facial tissue *to prevent contamination of the lubricant supply.* Put on gloves.
- Lubricate about ½″ (1.3 cm) of the thermometer tip for an infant, 1″ (2.5 cm) for a child, or about 1½″ (3.8 cm) for an adult. *Lubrication reduces friction and thus eases insertion.* This step may be unnecessary when using disposable rectal sheaths *because they're prelubricated.*
- Lift the patient's upper buttock, and ask the patient to take a slow, deep breath. *This helps relax the anal sphincter to ease insertion of the thermometer.* Insert the thermometer about ½″ for an infant or 1½″ for an adult. Gently direct the thermometer along the rectal wall toward the umbilicus. *This will avoid perforating the anus or rectum or breaking the thermometer. It will also help ensure an accurate reading because the thermometer will register hemorrhoidal artery temperature instead of fecal temperature.*
- Hold the electronic thermometer in place until the maximum temperature is displayed. *Holding the thermometer prevents damage to rectal tissues caused by displacement or loss of the thermometer into the rectum.*
- Carefully remove the thermometer, wiping it as necessary. Then wipe the patient's anal area *to remove any lubricant or feces.* Remove and dispose of the rectal sheath. Remove and discard your gloves. Wash your hands.

Taking an axillary temperature

- Position the patient with the axilla exposed.
- Gently pat the axilla dry with a facial tissue *because moisture conducts heat.* Avoid harsh rubbing, *which generates heat.*
- Ask the patient to reach across his chest and grasp his opposite shoulder, lifting his elbow.
- Position the thermometer in the center of the axilla, with the tip pointing toward the patient's head.
- Tell him to keep grasping his shoulder and to lower his elbow and hold it against his chest. *This promotes skin contact with the thermometer.*
- Remove an electronic thermometer when it displays the maximum temperature. Axillary temperature takes longer to register than oral or rectal temperature *because the thermometer isn't enclosed in a body cavity.*
- Grasp the end of the thermometer and remove it from the axilla.

Special considerations

- Oral measurement is contraindicated in patients who are unconscious, disoriented, or seizure-prone; in young children and infants; and in patients who must breathe through their mouths. Rectal measurement is contraindicated in patients with diarrhea, recent rectal or prostatic surgery or injury *because it may injure inflamed tissue,* or recent myocardial infarction *because anal manipulation may stimulate the vagus nerve, causing bradycardia or another rhythm disturbance.*
- Use the same thermometer for repeated temperature taking *to avoid spurious variations caused by equipment differences.* Store chemical-dot thermometers in a cool area *because exposure to heat activates the dye dots.*
- Don't avoid taking an oral temperature when the patient is receiving nasal oxygen *because oxygen administration raises oral temperature by only about 0.3° F (0.17° C).*

Documentation

Record the time, route, and temperature on the patient's chart.

SELECTED REFERENCES

Craven, R.F., and Hirnle, C.J. *Fundamentals of Nursing: Human Health and Function*, 5th ed. Philadelphia: Lippincott Williams & Wilkins, 2006.

Khorshid, L. "Comparing Mercury-in-Glass, Tympanic and Disposable Thermometers in Measuring Body Temperature in Healthy Young People," *Journal of Clinical Nursing* 14(4):496-500, April 2005.

Quatrara, B., et al. "The Effect of Respiratory Rate and Ingestion of Hot and Cold Beverages on the Accuracy of Oral Temperature Measured by Electronic Thermometers," *MedSurg Nursing* 16(2):105-108, April 2007.

"Take Care with Tympanic Temperature Readings," *Nursing* 37(4):52-53, April 2007.

PULSE

Blood pumped into an already-full aorta during ventricular contraction creates a fluid wave that travels from the heart to the peripheral arteries. This recurring wave—called a pulse—can be palpated at locations on the body where an artery crosses over bone on firm tissue. In adults and children over age 3, the radial artery in the wrist is the most common palpation site. (See *Pulse points.*) In infants and children under age 3, a stethoscope is used to listen to the heart itself rather than palpating a pulse. Because auscultation is done at the heart's apex, this is called the *apical pulse.*

An apical-radial pulse is taken by simultaneously counting apical and radial beats—the first by auscultation at the apex of the heart, the second by palpation at the radial artery. Some heartbeats detected at the apex can't be detected at peripheral sites. When this occurs, the apical pulse rate is higher than the radial; the difference is the pulse deficit.

Pulse points

Shown at right are anatomic locations where an artery crosses bone or firm tissue and can be palpated for a pulse.

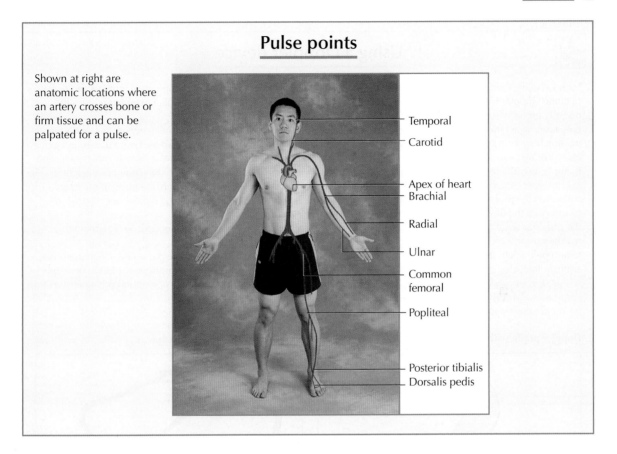

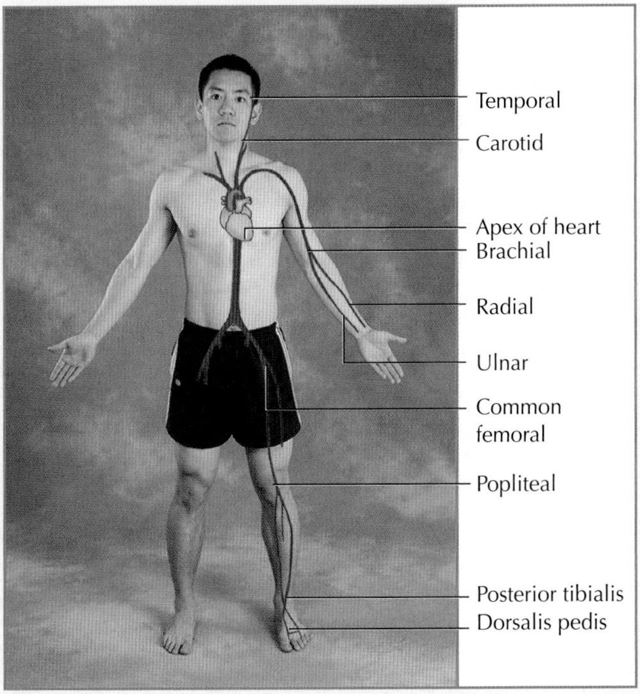

Pulse taking involves determining the rate (number of beats per minute), rhythm (pattern or regularity of the beats), and volume (amount of blood pumped with each beat). If the pulse is faint or weak, use a Doppler ultrasound blood flow detector if available. (See *Using a Doppler device,* page 16.)

Equipment

Watch with a second hand ▪ stethoscope (for auscultating an apical pulse) ▪ alcohol pad ▪ Doppler ultrasound blood flow detector if necessary.

Preparation of equipment

If you aren't using your own stethoscope, disinfect the earpieces with an alcohol pad before and after use *to prevent cross-contamination.*

Implementation

- Confirm the patient's identity using two patient identifiers according to your facility's policy.
- Wash your hands, and tell the patient that you intend to take his pulse.
- Make sure the patient is comfortable and relaxed *because an awkward, uncomfortable position may affect the heart rate.*

Taking a radial pulse

- Place the patient in a sitting or supine position, with his arm at his side or across his chest.
- Gently press your index, middle, and ring fingers on the radial artery, inside the patient's wrist, as shown below. You should feel a pulse with only moderate pressure; *excessive pressure may obstruct blood flow distal to the pulse site.* Don't use your thumb to take the patient's pulse *because your thumb's own strong pulse may be confused with the patient's pulse.*

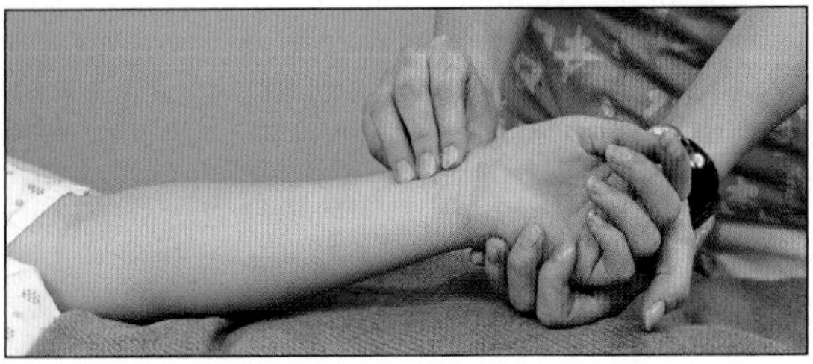

EQUIPMENT

Using a Doppler device

More sensitive than palpation for determining pulse rate, the Doppler ultrasound blood flow detector is especially useful when a pulse is faint or weak. Unlike palpation, which detects arterial wall expansion and retraction, this instrument detects the motion of red blood cells (RBCs).

■ Apply a small amount of coupling gel or transmission gel (not water-soluble lubricant) to the ultrasound probe.

■ Position the probe on the skin directly over the selected artery. In the illustration below left, the probe is over the posterior tibial artery.

■ When using a Doppler model like the one in the illustration below left, turn the instrument on and, moving counterclockwise, set the volume control to the lowest setting. If your model doesn't have a speaker, plug in the earphones and slowly raise the volume. The Doppler ultrasound stethoscope shown in the illustration below right is basically a stethoscope fitted with an audio unit, volume control, and transducer, which amplifies the movement of RBCs.

■ *To obtain the best signals with either device,* tilt the probe 45 degrees from the artery, being sure to put gel between the skin and the probe. Slowly move the probe in a circular motion to locate the center of the artery and the Doppler signal—a hissing noise at the heartbeat. Avoid moving the probe rapidly *because this distorts the signal.*

■ Count the signals for 60 seconds to determine the pulse rate.

■ After you've measured the pulse rate, clean the probe with a soft cloth soaked in antiseptic solution or soapy water. Don't immerse the probe or bump it against a hard surface.

Doppler probe with amplifier

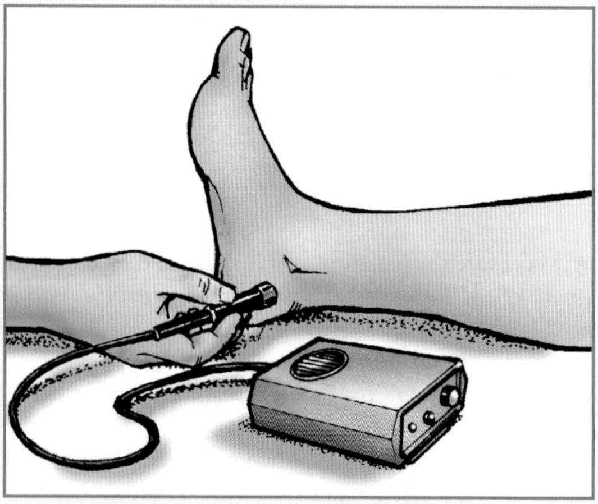

Doppler ultrasound stethoscope

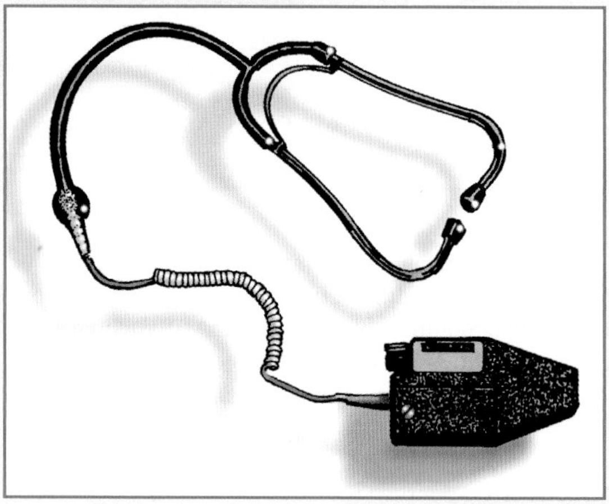

■ After locating the pulse, count the beats for 60 seconds, or count for 30 seconds and multiply by 2. *Counting for a full minute provides a more accurate picture of irregularities.* While counting the rate, assess pulse rhythm and volume by noting the pattern and strength of the beats. If you detect an irregularity, repeat the count, and note whether it occurs in a pattern or randomly. If you're still in doubt, take an apical pulse. (See *Identifying pulse patterns.*)

Taking an apical pulse

■ Help the patient to a supine position, and drape him if necessary.

■ Warm the diaphragm or bell of the stethoscope in your hand. *Placing a cold stethoscope against the skin may startle the patient and momentarily increase the heart rate.* Keep in mind that the bell transmits low-pitched sounds more effectively than the diaphragm.

■ Place the diaphragm or bell of the stethoscope over the apex of the heart (normally located at the fifth intercostal space left of the midclavicular line). Then insert the earpieces

Identifying pulse patterns

TYPE	RATE	RHYTHM (PER 3 SECONDS)	CAUSES AND INCIDENCE
Normal	60 to 80 beats/ minute; in neonates, 120 to 140 beats/ minute	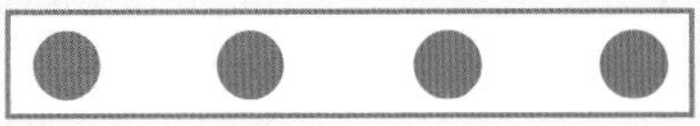	■ Varies with such factors as age, physical activity, and sex (males usually have lower pulse rates than females)
Tachycardia	More than 100 beats/minute	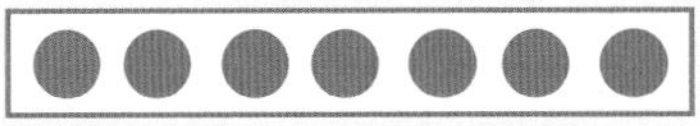	■ Accompanies stimulation of the sympathetic nervous system by emotional stress, such as anger, fear, or anxiety, or by the use of certain drugs such as caffeine ■ May result from exercise and from certain health conditions, such as heart failure, anemia, and fever (which increases oxygen requirements and therefore pulse rate)
Bradycardia	Less than 60 beats/minute	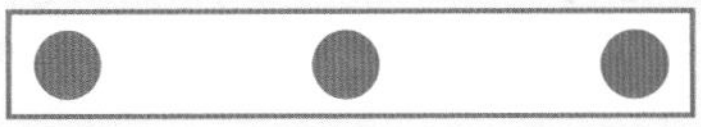	■ Accompanies stimulation of the parasympathetic nervous system by drug use, especially cardiac glycosides, and such conditions as cerebral hemorrhage and heart block ■ May also be present in fit athletes
Irregular	Uneven time intervals between beats (for example, periods of regular rhythm interrupted by pauses or premature beats)	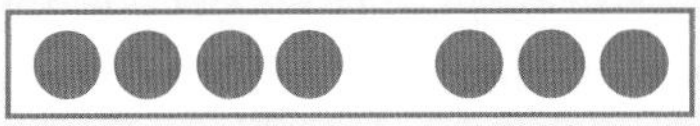	■ May indicate cardiac irritability, hypoxia, digoxin toxicity, potassium imbalance or, sometimes, more serious arrhythmias if premature beats occur frequently ■ Occasional premature beats normal

into your ears. Count the beats for 30 seconds and multiply by 2 (or count for 60 seconds if the rhythm is irregular), and note their rhythm, volume, and intensity (loudness).

■ Remove the stethoscope and make the patient comfortable.

■ Clean the stethoscope with an alcohol pad *to prevent cross-contamination.*

Taking an apical-radial pulse

■ Two nurses work together to obtain the apical-radial pulse; one palpates the radial pulse while the other auscultates the apical pulse with a stethoscope. Both must use the same watch when counting beats.

■ Help the patient to a supine position and drape him if necessary.

■ Locate the apical and radial pulses.

■ Determine a time to begin counting. Then each nurse should count beats for 60 seconds.

Special considerations

■ When the peripheral pulse is irregular, take an apical pulse to measure the heartbeat more directly. If the pulse is faint or weak, use a Doppler ultrasound blood flow detector if available.

- If another nurse isn't available for an apical-radial pulse, hold the stethoscope in place with the hand that holds the watch while palpating the radial pulse with the other hand. You can then feel any discrepancies between the apical and radial pulses.

Documentation

Record pulse rate, rhythm, and volume as well as the time of measurement. "Full" or "bounding" describes a pulse of increased volume; "weak" or "thready," decreased volume. When recording an apical pulse, include the intensity of the heart sounds. When recording an apical-radial pulse, chart the rate according to the pulse site—for example, A/R pulse of 80/76.

SELECTED REFERENCES

Craven, R.F., and Hirnle, C.J. *Fundamentals of Nursing: Human Health and Function*, 5th ed. Philadelphia: Lippincott Williams & Wilkins, 2006.

Docherty, B., and Coote, S. "Monitoring the Pulse as Part of Track and Trigger," *Nursing Times* 102(43):28-29, October 2006.

Thayer, J.F., et al. "Ethnic Differences in Heart Rate Variability: Does Ultralow-Frequency Heart Rate Variability Really Measure Autonomic Tone?" *American Heart Journal* 152(3):e27, September 2006.

BLOOD PRESSURE

Defined as the lateral force exerted by blood on the arterial walls, blood pressure depends on the force of ventricular contractions, arterial wall elasticity, peripheral vascular resistance, and blood volume and viscosity. Systolic, or maximum, pressure occurs during left ventricular contraction and reflects the integrity of the heart, arteries, and arterioles. Diastolic, or minimum, pressure occurs during left ventricular relaxation and directly indicates blood vessel resistance.

Pulse pressure—the difference between systolic and diastolic pressures—varies inversely with arterial elasticity. Rigid vessels, incapable of distention and recoil, produce high systolic pressure and low diastolic pressure. Normally, systolic pressure exceeds diastolic pressure by about 40 mm Hg. Narrowed pulse pressure—a difference of less than 30 mm Hg—occurs when systolic pressure falls and diastolic rises. These changes reflect reduced stroke volume, increased peripheral resistance, or both. Widened pulse pressure—a difference of more than 50 mm Hg between systolic and diastolic pressures—occurs when systolic pressure rises and diastolic pressure remains constant, or when systolic pressure rises and diastolic pressure falls. These changes reflect increased stroke volume, decreased peripheral resistance, or both.

Frequent blood pressure measurement is critical after serious injury, surgery, or anesthesia, and during any illness or condition that threatens cardiovascular stability. (Frequent measurement may be done with an automated vital signs monitor.) Regular measurement is indicated for patients with a history of hypertension or hypotension, and yearly screening is recommended for all adults.

Blood pressure should be measured using the recommendations set by the Seventh Report of the Joint National Committee on Prevention, Detection, Evaluation, and Treatment of High Blood Pressure (JNC VII). Until recently, patients with hypertension were stratified based on blood pressure readings alone. The JNC VII, however, also considers the patient's individual risk factors so that those with more risk factors are treated more aggressively. (See *Classification of blood pressure.*) The JNC VII has developed an innovative flowchart to guide the treatment of patients with hypertension. (See *Algorithm for treatment of hypertension,* page 20.)

Equipment

Mercury or aneroid sphygmomanometer ▪ stethoscope ▪ alcohol pad ▪ automated vital signs monitor (if available).

The sphygmomanometer consists of an inflatable compression cuff linked to a manual air pump and a mercury manometer or an aneroid gauge. The JNC VII recommends using a mercury sphygmomanometer *because it's more accurate and requires calibration less frequently than the aneroid model.* However, a recently calibrated aneroid manometer may be used. To obtain an accurate reading from a mercury sphygmomanometer, you must rest its gauge on a level surface and view the meniscus at eye level; you can rest an aneroid gauge in any position but must view it directly from the front.

Cuffs come in sizes ranging from neonate to extra-large adult. Disposable cuffs and thigh cuffs are available.

The automated vital signs monitor is a noninvasive device that measures pulse rate, systolic and diastolic pressures, and mean arterial pressure at preset intervals. (See *Using an electronic vital signs monitor,* page 21.)

Preparation of equipment

Carefully choose a cuff of appropriate size for the patient; the bladder should encircle at least 80% of the upper arm. *An excessively narrow cuff may cause a false-high pressure reading; an excessively wide one, a false-low reading.* If you aren't using your own stethoscope, disinfect the earpieces with an alcohol pad before placing them in your ears *to avoid cross-contamination.*

Classification of blood pressure

The Seventh Report of the Joint National Committee on Prevention, Detection, Evaluation, and Treatment of High Blood Pressure recommends that a person's risk factors be considered in the treatment of hypertension. The patient with more risk factors should be treated more aggressively.

CATEGORY	SBP MM HG		DBP MM HG
Normal	< 120	And	< 80
Prehypertension	120 to 139	Or	80 to 89
Hypertension, stage 1	140 to 159	Or	90 to 99
Hypertension, stage 2	≥ 160	Or	≥ 100

Key: SBP = systolic blood pressure; DBP = diastolic blood pressure

Adapted from the Seventh Report of the Joint National Committee on Prevention, Detection, Evaluation, and Treatment of High Blood Pressure. NIH Publication No. 03-5231. Bethesda, Md.: National Institutes of Health; National Heart, Lung, and Blood Institute; National High Blood Pressure Education Program, May 2003.

To use an automated vital signs monitor, collect the monitor, dual air hose, and pressure cuff. Then make sure the monitor unit is firmly positioned near the patient's bed.

Implementation

■ Confirm the patient's identity using two patient identifiers according to your facility's policy.

■ Tell the patient that you're going to take his blood pressure.

■ Have the patient rest for at least 5 minutes before measuring his blood pressure. Make sure that he hasn't had caffeine or smoked for at least 30 minutes.

■ The patient can lie supine or sit erect during blood pressure measurement. If the patient is sitting erect, make sure that he has both feet flat on the floor *because crossing the legs may elevate blood pressure.* His arm should be extended at heart level and be well supported. *If the artery is below heart level, you may get a false-high reading.* Make sure the patient is relaxed and comfortable when you take his blood pressure *so it stays at its normal level.*

■ Wrap the deflated cuff snugly around the upper arm. (See *Positioning the blood pressure cuff,* page 22.)

■ If the arm is very large or misshapen, and the conventional cuff won't fit properly, take leg or forearm measurement.

■ To obtain a thigh blood pressure, apply the appropriate-sized cuff to the thigh, and auscultate the pulsations over the popliteal artery, as shown below. To obtain a forearm blood pressure, apply the appropriate-sized cuff to the forearm 5″ (13 cm) below the elbow.

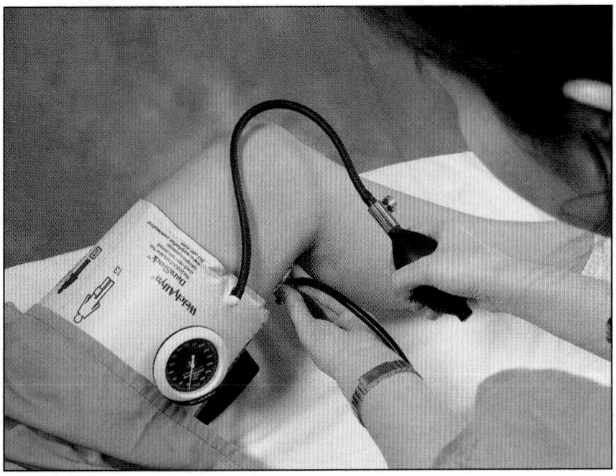

■ If necessary, connect the appropriate tube to the rubber bulb of the air pump and the other tube to the manometer. Then insert the stethoscope earpieces into your ears.

(Text continues on page 22.)

Algorithm for treatment of hypertension

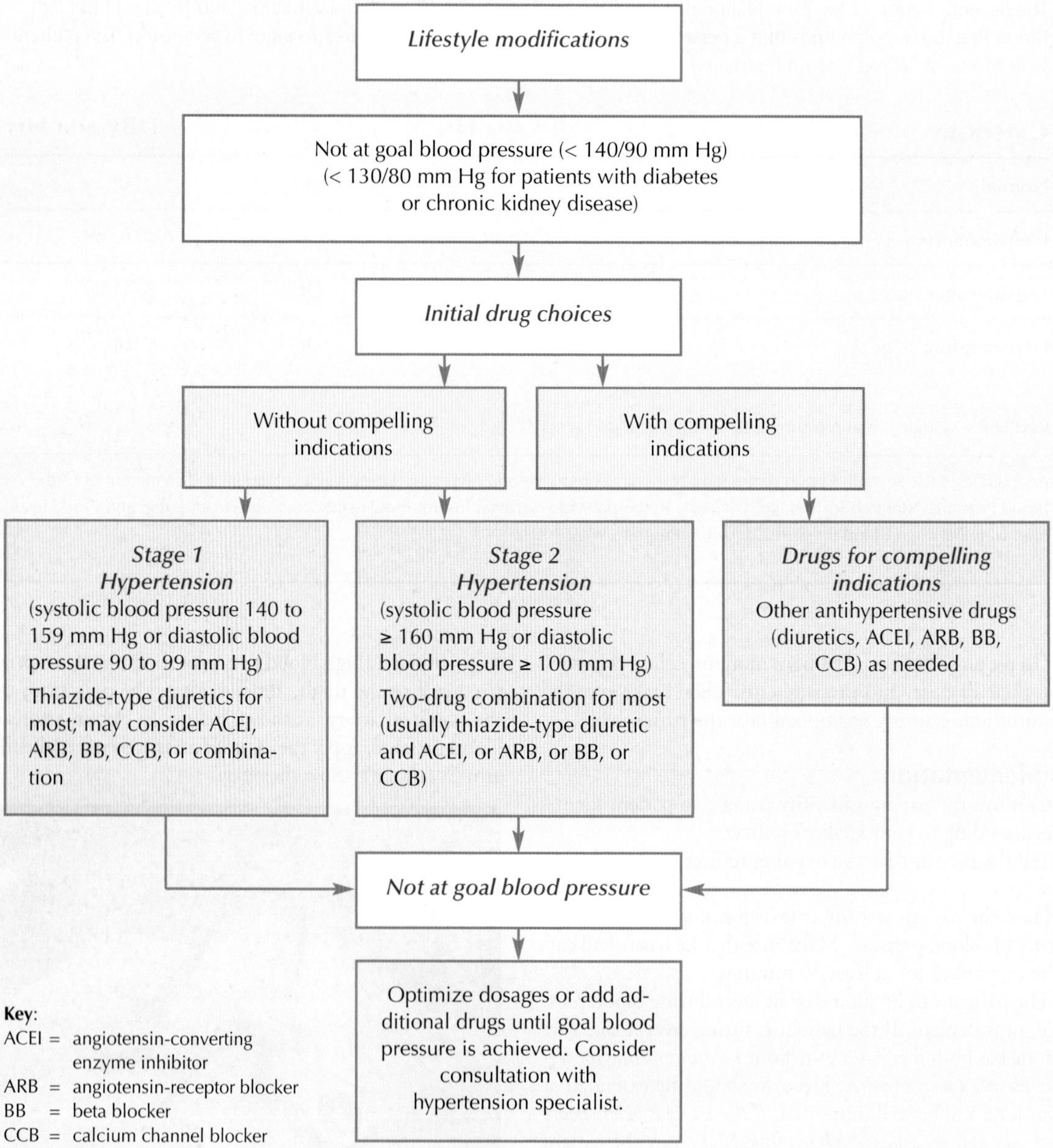

Adapted from the Seventh Report of the Joint National Committee on Prevention, Detection, Evaluation, and Treatment of High Blood Pressure. NIH Publication No. 03-5231. Bethesda, Md.: National Institutes of Health; National Heart, Lung, and Blood Institute; National High Blood Pressure Education Program, May 2003.

EQUIPMENT

Using an electronic vital signs monitor

An electronic vital signs monitor allows you to track a patient's vital signs continually, without having to reapply a blood pressure cuff each time. In addition, the patient won't need an invasive arterial line to gather similar data.

Some automated vital signs monitors are lightweight and battery-operated and can be attached to an I.V. pole for continual monitoring, even during patient transfers. Some models can also display patient temperature and pulse oximetry as well as blood pressure. A built-in printer is also available on certain models. Make sure that you know the capacity of the monitor's battery, and plug the machine in whenever possible *to keep it charged.* Regularly calibrate the monitor *to ensure accurate readings.*

Before using any monitor, check its accuracy. Determine the patient's pulse rate and blood pressure manually, using the same arm you'll use for the monitor cuff. Compare your results when you get initial readings from the monitor. If the results differ, call your supply department or the manufacturer's representative.

Check the manufacturer's guidelines *because most automated monitoring devices are intended for serial monitoring only and may be inaccurate for a one-time measurement.*

Preparing the device

- Explain the procedure to the patient. Describe the alarm system *so he won't be frightened if it's triggered.*
- Make sure that the power switch is off. Then plug the monitor into a properly grounded wall outlet. Secure the dual air hose to the front of the monitor.
- Connect the pressure cuff's tubing into the other ends of the dual air hose, and tighten connections *to prevent air leaks.* Keep the air hose away from the patient *to avoid accidental dislodgment.*
- Squeeze all air from the cuff, and wrap the cuff loosely around the patient's arm—about 1" (2.5 cm) above the antecubital fossa. Never apply the cuff to a limb that has an I.V. line in place. Position the cuff's "artery" arrow over the palpated brachial artery. Then secure the cuff for a snug fit.

Selecting parameters

- When you turn on the monitor, it will default to a manual mode. (In this mode, you can obtain vital signs yourself before switching to the automatic mode.) Press the AUTO/MANUAL button to select the automatic mode.

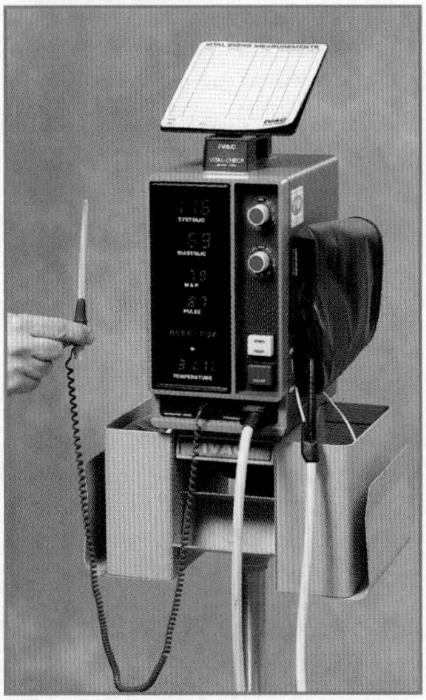

The monitor will give you baseline data for the pulse rate, systolic and diastolic pressures, and mean arterial pressure.

- Compare your previous manual results with these baseline data. If they match, you're ready to set the alarm parameters. Press the SELECT button to blank out all displays except systolic pressure.
- Use the HIGH and LOW limit buttons to set the specific parameters for systolic pressure. (These limits range from a high of 240 to a low of 0.) You'll also do this three more times for mean arterial pressure, pulse rate, and diastolic pressure. After you've set the parameters for diastolic pressure, press the SELECT button again to display all current data. Even if you forget to do this last step, the monitor will automatically display current data 10 seconds after you set the last parameters.

Collecting data

- You also need to tell the monitor how often to obtain data. Press the SET button until you reach the desired time interval in minutes. If you've chosen the automatic mode, the monitor will display a default cycle time of 3 minutes. You can override the default cycle time to set the interval you prefer.
- You can obtain a set of vital signs at any time by pressing the START button. Also, pressing the CANCEL button will stop the interval and deflate the cuff. You can retrieve stored data by pressing the PRIOR DATA button. The monitor will display the last data obtained along with the time elapsed since then. Scrolling backward, you can retrieve data from the previous 99 minutes. Make sure that the patient's vital signs are documented frequently on a vital signs assessment sheet.

Positioning the blood pressure cuff

Palpate the brachial artery. Position the cuff 1" (2.5 cm) above the site of pulsation, center the bladder above the artery with the cuff fully deflated, and wrap the cuff evenly and snugly around the upper arm.

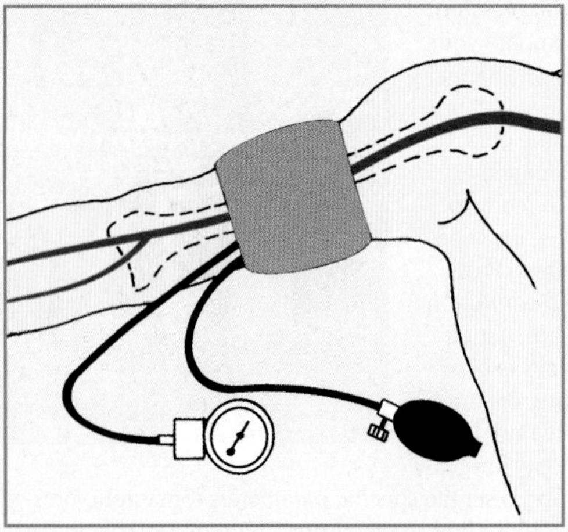

■ *To determine how high to pump the blood pressure cuff,* first estimate the systolic blood pressure by palpation. As you feel the radial artery with the fingers of one hand, inflate the cuff with your other hand until the radial pulse disappears. Read this pressure on the manometer and add 30 mm Hg to it. Use this sum as the target inflation *to prevent discomfort from overinflation.* Deflate the cuff and wait at least 2 minutes.
■ Locate the brachial artery by palpation. Center the bell of the stethoscope over the part of the artery where you detect the strongest beats, and hold it in place with one hand. *The bell of the stethoscope transmits low-pitched arterial blood sounds more effectively than does the diaphragm.*
■ Using the thumb and index finger of your other hand, turn the thumbscrew on the rubber bulb of the air pump clockwise to close the valve.
■ Pump up the cuff to the predetermined level.
■ Carefully open the valve of the air pump, and then slowly deflate the cuff—no faster than 2 to 3 mm Hg per second. While releasing air, watch the mercury column or aneroid gauge, and auscultate for the sound over the artery.
■ When you hear the first beat or clear tapping sound, note the pressure on the column or gauge. This is the systolic pressure. (The beat or tapping sound is the first of five Korotkoff sounds. The second sound resembles a murmur or swish; the third sound, crisp tapping; the fourth sound, a soft, muffled tone; and the fifth, the last sound heard.)
■ Continue to release air gradually while auscultating for the sound over the artery.
■ Note the pressure where the sound disappears. This is the diastolic pressure—the fifth Korotkoff sound.
■ After you hear the last Korotkoff sound, deflate the cuff slowly for at least another 10 mm Hg *to ensure that no further sounds are audible.*
■ Rapidly deflate the cuff. Record the pressure, wait 2 minutes, and then repeat the procedure. If the average of the readings is greater than 5 mmHg, take the average of two more readings. After doing so, remove and fold the cuff, and return it to storage.
■ Document the blood pressure results.

Special considerations

■ If you can't auscultate blood pressure, you may estimate systolic pressure. To do this, first palpate the brachial or radial pulse. Then inflate the cuff until you no longer detect the pulse. Slowly deflate the cuff and, when you detect the pulse again, record the pressure as the palpated systolic pressure.
■ Palpation of systolic blood pressure may also be important *to avoid underestimating blood pressure in patients with an auscultatory gap.* This gap is a loss of sound between the first and second Korotkoff sounds that may be as great as 40 mm Hg. You may find this in patients with venous congestion or hypotension.
■ Another alternative to auscultating with a stethoscope is to use Doppler ultrasound to hear Korotkoff sounds. This is useful when the blood pressure is diminished or when the pulse is nonpalpable.
■ If the patient is crying or anxious, delay blood pressure measurement, if possible, until he becomes calm *to avoid falsely elevated readings.*
■ Remember that malfunction in an aneroid sphygmomanometer can be identified only by checking it against a mercury manometer of known accuracy. Be sure to check your aneroid manometer this way periodically. Malfunction in a mercury manometer is evident in abnormal behavior of the mercury column. Don't attempt to repair either type yourself; instead, send it to the appropriate service department. (For information on other situations that can cause false-high or false-low readings, see *Correcting problems of blood pressure measurement.*)
■ Occasionally, blood pressure must be measured in both arms or with the patient in two different positions (such as lying and standing or sitting and standing). In such cases, observe and record any significant difference between the

TROUBLESHOOTING

Correcting problems of blood pressure measurement

Blood pressure readings can be falsely high or falsely low due to various causes. You'll need to assess the situation and respond accordingly.

REACTION AND CAUSES	NURSING ACTIONS
FALSE-HIGH READING	
■ Cuff too small	■ Make sure that the cuff bladder is 20% wider than the circumference of the arm or leg being used for measurement.
■ Cuff wrapped too loosely, reducing its effective width	■ Tighten the cuff.
■ Slow cuff deflation, causing venous congestion in the arm or leg	■ Never deflate the cuff more slowly than 2 mm Hg/heartbeat.
■ Tilted mercury column	■ Read pressures with the mercury column vertical.
■ Poorly timed measurement—after patient has eaten, ambulated, appeared anxious, or flexed arm muscles	■ Postpone blood pressure measurement or help the patient relax before taking pressures.
FALSE-LOW READING	
■ Incorrect position of arm or leg	■ Make sure the arm or leg is level with the patient's heart.
■ Mercury column below eye level	■ Read the mercury column at eye level.
■ Failure to notice auscultatory gap (sound fades out for 10 to 15 mm Hg, then returns)	■ Estimate systolic pressure by palpation before actually measuring it. Then check this pressure against the measured pressure.
■ Inaudible low-volume sounds	■ Before reinflating the cuff, instruct the patient to raise the arm or leg *to decrease venous pressure and amplify low-volume sounds.* After inflating the cuff, tell the patient to lower the arm or leg. Then deflate the cuff and listen. If you still fail to detect low-volume sounds, chart the palpated systolic pressure.

two readings, and record the blood pressure and the extremity and position used.

■ Measure the blood pressure of a patient taking antihypertensive medication while he's in a sitting position *to ensure accurate measurements.*

Complications

Don't take a blood pressure in the arm on the affected side of a mastectomy patient *because it may decrease already compromised lymphatic circulation, worsen edema, and damage the arm.* Likewise, don't take a blood pressure on an arm with an arteriovenous fistula or hemodialysis shunt *because blood flow through the vascular device may be compromised.*

Documentation

On the patient's chart, record blood pressure as systolic over diastolic pressures, such as 120/78 mm Hg. Chart an auscultatory gap if present. If required by your facility, chart blood pressures on a graph, using dots or checkmarks. Document the extremity used and the patient's position. If the blood pressure was palpated or auscultated using a Doppler device, record this as well. Include patient teaching about lifestyle modifications, drug therapy, and follow-up care. Record the name of any practitioner notified of blood pressure results and any orders given.

SELECTED REFERENCES

Craven, R.F., and Hirnle, C.J. *Fundamentals of Nursing: Human Health and Function*, 5th ed. Philadelphia: Lippincott Williams & Wilkins, 2006.

Eser, I. "The Effect of Different Body Positions on Blood Pressure," *Journal of Clinical Nursing* 16(1):137-140, January 2007.

O'Rourke, M.F., and Seward, J.B. "Central Arterial Pressure and Arterial Pressure Pulse: New Views Entering the Second Century after Korotkoff," *Mayo Clinic Proceedings* 81(8):1057-68, August 2006.

Schell, K.A. "Evidence-Based Practice: Noninvasive Blood Pressure Measurement in Children," *Pediatric Nursing* 32(3):263-67, May-June 2006.

The Seventh Report of the Joint National Committee on Prevention, Detection, and Treatment of High Blood Pressure. NIH Publication No. 03-5233. Bethesda, Md.: National Institutes of Health; National Heart, Lung, and Blood Institute; National High Blood Pressure Education Program. December 2003. Available at *www.nhlbi.nih.gov/guidelines/hypertension/express.pdf.*

RESPIRATION

Controlled by the respiratory center in the lateral medulla oblongata, respiration is the exchange of oxygen and carbon dioxide between the atmosphere and body cells. External respiration, or breathing, is accomplished by the diaphragm and chest muscles and delivers oxygen to the lower respiratory tract and alveoli.

Four measures of respiration—rate, rhythm, depth, and sound—reflect the body's metabolic state, diaphragm and chest-muscle condition, and airway patency. Respiratory rate is recorded as the number of cycles (with inspiration and expiration comprising one cycle) per minute; rhythm, as the regularity of these cycles; depth, as the volume of air inhaled and exhaled with each respiration; and sound, as the audible digression from normal, effortless breathing.

Equipment

Watch with second hand.

Implementation

- The best time to assess the patient's respirations is immediately after taking his pulse rate. Keep your fingertips over the radial artery, and don't tell the patient you're counting respirations. *If you tell him, he'll become conscious of his respirations, and the rate may change.*
- Count respirations by observing the rise and fall of the patient's chest as he breathes. Alternatively, position the patient's opposite arm across his chest and count respirations by feeling its rise and fall. Consider one rise and one fall as one respiration.
- Count respirations for 30 seconds and multiply by 2 or count for 60 seconds if respirations are irregular *to account for variations in respiratory rate and pattern.*
- As you count respirations, be alert for and record such breath sounds as stertor, stridor, wheezing, and an expiratory grunt. *Stertor* is a snoring sound resulting from secretions in the trachea and large bronchi. Listen for it in patients with neurologic disorders and in those who are comatose. *Stridor* is an inspiratory crowing sound that occurs with upper airway obstruction in laryngitis, croup, or the presence of a foreign body.

PEDIATRIC ALERT *When listening for stridor in infants and children with croup, also observe for sternal, substernal, or intercostal retractions.*

- *Wheezing* is caused by partial obstruction in the smaller bronchi and bronchioles. This high-pitched, musical sound is common in patients with emphysema or asthma.

PEDIATRIC ALERT *In infants, an expiratory grunt indicates imminent respiratory distress.*

ELDER ALERT ***In older patients, an expiratory grunt may result from partial airway obstruction or neuromuscular reflex.***

- Watch the patient's chest movements, and listen to his breathing to determine the rhythm and sound of respirations. (See *Identifying respiratory patterns.*)
- To detect other breath sounds—such as crackles and rhonchi—or the lack of sound in the lungs, you'll need a stethoscope.
- Observe chest movements for depth of respirations. If the patient inhales a small volume of air, record this as shallow; if he inhales a large volume, record this as deep.
- Observe the patient for use of accessory muscles, such as the scalene, sternocleidomastoid, trapezius, and latissimus dorsi. Using these muscles reflects weakness of the diaphragm and the external intercostal muscles—the major muscles of respiration.

Special considerations

- Respiratory rates of less than 8 or more than 40 breaths per minute are usually considered abnormal; report the sudden onset of such rates promptly. Observe the patient for signs of dyspnea, such as an anxious facial expression, flaring nostrils, a heaving chest wall, and cyanosis. To detect cyanosis, look for characteristic bluish discoloration in the nail beds or the lips, under the tongue, in the buccal mucosa, or in the conjunctiva.
- In assessing the patient's respiratory status, consider his personal and family history. Ask whether he smokes and, if so, for how many years and how many packs per day.

Identifying respiratory patterns

The table below shows several common types of respiratory patterns and their possible causes. It's important to assess the patient for the underlying cause and the effect on the patient.

TYPE	CHARACTERISTICS	PATTERN	POSSIBLE CAUSES
Apnea	Periodic absence of breathing	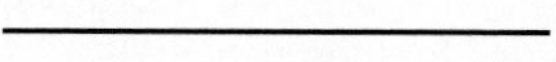	■ Mechanical airway obstruction ■ Conditions affecting the brain's respiratory center in the lateral medulla oblongata
Apneustic	Prolonged, gasping inspiration followed by extremely short, inefficient expiration	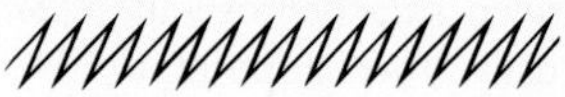	■ Lesions of the respiratory center
Bradypnea	Slow, regular respirations of equal depth	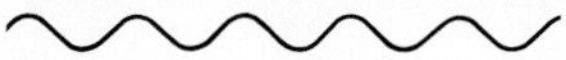	■ Normal pattern during sleep ■ Conditions affecting the respiratory center: tumors, metabolic disorders, respiratory decompensation, and use of opiates or alcohol
Cheyne-Stokes	Fast, deep respirations of 30 to 170 seconds punctuated by periods of apnea lasting 20 to 60 seconds	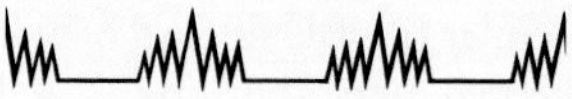	■ Increased intracranial pressure, severe congestive heart failure, renal failure, meningitis, drug overdose, and cerebral anoxia
Eupnea	Normal rate and rhythm	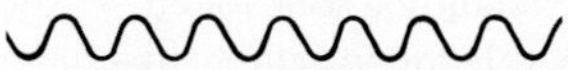	■ Normal respiration
Kussmaul's	Fast (over 20 breaths/minute), deep (resembling sighs), labored respirations without pause	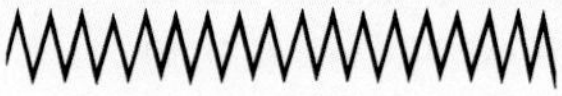	■ Renal failure and metabolic acidosis, particularly diabetic ketoacidosis
Tachypnea	Rapid respirations; rate rising with body temperature—about four breaths/minute for every degree Fahrenheit above normal	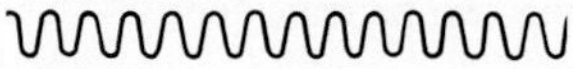	■ Pneumonia, compensatory respiratory alkalosis, respiratory insufficiency, lesions of the respiratory center, and salicylate poisoning

PEDIATRIC ALERT *A child's respiratory rate may double in response to exercise, illness, or emotion. Normally, the rate for neonates is 30 to 80 breaths/minute; for toddlers, 20 to 40; and for children of school age and older, 15 to 25. Children usually reach the adult rate (12 to 20) at about age 15.*

Documentation

Record the rate, depth, rhythm, and sound of the patient's respirations.

SELECTED REFERENCES

Aylott, M. "Observing the Sick Child: Part 2a. Respiration Assessment," *Paediatric Nursing* 18(9):38-44, November 2006.

Craven, R.F., and Hirnle, C.J. *Fundamentals of Nursing: Human Health and Function,* 5th ed. Philadelphia: Lippincott Williams & Wilkins, 2006.
Hogan, J. "Why Don't Nurses Monitor the Respiratory Rates of Patients?" *British Journal of Nursing* 15(9):489-92, May 2006.

HEIGHT AND WEIGHT

Height and weight are routinely measured for most patients during admission to a health care facility. An accurate record of the patient's height and weight is essential for calculating dosages of drugs, anesthetics, and contrast agents; assessing the patient's nutritional status; and determining the height-weight ratio. Because body weight provides the best overall picture of fluid status, monitoring it daily proves important for patients receiving sodium-retaining or diuretic medications. Rapid weight gain may signal fluid retention; rapid weight loss may indicate diuresis.

Weight can be measured with a standing scale, chair scale, or bed scale; height can be measured with the measuring bar on a standing scale, using a ruler, or with a tape measure for a supine patient. (See *Types of scales.*)

Equipment

Standing scale or chair or bed scale ■ ruler (if scale doesn't have measuring bar) ■ wheelchair (if needed to transport patient) ■ tape measure if needed.

Preparation of equipment

Select the appropriate scale—usually, a standing scale for an ambulatory patient or a chair or bed scale for an acutely ill or debilitated patient. Then check to make sure the scale is balanced. *Standing scales and, to a lesser extent, bed scales may become unbalanced when transported.*

Implementation

■ Confirm the patient's identity using two patient identifiers according to your facility's policy.
■ Explain the procedure to the patient.

Using a standing scale

■ Place a paper towel on the scale's platform.
■ Ask the patient to remove his robe and slippers or shoes. If the scale has wheels, lock them before the patient steps on. Assist the patient onto the scale, and remain close to him *to prevent falls.*
■ If you're using an upright balance (gravity) scale, slide the lower rider to the groove representing the largest increment below the patient's estimated weight. Grooves represent 50, 100, 150, and 200 lb. Then slide the small upper rider until the beam balances. Add the upper and lower rider figures *to determine the weight.* (The upper rider is calibrated to eighths of a pound.)
■ Return the weight holder to its proper place.
■ If you're using a digital scale, make sure the display reads 0 before use. Read the display with the patient standing as still as possible.
■ Help the patient off the scale, and give him his robe and slippers or shoes.

Using a chair scale

■ Transport the patient to the weighing area or the scale to the patient's bedside.
■ Lock the scale in place *to prevent it from moving accidentally.*
■ If you're using a scale with a swing-away chair arm, unlock the arm. When unlocked, the arm swings back 180 degrees *to permit easy access.*
■ Position the scale beside the patient's bed or wheelchair with the chair arm open. Transfer the patient onto the scale, swing the chair arm to the front of the scale, and lock it in place.
■ If the chair scale is digital, make sure the display reads 0 before use. Press the button and record the weight. If using a multiple-weight chair scale, use the same process as used with a standing scale to determine the weight.
■ Unlock the swing-away chair arm as before, and transfer the patient back to his bed or wheelchair.
■ Lock the main beam *to avoid damaging the scale during transport.* Then unlock the wheels and remove the scale from the patient's room.

Using a digital bed scale

■ Provide privacy, and tell the patient that you're going to weigh him on a special bed scale. Demonstrate its operation if appropriate.
■ Place the protective plastic covering over the stretcher, and confirm that the scale is balanced.
■ Release the stretcher to the horizontal position; then lock it in place. Turn the patient on his side, facing away from the scale.
■ Roll the base of the scale under the patient's bed. Adjust the lever *to widen the base of the scale, providing stability.* Then lock the scale's wheels.
■ Center the stretcher above the bed, lower it onto the mattress, and roll the patient onto the stretcher. Then position the circular weighing arms of the scale over the patient, and attach them securely to the stretcher bars.
■ Pump the handle with long, slow strokes *to raise the patient a few inches off the bed.* Make sure the patient doesn't lean on or touch the headboard, side rails, or other bed equip-

EQUIPMENT

Types of scales

Patient status determines the type of scale selected. Selection of scales varies, and the selection is influenced by the status of the patient.

For ambulatory patients **For acutely ill or debilitated patients**

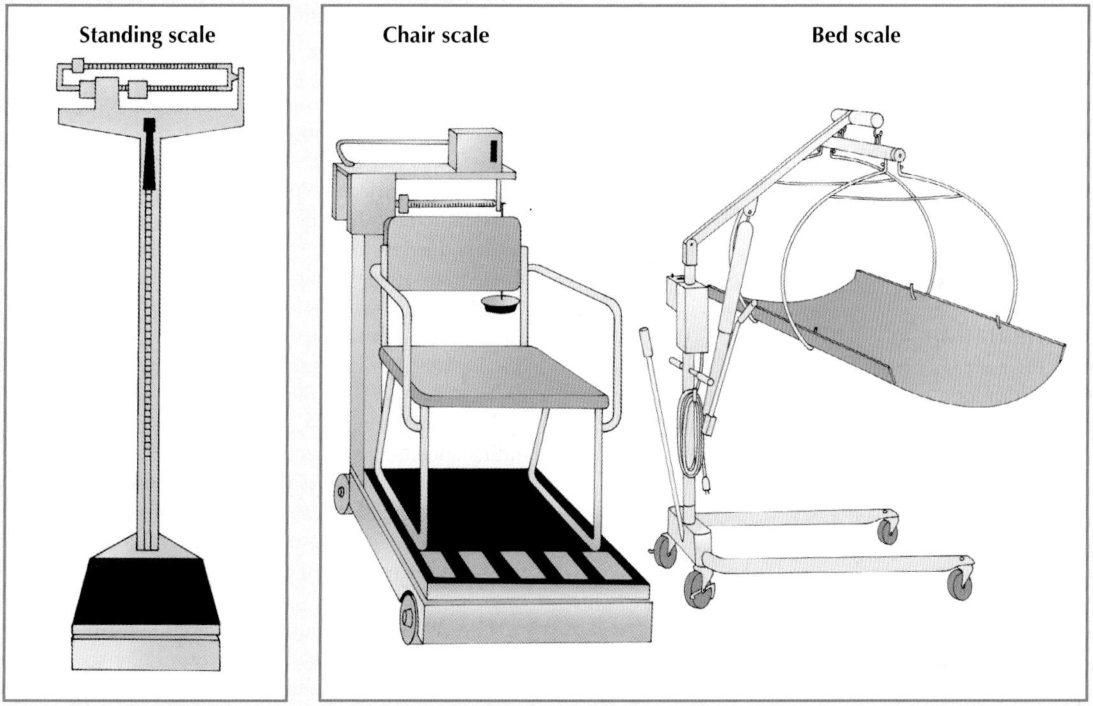

ment, and that nothing is pulling on the scale (such as I.V. or catheter tubing) *because these types of pressure will affect the weight measurement.*

- Depress the operate button, and read the patient's weight on the digital display panel. Then press in the scale's handle *to lower the patient.*
- Detach the circular weighing arms from the stretcher bars, roll the patient off the stretcher and remove it, and position him comfortably in bed.
- Release the wheel lock and withdraw the scale. Dispose of the protective plastic covering, and return the stretcher to its vertical position.

Height measurement

- If you're using a standing scale to measure height, tell the patient to stand erect on the platform of the scale. Raise the measuring bar beyond the top of the patient's head, extend the horizontal arm, and lower the bar until it touches the top of the patient's head. Then read the patient's height.
- Without a scale, have the patient remove his shoes. Have him stand against a wall with his back and heels touching the wall. Using a straight, level object (such as a ruler), place it on top of the patient's head parallel to the floor. Mark the location of the ruler on the wall. Measure the distance between the mark and the floor.

PEDIATRIC ALERT *When measuring the height of a child younger than age 2, measure the length of the child in a supine position, while holding the head in the midline position and gently holding the legs in full extension.*

Special considerations

- Reassure and steady patients who are at risk for losing their balance on a scale.
- Weigh the patient at the same time each day (usually before breakfast), in similar clothing, and using the same scale. If the patient uses crutches, weigh him with the crutches. Then weigh the crutches and any heavy clothing, and subtract their weight from the total to determine the patient's weight.
- Before using a bed scale, cover its stretcher with a drawsheet. Balance the scale with the drawsheet in place *to ensure accurate weighing.*
- When rolling the patient onto the stretcher, be careful not to dislodge I.V. lines, indwelling catheters, and other supportive equipment.
- Bed and dialysis scales, with platforms that are placed under the castors of the bed, are useful if frequent weights are needed or the patient is too critically ill to move.

Documentation

Record the patient's height and weight on the nursing assessment form and other medical records, as required by your facility.

SELECTED REFERENCES

Craven, R.F., and Hirnle, C.J. *Fundamentals of Nursing: Human Health and Function*, 5th ed. Philadelphia: Lippincott Williams & Wilkins, 2006.

Fransozi, F.G. "Should We Continue to Use BMI as a Cardiovascular Risk Factor?" *Lancet* 368(9536):624-25, August 2006.

Hendershot, K.M., et al. "Estimated Height, Weight, and Body Mass Index: Implications for Research and Patient Safety," *Journal of the American College of Surgeons* 203(6):887-93, December 2006.

Stoner, A., and Walker, J. "Growth Assessment: How Do We Measure Up?" *Paediatric Nursing* 18(7):26-28, September 2006.

ASSESSMENT TECHNIQUES

To perform physical assessment, a nurse uses four basic techniques: inspection, palpation, percussion, and auscultation. Performing these techniques correctly helps elicit valuable information about the patient's condition.

Inspection requires the use of vision, hearing, touch, and smell. Special lighting and various equipment—such as an otoscope, a tongue blade, or an ophthalmoscope—may be used to enhance vision or examine an otherwise hidden area. Inspection begins during the first patient contact and continues throughout the assessment.

Palpation usually follows inspection, except when examining the abdomen or assessing infants and children. Palpation involves touching the body to determine the size, shape, and position of structures; to detect and evaluate temperature, pulsations, and other movement; and to elicit tenderness.

The four palpation techniques include light palpation, deep palpation, light ballottement, and deep ballottement. Ballottement is the technique used to evaluate a flowing or movable structure. The nurse gently bounces the structure being assessed by applying pressure against it and then waits to feel it rebound. This technique may be used, for example, to check the position of an organ or a fetus.

Percussion uses quick, sharp tapping of the fingers or hands against body surfaces to produce sounds, detect tenderness, or assess reflexes. Percussing for sound helps locate organ borders, identify organ shape and position, and determine whether an organ is solid or filled with fluid or gas.

Organs and tissues produce sounds of varying loudness, pitch, and duration, depending on their density. For example, air-filled cavities, such as the lungs, produce markedly different sounds from those produced by the liver and other dense organs and tissues. Percussion techniques include indirect percussion, direct percussion, and blunt percussion.

Auscultation involves listening to various sounds of the body—particularly those produced by the heart, lungs, vessels, stomach, and intestines. Most auscultated sounds result from the movement of air or fluid through these structures.

Usually, the nurse auscultates after performing the other assessment techniques. When examining the abdomen, however, auscultation should occur after inspection but before percussion and palpation. This way, bowel sounds can be heard before palpation disrupts them. Auscultation is best performed first on infants and young children, who may start to cry when palpated or percussed. Auscultation is most successful when performed in a quiet environment with a properly fitted stethoscope.

Equipment

Flashlight or gooseneck lamp, as appropriate ▪ patient drape ▪ ophthalmoscope ▪ otoscope ▪ stethoscope.

Implementation

- Confirm the patient's identity using two patient identifiers according to your facility's policy.
- Explain the procedure to the patient, have him undress, and drape him appropriately.
- Make sure the room is warm and adequately lit *to make the patient comfortable and aid visual inspection.*
- Warm your hands and the stethoscope.

Inspection

■ Focus on areas related to the patient's chief complaint. Use your eyes, ears, and sense of smell to observe the patient.

■ To inspect a specific body area, first make sure the area is sufficiently exposed and adequately lit. Then survey the entire area, noting key landmarks and checking its overall condition. Next, focus on specifics—color, shape, texture, size, and movement. Note any unusual findings as well as predictable ones.

Palpation

■ Explain the procedure to the patient, and tell him what to expect such as occasional discomfort as pressure is applied. Encourage him to relax *because muscle tension or guarding can interfere with performance and results of palpation.*

■ Use the flattened fingerpads for palpating tender tissues, feeling for crepitus (crackling) at the joints, and lightly probing the abdomen. Use the thumb and index finger for assessing hair texture, grasping tissues, and feeling for lymph node enlargement. Use the back, or dorsal, surface of the hand when feeling for warmth.

■ Provide just enough pressure to assess the tissue beneath one or both hands. Then release pressure and gently move to the next area, systematically covering the entire surface to be assessed. (See *Performing palpation*, page 30.)

■ To perform light palpation, depress the skin, indenting ½" to ¾" (1 to 2 cm). Use the lightest touch possible *because excessive pressure blunts your sensitivity.*

■ If the patient tolerates light palpation, and you need to assess deeper structures, palpate deeply by increasing your fingertip pressure, indenting the skin about 1½" (4 cm). Place your other hand on top of the palpating hand to control and guide your movements.

■ To perform light ballottement, apply light, rapid pressure from quadrant to quadrant on the patient's abdomen. Keep your hand on the skin *to detect tissue rebound.*

■ To perform deeper ballottement, apply abrupt, deep pressure and then release it. Maintain fingertip contact.

■ Use both hands (bimanual palpation) to trap a deep, underlying, hard-to-palpate organ (such as the kidney or spleen) or to fix or stabilize an organ (such as the uterus) with one hand while you palpate it with the other.

Percussion

■ First, decide which of the percussion techniques best suits your assessment needs. Indirect percussion helps reveal the size and density of underlying thoracic and abdominal organs and tissues. Direct percussion helps assess an adult's sinuses for tenderness and elicits sounds in a child's thorax. Blunt percussion aims to elicit tenderness over organs, such as the kidneys, gallbladder, or liver. When percussing, note the characteristic sounds produced. (See *Identifying percussion sounds*, page 31.)

■ To perform indirect percussion, place one hand on the patient and tap the middle finger with the middle finger of the other hand. (See *Performing indirect percussion,* page 31.)

■ To perform direct percussion, tap your hand or fingertip directly against the body surface.

■ To perform blunt percussion, strike the ulnar surface of your fist against the body surface. Or place the palm of one hand against the body, make a fist with the other hand, and strike the back of the first hand.

Auscultation

■ First, determine whether to use the bell or diaphragm of your stethoscope. Use the diaphragm to detect high-pitched sounds, such as breath and bowel sounds. Use the bell to detect lower-pitched sounds, such as heart and vascular sounds.

■ Place the diaphragm or bell of the stethoscope over the appropriate area of the patient's body. Place the earpieces in your ears, listen intently to individual sounds, and try to identify their characteristics. Determine the intensity, pitch, and duration of each sound, and check the frequency of recurring sounds.

Special considerations

■ Avoid palpating or percussing an area of the body known to be tender at the start of your examination. Instead, work around the area; then gently palpate or percuss it at the end of the examination. *This progression minimizes the patient's discomfort and apprehension.*

■ To assess the abdomen, inspect visually first. Then auscultate bowel sounds before palpation and percussion, *which alter these sounds.*

■ To pinpoint an inflamed area deep within the patient's body, perform a variation on deep palpation: Press firmly with one hand over the area you suspect is involved, and then lift your hand away quickly. If the patient reports that pain increases when you release the pressure, then you've identified rebound tenderness.

NURSING ALERT *Suspect peritonitis if you elicit rebound tenderness when examining the abdomen.*

■ If you can't palpate because the patient fears pain, try distracting him with conversation. Then perform auscultation and gently press your stethoscope into the affected area *to try to elicit tenderness.*

Complications

Palpation may cause an enlarged spleen or infected appendix to rupture.

(Text continues on page 32.)

Performing palpation

You should be familiar with four palpation techniques: light palpation, deep palpation, light ballottement, and deep ballottement.

Light palpation

With the tips of two or three fingers held close together, press gently on the skin to a depth of ½″ to ¾″ (1 to 2 cm). Use the lightest touch possible; *too much pressure blunts your sensitivity.*

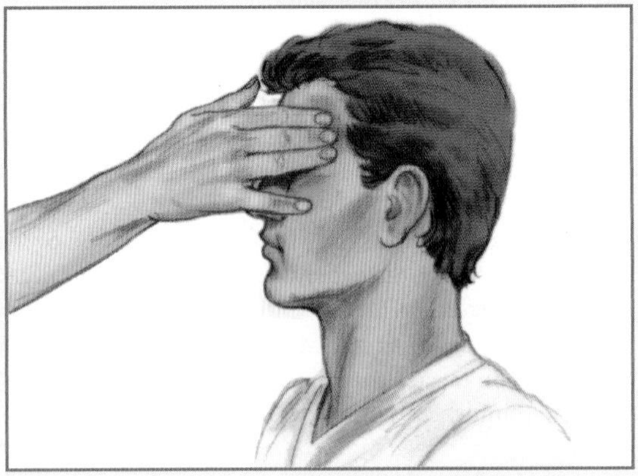

Light ballottement

Apply light, rapid pressure to the abdomen, moving from one quadrant to another. Keep your hand on the skin surface *to detect tissue rebound.*

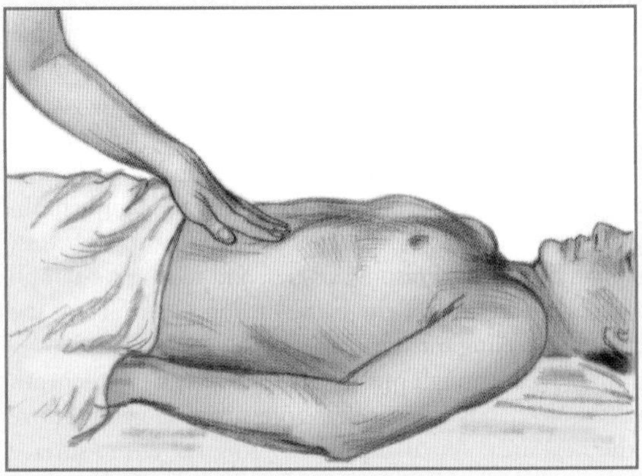

Deep palpation (bimanual palpation)

Place one hand on top of the other. Then press down about 1½″ to 2″ (4 to 5 cm) with the fingertips of both hands.

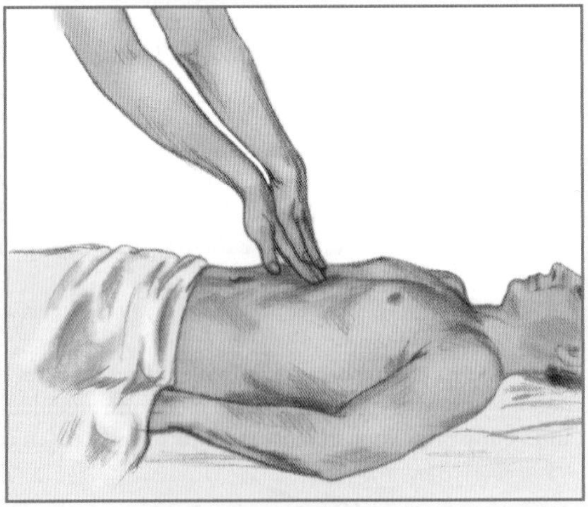

Deep ballottement

Apply abrupt, deep pressure on the patient's abdomen. Release the pressure completely, but maintain fingertip contact with the skin.

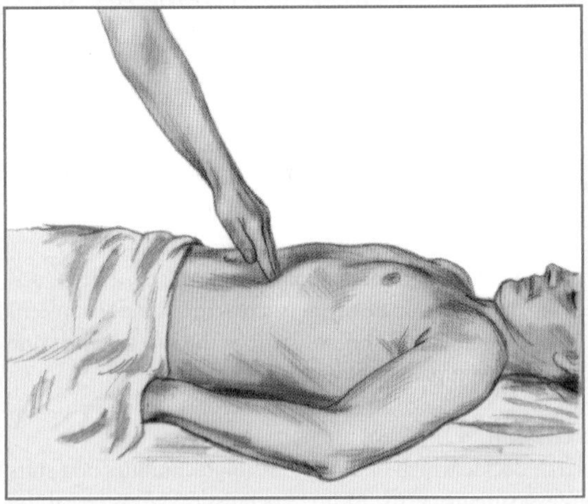

Identifying percussion sounds

Percussion produces sounds that vary according to the tissue being percussed. This table lists important percussion sounds along with their characteristics and typical sources.

SOUND	INTENSITY	PITCH	DURATION	QUALITY	SOURCE
Resonance	Moderate to loud	Low	Long	Hollow	Normal lung
Tympany	Loud	High	Moderate	Drumlike	Gastric air bubble, intestinal air
Dullness	Soft to moderate	High	Moderate	Thudlike	Liver, full bladder, pregnant uterus
Hyperresonance	Very loud	Very low	Long	Booming	Hyperinflated lung (as in emphysema)
Flatness	Soft	High	Short	Flat	Muscle

Performing indirect percussion

To perform indirect percussion, use the middle finger of your nondominant hand as the pleximeter (the mediating device used to receive the taps) and the middle finger of your dominant hand as the plexor (the device used to tap the pleximeter).

Place the pleximeter finger firmly against a body surface such as the upper back. With your wrist flexed loosely, use the tip of your plexor finger to deliver a crisp blow just beneath the distal joint of the pleximeter.

Be sure to hold the plexor perpendicular to the pleximeter. Tap lightly and quickly, removing the plexor as soon as you have delivered each blow. Move your nondominant hand to cover the entire area to be percussed.

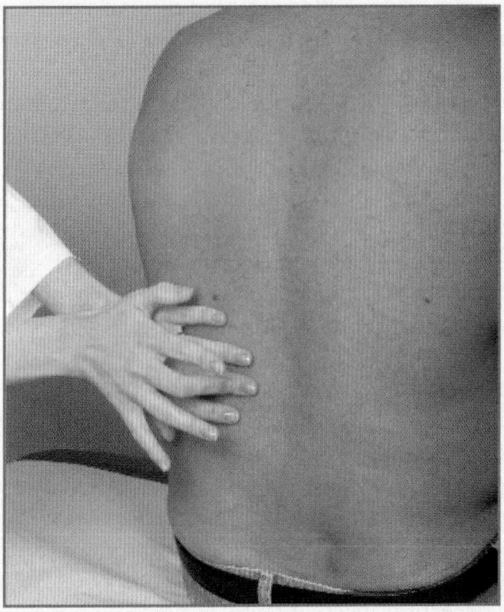

Documentation

Document your assessment findings and the technique used to elicit those findings—for example, "right lower quadrant tenderness on deep palpation, no rebound tenderness."

SELECTED REFERENCES

Bickley, L.S., and Szilagyi, P.G. *Bates' Guide to Physical Examination and History Taking,* 9th ed. Philadelphia: Lippincott Williams & Wilkins, 2007.

Craven, R.F., and Hirnle, C.J. *Fundamentals of Nursing: Human Health and Function,* 5th ed. Philadelphia: Lippincott Williams & Wilkins, 2006.

Jevon, P. "Chest Examination Part 1—Chest Palpation," *Nursing Times* 102(44):26-27, October-November 2006.

Jevon, P. "Chest Examination Part 2—Chest Percussion," *Nursing Times* 102(45):26-27, November 2006.

Jevon, P., and Cunnington, A. "Chest Examination Part 3—Chest Auscultation," *Nursing Times* 102(46):26-27, November 2006.

PHYSICAL ASSESSMENT

Nurses perform a complete physical assessment when the patient is admitted to the facility and partial reassessments as the patient's condition warrants. A complete assessment includes a thorough health history and physical examination. The health history includes the chief complaint, a history of the current illness, general medical and surgical histories, a family history, a social history, and a review of systems.

Typically, the physical examination follows a methodical, head-to-toe format. Patient preparation includes providing a clear explanation of the examination as well as proper positioning and draping before and during the examination. During this procedure, the nurse must make every effort to recognize and respect the patient's feelings (particularly embarrassment and anxiety) as well as to provide comfort measures and follow appropriate safety precautions.

Equipment

Although equipment varies with the examination's focus, the following may be included: Scale with height measurement bar ■ urine specimen container and laboratory request form (if ordered) ■ sphygmomanometer ■ watch with second hand ■ stethoscope ■ thermometer ■ gown (for patient) ■ examining table (with stirrups if necessary) ■ gloves ■ drapes (sheet, bath blanket, or towel, as needed) ■ adhesive tape ■ spotlight or gooseneck lamp ■ flashlight ■ laryngeal mirror ■ tongue blades ■ percussion (reflex) hammer ■ otoscope ■ tuning fork ■ tape measure ■ visual acuity chart ■ ophthalmoscope ■ test tubes of hot and cold water ■ containers of odorous materials (such as coffee or chocolate) ■ substances for taste assessment (sugar, salt, vinegar) ■ coin ■ pin and cotton ■ paper clip ■ fecal occult blood test kit ■ linen-saver pad ■ water-soluble lubricant ■ facial tissues ■ cotton-tipped applicators ■ nursing assessment form.

Preparation of equipment

Adjust the temperature in the examining room, and close the doors *to prevent drafts and provide privacy.* Cover the examination table with a clean sheet or disposable paper. Then assemble the appropriate equipment for the examination.

Implementation

- Review the patient's health history *to obtain subjective data about the patient and insight into problem areas and subtle physical changes.* Investigate the patient's chief complaint. (See *Exploring a patient's symptoms.*)
- Obtain biographical data, including the patient's name, address, telephone number, contact person, gender, age and birth date, birthplace, Social Security number, marital status, education, religion, occupation, race, nationality, and cultural background as well as the names of persons living with the patient.
- Ask about health and illness patterns, the chief complaint, current and past health status, family health status, and condition of body systems.
- Ask about any medications the patient is taking, including prescription, over-the-counter, and herbal medications. Write down the name of the medication along with the dose, frequency, and route. Determine the purpose of the medication and when the patient last took it.
- Ask about health promotion and protection patterns, including health beliefs, personal habits, sleep and wake cycles, exercise, recreation, nutrition, stress level and coping skills, socioeconomic status, environmental health conditions, and occupational health hazards.
- Explore the patient's role and relationship patterns, including self-concept, cultural and religious influences, family roles and relationships, sexuality and reproductive patterns, social support systems, and any other psychosocial considerations.
- Explain the physical examination and answer questions.
- Instruct the patient to void if possible. Collect a urine specimen if ordered. *Emptying the bladder increases patient comfort during the examination.*
- Help the patient undress, and provide a gown. Then measure and record height, weight, and vital signs.
- Assist the patient onto the examination table. Requirements for positioning and draping vary with the body system and region being assessed. To examine the head, neck, and anterior and posterior thorax, have the patient sit on

Exploring a patient's symptoms

A clear understanding of the patient's symptoms is essential to a complete physical assessment. One method of gaining that understanding involves using the mnemonic device PQRST as a guide.

Provocative or palliative

What causes the symptom? What makes it better or worse?

- What were you doing when you first noticed it?
- What seems to trigger it? Stress? Position? Certain activities? An argument? (For a sign such as an eye discharge: What seems to cause it or make it worse? For a psychological symptom such as depression: Does the depression occur after specific events?)
- What relieves the symptom? Changing diet? Changing position? Taking medication? Being active?
- What makes the symptom worse?

Quality or quantity

How does the symptom feel, look, or sound? How much of it are you experiencing now?

- How would you describe the symptom—how it feels, looks, or sounds?
- How much are you experiencing now? Is it so much that it prevents you from performing any activities? Is it more or less than you experienced at any other time?

Region or radiation

Where's the symptom located? Does it spread?

- Where does the symptom occur?
- In the case of pain, does it travel down your back or arms, up your neck, or down your legs?

Severity

How does the symptom rate on a scale of 1 to 10, with 10 being the most severe?

- How bad is the symptom at its worst? Does it force you to lie down, sit down, or slow down?
- Does the symptom seem to be getting better, getting worse, or staying about the same?

Timing

When did the symptom begin? Did it occur suddenly or gradually? How often does it occur?

- On what date and time did the symptom first occur?
- How did the symptom start? Suddenly? Gradually?
- How often do you experience the symptom? Hourly? Daily? Weekly? Monthly?
- When do you usually experience the symptom? During the day? At night? In the early morning? Does it awaken you? Does it occur before, during, or after meals? Does it occur seasonally?
- How long does an episode of the symptom last?

the edge of the examination table or the bed. For the abdomen and cardiovascular system, place the patient in a supine position, and stand to his right. For a female patient, place a towel over her breasts and upper thorax during abdominal assessment. Pull the sheet down as far as her symphysis pubis, but no farther.

- Perform a physical examination. (See *Performing a head-to-toe assessment,* pages 34 to 45.)

Documentation

Document significant normal and abnormal findings in an organized manner according to the related body systems.

SELECTED REFERENCES

"Assessing the Cranial Nerves," *Nursing* 36(11):47-49, November 2006.

Baid, H. "The Process of Conducting a Physical Assessment: A Nursing Perspective," *British Journal of Nursing* 15(13):710-14, July 2006.

Bickely, L.S., and Szilagyi, P.G. *Bates' Guide to Physical Examination and History Taking,* 9th ed. Philadelphia: Lippincott Williams & Wilkins, 2007.

Dulak, S.B. "Hands-On Help: Assessing Heart Sounds," *RN* 67(8):24ac1-4, August 2004.

The Joint Commission. *The Comprehensive Accreditation Manual for Hospitals: The Official Handbook.* Standard PC.2.20, 2007.

The Joint Commission. *The Comprehensive Accreditation Manual for Hospitals: The Official Handbook.* Standards PC.2.120 to PC.2.150, 2007.

Madsen, D., et al. "Listening to Bowel Sounds: An Evidence-Based Practice Project: Nurses Find That a Traditional Practice Isn't the Best Indicator of Returning Gastrointestinal Motility in Patients Who've Undergone Abdominal Surgery," *AJN* 105(12):40-49, December 2005.

Roper, J.D. "The Abdomen: The Complete Examination," *School Nurse News* 23(3):41-42, May 2006.

Simpson, H. "Respiratory Assessment," *British Journal of Nursing* 15(9):484-88, May 2006.

(Text continues on page 45.)

Performing a head-to-toe assessment

The table on the following pages provides guidelines for a systematic head-to-toe assessment. It groups assessment techniques by body region and nurse-patient positioning *to make the assessment as efficient as possible and to avoid tiring the patient.* The first column describes the assessment technique to use for each body system or region. The second column lists normal findings for adults. The third column reviews special considerations, including the purpose of the technique as well as nursing and developmental considerations.

TECHNIQUE	NORMAL FINDINGS	SPECIAL CONSIDERATIONS
HEAD AND NECK		
Inspect the patient's head. Note hair color, texture, and distribution. Palpate from the forehead to the posterior triangle of the neck for the posterior cervical lymph nodes.	Symmetrical, rounded normocephalic head positioned at midline and erect with no lumps or ridges	■ This technique can detect asymmetry, size changes, enlarged lymph nodes, and tenderness. ■ Wear gloves for palpation if the patient has scalp lesions. ■ Inspect and gently palpate the fontanels and sutures in an infant.
Palpate in front of and behind the ears, under the chin, and in the anterior triangle for the anterior cervical lymph nodes.	Nonpalpable lymph nodes or small, round, soft, mobile, nontender lymph nodes	■ This technique can detect enlarged lymph nodes. ■ Palpable lymph nodes may be normal in a patient younger than age 12.
Palpate the left and then the right carotid artery.	Bilateral equality in pulse amplitude and rhythm	■ This technique evaluates circulation through the carotid pulse. ■ Don't palpate both arteries at the same time *to avoid occluding blood flow to the brain.*
Auscultate the carotid arteries.	No bruit on auscultation	■ Auscultation in this area can detect a bruit, a sign of turbulent blood flow.
Palpate the trachea.	Straight, midline trachea	■ This technique evaluates trachea position.
Palpate the suprasternal notch.	Palpable pulsations with an even rhythm	■ Palpation in this area allows evaluation of aortic arch pulsations.
Palpate the supraclavicular area.	Nonpalpable lymph nodes	■ This technique can detect enlarged lymph nodes.
Palpate the thyroid gland, and auscultate for bruits.	Thin, mobile thyroid isthmus; nonpalpable thyroid lobes	■ Palpation detects thyroid enlargement, tenderness, or nodules.
Have the patient touch his chin to his chest and to each shoulder, each ear to the corresponding shoulder, then tip his head back as far as possible.	Symmetrical strength and movement of neck muscles	■ These maneuvers evaluate range of motion (ROM) in the neck.

Performing a head-to-toe assessment *(continued)*

TECHNIQUE	NORMAL FINDINGS	SPECIAL CONSIDERATIONS
HEAD AND NECK *(continued)*		
Place your hands on the patient's shoulders while the patient shrugs them against resistance. Then place your hand on the patient's left cheek, then the right, and have the patient push against it.	Symmetrical strength and movement of neck muscles	■ This procedure checks cranial nerve XI (accessory nerve) functioning and trapezius and sternocleidomastoid muscle strength.
Have the patient smile, frown, wrinkle the forehead, and puff out the cheeks.	Symmetrical smile, frown, and forehead wrinkles; equal puffing out of the cheeks	■ This maneuver evaluates the motor portion of cranial nerve VII (facial nerve).
Occlude one nostril externally with your finger while the patient breathes through the other. Repeat on the other nostril.	Patent nostrils	■ This technique checks the patency of the nasal passages.
Inspect the internal nostrils using a nasal speculum or an ophthalmoscope handle with a nasal attachment.	Moist, pink to red nasal mucosa without deviated septum, lesions, or polyps	■ This technique can detect edema, inflammation, and excessive drainage. ■ Use only a flashlight to inspect an infant's or toddler's nostrils; a nasal speculum is too sharp.
Palpate the nose.	No bumps, lesions, edema, or tenderness	■ This technique assesses for structural abnormalities in the nose. ■ An infant's nose usually is slightly flattened.
Palpate and percuss the frontal and maxillary sinuses. If palpation and percussion elicit tenderness, assess further by transilluminating the sinuses.	No tenderness on palpation or percussion	■ These techniques are used to elicit tenderness, which may indicate sinus congestion or infection. ■ In a child under age 8, frontal sinuses commonly are too small to assess.
Palpate the temporomandibular joints as the patient opens and closes the jaws.	Smooth joint movement without pain; correct approximation	■ This action assesses the temporomandibular joints and the motor portion of cranial nerve V (trigeminal nerve).
Inspect the oral mucosa, gingivae, teeth, and salivary gland openings, using a tongue blade and a penlight.	Pink, moist, smooth oral mucosa without lesions or inflammation; pink, moist slightly irregular gingivae without sponginess or edema; 32 teeth with correct occlusion	■ This technique evaluates the condition of several oral structures. ■ A child may have up to 20 temporary (baby) teeth. ■ Slight gingival swelling may be normal during pregnancy.

(continued)

Performing a head-to-toe assessment *(continued)*

Technique	Normal findings	Special considerations
Head and neck *(continued)*		
Observe the tongue and the hard and soft palates.	Pink, slightly rough tongue with a midline depression; pink to light red palates with symmetrical lines	■ Observation provides information about the patient's hydration status and the condition of these oral structures.
Ask the patient to stick out his tongue.	Midline tongue without tremors	■ This procedure tests cranial nerve XII (hypoglossal nerve).
Ask the patient to say "Ahh" while sticking out his tongue. Inspect the visible oral structures.	Symmetrical rise in soft palate and uvula during phonation; pink, midline, cone-shaped uvula; +1 tonsils (both tonsils behind the pillars)	■ Phonation ("Ahh") checks portions of cranial nerves IX and X (glossopharyngeal and vagus nerves). Lowering the tongue aids viewing.
Test the gag reflex using a tongue blade.	Gagging	■ Gagging during this procedure indicates that cranial nerves IX and X are intact.
Place the tongue blade at the side of the tongue while the patient pushes it to the left and right with the tongue.	Symmetrical ability to push tongue blade to left and right	■ This action tests cranial nerve XII.
Test the sense of smell using a test tube of coffee, chocolate, or another familiar substance.	Correct identification of smells in both nostrils	■ This action tests cranial nerve I (olfactory nerve). ■ Make sure the patient keeps both eyes closed during the test.
Eyes and ears		
Perform a visual acuity test using the standard Snellen eye chart or another visual acuity chart, with the patient wearing corrective lenses, if needed.	20/20 vision	■ This test assesses the patient's distance vision (central vision) and evaluates cranial nerve II (optic nerve).
Ask the patient to identify the pattern in a specially prepared page of color dots or plates.	Correct identification of pattern	■ This test assesses the patient's color perception.
Test the six cardinal positions of gaze.	Bilaterally equal eye movement without nystagmus	■ This test evaluates the function of each of the six extraocular muscles and tests cranial nerves III, IV, and VI (oculomotor, trochlear, and abducens nerves).

Performing a head-to-toe assessment *(continued)*

TECHNIQUE	NORMAL FINDINGS	SPECIAL CONSIDERATIONS
EYES AND EARS *(continued)*		
Inspect the external structures of the eyeball (eyelids, eyelashes, and lacrimal apparatus).	Bright, clear, symmetrical eyes free from nystagmus; eyelids close completely; no lesions, scaling, or inflammation	■ This inspection allows detection of such problems as ptosis, ectropion (outward-turning eyelids), entropion (inward-turning eyelids), and styes.
Inspect the conjunctiva and sclera.	Pink palpebral conjunctiva and clear bulbar conjunctiva without swelling, drainage, or hyperemic blood vessels; white, clear sclera	■ Inspection detects conjunctivitis and the scleral color changes that may occur with systemic disorders.
Inspect the cornea, iris, and anterior chamber by shining a penlight tangentially across the eye.	Clear, transparent cornea and anterior chamber; illumination of total iris	■ This technique assesses anterior chamber depth and the condition of the cornea and iris. ■ An elderly patient may exhibit a thin, grayish ring in the cornea (called arcus senilis).
Examine the pupils for equality of size, shape, reaction to light, and accommodation.	Pupils equal, round, reactive to light and accommodation (PERRLA), directly and consensually	■ Testing the pupillary response to light and accommodation assesses cranial nerves III, IV, and VI.
Observe the red reflex using an ophthalmoscope.	Sharp, distinct orange-red glow	■ Presence of the red reflex indicates that the cornea, anterior chamber, and lens are free from opacity and clouding.
Inspect the ear. Perform an otoscopic examination, if indicated.	Nearly vertically positioned ears that line up with the eye, match the facial color, are similarly shaped, and are in proportion to the face; no drainage, nodules, or lesions	■ A dark-skinned patient may have darker orange or brown cerumen (earwax); a fair-skinned patient typically will have yellow cerumen.
Palpate the ear and mastoid process.	No pain, swelling, nodules, or lesions	■ This assessment technique can detect inflammation or infection. It may also uncover other abnormalities, such as nodules or lesions.
Perform the whispered voice test or the watch-tick test on one ear at a time.	Whispered voice heard at a distance of 1′ to 2′ (30 to 61 cm); watch-tick heard at a distance of 5″ (13 cm)	■ This test provides a gross assessment of cranial nerve VIII (acoustic nerve).

(continued)

Performing a head-to-toe assessment *(continued)*

TECHNIQUE	NORMAL FINDINGS	SPECIAL CONSIDERATIONS
EYES AND EARS *(continued)*		
Perform Weber's test using a 512 or 1024 hertz (Hz) tuning fork.	Tuning fork vibrations heard equally in both ears or in the middle of the head	■ This test differentiates conductive from sensorineural hearing loss. ■ The sound is heard best in the ear with a conductive loss.
Perform the Rinne test using a 512 or 1024 Hz tuning fork.	Tuning fork vibrations heard in front of the ear for as long as they are heard on the mastoid process	■ This test helps differentiate conductive from sensorineural hearing loss.
POSTERIOR THORAX		
Observe the skin, bones, and muscles of the spine, shoulder blades, and back as well as symmetry of expansion and accessory muscle use.	Even skin tone; symmetrical placement of all structures; bilaterally equal shoulder height; symmetrical expansion with inhalation; no accessory muscle use	■ Observation provides information about lung expansion and accessory muscle use during respiration. It may also detect a deformity that can alter ventilation, such as scoliosis.
Assess the anteroposterior and lateral diameters of the thorax.	Lateral diameter up to twice the anteroposterior diameter (2:1)	■ This assessment may detect abnormalities, such as an increased anteroposterior diameter (barrel chest may be as low as 1:1). ■ Normal anteroposterior diameters vary with age. ■ Measure an infant's chest circumference at the nipple line.
Palpate down the spine.	Properly aligned spinous processes without lesions or tenderness; firm, symmetrical, evenly spaced muscles	■ This technique detects pain in the spine and paraspinous muscles. It also evaluates the muscles' consistency.
Palpate over the posterior thorax.	Smooth surface; no lesions, lumps, or pain	■ This technique helps detect musculoskeletal inflammation.
Assess respiratory excursion.	Symmetrical expansion and contraction of the thorax	■ This technique checks for equal expansion of the lungs.
Palpate for tactile fremitus as the patient repeats the word "ninety-nine."	Equally intense vibrations of both sides of the chest	■ Palpation provides information about the content of the lungs; vibrations increase over consolidated or fluid-filled areas and decrease over gas-filled areas.

Performing a head-to-toe assessment *(continued)*

TECHNIQUE	NORMAL FINDINGS	SPECIAL CONSIDERATIONS
POSTERIOR THORAX *(continued)*		
Percuss over the posterior and lateral lung fields.	Resonant percussion note over the lungs that changes to a dull note at the diaphragm	■ This technique helps identify the density and location of the lungs, diaphragm, and other anatomic structures. ■ Percussion may produce hyperresonant sounds in a patient with chronic obstructive pulmonary disease or an elderly patient *because of hyperinflation of lung tissue*.
Percuss for diaphragmatic excursion on each side of the posterior thorax.	Excursion from 1¼″ to 2¼″ (3 to 6 cm)	■ This technique evaluates diaphragm movement during respiration.
Auscultate the lungs through the posterior thorax as the patient breathes slowly and deeply through the mouth. Also auscultate lateral areas.	Bronchovesicular sounds (soft, breezy sounds) between the scapulae; vesicular sounds (soft, swishy sounds about two notes lower than bronchovesicular sounds) in the lung periphery	■ Lung auscultation helps detect abnormal fluid or mucus accumulation as well as obstructed passages. ■ Auscultate a child's lungs before performing other assessment techniques that may cause crying, which increases the respiratory rate and interferes with clear auscultation. ■ A child's breath sounds are normally harsher or more bronchial than an adult's.
ANTERIOR THORAX		
Observe the skin, bones, and muscles of the anterior thoracic structures as well as symmetry of expansion and accessory muscle use during respiration.	Even skin tone; symmetrical placement of all structures; symmetrical costal angle of less than 90 degrees; symmetrical expansion with inhalation; no accessory muscle use	■ Observation provides information about lung expansion and accessory muscle use. ■ It may also detect a deformity that can prevent full lung expansion, such as pigeon chest.
Inspect the anterior thorax for lifts, heaves, or thrusts. Also check for the apical impulse.	No lifts, heaves, or thrusts; apical impulse not usually visible	■ Apical impulse may be visible in a thin or young patient.
Palpate over the anterior thorax.	Smooth surface; no lesions, lumps, or pain	■ This technique helps detect musculoskeletal inflammation.
Assess respiratory excursion.	Symmetrical expansion and contraction of the thorax	■ This technique checks for equal expansion of the lungs.

(continued)

Performing a head-to-toe assessment *(continued)*

TECHNIQUE	NORMAL FINDINGS	SPECIAL CONSIDERATIONS
ANTERIOR THORAX *(continued)*		
Palpate for tactile fremitus as the patient repeats the word "ninety-nine."	Equally intense vibrations of both sides of the chest, with more vibrations in the upper chest than in the lower chest	■ Palpation provides information about the content of the lungs.
Percuss over the anterior thorax.	Resonant percussion note over lung fields that changes to a dull note over ribs and other bones	■ This technique helps identify the density and location of the lungs, diaphragm, and other anatomic structures. ■ Percussion is unreliable in an infant *because of the infant's small chest size.* ■ Percussion may produce hyperresonant sounds in an elderly patient *because of hyperinflation of lung tissue.*
Auscultate the lungs through the anterior thorax as the patient breathes slowly and deeply through the mouth. Also auscultate lateral areas.	Bronchovesicular sounds (soft, breezy sounds) between the scapulae; vesicular sounds (soft, swishy sounds about two notes lower than bronchovesicular sounds) in the lung periphery	■ Lung auscultation helps detect abnormal fluid or mucus accumulation. ■ Auscultate a child's lungs before performing other assessment techniques that may cause crying. ■ Breath sounds are normally harsher or more bronchial in a child.
Inspect the breasts and axillae with the patient's hands resting at the sides of the body, placed on the hips, and raised above the head.	Symmetrical, convex, similar-looking breasts with soft, smooth skin and bilaterally similar venous patterns; symmetrical axillae with varying amounts of hair, but no lesions; nipples at same level on chest and of same color	■ This technique evaluates the general condition of the breasts and axillae and detects such abnormalities as retraction, dimpling, and flattening. ■ Expect to see enlarged breasts with darkened nipples and areolae and purplish linear streaks if the patient is pregnant.
Palpate the axillae with the patient's arms resting against the side of the body.	Nonpalpable nodes	■ This technique detects nodular enlargements and other abnormalities.
Palpate the breasts and nipples with patient lying supine.	Smooth, relatively elastic tissue without masses, cracks, fissures, areas of induration (hardness), or discharge	■ This technique evaluates the consistency and elasticity of the breasts and nipples and may detect nipple discharge. ■ The premenstrual patient may exhibit breast tenderness, nodularity, and fullness. ■ A pregnant patient may discharge colostrum from the nipple and may exhibit nodular breasts with prominent venous patterns.

Performing a head-to-toe assessment *(continued)*

TECHNIQUE	NORMAL FINDINGS	SPECIAL CONSIDERATIONS
ANTERIOR THORAX *(continued)*		
Inspect the neck for jugular vein distention with patient lying supine at a 45-degree angle.	No visible pulsations	■ This technique assesses right-sided heart pressure.
Palpate the precordium for the apical impulse.	Apical impulse present in the apical area (fifth intercostal space at the midclavicular line)	■ This action evaluates the size and location of the left ventricle.
Auscultate the aortic, pulmonic, tricuspid, and mitral areas for heart sounds.	S_1 and S_2 heart sounds with a regular rhythm and an age-appropriate rate	■ Auscultation over the precordium evaluates the heart rate and rhythm and can detect other abnormal heart sounds. ■ A child or a pregnant woman in the third trimester may have functional (innocent) heart murmurs.
ABDOMEN		
Observe the abdominal contour.	Symmetrical flat or rounded contour	■ This technique determines whether the abdomen is distended or scaphoid. ■ An infant or a toddler will have a rounded abdomen.
Inspect the abdomen for skin characteristics, symmetry, contour, peristalsis, and pulsations.	Symmetrical contour with no lesions, striae, rash, or visible peristaltic waves	■ Inspection can detect an incisional or umbilical hernia or an abnormality caused by bowel obstruction.
Auscultate all four quadrants of the abdomen.	Normal bowel sounds in all four quadrants; no bruits	■ Abdominal auscultation can detect abnormal bowel sounds.
Percuss from below the right breast to the inguinal area down the right midclavicular line.	Dull percussion note over the liver; tympanic note over the rest of the abdomen	■ Percussion in this area helps evaluate the size of the liver.
Percuss from below the left breast to the inguinal area down the left midclavicular line.	Tympanic percussion note	■ Percussion that elicits a dull note in this area can detect an enlarged spleen.
Palpate all four abdominal quadrants.	Nontender organs without masses	■ Palpation provides information about the location, size, and condition of the underlying structures.
Palpate for the kidneys on each side of the abdomen.	Nonpalpable kidneys or solid, firm, smooth kidneys (if palpable)	■ This technique evaluates the general condition of the kidneys.

(continued)

Performing a head-to-toe assessment *(continued)*

TECHNIQUE	NORMAL FINDINGS	SPECIAL CONSIDERATIONS
ABDOMEN *(continued)*		
Palpate the liver at the right costal border.	Nonpalpable liver or smooth, firm, nontender liver with a rounded, regular edge (if palpable)	▪ This technique evaluates the general condition of the liver.
Palpate for the spleen at the left costal border.	Nonpalpable spleen	▪ This procedure detects splenomegaly (spleen enlargement).
Palpate the femoral pulses in the groin.	Strong, regular pulse	▪ Palpation assesses vascular patency.
UPPER EXTREMITIES		
Observe the skin and muscle mass of the arms and hands.	Uniform color and texture with no lesions; elastic turgor; bilaterally equal muscle mass	▪ The skin provides information about hydration and circulation. Muscle mass provides information about injuries and neuromuscular disease.
Ask the patient to extend the arms forward and then rapidly turn the palms up and down.	Steady hands with no tremor or pronator drift	▪ This maneuver tests proprioception and cerebellar function.
Place your hands on the patient's upturned forearms while the patient pushes up against resistance. Then place your hands under the forearms while the patient pushes down.	Symmetrical strength and ability to push up and down against resistance	▪ This procedure checks the muscle strength of the arms.
Inspect and palpate the fingers, wrists, and elbow joints.	Smooth, freely movable joints with no swelling	▪ An elderly patient may exhibit osteoarthritic changes.
Palpate the patient's hands to assess skin temperature.	Warm, moist skin with bilaterally even temperature	▪ Skin temperature assessment provides data about circulation to the area.
Palpate the radial and brachial pulses.	Bilaterally equal rate and rhythm	▪ Palpation of pulses helps evaluate peripheral vascular status.
Inspect the color, shape, and condition of the patient's fingernails, and test for capillary refill.	Pink nail beds with smooth, rounded nails; brisk capillary refill; no clubbing	▪ Nail assessment provides data about the integumentary, cardiovascular, and respiratory systems.
Place two fingers in each of the patient's palms while the patient squeezes your fingers.	Bilaterally equal hand strength	▪ This maneuver tests muscle strength in the hands.

Performing a head-to-toe assessment *(continued)*

TECHNIQUE	NORMAL FINDINGS	SPECIAL CONSIDERATIONS
LOWER EXTREMITIES		
Inspect the legs and feet for color, lesions, varicosities, hair growth, nail growth, edema, and muscle mass.	Even skin color; symmetrical hair and nail growth; no lesions, varicosities, or edema; bilaterally equal muscle mass	■ Inspection assesses adequate circulatory function.
Test for pitting edema in the pretibial area.	No pitting edema	■ This test assesses for excess interstitial fluid.
Palpate for pulses and skin temperature in the posterior tibial, dorsalis pedis, and popliteal areas.	Bilaterally even pulse rate, rhythm, and skin temperature	■ Palpation of pulses and temperature in these areas evaluates the patient's peripheral vascular status.
Perform the straight leg test on one leg at a time.	Painless leg lifting	■ This test checks for vertebral disk problems.
Palpate for crepitus as the patient abducts and adducts the hip. Repeat on the opposite leg.	No crepitus; full ROM without pain	■ Perform Ortolani's maneuver on an infant to assess hip abduction and adduction.
Ask the patient to raise his thigh against the resistance of your hands. Repeat this procedure on the opposite thigh.	Each thigh lifts easily against resistance	■ This maneuver tests the motor strength of the upper legs.
Ask the patient to push outward against the resistance of your hands.	Each leg pushes easily against resistance	■ This maneuver tests the motor strength of the lower legs.
Ask the patient to pull backward against the resistance of your hands.	Each leg pulls easily against resistance	■ This maneuver tests the motor strength of the lower legs.
NERVOUS SYSTEM		
Lightly touch the ophthalmic, maxillary, and mandibular areas on each side of the patient's face with a cotton-tipped applicator and a pin.	Correct identification of sensation and location	■ This test evaluates the function of cranial nerve V (trigeminal nerve).
Touch the dorsal and palmar surfaces of the arms, hands, and fingers with a cotton-tipped applicator and a pin.	Correct identification of sensation and location	■ This test evaluates the function of the ulnar, radial, and medial nerves.
Touch several nerve distribution areas on the legs, feet, and toes with a cotton-tipped applicator and a pin.	Correct identification of sensation and location	■ This test evaluates the function of the dermatome areas randomly.

(continued)

Performing a head-to-toe assessment *(continued)*

TECHNIQUE	NORMAL FINDINGS	SPECIAL CONSIDERATIONS
NERVOUS SYSTEM *(continued)*		
Place your fingers above the patient's wrist, and tap them with a reflex hammer. Repeat on the other arm.	Normal reflex reaction	■ This procedure elicits the brachioradialis deep tendon reflex (DTR).
Place your fingers over the antecubital fossa, and tap them with a reflex hammer. Repeat on the other arm.	Normal reflex reaction	■ This procedure elicits the biceps DTR.
Place your fingers over the triceps tendon area, and tap them with a reflex hammer. Repeat on the other arm.	Normal reflex reaction	■ This procedure elicits the triceps DTR.
Tap just below the patella with a reflex hammer. Repeat this procedure on the opposite patella.	Normal reflex reaction	■ This procedure elicits the patellar DTR.
Tap over the Achilles tendon area with a reflex hammer. Repeat this procedure on the opposite ankle.	Normal reflex reaction	■ This procedure elicits the Achilles DTR.
Stroke the sole of the patient's foot with the end of the reflex hammer handle.	Plantar reflex	■ This procedure elicits plantar flexion of all toes. ■ Expect Babinski's sign in children age 2 and under.
Ask the patient to demonstrate dorsiflexion by bending both feet upward against resistance.	Both feet lift easily against resistance	■ This procedure tests foot strength and ROM.
Ask the patient to demonstrate plantar flexion by bending both feet downward against resistance.	Both feet push down easily against resistance	■ This procedure tests foot strength and ROM.
Using your finger, trace a one-digit number in the palm of the patient's hand.	Correct identification of traced number	■ This procedure evaluates the patient's tactile discrimination through graphesthesia.
Place a familiar object, such as a key or a coin, in the patient's hand.	Correct identification of object	■ This procedure evaluates the patient's tactile discrimination.
Observe the patient while he walks with a regular gait, on the toes, on the heels, and heel to toe.	Steady gait, good balance, and no signs of muscle weakness or pain in any style of walking	■ This technique evaluates the cerebellum and motor system and checks for vertebral disk problems.

Performing a head-to-toe assessment *(continued)*

TECHNIQUE	NORMAL FINDINGS	SPECIAL CONSIDERATIONS
NERVOUS SYSTEM *(continued)*		
Inspect the scapulae, spine, back, and hips as the patient bends forward, backward, and from side to side.	Full ROM, easy flexibility, and no signs of scoliosis or varicosities	■ Inspection evaluates the patient's ROM and detects musculoskeletal abnormalities such as scoliosis.
Perform the Romberg test. Ask the patient to stand straight with both eyes closed and both arms extended, with hands palms up.	Steady stance with minimal weaving	■ This test checks cerebellar functioning and evaluates balance and coordination.

CARE PLAN PREPARATION

A care plan directs the patient's nursing care from admission to discharge. This written action plan is based on nursing diagnoses that have been formulated after reviewing assessment findings. (See *Elements of a nursing diagnosis,* page 46.) The care plan consists of three parts: *goals* (or *expected outcomes*), which describe behaviors or results to be achieved within a specified time; appropriate *nursing actions* or *interventions* needed to achieve these goals; and *evaluations of the established goals.*

A nursing care plan should be written for each patient, preferably within 24 hours of admission. It's usually begun by the patient's primary nurse or the nurse who admits the patient. If the care plan contains more than one nursing diagnosis, the nurse must assign priorities to each one and implement those with the highest priority first. Nurses update and revise the plan throughout the patient's stay, and the document becomes part of the permanent patient record.

Some health care facilities use standardized care plans that can be modified to serve many patients. Others use computer programs to facilitate development of nursing care plans. Most have preprinted care plan forms that can be filled in as needed, typically on the nursing Kardex.

A nursing care plan serves as a database for planning assignments, giving change-of-shift reports, conferring with the practitioner or other members of the health care team, planning patient discharge, and documenting patient care. In addition, the care plan can be used as a management tool to determine staffing needs and assignments.

Equipment

Preprinted nursing care plan form ■ nursing care plan computer program if appropriate ■ patient record, including nursing assessment.

Implementation

■ Review the patient record, especially the nursing assessment completed on admission. Obtain from the patient any additional subjective or objective information needed to complete your assessment. Review diagnostic test results, the medical plan, and other information that may affect patient care. If the patient has just been admitted, complete a nursing history and physical assessment, and add it to the patient's record.

■ Based on an analysis of the data, determine which nursing diagnoses will guide your patient care. Be sure to address all of the patient's significant needs when determining nursing diagnoses.

■ Work with the patient to identify individualized short-term and long-term goals (expected outcomes) for each nursing diagnosis. Short-term goals can be achieved quickly; long-term goals take more time to achieve and usually involve prevention, patient teaching, and rehabilitation.

A correctly written goal expresses the desired patient behavior, criteria for measurement, appropriate time, and conditions under which the behavior will occur. For example, a goal containing all these elements might read: "By Monday, using crutches, Mary Ballin will be able to walk to the end of the hall and back." *Goals (or expected outcomes) serve as the basis for evaluating the effectiveness of your nursing interventions.*

■ Select interventions that will help the patient achieve the stated goals for each nursing diagnosis. Include specific in-

Elements of a nursing diagnosis

The following summary presents the key elements of a nursing diagnosis.

Human response or problem

After analyzing the patient's condition, choose a diagnostic label from a hospital-sanctioned list or create a label specific to the patient. For consistency, most hospitals use NANDA-I's list of nursing diagnoses. An example of a diagnostic label is *Excess fluid volume.*

Related factors

The second part of the nursing diagnosis lists factors that seem to influence the patient in a way that pertains to the diagnostic label. Connect these factors to the diagnostic label with the phrase *related to* or the abbreviation *R/T*. The previous example could read, *Excess fluid volume R/T increased sodium intake.*

Signs and symptoms

To complete the nursing diagnosis, list signs and symptoms uncovered during assessment that help define the diagnostic label. You may list them beneath the diagnosis and related factors, or you may add them to the diagnostic statement and connect them with the phrase *as evidenced by* or the abbreviation *AEB*. The example could read, *Excess fluid volume R/T increased sodium intake AEB edema, weight gain, shortness of breath, and* S_3 *heart sounds.*

Tips for writing an effective patient care plan

How do you write a care plan that's realistic, accurate, and helpful? Here are some guidelines.

Be systematic

Avoid setting an initial goal that's impossible to achieve. For example, suppose the goal for a newly admitted patient with a stroke was "Patient will ambulate without assistance." Although this goal is certainly appropriate in the long term, several short-term goals, such as "Patient maintains joint range of motion," need to be achieved first.

Be realistic

The nursing intervention should match staff resources and capabilities. For example, "Passive range-of-motion exercises to all extremities every 2 hours" may not be reasonable given the unit's staffing pattern and care requirements. The goals you set to correct a patient's problem should reflect what's reasonably possible in your setting—for example, "Passive range-of-motion exercises with a.m. care, p.m. care, and once during the night."

Be clear

Remember, you'll use goals to evaluate the care plan's effectiveness, so it's important to express them in measurable terms.

Be specific

"Give plenty of fluids" doesn't indicate much; the directive is nonspecific. In contrast, an intervention that says "Force fluids—1,000 ml/day shift, 1,000 ml/evening shift, 500 ml/night shift" allows another nurse to carry out the intervention with some assurance of having done what you ordered.

Be brief

An intervention that says "Follow turning schedule posted at bedside" is more readable and useful than writing the entire schedule on the nursing care plan.

formation, such as the frequency or particular intervention technique. *Goals establish criteria against which you'll judge further nursing actions.* (See *Tips for writing an effective patient care plan.*)

Special considerations

- Always fill out the nursing care plan in ink *because the document is part of the permanent medical record.* If you must revise your plan as the patient's condition changes, fill out a new care plan and add it to the medical record.

- Sign and date the care plan whenever you make new entries *to keep the plan current and to maintain accountability for planning the patient's care.*
- Customize a standardized care plan *to avoid "standardizing" the patient's care and to allow you to address the patient's individual concerns.*
- Long-term goals may not be met during hospitalization, so your planning should address postdischarge and home care needs. Interventions may include coordinating home care services.
- Some agencies use critical pathways to address standardized desired outcomes of care. Critical pathways are multidisciplinary documents that may be viewed as replacements for care plans. If nursing diagnoses are included, these agencies use only the diagnostic statements that are most frequently observed.

Documentation

Documentation of the patient's progress (or lack of it) is required by the Joint Commission and other regulatory agencies that monitor health care quality. Document all pertinent nursing diagnoses, expected outcomes, nursing interventions, and evaluations of expected outcomes. Write the care plan clearly and concisely *so that other members of the health care team can understand it.*

SELECTED REFERENCES

American Nurses Association. *Nursing: Scope and Standards of Practice.* Washington, D.C., 2004.

Carpenito-Moyet, L.J. *Nursing Diagnosis: Application to Clinical Practice,* 11th ed. Philadelphia: Lippincott Williams & Wilkins, 2006.

Clemow, R. "Care Plans as the Main Focus of Nursing Handover: Information Exchange Model," *Journal of Clinical Nursing* 15(11):1463-65, November 2006.

The Joint Commission. *Comprehensive Accreditation Manual for Hospitals: The Official Handbook.* Standard PC.4.10 Oakbrook Terrace, Ill.: 2005.

Lee, T.T. "Nursing Diagnoses: Factors Affecting Their Use in Charting Standardized Care Plans," *Journal of Clinical Nursing* 14(5):640-47, May 2005.

Mills, C., et al. "Care Planning with the Electronic Patient Record," *Nursing Times* 101(37):26-27, September 2005.

SEXUAL ASSAULT EXAMINATION

Each facility or agency has a specific protocol for specimen collection in cases involving sexual assault. Specimens can be collected from various sources, including blood, hair, nails, tissues, and body fluids such as urine, semen, saliva, and vaginal secretions. In addition, evidence can be obtained from the results of diagnostic tests, such as computed tomography and radiography. Regardless of the protocol or specimen source, accurate and precise specimen collection is essential in conjunction with thorough, objective documentation because in many cases, this information will be used as evidence in legal proceedings.

Many institutions have a Sexual Assault Nurse Examiner (SANE) available to care for patients who are victims of sexual assault. SANEs are skilled rape crisis professionals who can evaluate the victim and collect specimens. They may also be called upon at a later date to testify in legal proceedings.

If you're responsible for collecting specimens in a sexual assault, follow these important guidelines:

- Be knowledgeable about your facility's policy and procedures for specimen collection in sexual assault cases.
- When obtaining specimens, be sure to collect them from the victim and, if possible, from the suspect.
- Check with local law enforcement agencies about additional specimens that may be needed; for example, trace evidence, such as soot, grass, gravel, glass, or other debris.
- Wear gloves and change them frequently; use disposable equipment and instruments if possible.
- Avoid coughing, sneezing, or talking over specimens or touching your face, nose, or mouth when collecting specimens.
- Include the victim's clothing as part of the collection procedure.
- Place all items collected in a paper bag.

NURSING ALERT *Never allow a specimen or item considered as evidence to be left unattended.*

- Document each item or specimen collected; have another person witness each collection and document it.
- Obtain photographs of all injuries for documentation.
- Include written documentation of the victim's physical and psychological condition on first encounter, throughout specimen collection, and afterward.

Equipment

Gloves ▪ Wood's lamp ▪ examination paper ▪ clean paper bag (one for each article of clothing) ▪ swabs for collecting specimens ▪ comb ▪ EDTA tube ▪ supplies for venipuncture ▪ straight catheter kit ▪ camera for photographs ▪ optional: tetanus shot, antibiotics.

When possible, obtain a special Sexual Assault Evidence Collection Kit, which contains the necessary items for specimen collection based on the evidence required by the local crime laboratory. In addition, the kit contains a form that's to be completed, signed, and dated by the examiner. Keep in mind that when collecting specimens for moist secretions, typically a one-swab technique is used; if secretions are dry, then a two-swab technique is used.

Implementation

■ Ensure patient privacy throughout the collection procedure.
■ Assess the patient's ability to undergo the specimen collection procedure.
■ Explain the procedures that the patient will undergo, what specimens will be collected and from where, and provide emotional support throughout.
■ Ask if the patient would like someone, such as a family member, friend, or other person to stay during the specimen collection.
■ Before obtaining any specimens, inspect the genital area using a Wood's lamp. This device uses long wave ultraviolet light *to scan the area for secretions* and aids in identifying areas of trauma.

Clothing for specimen collection

■ Ask the patient to stand on a clean piece of examination paper if possible; if the patient can't stand, then have the patient remain on the examination table or bed.
■ Have the patient remove each article of clothing, one at a time, and place each article in a separate, clean paper bag.
■ If the clothing is wet, allow it to dry first before placing the item into the paper bag.

NURSING ALERT *Never use plastic bags to collect clothing. Plastic promotes bacterial growth and can destroy DNA.*

■ Fold the examination paper onto itself, and place it into a clean paper bag.
■ Fold over, seal, label, and initial each bag.

Vaginal or cervical secretion collection

■ Swab the vaginal area thoroughly with four swabs; swab the cervical area with two swabs, being sure to keep the vaginal swabs separate from the cervical swabs.
■ Run the vaginal swabs over a slide (supplied in the kit), and allow the slide and swabs to air dry; do the same for the cervical swabs.
■ Place the vaginal swabs in the swab container and close it; place the slide in the cardboard sleeve, close it and tape it shut; repeat this procedure for the cervical swabs.
■ Place the swab container and cardboard sleeve into the envelope, and seal it securely.
■ Complete the information as provided on the front of the envelope; if both vaginal and cervical swabs are obtained, use a separate envelope for each.

Anal secretion collection

■ Moisten a single swab with sterile water.
■ Insert the swab gently into the patient's rectum approximately 1¼″ (3 cm).
■ Rotate the swab gently, and then remove it.
■ Allow the swab to air dry, and then place it in an envelope.
■ Seal and label the envelope appropriately.

Penile secretion collection

■ Moisten a single swab with sterile water.
■ Swab the entire external surface of the penis.
■ Repeat this at least one more time (so that at least two swabs are obtained).
■ Allow the swab to air dry, and then place it in an envelope.
■ Seal and label the envelope appropriately.

Pubic hair collection

■ Use the comb provided in the kit, and comb through the pubic hair.
■ Collect approximately 20 to 30 pubic hairs, and place them in the envelope.
■ Alternatively, obtain 20 to 30 plucked hairs from the patient; allow the patient the option of plucking the pubic hair.
■ Place the hair in the envelope, seal and label it appropriately.

Blood samples

■ After performing a venipuncture, obtain at least 5 ml of blood in an EDTA tube.
■ Write the patient's name and date on the label of the tube.
■ Remove the DNA stain card from the kit, and label it with the patient's name.
■ Using the blood collected in this tube, withdraw 1 ml of blood, and apply blood to each of the four circles on the card, completely filling each circle if possible.
■ Let the card air dry, and then place the card in the envelope.
■ Seal and label the envelope appropriately.
■ Place the blood tube into the tube holder supplied in the kit, and seal the holder with the tape supplied in the kit (may be referred to as evidence tape).
■ Place the tube and holder in the zippered bag provided.
■ Collect additional blood samples to test for pregnancy; sexually transmitted diseases, such as gonorrhea, Chlamydia, and syphilis; or toxicology as appropriate, and send to the laboratory immediately.

Urine specimens

■ Obtain a random urine specimen from the patient; if necessary, obtain the urine specimen via catheterization.

Specimen storage and transport

- Refrigerate blood samples obtained.
- Place all other specimens in the specimen kit, and keep the kit at room temperature.
- Give all the specimens to the police when they arrive.

Special considerations

- Be sure to follow the directions in the kit precisely *to ensure that the chain of evidence is followed.*
- Provide follow-up counseling and support to the patient.
- If necessary, administer ordered medications, such as tetanus or antibiotics.
- Make sure that the patient has a support person to accompany the patient home.
- Arrange for referral to local support group, or follow up with a trained counselor.

Documentation

Document all specimens collected, including type, location, time, and patient's name, identification number, and any other relevant information. Include photographs as appropriate, being sure to also include relevant information on the photo.

SELECTED REFERENCES

Anderson, S., et al. "Genital Findings of Women after Consensual and Nonconsensual Intercourse," *Journal of Forensic Nursing* 2(2):59-65, Summer 2006.

Boykins, A.D. "The Forensic Exam: Assessing Health Characteristics of Adult Female Victims of Recent Sexual Assault," *Journal of Forensic Nursing* 1(4):166-71, Winter 2005.

Eckert, L.O., et al. "Factors Impacting Injury Documentation after Sexual Assault: Role of Examiner Experience and Gender," *American Journal of Obstetrics and Gynecology* 190(6): 1739-43, June 2004.

Johnston, B.J. "Outcome Indicators for Sexual Assault Victims," *Journal of Forensic Nursing* 1(3):118-23, Fall 2005.

FUNCTIONAL ASSESSMENT

A functional assessment is used to evaluate the older adult's overall well-being and self-care abilities. It will help you identify individual needs and care deficits, provide a basis for developing a plan of care that enhances the abilities of the older adult with coexisting disease and chronic illness, and provide feedback about treatment and rehabilitation. You can use the information to identify and match the older adult's needs with such services as housekeeping, home health care, and day care to help the patient maintain independence.

Numerous tools are available to help you perform a methodical functional assessment. Some widely used methods are discussed here.

Katz index

The Katz Index of Activities of Daily Living is a widely used tool for evaluating a person's ability to perform six daily personal care activities: bathing, dressing, toileting, transfer, continence, and feeding. It describes his functional level at a specific point in time and objectively scores his performance. (See *Katz index of activities of daily living,* page 50.)

Lawton scale

Another widely used tool, the Lawton Scale for Instrumental Activities of Daily Living, evaluates the ability to perform more complex personal care activities. It addresses the activities needed to support independent living, such as the ability to use the telephone, cook, shop, do laundry, manage finances, take medications, and prepare meals. The activities are rated on a three-point scale, ranging from independence to needing some help to complete disability. (See *Lawton scale for instrumental activities of daily living,* page 51.)

Barthel index and scale

The Barthel Index evaluates the following 10 self-care functions: feeding, moving from wheelchair to bed and returning, performing personal toilet, getting on and off the toilet, bathing, walking on a level surface or propelling a wheelchair, going up and down stairs, dressing and undressing, maintaining bowel continence, and controlling the bladder. Each item is scored according to the degree of assistance needed; over time, results reveal improvement or decline.

A similar scale—called the Barthel Self-Care Rating Scale—is a more detailed scale to evaluate function. Both tools provide information to help you determine the type of assistance needed.

OARS Social Resource Scale

The Older Americans Research and Service Center (OARS) Social Resource Scale is an assessment tool developed at Duke University in 1978. A multidimensional tool, it evaluates level of function in the following five areas:

- social resources
- economic resources
- physical health
- mental health
- activities of daily living.

The primary activities of daily living (ADLs) include mobility, dressing, personal hygiene, eating, and toileting or continence factors. However, ADLs may be expanded to in-

Katz index of activities of daily living

Evaluation form Name *Henry Collins* Date *January 2, 2008*

For each area of functioning listed below, check the description that applies. (The word "assistance" means supervision, direction, or personal assistance.)

Bathing: Sponge bath, tub bath, or shower

☑ Receives no assistance (gets into and out of tub by self, if tub is usual means of bathing)	☐ Receives assistance in bathing only one part of the body (such as the back or leg)	○ Receives assistance in bathing more than one part of the body (or not bathed)

Dressing: Gets outer garments and underwear from closets and drawers and uses fasteners, including suspenders, if worn

☑ Gets clothes and gets completely dressed without assistance	☐ Gets clothes and gets dressed without assistance except for tying shoes	○ Receives assistance in getting clothes or in getting dressed, or stays partly or completely undressed

Toileting: Goes to the room termed "toilet" for bowel movement and urination, cleans self afterward, and arranges clothes

☑ Goes to toilet room, cleans self, and arranges clothes without assistance (may use object for support, such as cane, walker, or wheelchair and may manage night bedpan or commode, emptying it in the morning)	○ Receives assistance in going to toilet room or in cleaning self or arranging clothes after elimination or in use of night bedpan or commode	○ Doesn't go to toilet room for the elimination process

Transfer

☑ Moves into and out of bed and chair without assistance (may use object, such as cane or walker for support)	○ Moves into or out of bed or chair with assistance	○ Doesn't get out of bed

Continence

☐ Controls urination and bowel movement completely by self	✓○ Has occasional accidents	○ Needs supervision to help keep control of urination or bowel movement or catheter is used or is incontinent

Feeding

☑ Feeds self without assistance	☐ Feeds self except for assistance in cutting meat or buttering bread	○ Receives assistance in feeding or is fed partly or completely through tubes or by I.V. fluids

Key ☐ Indicates independence ○ Indicates dependence

A: Independent in all six functions
B: Independent in all but one of these functions
C: Independent in all but bathing and one additional function
D: Independent in all but bathing, dressing, and one additional function
E: Independent in all but bathing, dressing, toileting, and one additional function
F: Independent in all but bathing, dressing, toileting, transferring, and one additional function
G: Dependent in all six functions
Other: Dependent in at least two functions but not classifiable as C, D, E, or F

Evaluation form *P. Rastelli, RN*

Lawton scale for instrumental activities of daily living

The Lawton scale evaluates more sophisticated functions than the Katz index. Patients or caregivers can complete the form in a few minutes. The first answer in each case—except for 8a—indicates independence, the second indicates capability with assistance, and the third indicates dependence. In this version, the maximum score is 29, although scores have meaning only for an individual patient, as when declining scores over time reveal deterioration. Questions 4 to 7 tend to be gender-specific; modify them as necessary.

Name *Mary Stevens* **Rated by** *Joan Masterson, RN* **Date** *April 23, 2008*

1. Can you use the telephone?

without help	(3)
with some help	2
completely unable	1

2. Can you get to places beyond walking distance?

without help	(3)
with some help	2
not without special arrangements	1

3. Can you go shopping for groceries?

without help	(3)
with some help	2
completely unable	1

4. Can you prepare your own meals?

without help	(3)
with some help	2
completely unable	1

5. Can you do your own housework?

without help	3
with some help	(2)
completely unable	1

6. Can you do your own handyman work?

without help	3
with some help	(2)
completely unable	1

7. Can you do your own laundry?

without help	(3)
with some help	2
completely unable	1

8a. Do you take medicines or use any medications?

Yes (If yes, answer Question 8b.)	(1)
No (If no, answer Question 8c.)	2

8b. Do you take your own medicine?

without help (in the right doses at the right times)	(3)
with some help (if someone prepares it for you and/or reminds you to take it)	2
completely unable	1

8c. If you had to take medicine, could you do it?

without help (in the right doses at the right time)	3
with some help (if someone prepared it for you and reminded you to take it)	(2)
completely unable	1

9. Can you manage your own money?

without help	(3)
with some help	2
completely unable	1

Adapted with permission from Lawton, M.P., and Brody, E.M. "Assessment of Older People: Self-Maintaining and Instrumental Activities of Daily Living," *The Gerontologist* 9(3):179-86, Autumn 1969.

clude instrumental activities (shopping, household maintenance, using the telephone, paying bills, administering medications, cooking and laundry) and advanced activities (voluntary social activities, occupational activities, and recreational activities). Each area is scored on a scale of 1 to 6. At the end of the assessment, a cumulative impairment score is determined. The lower the score, the less the degree of impairment.

Minimum Data Set

In an attempt to improve the quality of care in extended-care facilities, the federal government instituted major reforms through the Omnibus Budget Reconciliation Act (OBRA) of 1981 and its amendments. A standardized assessment tool called the Minimum Data Set was developed to make patient assessments more consistent and reliable throughout the country. The government requires all extended-care facilities that receive federal funding to use this assessment method.

Equipment

Whichever functional assessment tool your facility uses.

Implementation

- Explain the test to the patient, and tell him where it will take place (hospital room or treatment room).
- Review the patient's health history *to obtain subjective data about the patient and insight into problem areas and subtle physical changes.*
- Obtain biographical data, including the patient's name, age, birth date, and so forth, if not provided.
- Using the functional assessment tool, ask the patient to answer the questions. If the patient can't answer, have his caregiver provide the answers.

Special considerations

- According to OBRA, the physical portion of the assessment must be complete by a licensed nurse within 24 hours of a patient's admission. The entire assessment must be completed within 4 days. OBRA also mandates that the total assessment be revised and updated whenever a significant change occurs in a resident's mental or physical condition.
- When using the Lawton scale, make sure you evaluate the patient in terms of safety. For example, a person may be able to cook a small meal for himself but may leave the stove burner on after cooking.
- Both the Barthel Index and the Barthel Self-Care Rating Scale are used more commonly in rehabilitation and long-term care settings as tools to document improvement in a patient's abilities.

Documentation

Document all assessment findings according to your facility's policy.

SELECTED REFERENCES

Fukuse, T., et al. "Importance of a Comprehensive Geriatric Assessment in Prediction of Complications following Thoracic Surgery in Elderly Patients," *Chest* 127(3):886-91, March 2005.

Rozzini, R., et al. "Relationship between Functional Loss before Hospital Admission and Mortality in Elderly Persons with Medical Illness," *The Journals of Gerontology* 60(9):1180-83, September 2005.

DOCUMENTATION

Documentation is the process of preparing a complete record of a patient's care and is a vital tool for communication among health care team members. Accurate, detailed charting shows the extent and quality of the care that nurses provide, the outcomes of that care, and treatment and education that the patient still needs. Thorough, accurate documentation decreases the potential for miscommunication and errors.

Documentation is a valuable method for demonstrating that the nurse has applied nursing knowledge, skills, and judgment according to professional nursing standards. In a court of law, the patient's health record serves as the legal record of the care provided to that patient. Accrediting agencies and risk managers use the medical record to evaluate the quality of care a patient receives. Insurance companies use documentation systems to verify the care received. Nursing documentation in the medical record may also be utilized for research and education as well as used for quality improvement programs.

Equipment

Medical record (electronic or written) ■ pen with black or blue ink, if using a written medical record.

Preparation of equipment

There are various charting systems used for documentation. Since each documentation system follows specific policies and procedures for charting, familiarize yourself with the requirements of each system. (See *Comparing charting systems.*)

Implementation

- Write legibly *because illegible entries can result in misinterpretation of information and possible patient harm.*
- Use ink *because the medical record is a permanent document, and ink can't be erased.*
- Sign all entries using your first and last name and title *to clearly identify who wrote the entry.*
- When signing your initials on a form, use your full signature in the appropriate place on the form *to identify yourself as the care provider.*
- Stamp each sheet of the medical record with the patient's identifying information *to avoid charting on the wrong patient or mistaking the patient for another patient.*
- Use correct spelling and grammar in your entries *because misspelled words and poor grammar look unprofessional and can lead to errors.*
- If you make an error, draw a single line through the mistake and make a notation, such as "charting error," and initial it along with the date and time according to your facility's policy. Then record the correct entry. Don't use white-out, erasures, or entries between lines.
- Don't leave blank lines within and between entries. Draw a line through the blank line *to ensure that no further entries may be made.*
- Document in chronological order using the correct time and date. Avoid block charting, *which is vague, implies inat-*

Comparing charting systems

The table below compares elements of the different charting systems used today. Note that the second column provides information on which systems work best in which settings.

SYSTEM	USEFUL SETTINGS	PARTS OF RECORD	ASSESSMENT	CARE PLAN	OUTCOMES AND EVALUATIONS	PROGRESS NOTES FORMAT
Narrative	■ Acute care ■ Long-term care ■ Home care ■ Ambulatory care	■ Progress notes ■ Flow sheets to supplement care plan	■ *Initial:* history and admission form ■ *Ongoing:* progress notes	■ Care plan	■ Progress notes ■ Discharge summaries	■ Narration at time of entry
Problem-oriented medical record (POMR)	■ Acute care ■ Long-term care ■ Home care ■ Rehabilitation ■ Mental health facilities	■ Database ■ Care plan ■ Problem list ■ Progress notes ■ Discharge summary	■ *Initial:* database and care plan ■ *Ongoing:* progress notes	■ Database ■ Nursing care plan based on problem list	■ Progress notes (section E of SOAPIE and SOAPIER)	■ SOAP, SOAPIE, SOAPIER
Problem-intervention-evaluation (PIE)	■ Acute care	■ Assessment flow sheets ■ Progress notes ■ Problem list	■ *Initial:* assessment form ■ *Ongoing:* assessment form every shift	■ None; included in progress notes (section P)	■ Progress notes (section E)	■ Problem ■ Intervention ■ Evaluation
FOCUS	■ Acute care ■ Long-term care	■ Progress notes ■ Flow sheets ■ Checklists	■ *Initial:* patient history and admission assessment ■ *Ongoing:* assessment form	■ Nursing care plan based on problems or nursing diagnoses	■ Progress notes (section R)	■ Data ■ Action ■ Response
Charting by exception (CBE)	■ Acute care ■ Long-term care	■ Care plan ■ Flow sheets, including patient-teaching records and patient discharge notes ■ Graphic record ■ Progress notes	■ *Initial:* database assessment sheet ■ *Ongoing:* nursing and medical order flow sheets	■ Nursing care plan based on nursing diagnoses	■ Progress notes (section E)	■ SOAPIE or SOAPIER

(continued)

Comparing charting systems *(continued)*

System	Useful settings	Parts of record	Assessment	Care plan	Outcomes and evaluations	Progress notes format
Flow sheet, assessment, concise, timely (FACT)	▪ Acute care ▪ Long-term care	▪ Assessment sheet ▪ Flow sheets ▪ Progress notes	▪ *Initial:* baseline assessment ▪ *Ongoing:* flow sheets and progress notes	▪ Nursing care plan based on nursing diagnoses	▪ Flow sheets (section R)	▪ Data ▪ Action ▪ Response
Core	▪ Acute care ▪ Long-term care	▪ Kardex ▪ Flow sheets ▪ Progress notes	▪ *Initial:* baseline assessment ▪ *Ongoing:* progress notes	▪ Care plan	▪ Progress notes (section E)	▪ Data ▪ Action ▪ Evaluation
Computerized	▪ Acute care ▪ Long-term care ▪ Home care ▪ Ambulatory care	▪ Progress notes ▪ Flow sheets ▪ Nursing care plan ▪ Database ▪ Teaching plan	▪ *Initial:* baseline assessment ▪ *Ongoing:* progress notes	▪ Database ▪ Care plan	▪ Outcome-based care plan	▪ Evaluative statements ▪ Expected outcomes ▪ Learning outcomes

tention to the patient, and makes it hard to determine when specific events occurred.

▪ Document time according to your facility's policy using 24-hour military time or including a.m. or p.m.

▪ Chart information as soon as possible *to ensure the accuracy of the information and to reflect ongoing care. Delayed charting increases the potential for omissions, error, and inaccuracy due to memory lapse.*

▪ Describe observations and behavior of the client rather than "labeling" the patient. Don't offer opinions or use subjective statements or judgments.

▪ Use only approved abbreviations. (See *Abbreviations to avoid.*)

Special considerations

▪ If your facility uses computerized charting, most computer systems record the date and time that entries are made. Therefore, it's important to state specifically in the body of your note the time that events occurred and the action taken.

▪ Maintain the confidentiality of the medical record at all times. Keep the medical record closed when not in use, and store it in a secure place. If charting on a computer, make sure that no one else can read the screen, and log off when you are done charting. Never share your password with anyone else.

▪ At times, you may need to add a late entry, such as an event that you forgot to chart earlier or when the medical record wasn't available. Late entries, however, can look suspicious. Add the entry on the next available line, and label it as a "late entry" to show it's out of sequence. Then record the date and time of the entry as well as the date and time when the entry should have been made. Be sure to check if your facility has a policy for charting late entries.

▪ When charting continues from one page to the next, sign the bottom of the first page. At the top of the next page, write the date, time, and "continued from previous page."

▪ If information listed on a form doesn't apply to your patient, write N/A (not applicable) rather than leaving the space blank. *This shows that you read the question and that it doesn't apply rather than that you forgot to gather the data. It also prevents someone else from adding the information at a later date.*

▪ If your facility uses computerized records, know that most software programs establish an electronic signature based on your personal user password.

Abbreviations to avoid

To reduce the risk of medical errors, the Joint Commission has created a "minimum list" of abbreviations to avoid.

ABBREVIATION	POTENTIAL PROBLEM	PREFERRED TERM
U (for "unit")	Mistaken as zero, four, or cc	Write "unit."
IU (for "international unit")	Mistaken as IV (intravenous) or 10 (ten)	Write "international unit."
Q.D., Q.O.D, QD, QOD, q.d., q.o.d., qd, qod (Latin abbreviation for "once daily" and "every other day")	Mistaken for each other; period after "Q" can be mistaken for an "I" and "O" can be mistaken for "I"	Write "daily" and "every other day."
Trailing zero (X.0 mg) (Note: Prohibited only for medication-related notations); lack of leading zero (.X mg)	Decimal point is missed	Never write a zero by itself after a decimal point (X mg), and always use a zero before a decimal point (0.X mg).
MS MSO_4 $MgSO_4$	Confused for one another; can mean "morphine sulfate" or "magnesium sulfate"	Write "morphine sulfate" or "magnesium sulfate."
In addition to the Joint Commission's minimum "Do Not Use" list, the following items should be considered when evaluating which abbrevations to avoid.		
μg (for "microgram")	Mistaken for mg (milligrams), resulting in 1,000-fold dosing overdose	Write "mcg."
H.S. (for "half-strength" or Latin abbreviation for "at bedtime"	Mistaken for either "half-strength" or "hour of sleep" (at bedtime)	Write out "half-strength" or "at bedtime."
q.H.S.	Mistaken for "every hour"; can result in a dosing error	Write out "at bedtime."
T.I.W. (for "three times a week")	Mistaken for "three times a day" or "twice weekly," resulting in an overdose	Write "3 times weekly" or "three times weekly."
S.C or S.Q. (for "subcutaneous")	Mistaken for SL for "sublingual," or "5 every"	Write "Sub-Q", "subQ," or "subcutaneously."
D/C (for "discharge")	Interpreted as "discontinue" whatever medications follow (typically discharge meds)	Write "discharge."
c.c. (for "cubic centimeters")	Mistaken for U (units) when poorly written	Write "ml" for milliliters.
AS, AD, AU (Latin abbreviation for "left ear," "right ear," or "both ears")	Mistaken for OS, OD, and OU	Write "left ear," "right ear," or "both ears."

Guidelines for facilitating communication

- Speak in a normal tone.
- Don't raise your voice or shout.
- Realize that speaking louder doesn't increase comprehension.
- Speak to the patient on an adult level.
- Remember that impaired communication doesn't indicate impaired intelligence.
- Avoid carrying on more than one conversation at a time.
- Ask simple questions that require simple answers.
- Keep the atmosphere quiet and relaxed.
- Reduce or eliminate environmental noises.
- Make sure you have the patient's attention before you speak.
- Maintain eye contact with the patient throughout the conversation.
- Assume that the patient can understand you. Don't discuss his case or other inappropriate topics in front of him.
- Don't rush the patient. Give him adequate time to respond.
- Don't correct mistakes.
- If you don't understand, ask the patient to repeat what he said.
- Praise the patient for attempts at speech.

Adapted with permission from Craven, R.F., and Hirnle, C.J. *Fundamentals of Nursing: Human Health and Function,* 5th ed. Philadelphia: Lippincott Williams & Wilkins, 2006.

SELECTED REFERENCES

Alford, D.M. "The Clinical Record: Recognizing Its Value in Litigation," *Geriatric Nursing* 24(4):228-230, July-August 2003.

Austin, S. "Ladies and Gentlemen of the Jury, I Present…The Nursing Documentation," *Nursing* 36(1):56-62, January 2006.

Birmingham, J. "Documentation: A Guide for Case Managers," *Lippincott's Case Management* 9(3):155-157, May/June, 2004.

Helleso, R. "Information Handling in the Nursing Discharge Note," *Journal of Clinical Nursing* 15(1):11-21, January 2006.

The Joint Commission. *Comprehensive Accreditation Manual for Hospitals: The Official Handbook.* Standard IM.6.20. 2007.

The Joint Commission. Official "Do Not Use" List. Accessed August 2007 via the Web at *www.jointcommission.org.*

Roberts, D. "The Legal Side of Nursing," *MedSurg Nursing* 13(4):210, 225, August 2004.

COMMUNICATING WITH DIFFICULT PATIENTS

Nurses make every effort to communicate with their patients in a therapeutic manner. Communicating with the difficult patient can be a challenge. The difficult patient is one whose behavior makes it hard for the nurse to provide quality nursing care. Understanding why some patients are difficult and then using therapeutic communication techniques to diffuse the difficult behavior will help the nurse to develop a therapeutic working relationship with the patient. A patient may exhibit difficult behavior for various reasons such as pain or discomfort, frustration, grieving, hopelessness, difficulty expressing feelings, poor coping skills, effects of medications, fear, psychiatric illness, and delirium.

Equipment

Medical record ■ quiet environment.

Preparation of equipment

Before meeting with the patient, if possible, review the medical record *to determine if the patient's condition may be contributing to his behavior.* Attempt to determine the contributing diagnoses or reasons for the behavior *so they can be corrected.* If possible, talk with the patient in a quiet environment that's conducive to communication and free from distractions.

Implementation

- Always greet your patient by his full name *to show respect.*
- Introduce yourself, using your first and last name and your title *so the patient knows who you are and your role in his care.*
- Allow the patient to express his feelings and let him know that you're willing to listen. (See *Guidelines for facilitating communication.*)
- Don't interrupt; let the patient tell his story.
- Summarize your understanding of what the patient said, and ask for clarification *so the patient knows you're trying to understand and help him.* (See *Therapeutic communication techniques.)*
- Express empathy *to let the patient know you're trying to understand his feelings and what they mean to him.*

Therapeutic communication techniques

TECHNIQUE	DEFINITION
Offering self	Making self available to listen to the patient
Open-ended questions	Asking neutral questions that encourage the patient to express concerns
Opening remarks	Using general statements based on observations and assessments about the patient
Restatement	Repeating to the patient the main content of his or her communication
Reflection	Identifying the main emotional themes contained in a communication and directing these back to the patient
Focusing	Asking goal-directed questions to help the patient focus on key concerns
Encouraging elaboration	Helping the patient describe more fully the concerns or problems under discussion
Seeking clarification	Helping the patient put into words unclear thoughts or ideas
Giving information	Sharing with the patient relevant information for his or her health care and well-being
Looking at alternatives	Helping the patient see options and participate in the decision-making process related to his or her health care and well-being
Silence	Allowing for a pause in communications that permits nurse and patient time to think about what has taken place
Summarizing	Highlighting the important points of a conversation by condensing what was said

Adapted with permission from Craven, R.F., and Hirnle, C.J. *Fundamentals of Nursing: Human Health and Function,* 5th ed. Philadelphia: Lippincott Williams & Wilkins, 2006.

- Acknowledge the patient's feelings *so he knows you're listening.*
- Confirm your willingness to work with the patient *to show that you care and want to help resolve the problem.*
- Allow the patient to make choices, when possible, *to give him a sense of control.*
- Provide for continuity of caregivers *to allow a consistent and trusting relationship to develop.*
- Ask the patient what you can do to make the situation better *to show him you're concerned and want to help.*
- Tell the patient your expectations, and set limits *so the patient understands what's expected of him.*
- Consider a behavioral contract, which outlines expected behaviors.
- Obtain a psychiatric consultation if the patient's behaviors become unmanageable.

Protecting yourself and others

- Be alert for escalating behavior, such as clenched jaw or fist, agitation, pacing, loud or profane speech, flushed face, enlarged eyes, flaring nostrils, and rapid respirations *so that you can provide measures to calm the patient and call for help, if necessary.*
- Observe for signs of imminent violent behavior, such as verbal threats, demands of immediate attention, and encroaching on your personal space *so that you can remove yourself and others from the immediate area and obtain help.*

Nine rules for the verbal de-escalation of anger

RULE	EXPLANATION
1. Respect personal space	Stay two arms' lengths away from the patient. Maintain usual social eye contact—neither staring nor averting your gaze. Don't block an escape route for either you or the patient.
2. Don't provoke patient	Maintain a calm demeanor and stance. Speak softly and don't threaten.
3. Be concise and repeat yourself	Use short phrases or sentences. Use a simple vocabulary. Repeat yourself as often as necessary.
4. Recognize patient's wants and feelings	"You seem angry…do you want something you're not getting?" or "You seem afraid…do you think something bad will happen?"
5. Listen	Try to understand what the patient is saying. "Let me see if I understand correctly." Don't argue. Don't respond to insults.
6. Agree with patient	Do this without lying or furthering a delusion.
7. Set limits	Be clear about acceptable and unacceptable behavior. Be honest. State positive and negative consequences.
8. Offer choices	"Would you like some medicine to help you calm down?" or "Would you like to call someone?"
9. Debrief patient and staff	After the patient is calm, ask about his or her reaction and explain why you took certain steps. Meet with staff as well.

Adapted with permission from Craven, R.F., and Hirnle, C.J. *Fundamentals of Nursing: Human Health and Function,* 5th ed. Philadelphia: Lippincott Williams & Wilkins, 2006.

- If a patient becomes verbally abusive, remove yourself from the room. Tell the patient you won't stay with him when he uses abusive language but that you'll be back in 15 minutes. This allows the patient time to calm down and get control of his feelings. (See *Nine rules for the verbal de-escalation of anger*.)
- Avoid turning your back on a potentially violent patient, *so that you can observe the patient's actions at all times and move defensively if he becomes violent.*
- Position yourself so the patient isn't between you and the door *to provide an escape route if the patient does become violent.*
- Stand back from the patient, and avoid entering his personal space *to remain out of his reach and to prevent the patient from feeling physically threatened.*
- Don't touch the patient *because this may be misinterpreted as an aggressive gesture.*
- Remain composed *to show you're in control.*
- Avoid arguing or being confrontational *as this may escalate the patient's behaviors.*

Special considerations

- Be aware of your own feelings, and recognize when you're tense, angry, or uncomfortable in a situation. If you're feeling uneasy, leave the room and examine your own feelings and what's making you feel this way. If you can't calmly and objectively meet the needs of your patient, ask the help of your colleagues.
- Document interventions that are successful in the plan of care, *so that the information is communicated to all members*

of the health care team and all team members respond to the patient using a consistent approach.

Documentation

Record the date and time of the difficult patient encounter. Document the patient's behaviors objectively. Note his complaints using the patient's own words, in quotes, if possible. Record the specific care given to the patient in direct response to the situation and his response to that care. Record details of your contacts with the patient. Note the times and names of any people you notified of the patient's behavior and their response. Record whether or not they came to see the patient.

SELECTED REFERENCES

Distasio, C.A. Protecting Yourself from Violence, *Nursing* 32(6):58-93, June 2002.

Essary, A.C., and Symington, S.L. "How to Make the 'Difficult' Patient Encounter Less Difficult," *JAAPA* 18(5): 49-54, May 2005.

Haas, L.J., Leiser, et al. "Management of the Difficult Patient," *American Family Physician* 72(10):2063-2068, November 2005.

White, M.K., and Keller, V.F. "Difficult Clinician-Patient Relationships," *CRICO/RMF* 20(6):4-7, December 2000.

SAFETY AND MOBILITY

RESTRAINT APPLICATION

Restraint is a method of physically restricting a person's freedom of movement, physical activity, or normal access to his body. This includes not only traditional restraints, such as limb or vest restraints, but also tightly tucked sheets or the use of side rails to prevent a patient from getting out of bed.

The Joint Commission has issued standards regarding the use of restraints. According to these standards, restraints are to be limited to emergencies in which the patient is at risk for harming himself or others and when other less-restrictive measures have proved ineffective. The standards vary based on the setting and the reason for restraint. Restraints that are applied for patient safety or any reason other than behavioral health reasons have less strict standards than those applied for behavioral health care. Most restraints applied in a hospital are for patient safety. The Centers for Medicare and Medicaid Services (CMS) doesn't specify standards based on setting. Their standards are based on patient behavior and risk of injury. Always check your facility's policy for its definition of restraints for safety and behavioral health restraints. One purpose of the revisions is to reduce the use of restraints. (See *Alternatives to restraints.*) Restraints can cause numerous problems, including limited mobility, skin breakdown, impaired circulation, incontinence, psychological distress, and strangulation.

Alternatives to restraints

Restraints must be used only after all other measures have failed to keep the patient from harming himself or others. They should be applied in the least restrictive manner and for as short a time as possible.

To reduce the need for restraints, take an individualized approach that seeks to prevent behavior problems. Look for an underlying problem that may be causing your patient's behavior—such as adverse drug effects, infection, electrolyte imbalance, or hypoxia—and take measures to correct the problem.

Look for "agenda behaviors" in which the patient's behavior may be an attempt to correct a problem, such as pain, hunger, fatigue, heat, cold, or the need for toileting.

Create an environment that's free from restraints and encourages patient mobility. This requires a unit and facility commitment because policy changes and even structural changes may be required.

If the problem behavior continues after you've identified and corrected conditions that may be the cause, consider alternatives to restraints, such as:

- reorienting the patient as needed
- providing explanations for procedures
- keeping the patient warm, dry, and comfortable
- establishing eye contact and talking to the patient
- listening and validating the patient's concerns
- determining the patient's routines and habits and trying to adhere to them
- wrapping elastic compression bandages around I.V. sites, other tubing, or dressings
- switching to a capped I.V. line if possible
- determining whether equipment or treatment is really necessary
- moving tubing or equipment out of the patient's sight
- using an abdominal binder to cover abdominal drains, tubes, and dressings and urinary catheters.

EQUIPMENT

Types of child restraints

You may need to restrain an infant or a child to prevent injury or to facilitate examination, diagnostic tests, or treatment. If so, follow these steps:

- Provide a simple explanation, reassurance, and constant observation *to minimize the child's fear.*
- Explain the restraint to the parents and enlist their help.
- Reassure them that it won't hurt the child.
- Make sure that the restraint ties or safety pins are secured outside the child's reach *to prevent injury.*
- When using a mummy restraint, secure the infant's arms in proper alignment with the body *to avoid dislocation and other injuries.*

Vest

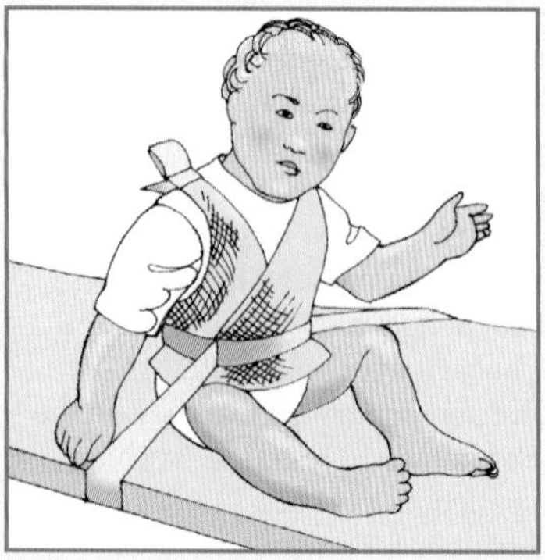

Elbow

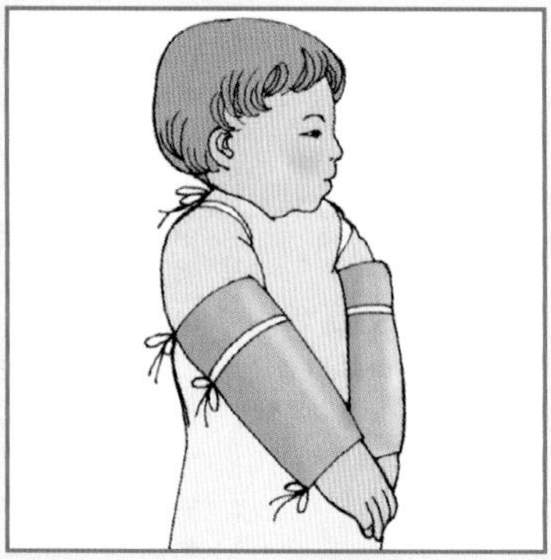

Mummy

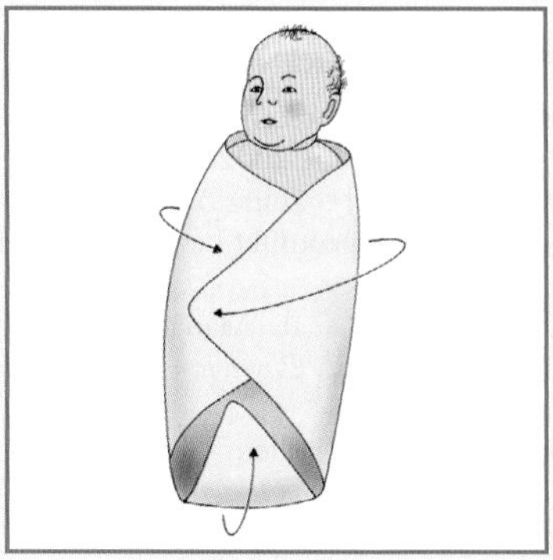

Belt

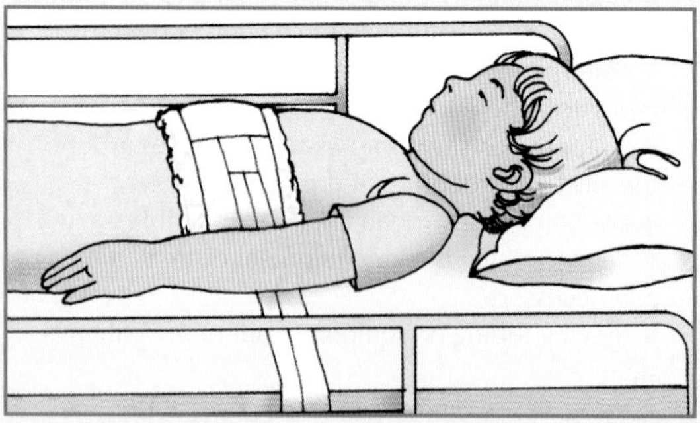

Limb

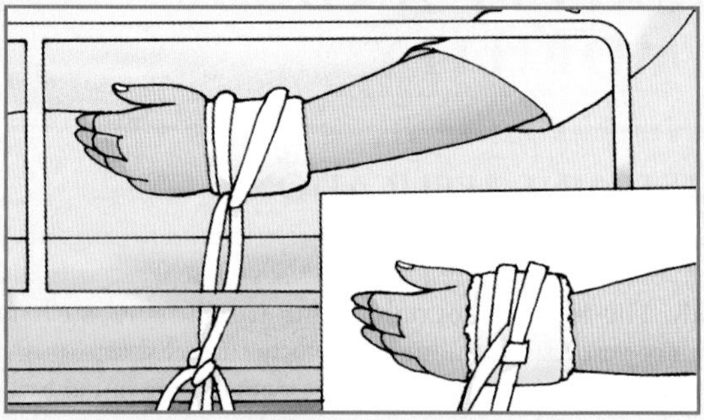

Crib with net

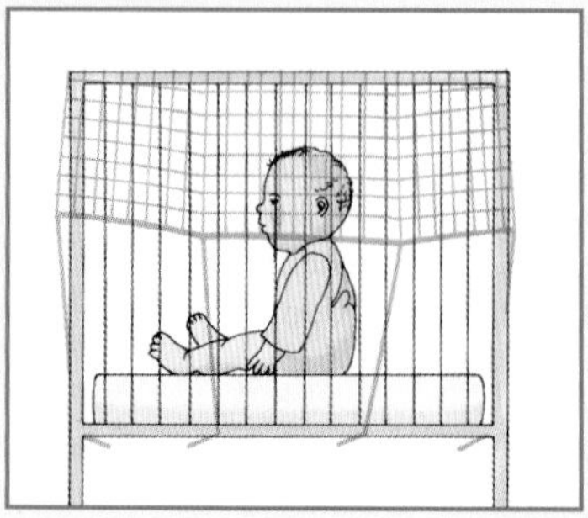

Mitt

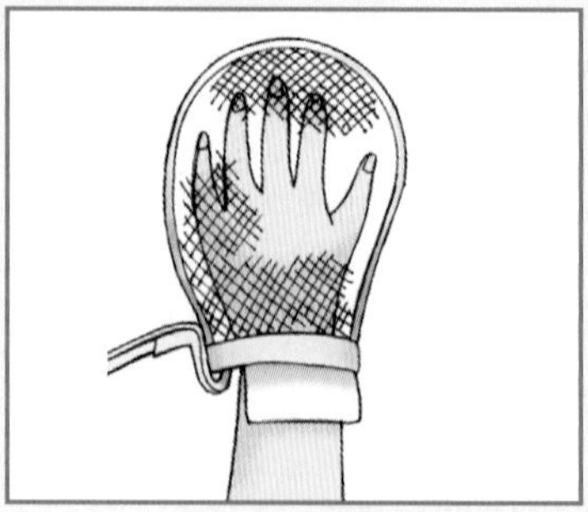

Restraining board

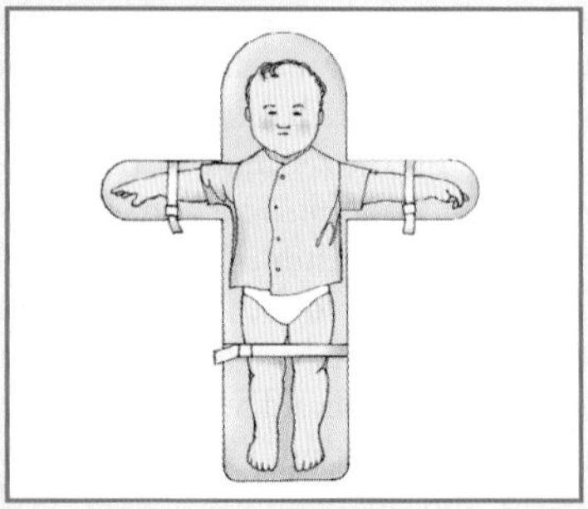

Equipment

For soft restraints: Restraint (vest, limb, mitt, or belt, as needed) ■ padding if needed ■ restraint flow sheet.

For leather restraints: Two wrist and two ankle leather restraints ■ four straps ■ key ■ large gauze pads to cushion each extremity ■ restraint flow sheet.

Preparation of equipment

Before entering the patient's room, make sure the restraints are the correct size, using the patient's build and weight as a guide. If you use leather restraints, make sure the straps are unlocked and the key fits the locks.

PEDIATRIC ALERT *For children, who are typically too small for standard restraints, use a child restraint. (See* Types of child restraints.*)*

Implementation

■ Follow Joint Commission and CMS standards for applying restraints. Make sure that less-restrictive measures have been tried before applying restraints.

■ When all the other methods have failed to keep the patient from harming himself or others, apply restraints for as short a time as possible. Choose a restraint that's least restrictive to the patient.

■ Tell the patient what you're about to do, and describe the restraints to him. Assure him that they're being used to protect him from injury rather than to punish him.

■ If necessary, obtain adequate assistance to restrain the patient before entering his room. Enlist the aid of several coworkers and organize their effort, giving each person a specific task; for example, one person explains the procedure to the patient and applies the restraints while the others immobilize the patient's arms and legs.

■ When applying restraints for patient safety, inform the licensed independent practitioner within 12 hours of placing the patient in restraints and obtain a written or verbal order for the restraints. The patient must be examined by the practitioner within 24 hours of the initiation of restraints. Assess the patient every 2 hours or according to your facility's policy.

■ When applying restraints for behavioral health reasons, obtain a written or verbal order from a licensed independent practitioner immediately. A licensed independent practitioner must evaluate the patient in person within 1 hour. A new order must be obtained every 4 hours, and an in-person evaluation must take place every 8 hours. Assess the patient every 15 minutes or according to your facility's policy.

■ If the patient consented to have his family informed of his care, notify them of the use of restraints.

Knots for securing soft restraints

When securing soft restraints, use knots that can be released quickly and easily, like those shown below. Remember, never secure restraints to the bed's side rails.

Magnus hitch

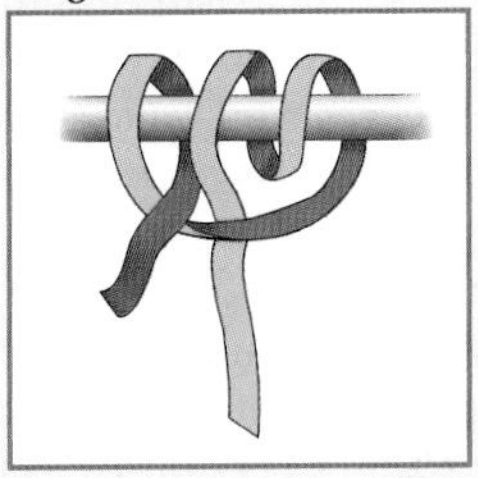

Clove hitch

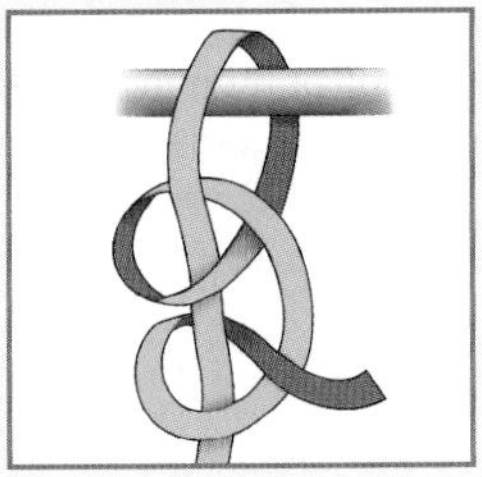

Loop

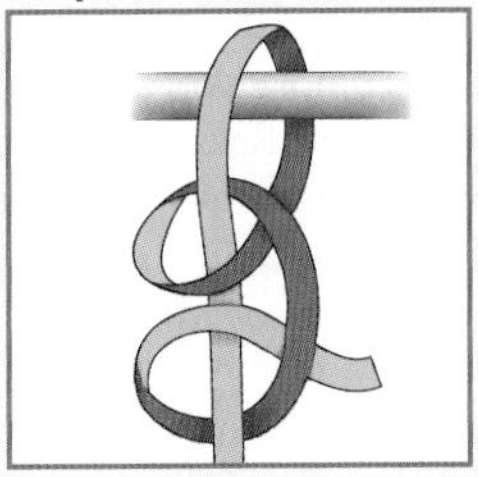

Applying a vest restraint

■ Assist the patient to a sitting position if his condition permits. Then slip the vest over his gown. Crisscross the cloth flaps at the front, placing the V-shaped opening at the patient's throat. Never crisscross the flaps in the back *because this may cause the patient to choke if he tries to squirm out of the vest.*

■ Pass the tab on one flap through the slot on the opposite flap. Then adjust the vest for the patient's comfort. You should be able to slip your fist between the vest and the patient. Avoid wrapping the vest too tightly *because it may restrict respiration.*

■ Tie all restraints securely to the frame of the bed, chair, or wheelchair and out of the patient's reach. Never secure the restraint to a bed rail or other movable part of the equipment. Use a bow or a knot that can be released quickly and easily in an emergency. (See *Knots for securing soft restraints.*) Never tie a regular knot to secure the straps. Leave 1″ to 2″ (2.5 to 5 cm) of slack in the straps *to allow room for movement.*

- After applying the vest, check the patient's respiratory rate and breath sounds regularly. Be alert for signs of respiratory distress. Also, make sure the vest hasn't tightened with the patient's movement. Loosen the vest frequently, if possible, *so the patient can stretch, turn, and breathe deeply.*

Applying a limb restraint

- Wrap the patient's wrist or ankle with a padded restraint.
- Pass the strap on the narrow end of the restraint through the slot in the broad end, and adjust for a snug fit. Alternatively, fasten the buckle or Velcro cuffs to fit the restraint. You should be able to slip one or two fingers between the restraint and the patient's skin. Avoid applying the restraint too tightly *because it may impair circulation distal to the restraint.*
- Tie the restraint as above.
- After applying limb restraints, be alert for signs of impaired circulation, movement, or sensation in the extremity distal to the restraint. Check the patient's distal extremities for color, temperature, and pulse according to your facility's policy. If the skin appears blue or feels cold, or if the patient complains of a tingling sensation or numbness, loosen the restraint. Release the restraint every 2 hours *to assess the skin,* and perform range-of-motion (ROM) exercises regularly *to stimulate circulation and prevent contractures and resultant loss of mobility.*

Applying a mitt restraint

- Wash and dry the patient's hands.
- Roll up a washcloth or gauze pad, and place it in the patient's palm. Have him form a loose fist, if possible; then pull the mitt over it and secure the closure.
- *To restrict the patient's arm movement,* attach the strap to the mitt and tie it securely, using a bow or a knot that can be released quickly and easily in an emergency.
- When using mitts made of transparent mesh, check hand movement and skin color frequently *to assess circulation.* Remove the mitts regularly *to stimulate circulation,* and perform passive ROM exercises *to prevent contractures.*

Applying a belt restraint

- Center the flannel pad of the belt on the bed. Then wrap the short strap of the belt around the bed frame and fasten it under the bed.
- Position the patient on the pad. Then have him roll slightly to one side while you guide the long strap around his waist and through the slot in the pad.
- Wrap the long strap around the bed frame, and fasten it under the bed.
- After applying the belt, slip your hand between the patient and the belt to ensure a secure but comfortable fit. A loose belt can be raised to chest level; a tight one can cause abdominal discomfort.

Applying leather restraints

- Position the patient supine on the bed, with each arm and leg securely held down *to minimize combative behavior and to prevent injury to the patient and others.* Immobilize the patient's arms and legs at the joints—knee, ankle, shoulder, and wrist—*to minimize his movement without exerting excessive force.*
- Apply pads to the patient's wrists and ankles *to reduce friction between his skin and the leather, preventing skin irritation and breakdown.*
- Wrap the restraint around the gauze pads. Then insert the metal loop through the hole that gives the best fit. Apply the restraints securely but not too tightly. You should be able to slip one or two fingers between the restraint and the patient's skin. *A tight restraint can compromise circulation; a loose one can slip off or move up the patient's arm or leg, causing skin irritation and breakdown.*
- Thread the strap through the metal loop on the restraint, close the metal loop, and secure the strap to the bed frame, out of the patient's reach.
- Lock the restraint by pushing in the button on the side of the metal loop, and tug it gently to *make sure it's secure.* Once the restraint is secure, a coworker can release the arm or leg. Flex the patient's arm or leg slightly before locking the strap *to allow room for movement and to prevent frozen joints and dislocations.*
- Place the key in an accessible location at the nurse's station.
- After applying leather restraints, observe the patient regularly *to give emotional support and to reassess the need for continued use of the restraint.* Check his pulse rate and vital signs according to your facility's policy. Remove or loosen the restraints one at a time, every 2 hours, and perform passive ROM exercises if possible. Watch for signs of impaired peripheral circulation, such as cool, cyanotic skin. To unlock the restraint, insert the key into the metal loop, opposite the locking button. This releases the lock, and the metal loop can be opened.

Special considerations

- Know the latest Joint Commission and CMS standards for restraint applications. Implement alternative strategies to reduce the need for restraints. Choose the least restrictive restraint, if necessary, for your patient.
- Provide for continuous patient monitoring in which a designated person can directly observe the patient at all times.
- Assess and assist the restrained patient according to your facility's policy, including injuries caused by the restraint, nutrition, hydration, circulation, ROM, vital signs, hygiene,

elimination, comfort, and physical and psychosocial status. Also assess whether the patient is ready to have restraints discontinued.

- The condition of the restrained patient must be continually monitored, assessed, and evaluated. Release the restraints every hour; assess the patient's pulse and skin condition, and perform ROM exercises. A restraint flow sheet must be used with hourly notations.
- When the patient is at high risk for aspiration, restrain him on his side. Never secure all four restraints to one side of the bed *because the patient may fall out of bed.*
- When loosening restraints, have a coworker on hand *to assist in restraining the patient if necessary.*
- Don't apply a limb restraint above an I.V. site *because the constriction may occlude the infusion or cause infiltration into surrounding tissue.*
- Never secure restraints to the side rails *because someone might inadvertently lower the rail before noticing the attached restraint. This may jerk the patient's limb or body, causing him discomfort and trauma.* Never secure restraints to the fixed frame of the bed if the patient's position is to be changed.
- Don't restrain a patient in the prone position. *This position limits his field of vision, intensifies feelings of helplessness and vulnerability, and impairs respiration, especially if the patient has been sedated.*
- *Because the restrained patient has limited mobility,* his nutrition, elimination, and positioning become your responsibility. *To prevent pressure ulcers,* reposition the patient every 2 hours, and massage and pad bony prominences and other vulnerable areas.

Complications

Excessively tight limb restraints can reduce peripheral circulation; tight vest restraints can impair respiration. Apply restraints carefully and check them according to standards.

Skin breakdown can also occur under limb restraints. To prevent this, pad the patient's wrists and ankles, loosen or remove the restraints frequently, and provide regular skin care.

Long periods of immobility can predispose the patient to pneumonia, urine retention, constipation, and sensory deprivation. Reposition the patient, and attend to his elimination requirements as needed.

Some patients resist restraints by biting, kicking, scratching, or head butting, in the course of which they may injure themselves or others.

Documentation

Document each episode of the use of restraints, including the date and time they were initiated. Record the circumstances resulting in the use of restraints and the nonphysical interventions tried first. Describe the rationale for the specific type of restraint used. Include the conditions or behaviors necessary for discontinuing the restraint and whether these conditions were communicated to the patient.

Chart the name of the licensed independent practitioner who ordered the restraint and each in-person evaluation by the licensed independent practitioner.

Record 15-minute assessments of the patient, including signs of injury, nutrition, hydration, circulation, ROM, vital signs, hygiene, elimination, comfort, physical and psychological status, and readiness for removing restraints. Record your interventions to help the patient meet the conditions for removing the restraints. Note that the patient was continuously monitored. Document any injuries or complications, the time and name of the practitioner notified of your interventions, and your actions.

SELECTED REFERENCES

Amato, S., et al. "Physical Restraint Reduction in the Acute Rehabilitation Setting: A Quality Improvement Study," *Rehabilitation Nursing* 31(6):235-41, November-December 2006.

The Joint Commission. *Comprehensive Accreditation Manual for Hospitals: An Official Handbook.* Standard PC.11.10 to PC.11.100 and PC.12.10 to PC.12.190, 2007.

Kowk, T., et al. "Does Access to Bed-Chair Pressure Sensors Reduce Physical Restraint Use in the Rehabilitative Care Setting?" *Journal of Clinical Nursing* 15(5):581-87, May 2006.

McBeth, S. "Get a Firmer Grasp on Restraints," *Nursing Management* 35(10):20, 22, October 2004.

Saulf, N.M. "Restraints Use and Falls Prevention," *Journal of Perianesthesia Nursing* 19(6):433-36, December 2004.

Suen, L.K., et al. "Use of Physical Restraints in Rehabilitation Settings: Staff Knowledge, Attitudes and Predictors," *Journal of Advanced Nursing* 55(1):20-28, July 2006.

FALL PREVENTION AND MANAGEMENT

Falls are a major cause of injury and death among elderly people. In fact, the older the person, the more likely he is to die of a fall or its complications. In people age 65 or older, falls account for three times as many accidental deaths as motor vehicle accidents.

Factors that contribute to falls among elderly patients include lengthy convalescent periods, a greater risk of incomplete recovery, medications, increasing physical disability, and impaired vision or hearing. For example, once impaired, equilibrium takes longer to be restored in elderly people than in younger adults. Naturally, loss of balance increases the risk of falling. Besides causing physical harm, injuries from falls can trigger psychological problems, leading to a loss of self-confidence and hastening dependence and a move to a long-term care facility or nursing home.

Determining a patient's risk of falling

The Morse Fall Scale is one method of rapidly assessing a patient's likelihood of falling. It's widely used in hospital and long-term care inpatient settings.

To use the scale, score each item and total the number of points. A score between 0 and 24 indicates no risk, 25 to 50 indicates low risk, and a score greater than 50 indicates a high risk of falling.

ITEM		SCALE	SCORING
History of falling; immediate or within 3 months	No	0	0
	Yes	25	
Secondary diagnosis	No	0	0
	Yes	15	
Ambulatory aid			15
■ Bed rest/nurse assist		0	
■ Crutches/cane/walker		15	
■ Furniture		30	
I.V./Saline lock	No	0	20
	Yes	20	
Gait/Transferring			
■ Normal/bed rest/immobile		0	20
■ Weak		10	
■ Impaired		20	
Mental status			
■ Oriented to own ability		0	0
■ Forgets limitations		15	
TOTAL			55

Adapted with permission from Morse, J.M. *Preventing Patient Falls.* Thousand Oaks, Calif.: Sage Publications, 1997.

Falls may be caused by extrinsic or environmental factors, such as poor lighting, slippery throw rugs, highly waxed floors, unfamiliar surroundings, or misuse of assistive devices. However, they usually result from intrinsic or physiologic factors, such as temporary muscle paralysis, vertigo, orthostatic hypotension, central nervous system lesions, dementia, failing eyesight, osteoporosis, and decreased strength or coordination.

In a hospital or other health care facility, an accidental fall can change a short stay for a minor problem into a prolonged stay for serious—and possibly life-threatening—problems. The risk of falling is highest during the first week of a stay in a hospital or nursing home. The adage "an ounce of prevention is worth a pound of cure" is worth remembering when working with elderly patients. (See *Determining a patient's risk of falling.*)

Recommendations from the Centers for Disease Control and Prevention for preventing falls in elderly patients include:

- physical condition, rehabilitation, or physical therapy that include exercise to improve endurance and strength
- environmental assessments and modifications to improve mobility such as installing handrails in hallways, raised toilet seats, and grab bars in showers
- review of prescribed medications to assess potential risks and benefits
- technological devices, such as alarm systems, that are activated when patients get out of bed.

Clinical practice guideline: Preventing falls

The following guideline was developed by a panel of health care professionals to help you assess the risk of falls in elderly patients.

Assessment

As part of routine care for older persons, ask patients (or caregivers) about falls in the past year.

For the patient who reports a single fall:
- have the patient stand up from a chair without using his arms, walk several paces, turn, return to the chair, and sit down
- if the patient has no difficulty, he needs no further assessment.

For the patient who reports more than one fall or has an abnormal gait or balance, perform a fall evaluation, including:
- a history of fall circumstances, medical problems, and mobility
- a medication review and modification, as needed, especially when the patient is taking more than four drugs
- examination of vision, gait, balance, lower extremity function, neurologic function, cerebellar function, and cardiovascular status
- a home environmental assessment.

Recommended interventions

For patients living in their own homes:
- gait training and advice on assistive devices
- medication review and modification, as needed
- exercise programs with balance training
- treatment of orthostatic hypotension
- correction of environmental hazards
- treatment of cardiovascular disorders and arrhythmias.

For patients in long-term care or assisted-living settings:
- staff education programs
- gait training and advice on assistive devices
- medication review and modification, as needed.

For patients in acute hospital settings, evidence is insufficient to recommend interventions.

Reprinted from American Geriatrics Society, British Geriatrics Society, and American Academy of Orthopaedic Surgeons Panel on Falls Prevention. "Guideline for the Prevention of Falls in Older Persons," *Journal of the American Geriatrics Society* 49(5):664-72, May 2001, with permission of the publisher.

Nursing interventions to reduce falls should follow the clinical practice guidelines endorsed by the American Geriatrics Society, British Geriatrics Society, and the American Academy of Orthopaedic Surgeons. (See *Clinical practice guideline: Preventing falls.*)

Equipment

Stethoscope ▪ sphygmomanometer ▪ analgesics ▪ cold and warm compresses ▪ pillows ▪ blankets ▪ emergency resuscitation equipment (crash cart) if needed ▪ electrocardiograph (ECG) monitor if needed.

Preparation of equipment

If you're helping a fallen patient, send an assistant to collect the assessment or resuscitation equipment you need.

Implementation

- Whether your plan of care focuses on preventing a fall or managing one in an elderly patient, you'll need to proceed with patience and caution.

Preventing falls

- Assess your patient's risk of falling on admission and regularly thereafter using a standardized assessment tool. Note any changes in his condition—such as decreased mental status—that increase his chances of falling. If you decide that he's at risk, take steps to reduce the danger.
- Orient the patient to the room and nursing unit. Show him how to use the call bell, and assess his ability to use it. Place the call bell within reach.
- Correct potential dangers in the patient's room. Provide adequate nighttime lighting.
- Place the patient's personal belongings and aids (purse, wallet, books, tissues, urinal, commode, cane, or walker) within easy reach.
- Instruct him to rise slowly from a supine position *to avoid possible dizziness and loss of balance.*
- Keep the bed in its lowest position *so the patient can easily reach the floor when he gets out of bed. This also reduces the distance to the floor in case he falls.* Lock the bed's wheels. If side rails are to be raised, observe the patient frequently.

Medications associated with falls

This table highlights some classes of drugs that are commonly prescribed for older patients and the possible adverse effects of each that may increase a patient's risk of falling.

DRUG CLASS	ADVERSE EFFECTS
Antidiabetics	Acute hypoglycemia
Antihistamines and benzodiazepines	Excessive sedation Confusion Paradoxical agitation Loss of balance
Antihypertensives	Hypotension
Antipsychotics	Excessive sedation Confusion Paradoxical agitation Loss of balance
Diuretics	Hypovolemia Orthostatic hypotension Electrolyte imbalance Urinary incontinence
Hypnotics	Excessive sedation Ataxia Poor balance Confusion Paradoxical agitation
Opioids	Hypotension Sedation Motor incoordination Agitation
Tricyclic antidepressants	Orthostatic hypotension

- Advise the patient to wear nonskid footwear.
- Respond promptly to the patient's call bell *to help limit the number of times he gets out of bed without help.*
- Check the patient at least every 2 hours. Check a high-risk patient every 15 to 30 minutes.
- Alert other caregivers to the patient's risk of falling and to the interventions you've implemented.
- Consider other precautions, such as placing two high-risk patients in the same room and having someone with them at all times.
- Encourage the patient to perform active range-of-motion (ROM) exercises *to improve flexibility and coordination.*
- Encourage the patient to use handrails and grab bars whenever possible.
- Educate the patient and his family about mobility limitations and fall reduction measures.

Managing falls

- If you're with a patient as he falls, try to break his fall with your body.
- As you gently guide him to the floor, support his body, particularly his head and trunk. If possible, help him to a supine position.
- While guiding the patient, concentrate on maintaining proper body alignment yourself *to keep the center of gravity within your support base.* Spread your feet *to widen your support base.* Remember, the wider the base, the better your balance will be. Bend your knees—rather than your back—*to support the patient and to avoid injuring yourself.*
- Remain calm and stay with the patient *to prevent any further injury.*
- Ask another nurse to collect any tools you may need, such as a stethoscope, a sphygmomanometer and, if necessary, an ECG monitor.
- Assess the patient's airway, breathing, and circulation *to make sure the fall wasn't caused by respiratory or cardiac arrest.* If you don't detect respirations or a pulse, call a code and begin emergency resuscitation measures. Also note his level of consciousness (LOC), and assess pupil size, equality, and reaction to light.
- *To determine the extent of the patient's injuries,* look for lacerations, abrasions, and obvious deformities. Note any deviations from the patient's baseline condition. Notify the practitioner. Determine if there was head trauma, which requires further diagnostic evaluation to rule out subdural hematoma.

NURSING ALERT *Patients taking anticoagulants or aspirin therapy who experience head trauma are at increased risk for subdural hematoma.*

- If you weren't present during the fall, ask the patient or a witness what happened. Ask if the patient experienced pain or a change in LOC.
- Don't move the patient until you evaluate his status fully. Provide reassurance as needed, and observe for such signs and symptoms as confusion, tremor, weakness, pain, and dizziness.
- Assess the patient's limb strength and motion. Don't perform ROM exercises if you suspect a fracture or if the patient complains of any odd sensations or limited movement.

If you suspect a disorder, don't move the patient until a practitioner examines him.

- While the patient lies on the floor until the practitioner arrives, offer pillows and blankets for comfort. If you suspect a spinal cord injury, however, don't place a pillow under his head.
- If you don't detect any problems, return the patient to his bed with the help of another staff member. Never try to lift a patient alone *because you may injure yourself or the patient.*
- Take steps to control bleeding (if indicated) and to obtain an X-ray if you suspect a fracture. Provide first aid for minor injuries as needed. Then monitor the patient's status for the next 24 hours.
- Even if the patient shows no signs of distress or has sustained only minor injuries, monitor his vital signs every 15 minutes for 1 hour, then every 30 minutes for 1 hour, then every hour for 2 hours, or until his condition stabilizes. Monitor neurologic assessments with vital signs as per your facility's protocol. Notify the practitioner if you note any change from the baseline.
- Perform necessary measures to relieve the patient's pain and discomfort. Give analgesics as ordered. Apply cold compresses for the first 24 hours and warm compresses thereafter.
- Reassess the patient's environment and his risk of falling. Talk to him about the fall. Discuss why it occurred and how he thinks it could have been prevented. Review the events that preceded the fall. Did the patient change position abruptly? Does he wear corrective lenses, and was he wearing them when he fell? Had he been drinking alcohol? Review medications that may have contributed to the fall, such as tranquilizers and opioids. (See *Medications associated with falls.*) In addition, assess gait disturbances or improper use of canes, crutches, or a walker.

Special considerations

- After a fall, review the patient's medical history to determine whether he's at risk for other complications. For example, if he hit his head, check his history to see whether he takes anticoagulants. If he does, he's at greater risk for intracranial bleeding, and you'll need to monitor him accordingly.
- Develop an individualized fall prevention program with multiple interventions.

NURSING ALERT *Perform a risk assessment for falls on all admitted patients.*

- Devise an alternative to restraints for a high-risk patient. For example, consider using a device such as a pressure-pad alarm for chairs and beds. The pressure sensor pad lies under the bed linens or the chair pad. The reduced pressure that results as the patient gets out of bed triggers an alarm at the nurses' station. One such system consists of a lightweight plastic sensor sheet and a control unit. The system adapts to both bed and chair, and setting it up according to the manufacturer's directions prevents false alarms. An alternative alarm device can be worn by the patient just above the knee. The alarm sounds when the patient moves his leg to a vertical position.
- *To promote patient safety,* add an appropriate notation (such as "Risk for falls") to the Kardex and chart.
- Provide emotional support, whether you're managing a fall or preventing one. Let the elderly patient know that you recognize his limitations and acknowledge his fears. Point out measures that you'll take to provide a safe environment.
- Teach the patient how to fall safely. Show him how to protect his hands and face. If he uses a walker or a wheelchair, demonstrate how to cope with and recover from a fall. Instruct him to survey the room for a low, sturdy, supportive piece of furniture (such as a coffee table). Then review the proper procedure for lifting himself off the floor and either standing up with the walker or getting into the wheelchair.

Home care

- Before discharge, teach the patient and his family how to prevent accidental falls at home by correcting common household hazards. Encourage them to take steps to ensure safety. (See *Promoting safety in the home,* page 68.) As needed, refer the patient to the local visiting nurse association so that nursing services can continue after discharge and during convalescence.

Documentation

After a fall, complete a detailed incident report *to help track frequent patient falls so that prevention measures can be used with high-risk patients.* Primarily for your facility's insurance carrier, this report isn't considered part of the patient's record. A copy, however, will go to the facility's administrator, who will evaluate care given on the unit and propose new safety policies as appropriate. It may also go to other patient care teams, such as fall prevention teams.

The incident report should note where and when the fall occurred, how the patient was found, and in what position. Include the events preceding the fall, the names of witnesses, the patient's reaction to the fall, and a detailed description of his condition based on assessment findings. The patient's statement of the event is also included. Note any interventions taken and the names of other staff members who helped care for him after the fall. Record the practitioner's name, and the date and time that he was notified as well as the patient's power of attorney's name and the date and time notified. Include a copy of the practitioner's report. Note too whether the patient was sent for diagnostic tests or transferred to another unit.

HOME CARE

Promoting safety in the home

Before your patient leaves the health care facility, provide him with the following tips for ensuring a safe home environment:

- Secure all carpets and floor coverings around the edges, and tack down worn spots. Never use lightweight, loose mats or rugs on bare floors.
- Make sure potential hazards such as stairs are well lighted. White paint on either side of a staircase can enhance visibility.
- Install strong banisters along all indoor and outdoor steps.
- Use a bedside lamp or low-wattage nightlight in the bedroom *to avoid having to grope in the dark when getting out of bed.*
- Fit secure handrails in convenient places in the shower, bathtub, and toilet. Use nonskid mats inside and alongside every tub or shower.
- Minimize clutter. Store children's toys, especially those on wheels, when not in use.
- Walk carefully if a pet, such as a dog or a cat, is present.
- Secure wires from electrical appliances to walls or moldings.
- Store frequently used clothing and other items in places where they can be reached without standing on a stool or chair.
- Reduce the risk of accidental slips and falls by selecting well-fitting shoes with nonskid soles, by avoiding long robes, and by wearing glasses if needed.
- Sit on the edge of a bed or chair for a few minutes before rising.
- Use a walking stick, cane, or walker whenever an unsteady feeling arises—but always inspect the condition of assistive devices before use.

Include all of the information about the fall in the patient's record. Also, document his vital signs. If you're monitoring the patient for a severe complication, record this as well.

SELECTED REFERENCES

A Guide to Bed Safety: Bed Rails in Hospitals, Nursing Homes, and Home Health Care: The Facts. U.S. Food and Drug Administration, March 25, 2005. Available at *www.fda.gov/cdrh/beds/.*

American Geriatrics Society, British Geriatrics Society, and American Academy of Orthopaedic Surgeons Panel on Falls Prevention. "Guidelines for the Prevention of Falls in Older Persons," *Journal of the American Geriatrics Society* 29(5):664-72, May 2001.

Currie, L.M. "Fall and Injury Prevention," *Annual Review of Nursing Research* 24:39-74, 2006.

Ganz, D.A. "Will My Patient Fall?" *Journal of the American Medical Association* 297(1):77-86, January 2007.

The Joint Commission. "National Patient Safety Goals," 2005. Available at *www.jointcommission.org.*

Lyons, S.S. "Evidence-Based Protocol: Fall Prevention for Older Adults," *Journal of Gerontological Nursing* 31(11):9-14, November 2005.

National Center for Injury Prevention and Control: US. Fall Prevention Program for Seniors. Available at *www.cdc.gov/ncipc/falls/default.htm.*

ALIGNMENT AND PRESSURE-REDUCING DEVICES

Various assistive devices can be used to maintain correct body positioning and to help prevent complications that commonly arise when a patient must be on prolonged bed rest. These devices include cradle boots to protect the heels and help prevent skin breakdown and footdrop; abduction pillows to help prevent internal hip rotation after femoral fracture, hip fracture, or surgery; trochanter rolls to help prevent external hip rotation; and hand rolls to help prevent hand contractures.

Several of these devices—cradle boots, trochanter rolls, and hand rolls—are especially useful when caring for patients who have a loss of sensation, mobility, or consciousness.

Equipment

Cradle boots or substitute ▪ abduction pillow ▪ trochanter rolls ▪ hand rolls. (See *Common preventive devices.*)

Cradle boots, made of sponge rubber with heel cutouts, cushion the ankle and foot without completely enclosing it. Other commercial boots are available, but not all help to prevent external hip rotation. Footboards with antirotation blocks help prevent footdrop and external hip rotation but don't prevent heel pressure. High-topped sneakers may be used to help prevent footdrop, but they don't prevent external hip rotation or heel pressure.

The abduction pillow is a wedge-shaped piece of sponge rubber with lateral indentations for the patient's thighs. Its straps wrap around the thighs to maintain correct positioning. Although a properly shaped bed pillow may temporarily substitute for the commercial abduction pillow, it's dif-

EQUIPMENT

Common preventive devices

Equipment is available to reduce pressure or help maintain positioning, depending upon the patient's needs.

Cradle boot
Prevents footdrop, skin breakdown, and external hip rotation

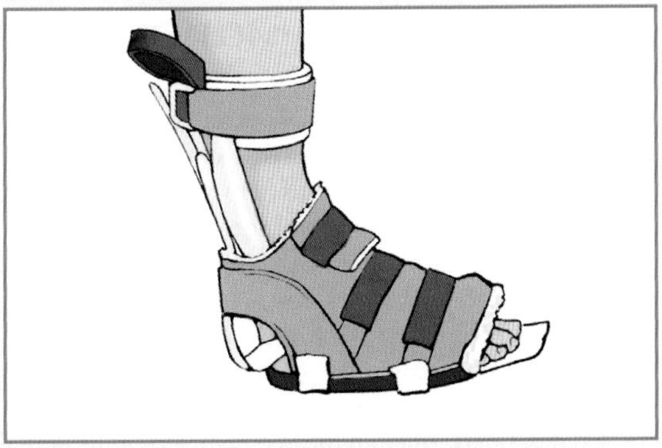

Trochanter roll
Prevents external hip rotation

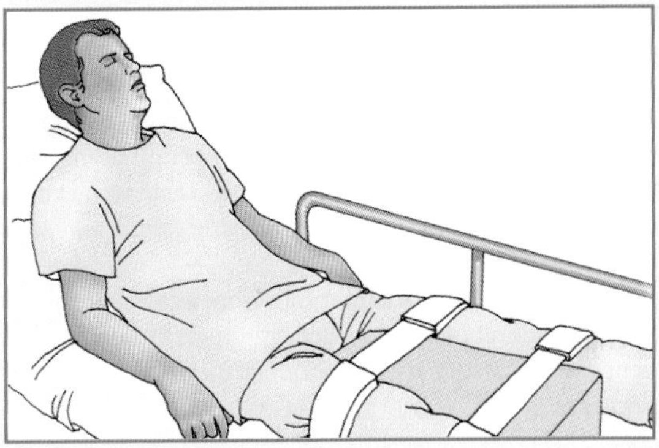

Abduction pillow
Prevents internal hip rotation and hip abduction

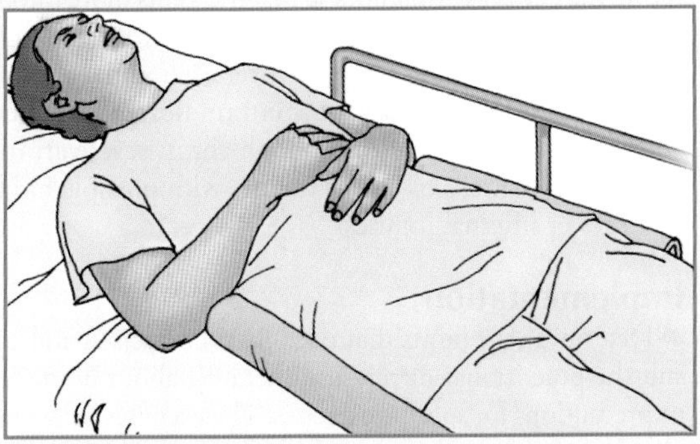

Hand roll
Prevents hand contractures

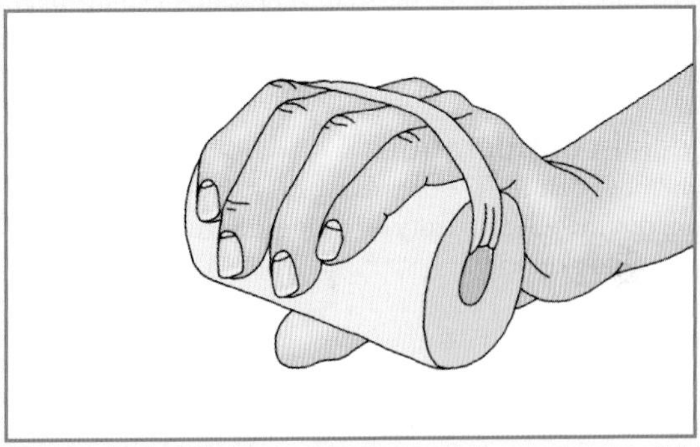

ficult to apply and fails to maintain the correct lateral alignment.

The commercial trochanter roll is made of sponge rubber, but you can also improvise one from a rolled blanket or towel. The hand roll, available in hard and soft materials, is held in place by fixed or adjustable straps. It can be improvised from a rolled washcloth secured with roller gauze and adhesive tape.

Preparation of equipment
If you're using a device that's available in different sizes, select the appropriate size for the patient.

Implementation
- Confirm the patient's identity using two patient identifiers according to your facility's policy.
- Explain the purpose and steps of the procedure to the patient.

Applying a cradle boot
- Open the slit on the superior surface of the boot. Then place the patient's heel in the circular cutout area. If the patient is positioned laterally, you may apply the boot only to the bottom foot and support the flexed top foot with a pillow.
- If appropriate, insert the other foot in the second boot.

■ Position the patient's legs in alignment *to prevent strain on hip ligaments and pressure on bony prominences.*

Applying an abduction pillow

■ Place the patient in a supine position, and put the pillow between his legs. Slide it toward the groin so that it touches his legs all along its length.
■ Place the upper part of both legs in the pillow's lateral indentations, and secure the straps *to prevent the pillow from slipping.*

Applying a trochanter roll

■ Position one roll along the outside of the thigh, from the iliac crest to midthigh. Then place another roll along the other thigh. Make sure neither roll extends as far as the knee *to avoid peroneal nerve compression and palsy, which can lead to footdrop.*
■ If you've fashioned trochanter rolls from a towel or rolled sheet, leave several inches unrolled, and tuck this under the patient's thigh *to hold the device in place and maintain the patient's position.*

Applying a hand roll

■ Place one roll in the patient's hand to maintain the neutral position. Then secure the strap, if present, or apply roller gauze and secure with hypoallergenic or adhesive tape.
■ Place another roll in the other hand.

Special considerations

Remember that the use of assistive devices doesn't preclude regularly scheduled patient positioning, range-of-motion exercises, and skin care.

Home care

Explain the use of appropriate devices to the patient and caregiver. Demonstrate how to use each device, emphasizing proper alignment of extremities, and have the patient or caregiver give a return demonstration *so you can check for proper technique.* Emphasize measures needed to prevent pressure ulcers.

Complications

Contractures and pressure ulcers may occur with the use of a hand roll and possibly with other assistive devices. *To avoid these problems,* remove hand rolls every 2 hours.

Documentation

Record the use of these devices in the patient's chart and the nursing care plan, include the reason for the device, and indicate assessment for complications. Document any patient teaching performed and the patient's understanding. Reevaluate your patient care goals as needed.

Selected references

Baranoski, S., and Ayello, E. *Wound Care Essentials Practice and Principles,* 2nd ed. Philadelphia: Lippincott Williams & Wilkins, 2008.

Jones, J. "Evaluation of Pressure Ulcer Prevention Devices: A Critical Review of the Literature," *Journal of Wound Care* 14(9):422-25, October 2005.

National Pressure Ulcer Advisory Panel: *www.npuap.org.*

Passive range-of-motion exercises

Used to move the patient's joints through as full a range of motion (ROM) as possible, passive ROM exercises improve or maintain joint mobility and help prevent contractures. Performed by a nurse, a physical therapist, or a caregiver of the patient's choosing, these exercises are indicated for the patient with temporary or permanent loss of mobility, sensation, or consciousness. Performed properly, passive ROM exercises require recognition of the patient's limits of motion and support of all joints during movement.

Exercises performed in the bed help with joint mobility, strength, and endurance, and they prepare the patient for ambulating. During passive ROM exercises, another person moves the patient's extremities so that the joints move through a complete range of movement, maximally stretching all muscle groups within each plane over each joint.

Passive ROM exercises are contraindicated in patients with septic joints, acute thrombophlebitis, severe arthritic joint inflammation, or recent trauma with possible hidden fractures or internal injuries.

Implementation

■ Determine the joints that need ROM exercises, and consult the practitioner or physical therapist about limitations or precautions for specific exercises. The exercises below treat all joints, but they don't have to be performed in the order given or all at once. You can schedule them over the course of a day, whenever the patient is in the most convenient position. Remember to perform all exercises slowly, gently, and to the end of the normal ROM or to the point of pain, but no further. Hold this position for 1 to 2 seconds, then slowly release. (See *Glossary of joint movements.*)
■ Confirm the patient's identity using two patient identifiers according to your facility's policy.
■ Before you begin, raise the bed to a comfortable working height, and provide privacy for the patient.

Exercising the neck

■ Support the patient's head with your hands, and extend the neck, flex the chin to the chest, and tilt the head laterally toward each shoulder.

Glossary of joint movements

Joints should be exercised to the point of discomfort, but not pain. Joints should also be moved in the intended direction of function, holding the position for a few seconds, and then returning to the rest position.

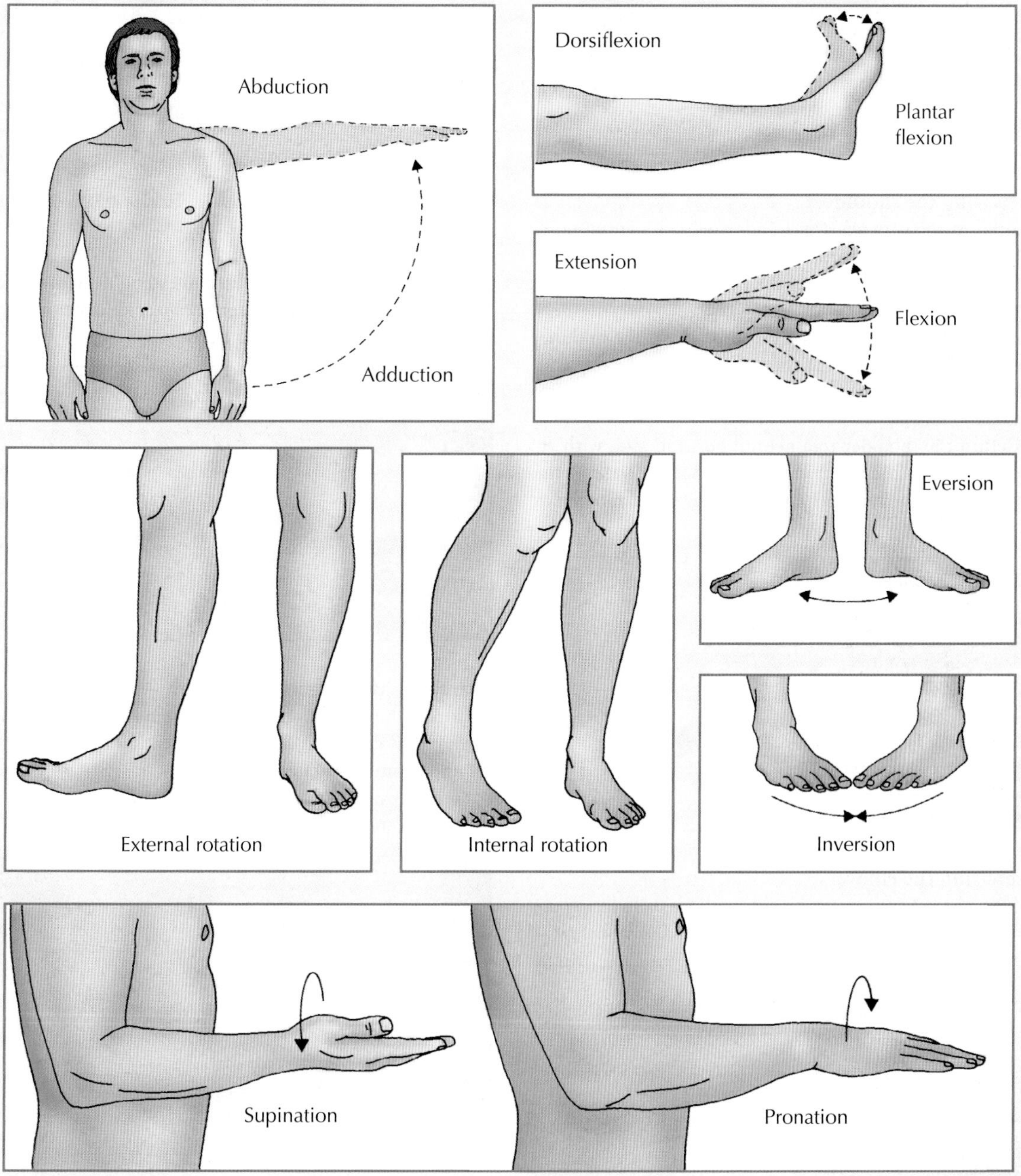

■ Rotate the head from right to left as shown below.

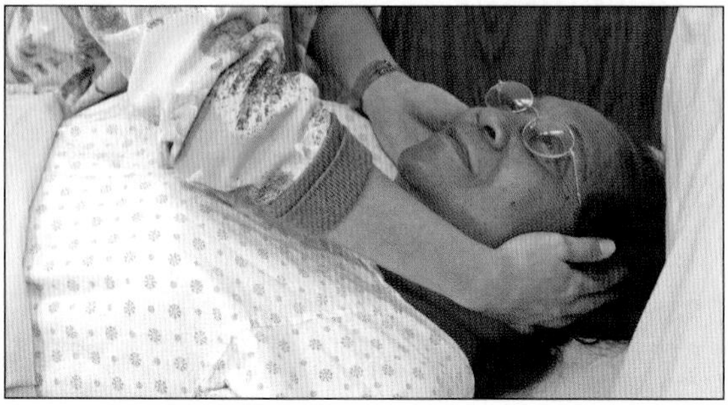

Exercising the shoulders

■ Support the patient's arm in an extended, neutral position; then extend the forearm, and flex it back. Abduct the arm outward from the side of the body, and adduct it back to the side.

■ Rotate the shoulder so that the arm crosses the midline, and bend the elbow so that the hand touches the opposite shoulder, then touches the mattress of the bed *for complete internal rotation.*

■ Return the shoulder to a neutral position and, with elbow bent, push the arm backward so that the back of the hand touches the mattress *for complete external rotation* as shown below.

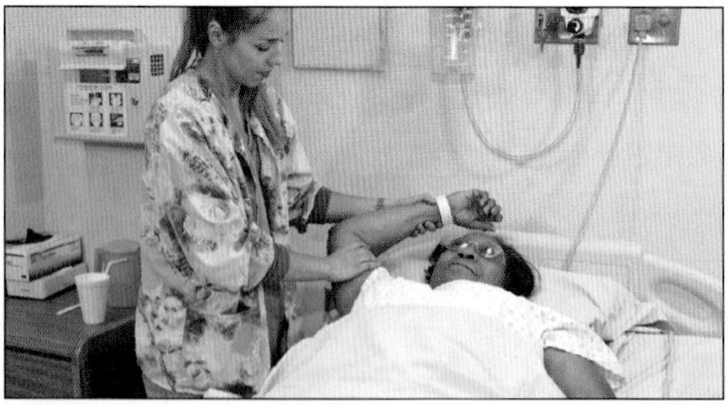

Exercising the elbow

■ Place the patient's arm at his side with his palm facing up.

■ Flex and extend the arm at the elbow as shown below.

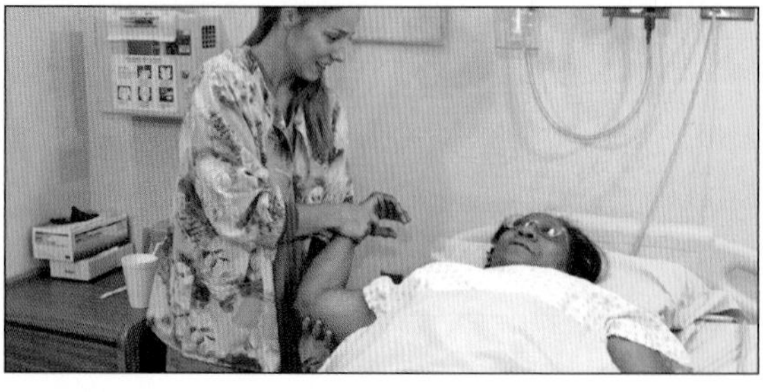

Exercising the forearm

■ Stabilize the patient's elbow, and then twist the hand to bring the palm up (supination) as shown below.

■ Twist it back again to bring the palm down (pronation).

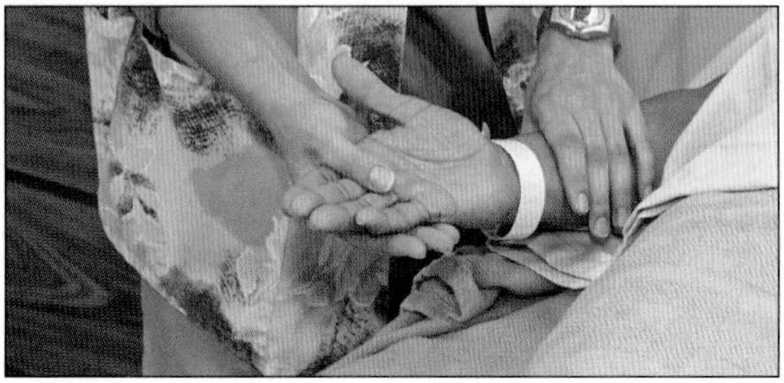

Exercising the wrist

■ Stabilize the forearm, and flex and extend the wrist. Then rock the hand sideways *for lateral flexion,* and rotate the hand in a circular motion as shown below.

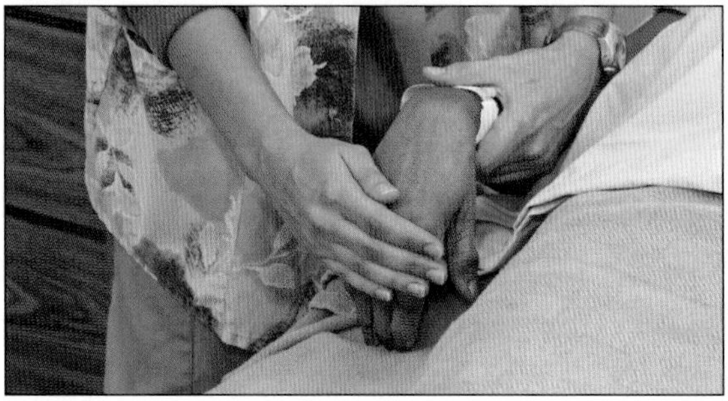

Exercising the fingers and thumb

■ Extend the patient's fingers, and then flex the hand into a fist; repeat extension and flexion of each joint of each finger and thumb separately.

■ Spread two adjoining fingers apart (abduction) as shown below, and then bring them together (adduction).

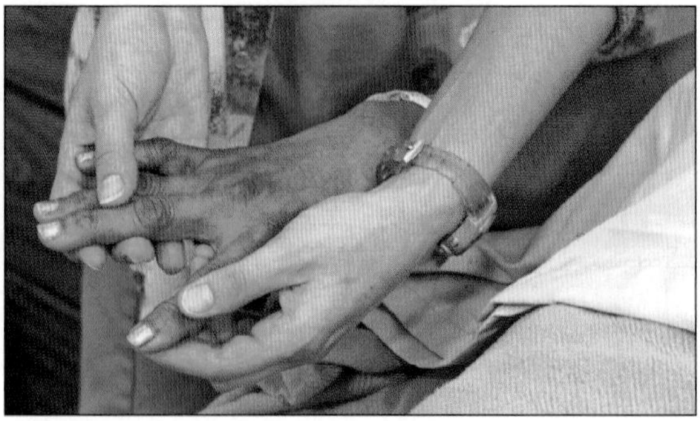

■ Oppose each fingertip to the thumb, and rotate the thumb and each finger in a circle.

Exercising the hip and knee

- Fully extend the patient's leg, bend the hip and knee toward the chest, allowing full joint flexion, and then return to the extended position.
- Next, move the straight leg sideways, out and away from the other leg (abduction), and then back, over, and across it (adduction).
- Rotate the straight leg internally toward the midline, and then externally away from the midline as shown below.

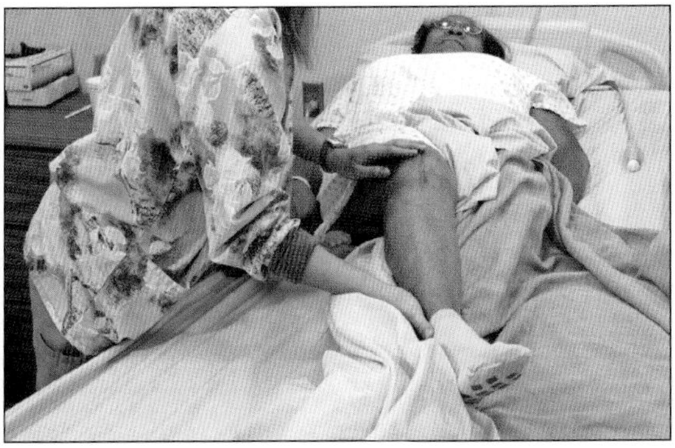

Exercising the ankle

- Bend the patient's foot so that the toes push upward (dorsiflexion), and then bend the foot so that the toes push downward (plantar flexion).
- Rotate the ankle in a circular motion.
- Invert the ankle so that the sole of the foot faces the midline as shown below, and then evert the ankle so that the sole faces away from the midline.

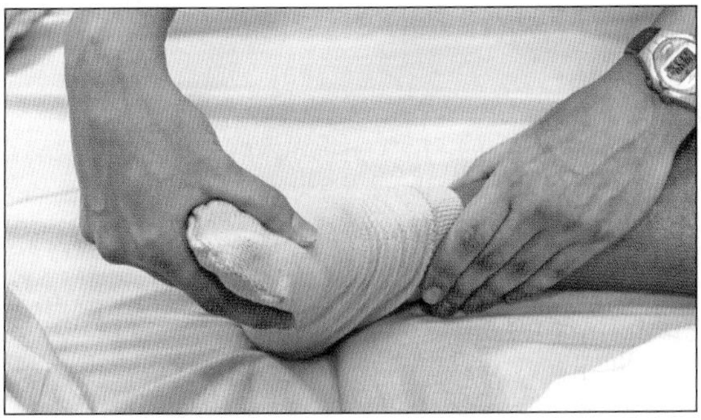

Exercising the toes

- Flex the patient's toes toward the sole, and then extend them back toward the top of the foot.
- Spread two adjoining toes apart (abduction) as shown top of next column, and then bring them together (adduction).

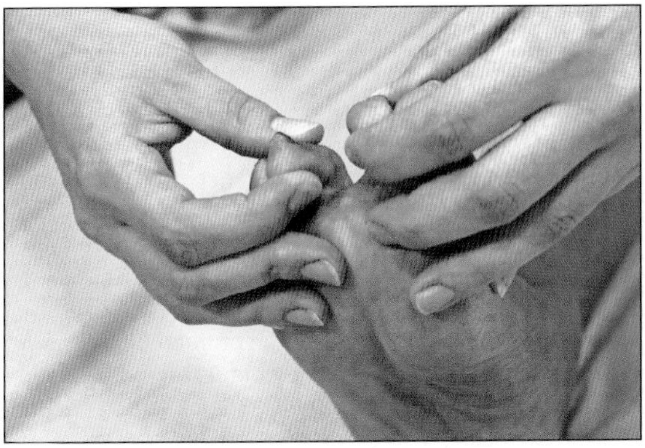

Special considerations

- *Because joints begin to stiffen within 24 hours of disuse,* start passive ROM exercises as soon as possible, and perform them at least every 4 hours. Passive ROM exercises can be performed while bathing or turning the patient. Use proper body mechanics, and repeat each exercise at least three times.
- Patients who experience prolonged bed rest or limited activity without profound weakness can be taught to perform ROM exercises on their own (called active ROM), or they may benefit from isometric exercises. (See *Learning about isometric exercises,* page 74.)
- If a disabled patient requires long-term rehabilitation after discharge, consult with a physical therapist and teach a family member or caregiver to perform passive ROM exercises.

Documentation

Record which joints were exercised, the presence of edema or pressure areas, any pain resulting from the exercises, any limitation of ROM, and the patient's tolerance of the exercises.

SELECTED REFERENCES

Craven, R.F., and Hirnle, C.J. *Fundamentals of Nursing: Human Health and Function*, 5th ed. Philadelphia: Lippincott Williams & Wilkins, 2006.

"Performing Passive Range-of-Motion Exercises," *Nursing* 36(3):50-51, March 2006.

Winkleman, C., et al. "Activity in the Chronically Critically Ill," *Dimensions in Critical Care Nursing* 24(6):281-90, November-December 2005.

PROGRESSIVE AMBULATION

After surgery or a period of bed rest, patients must begin the gradual return to full ambulation. When it's begun promptly and properly, this process—called progressive ambula-

Learning about isometric exercises

Patients can strengthen and increase muscle tone by contracting muscles against resistance (from other muscles or from a stationary object, such as a bed or a wall) without joint movement. These exercises require only a comfortable position—standing, sitting, or lying down—and proper body alignment. For each exercise, instruct the patient to hold each contraction for 2 to 5 seconds and to repeat it three or four times daily, below peak contraction level for the first week and at peak level thereafter.

Neck rotators
The patient places the heel of his hand above one ear. Then he pushes his head toward the hand as forcefully as possible, without moving the head, neck, or arm. He repeats the exercise on the other side.

Neck flexors
The patient places both palms on his forehead. Without moving his neck, he pushes the head forward while resisting with the palms.

Neck extensors
The patient clasps his fingers behind his head and then pushes the head against the clasped hands without moving his neck.

Shoulder elevators
Holding the right arm straight down at the side, the patient grasps his right wrist with his left hand. He then tries to shrug his right shoulder, but prevents it from moving by holding his arm in place. He repeats this exercise, alternating arms.

Shoulder, chest, and scapular musculature
The patient places his right fist in his left palm and raises both arms to shoulder height. He pushes the fist into the palm as forcefully as possible without moving either arm. Then, with his arms in the same position, he clasps the fingers and tries to pull the hands apart. He repeats the pattern, beginning with the left fist in the right palm.

Elbow flexors and extensors
With his right elbow bent 90 degrees and his right palm facing upward, the patient places his left fist against his right palm. He tries to bend the right elbow further while resisting with the left fist. He repeats the pattern, bending the left elbow.

Abdomen
The patient assumes a sitting position and bends slightly forward, with his hands in front of the middle of his thighs. He tries to bend forward further, resisting by pressing the palms against the thighs.

Alternatively, in the supine position, he clasps his hands behind his head. Then he raises his shoulders about 1" (2.5 cm), holding this position for a few seconds.

Back extensors
In a sitting position, the patient bends forward and places his hands under his buttocks. He tries to stand up, resisting with both hands.

Hip abductors
While standing, the patient squeezes his inner thighs together as tightly as possible. Placing a pillow between the knees supplies resistance and increases the effectiveness of this exercise.

Hip extensors
The patient squeezes his buttocks together as tightly as possible.

Knee extensors
The patient straightens his knee fully. Then he vigorously tightens the muscle above the knee so that it moves the kneecap upward. He repeats this exercise, alternating legs.

Ankle flexors and extensors
The patient pulls his toes upward, holding briefly. Then he pushes them down as far as possible, again holding briefly.

tion—thwarts many of the complications of prolonged inactivity.

Complications prevented by early progressive ambulation include respiratory stasis and hypostatic pneumonia; circulatory stasis, thrombophlebitis, and emboli; urine retention, urinary tract infection, urinary stasis, and calculus formation; abdominal distention, constipation, and decreased appetite; and sensory deprivation. Progressive ambulation also helps restore the patient's sense of equilibrium and enhances his self-confidence and self-image.

Progressive ambulation begins with dangling the patient's feet over the edge of the bed and progresses to seating him in an armchair or wheelchair, walking around the room with him, and then walking with him in the halls until he can walk by himself. The patient's progress depends on his physical condition and his tolerance. Successful return to full ambulation requires correct body mechanics, careful patient observation, and open communication among the patient, practitioner, and nurse.

Equipment

Robe ■ chair or wheelchair ■ slippers for sitting; hard-soled shoes for walking ■ assistive device (cane, crutches, walker) if necessary.

Implementation

■ If the patient requires an assistive device, the physical therapist usually selects the appropriate one and teaches its use.
■ Check the patient's history, diagnosis, and therapeutic regimen. Ask him whether he's in pain or feels weak; if necessary, give an analgesic and wait 30 to 60 minutes for it to take effect before trying ambulation. Remember that a medicated patient may develop hypotension, dizziness, or drowsiness.
■ Explain the goal of ambulation. (See *Helping the patient regain mobility.*) Provide encouragement *because he may be hesitant or fearful;* reassure him that he need not attempt more than he can reasonably do. If he fears pain in an incision, show him how to support it by placing a hand alongside or gently over the dressing site, or splint the incision for him.
■ Remove equipment or other objects *to provide a clear path and prevent falls.*
■ Lock the wheels on the bed or chair, if appropriate.

Dangling the patient's legs

■ Position the bed horizontally and the patient laterally, facing you. Move his legs over the side of the bed, and grasp his shoulders, standing with your feet apart *so you have a wide base of support.* Ask him to help by pushing up from the bed with his arms. Then shift your weight from the foot closest to his head to the other foot as you steadily raise him to the sitting position. Pull with your whole body, not just your arms, *to avoid straining your back and jostling the patient.*

Alternatively, you can raise the head of the bed to a 45-degree angle *to allow easier elevation of the patient.* Don't use this method if the patient has trouble balancing himself while sitting. Ask a coworker for assistance whenever necessary.
■ While the patient adjusts to an upright position, continue to stand facing him *to keep him from falling,* and observe him closely. Be alert for signs and symptoms of orthostatic

Helping the patient regain mobility

Dangling legs

To help the patient support himself in a dangling position, move an overbed table in front of him and place a pillow on it.

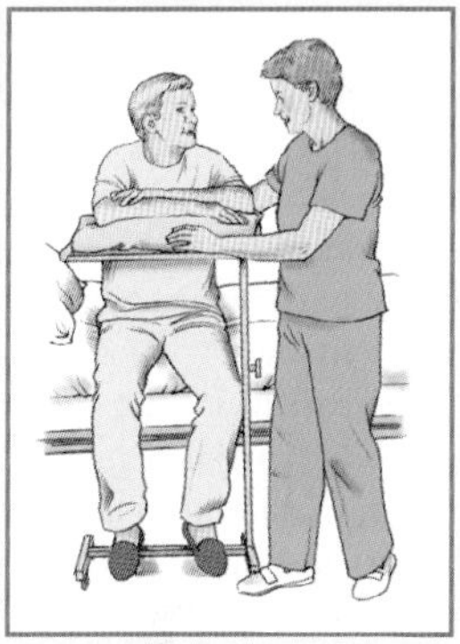

Sitting

Seat the patient in a chair with armrests and a straight back, with his lower back against the rear of the chair, feet flat on the floor, hips and knees at right angles, and upper body straight. Rest his forearms on the armrests.

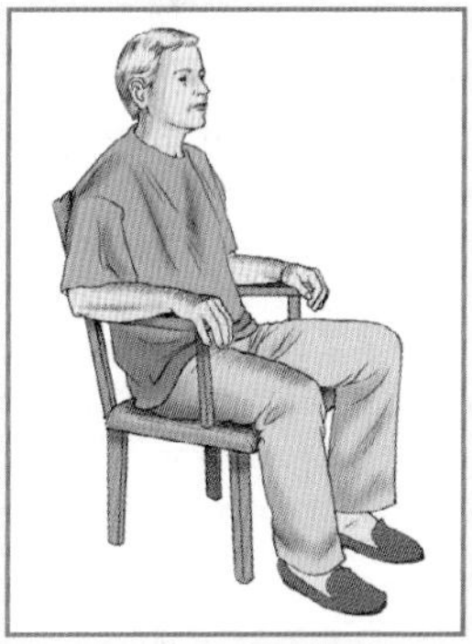

Walking

Provide a path unimpeded by equipment and other objects, and avoid overexertion. If necessary, hold the patient so you can control his upper and lower body and any lateral movements.

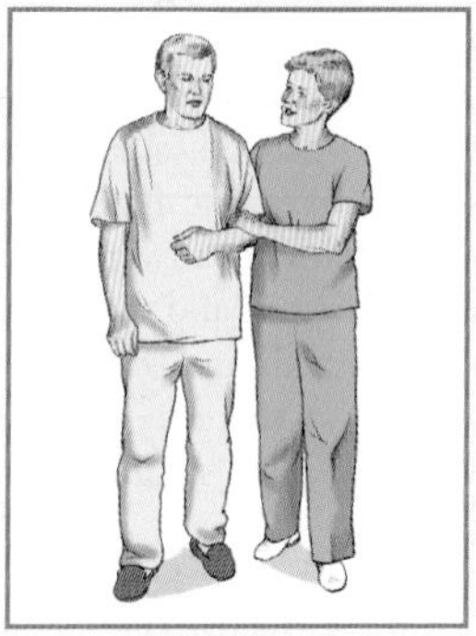

hypotension, such as fainting, dizziness, and complaints of blurred vision. If desired, check the patient's pulse rate and blood pressure. If the pulse rate increases more than 20 beats per minute, allow the patient to rest before progressing slowly.

Helping the patient stand

- After the patient can dangle his legs and support his weight on them, have him attempt the standing position. Help him put on a robe and nonskid slippers or shoes.
- If you plan to use a walking belt, apply it now. Don't allow a robe, a drainage tube, or anything else to dangle around the patient's feet.
- If the patient is alert and fairly strong, place his feet flat on the floor, and allow him to stand by himself. As he stands, place one hand under his axilla and the other hand around his waist *to prevent falls.* Help him stand fully erect. Encourage him to look forward and not at the floor *to help maintain his balance.*
- If the patient needs help standing up, face him and position your knees at either side of his. Bend your knees, put your arms around his waist, and instruct him to push up from the bed with his arms. Then straighten your knees, and pull the patient with you while rising to an erect position. *This technique helps you avoid back strain.*

Helping the patient sit or walk

- After the patient stands, you can pivot and lower him into an armchair or wheelchair, or you can begin to walk with him.
- If you've decided to seat him, make sure the chair is secure and won't slip as you lower the patient into it. Place his lower back against the rear of the chair and his feet flat on the floor. Position his hips and knees at right angles, and keep his upper body straight. Then flex his elbows, and place his forearms on the arms of the chair.
- If the patient can walk safely only with your assistance, stand to the side and slightly behind him, placing one hand under his axilla and the other hand around his waist. If the patient has weakness or paralysis on one side, stand on the affected side and stabilize him by putting one arm around his waist.
- If necessary, ask a coworker to help you. Stand on opposite sides of the patient, and place one hand under his arm or on his elbow, or grasp the walking belt.
- Give the patient verbal and tactile cues *to encourage him.* Stay close to a railed wall or another supportive structure and, if necessary, allow the patient to rest in a chair before attempting to walk back to his room. If he can't walk back, tell him to remain seated while you summon assistance or obtain a wheelchair. Don't leave the patient unattended if you have any reason to think he may fall. If you can't find a chair nearby, have the patient lean against the wall, and call for assistance as you help support him. If necessary, steady him as he slides down the wall to sit on the floor.

Special considerations

- Patients on medications such as beta-adrenergic blockers and vasodilators may be subject to episodes of bradycardia and hypotension.
- If early ambulation is impossible, encourage bed exercises. Don't let the use of catheters and infusion containers discourage ambulation; secure these devices so they're easily portable, and check dressings and tubes carefully afterward for proper position and changes in drainage. If appropriate, measure pulse, respiratory rate, and blood pressure. When leaving the patient sitting up in a chair, make certain that he has a call bell or signal device.
- If the patient begins to fall, try to break his fall by easing him to the bed, chair, or floor, making sure that he doesn't strike his head. Then summon help. Don't leave the patient alone—he needs your comfort and reassurance.
- If the patient experiences dyspnea, diaphoresis, or orthostatic hypotension, stabilize his position and take his vital signs. Place him in semi-Fowler's position *to facilitate breathing.* If his condition doesn't improve rapidly, notify the practitioner.

Documentation

Record the type of transfer and assistance needed; the duration of sitting, standing, or walking; the distance walked, if appropriate; the patient's response to ambulation; and any significant changes in blood pressure, pulse, and respiration.

SELECTED REFERENCES

Autar, R. "Evidence for the Prevention of Venous Thromboembolism," *British Journal of Nursing* 15(18):980-86, October 2006.

Kehl-Pruett, W. "Deep Vein Thrombosis in Hospitalized Patients: A Review of Evidence-Based Guidelines for Prevention," *American Journal of Nursing* 25(2):53-59, March-April 2006.

Killey, B., and Watt, E. "The Effect of Extra Walking on the Mobility, Independence and Exercise Self-Efficacy of Elderly Hospital In-Patients: A Pilot Study," *Contemporary Nursing* 22(1):120-33, July 2006.

TILT TABLE

The tilt table, a padded table or bedlength board that can be raised gradually from a horizontal to a vertical position, can help prevent the complications of prolonged bed rest.

Used for the patient with a spinal cord injury, brain damage, orthostatic hypotension, or any other condition that prevents free standing, the tilt table increases tolerance of the upright position, conditions the cardiovascular system, stretches muscles, and helps prevent contractures, bone demineralization, and urinary calculus formation. This procedure is performed once or twice per day, depending on the patient's tolerance.

Equipment

Tilt table with footboard and restraining straps ■ sphygmomanometer ■ stethoscope ■ antiembolism stockings or elastic bandages ■ optional: abdominal binder, wooden block.

Preparation of equipment

Common types of tilt tables include the electric table, which moves at a slow, steady rate; the manual table, which is raised by a handle; and the spring assisted table, which is raised by a pedal. Familiarize yourself with operating instructions for the model you'll be using.

Implementation

■ Explain the use and benefits of the tilt table to the patient or his family.
■ Apply antiembolism stockings *to restrict vessel walls and help prevent blood pooling and edema.* If necessary, apply an abdominal binder *to avoid pooling of blood in the splanchnic region, which contributes to insufficient cerebral circulation and orthostatic hypotension.*
■ Make sure the tilt table is locked in the horizontal position. Then summon assistance and transfer the patient to the table, placing him in the supine position with his feet flat against the footboard.
■ If the patient can't bear weight on one leg, place a wooden block between the footboard and the weight-bearing foot, permitting the non-weight-bearing leg to dangle freely.
■ Fasten the safety straps, then take the patient's blood pressure and pulse rate.
■ Tilt the table slowly in 15 to 30 degree increments, evaluating the patient constantly. Take his blood pressure every 3 to 5 minutes *because movement from the supine to the upright position decreases systolic pressure.* Be alert for signs and symptoms of insufficient cerebral circulation, including dizziness, nausea, pallor, diaphoresis, tachycardia, or a change in mental status. If the patient experiences any of these signs or symptoms, or hypotension or seizures, return the table immediately to the horizontal position.
■ If the patient tolerates the position shift, continue to tilt the table until reaching the desired angle, usually between 45 degrees and 80 degrees. A 60 degree tilt gives the patient the physiologic effects and sensations of standing upright.
■ Gradually return the patient to the horizontal position, and check his vital signs. Then obtain assistance, and transfer the patient onto the stretcher for transport back to his room.

Special considerations

Let the patient's response determine the angle of tilt and duration of elevation, but avoid prolonged upright positioning (greater than 45 minutes) *because it may lead to venous stasis.*

NURSING ALERT ***Never leave the patient unattended on the tilt table*** **because marked physiologic changes, such as hypotension or severe headache, can occur suddenly.**

Complications

Use of a tilt table can lead to sudden hypotension, severe headache, and other dramatic physiologic changes.

Documentation

Record the angle and duration of elevation; changes in the patient's pulse rate, blood pressure, and physical and mental status; and his response to treatment.

SELECTED REFERENCES

Chang, A.T., et al. "Standing with the Assistance of a Tilt Table Improves Minute Ventilation in Chronic Critically Ill Patients," *Archives of Physical Medicine and Rehabilitation* 85(12):1972-76, December 2004.
Claydon, V.E., and Hayworth, R. "Postural Sway in Patients with Syncope and Poor Orthostatic Tolerance," *Heart* 92(11):1688-89, November 2006.

CANES

Indicated for the patient with one-sided weakness or injury, occasional loss of balance, or increased joint pressure, a cane provides balance and support for walking and reduces fatigue and strain on weight-bearing joints. Available in various sizes, the cane should extend from the greater trochanter to the floor and have a rubber tip to prevent slipping. Canes are contraindicated for the patient with bilateral weakness; such a patient should use crutches or a walker.

Equipment

Rubber-tipped cane ■ optional: walking belt.

Although wooden canes are available, three types of aluminum canes are used most commonly. The standard aluminum cane (used by the patient who needs only slight assistance with walking) provides the least support; its half-circle handle allows it to be hooked over chairs. The T-handle cane (used by the patient with hand weakness) has a straight-shaped handle with grips and a bent shaft. It provides greater stability than the standard cane. Three- or four-pronged (quad) canes are used by the patient with poor balance or one-sided weakness and an inability to hold onto a walker with both hands. The base of these types of canes splits into three or four short, splayed legs and provides greater stability than a standard cane, but considerably less than a walker.

Preparation of equipment

Ask the patient to hold the cane on the uninvolved side 6″ (15.2 cm) from the base of the little toe. If the cane is made of aluminum, adjust its height by pushing in the metal button on the shaft and raising or lowering the shaft; if it's wood, the rubber tip can be removed and excess length sawed off. At the correct height, the handle of the cane is level with the greater trochanter and allows approximately 30-degree flexion at the elbow. If the cane is too short, the patient will have to drop his shoulder to lean on it; if it's too long, he'll have to raise his shoulder and will have difficulty supporting his weight.

Implementation

- Explain the mechanics of cane walking to the patient. Demonstrate the technique; then have the patient return the demonstration. Coordinate practice sessions in the physical therapy department if necessary.
- Tell the patient to hold the cane on the uninvolved side *to promote a reciprocal gait pattern and to distribute weight away from the involved side.*
- Instruct the patient to hold the cane close to his body *to prevent leaning* and to move the cane forward 4″ to 8″ (10 to 20 cm) and the involved leg simultaneously, followed by the uninvolved leg.
- Encourage the patient to keep the stride length of each leg and the timing of each step (cadence) equal.

Negotiating stairs

- Instruct the patient to always use a railing, if present, when going up or down stairs. Tell him to hold the cane with the other hand or to keep it in the hand grasping the railing. To ascend stairs, the patient should lead with the uninvolved leg and follow with the involved leg; to descend, he should lead with the involved leg and follow with the uninvolved one. Help the patient remember by telling him to use this mnemonic device: "The good goes up; the bad goes down" (as shown top of next column)

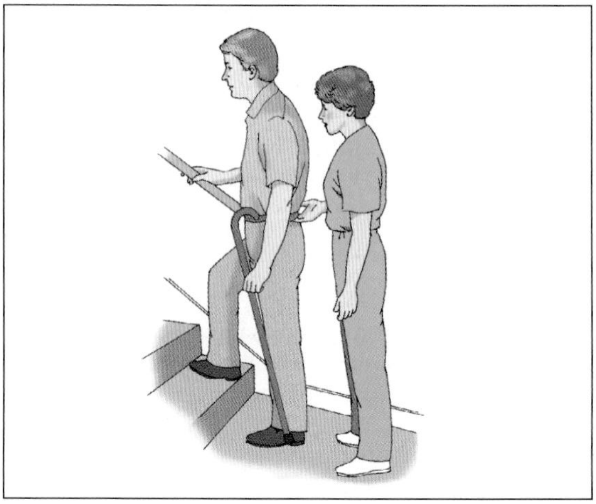

- To negotiate stairs without a railing, the patient should use the walking technique to ascend and descend the stairs, but should move the cane just before the involved leg. Thus, to ascend stairs, the patient should hold the cane on the uninvolved side, step with the uninvolved leg, advance the cane, and then move the involved leg. To descend, he should hold the cane on the uninvolved side, lead with the cane, advance the involved leg, and then, finally, move the uninvolved leg.

Using a chair

- To teach the patient to sit down, stand by his affected side, and tell him to place the backs of his legs against the edge of the chair seat. Then tell him to move the cane out from his side and to reach back with both hands to grasp the chair's armrests as shown below. Supporting his weight on the armrests, he can then lower himself onto the seat. While he's seated, he should keep the cane hooked on the armrest or the chair back.

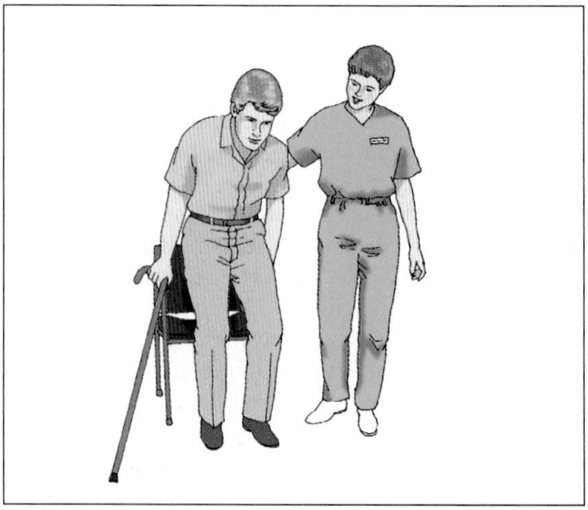

Fitting a patient for a crutch

To measure for an axilla crutch, position the crutch so that it extends from a point 4″ to 6″ (10 to 15 cm) to the side and 4″ to 6″ in front of the patient's feet to 1½″ to 2″ (4 to 5 cm) below the axillae (about the width of two fingers). Then adjust the handgrips so that the patient's elbows are flexed at a 30-degree angle when he's standing with the crutches in the resting position and the wrists at a 15-degree angle.

To fit a forearm crutch, have the patient flex his elbow so the crease in his wrist is at his hip. Then measure his forearm from 3″ (7.6 cm) below the elbow, and add the distance between his wrist and the floor.

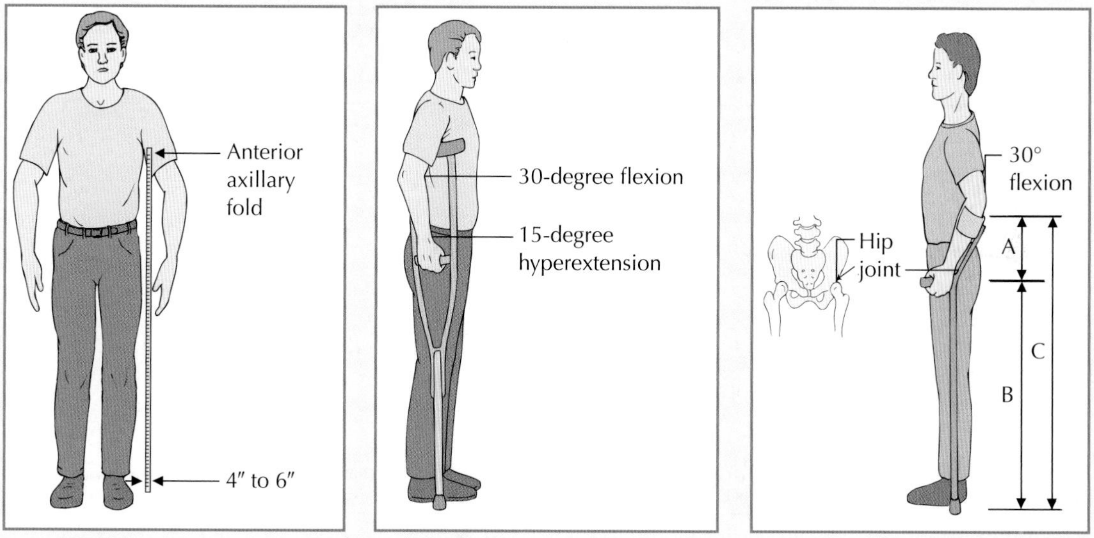

■ To teach the patient to get up, stand by his affected side, and tell him to unhook the cane from the chair and hold it in his stronger hand as he grasps the armrests. Then tell him to move his uninvolved foot slightly forward, to lean slightly forward, and to push against the armrests to raise himself upright.

■ Instruct the patient not to lean on the cane when sitting or rising from the chair *to prevent falls.*

■ Supervise the patient each time he gets in or out of a chair until you're both certain he can do it alone.

Special considerations

To prevent falls during the learning period, guard the patient carefully by standing behind him slightly to his stronger side and putting one foot between his feet and your other foot to the outside of the uninvolved leg. If necessary, use a walking belt.

Complications

A poorly fitted cane can cause the patient to lose his balance and fall.

Documentation

Record the type of cane used, the amount of guarding required, the distance walked, and the patient's understanding and tolerance of cane walking.

SELECTED REFERENCES

Bateni, H., and Maki, B.E. "Assistive Devices for Balance and Mobility: Benefits, Demands, and Adverse Consequences," *Archives of Physical Medicine and Rehabilitation* 86(1):134-45, January 2005.

Craven, R.F., and Hirnle, C.J. *Fundamentals of Nursing Human Health and Function,* 5th ed. Philadelphia: Lippincott Williams & Wilkins, 2006.

Youdas, J.W., et al. "Partial Weight-Bearing Gait Using Conventional Assistive Devices," *Archives of Physical Medicine and Rehabilitation* 86(3):394-98, March 2005.

Crutch gaits

Guide for using the 4-point, 3-point, 2-point, swing-to, and swing-through gaits. Start at the bottom and move forward. *Note:* Shaded areas indicate weight bearing.

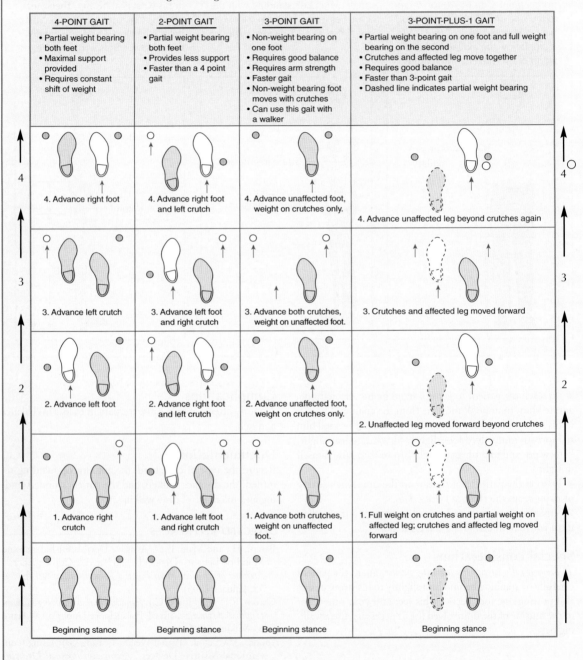

4-POINT GAIT	2-POINT GAIT	3-POINT GAIT	3-POINT-PLUS-1 GAIT
• Partial weight bearing both feet • Maximal support provided • Requires constant shift of weight	• Partial weight bearing both feet • Provides less support • Faster than a 4 point gait	• Non-weight bearing on one foot • Requires good balance • Requires arm strength • Faster gait • Non-weight bearing foot moves with crutches • Can use this gait with a walker	• Partial weight bearing on one foot and full weight bearing on the second • Crutches and affected leg move together • Requires good balance • Faster than 3-point gait • Dashed line indicates partial weight bearing
4. Advance right foot	4. Advance right foot and left crutch	4. Advance unaffected foot, weight on crutches only.	4. Advance unaffected leg beyond crutches again
3. Advance left crutch	3. Advance left foot and right crutch	3. Advance both crutches, weight on unaffected foot.	3. Crutches and affected leg moved forward
2. Advance left foot	2. Advance right foot and left crutch	2. Advance unaffected foot, weight on crutches only.	2. Unaffected leg moved forward beyond crutches
1. Advance right crutch	1. Advance left foot and right crutch	1. Advance both crutches, weight on unaffected foot.	1. Full weight on crutches and partial weight on affected leg; crutches and affected leg moved forward
Beginning stance	Beginning stance	Beginning stance	Beginning stance

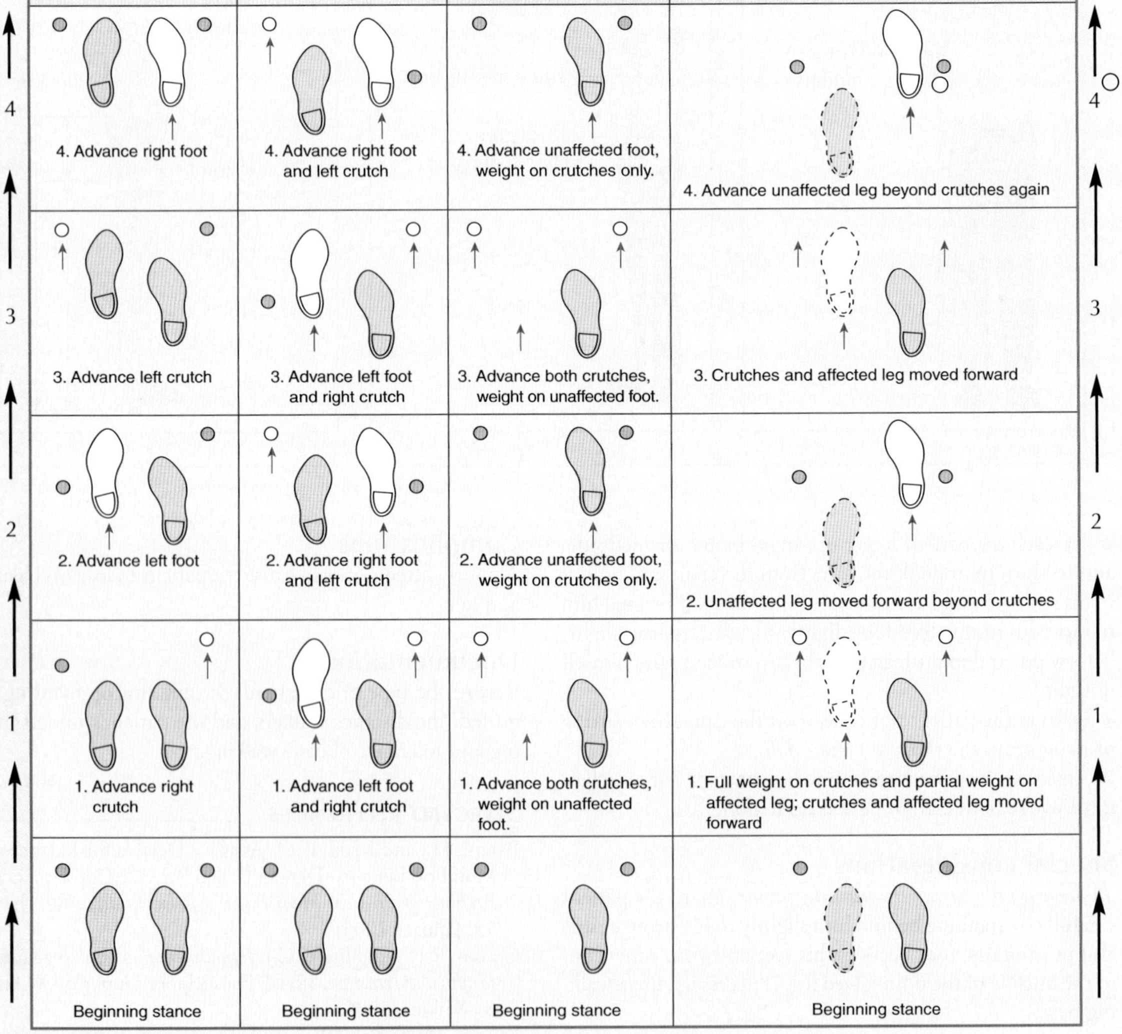

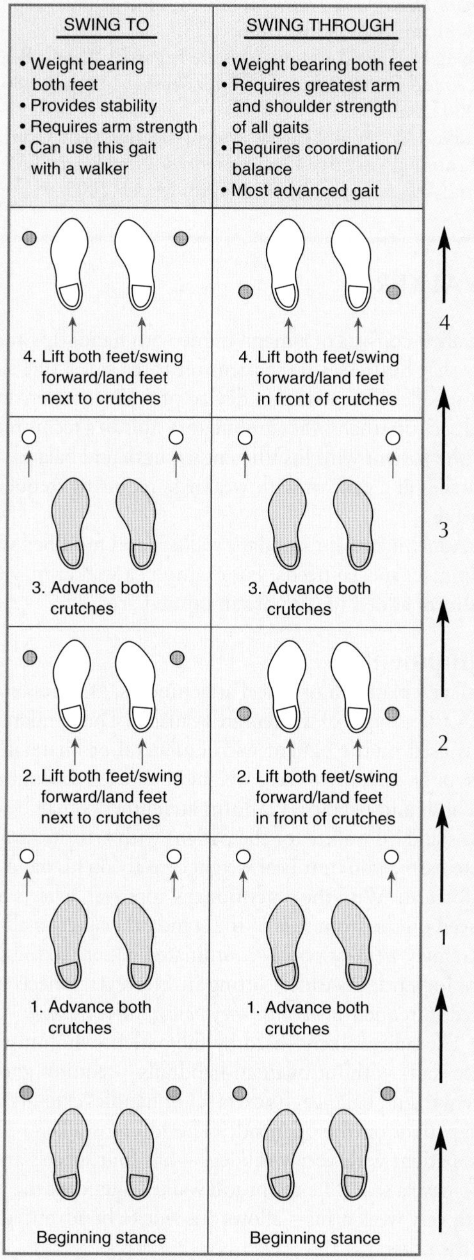
SWING TO
• Weight bearing both feet
• Provides stability
• Requires arm strength
• Can use this gait with a walker
SWING THROUGH
• Weight bearing both feet
• Requires greatest arm and shoulder strength of all gaits
• Requires coordination/ balance
• Most advanced gait
4. Lift both feet/swing forward/land feet next to crutches
4. Lift both feet/swing forward/land feet in front of crutches
4
3. Advance both crutches
3. Advance both crutches
3
2. Lift both feet/swing forward/land feet next to crutches
2. Lift both feet/swing forward/land feet in front of crutches
2
1. Advance both crutches
1. Advance both crutches
1
Beginning stance
Beginning stance

CRUTCHES

Crutches remove weight from one or both legs, enabling the patient to support himself with his hands and arms. Typically prescribed for a patient with lower-extremity injury or weakness, crutches require balance, stamina, and upper-body strength for successful use. Crutch selection and walking gait depend on the patient's condition. A patient who can't use crutches may be able to use a walker.

Equipment

Crutches with axillary pads, handgrips, and rubber suction tips ▪ optional: walking belt.

Three types of crutches are commonly used. Standard aluminum or wooden crutches are used by the patient with a sprain, strain, or cast. They require stamina and upper-body strength. Aluminum forearm crutches are used by the paraplegic or other patient using the swing-through gait. They have a collar that fits around the forearm and a horizontal handgrip that provides support. Platform crutches are used by the arthritic patient who has an upper-extremity deficit that prevents weight bearing through the wrist. They provide padded surfaces for the upper extremities.

Preparation of equipment

After choosing the appropriate crutches, adjust their height with the patient standing or, if necessary, recumbent. (See *Fitting a patient for a crutch,* page 79.)

Implementation

▪ Consult with the patient's practitioner and physical therapist *to coordinate rehabilitation orders and teaching.*

▪ Describe the gait you'll teach and the reason for your choice. Then demonstrate the gait as necessary. Have the patient give a return demonstration.

▪ Place a walking belt around the patient's waist, if necessary, *to help prevent falls.* Tell the patient to position the crutches and to shift his weight from side to side. Then place him in front of a full-length mirror *to facilitate learning and coordination.*

▪ Teach the four-point gait to the patient who can bear weight on both legs. Although this is the safest gait *because three points are always in contact with the floor,* it requires greater coordination than others *because of its constant shifting of weight.* Use this sequence: right crutch, left foot, left crutch, right foot. Suggest counting *to help develop rhythm,* and make sure each short step is of equal length. If the patient gains proficiency at this gait, teach him the faster two-point gait. (See *Crutch gaits.*)

▪ Teach the three-point gait to the patient who can bear only partial or no weight on one leg. Instruct him to advance both crutches 6″ to 8″ (15 to 20 cm) along with the involved leg. Then tell him to bring the uninvolved leg forward and to bear the bulk of his weight on the crutches, but some of it on the involved leg, if possible. Stress the importance of taking steps of equal length and duration with no pauses.

- Teach the two-point gait to the patient with weak legs but good coordination and arm strength. This is the most natural crutch-walking gait *because it mimics walking, with alternating swings of the arms and legs.* Instruct the patient to advance the right crutch and left foot simultaneously, followed by the left crutch and right foot.
- Teach the swing-to or swing-through gaits—the fastest ones—to the patient with complete paralysis of the hips and legs. Instruct him to advance both crutches simultaneously and to swing the legs parallel to (swing-to) or beyond the crutches (swing-through).
- To teach the patient who uses crutches to get up from a chair, tell him to hold both crutches in one hand, with the tips resting firmly on the floor. Then instruct him to push up from the chair with his free hand, supporting himself with the crutches.
- To sit down, the patient reverses the process: Tell him to support himself with the crutches in one hand and to lower himself with the other.
- To teach the patient to ascend stairs using the three-point gait, tell him to lead with the uninvolved leg and to follow with both the crutches and the involved leg. To descend stairs, he should lead with the crutches and the involved leg and follow with the good leg. He may find it helpful to remember "The good goes up; the bad goes down."

Special considerations

Encourage arm- and shoulder-strengthening exercises to prepare the patient for crutch walking. If possible, consult with physical therapy to teach the patient two techniques—one fast and one slow—*so he can alternate between them to prevent excessive muscle fatigue and can adjust more easily to various walking conditions.*

Complications

When used with chronic conditions, the swing-to and swing-through gaits can lead to atrophy of the hips and legs if appropriate therapeutic exercises aren't performed routinely. Caution the patient against habitually leaning on his crutches *because prolonged pressure on the axillae can damage the brachial nerves, causing brachial nerve palsy.*

Documentation

Record the type of gait the patient used, the amount of assistance required, the distance walked, and the patient's tolerance of the crutches and gait.

Selected references

Clark, B.C., et al. "Leg Muscle Activity during Walking with Assistive Devices at Varying Levels of Weight Bearing," *Archives of Physical Medicine and Rehabilitation* 85(9):1555-60, September 2004.

Craven, R.F., and Hirnle, C.J. *Fundamentals of Nursing: Human Health and Function*, 5th ed. Philadelphia: Lippincott Williams & Wilkins, 2006.

Dabke, H.V., et al. "How Accurate Is Partial Weight Bearing?" *Clinical Orthopaedics and Related Research* (421):282-86, April 2004.

Youdas, J.W., et al. "Partial Weight-Bearing Gait Using Conventional Assistive Devices," *Archives of Physical Medicine and Rehabilitation* 86(3):394-98, March 2005.

Walkers

A walker consists of a metal frame with handgrips and four legs that buttresses the patient on three sides; one side remains open. Because this device provides greater stability and security than other ambulatory aids, it's recommended for the patient with insufficient strength and balance to use crutches or a cane or with weakness requiring frequent rest periods.

Attachments for standard walkers and modified walkers help meet special needs. For example, a walker may have a platform added to support an injured arm.

Equipment

Walker ▪ platform or wheel attachments, as necessary.

Various types of walkers are available. The standard walker is used by the patient with unilateral or bilateral weakness or an inability to bear weight on one leg. It requires arm strength and balance. Platform attachments may be added to a standard walker for the patient with arthritic arms or a casted arm, who can't bear weight directly on his hand, wrist, or forearm. With the practitioner's approval, wheels may be placed on the front legs of the standard walker to allow the extremely weak or poorly coordinated patient to roll the device forward, instead of lifting it. However, wheels are applied infrequently *because they pose a safety hazard.*

The stair walker—used by the patient who must negotiate stairs without bilateral handrails—requires good arm strength and balance. Its extra set of handles extends toward the patient on the open side. The rolling walker—used by the patient with very weak legs—has four wheels and may also have a seat. The reciprocal walker—used by the patient with very weak arms—allows one side to be advanced ahead of the other.

Teaching safe use of a walker

Sitting down

- First, tell the patient to stand with the back of his stronger leg against the front of the chair, his weaker leg slightly off the floor, and the walker directly in front.
- Tell him to grasp the armrests on the chair one arm at a time while supporting most of his weight on the stronger leg. (In the illustrations, the patient has left leg weakness.)
- Tell the patient to lower himself into the chair and slide backward. After he's seated, he should place the walker beside the chair.

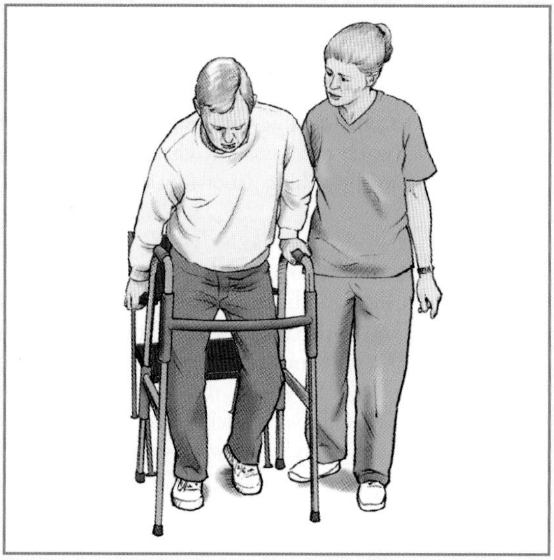

Getting up

- After bringing the walker to the front of his chair, tell the patient to slide forward in the chair. Placing the back of his stronger leg against the seat, he should then advance the weaker leg.
- Next, with both hands on the armrests, the patient can push himself to a standing position. Supporting himself with the stronger leg and the opposite hand, the patient should grasp the walker's handgrip with his free hand.
- Then the patient should grasp the free handgrip with his other hand.

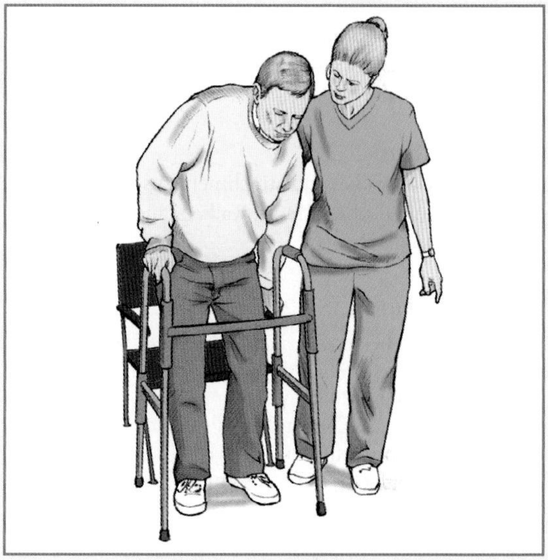

Preparation of equipment

Obtain the appropriate walker with the advice of a physical therapist, and adjust it to the patient's height: His elbows should be flexed at a 15- to 30-degree angle when standing comfortably within the walker with his hands on the grips. To adjust the walker, turn it upside down, and change the leg length by pushing in the button on each shaft and releasing it when the leg is in the correct position. Make sure the walker is level before the patient attempts to use it.

Implementation

- Help the patient stand within the walker, and instruct him to hold the handgrips firmly and equally. Stand behind him, closer to the involved leg.
- If the patient has one-sided leg weakness, tell him to advance the walker 6″ to 8″ (15 to 20 cm) and to step forward with the involved leg and follow with the uninvolved leg, supporting himself on his arms. Encourage him to take equal strides. If he has equal strength in both legs, instruct him to advance the walker 6″to 8″ and to step forward with either leg. If he can't use one leg, tell him to advance the walker 6″to 8″ and to swing onto it, supporting his weight on his arms.
- If the patient is using a reciprocal walker, teach him the two-point gait. Instruct the patient to stand with his weight evenly distributed between his legs and the walker. Stand behind him, slightly to one side. Tell him to simultaneously advance the walker's right side and his left foot. Then have the patient advance the walker's left side and his right foot.

- If the patient is using a reciprocal walker, you may also teach him the four-point gait. Instruct the patient to evenly distribute his weight between his legs and the walker. Stand behind him and slightly to one side. Have him move the right side of the walker forward. Then have the patient move his left foot forward. Next, instruct him to move the left side of the walker forward. Finally, have him move his right foot forward.
- If the patient is using a wheeled or stair walker, reinforce the physical therapist's instructions. Stress the need for caution when using a stair walker.
- Teach the patient how to sit down and get up from a chair safely. (See *Teaching safe use of a walker,* page 83.)

Special considerations

If the patient starts to fall, support his hips and shoulders *to help him maintain an upright position if possible.* If unsuccessful, ease him slowly to the closest surface—bed, floor, or chair.

Documentation

Record the type of walker and attachments used, the degree of guarding required, the distance walked, and the patient's tolerance of ambulation.

SELECTED REFERENCES

Craven, R.F., and Hirnle, C.J. *Fundamentals of Nursing: Human Health and Function,* 5th ed. Philadelphia: Lippincott Williams & Wilkins, 2006.

Haubert, L.L., et al. "A Comparison of Shoulder Joint Forces during Ambulation with Crutches Versus a Walker in Persons with Incomplete Spinal Cord Injury," *Archives of Physical Medicine and Rehabilitation* 87(1):63-70, January 2006.

SUPPLEMENTAL BED EQUIPMENT

Certain equipment can promote the bedridden patient's comfort and help prevent pressure ulcers and other complications of immobility. A wood or hard plastic footboard prevents footdrop by maintaining proper alignment. It also raises bed linens off the patient's feet. A foot cradle—a horizontal or arched bar over the end of the bed—keeps bed linens off the patient's feet, preventing skin irritation and breakdown, especially in patients with peripheral vascular disease or neuropathy. A bed board, made of wood or wood covered with canvas, firms the mattress and is especially useful for the patient with spinal injuries. A basic metal frame and a metal trapeze (a triangular piece attached to this frame) allow the patient with arm mobility and strength to lift himself off the bed, facilitating bedmaking and bedpan positioning. A metal overbed cradle, a cagelike frame placed on top of the mattress, keeps bed linens off the patient with burns, open wounds, or a wet cast.

A vinyl water mattress, used to prevent or treat pressure ulcers, exerts less pressure on the skin than the standard hospital mattress. An alternating pressure pad (a vinyl pad divided into chambers filled with air or water and attached to an electric pump) serves the same purpose, but it also stimulates circulation by alternately inflating and deflating its chambers.

Reusable and disposable water mattresses are also available. The reusable water mattress replaces the standard hospital mattress and rests on a sheet of heavy cardboard placed over the bedsprings; the smaller, less bulky disposable mattress rests on top of the standard hospital mattress. All supplemental bed equipment is optional, depending on the patient's needs. (See *Types of supplemental bed equipment.*)

Equipment

Footboard and cover ▪ drawsheet ▪ bath blanket ▪ foot cradle ▪ bed board ▪ basic frame with trapeze ▪ overbed cradle ▪ roller gauze ▪ water mattress ▪ stretcher ▪ alternating pressure pad ▪ pump and tubing ▪ footstool ▪ linen-saver pad ▪ safety pins.

Preparation of equipment

If you're preparing a footboard for use, place a cover over it *to provide padding,* or pad it with a folded drawsheet or bath blanket; bring the top and side edges of the sheet or blanket to the back of the footboard, miter the corners, and secure them at the center with safety pins. *Padding cushions the patient's feet against pressure from the hard footboard, helping to prevent skin irritation and breakdown.* Avoid wrinkles *to prevent skin irritation.*

Implementation

- Tell the patient what you're going to do, and describe the equipment.
- Wash your hands.

Using a footboard

- Move the patient up in the bed *to allow room for the footboard.* Loosen the top linens at the foot of the bed, and then fold them back over the patient *to expose his feet.*
- Lift the mattress at the foot of the bed, and place the lip of the footboard between the mattress and the bedsprings. Alternatively, secure the footboard under both sides of the mattress.
- Adjust the footboard so that the patient's feet rest comfortably against it. If the footboard isn't adjustable, tuck a folded bath blanket between the board and the patient's feet.

Types of supplemental bed equipment

Adjustable footboard

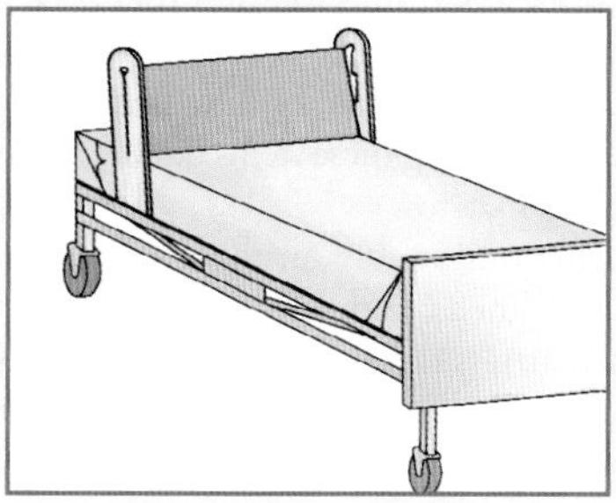

Section cradle with one side arm

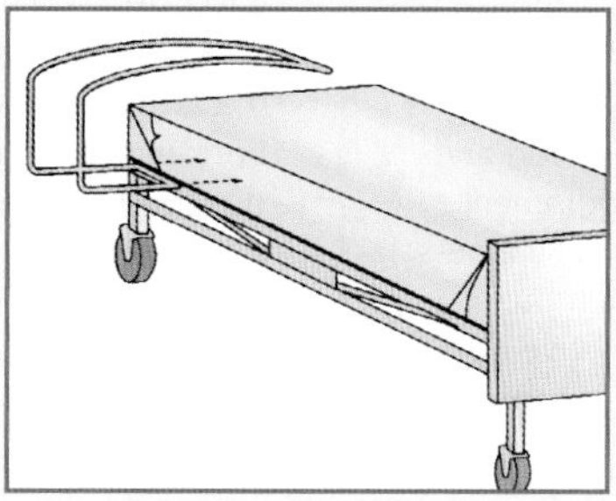

Overbed cradle

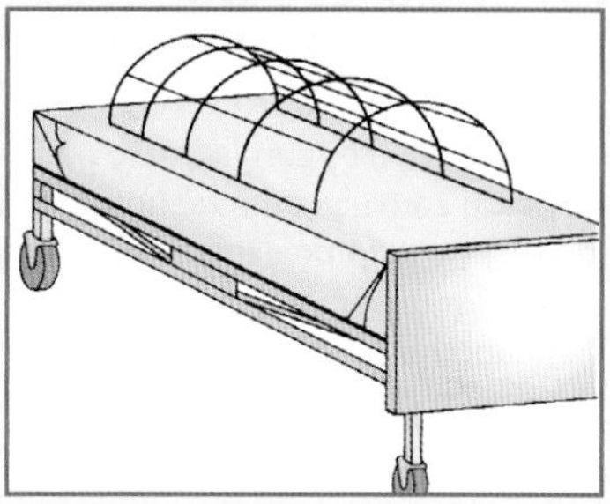

Alternating pressure mattress

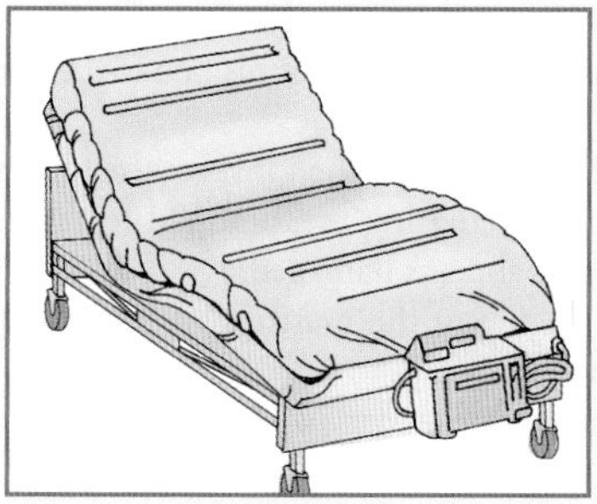

Trapeze and basic frame

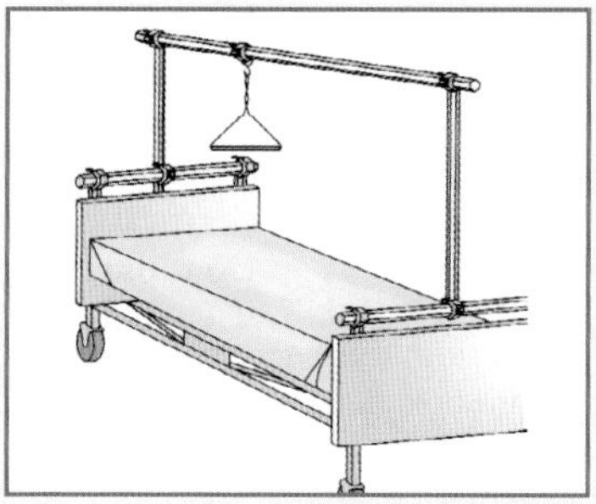

Alternating pressure pad

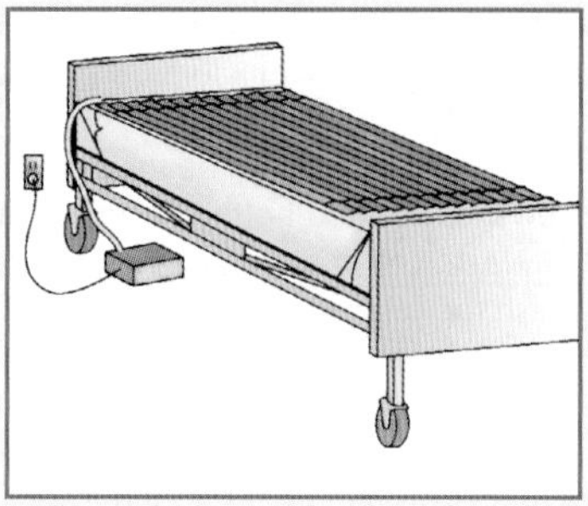

■ Unless the footboard has side supports, place a sandbag, a folded bath blanket, or a pillow alongside each foot *to maintain 90-degree foot alignment.*
■ Fold the top linens over the footboard, tuck them under the mattress, and miter the corners.

Using a foot cradle

■ Loosen the top linens at the foot of the bed, and fold them over the patient or to one side.
■ When using a one-piece cradle, place one side arm under the mattress, carefully extend the arch over the bed, and place the other side arm under the mattress on the opposite side. Then adjust the tension rods *so that they rest securely over the edge of the mattress.*
■ When using a sectional cradle with two side arms, first place the side arms under the mattress. Secure the tension rods over the edge of the mattress. Then carefully place the arch over the bed and connect it to the side arms. When using a sectional cradle with one side arm, connect the side arm and horizontal cradle bar before placement. Then place the side arm under the mattress on one side of the bed.
■ Cover the cradle with the top linens, tuck them under the mattress at the foot of the bed, and miter the corners.

Using a bed board

■ Transfer the patient from his bed to a stretcher or a chair. Obtain assistance if necessary.
■ Strip the linens from the bed. If you plan to reuse them, fold each piece neatly and hang it over the back of a chair. Otherwise, place soiled linens in a laundry bag.
■ If the bed board consists of wooden slats encased in canvas, lift the mattress at the head of the bed, and center the board over the bedsprings *to prevent it from jutting out and causing accidental injury.* Unroll the slats to cover the bedsprings at the head of the bed. Then lift the mattress at the foot of the bed, and unroll the remaining slats.
■ If the bed board consists of one solid or two hinged pieces of wood, lift the mattress on one side of the bed, and center the board over the bedsprings.
■ After positioning the bed board, replace the linens. Then return the patient to bed.

Using a basic frame with trapeze

■ If an orthopedic technician isn't available to secure the frame and trapeze to the patient's bed, get assistance to attach these devices to the bed as necessary. Be sure to hang

HOME CARE

Helping patients improvise assistive devices at home

Assistive devices can increase patient comfort and improve care given in the home. This equipment doesn't need to be expensive. If the patient's illness is brief or financial constraints exist, teach the patient and his caregivers to improvise assistive devices with common household items. For example:

- Side rails can be made by placing kitchen chairs along the sides of a bed and securing their legs to the bed frame.
- Linen-saver pads can be fashioned from shower curtains, plastic tablecloths, a plastic raincoat, or trash bags.
- Absorbent pads can be made by placing sheets of newspaper and a bottom layer of plastic inside a pillowcase. When damp, discard the newspaper and wash the pillowcase.
- An ironing board, a wooden crate with two sides removed, a child's table, or a sturdy cardboard box can serve as an over-the-bed table or a bed cradle.
- Backrests can be fashioned from a large item such as a cutting board padded on top and supported underneath by pillows.
- A pull rope to assist the patient in turning or sitting up can be made by braiding nylon stockings together and fastening the rope to the side or end of the bed.

the trapeze within the patient's easy reach *so he won't need to strain to reach it.*

Using an overbed cradle

- Loosen and remove the top linens.
- Carefully lower the cradle onto the patient's bed and secure it in place. Wrap roller gauze around both sides of the cradle. Then pull the gauze taut and attach it to the bedsprings.
- Cover the cradle with the top linens, tuck them under the mattress at the foot of the bed, and miter the corners.

Using a portable water mattress

- *Because this mattress is heavy and bulky,* you'll need several coworkers to help you transfer it from the stretcher to the patient's bed. Check with the maintenance department before transferring the mattress *because its weight may rule out use on some electric beds.* Also, ensure that the patient isn't prone to motion sickness *because the movement of the water in the mattress may cause nausea.*
- Position the mattress on the bed, and place the protective cover over it. Then place a bottom sheet over the cover, and tuck it in loosely.
- Place a sheepskin, linen-saver pad, or drawsheet over the bottom sheet as needed. Adding these items doesn't decrease the effectiveness of this mattress.
- Position the patient comfortably on the mattress. Then cover him with the top linens, and tuck them in loosely.
- Check the water mattress daily *to ensure adequate flotation.* To do so, place your hand under the patient's thighs. If you can feel the bottom of the mattress, arrange to have water added.

Using an alternating pressure pad

- If possible, transfer the patient from his bed to a chair or stretcher. Get help if necessary.
- Strip the linens from the bed. Then inspect the plug and electrical cord of the alternating pressure pad for defects. Don't use the unit if it appears damaged.
- Unfold the pad on top of the mattress with the appropriate side facing up.
- Place the motor on a linen-saver pad on the floor or on a footstool near the mattress outlets. Connect the tubing securely to the motor and to the mattress outlets, and plug the cord into an electrical outlet. Turn the motor on.
- After several minutes, observe the emptying and filling of the pad's chambers, and check the tubing for kinks *because they could interfere with the pad's function.*
- Place a bottom sheet over the pad, and tuck it in loosely. *To avoid tube constriction,* don't miter the corner where the tubing is attached.
- Position the patient comfortably on the pad, cover him with the top linens, and tuck them in loosely.
- If the pad becomes soiled, clean it with a damp cloth and mild soap, then dry it well. *To avoid damaging the pad's surface,* don't use alcohol.
- When the patient no longer needs the pad or is discharged, turn the motor off, disconnect the tubing, and unplug the cord from the wall outlet. Remove the pad from the patient's bed, and fold and discard it. If applicable, give the pad to the patient to take home. Inform him that the motor needed to power the pad can usually be rented from a surgical supply store. Explain to the patient or a caregiver how to operate the pad at home. (See *Helping patients improvise assistive devices at home.*)
- Coil the tubing and electrical cord, and then strap them to the motor. Return the motor unit to the central supply department.

Special considerations

- Place the patient in bed before positioning and securing an overbed or foot cradle *to ensure its proper placement and to prevent patient injury.* Similarly, remove the cradle before the patient gets out of bed. When turning or positioning the patient on his side, make sure the foot cradle's tension rod doesn't rest against his skin *because this may cause pressure and predispose him to skin breakdown.*
- Exercise caution when turning the obese patient on a water mattress *because turning displaces a large volume of water.* Be sure to keep the side rails raised during turning *to prevent falls.*
- Avoid placing excessive layers of drawsheets or linen-saver pads between the alternating pressure pad and the patient *because these decrease the pad's effectiveness.* Avoid using pins or sharp instruments near an alternating pressure pad or water mattress *to prevent accidental puncture.*

NURSING ALERT **Because a plastic-covered mattress slides off a bed board easily,** ***make sure a coworker stands on the opposite side of the bed when you're transferring the patient from stretcher to bed.***

- If the bottom sheet isn't wide enough to cover both the standard and the specialty mattress (such as a foam mattress), use two bottom sheets. Cover the standard mattress with one sheet, then cover the foam mattress with a second sheet, and tuck it between the standard and foam mattresses. Two top sheets may be needed to cover the patient when a footboard, foot cradle, or bed cradle is used.

Documentation

In your notes and care plan, record the type of supplemental bed equipment used, the time and date of use, and the patient's response to treatment.

Selected references

Craven, R.F., and Hirnle, C.J. *Fundamentals of Nursing: Human Health and Function,* 5th ed. Philadelphia: Lippincott Williams & Wilkins, 2007.

Roelands, M., et al. "Clinical Practice Guidelines to Improve Shared Decision-Making about Assistive Device Use in Home Care: A Pilot Intervention Study," *Patient Education and Counseling* 55(2):252-64, November 2004.

Roelands, M., et al. "Introduction of Assistive Devices: Home Nurses' Practices and Beliefs," *Journal of Advanced Nursing* 54(2):180-88, April 2006.

Taylor, C., et al. *Fundamentals of Nursing: The Art and Science of Nursing Care,* 6th ed. Philadelphia: Lippincott Williams & Wilkins, 2008.

BODY MECHANICS AND TRANSFER TECHNIQUES

Body mechanics

Body mechanics is the term used to describe the efficient, coordinated, and safe use of muscle groups to maintain balance, reduce fatigue, reduce energy requirements, and decrease the risk of injury while moving objects and carrying out activities of daily living. It involves the concepts of *center of gravity, line of gravity,* and *base of support* in relation to body alignment and balance.

The center of gravity is a point in the center of the body at navel level that's the pivot point for forward, back, and lateral balance. The line of gravity is located midline and forms a vertical line from the middle of the forehead to the midpoint between the feet, which form the base of support. When a person moves, the center of gravity moves continuously in the same direction as the body. Balance depends on the interrelationship of the center of gravity, line of gravity, and base of support. During movement, the closer the line of gravity is to the center of the base of support, the more stable the balance. The closer the line of gravity is to the edge of the base of support, the more precarious the balance. If the line of gravity falls outside the base of support, balance is lost.

The broader the base of support and the lower the center of gravity, the greater the stability and balance. Body balance, therefore, can be greatly enhanced by widening the base of support and lowering the center of gravity, bringing it closer to the base of support.

The best practice for body mechanics can be summed up in three principles. First, *keep a low center of gravity* by flexing the hips and knees instead of bending at the waist. This position distributes weight evenly between the upper and lower body, helps maintain balance, and decreases the load on the back muscles by transferring the weight to the stronger leg muscles. Second, *create a wide base of support* by spreading the feet apart. This tactic provides lateral stability and lowers the body's center of gravity. Finally, *maintain proper body alignment*—spine straight, head in neutral position, and all extremities in functional position—and keep the center of gravity directly over the base of support by moving the feet rather than twisting and bending at the waist.

Many patient care activities require the nurse to push, pull, lift, and carry. Application of proper body mechanics enables her to use the appropriate muscle groups when performing nursing care and can prevent musculoskeletal injury and fatigue and reduce the risk of injuring patients.

Implementation

Follow the directions below to push, pull, stoop, lift, and carry correctly.

Pushing and pulling correctly

- Stand close to the object, and place one foot slightly ahead of the other, as in a walking position. Tighten the leg muscles and set the pelvis by simultaneously contracting the abdominal and gluteal muscles.
- To push, place your hands on the object and flex your elbows. Lean into the object by shifting weight from the back leg to the front leg, and apply smooth, continuous pressure, using your leg muscles as shown below.

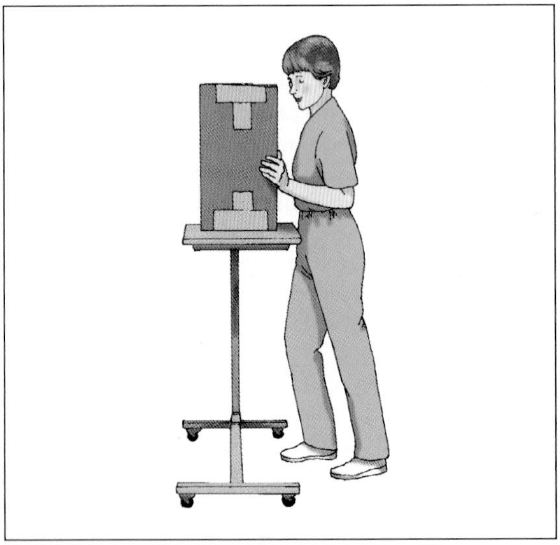

- To pull, grasp the object and flex your elbows. Lean away from the object by shifting weight from the front leg to the back leg. Pull smoothly, avoiding sudden, jerky movements.
- After you've started to move the object, keep it in motion; *stopping and starting uses more energy.*

Stooping correctly

- Stand with your feet 10″ to 12″ (25 to 30 cm) apart and one foot slightly ahead of the other *to widen the base of support.*
- Lower yourself by flexing your knees, and place more weight on the front foot than on the back foot. Keep the upper body straight by not bending at the waist as shown top of next column.

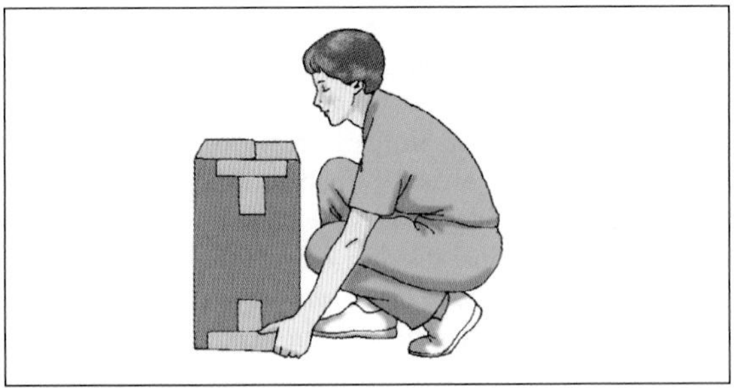

- To stand up again, straighten the knees and keep the back straight.

Lifting and carrying correctly

- Assume the stooping position directly in front of the object *to minimize back flexion and avoid spinal rotation when lifting.*
- Grasp the object, and tighten your abdominal muscles.
- Stand up by straightening the knees, using the leg and hip muscles. Always keep your back straight *to maintain a fixed center of gravity* as shown below.

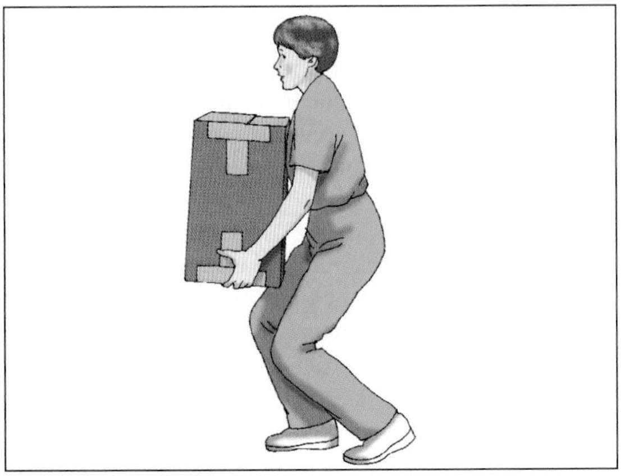

- Carry the object close to your body at waist height—near the body's center of gravity—*to avoid straining the back muscles.*

Special considerations

- Wear shoes with low heels, flexible nonslip soles, and closed backs *to promote correct body alignment, facilitate proper body mechanics, and prevent accidents.*
- When possible, pull rather than push an object *because the elbow flexors are stronger than the extensors. Pulling an object allows the use of hip and leg muscles and avoids the use of lower back muscles.*

■ When doing heavy lifting or moving, remember to use assistive or mechanical devices, if available, or obtain assistance from coworkers; know your limitations and use sound judgment.
■ Mechanical and other assistive devices have been shown to significantly decrease incidences of lower back injury in nursing personnel.

SELECTED REFERENCES

Craven, R.F., and Hirnle, C.J. *Fundamentals of Nursing: Human Health and Function*, 5th ed. Philadelphia: Lippincott Williams & Wilkins, 2006.

Nelson, A., and Baptiste, A.S. "Evidence-Based Practices for Safe Patient Handling and Movement," *Online Journal of Issues in Nursing* 9(3):4, September 2004.

Pellino, T.A., et al. "The Evaluation of Mechanical Devices for Lateral Transfers on Perceived Exertion and Patient Comfort," *Orthopaedic Nursing* 25(1):4-10, January-February 2006.

Viera, E.R., et al. "Low Back Problems and Possible Improvements in Nursing Jobs," *Journal for Advanced Nursing* 55(1):79-89, July 2006.

TRANSFER FROM BED TO STRETCHER

Transfer from bed to stretcher, one of the most common transfers, can require the help of one or more coworkers, depending on the patient's size and condition and the primary nurse's physical abilities. Techniques for achieving this transfer include the straight lift, carry lift, lift sheet, and sliding board.

The nurse should always remember to maintain good body mechanics—a wide base of support and bent knees—when transferring a patient, to reduce the risk of injury to the patient and herself. To reduce the risk of injury to the patient during transfer, the nurse should make sure that the patient maintains proper body alignment—back straight, head in neutral position, and extremities in a functional position

In the straight (or patient-assisted) lift—used to move a child, a very light patient, or a patient who can assist transfer—the transfer team members place their hands and arms under the patient's buttocks and, if necessary, his shoulders. Other patients may require a four-person straight lift, detailed below. In the carry lift, team members roll the patient onto their upper arms and hold him against their chests. In the lift sheet transfer, they place a sheet under the patient and lift or slide him onto the stretcher. In the sliding-board transfer, two team members slide him onto the stretcher.

Equipment

Stretcher ■ sliding board or lift sheet if necessary.

Preparation of equipment

Adjust the bed to the same height as the stretcher.

Implementation

■ Tell the patient that you're going to move him from the bed to the stretcher, and place him in the supine position.
■ Ask team members to remove watches and rings *to avoid scratching the patient during transfer.*

Four-person straight lift

■ Place the stretcher parallel to the bed, and lock the wheels of both *to ensure the patient's safety.*
■ Stand at the center of the stretcher, and have another team member stand at the patient's head. The two other team members should stand next to the bed, on the other side—one at the center and the other at the patient's feet.
■ Slide your arms, palms up, beneath the patient, while the other team members do the same. In this position, you and the team member directly opposite support the patient's buttocks and hips; the team member at the head of the bed supports the patient's head and shoulders; the one at the foot supports the patient's legs and feet.
■ On a count of three, the team members lift the patient several inches, move him onto the stretcher, and slide their arms out from under him. Keep movements smooth *to minimize patient discomfort and avoid muscle strain by team members.*

Four-person carry lift

■ Place the stretcher perpendicular to the bed, with the head of the stretcher at the foot of the bed. Lock the bed and stretcher wheels *to ensure the patient's safety.*
■ Raise the bed to a comfortable working height.
■ Line up all four team members on the same side of the bed as the stretcher, with the tallest member at the patient's head and the shortest at his feet. The member at the patient's head is the leader of the team and gives the lift signals.
■ Tell the team members to flex their knees and slide their hands, palms up, under the patient until he rests securely on their upper arms. Make sure the patient is adequately supported at the head and shoulders, buttocks and hips, and legs and feet.
■ On a count of three, the team members straighten their knees and roll the patient onto his side, against their chests. *This reduces strain on the lifters and allows them to hold the patient for several minutes if necessary.*
■ Together, the team members step back, with the member supporting the feet moving the farthest. The team members move forward to the stretcher's edge and, on a count of three, lower the patient onto the stretcher by bending at the knees and sliding their arms out from under the patient.

Four-person lift sheet transfer

■ Position the bed, stretcher, and team members for the straight lift. Then instruct the team to hold the edges of the sheet under the patient, grasping them close to the patient *to obtain a firm grip, provide stability, and spare the patient undue feelings of instability.*

■ On a count of three, the team members lift or slide the patient onto the stretcher in a smooth, continuous motion *to avoid muscle strain and minimize patient discomfort.*

Sliding-board transfer

■ Place the stretcher parallel to the bed, and lock the wheels of both *to ensure the patient's safety.*

■ Stand next to the bed, and instruct a coworker to stand next to the stretcher.

■ Reach over the patient and pull the far side of the bedsheet toward you to turn the patient slightly on his side. Your coworker then places the sliding board beneath the patient, making sure the board bridges the gap between stretcher and bed as shown below.

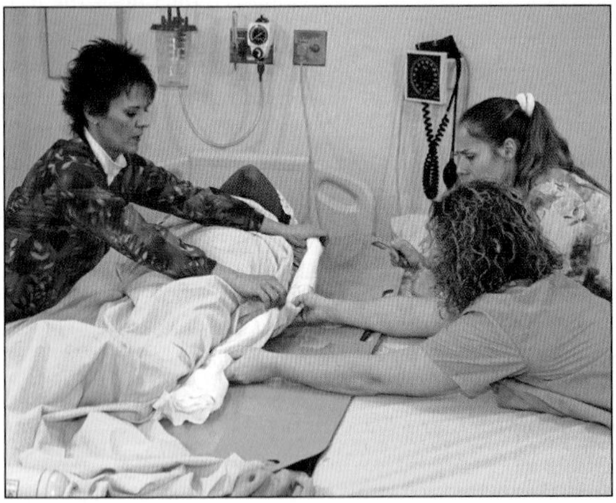

■ Ease the patient onto the sliding board and release the sheet. Your coworker then grasps the near side of the sheet at the patient's hips and shoulders and pulls him onto the stretcher in a smooth, continuous motion. She then reaches over the patient, grasps the far side of the sheet, and logrolls him toward her.

■ Remove the sliding board as your coworker returns the patient to the supine position.

After all transfers

■ Position the patient comfortably on the stretcher, apply safety straps, and raise and secure the side rails.

Special considerations

When transferring an immobile or markedly obese patient from bed to stretcher, first lift and move him, in increments, to the edge of the bed. Then rest for a few seconds, repositioning the patient if necessary, and lift him onto the stretcher. If the patient can bear weight on his arms or legs, two or three coworkers can perform this transfer: One can support the buttocks and guide the patient, another can stabilize the stretcher by leaning over it and guiding the patient into position, and a third can transfer any attached equipment. If a team member isn't available to guide equipment, move I.V. lines and other tubing first *to make sure it's out of the way and not in danger of pulling loose* (disconnect tubes if possible). If the patient is light, three coworkers can perform the carry lift; however, no matter how many team members are present, one must stabilize the patient's head if he can't support it himself, has cervical instability or injury, or has undergone surgery.

Depending on the patient's size and condition, a lift sheet transfer can require two to seven people.

Documentation

Record the time and, if necessary, the type of transfer in your notes. Complete other required forms as necessary.

SELECTED REFERENCES

Craven, R.F., and Hirnle, C.J. *Fundamentals of Nursing: Human Health and Function*, 5th ed. Philadelphia: Lippincott Williams & Wilkins, 2006.

Kjellberg, K., et al. "Patient Safety and Comfort during Transfers in Relation to Nurses' Work Technique," *Journal of Advanced Nursing* 47(3):251-59, August 2004.

Lloyd, J.D., and Baptiste, A. "Friction-Reducing Devices for Lateral Patient Transfers: A Biomechanical Evaluation," *AAOHN Journal* 54(3):113-19, March 2006.

TRANSFER FROM BED TO WHEELCHAIR

For the patient with diminished or absent lower-body sensation or one-sided weakness, immobility, or injury, transfer from bed to wheelchair may require partial support to full assistance—initially by at least two persons. Subsequent transfer of the patient with generalized weakness may be performed by one nurse. After transfer, proper positioning helps prevent excessive pressure on bony prominences, which predisposes the patient to skin breakdown.

Equipment

Wheelchair with locks (or sturdy chair) ■ pajama bottoms (or robe) ■ shoes or slippers with nonslip soles ■ watch with

Teaching the patient to use a transfer board

For the patient who can't stand, a transfer board allows safe transfer from bed to wheelchair. To perform this transfer, take the following steps:

- First, explain and demonstrate the procedure. Eventually, the patient may become proficient enough to transfer himself independently or with supervision.
- Help the patient put on pajama bottoms or a robe and shoes or nonslip slippers.
- Lock the bed wheels.
- Place the wheelchair angled slightly and facing the foot of the bed. Lock the wheels, and remove the armrest closest to the patient. Make sure that the bed is flat, and adjust its height so that it's level with the wheelchair seat.
- Assist the patient to a sitting position on the edge of the bed, with his feet resting on the floor. Make sure that the front edge of the wheelchair seat is aligned with the back of the patient's knees (as shown below left). Although it's important that the patient have an even surface on which to transfer, he may find it easier to transfer to a slightly lower surface.
- Ask the patient to lean away from the wheelchair while you slide one end of the transfer board under him.
- Now place the other end of the transfer board on the wheelchair seat, and help the patient return to the upright position.
- Stand in front of the patient *to prevent him from sliding forward.* Tell him to push down with both arms, lifting the buttocks up and onto the transfer board. The patient then repeats this maneuver, edging along the board, until he's seated in the wheelchair. If the patient can't use his arms to assist with the transfer, stand in front of him, put your arms around him and, if he's able, have him put his arms around you. Gradually slide him across the board until he's safely in the chair (as shown below right).
- When the patient is in the chair, fasten a seat belt, if necessary, *to prevent falls.*
- Then remove the transfer board, replace the wheelchair armrest and footrest, and reposition the patient in the chair.

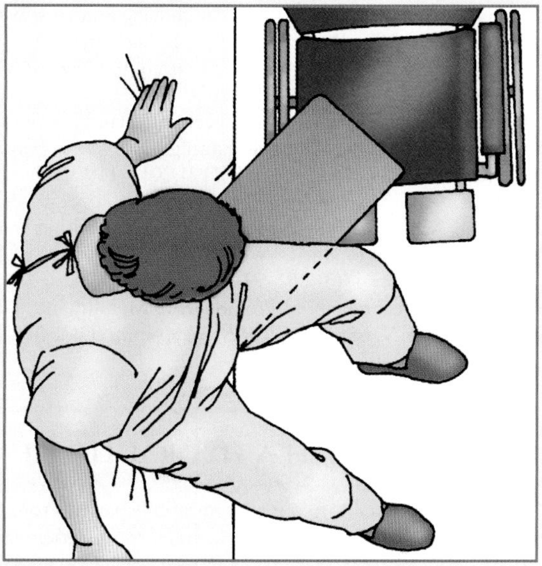

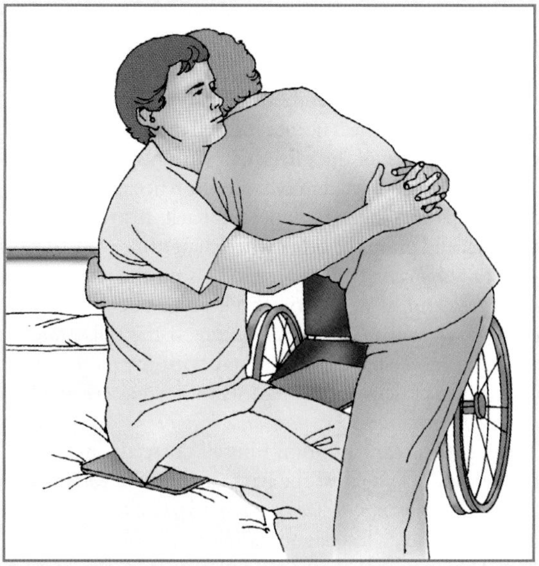

a second hand ▪ stethoscope ▪ sphygmomanometer ▪ optional: transfer board if appropriate. (See *Teaching the patient to use a transfer board.*)

Implementation

- Explain the procedure to the patient and demonstrate his role.
- Use good body mechanics during the transfer *to prevent injury.*

- Place the wheelchair parallel to the bed, facing the foot of the bed, and lock its wheels. Raise the wheelchair footrests *to avoid interfering with the transfer.* Make sure the bed wheels are also locked and the bed is in the lowest position in relation to the floor *to prevent an accident.*
- Check pulse rate and blood pressure with the patient supine *to obtain a baseline.* Then help him put on the pajama bottoms and slippers or shoes with nonslip soles *to prevent falls.*
- Raise the head of the bed, and allow the patient to rest briefly *to adjust to posture changes.* Then bring him to the dangling position (see "Progressive ambulation," page 73). Recheck pulse rate and blood pressure if you suspect cardiovascular instability. Don't proceed until the patient's pulse rate and blood pressure are stabilized *to prevent falls.*
- Tell the patient to move toward the edge of the bed and, if possible, to place his feet flat on the floor. Stand in front of the patient, blocking his toes with your feet and his knees with yours *to prevent his knees from buckling.*
- Flex your knees slightly, place your arms around the patient's back above the level of the axilla, and tell him to place his hands on the edge of the bed. Avoid bending at your waist *to prevent back strain.*
- Ask the patient to push himself off the bed and to support as much of his own weight as possible. At the same time, straighten your knees and hips, raising the patient as you straighten your body.
- Supporting the patient as needed, pivot toward the wheelchair, keeping your knees next to his. Tell the patient to grasp the farthest armrest of the wheelchair with his closest hand.
- Help the patient lower himself into the wheelchair by flexing your hips and knees, but not your back. Instruct him to reach back and grasp the other wheelchair armrest as he sits *to avoid abrupt contact with the seat.* Fasten the seat belt *to prevent falls* and, if necessary, check pulse rate and blood pressure *to assess cardiovascular stability.* If the pulse rate is 20 beats or more above baseline, stay with the patient and monitor him closely until it returns to normal *because he's experiencing orthostatic hypotension.*
- If the patient can't position himself correctly, help him move his buttocks against the back of the chair *so that the ischial tuberosities, not the sacrum, provide the base of support.*
- Place the patient's feet flat on the footrests, pointed straight ahead. Then position the knees and hips with the correct amount of flexion and in appropriate alignment. If appropriate, use elevating leg rests to flex the patient's hips at more than 90 degrees; *this position relieves pressure on the popliteal space and places more weight on the ischial tuberosities.*
- Position the patient's arms on the wheelchair's armrests with shoulders abducted, elbows slightly flexed, forearms pronated, and wrists and hands in the neutral position. If necessary, support or elevate the patient's hands and forearms with a pillow *to prevent dependent edema.*

Special considerations

- If the patient starts to fall during transfer, ease him to the closest surface—bed, floor, or chair. Never stretch to finish the transfer. *Doing so can cause loss of balance, falls, muscle strain, and other injuries to you and the patient.*
- If the patient has one-sided weakness, follow the preceding steps, but place the wheelchair on the patient's unaffected side. Instruct the patient to pivot and bear as much weight as possible on the unaffected side. Support the affected side *because the patient will tend to lean to this side.* Use pillows to support the hemiplegic patient's affected side *to prevent slumping in the wheelchair.*

Documentation

If necessary, record the time of transfer, the extent of assistance, and note how the patient tolerated the transfer.

SELECTED REFERENCES

Craven, R.F., and Hirnle, C.J. *Fundamentals of Nursing Human: Health and Function*, 5th ed. Philadelphia: Lippincott Williams & Wilkins, 2006.

Johnsonn, A.C., et al. "Evaluation of Nursing Students' Work Technique After Proficiency Training in Patient Transfer Methods During Undergraduate Education," *Nurse Education Today* 26(4):322-31, May 2006.

Kirby, R.L., et al. "The Manual Wheelchair-Handling Skills of Caregivers and the Effect of Training," *Archives of Physical Medicine and Rehabilitation* 85(12):2011-119, December 2004.

Kjellberg, K., et al. "Patient Safety and Comfort during Transfers in Relation to Nurses' Work Technique," *Journal of Advanced Nursing* 47(3):251-59, August 2004.

Nelson, A. "Technology to Promote Safe Mobility in the Elderly," *The Nursing Clinics of North America* 39(3):649-71, September 2004.

TRANSFER WITH A HYDRAULIC LIFT

Using a hydraulic lift to raise the immobile patient from the supine to the sitting position allows safe, comfortable transfer between bed and chair. It's indicated for the obese or immobile patient for whom manual transfer poses the potential for nurse or patient injury. Although most hydraulic lift models can be operated by one person, it's better to have two staff members present during transfer to stabilize and support the patient.

Equipment

Hydraulic lift, with sling, chains or straps, and hooks ■ chair or wheelchair.

Preparation of equipment

Because hydraulic lift models may vary in weight capacity, check the manufacturer's specifications before attempting patient transfer. Make sure the bed and wheelchair wheels are locked before beginning the transfer.

Implementation

- Explain the procedure to the patient, and reassure him that the hydraulic lift can safely support his weight and won't tip over.
- Ensure the patient's privacy. If the patient has an I.V. line or urinary drainage bag, move it first. Arrange tubing securely *to prevent dangling during transfer.* If the tubing of the urinary drainage bag isn't long enough to permit the transfer, clamp the tubing and drainage bag and place it on the patient's abdomen during transfer. After the transfer, place the drainage bag in a dependent position and unclamp the tubing.
- Make sure the side rail opposite you is raised and secure. Then roll the patient toward you, onto his side, and raise the side rail. Walk to the opposite side of the bed and lower the side rail.
- Place the sling under the patient's buttocks with its lower edge below the greater trochanter. Then fanfold the far side of the sling against the back and buttocks.
- Roll the patient toward you onto the sling, and raise the side rail. Then lower the opposite side rail.
- Slide your hands under the patient and pull the sling from beneath him, smoothing out all wrinkles. Then roll the patient onto his back and center him on the sling.
- Place the appropriate chair next to the head of the bed, facing the foot.
- Lower the side rail next to the chair, and raise the bed only until the base of the lift can extend under the bed. *To avoid alarming and endangering the patient,* don't raise the bed completely.
- Set the lift's adjustable base to its widest position *to ensure optimal stability.* Then move the lift so that its arm lies perpendicular to the bed, directly over the patient.
- Connect one end of the chains (or straps) to the side arms on the lift; connect the other hooked end to the sling. Face the hooks away from the patient *to prevent them from slipping and to avoid the risk of their pointed edges injuring the patient.* The patient may place his arms inside or outside the chains (or straps), or he may grasp them once the slack is gone *to avoid injury.* (See *Using a hydraulic lift.*)

EQUIPMENT

Using a hydraulic lift

After placing the patient supine in the center of the sling, position the hydraulic lift above her (as shown below). Then attach the chains to the hooks on the sling.

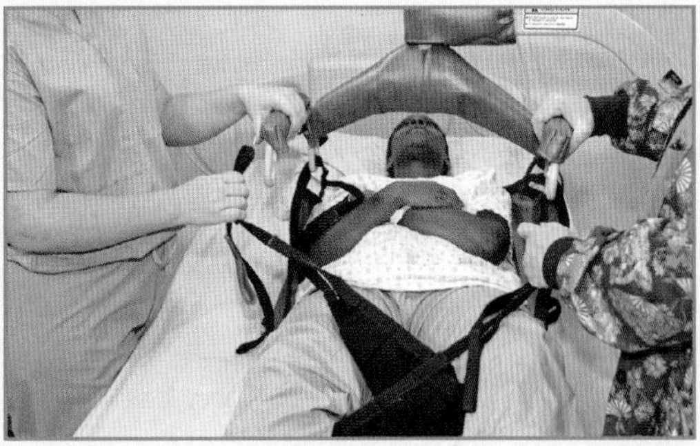

Turn the lift handle clockwise to raise the patient to the sitting position. If she's positioned properly, continue to raise her until he's suspended just above the bed.

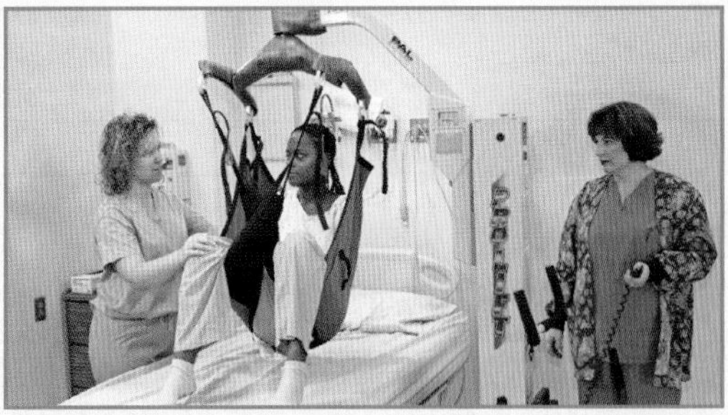

After positioning the patient above the wheelchair, turn the lift handle counterclockwise to lower her onto the seat. When the chains become slack, stop turning and unhook the sling from the lift.

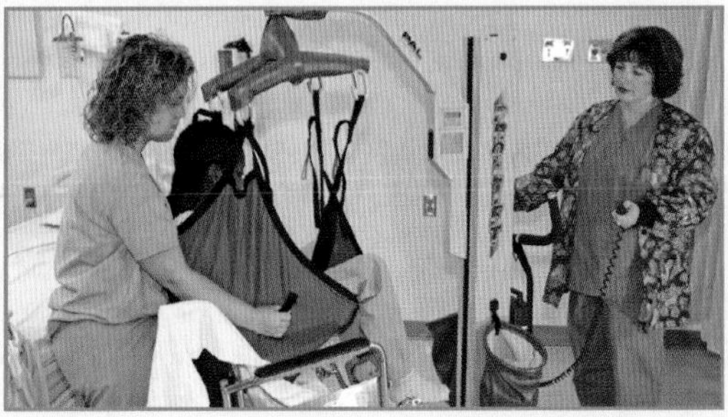

Low-air-loss therapy bed

The low-air-loss therapy bed reduces pressure on skin surfaces and may be used for patients with conditions such as immobility, malnutrition, incontinence, contractures, fractures, or amputations. Some models come with special features, such as rotational or percussion options.

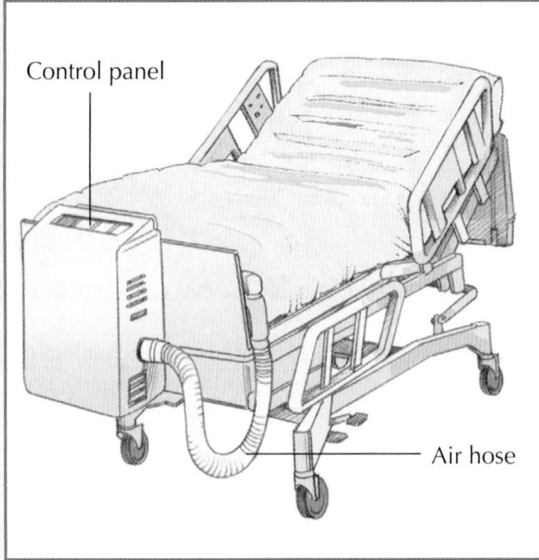

■ Tighten the turnscrew on the lift. Then, depending on the type of lift you're using, pump the handle or turn it clockwise until the patient has assumed a sitting position and his buttocks clear the bed surface by 1″ to 2″ (2.5 to 5 cm). Momentarily suspend him above the bed until he feels secure in the lift and sees that it can bear his weight.
■ Steady the patient as you move the lift or, preferably, have another coworker guide the patient's body while you move the lift. Depending on the type of lift you're using, the arm should now rest in front of or to one side of the chair.
■ Release the turnscrew. Then depress the handle or turn it counterclockwise *to lower the patient into the chair.* While lowering the patient, push gently on his knees *to maintain the correct sitting posture.* After lowering the patient into the chair, fasten the seat belt *to ensure his safety.*
■ Remove the hooks or straps from the sling, but leave the sling in place under the patient so you'll be able to transfer him back to the bed from the chair. Then move the lift away from the patient.
■ To return the patient to bed, reverse the procedure.

Special considerations

■ If the patient has an altered center of gravity (caused by a halo vest or a lower-extremity cast, for example), obtain help from a coworker before transferring him with a hydraulic lift.
■ If the patient will require the use of a hydraulic lift for transfers after discharge, teach his family how to use this device correctly and allow them to practice with supervision.

Documentation

Record the time of transfer in your notes, and note how the patient tolerated the activity.

SELECTED REFERENCES

Craven, R.F., and Hirnle, C.J. *Fundamentals of Nursing: Human Health and Function,* 5th ed. Philadelphia: Lippincott Williams & Wilkins, 2006.

Kjellberg, K., et al. "Patient Safety and Comfort during Transfers in Relation to Nurses' Work Technique," *Journal of Advanced Nursing* 47(3):251-59, August 2004.

SPECIAL BEDS

LOW-AIR-LOSS THERAPY BEDS

Low-air-loss therapy beds, composed of segmented cushions that provide surface area for pressure relief, help prevent and treat skin breakdown as well as minimize pain. These beds are indicated for patients with skin grafts and surgical flaps, pressure ulcers, edema, and malnutrition, as well as oncology, transplant, and orthopedic patients. The segmented air cushions, covered by a low-friction fabric, inflate and rest on a bed frame (similar to a standard bed frame), reducing pressure on skin surfaces and diminishing shearing forces when repositioning the patient. (*Note:* A maximum-inflate feature allows the entire surface to become firm for patient repositioning. The system is also capable of deflating quickly in emergencies.) As with a standard bed frame, the head and foot of the bed can be adjusted. Low-air-loss therapy beds circulate cool air, which helps to evaporate moisture and reduce temperature, thereby reducing excess skin moisture and preventing maceration. (See *Low-air-loss therapy bed.*)

Some models are equipped with pulsation or rotational capability. Pulsation promotes circulation, thus improving healing; and rotational capability better facilitates turning, thus mobilizing secretions and preventing pulmonary complications. Larger beds are available for patients who weigh more than 300 lb (135 kg). Further, pressure zones may be adjusted, and adjustable lumbar supports are available in some models.

The low-air-loss therapy bed is contraindicated for patients with an unstable cervical, thoracic, or lumbar fracture. Patients with uncontrolled diarrhea, hemodynamic instability, severe agitation, or uncontrolled claustrophobia may not benefit from this bed.

Equipment

Low-air-loss therapy bed ■ turning sheet.

Preparation of equipment

Usually the manufacturer's representative or a trained staff member prepares the bed for use. The unit is plugged in and turned on to inflate the bed. Make sure the bed inflates properly, and the equipment is in working order. The settings are adjusted as appropriate (such as degrees of rotation). Fully inflate until the patient is moved onto it.

Implementation

- Explain and, if possible, demonstrate the operation of the low-air-loss therapy bed. Tell the patient the reason for its use. Explain any special features of the bed (lumbar supports, rotation, and so forth).
- With the help of three or more coworkers, transfer the patient to the bed using a lift sheet.
- Resume the settings, as set by the representative, monitor the patient for comfort and proper body alignment, and ensure proper functioning of the bed.
- Adjust the inflation settings on the control panel according to the patient's comfort and therapeutic use.

Special considerations

- Encourage coughing and deep breathing every 2 hours.
- If the bed doesn't rotate, turn the patient at least every 2 hours, and reposition using an approved turning sheet. Some beds come with special foam wedges that are used for repositioning.
- To turn and reposition the patient, use the maximum inflate feature to fully inflate the bed. Use the turning sheet to position the patient and place the pillows or foam wedges. Then return the bed to the correct patient settings.
- If the bed is rotational, verify that invasive lines and tubes are secured at the correct angle *to minimize the risk of binding, disconnecting, or dislodging them.*
- To position a bedpan, deflate the seat portion of the bed, roll the patient away from you, and place the bedpan on the turning sheet. Then reposition the patient. To remove the bedpan, hold it steady, roll the patient away from you, and remove the bedpan. Then reinflate the seat portion of the bed.
- Don't use pins or clamps to secure sheets or tubing, *which may puncture the bed and result in air loss.* Take care to avoid puncturing the bed when giving injections.
- Assess the patient's skin every 2 hours.

Documentation

Record the duration of therapy and the patient's response to it. Document the condition of the patient's skin, including the presence of pressure ulcers and other wounds. Document the patient's comfort level and tolerance of rotational angles, as applicable.

SELECTED REFERENCES

Brienza, D.M., and Geyer, M.J. "Using Support Surfaces to Manage Tissue Integrity," *Advances in Skin & Wound Care* 18(3):151-57, April 2005.

Collins, F. "Russka Pressure-Relieving Low Air-Loss Mattress System," *British Journal of Nursing* 13(6 Suppl):S50-4, March 2004.

Ochs, R.F., et al. "Comparison of Air-Fluidized Therapy with Other Support Surfaces Used to Treat Pressure Ulcers in Nursing Home Residents," *Ostomy Wound Management* 51(2):38-68, February 2005.

BARIATRIC BEDS

Obesity affects nearly one-third of all Americans. A patient is considered obese if his body mass index is 30 kg/m^2 or greater. Bariatric patients may be hospitalized for medical issues or for surgery, including gastric bypass. Typical hospital beds are designed to hold patients weighing up to 450 pounds and who don't have a wide abdominal girth. Bariatric beds are a recent addition to hospital equipment designed to accommodate these larger patients. Various bariatric beds are available, ranging from simply being a larger version of a standard bed to a low-air-loss mattress that provides pressure relief.

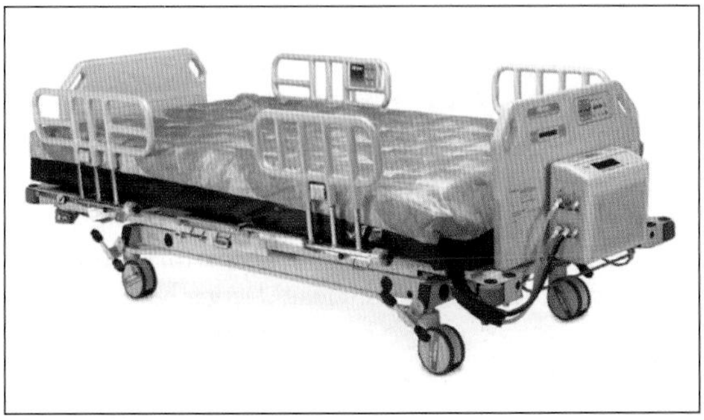

Use of a bariatric bed provides more comfort for obese patients than a standard-sized bed. It preserves self-esteem by providing these patients with a bed that easily fits their larger body size as well as special side rails that help them turn and reposition themselves. Bariatric beds also allow caregivers to perform routine care, such as boosting, turning, and transferring in and out of bed, with greater ease and less risk of injury. Most bariatric beds have a built-in scale that allows the nurse to more easily weigh the patient. Some bariatric beds easily convert to a cardiac chair.

Equipment
Bariatric bed ■ optional: overhead trapeze, special sheets.

Preparation of equipment
Prepare the bed according to the manufacturer's guidelines. A company representative may be involved in the patient assessment to ensure that the appropriate type and size of bed are provided. Choose the appropriate type of mattress to meet your patient's needs. Specialized sheets may be necessary. Attach an overhead trapeze if indicated.

Implementation
- Discuss the need for a specialized bed with the patient *so that he understands its benefits and therapeutic effects.*
- Consult with other health care team members, such as the practitioner, surgical team, physical therapy, occupational therapy, wound care, and respiratory therapy, to choose the appropriate type of bed for the patient's needs.
- Verify the practitioner's order for the bariatric bed.
- Obtain the bariatric bed from central supply, or contact the company representative to have the bed delivered, according to facility protocol.
- If the bed is rented, ask the company representative for an in-service *so that all health care team members understand its use and provide safe care.*
- Make sure that written instructions come with the bed, and keep them at the bedside.
- Provide the patient with any product information, and orient him to the bed functions and controls *so that he understands its many features and safe use.*

Special considerations
- Provide for other bariatric equipment, such as hospital gowns, commodes, wheelchairs, lifts, scales, and stretchers for patient comfort and safety.
- When sending the patient to other departments, call first to make sure they can accommodate a larger bed and are familiar with its use.

Documentation
Document the type of bed ordered and the date and time it was delivered. Indicate that staff was oriented to the use of the bed by the representative. Include that the patient was oriented to the safe use of the bed and that he gave a return demonstration. Note if written information was given to the patient or left at the bedside. Record any other equipment provided, such as an overhead trapeze or special sheets. Note the type of mattress on the bed. Document skin condition when patient is placed on the bed. Record the patient's response to the bed.

SELECTED REFERENCES

Arzouman, J., et al. "Developing a Comprehensive Bariatric Protocol: A Template for Improving Patient Care," *MedSurg Nursing* 15(1):21-26, February 2006.

Barth, M.M., and Jensen, C.E. "Postoperative Nursing Care of Gastric Bypass Patients," *American Journal of Critical Care,* 15(4):378-87, July 2006.

Grindel, M.E., and Grindel, C.G. "Nursing Care of the Person Having Bariatric Surgery," *MedSurg Nursing* 15(3):129-145, June 2006.

National Institutes of Health: Clinical Guidelines on the Identification, Evaluation and Treatment of Overweight and Obesity in Adults—Executive Summary: Evidence-Based Guidelines. Available at *www.nhlbi.nih.gov/guidelines/obesity/sum_evid.htm.*

Wright, W., and Bauer, C. "Meeting Bariatric Patient Care Needs. Procedures and Protocol Development," *Journal of Wound, Ostomy, and Continence Nursing* 32(6):402-405, November-December 2005.

ROTATION BEDS

Because of their constant motion, rotation beds—such as the Roto Rest—promote postural drainage and peristalsis and help prevent the complications of immobility. These beds rotate from side to side in a cradlelike motion, achieving a maximum elevation of 62 degrees and full side-to-side turning approximately every 4½ minutes.

Because the bed holds the patient motionless, it's especially helpful for patients with spinal cord injury, multiple trauma, stroke, multiple sclerosis, coma, severe burns, hypostatic pneumonia, atelectasis, or other unilateral lung involvement causing poor ventilation and perfusion.

Rotation beds such as the Roto Rest bed can accommodate cervical traction devices and tongs. One type of Roto Rest bed has an access hatch underneath for the perineal area; another type has access hatches for the perineal, cervical, and thoracic areas. Both have arm and leg hatches that fold down to allow range-of-motion (ROM) exercises. Other features include variable angles of rotation, a fan, access for X-rays, and supports and clips for chest tubes, catheters,

Roto Rest bed

Driven by a silent motor, the Roto Rest bed turns the immobilized patient slowly and continuously—more than 300 times daily. The motion provides constant passive exercise and peristaltic stimulation without depriving the patient of sleep or risking further injury. The bed is radiolucent, permitting X-rays to be taken through it without moving the patient. It also has a built-in cooling fan and allows access for surgery on multiple-trauma patients without disrupting spinal alignment or traction.

The bed's hatches provide access to various parts of the patient's body. Arm hatches permit full range of motion and have holes for chest tubes. Leg hatches allow full hip extension. The perineal hatch provides access for bowel and bladder care, the thoracic hatch for chest auscultation and lumbar puncture, and the cervical hatch for wound care, bathing, and shampooing.

Top view

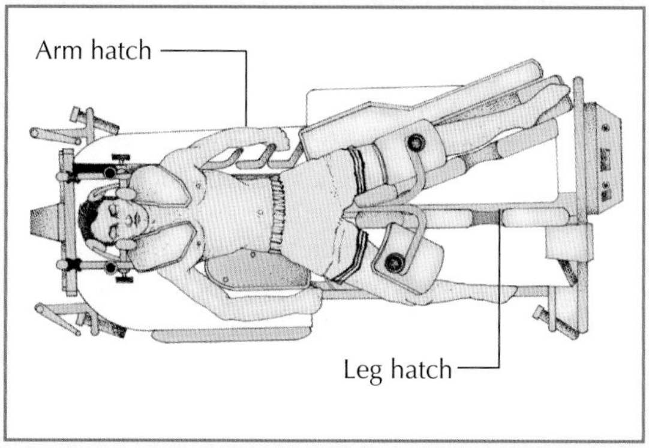

Back view

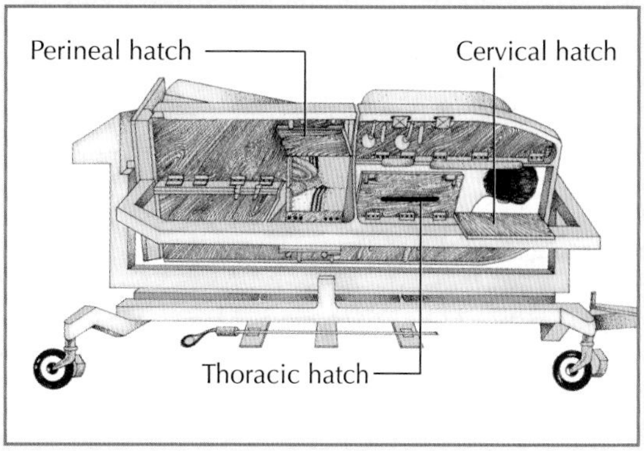

and drains. Racks beneath the bed hold X-ray plates in place for chest and spinal films. (See *Roto Rest bed.*)

Rotation beds are contraindicated for the patient who has severe claustrophobia or who has an unstable cervical fracture without neurologic deficit and the complications of immobility. Patient transfer and positioning on the bed should be performed by at least two persons to ensure the patient's safety.

The instructions given below apply to the Roto Rest bed.

Equipment

Rotation bed with appropriate accessories ▪ pillowcases or linen-saver pads ▪ flat sheet or padding.

Preparation of equipment

When using the Roto Rest bed, carefully inspect the bed, and run it through a complete cycle in both automatic and manual modes *to ensure that it's working properly.* If you're using the Mark I model, check the tightness of the set screws at the head of the bed.

To prepare the bed for the patient, remove the counterbalance weights from the keel, and place them in the base frame's storage area. Release the connecting arm by pulling down on the cam handle and depressing the lower side of the footboard. Next, lock the table in the horizontal position, and place all side supports in the extreme lateral position by loosening the cam handles on the underside of the table. Slide the supports off the bed. Note that all supports and packs are labeled RIGHT or LEFT on the bottom *to facilitate reassembly.*

Remove the knee packs by depressing the snap button and rotating and pulling the packs from the tube. Then remove the abductor packs (the Mark III model has only one) by depressing and sliding them toward the head of the bed. Next, loosen the foot and knee assemblies by lifting the cam handle at its base, and slide them to the foot of the bed. Finally, loosen the shoulder clamp assembly and knobs, swing the shoulder clamps to the vertical position, and retighten them.

If you're using the Mark I model, remove the cervical, thoracic, and perineal packs. Cover them with pillowcases or linen-saver pads, smooth all wrinkles, and replace the packs. If you're using the Mark III model, remove the perineal pack, cover, and replace. Cover the upper half of the bed, which is a solid unit, with padding or a sheet. Install new disposable foam cushions for the patient's head, shoulders, and feet.

Implementation

■ If possible, show the patient the bed before use. Explain and demonstrate its operation, and reassure the patient that the bed will hold him securely.
■ Before positioning the patient on the bed, make sure it's turned off. Then place and lock the bed in the horizontal position, out of gear. Latch all hatches and lock the wheels.
■ Obtain assistance and transfer the patient. Move him gently to the center of the bed *to prevent contact with the pillar posts and to ensure proper balance during bed operation.* Smooth the pillowcase or linen-saver pad beneath his hips. Then place any tubes through the appropriate notches in the hatches and ensure that any traction weights hang freely.
■ Insert the thoracic side supports in their posts. Adjust the patient's longitudinal position to allow a 1" (2.5 cm) space between the axillae and the supports, *thereby avoiding pressure on the axillary blood vessels and the brachial plexus.* Push the supports against his chest, and lock the cam arms securely *to provide support and ensure patient safety.*
■ Place the disposable supports under his legs *to remove pressure from his heels and prevent pressure ulcers.*
■ Install and adjust the foot supports so that the patient's feet lie in the normal anatomic position, *thereby helping to prevent footdrop.* The foot supports should be in position for only 2 hours of every shift *to prevent excessive pressure on the soles and toes.*
■ Place the abductor packs in the appropriate supports, allowing a 6" (15 cm) space between the packs and the patient's groin. Tighten the knobs on the bed's underside at the base of the support tubes.
■ Install the leg side supports snugly against the patient's hips, and tighten the cam arms. Position the knee assemblies slightly above his knees, and tighten the cam arms. Then place your hand on the patient's knee, and move the knee pack until it rests lightly on the top of your hand. Repeat for the other knee.
■ Loosen the retaining rings on the crossbar, and slide the head and shoulder assembly laterally. The retaining rings maintain correct lateral position of the shoulder clamp assembly and head support pack.
■ Carefully lower the head and shoulder assembly into place, and slide it to touch the patient's head.
■ Place your hand on the patient's shoulder, and move the shoulder pack until it touches your hand. Tighten it in place. Repeat for the other shoulder. *The 1" clearance between the shoulders and the packs prevents excess pressure, which can lead to pressure ulcers.*
■ Place the head pack close to, but not touching, the patient's ears (or tongs).
■ Tighten the head and shoulder assembly securely *so it won't lift off the bed.* Position the restraining rings next to the shoulder assembly bracket and tighten them.
■ Place the patient's arms on the disposable supports. Install the side arm supports and secure the safety straps, placing one across the shoulder assembly and the other over the thoracic supports. If necessary, cover the patient with a flat sheet.
■ Make sure all tubing is intact and secured *so it won't be pulled out upon turning.*

Balancing the bed

■ Place one hand on the footboard *to prevent the bed from turning rapidly if it's unbalanced.* Then remove the locking pin. If the bed rotates to one side, reposition the patient in its center; if it tilts to the right, gently turn it slightly to the left and slide the packs on the right side toward the patient; if it tilts to the left, reverse the process. If a large imbalance exists, you may have to adjust the packs on both sides.
■ After the patient is centered, gently turn the bed to the 62-degree position.
■ Measure the space between the patient's chest, hip, and thighs and the inside of the packs. If this space exceeds ½" (1.3 cm) for the Mark III model or 1" (2.5 cm) for the Mark I, return the bed to horizontal position, lock it in place, and slide the packs inward on both sides. If the space appears too tight, proceed as above, but slide both packs outward. *Excessively loose packs cause the patient to slide from side to side during turning, possibly resulting in unnecessary movement at fracture sites, skin irritation from shearing force, and bed imbalance. Overly tight packs can place pressure on the patient during turning.*
■ After adjusting the packs, check the bed; balance it and make any necessary adjustments.
■ If you're using the Mark III model bed, and the patient weighs more than 160 lb (72.5 kg), the bed may become top-heavy. *To correct this,* place counterbalance weights in the appropriate slots in the keel of the bed. Add one weight for every 20 lb (9 kg) over 160, but remember that placement of weights doesn't replace correct patient positioning.
■ If you're using the Mark I model, it may be necessary to add weights for the patient weighing less than 160 lb. Place one weight for each 20 lb less than 160 in the proper bracket at the foot of the bed.

Initiating automatic bed rotation

■ Ensure that all packs are securely in place. Then hold the footboard firmly, and remove the locking pin *to start the bed's motor.* The bed will continue to rotate until the pin is reinserted.

■ Raise the connecting arm cam handle until the connecting assembly snaps into place, locking the bed into automatic rotation.

■ Remain with the patient for at least three complete turns from side to side *to evaluate his comfort and safety.* Observe his response and offer him emotional support.

Special considerations

■ If the patient develops cardiac arrest while on the bed, perform cardiopulmonary resuscitation after taking the bed out of gear, locking it in the horizontal position, removing the side arm support and the thoracic pack, lifting the shoulder assembly, and dropping the arm pack. Doing all these steps takes only 5 to 10 seconds. You won't need a cardiac board *because of the bed's firm surface.*

■ If the electricity fails, lock the bed in the horizontal or lateral position, and rotate it manually every 30 minutes *to prevent pressure ulcers.* If cervical traction causes the patient to slide upward, place the bed in reverse Trendelenburg's position; if extremity traction causes the patient to migrate toward the foot of the bed, use Trendelenburg's position.

■ Lock the bed in the extreme lateral position for access to the back of the head, thorax, and buttocks through the appropriate hatches. Clean the mattress and nondisposable packs during patient care, and rinse them thoroughly *to remove all soap residue.* When replacing the packs and hatches, take care not to pinch the patient's skin between the packs. *This can cause pain and tissue necrosis.*

■ Expect increased drainage from any pressure ulcers for the first few days the patient is on the bed *because the motion helps debride necrotic tissue and improves local circulation.*

■ Perform or schedule daily ROM exercises, as ordered, *because the bed allows full access to all extremities without disturbing spinal alignment.* Drop the arm hatch for shoulder rotation, remove the thoracic packs for shoulder abduction, and drop the leg hatch and remove leg and knee packs for hip rotation and full leg motion.

■ For female patients, tape an indwelling urinary catheter to the thigh before bringing it through the perineal hatch. For the male patient with spinal cord lesions, tape the catheter to the abdomen and then to the thigh *to facilitate gravity drainage.* Hang the drainage bag on the clips provided, and make sure it doesn't become caught between the bed frames during rotation.

■ If the patient has a tracheal or endotracheal tube and is on mechanical ventilation, attach the tube support bracket between the cervical pack and the arm packs. Tape the connecting T tubing to the support, and run it beside the patient's head and off the center of the table *to help prevent reflux of condensation.*

■ For a patient with pulmonary congestion or pneumonia, suction secretions more often during the first 12 to 24 hours on the bed *because the motion will increase drainage.* A vibrator is available for use under the thoracic hatch of the Mark I to help mobilize pulmonary secretions more quickly.

Documentation

Record changes in the patient's condition and his response to therapy in your progress notes. Note turning times and ongoing care on the flowchart.

SELECTED REFERENCES

Anderson, C., and Rappl, L. "Lateral Rotation Mattresses for Wound Healing," *Ostomy Wound Management* 50(4):50-58, April 2004.

Goldhill, D.R., et al. "Rotational Bed Therapy to Prevent and Treat Respiratory Complications: A Review and Meta-Analysis," *American Journal of Critical Care* 16(1):50-61 January 2007.

Marlew, A. "Body Positioning and Its Effects on Oxygenation: A Literature Review," *Nursing in Critical Care* 11(1):16-22, January-February 2006.

McCool, F.D., and Rosen, M.J. "Nonpharmacologic Airway Clearance Therapies: AACP Evidence-Based Clinical Practice Guidelines," *Chest* 129(1 Suppl):2505-595, January 2006.

AIR-FLUIDIZED THERAPY BEDS

Originally designed for managing burns, the air-fluidized therapy bed is now used for patients with other conditions, such as pressure ulcers, wounds, and surgical flaps and grafts. By allowing harmless contact between the bed's surface and grafted sites, the bed promotes comfort and healing.

The traditional bed is actually a large tub that supports the patient on a thick layer of silicone-coated microspheres. Another version combines the air-fluidized section with a low-air-loss or cushioned section. (See *Air-fluidized therapy bed,* page 100.) A monofilament polyester filter sheet covers the microsphere-filled area, allowing moisture to pass through. Warmed air, propelled by a blower beneath the bed, passes through it. The resulting fluidlike surface reduces pressure on the skin to avoid obstructing capillary blood flow, thereby helping to prevent pressure ulcers and to promote wound healing. The bed's air temperature can be adjusted to help control hypothermia and hyperthermia. The

Air-fluidized therapy bed

The air-fluidized therapy bed is a large tub filled with microspheres that are suspended by air pressure and give the patient fluidlike support. The bed provides the advantages of flotation without the disadvantages of instability, patient positioning difficulties, and immobility.

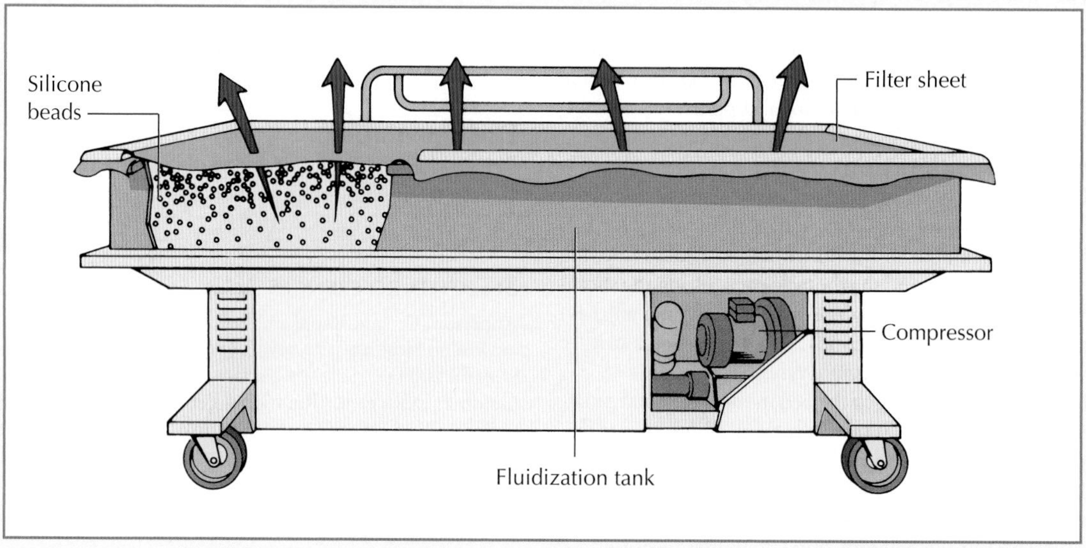

microprocessor technology also allows manipulation of various sections of the unit for optimum patient adjustment.

The air-fluidized therapy bed is contraindicated for patients with an unstable spine. The fully air-fluidized therapy bed may also be contraindicated for the patient unable to mobilize and expel pulmonary secretions *because the lack of back support impairs productive coughing.* Some models come with adjustable back and leg supports to promote positioning.

Equipment

Air-fluidized therapy bed with microspheres (about 1,650 lb [748 kg]) ▪ filter sheet ▪ flat sheet ▪ elastic cord.

Preparation of equipment

Usually, a manufacturer's representative or a trained staff member prepares the bed for use. If you must help with the preparation, make sure the microspheres reach to within ½″ (1.3 cm) of the top of the filter sheet. Then position the filter sheet on the bed with its printed side facing up. Match the holes in the sheet to the holes in the edge of the bed's frame. If the bed has detachable aluminum rails, place them on the frame, with the studs in the proper holes. Depress the rails firmly, and secure them by tightening the knurled knobs to seal the filter sheet. Place a flat hospital sheet over the filter sheet or specialized sheet provided by the bed company, and secure it with the elastic cord. Turn on the air current *to activate the microspheres and to ensure that the bed is working properly;* then turn it off.

Implementation

- Explain and, if possible, demonstrate the operation of the air-fluidized therapy bed. Tell the patient the reason for its use and that he'll feel as though he's floating.
- With the help of three or more coworkers, transfer the patient to the bed using a lift sheet.
- Turn on the air pressure to activate the bed.
- Adjust the air temperature as necessary. *Because the bed usually operates within 10° to 12° F (5.6° to 6.7° C) of ambient air temperature,* set the room temperature to 75° F (23.9° C). If microsphere temperature reaches 105° F (40.6° C), the bed automatically shuts off. It restarts automatically after 30 minutes.

Special considerations

■ Monitor fluid and electrolyte status *because the air-fluidized bed promotes evaporative water loss.* Because of this drying effect, always cover a mesh graft for the first 2 to 8 days as ordered. If the patient has excessive upper respiratory tract dryness, use a humidifier and mask as ordered. Encourage coughing and deep breathing every 2 hours or as per your facility's policy.

NURSING ALERT *Observe patients on prolonged bed rest for hypocalcemia and hypophosphatemia.*

■ To position a bedpan, roll the patient away from you, place the bedpan on the flat sheet, and push it into the microspheres. Then reposition the patient. To remove the bedpan, hold it steady and roll the patient away from you. Turn off the air pressure, and remove the bedpan. Then turn the air on, and reposition the patient.

■ Don't secure the filter sheet with pins or clamps, *which may puncture the sheet and release microspheres.* Take care to avoid puncturing the bed when giving injections. Holes or tears may be repaired with iron-on patching tape. Sieve the microspheres monthly or between patients *to remove any clumped microspheres.* Handle them carefully to avoid spills; *spilled microspheres may cause falls.* Treat a soiled filter sheet and clumped microspheres as contaminated items; handle according to policy. Change the filter sheet, and operate the unit unoccupied for 24 hours between patients.

■ Assess the patient's skin, and reposition him every 2 hours. *Specialty beds don't eliminate the need for frequent assessment and position changes.*

■ For cardiopulmonary resuscitation, an emergency STOP/DEFLATE button immediately stops the action of the bed.

■ Use the foam wedge to elevate the head of the bed for patients with tube feedings *to prevent aspiration.*

Documentation

Record the duration of therapy and the patient's response to it. Document the condition of the patient's skin, pressure ulcers, and other wounds.

SELECTED REFERENCES

Edlich, R.F., et al. "Pressure Ulcer Prevention," *Journal of Long Term Effects of Medical Implants* 14(4):285-304, 2004.

Hickerson, W.L. "Comparison of Total Body Tissue Interface Pressure of Specialized Pressure-Relieving Mattresses," *Journal of Long Term Effects of Medical Implants* 14(2):81-94, 2004.

Ochs, R.F., et al. "Comparison of Air-Fluidized Therapy with Other Support Surfaces Used to Treat Pressure Ulcers in Nursing Home Residents," *Ostomy Wound Management* 51(2):38-68, February 2005.

PERSONAL HYGIENE AND COMFORT

MAKING AN UNOCCUPIED BED

Although considered routine, daily changing and periodic straightening of bed linens promotes patient comfort and prevents skin breakdown. When preceded by hand washing, performed using clean technique, and followed by proper handling and disposal of soiled linens, this procedure helps control nosocomial infections.

Equipment

Two sheets (one fitted, if available) ■ pillowcase ■ bedspread ■ gloves ■ optional: bath blanket, laundry bag, linen-saver pads, drawsheet.

Preparation of equipment

Obtain clean linen, which should be folded in half lengthwise and then folded again. If the linen is folded incorrectly, refold it. The bottom sheet should be folded so the rough side of the hem is facedown when placed on the bed; *this helps prevent skin irritation caused by the rough hem edge rubbing against the patient's heels.* The top sheet should be folded similarly so that the smooth side of the hem is face up when folded over the spread, *to give the bed a finished appearance.*

Implementation

■ Wash your hands thoroughly, put on gloves, and bring clean linen to the patient's bedside. If the patient is present, tell him that you're going to change his bed. Help him to a chair if necessary.

■ Move any furniture away from the bed *to provide ample working space.*

■ Lower the head of the bed to make the mattress level and ensure tight-fitting, wrinkle-free linens. Then raise the bed to a comfortable working height *to prevent back strain.*

■ When stripping the bed, watch for any belongings that may have fallen among the linens.

■ Remove the pillowcase and place it in the middle of the bed, or use it, hooked over the back of a chair, as a laundry bag. Set the pillow aside.

■ Lift the mattress edge slightly and work around the bed, untucking the linens. If you plan to reuse the top linens, fold the top hem of the spread down to the bottom hem. Then pick up the hemmed corners, fold the spread into quarters, and hang it over the back of the chair. Do the same for the top sheet. Otherwise, carefully remove and place the top linens in the laundry bag or pillowcase. *To avoid spreading microorganisms,* don't fan the linens, hold them against your clothing, or place them on the floor.

- Remove the soiled bottom linens, and place them in the laundry bag.
- If the mattress has slid downward, push it to the head of the bed. *Adjusting it after bed making loosens the linens.*
- Place the bottom sheet with its center fold in the middle of the mattress.
- For a fitted sheet, secure the top and bottom corners over the mattress corners on the side of the bed nearest you. For a flat sheet, align the end of the sheet with the foot of the mattress, and miter the top corner *to keep the sheet firmly tucked under the mattress.* To miter the corner, first tuck the top end of the sheet evenly under the mattress at the head of the bed. Then lift the side edge of the sheet about 12″ (30 cm) from the mattress corner, and hold it at a right angle to the mattress. Tuck in the bottom edge of the sheet hanging below the mattress. Finally, drop the top edge and tuck it under the mattress. (See *Making a mitered corner.*)
- After tucking under one side of the bottom sheet, place the drawsheet (if needed) about 15″ (38 cm) from the top of the bed, with its center fold in the middle of the bed. Then tuck in the entire edge of the drawsheet on that side of the bed.
- Place the top sheet with its center fold in the middle of the bed and its wide hem even with the top of the bed. Position the rough side of the hem face up *so that the smooth side shows after folding.* Allow enough sheet at the top of the bed to form a cuff over the spread.
- Place the spread over the top sheet, with its center fold in the middle of the bed. (If the patient will be returning from surgery, use the alternative technique described in *Making a surgical bed,* page 104.)
- Make a 3″ (7.6-cm) toe pleat, or vertical tuck, in the top linens *to allow room for the patient's feet and to prevent pressure that can cause discomfort, skin breakdown, and footdrop.*
- Tuck the top sheet and spread under the foot of the mattress. Then miter the bottom corners.
- Move to the opposite side of the bed, and repeat the procedure.
- After fitting all corners of the bottom sheet or tucking them under the mattress, pull the sheet at an angle from the head toward the foot of the bed. *This tightens the linens, making the bottom sheet taut and wrinkle-free and promoting patient comfort.*
- Fold the top sheet over the spread at the head of the bed *to form a cuff and to give the bed a finished appearance.* When making an open bed, fanfold the top linens to the foot of the bed. If a linen-saver pad is needed, place it on top of the bottom sheets.
- Slip the pillow into a clean case, tucking in the corners. Then place the pillow with its seam toward the top of the bed *to prevent it from rubbing against the patient's neck, causing irritation,* and its open edge facing away from the door *to give the bed a finished appearance.*
- Lower the bed and lock its wheels *to ensure the patient's safety.*
- Return furniture to its proper place, and place the call bell within the patient's easy reach. Carry away soiled linens in outstretched arms *to avoid contaminating your uniform.*
- After disposing of the linens, remove gloves if used, and wash your hands thoroughly *to prevent the spread of microorganisms.*

Special considerations

- *Because a hospital mattress is usually covered with plastic to protect it and to facilitate cleaning between patients,* a flat bottom sheet tends to loosen and become untucked. Use a fitted sheet, if available, *to prevent this.*
- If a fitted sheet isn't available, the top corners of a flat sheet may be tied together under the top of the mattress *to prevent the sheet from becoming dislodged.*
- A bath blanket placed on top of the mattress, under the bottom sheet, *helps to absorb moisture and prevent dislodgment of the bottom sheet.*

Documentation

Although linen changes aren't usually documented, record their dates and times in your notes for patients with incontinence, excessive wound drainage, or diaphoresis.

SELECTED REFERENCES

Craven, R.F., and Hirnle, C.J. *Fundamentsl of Nursing: Human Health and Function,* 5th ed. Philadelphia: Lippincott Williams & Wilkins, 2007.

Edlich, R.F., et al. "Pressure Ulcer Prevention," *Journal of Long Term Effects of Medical Implants* 14(4):285-304, 2004.

Taylor, C., et al. *Fundamentals of Nursing: The Art and Science of Nursing Care,* 6th ed. Philadelphia: Lippincott Williams & Wilkins, 2008.

Thomas, D.R. "Prevention and Treatment of Pressure Ulcers," *Journal of American Medical Directors Association* 7(1):46-49, January 2006.

Thompson, P., et al. "Skin Care Protocol for Pressure Ulcers and Incontinence in Long Term Care: a Quasi-Experimental Study," *Advances in Skin & Wound Care* 18(8):422-29, October 2005.

Making a mitered corner

To make a mitered corner, after placing the sheet on the bed, grasp the side edge of the sheet, and lift it up to form a triangle.

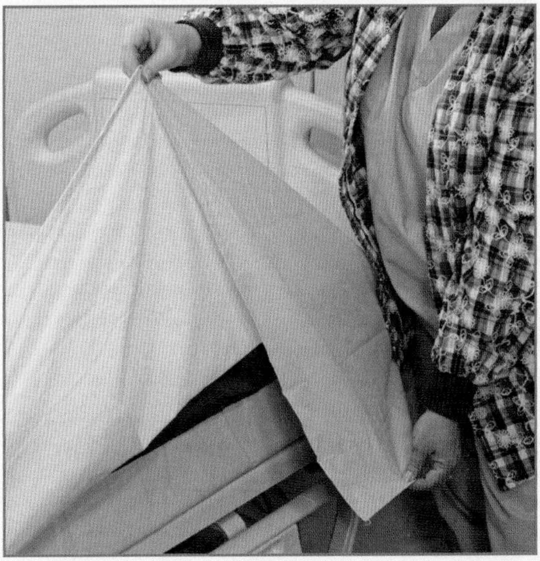

Then place the sheet on the top of the bed, making a flat triangular fold.

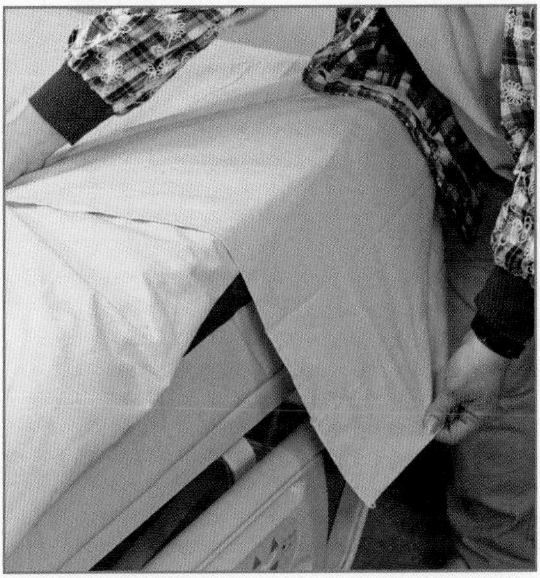

While holding the point of the triangle on the bed, tuck the sheet under the mattress.

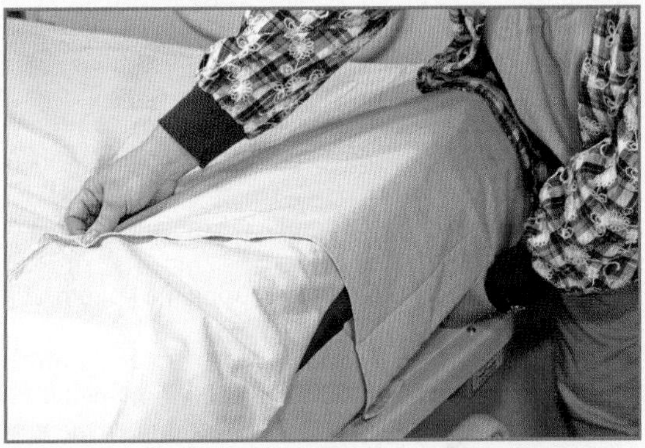

Take the triangular fold from the mattress, and place it over the side of the mattress.

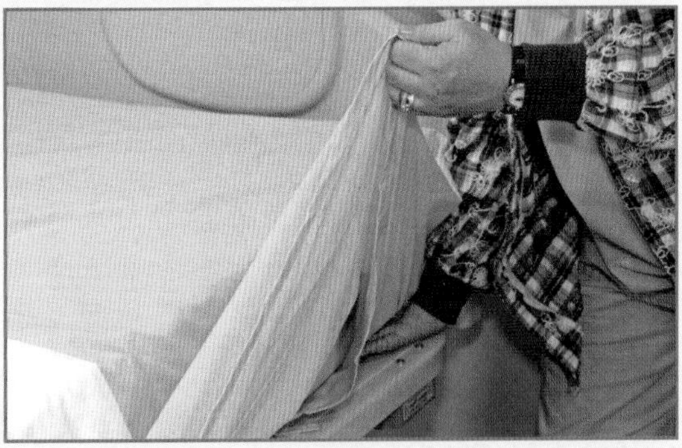

Tuck the remaining end of the triangular linen fold under the mattress.

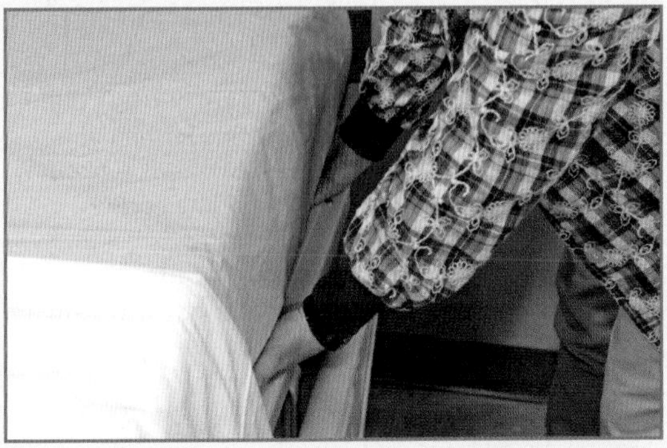

Making a surgical bed

Preparation of a surgical bed permits easy patient transfer from surgery and promotes cleanliness and comfort. To make such a bed, take the following steps:

- Assemble linens as you would for making an unoccupied bed, including two clean sheets (one fitted, if available), a drawsheet, a bath blanket, a spread or sheet, a pillowcase, facial tissues, a trash bag, and linen-saver pads. Raise the bed to a comfortable working height *to prevent back strain.*
- Slip the pillow into a clean pillowcase, and place it on a nearby table or chair.
- Make the foundation of the bed using the bottom sheet and drawsheet.
- Place an open bath blanket about 15" (38 cm) from the head of the bed, with its center fold positioned in the middle of the bed. *The blanket warms the patient and counteracts the decreased body temperature caused by anesthesia.*
- Place a top sheet or spread on the bath blanket, and position it as you did the blanket. Then fold the blanket and sheet back from the top so that the blanket shows over the sheet. Similarly, fold the sheet and blanket up from the bottom (as shown in illustration 1).
- On the side of the bed where you'll receive the patient, fold up the two outer corners of the sheet and blanket so they meet in the middle of the bed (as shown in illustration 2).
- Pick up the point hanging over this side of the bed, and fanfold the linens back to the other side of the bed *so the linens won't interfere with patient transfer* (as shown in illustration 3).
- Raise the bed to the high position if you haven't already done so. Then lock the wheels and lower the side rails. Make sure that the side rails work properly. Move the bedside stand and other objects out of the stretcher's path *to facilitate easy transfer when the patient arrives.*
- After the patient is transferred to the bed, position the pillow for his comfort and safety. Cover him by pulling the top point of the sheet and blanket over him and opening the folds. After covering the patient, tuck in the linens at the foot of the bed and miter the corners.
- *To make the patient comfortable and prevent unnecessary movement and linen changes,* try to anticipate and be ready for his special needs. For nausea, keep an emesis basin, facial tissues, and linen-saver pads at the bedside. Also, remove all liquids from the bedside. If you expect bleeding or discharge, place one or more pads on the bed.
- Keep extra pillows handy *to elevate arms and legs and to promote circulation, thereby preventing edema.* If necessary, have I.V. equipment, suction apparatus, roller for patient transfer, or other special equipment ready.

1.

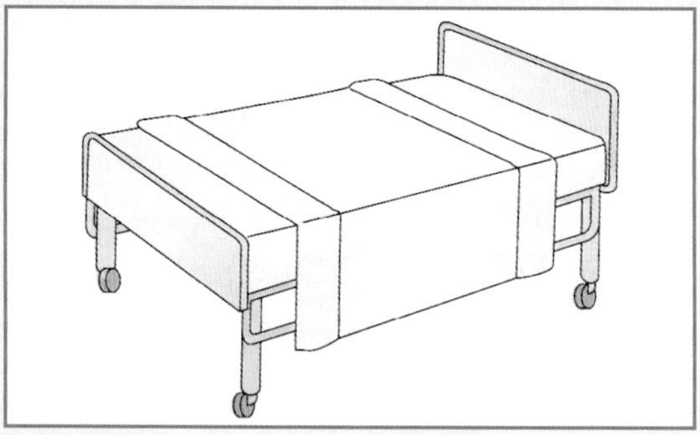

2.

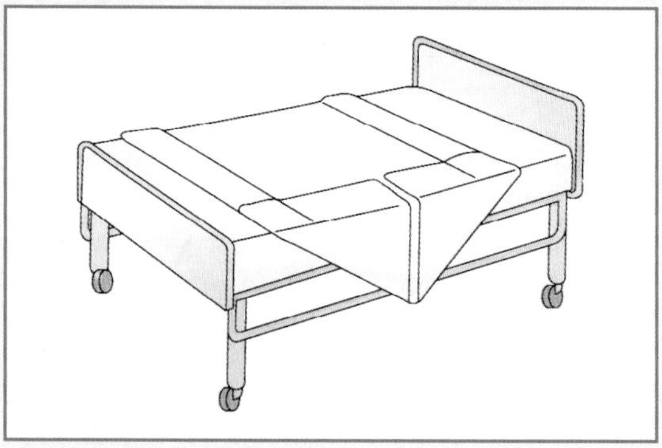

3.

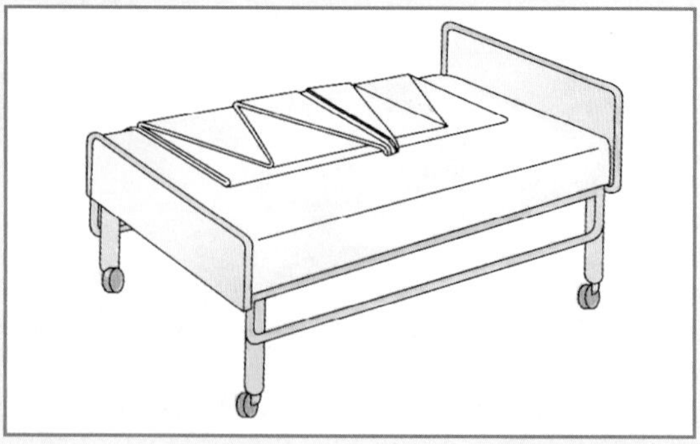

MAKING AN OCCUPIED BED

For the bedridden patient, linen changes promote comfort and help prevent skin breakdown and nosocomial infection. Such changes necessitate the use of side rails to prevent the patient from rolling out of bed and, depending on the patient's condition, the use of a turning sheet to move him from side to side.

Making an occupied bed may require more than one person. It also entails loosening the bottom sheet on one side and fanfolding it to the center of the mattress instead of loosening the bottom sheet on both sides and removing it, as in an unoccupied bed. Also, the foundation of the bed must be made before the top sheet is applied instead of both the foundation and top being made on one side before being completed on the other side. (See *Making a traction bed,* page 106.)

Equipment

Two sheets (one fitted, if available) ▪ pillowcase ▪ one or two drawsheets ▪ spread ▪ one or two bath blankets ▪ gloves ▪ sheepskin or other comfort-enhancing device, as needed ▪ optional: laundry bag, linen-saver pad.

Preparation of equipment

Obtain clean linen and make sure it's folded properly, as for an unoccupied bed.

Implementation

- Wash your hands, put on gloves, and bring clean linen to the patient's room.
- Identify the patient, and tell him you'll be changing his bed linens. Explain how he can help if he's able, adjusting the plan according to his abilities and needs. Provide privacy.
- Move any furniture away from the bed *to ensure ample working space.*
- Raise the side rail on the far side of the bed *to prevent falls.* Adjust the bed to a comfortable working height *to prevent back strain.*
- If allowed, lower the head of the bed to ensure tight-fitting, wrinkle-free linens.
- When stripping the bed, watch for belongings among the linens.
- Cover the patient with a bath blanket *to avoid exposure and provide warmth and privacy.* Then fanfold the top sheet and spread from beneath the bath blanket, and bring them back over the blanket. Loosen the top linens at the foot of the bed, and remove them separately. If reusing the top linens, fold each piece, and hang it over the back of the chair. Otherwise, place it in the laundry bag. *To avoid dispersing microorganisms,* don't fan the linens, hold them against your clothing, or place them on the floor.
- If the mattress slides down when the head of the bed is raised, pull it up again. *Adjusting the mattress after the bed is made loosens the linens.* If the patient is able, ask him to grasp the head of the bed and pull with you; otherwise, ask a coworker to help you.
- Roll the patient to the far side of the bed, and turn the pillow lengthwise under his head *to support his neck.* Ask him to help (if he can) by grasping the far side rail as he turns *so that he's positioned at the far side of the bed.*
- Loosen the soiled bottom linens on the side of the bed nearest you. Then roll the linens toward the patient's back in the middle of the bed as shown below.

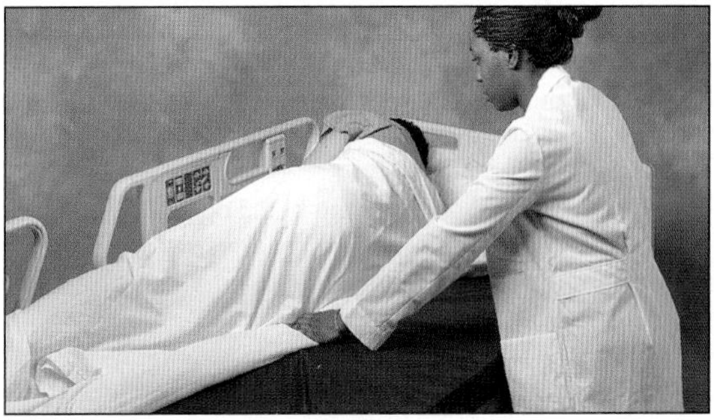

- Place a clean bottom sheet on the bed, with its center fold in the middle of the mattress. For a fitted sheet, secure the top and bottom corners over the side of the mattress nearest you. For a flat sheet, place its end even with the foot of the mattress. Miter the top corner as you would for an unoccupied bed *to keep linens firmly tucked under the mattress, preventing wrinkling.*
- Fanfold the remaining clean bottom sheet toward the patient, and place the drawsheet, if needed, about 15″ (38 cm) from the top of the bed, with its center fold in the middle of the mattress. Tuck in the entire edge of the drawsheet on the side nearest you. Fanfold the remaining drawsheet toward the patient as shown below.

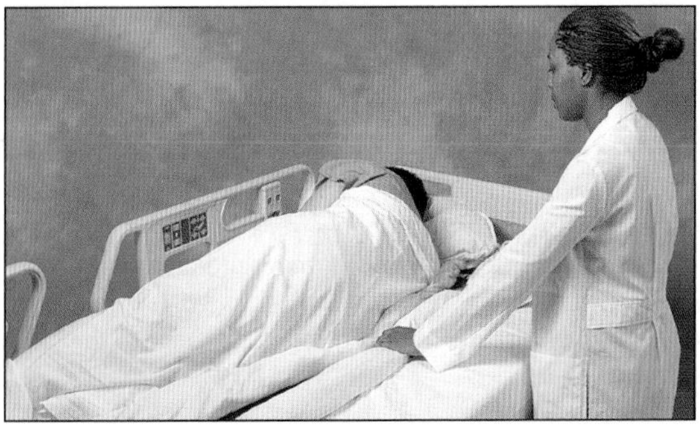

Making a traction bed

For a patient in traction, obtain help from a coworker to make the bed. Work from head to toe *to minimize the risk of traction misalignment.*

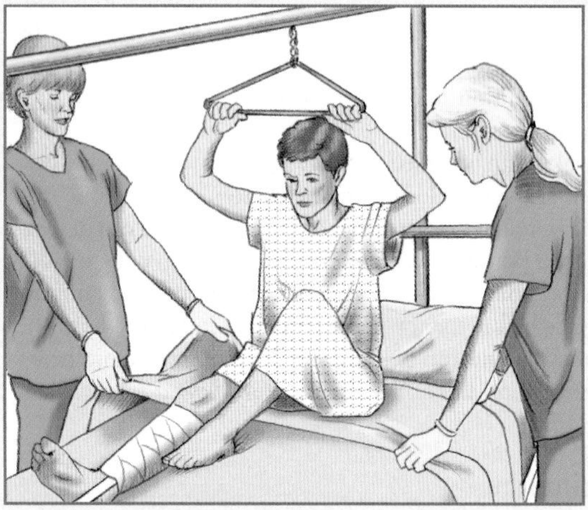

Preparation

■ Wash your hands. Put on gloves, if necessary. Bring clean linen and arrange it in the order of use on the bedside stand or a chair.
■ Explain the procedure, provide privacy, and remove unnecessary furniture.

Changing the linens

■ Lower both side rails. Stand near the headboard, opposite your coworker.
■ Gently pull the mattress to the head of the bed. Avoid sudden movements *because they can misalign traction and cause patient discomfort.*
■ Remove the pillow from the bed. Loosen the bottom linens, and roll them from the headboard toward the patient's head. Then remove the soiled pillowcase, and replace it with a clean one.
■ Fold a clean bottom sheet crosswise, and place the sheet across the head of the bed. Tell the patient to raise her head and upper shoulders by grasping the trapeze above the bed (as shown at right). With your coworker, quickly fanfold the bottom sheet from the head of the bed under the patient's shoulders, so that it meets the soiled linen. Tuck at least 12″ (30 cm) of the bottom sheet under the head of the mattress. Miter the corners and tuck in the sides.
■ Tell the patient to raise her buttocks by grasping the trapeze. As a team, move toward the foot of the bed and, in one movement, quickly and carefully roll soiled linens and clean linens under the patient.
■ Instruct the patient to release the trapeze and to rest. Place a pillow under her head for comfort.
■ If allowed, remove any pillows from under the patient's extremity. If pillow removal is contraindicated, continue to move linens toward the foot of the bed and under the patient's legs and traction while your coworker lifts the pillows and supports the patient's extremity.
■ Put soiled linens in a laundry bag or pillowcase.
■ Tuck the remaining loose linens securely under the mattress. *To ensure a tight-fitting bottom sheet,* have the patient raise herself off the bed by simultaneously grasping the trapeze and raising her buttocks while you pull the sheet tight. As needed, place a drawsheet, linen-saver pad, or sheepskin under her. Complete the bed-making alone.
■ If the bottom sheet doesn't cover the foot of the mattress, cover it with a drawsheet. Miter its corners and tuck in the sides.
■ Replace the pillows under the patient's extremity, then cover her with a clean top sheet. Fold over the top hem of the sheet approximately 8″ (20 cm). If one or both legs are in traction, fit the lower end of the sheet loosely over the traction apparatus; don't press on the traction ropes. To secure the sheet, tuck in the corner opposite the traction under the foot of the bed, and miter the corner. Neatly tuck in the lower corner of the sheet on the traction side to expose the leg and foot.
■ If the traction equipment exposes the patient's sides, cover her with a drawsheet, not a full sheet or spread.
■ Lower the bed, but don't allow the traction weights to touch the floor. Raise the side rails to prevent falls. If allowed, however, leave one side rail down so the patient can reach the bedside stand.

■ If necessary, position a linen-saver pad on the drawsheet *to absorb excretions or surgical drainage*, and fanfold it toward the patient.
■ Raise the other side rail, and roll the patient to the clean side of the bed.
■ Move to the unfinished side of the bed, and lower the side rail nearest you. Then loosen and remove the soiled bottom linens separately and place them in the laundry bag.
■ Pull the clean bottom sheet taut. Secure the fitted sheet or place the end of a flat sheet even with the foot of the bed,

and miter the top corner. Pull the drawsheet taut, and tuck it in. Unfold and smooth the linen-saver pad, if used.

- Assist the patient to the supine position if his condition permits.
- Remove the soiled pillowcase, and place it in the laundry bag. Then slip the pillow into a clean pillowcase, tucking its corners well into the case *to ensure a smooth fit.* Place the pillow beneath the patient's head, with its seam toward the top of the bed *to prevent it from rubbing against the patient's neck, causing irritation.* Place the pillow's open edge away from the door *to give the bed a finished appearance.*
- Unfold the clean top sheet over the patient with the rough side of the hem facing away from the bed *to avoid irritating the patient's skin.* Allow enough sheet to form a cuff over the spread.
- Remove the bath blanket from beneath the sheet, and center the spread over the top sheet.
- Make a 3″ (7.6 cm) toe pleat, or vertical tuck, in the top linens to allow room for the patient's feet and prevent pressure that can cause discomfort, skin breakdown, and footdrop.
- Tuck the top sheet and spread under the foot of the bed, and miter the bottom corners. Fold the top sheet over the spread *to give the bed a finished appearance.*
- Raise the head of the bed to a comfortable position, make sure both side rails are raised, and then lower the bed and lock its wheels *to ensure the patient's safety.* Assess the patient's body alignment and his mental and emotional status.
- Place the call bell within the patient's easy reach. Remove the laundry bag from the room.
- Remove and discard gloves, and wash your hands to prevent the spread of nosocomial infections.

Special considerations

- Use a fitted sheet, when available, *because a flat sheet slips out from under the mattress easily, especially if the mattress is plastic-coated.*
- *To prevent the patient from sliding down in bed,* tuck a tightly rolled pillow under the top linens at the foot of the bed.
- For the diaphoretic or bedridden patient, fold a bath blanket in half lengthwise, and place it between the bottom sheet and the plastic mattress cover; *the blanket acts as a cushion and helps absorb moisture. To help prevent sheet burns on the heels and bony prominences,* center a bath blanket or sheepskin over the bottom sheet, and tuck the blanket under the mattress.
- If the patient can't help you move or turn him, devise a turning sheet *to facilitate bed making and repositioning.* To do this, first fold a drawsheet or bath blanket, and place it under the patient's buttocks. Make sure the sheet extends from the shoulders to the knees *so that it supports most of the patient's weight.* Roll the sides of the sheet to form handles. Next, ask a coworker to help you lift and move the patient. With one person holding each side of the sheet, you can move the patient without wrinkling the bottom linens. If you can't get help and must turn the patient yourself, stand at the side of the bed. Turn the patient toward the rail, and, if he's able, ask him to grasp the opposite rolled edge of the turning sheet. Pull the rolled edge carefully toward you, and turn the patient.

Documentation

Although linen changes aren't usually documented, record their dates and times in your notes for patients with incontinence, excessive wound drainage, pressure ulcers, or diaphoresis.

SELECTED REFERENCES

Craven, R.F., and Hirnle, C.J. *Fundamentsl of Nursing: Human Health and Function,* 5th ed. Philadelphia: Lippincott Williams & Wilkins, 2007.

Edlich, R.F., et al. "Pressure Ulcer Prevention," *Journal of Long Term Effects of Medical Implants* 14(4):285-304, 2004.

Taylor, C., et al. *Fundamentals of Nursing: The Art and Science of Nursing Care,* 6th ed. Philadelphia: Lippincott Williams & Wilkins, 2008.

Thomas, D.R. "Prevention and Treatment of Pressure Ulcers," *Journal of American Medical Directors Association* 7(1):46-49, January 2006.

Thompson, P., et al. "Skin Care Protocol for Pressure Ulcers and Incontinence in Long Term Care: a Quasi-Experimental Study," *Advances in Skin & Wound Care* 18(8):422-29, October 2005.

BED BATH

A complete bed bath cleans the skin, stimulates circulation, provides mild exercise, and promotes comfort. Bathing also allows assessment of skin condition, joint mobility, and muscle strength. Depending on the patient's overall condition and duration of hospitalization, he may have a complete or partial bath daily. A partial bath—including hands, face, axillae, back, genitalia, and anal region—can replace the complete bath for the patient with dry, fragile skin or extreme weakness, and can supplement the complete bath for the diaphoretic or incontinent patient.

Equipment

Bath basin ▪ bath blanket ▪ soap ▪ towel ▪ washcloth ▪ skin lotion ▪ orangewood stick ▪ gloves ▪ deodorant ▪ optional: bath oil, perineal pad, abdominal pad, linen-saver pad.

Preparation of equipment

Adjust the temperature of the patient's room, and close any doors or windows to prevent drafts and provide privacy. Determine the patient's preference for soap or other hygiene aids *because some patients are allergic to soap or prefer bath oil or lotions.* Assemble the equipment on an overbed table or bedside stand.

Implementation

- Tell the patient you'll be giving him a bath, and provide privacy. If the patient's condition permits, encourage him to assist with bathing *to provide exercise and promote independence.*
- Raise the patient's bed to a comfortable working height *to avoid back strain.* Offer him a bedpan or urinal.
- Fill the bath basin two-thirds full of warm water (about 115° F [46.1° C]), and bring it to the patient's bedside. If a bath thermometer isn't available, test the water temperature carefully with your elbow *to avoid scalding or chilling the patient*; the water should feel comfortably warm.
- If the bed will be changed after the bath, remove the top linen. If not, fanfold it to the foot of the bed.
- Put on gloves. Position the patient supine if possible.
- Remove the patient's gown and other articles, such as elastic stockings, elastic bandages, and restraints (as ordered). Cover him with a bath blanket *to provide warmth and privacy.*
- Place a towel under the patient's chin. To wash his face, begin with the eyes, working from the inner to the outer canthus without soap. Use a separate section of the washcloth for each eye *to avoid spreading ocular infection.*
- If the patient tolerates soap, apply it to the cloth, and wash the rest of his face, ears, and neck, using firm, gentle strokes. Rinse thoroughly *because residual soap can cause itching and dryness.* Then dry the area thoroughly, taking special care in skin folds and creases. Observe the skin for irritation, scaling, or other abnormalities.
- Turn down the bath blanket, and drape the patient's chest with a bath towel. While washing, rinsing, and drying the chest and axillae, observe the patient's respirations. Use firm strokes *to avoid tickling the patient.* If the patient tolerates deodorant, apply it.
- Place a bath towel beneath the patient's arm farthest from you. Then bathe his arm, using long, smooth strokes and moving from wrist to shoulder, *to stimulate venous circulation.* If possible, soak the patient's hand in the basin *to remove dirt and soften nails.* Clean the patient's fingernails with the orangewood stick if necessary. Observe the color of his hand and nail beds to *assess peripheral circulation.* Follow the same procedure for the other arm and hand.
- Turn down the bath blanket to expose the patient's abdomen and groin, keeping a bath towel across his chest *to prevent chills.* Bathe, rinse, and dry the abdomen and groin while checking for abdominal distention or tenderness. Then turn back the bath blanket to cover the patient's chest and abdomen.
- Uncover the leg farthest from you, and place a bath towel under it. Flex this leg and bathe it, moving from ankle to hip *to stimulate venous circulation.* Don't massage the leg, however, *to avoid dislodging any existing thrombus, possibly causing a pulmonary embolus.* Rinse and dry the leg.
- If possible, place a basin on the patient's bed, flex the leg at the knee, and place the foot in the basin. Soak the foot, and then wash and rinse it thoroughly. Remove the foot from the basin, dry it, and clean the toenails. Observe skin condition and color during cleaning *to assess peripheral circulation.* Repeat the procedure for the other leg and foot.
- Cover the patient with the bath blanket *to prevent chilling.* Then lower the bed and raise the side rails *to ensure patient safety while you change the bath water.*
- When you return, roll the patient on his side or stomach, place a towel beneath him, and cover him *to prevent chilling.* Bathe, rinse, and dry his back and buttocks.
- Massage the patient's back with lotion. Check for redness, abrasions, and pressure ulcers.
- Bathe the anal area from front to back *to avoid contaminating the perineum.* Rinse and dry the area well.
- After lowering the bed and raising the side rails *to ensure the patient's safety,* change the bath water again. Then turn the patient on his back, and bathe the genital area thoroughly but gently, using a different section of the washcloth for each downward stroke. Bathe from front to back, avoiding the anal area. Rinse thoroughly and pat dry.
- If applicable, perform indwelling urinary catheter care. Apply perineal pads or scrotal supports as needed.
- Dress the patient in a clean gown, and reapply any elastic bandages, elastic stockings, or restraints removed before the bath.
- Remake the bed or change the linens, and remove the bath blanket.
- Place a bath towel beneath the patient's head *to catch loose hair,* and then brush and comb his hair.
- Return the bed to its original position, and make the patient comfortable.
- Carry soiled linens to the hamper with outstretched arms. *To avoid spreading microorganisms,* don't let soiled linens touch your clothing. Remove gloves.

Special considerations

- Fold the washcloth around your hand to form a mitt while bathing the patient. *This keeps the cloth warm longer and avoids dribbling water on the patient from the cloth's loose ends.* Change the water as often as necessary to keep it warm and clean.

■ Carefully dry creased skin-fold areas—for example, under breasts, in the groin area, and between fingers, toes, and buttocks. Dust these areas lightly with powder after drying *to reduce friction.* Use powder sparingly *to avoid caking and irritation and to avoid provoking coughing in patients with respiratory disorders.*

■ If the patient has very dry skin, use bath oil instead of soap unless contraindicated. No rinsing is necessary. Warm the lotion before using it for back massage *because cold lotion can startle the patient and induce muscle tension and vasoconstriction.* (See "Back care," page 119.)

■ A bag bath involves the use of 8 or 10 premoistened, warmed, disposable cloths (in a plastic bag or prepackaged pouch container) that contain a no-rinse surfactant instead of soap. Before use, the prepackaged cloths are warmed in a microwave or special warming unit supplied by the manufacturer. A separate cloth is used to wash each part of the body. *A bag bath saves time compared with the conventional bed bath because no rinsing is required.*

■ *To improve circulation, maintain joint mobility, and preserve muscle tone,* move the body joints through their full range of motion during the bath.

■ If the patient is incontinent, loosely tuck an abdominal pad between his buttocks, and place a linen-saver pad under him *to absorb fecal drainage. Together these pads will help prevent skin irritation and reduce the number of linen changes.*

NURSING ALERT *Don't wash a trauma or rape victim until she has been examined by the physician and, possibly, the police.* Washing may remove important evidence (powder burns or body fluids) that may be needed later in court.

Documentation

Record the date and time of the bed bath on the flowchart. Note the patient's tolerance for the bath, his range of motion, and his self-care abilities, and report any unusual findings.

SELECTED REFERENCES

Celik, S., et al. "Sleep Disturbance: The Patient Care Activities Applied at the Night Shift in the Intensive Care Unit," *Journal of Clinical Nursing* 14(1):102-106, January 2005.

Craven, R.F., and Hirnle, C.J. *Fundamentals of Nursing: Human Health and Function,* 5th ed. Philadelphia: Lippincott Williams & Wilkins, 2007.

Holloway, S., and Jones, V. "The Importance of Skin Care and Assessment," *British Journal of Nursing* 14(22):1172-76, December 2005-January 2006.

Larson, E.L., et al. "Comparison of Traditional and Disposable Bed Baths in Critically Ill Patients," *American Journal of Critical Care* 13(3):235-41, May 2004.

Using a hydraulic bath lift

For the debilitated patient who can't ambulate to the shower or tub, a hydraulic bath lift can facilitate transfer and eliminate strain on the nurse's back. The bath lift typically is used in a rehabilitation or geriatric setting.

To accomplish patient transfer, lower the lift (a chair or stretcher) to the patient's bed level. Suspend the patient, position him above a height-adjustable tub set to your most comfortable working height, and then lower him into the tub. Because the patient remains on the lift throughout his bath, simply reverse the procedure when taking the patient out of the tub.

When using a hydraulic lift for the first time, most patients feel somewhat insecure and fearful. With experience, however, most find the bathing system comfortable and relaxing.

TUB BATHS AND SHOWERS

Tub baths and showers provide personal hygiene, stimulate circulation, and reduce tension for the patient. They also allow you to observe skin conditions and assess joint mobility and muscle strength. If not precluded by the patient's condition or safety considerations, privacy during bathing promotes the patient's sense of well-being by allowing him to assume responsibility for his own care.

Patients who are recovering from recent surgery, who are emotionally unstable, or who have casted extremities or dressings in place usually require the practitioner's permission for a tub bath or shower. (For an alternative bathing method, see *Using a hydraulic bath lift.*)

Equipment

One or two washcloths ■ bath towel ■ bath blanket ■ soap (or hypoallergenic equivalent) ■ nonskid bath mat, if tub lacks nonskid strips ■ towel mat ■ bath thermometer ■ clean clothing or hospital gown ■ optional: chair, shower cap, bath oil, shampoo, or mild castile soap.

Preparation of equipment

Prepare the bathing area before the patient arrives. Close any doors or windows, and adjust the room temperature *to avoid chilling the patient.* Check that the bathtub or shower is clean. Then assemble bathing articles, and observe appropriate safety measures.

For a bath: Position a chair next to the tub *to help the patient get in and out and to provide a seat if he becomes weak.* Place a bath blanket over the chair *to cover the patient if he becomes chilled.* Fill the tub halfway with water, and test the temperature with a bath thermometer. The temperature should range from 100° to 110° F (37.8° to 43.3° C). If you don't have a bath thermometer, test the temperature by immersing your elbow in the water; it should feel comfortable to the touch. Besides the obvious risk of scalding the patient, excessively hot water can cause cutaneous vasodilation, *which alters blood flow to the brain and may lead to dizziness or fainting.* Place a rubber mat in the tub and a towel mat on the floor in front of the tub *to prevent slipping.*

For a shower: Place a nonskid chair in the shower *to provide support.* The chair also allows the patient to sit down while washing his legs and feet, *reducing the risk of falling.* Cover the floor of the shower with a nonskid mat unless it already has nonskid strips. Next, place a towel mat next to the bathing area. Remove electrical appliances, such as hair driers and heaters, from the patient's reach *to prevent electrical accidents.* Adjust water flow and temperature just before the patient gets into the shower.

Implementation

- Escort the patient to the bathing area, explain the procedure, and help him undress as necessary. Offer him a shower cap if he wants to keep his hair dry. Otherwise, provide shampoo or mild castile soap.
- Help the patient into the tub or shower. Provide washcloths and soap. If he has dry skin, add bath oil to the water. Wait until after he gets into the tub before adding bath oil *because oil makes the tub slick and increases the risk of falling.*
- Taking care to respect his privacy, help the patient bathe, as needed; he may appreciate help washing his back. If you can safely leave the patient alone, place the call bell within easy reach and show him how to use it.
- Ask the patient to leave the door unlocked for his own safety, but assure him that you'll post an "Occupied" sign on the door. Stay nearby in case of emergency, and check on the patient every 5 to 10 minutes.
- When the patient finishes bathing, drain the tub or turn off the shower.
- Assist the patient onto the bath mat *to prevent him from falling.* Then help him to dry off and put on a clean gown or other clothing, as appropriate.
- Escort the patient to his room or to his bed.
- Dry the floor of the bathing area well *to prevent slipping.* Ensure that the tub or shower is cleaned and disinfected.
- Dispose of soiled towels, and return the patient's personal belongings to his bedside.

Special considerations

- If you're giving a tub bath to a patient with a cast or dressing on an arm or leg, wrap the extremity in a clear plastic bag. Secure the bag with tape, being careful not to constrict circulation. Instruct the patient to dangle the arm or leg over the edge of the tub, and keep it out of the water.
- Encourage the patient to use safety devices, bars, and rails when bathing.
- *Because bathing in warm water causes vasodilation,* the patient may feel faint. If so, open the drain or turn off the shower. Cover the patient's shoulders and back with a bath towel, and instruct him to lean forward in the tub and to lower his head. Alternatively, assist him out of the shower onto a chair, lower his head, and summon help. If you have an ampule of aromatic spirits of ammonia readily available, break it open and wave it under the patient's nostrils. Never leave the patient unattended to obtain an ampule. When the patient recovers, escort him to bed and monitor his vital signs.

Documentation

Describe the patient's skin condition, and record any discoloration or redness in your notes.

SELECTED REFERENCES

Craven, R.F., and Hirnle, C.J. *Fundamentals of Nursing: Human Health and Function,* 5th ed. Philadelphia: Lippincott Williams & Wilkins, 2007.

Draelous, Z.D. "Concepts in Skin Care Maintenance," *Cutis* 76(6suppl):19-25, December 2005.

Holloway, S., and Jones, V. "The Importance of Skin Care and Assessment," *British Journal of Nursing* 14(22):1172-76, December 2005-January 2006.

Subramanyan, K. "Role of Mild Cleansing in the Management of Patient Skin," *Dermatologic Therapy* 17(suppl 1):26-34, 2004.

HAIR CARE

Hair care includes combing, brushing, and shampooing. Combing and brushing stimulate scalp circulation, remove dead cells and debris, and distribute hair oils to produce a healthy sheen. Shampooing removes dirt and old oils and helps prevent skin irritation.

Frequency of hair care depends on the length and texture of the patient's hair, the duration of hospitalization, and the patient's condition. Usually, hair should be combed and brushed daily and shampooed according to the patient's normal routine. Typically, no more than 1 week, or perhaps 2 weeks, should elapse between washings. Shampooing is contraindicated in patients with a recent craniotomy, depressed skull fracture, conditions necessitating intracranial pressure monitoring, or other cranial involvement.

Equipment

Comb and brush ▪ hand towel ▪ liquid shampoo (or mild soap, such as castile) ▪ shampoo tray with tubing ▪ washcloth ▪ three bath towels ▪ two bath blankets ▪ cotton ▪ pail or plastic wastebasket ▪ two large pitchers or other large containers ▪ one small pitcher or beaker ▪ basin ▪ linen-saver pads ▪ gloves ▪ optional: hair conditioner or rinse, alcohol, oil, hair ties, footstool, drawsheet.

Preparation of equipment

The comb and brush should be clean. If necessary, wash them in hot, soapy water. The comb should have dull, even teeth *to prevent scratching the scalp.* The brush should have stiff bristles *to enhance vigorous brushing and stimulation of circulation.*

Before shampooing the patient's hair, adjust room temperature and eliminate drafts *to prevent chilling the patient.* Next, obtain a shampoo tray or devise a trough if necessary.

Implementation

■ Assemble the equipment on the patient's bedside stand.

Combing and brushing

■ Tell the patient you're going to comb and brush his hair. If possible, encourage him to do this himself, assisting him as necessary.
■ Adjust the bed to a comfortable working height *to prevent back strain.* If the patient's condition allows, help him to a sitting position by raising the head of the bed.
■ Provide privacy, and drape a bath towel over the patient's pillow and shoulders *to catch loose hair and dirt.* Put on gloves.
■ For short hair, comb and brush one side at a time. For long or curly hair, turn the patient's head away from you, and then part his hair down the middle from front to back. If the hair is tangled, rub alcohol or oil on the hair strands *to loosen them.* Comb and vigorously brush the hair on the side facing you. Then turn the patient's head and comb and brush the opposite side. Part hair into small sections for easier handling. Comb one section at a time, working from the ends toward the scalp *to remove tangles.* Anchor each section of hair above the area being combed *to avoid hurting the patient.* After combing, brush vigorously.
■ Style the hair as the patient prefers. Braiding long or curly hair helps prevent snarling. To braid, part hair down the middle of the scalp and begin braiding near the face. Don't braid too tightly *to avoid patient discomfort.* Fasten the ends of the braids with hair ties. Pin the braids across the top of the patient's head or let them hang, as the patient desires, *so the finished braids don't press against the patient's scalp.*
■ After styling the hair, carefully remove the towel by folding it inward. *This prevents loose hairs and debris from falling onto the pillow or into the patient's bed.*

Shampooing a bedridden patient's hair

■ Cover the patient with a bath blanket. Then fanfold the linens to the foot of the bed, or remove them if they're scheduled to be changed.
■ Place a wastebasket on a linen-saver pad on the floor or on a footstool near the head of the bed. *The pail or container catches wastewater from the shampoo tray.*
■ Fill large pitchers or containers with comfortably warm water and place them on the overbed table.
■ Lower the head of the bed until it's horizontal, and remove the patient's pillow, if allowed.
■ Fold the second bath blanket and tuck it under the patient's shoulders *to improve water drainage.*
■ Cover the bath blanket and the head of the bed with a linen-saver pad *to protect them from moisture.*
■ Place a bath towel and linen-saver pad together, and position them around the patient's neck and over his shoulders. *This protects the patient from moisture and pads his neck against the pressure of the shampoo tray.*
■ Place the shampoo tray under the patient's head with his neck in the U-shaped opening. Arrange the bath blanket and towel so the patient is comfortable.
■ Adjust the shampoo tray to carry wastewater away from the patient's head, and place the drainage tubing in the pail. Tuck a folded towel or drawsheet under the opposite side of the shampoo tray *to promote drainage, if necessary.* Put on gloves.
■ When shampooing, place cotton in the patient's ears *to prevent moisture from collecting in them.*
■ Fill the small pitcher or beaker by dipping it into the large pitcher. Carefully pour water over the patient's hair as shown below. *To avoid spills,* don't overfill the shampoo tray.

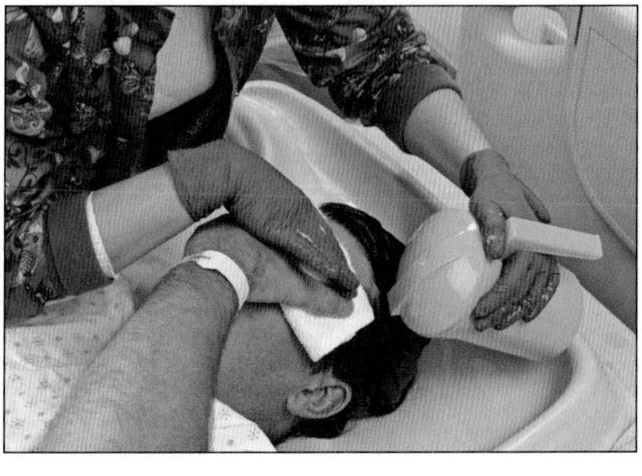

- Then with your fingertips, rub shampoo into the patient's hair. Massage his scalp well to emulsify hair oils. *Vigorous rubbing stimulates the scalp and also helps the patient relax.*
- Using the small pitcher or beaker, pour water over the patient's hair until it's free from shampoo. Then reapply shampoo and rinse again. Apply conditioner or a rinse, if desired.
- Remove the shampoo tray, and wrap the patient's hair in a towel. Remove the linen-saver pad from the bed, and return the bed to its original position.
- Dry the patient's hair by gently rubbing it with a towel. Then comb, brush, and style it.
- Remake the bed or change the linens, if needed, and remove the bath blanket.
- Reposition the patient comfortably.
- Remove and empty the pail. Clean the shampoo tray, and return it to storage. Remove pitchers from the bedside, and return the shampoo to the bedside stand. Remove gloves.

Special considerations

- When giving hair care, check the patient's scalp carefully for signs of scalp disorders or skin breakdown, particularly if the patient is bedridden. Make sure each patient has his own comb and brush *to avoid cross-contamination.*
- If you don't have a shampoo tray and can't devise a trough, place pillows under the patient's shoulders to elevate his head, and use a basin. Because a standard basin doesn't have a drainage spout, empty it frequently *to prevent overflow.*

Documentation

Record the date, time, and patient's response to the shampoo on the flowchart. Describe any scalp abnormalities in your notes.

SELECTED REFERENCES

Craven, R.F., and Hirnle, C.J. *Fundamentals of Nursing: Human Health and Function,* 5th ed. Philadelphia: Lippincott Williams & Wilkins, 2007.

Larson, E., and Nirenberg, A. "Evidence-Based Nursing Practice to Prevent Infection in Hospitalized Neutropenic Patients with Cancer," *Oncology Nursing Forum* 31(4):717-25, July 2004.

Lomborg, K. "Body Care Experienced by People Hospitalized with Severe Respiratory Disease," *Journal of Advanced Nursing* 50(3):262-71, May 2005.

Parker, L. "Infection Control: Maintaining the Personal Hygiene of Patients and Staff," *British Journal of Nursing* 13(8):474-78, April-May 2004.

SHAVING

Performed with a safety or electric razor, shaving is part of the male patient's usual daily care. Besides reducing bacterial growth on the face, shaving promotes patient comfort by removing whiskers that can itch and irritate the skin and produce an unkempt appearance. Because nicks and cuts occur most frequently with a safety razor, shaving with an electric razor is indicated for the patient with a clotting disorder or the patient undergoing anticoagulant therapy. Shaving may be contraindicated in the patient with a facial skin disorder or wound.

Equipment

For a safety razor: Shaving kit containing a razor and soap container ▪ gloves ▪ soap or shaving cream ▪ towel ▪ washcloth ▪ basin ▪ optional: after-shave lotion, talcum powder.

For an electric razor: Bath towel ▪ optional: preshave and aftershave lotions, mirror, grounded three-pronged plug.

Preparation of equipment

With a safety razor, make sure the blade is sharp, clean, even, and rust-free. If necessary, insert a new blade securely into the razor. A razor may be used more than once, but only by the same patient. If the patient is bedridden, assemble the equipment on the bedside stand or overbed table; if he's ambulatory, assemble it at the sink. When the patient is ready to shave, fill the basin or sink with warm water.

If you're using an electric razor, check its cord for fraying or other damage that could create an electrical hazard. If the razor isn't double-insulated or battery operated, use a grounded three-pronged plug. Examine the razor head for sharp edges and dirt. Read the manufacturer's instructions, if available, and assemble the equipment at the bedside.

Implementation

- Tell the patient that you're going to shave him, and provide privacy. Ask him to assist you as much as possible *to promote his independence.*
- Unless contraindicated, place the conscious patient in high Fowler's or semi-Fowler's position. If the patient is unconscious, elevate his head *to prevent soap and water from running behind it.*
- Direct bright light onto the patient's face, but not into his eyes.

Using a safety razor

- Drape a bath towel around the patient's shoulders, and tuck it under his chin *to protect the bed from moisture and to catch falling whiskers.*

■ Put on gloves, and fill the basin with warm water. Using the washcloth, wet the patient's entire beard with warm water. Let the warm cloth soak the beard for at least 1 minute *to soften whiskers.*
■ Apply shaving cream to the beard. If you're using soap, rub to form a lather.
■ Gently stretch the patient's skin taut with one hand and shave with the other, holding the razor firmly. Ask the patient to puff his cheeks or turn his head, as necessary, *to shave hard-to-reach areas.*
■ Begin at the sideburns and work toward the chin using short, firm, downward strokes in the direction of hair growth as shown below. *This reduces skin irritation and helps prevent nicks and cuts.*

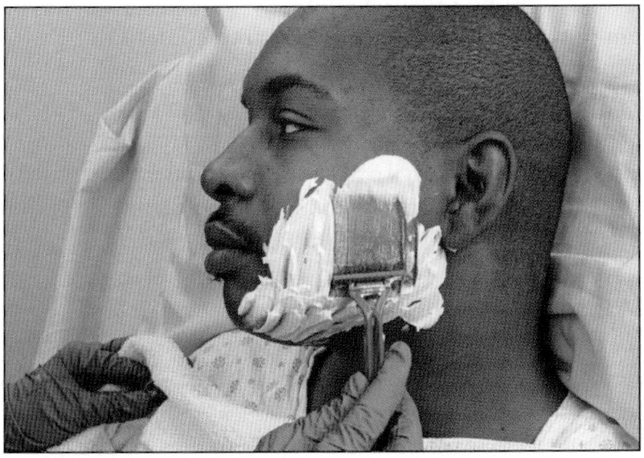

■ Rinse the razor often *to remove whiskers.* Apply more warm water or shaving cream to the face, as needed, *to maintain adequate lather.*
■ Shave across the chin and up the neck and throat. Use short, gentle strokes for the neck and the area around the nose and mouth *to avoid skin irritation.*
■ Change the water, and rinse any remaining lather and whiskers from the patient's face. Then dry his face with a bath towel and, if the patient desires, apply after-shave lotion or talcum powder.
■ Rinse the razor and basin, and then return the razor to its storage area.

Using an electric razor
■ Plug in the razor, and apply preshave lotion, if available, *to remove skin oils.* If the razor head is adjustable, select the appropriate setting.
■ Using a circular motion and pressing the razor firmly against the skin, shave each area of the patient's face until smooth.
■ If the patient desires, apply talcum powder or after-shave lotion.
■ Clean the razor head, and return the razor to its storage area.

Special considerations
■ If the patient is conscious, find out his usual shaving routine. *Although shaving in the direction of hair growth is most common, the patient may prefer the opposite direction.*
■ Don't interchange patients' shaving equipment *to prevent cross-contamination.*
■ Shaving may be contraindicated if the patient is on anticoagulant therapy (for example, post–tissue plasminogen activator, heparin infusion). Check your facility's policy.

Complications
Cuts and abrasions are the most common complications of shaving and can require the application of antiseptic lotion.

Documentation
If applicable, record nicks or cuts resulting from shaving.

SELECTED REFERENCES
Occupational Safety and Health Administration. Bloodborne Pathogens. Standard 1910-1030.
Taylor, C., et al. *Fundamentals of Nursing: The Art and Science of Nursing Care,* 6th ed. Philadelphia: Lippincott Williams & Wilkins, 2007.

EYE CARE

When paralysis or coma impairs or eliminates the corneal reflex, frequent eye care aims to keep the exposed cornea moist, preventing ulceration and inflammation. Application of saline-saturated gauze pads over the eyelids moistens the eyes. Commercially available eye ointments and artificial tears also lubricate the corneas, but a practitioner's order is required for their use.

Although eye care isn't a sterile procedure, asepsis should be maintained as much as possible.

Equipment
Sterile basin ■ gloves ■ sterile towel ■ sterile normal saline solution ■ sterile cotton balls or gauze pads ■ mineral oil ■ artificial tears or eye ointment (if ordered) ■ gauze or eyepads ■ hypoallergenic tape.

Preparation of equipment
Assemble the equipment at the patient's bedside. Pour a small amount of normal saline solution into the basin.

Implementation

- Wash your hands thoroughly, put on gloves, and tell the patient what you're about to do, even if he's comatose or appears unresponsive.
- To remove secretions or crusts adhering to the eyelids and eyelashes, first soak a cotton ball in sterile normal saline solution. Then gently wipe the patient's eye with the moistened cotton ball, working from the inner canthus to the outer canthus to *prevent debris and fluid from entering the nasolacrimal duct.*
- *To prevent cross-contamination,* use a fresh cotton ball for each wipe until the eye is clean. *To prevent irritation,* avoid using soap for cleaning the eyes. Repeat the procedure for the other eye.
- After cleaning the eyes, instill artificial tears or apply eye ointment, as ordered, *to keep them moist.*
- Close the patient's eyelids. Dab a small amount of mineral oil on each lid *to lubricate and protect fragile skin.*
- Soak gauze or eyepads in sterile normal saline solution, place them over the eyelids, and secure with hypoallergenic tape. Change gauze pads, as necessary, *to keep them well saturated.*
- After giving eye care, cover the basin with a sterile towel and dispose of your gloves. Change the eye care setup (basin, towel, and normal saline solution) at least daily.

Documentation

Record the time and type of eye care in your notes. If applicable, chart administration of eyedrops or ointment in the patient's medication record. Document unusual crusting or excessive or colored drainage.

SELECTED REFERENCES

Dawson, D. "Development of New Eye Care Guidelines for Critically Ill Patients," *Intensive and Critical Care Nursing* 21(2):119-22, April 2005.

Ubels, J.L., et al. "Pre-Clinical Investigation of Efficacy of an Artificial Tear Solution Containing Hydroxypropyl-Guar as a Gelling Agent," *Current Eye Research* 28(6):437-44, June 2004.

CONTACT LENS CARE

Illness or emergency treatment may require that you insert or remove and store a patient's contact lenses. Proper handling and lens care techniques help prevent eye injury and infection as well as lens loss or damage. Appropriate lens-handling techniques depend in large part on what type of lenses the patient wears.

All contact lenses float on the corneal tear layer. Rigid lenses typically have a smaller diameter than the cornea; soft lens diameter typically exceeds that of the cornea. Because they're larger and more pliable, soft lenses tend to mold themselves more closely to the eye for a more stable fit than rigid lenses.

Modes of lens wear vary widely. Although most patients remove and clean their lenses daily, some wear lenses overnight or for several days (sometimes up to a month) without removing them for cleaning. Still other patients wear disposable lenses, which means that they replace old lenses with new ones at regular intervals (a few days to a few months), possibly without removing them for cleaning between replacements.

Keep in mind that handling contact lenses improperly can provide a direct source of contamination to the eye.

Equipment

Lens storage case or two small medicine cups and adhesive tape ▪ gloves ▪ patient's equipment for contact lens care, if available ▪ sterile normal saline solution or soaking solution ▪ flashlight, if needed ▪ optional: suction cup.

Preparation of equipment

If a commercial lens storage case isn't available, place enough sterile normal saline solution into two small medicine cups to submerge a lens in each one. *To avoid confusing the left and right lenses,* which may have different prescriptions, mark one cup "L" and the other cup "R" and place the corresponding lens in each cup.

Implementation

- Tell the patient what you're about to do, wash your hands, and put on gloves *to help prevent ocular infection.*

Inserting rigid lenses

- Wet one lens with solution, and gently rub it between your thumb and index finger, or place it on your palm and rub it with your opposite index finger. Rinse well with the solution, leaving a small amount in the lens.
- Place the lens, convex side down, on the tip of the index finger of your dominant hand.
- Instruct the patient to gaze upward slightly. Separate the eyelids with your other thumb and index finger, and place the lens directly and gently on the cornea. You need not press it to the eye; *the tear film will attract it naturally at the first touch.* Using the same procedure, insert the opposite lens.

Inserting soft lenses

- To see if the lens is inside out, bend it between your thumb and index finger or fill it with saline or soaking solution. If the lens tends to roll inward or the edge points slightly inward, it's oriented correctly. If the edge points outward or the lens tends to collapse over your fingertip, it's probably inside out and should be reversed.

- Wet the lens with fresh normal saline solution, and rub it gently between your thumb and index finger, or place it on your palm and rub it with your opposite index finger. Rinse well.
- Place the lens, convex side down, on the tip of the index finger of your dominant hand.
- Instruct the patient to gaze upward slightly. Separate the eyelids with your other thumb and index finger, and place the lens on the sclera, just below the cornea. Then, slide the lens gently upward with your finger until it centers on the cornea. Using the same procedure, insert the opposite lens.

Removing rigid lenses

- Before removing a lens, position the patient supine *to prevent the lens from popping out onto the floor, risking loss or damage.*
- Place one thumb against the patient's upper eyelid and the other thumb against the lower eyelid. Move the lids toward each other while gently pressing inward against the eye *to trap the lens edge and break the suction.* Extract the lens from the patient's eyelashes.
- Depending on the lens type and thickness, it may pop out when the suction breaks. You may want to try to break the suction with one hand while cupping the other hand below the patient's eye *to catch the lens as it falls.*
- Sometimes the lens will pop out on its own if you ask the patient to blink after stretching the corner of the eyelids toward the temporal bone, thus tightening the lid edges against the globe of the eye.
- After removal, place the lens in the proper well of the storage case (L or R) with enough of the appropriate storage solution to cover it. Alternatively, place the lens in a labeled medicine cup with solution, and secure adhesive tape over the top of the cup *to prevent loss of the lens.*
- Remove and care for the opposite lens using the same technique.

Removing soft lenses

- Place the patient in the supine position. Using your nondominant hand, raise the patient's upper eyelid and hold it against the orbital rim as shown top of next column.

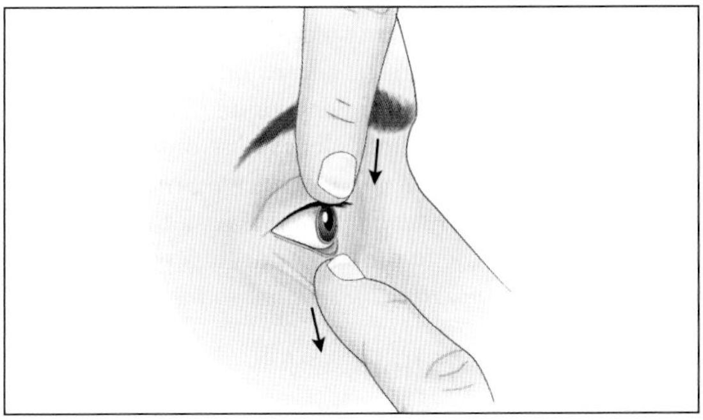

- Lightly place the forefinger of your other hand on the lens, and move it down onto the sclera below the cornea. Then pinch the lens between your forefinger and thumb; it should pop off as shown below.

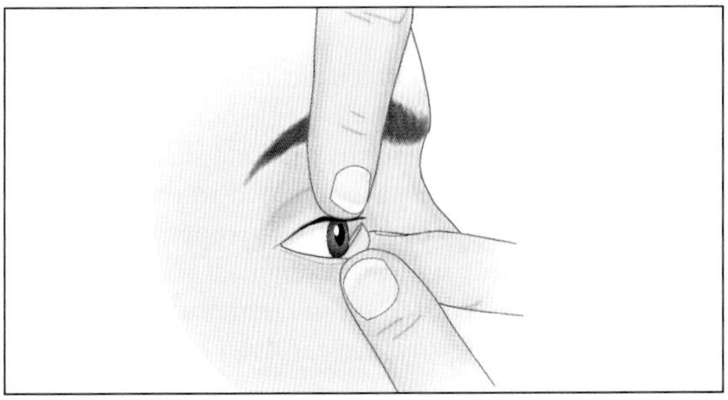

- Place the lens in the proper well of the storage case with enough of the appropriate storage solution to cover it. Alternatively, place the lens in a labeled medicine cup with solution, and secure adhesive tape over the top of the cup *to prevent loss of the lens.*
- Remove and care for the other lens using the same technique.

Cleaning lenses

- *Because lens-cleaning steps vary with lens type and with each manufacturer's and practitioner's instructions,* ask the patient to guide you step-by-step through his normal cleaning routine.
- If the patient can't tell you how to clean his lenses properly, remember that all lens types require two steps: cleaning and disinfection.
- Cleaning involves rubbing the lens with a surfactant solution designed to remove most surface deposits. For most patients, especially those who wear soft lenses, the cleaning step may also include use of an enzyme agent *to remove protein deposits against which surfactant cleaners are typically ineffective.* Enzyme cleaning involves soaking lenses overnight in a solution in which you've dissolved special enzyme tablets.

■ Disinfection, which doesn't require rubbing, may be accomplished through chemical means or by heat. *This step aims to rid the lens of infectious organisms.*

■ If you must clean a patient's lenses, use only his own solutions. *This minimizes the risk of allergic reactions to substances included in other solution brands.* Never touch the nozzle of a solution bottle to the lens, your fingers, or anything else *to avoid contaminating the solution in the bottle.*

Special considerations

■ If the patient's eyes appear dry, or you have trouble moving the lens on the eye, instill several drops of sterile normal saline solution, and wait a few minutes before trying again to remove the lens *to prevent corneal damage.* If you still can't remove the lens easily, notify the practitioner. Avoid instilling eye medication while the patient is wearing lenses. *The lenses could trap the medication, possibly causing eye irritation or lens damage.*

■ Don't allow soft lenses, which are 40% to 60% water, to dry out. If they do, soak them in sterile normal saline solution, and they may return to their natural shape.

■ If an unconscious patient is admitted to the emergency department, check for contact lenses by opening each eyelid and searching with a small flashlight. If you detect lenses, remove them immediately *because tears can't circulate freely beneath the lenses with eyelids closed, possibly leading to corneal oxygen depletion or infection.*

■ Advise contact lens wearers to carry appropriate identification *to speed lens removal and ensure proper care in an emergency.*

■ If a patient can't provide adequate care for his lenses during hospitalization, encourage him to send them home with a family member. If you aren't sure how to care for the lenses in the interim, store them in sterile normal saline solution until the family member can take them home.

Documentation

Record eye condition before and after removal of lenses; the time of lens insertion, removal, and cleaning; the location of stored lenses; and, if applicable, the removal of lenses from the facility by a family member.

SELECTED REFERENCES

Alfonso, E.C., et al. "Fungal Keratitis Associated with Nontherapeutic Soft Contact Lenses," *American Journal of Ophthalmology* 142(1):154-55, July 2006.

Cohen, E.J. "Fusarium Keratitis Associated with Soft Contact Lens Wear," *Archives of Ophthalmology* 1245(8):1183-84, August 2006.

Collins, M.J., et al. "The Biomechanics of Rigid Contact Lens Removal," *Contact Lens & Anterior Eye* 28(3):121-25, September 2005.

Foulks, G.N. "Prolonging Contact Lens Wear and Making Contact Lens Wear Safer," *American Journal of Ophthalmology* 141(2):369-373, February 2006.

Niyadurupola, N., and Illingworth, C.D. "Acanthamoeba Keratitis Associated with Misuse of Daily Disposable Contact Lenses," *Contact Lens & Anterior Eye* 29(5):269-71, December 2006.

MOUTH CARE

Given in the morning, at bedtime, or after meals, mouth care entails brushing and flossing the teeth and inspecting the mouth. It removes soft plaque deposits and calculus from the teeth, cleans and massages the gums, reduces mouth odor, and helps prevent infection. By freshening the patient's mouth, mouth care also enhances appreciation of food, thereby aiding appetite and nutrition.

Although the ambulatory patient can usually perform mouth care alone, the bedridden patient may require partial or full assistance. The comatose patient requires the use of suction equipment to prevent aspiration during oral care.

Equipment

Towel or facial tissues ■ emesis basin ■ trash bag ■ mouthwash ■ toothbrush and toothpaste ■ pitcher and glass ■ drinking straw ■ dental floss ■ gloves ■ small mirror, if necessary ■ optional: dental floss holder, oral irrigating device.

For the comatose or debilitated patient as needed: Linen-saver pad ■ bite-block ■ petroleum jelly ■ hydrogen peroxide ■ sponge-tipped mouth swab ■ oral suction equipment or gauze pads ■ optional: mouth-care kit, tongue blade, 4″ gauze pads, adhesive tape.

Preparation of equipment

Fill a pitcher with water and bring it and other equipment to the patient's bedside. If you'll be using oral suction equipment, connect the tubing to the suction bottle and suction catheter, insert the plug into an outlet, and check for correct operation. If necessary, devise a bite-block *to protect yourself from being bitten during the procedure.* Wrap a gauze pad over the end of a tongue blade, fold the edge in, and secure it with adhesive tape.

Implementation

■ Wash your hands thoroughly, put on gloves, explain the procedure to the patient, and provide privacy.

Supervising mouth care

■ For the bedridden patient capable of self-care, encourage him to perform his own mouth care.

Dealing with dentures

Prostheses made of acrylic resins, vinyl composites, or both, dentures replace some or all of the patient's natural teeth. Dentures require proper care to remove soft plaque deposits and calculus and to reduce mouth odor. Such care involves removing and rinsing dentures after meals, daily brushing and removal of tenacious deposits, and soaking in a commercial denture cleaner. Dentures must be removed from the comatose or presurgical patient *to prevent possible airway obstruction.*

Equipment and preparation

Start by assembling the following equipment at the patient's bedside: emesis basin ■ labeled denture cup ■ toothbrush or denture brush ■ gloves ■ toothpaste ■ commercial denture cleaner ■ paper towel ■ sponge-tipped mouth swab ■ mouthwash ■ gauze ■ optional: adhesive denture liner.

Wash your hands and put on gloves.

Removing dentures

■ To remove a full upper denture, grasp the front and palatal surfaces of the denture with your thumb and forefinger. Position the index finger of your opposite hand over the upper border of the denture, and press to break the seal between denture and palate. Grasp the denture with gauze *because saliva can make it slippery.*
■ To remove a full lower denture, grasp the front and lingual surfaces of the denture with your thumb and index finger, and gently lift up.
■ To remove partial dentures, first ask the patient or caregiver how the prosthesis is retained and how to remove it. If it's held in place with clips or snaps, then exert equal pressure on the border of each side of the denture. Avoid lifting the clasps, which easily bend or break.

Oral and denture care

■ After removing dentures, place them in a properly labeled denture cup. Add warm water and a commercial denture cleaner *to remove stains and hardened deposits.* Follow package directions. Avoid soaking dentures in mouthwash containing alcohol *because it may damage a soft liner.*
■ Instruct the patient to rinse with *mouthwash to remove food particles and reduce mouth odor.* Then stroke the palate, buccal surfaces, gums, and tongue with a soft toothbrush or sponge-tipped mouth swab *to clean the mucosa and stimulate circulation.* Inspect for irritated areas or sores *because they may indicate a poorly fitting denture.*
■ Carry the denture cup, emesis basin, toothbrush, and toothpaste to the sink. After lining the basin with a paper towel, fill it with water *to cushion the dentures in case you drop them.* Hold the dentures over the basin, wet them with warm water, and apply toothpaste to a denture brush or long-bristled toothbrush. Clean the dentures using only moderate pressure *to prevent scratches* and warm water *to prevent distortion.*
■ Clean the denture cup, and place the dentures in it. Rinse the brush, and clean and dry the emesis basin. Return all equipment to the patient's bedside stand.

Wearing dentures

■ If the patient desires, apply adhesive liner to the dentures. Moisten them with water, if necessary, *to reduce friction and ease insertion.*
■ Encourage the patient to wear his dentures *to enhance his appearance, facilitate eating and speaking, and prevent changes in the gum line that may affect denture fit.*

■ If allowed, place the patient in Fowler's position. Place the overbed table in front of the patient, and arrange the equipment on it. Open the table and set up the built-in mirror, if available, or position a small mirror on the table.
■ Drape a towel over the patient's chest *to protect his gown.* Tell him to floss his teeth while looking into the mirror.
■ Observe the patient *to make sure he's flossing correctly,* and correct him if necessary. Tell him to wrap the floss around the second or third fingers of both hands. Starting with his front teeth and without injuring the gums, he should insert the floss as far as possible into the space between each pair of teeth. Then he should clean the surfaces of adjacent teeth by pulling the floss up and down against the side of each tooth. After the patient flosses a pair of teeth, remind him to use a clean 1″ (2.5 cm) section of floss for the next pair.
■ After the patient flosses, mix mouthwash and water in a glass, place a straw in the glass, and position the emesis basin nearby. Then instruct the patient to brush his teeth and gums while looking into the mirror. Encourage him to rinse frequently during brushing, and provide facial tissues for him to wipe his mouth.

Using an oral irrigating device

An oral irrigating device, such as the Water Pik, directs a pulsating jet of water around the teeth to massage gums and remove debris and food particles. It's especially useful for cleaning areas missed by brushing, such as around bridgework, crowns, and dental wires. *Because this device enhances oral hygiene,* it benefits patients undergoing head and neck irradiation, which can damage teeth and cause severe caries. The device also maintains oral hygiene in a patient with a fractured jaw or with mouth injuries that limit standard mouth care.

Equipment and preparation

To use the device, first assemble the following equipment: oral irrigating device ■ towel ■ emesis basin ■ pharyngeal suction apparatus ■ salt solution or mouthwash, if ordered ■ soap.

Wash your hands, and put on gloves.

Implementation

■ Turn the patient to his side *to prevent aspiration of water.* Then place a towel under his chin and an emesis basin next to his cheek *to absorb or catch drainage.*

■ Insert the oral irrigating device's plug into a nearby electrical outlet. Remove the device's cover, turn it upside down, and fill it with lukewarm water or with a mouthwash or salt solution, as ordered. When using a salt solution, dissolve the salt beforehand in a separate container. Then pour the solution into the cover. (*Note:* Salt solution shouldn't be used in patients with oral dryness or dehydration *because salt exacerbates these conditions.*)

■ Secure the cover to the base of the device. Remove the water hose handle from the base, and snap the jet tip into place. If necessary, wet the grooved end of the tip *to ease insertion.* Adjust the pressure dial to the setting most comfortable for the patient. If his gums are tender and prone to bleed, choose a low setting.

■ Adjust the knurled knob on the handle to direct the water jet, place the jet tip in the patient's mouth, and turn on the device. Instruct the alert patient to keep his lips partially closed *to avoid spraying water.*

■ Direct the water at a right angle to the gum line of each tooth and between teeth. Avoid directing water under the patient's tongue *because this may injure sensitive tissue.*

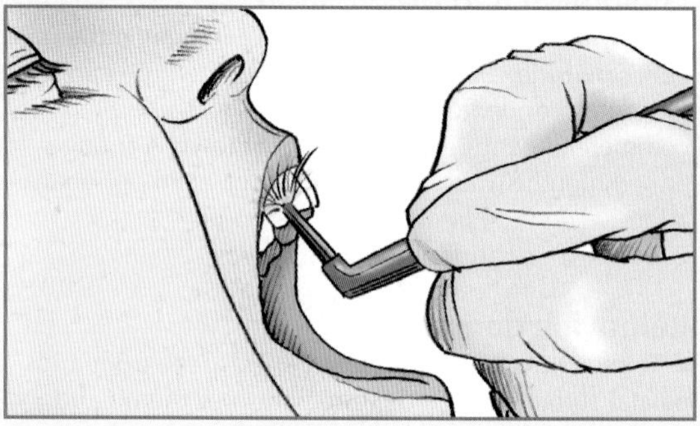

■ After irrigating each tooth, pause briefly and instruct the patient to expectorate the water or solution into the emesis basin. If he can't do so, suction it from the sides of the mouth with the pharyngeal suction apparatus. After irrigating all teeth, turn off the device, and remove the jet tip from the patient's mouth.

■ Empty the remaining water or solution from the cover, remove the jet tip from the handle, and return the handle to the base. Clean the jet tip with soap and water, rinse the cover, and dry them both and return them to storage.

Performing mouth care

■ For the comatose patient or the conscious patient incapable of self-care, you'll perform mouth care. If the patient wears dentures, clean them thoroughly. (See *Dealing with dentures,* page 117.) Some patients may benefit from using an oral irrigating device such as a Water Pik. (See *Using an oral irrigating device.*)

■ Arrange the equipment on the overbed table or bedside stand, including the oral suction equipment, if necessary. Turn on the machine. If a suction machine isn't available, wipe the inside of the patient's mouth frequently with a gauze pad.

■ Raise the bed to a comfortable working height *to prevent back strain.* Then lower the head of the bed, and position the patient on his side, with his face extended over the edge of the pillow *to facilitate oral drainage and prevent fluid aspiration.*

■ Place a linen-saver pad under the patient's chin and an emesis basin near his cheek *to absorb or catch oral drainage.*

■ Lubricate the patient's lips with petroleum jelly *to prevent dryness and cracking.* Reapply lubricant, as needed, during oral care.

■ If necessary, insert the bite-block to hold the patient's mouth open during oral care.
■ Using a dental floss holder, hold the floss against each tooth and direct it as close to the gum as possible without injuring the sensitive tissues around the tooth.
■ After flossing the patient's teeth, mix mouthwash and water in a glass, and place the straw in it.
■ Wet the toothbrush with water. If necessary, use hot water *to soften the bristles.* Apply toothpaste.
■ Brush the patient's lower teeth from the gum line up; the upper teeth, from the gum line down. Place the brush at a 45-degree angle to the gum line, and press the bristles gently into the gingival sulcus. Using short, gentle strokes *to prevent gum damage,* brush the facial surfaces (toward the cheek) and the lingual surfaces (toward the tongue) of the bottom teeth. Use just the tip of the brush for the lingual surfaces of the front teeth. Then, using the same technique, brush the facial and lingual surfaces of the top teeth. Next, brush the biting surfaces of the bottom and top teeth, using a back and forth motion. If possible, ask the patient to rinse frequently during brushing by taking the mouthwash solution through the straw. Hold the emesis basin steady under the patient's cheek, and wipe his mouth and cheeks with facial tissues as needed.
■ After brushing the patient's teeth, dip a sponge-tipped mouth swab into the mouthwash solution. Press the swab against the side of the glass *to remove excess moisture.* Gently stroke the gums, buccal surfaces, palate, and tongue *to clean the mucosa and stimulate circulation.* Replace the swab as necessary for thorough cleaning. Avoid inserting the swab too deeply *to prevent gagging and vomiting.*

After mouth care

■ Assess the patient's mouth for cleanliness and tooth and tissue condition.
■ Then remove your gloves, rinse the toothbrush, and clean the emesis basin and glass. Empty and clean the suction bottle, if used, and place a clean suction catheter on the tubing. Return reusable equipment to the appropriate storage location, and properly discard disposable equipment in the trash bag.

Special considerations

■ Use sponge-tipped mouth swabs to clean the teeth of a patient with sensitive gums. *These swabs produce less friction than a toothbrush but don't clean as well.*
■ Clean the mouth of a toothless comatose patient by wrapping a gauze pad around your index finger, moistening it with mouthwash, and gently swabbing the oral tissues.
■ Remember that *mucous membranes dry quickly in the patient breathing through his mouth or receiving oxygen therapy.* Moisten his mouth and lips regularly with moistened sponge-tipped swabs.

Documentation

Record the date and time of mouth care in your notes. Also note any unusual conditions, such as bleeding, edema, mouth odor, excessive secretions, or plaque on the tongue.

SELECTED REFERENCES

Allen Furr, L., et al. "Factors Affecting Quality of Oral Care in Intensive Care Units," *Journal of Advanced Nursing* 48(5):454-62, December 2004.

Berry, A.M., and Davidson, P.M. "Beyond Comfort: Oral Hygiene as a Critical Nursing Activity in the Intensive Care Unit," *Intensive and Critical Care Nursing* 22(6):318-28, December 2006.

Kinley, J., and Brennan, S. "Changing Practice: Use of Audit to Change Oral Care Practice," *International Journal of Palliative Nursing* 10(12):580-87, December 2004.

BACK CARE

Regular bathing and massage of the neck, back, buttocks, and upper arms promotes patient relaxation and allows assessment of skin condition. Particularly important for the bedridden patient, massage causes cutaneous vasodilation, helping to prevent pressure ulcers caused by prolonged pressure on bony prominences or by perspiration. Gentle back massage can be performed after myocardial infarction but may be contraindicated in patients with rib fractures, surgical incisions, or other recent traumatic injury to the back.

Equipment

Basin ■ soap ■ bath blanket ■ bath towel ■ washcloth ■ back lotion with lanolin base ■ gloves, if the patient has open lesions or has been incontinent.

Preparation of equipment

Fill the basin two-thirds full with warm water. Place the lotion bottle in the basin to warm it. Application of warmed lotion prevents chilling or startling the patient, thereby reducing muscle tension and vasoconstriction.

Implementation

■ Assemble the equipment at the patient's bedside.
■ Explain the procedure to the patient, and provide privacy. Ask him to tell you if you're applying too much or too little pressure.
■ Adjust the bed to a comfortable working height, and lower the head of the bed, if allowed. Wash your hands, and put on gloves, if applicable.

Making a washcloth mitt

To make a washcloth mitt, take a clean, dry washcloth, and fold it in thirds lengthwise around your hand. Fold the top of the wash cloth down, and tuck it in the bottom of the mitt.

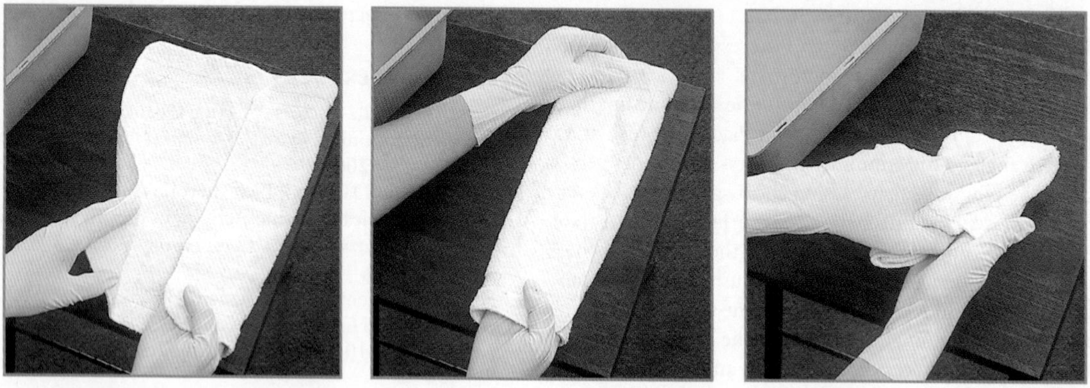

■ Place the patient in the prone position, if possible, or on his side. Position him along the edge of the bed nearest you *to prevent back strain.*

■ Untie the patient's gown, and expose his back, shoulders, and buttocks. Then drape the patient with a bath blanket *to prevent chills and minimize exposure.* Place a bath towel next to or under the patient's side *to protect bed linens from moisture.*

■ Fold the washcloth around your hand to form a mitt. *This prevents the loose ends of the cloth from dripping water onto the patient and keeps the cloth warm longer.* Then work up a lather with soap. (See *Making a washcloth mitt.)*

■ Using long, firm strokes, bathe the patient's back, beginning at the neck and shoulders and moving downward to the buttocks. Rinse and dry well *because moisture trapped between the buttocks can cause chafing and predispose the patient to formation of pressure ulcers.* While giving back care, closely examine the patient's skin, especially the bony prominences of the shoulders, the scapulae, and the coccyx, for redness or abrasions.

■ Remove the warmed lotion bottle from the basin, and pour a small amount of lotion into your palm. Rub your hands together *to distribute the lotion.* Then apply the lotion to the patient's back, using long, firm strokes. *The lotion reduces friction, making back massage easier.*

■ Massage the patient's back, beginning at the base of the spine and moving upward to the shoulders. *For a relaxing effect,* massage slowly; *for a stimulating effect,* massage quickly. Alternate the three basic strokes: effleurage, friction, and petrissage. (See *How to give a back massage.*) Add lotion as needed, keeping one hand on the patient's back *to avoid interrupting the massage.*

■ Compress, squeeze, and lift the trapezius muscle *to help relax the patient.*

■ Finish the massage by using long, firm strokes, and blot any excess lotion from the patient's back with a towel. Then retie the patient's gown, and straighten or change the bed linens, as necessary.

■ Return the bed to its original position, and make the patient comfortable. Empty and clean the basin. Dispose of gloves, if used, and return equipment to the appropriate storage area.

Special considerations

■ Before giving back care, assess the patient's body structure and skin condition, and tailor the duration and intensity of the massage accordingly. If you're giving back care at bedtime, have the patient ready for bed beforehand, *so the massage can help him fall asleep.*

■ Use separate lotion for each patient *to prevent cross-contamination.*

■ When massaging the patient's back, stand with one foot slightly forward and your knees slightly bent *to allow effective use of your arm and shoulder muscles.*

■ Give special attention to bony prominences because these areas are disposed to formation of pressure ulcers. Don't massage the patient's legs unless ordered *because reddened legs can signal clot formation, and massage can dislodge the clot,*

How to give a back massage

Effleurage, friction, and petrissage are the three strokes used commonly when giving a back massage. Start with effleurage, go on to friction, and then to petrissage. Perform each stroke at least six times before moving on to the next, and then repeat the whole series, if desired.

When performing effleurage and friction, keep your hands parallel to the vertebrae to avoid tickling the patient. For all three strokes, maintain a regular rhythm and steady contact with the patient's back to help him relax.

Effleurage

Using your palm, stroke from the buttocks up to the shoulders, over the upper arms, and back to the buttocks (as shown below). Use slightly less pressure on the downward strokes.

Friction

Use circular thumb strokes to move from buttocks to shoulders; then, using a smooth stroke, return to the buttocks (as shown below).

Petrissage

Using your thumb to oppose your fingers, knead and stroke half the back and upper arms, starting at the buttocks and moving toward the shoulder (as shown below). Then knead and stroke the other half of the back, rhythmically alternating your hands.

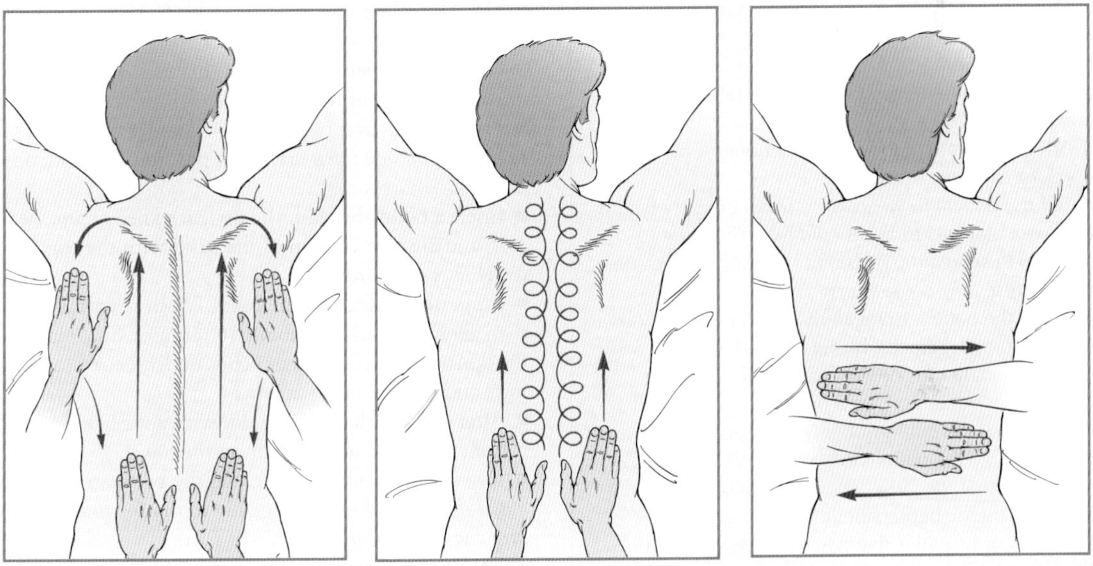

causing an embolus. Develop a turning schedule, and give back care at each position change.

Documentation

Chart back care on the flowchart. Record redness, abrasion, or change in skin condition in your notes.

SELECTED REFERENCES

Robinson, S.B., et al. "The Sh-h-h-h Project: Nonpharmacological Interventions," *Holistic Nursing Practice* 19(6):263-66, November-December 2005.

FOOT CARE

Daily bathing of feet and regular trimming of toenails promotes cleanliness, prevents infection, stimulates peripheral circulation, and controls odor by removing debris from between toes and under toenails. It's particularly important for bedridden patients and those especially susceptible to foot infection. Increased susceptibility may be caused by peripheral vascular disease, diabetes mellitus, poor nutritional status, arthritis, or any condition that impairs peripheral

Foot care for diabetic patients

Because diabetes mellitus can reduce blood supply to the feet, normally minor foot injuries can lead to dangerous infection. When caring for a diabetic patient, keep the following foot care guidelines in mind:

- Exercising the feet daily can help improve circulation. While the patient is sitting on the edge of the bed, ask him to point his toes upward, then downward, 10 times. Then have him make a circle with each foot 10 times.
- A diabetic patient's shoes must fit properly. Instruct the patient to break in new shoes gradually by increasing wearing time by 30 minutes each day. Also tell the patient to check old shoes frequently *in case they develop rough spots in the lining.*
- Tell the patient to wear clean socks daily and to avoid socks with holes, darned spots, or rough, irritating seams.
- Advise the patient to see a practitioner if he has corns or calluses.
- Tell the patient to wear warm socks or slippers and use extra blankets *to avoid cold feet.* The patient shouldn't use heating pads and hot water bottles *because these may cause burns.*
- Teach the patient to regularly inspect the skin on the feet for cuts, cracks, blisters, or red, swollen areas. Even slight cuts on the feet should receive a practitioner's attention. As a first-aid measure, tell him to wash the cut thoroughly and apply a mild antiseptic. Urge the patient to avoid harsh antiseptics, such as iodine, *because they can damage tissue.*
- Advise the diabetic patient to avoid tight-fitting garments or activities that can decrease circulation. He should especially avoid wearing elastic garters, sitting with knees crossed, picking at sores or rough spots on the feet, walking barefoot, or applying adhesive tape to the skin on the feet.

circulation. In such patients, proper foot care should include meticulous cleanliness and regular observation for signs of skin breakdown. (See *Foot care for diabetic patients.*)

Toenail trimming is contraindicated in patients with toe infections, diabetes mellitus, neurologic disorders, renal failure, or peripheral vascular disease, unless performed by a physician or podiatrist.

Equipment

Bath blanket ▪ large basin ▪ soap ▪ towel ▪ linen-saver pad ▪ pillow ▪ washcloth ▪ orangewood stick ▪ cotton-tipped applicator ▪ cotton ▪ lotion ▪ water-absorbent powder ▪ bath thermometer ▪ gloves, if the patient has open lesions.

Preparation of equipment

Fill the basin halfway with warm water. Test water temperature with a bath thermometer *because patients with diminished peripheral sensation could burn their feet in excessively hot water (over 105° F [40.6° C]) without feeling any warning pain.* If a bath thermometer isn't available, test the water by inserting your elbow. The water temperature should feel comfortably warm.

Implementation

- Assemble equipment at the patient's bedside. Wash your hands, and put on gloves if necessary.
- Tell the patient that you'll wash his feet and provide foot and toenail care.
- Cover the patient with a bath blanket. Fanfold the top linen to the foot of the bed.
- Place a linen-saver pad and a towel under the patient's feet *to keep the bottom linen dry.* Then position the basin on the pad.
- Insert a pillow beneath the patient's knee *to provide support,* and cushion the rim of the basin with the edge of the towel *to prevent pressure.*
- Immerse one foot in the basin. Wash it with soap, and then allow it to soak for about 10 minutes. Soaking softens the skin and toenails, loosens debris under toenails, and comforts and refreshes the patient.
- After soaking the foot, rinse it with a washcloth, remove it from the basin, and place it on the towel.
- Dry the foot thoroughly, especially between the toes, *to avoid skin breakdown.* Blot gently to dry *because harsh rubbing may damage the skin.*
- Empty the basin, refill it with warm water, and clean and soak the other foot.
- While the second foot is soaking, give the first one a pedicure. Using the cotton-tipped applicator, carefully clean the toenails. Using an orangewood stick, gently remove any dirt beneath the toenails; avoid injuring subungual skin.
- Consult a podiatrist if nails need trimming.
- Rinse the foot that has been soaking, dry it thoroughly, and give it a pedicure.
- Apply lotion *to moisten dry skin,* or lightly dust water-absorbent powder between the toes *to absorb moisture.*
- Remove and clean all equipment, and dispose of gloves.

Special considerations

- While providing foot care, observe the color, shape, and texture of the toenails. If you see redness, drying, cracking, blisters, discoloration, or other signs of traumatic injury, especially in patients with impaired peripheral circulation, notify the practitioner. *Because such patients are vulnerable to infection and gangrene,* they need prompt treatment.
- If a patient's toenail grows inward at the corners, tuck a wisp of cotton under it *to relieve pressure on the toe.*
- When giving the bedridden patient foot care, perform range-of-motion exercises unless contraindicated *to stimulate circulation and prevent foot contractures or muscle atrophy.* Tuck folded 2″ × 2″ gauze pads between overlapping toes *to protect the skin from the toenails.* Apply heel protectors or protective boots *to prevent skin breakdown.*

Documentation

Record the date and time of bathing and toenail trimming in your notes. Record and report any abnormal findings and any nursing actions you take.

SELECTED REFERENCES

American Orthopaedic Foot and Ankle Society: *www.aofas.org.*

American Podiatric Medical Association: *www.apma.org.*

Delmas, L. "Best Practice in the Assessment and Management of Diabetic Foot Ulcers," *Rehabilitation Nursing* 31(6):228-34, November-December 2006.

Frykberg, R.G., et al. "Diabetic Food Disorders: A Clinical Practice Guideline," *Journal of Foot and Ankle Surgery* 45(5 Suppl):S1-66, September-October 2006.

PERINEAL CARE

Perineal care, which includes care of the external genitalia and the anal area, should be performed during the daily bath and, if necessary, at bedtime and after urination and bowel movements. The procedure promotes cleanliness and prevents infection. It also removes irritating and odorous secretions, such as smegma, a cheeselike substance that collects under the foreskin of the penis and on the inner surface of the labia. For the patient with perineal skin breakdown, frequent bathing followed by application of an ointment or cream aids healing.

Standard precautions must be followed when providing perineal care, with due consideration given to the patient's privacy.

Equipment

Gloves ▪ washcloths ▪ clean basin ▪ mild soap ▪ bath towel ▪ bath blanket ▪ toilet tissue ▪ linen-saver pad ▪ trash bag ▪ optional: bedpan, peri bottle, antiseptic soap, petroleum jelly, zinc oxide cream, vitamin A and D ointment, and an abdominal pad.

Following genital or rectal surgery, you may need to use sterile supplies, including sterile gloves, gauze, and cotton balls.

Preparation of equipment

Obtain ointment or cream as needed. Fill the basin two-thirds full with warm water. Also fill the peri bottle with warm water if needed.

Implementation

- Assemble equipment at the patient's bedside and provide privacy.
- Wash your hands thoroughly, put on gloves, and explain to the patient what you're about to do.
- Adjust the bed to a comfortable working height *to prevent back strain,* and lower the head of the bed, if allowed.
- Provide privacy and help the patient to a supine position. Place a linen-saver pad under the patient's buttocks *to protect the bed from stains and moisture.*

Perineal care for the female patient

- *To minimize the patient's exposure and embarrassment,* place the bath blanket over her with corners head to foot and side to side. Wrap each leg with a side corner, tucking it under her hip. Then fold back the corner between her legs to expose the perineum.
- Ask the patient to bend her knees slightly and to spread her legs. Separate her labia with one hand and wash with the other, using gentle downward strokes from the front to the back of the perineum *to prevent intestinal organisms from contaminating the urethra or vagina.* Avoid the area around the anus, and use a clean section of washcloth for each stroke by folding each used section inward. *This prevents the spread of contaminated secretions or discharge.*
- Using a clean washcloth, rinse thoroughly from front to back *because soap residue can cause skin irritation.* Pat the area dry with a bath towel *because moisture can also cause skin irritation and discomfort.*
- Apply ordered ointments or creams.
- Turn the patient on her side to Sims' position, if possible, *to expose the anal area.*
- Clean, rinse, and dry the anal area, starting at the posterior vaginal opening and wiping from front to back.

Perineal care for the male patient

■ Drape the patient's legs *to minimize exposure and embarrassment* and expose the genital area.

■ Hold the shaft of the penis with one hand, and wash with the other, beginning at the tip and working in a circular motion from the center to the periphery (as shown below) *to avoid introducing microorganisms into the urethra.* Use a clean section of washcloth for each stroke *to prevent the spread of contaminated secretions or discharge.*

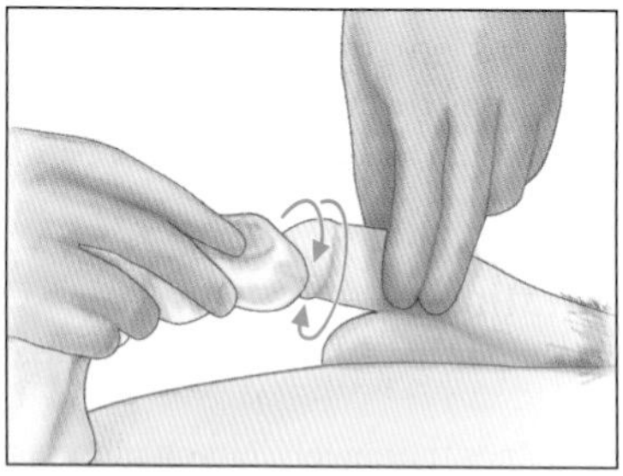

■ Rinse thoroughly, using the same circular motion.

■ For the uncircumcised patient, gently retract the foreskin and clean beneath it. Rinse well but don't dry *because moisture provides lubrication and prevents friction when replacing the foreskin.* Replace the foreskin *to avoid constriction of the penis, which causes edema and tissue damage.*

■ Wash the rest of the penis, using downward strokes toward the scrotum. Rinse well and pat dry with a towel.

■ Clean the top and sides of the scrotum; rinse thoroughly and pat dry. Handle the scrotum gently *to avoid causing discomfort.*

■ Turn the patient on his side. Clean the bottom of the scrotum and the anal area. Rinse well and pat dry.

After providing perineal care

■ Reposition the patient and make him comfortable. Remove the bath blanket and linen-saver pad, and then replace the bed linens.

■ Clean and return the basin and dispose of soiled articles including gloves.

Special considerations

■ Give perineal care to a patient of the opposite sex in a matter-of-fact way *to minimize embarrassment.*

■ If the patient is incontinent, first remove excess feces with toilet tissue. Then position him on a bedpan, and add a small amount of antiseptic soap to a peri bottle *to eliminate odor.* Irrigate the perineal area *to remove any remaining fecal matter.*

■ After cleaning the perineum, apply ointment or cream (petroleum jelly, zinc oxide cream, or vitamin A and D ointment) *to prevent skin breakdown by providing a barrier between the skin and excretions.*

■ To reduce the number of linen changes, tuck an abdominal pad between the patient's buttocks *to absorb oozing feces.*

Documentation

Record perineal care and any special treatment in your notes. Document the need for continued treatment, if necessary, in your care plan. Describe perineal skin condition and any odor or discharge.

Selected references

Grant, B.M., et al. "Vulnerable Bodies: Competing Discourses of Intimate Bodily Care," *Journal of Nursing Education* 44(11):498-504, November 2005.

Hansen, D., et al. "Perineal Dermatitis: A Consequence of Incontinence," *Advances in Skin and Wound Care* 19(5):246-50, June 2006.

Holloway, S., and Jones, V. "The Importance of Skin Care and Assessment," *British Journal of Nursing* 14(22):1172-76, December 2005-January 2006.

Kettle, C. "Perineal Care," *Clinical Evidence* 15:1905-18, June 2006.

Nix, D. "Prevention and Treatment of Perineal Skin Breakdown Due to Incontinence," *Ostomy/Wound Management* 52(4):26-28, April 2006.

Nix, D., and Ermer-Seltun, J. "A Review of Perineal Skin Care Protocols and Skin Barrier Product Use," *Ostomy/Wound Management* 50(12):59-67, December 2004.

Rader, J., et al. "The Bathing of Older Adults with Dementia," *AJN* 106(4):40-48, April 2006.

Wound, Ostomy, and Continence Nurses Society: *www.wocn.org.*

Hour of sleep care

Hour of sleep care meets the patient's physical and psychological needs in preparation for sleep. It includes providing for the patient's hygiene, making the bed clean and comfortable, and ensuring safety. For example, raising the bed's side rails can prevent the drowsy or sedated patient from falling out. Bedtime care also provides an opportunity to answer the patient's questions about the next day's tests and procedures and to discuss his worries and concerns.

Effective hour of sleep care prepares the patient for a good night's sleep. Ineffective care may contribute to sleeplessness, which can intensify patient anxiety and interfere with treatment and recuperation.

Equipment

Bedpan, urinal, or commode ■ basin ■ soap ■ towel ■ washcloth ■ toothbrush and toothpaste ■ denture cup and commercial denture cleaner, if necessary ■ lotion ■ clean linens, if necessary ■ blankets ■ facial tissues.

Preparation of equipment

Assemble the equipment at the patient's bedside. For the ambulatory patient who's capable of self-care, assemble soap, a washcloth, a towel, and oral hygiene items at the sink.

Implementation

■ Tell the patient you'll help him prepare for sleep, and provide privacy.

■ Offer the patient on bed rest a bedpan, urinal, or commode. Otherwise, assist the ambulatory patient to the bathroom.

■ Fill the basin with warm water and bring it to the patient's bedside. Immerse the lotion in the basin *to warm it for back massage.* Then wash the patient's face and hands and dry them well. Encourage the patient to do this himself, if possible, *to promote independence.*

■ Provide toothpaste or a properly labeled denture cup and commercial denture cleaner. Assist the patient with oral hygiene as necessary. (See "Mouth care," page 116.) If the patient prefers to wear dentures until bedtime, leave denture-care items within easy reach.

■ After providing mouth care, turn the patient on his side or stomach. Wash, rinse, and dry the patient's back and buttocks. Massage well with lotion *to help relax the patient.* (See "Back care," page 119, for complete information on massage.)

■ While providing back care, observe the skin for redness, cracking, or other signs of breakdown. If the patient's gown is soiled or damp, provide a clean one and help him put it on, if necessary.

■ Check dressings, binders, antiembolism stockings, or other aids, changing or readjusting them as needed.

■ Refill the water container, and place it and a box of facial tissues within the patient's easy reach *to prevent falls if the patient needs to reach for these items.*

■ Straighten or change bed linens, as necessary, and fluff the patient's pillow. Cover him with a blanket or place one within his easy reach *to prevent chills during the night.* Then position him comfortably. If he appears distressed, restless, or in pain, give ordered drugs, as needed.

■ After making the patient comfortable, evaluate his mental and physical condition. Place the bed in a low position, and raise the side rails according to your facility's policy. Place the call bell within the patient's easy reach, and instruct him to call you whenever necessary.

■ Next, tidy the patient's environment: Move all breakables from the overbed table out of his reach, and remove any equipment and supplies that could cause falls should the patient get up during the night.

■ Finally, put on the night-light and turn off the overhead light.

Special considerations

■ Ask the patient about his sleep routine at home and, whenever possible, let him follow it.

■ Also try to observe certain rituals, such as a bedtime snack, *which can aid sleep.* A back massage, tub bath, or shower may also help relax the patient and promote a restful night. If the patient normally bathes or showers before bedtime, let him do so if his condition and practitioner's orders permit it.

Documentation

Record the time and type of hour of sleep care in your notes. Include the use of any special procedurse, such as relaxation technique.

SELECTED REFERENCES

Béphage, G. "Promoting Quality Sleep in Older People: The Nursing Care Role," *British Journal of Nursing* 14(4):205-10, February 2005.

Carter, P.A. "A Brief Behavioral Sleep Intervention for Family Caregivers of Persons with Cancer," *Cancer Nursing* 29(2):95-103, March-April 2006.

Çelik, S., et al. "Sleep Disturbance: The Patient Care Activities Applied at the Night Shift in the Intensive Care Unit," *Journal of Clinical Nursing* 14(1):102-106, January 2005.

"Clinical Rounds: Does Sleep Ward Off Strokes?" *Nursing* 36(11):35, November 2006.

Craven, R.F., and Hirnle, C.J. *Fundamentals of Nursing: Human Health and Function,* 5th ed. Philadelphia: Lippincott Williams & Wilkins, 2007.

NUTRITION AND ELIMINATION

INTAKE AND OUTPUT

Many patients require fluid intake and output monitoring, such as surgical patients, patients on I.V. therapy or parenteral or enteral feedings, patients with fluid and electrolyte imbalances, those with nasogastric tubes connected to suction, and patients with burns, renal disease, heart disease, hemorrhage, vomiting, diarrhea, or edema. Intake and output assessment is also essential in monitoring a patient's response to treatment, particularly when treating dehydration or heart failure.

Fluid intake includes oral intake of fluids; I.V. fluids, medications, and flushes; tube feedings and flushes; liquid medications; and any other fluid installations or irrigations (such as bladder irrigations). Fluid output includes urine, liquid stool, vomitus, blood, and drainage from tubes, such as chest tubes, ileostomies, nephrostomy tubes, suction devices, and surgical drains. Approximately 100 ml of fluid or less is lost through the GI tract under normal conditions. Fluid is also lost through the skin and lungs, but these insensible sources of fluid loss aren't measurable.

Intake and output should be measured in milliliters and recorded on a 24-hour intake and output sheet. Intake and output may be recorded hourly or at the end of each shift, depending on the patient's condition. Total intake and output should be calculated at the end of 24 hours and recorded, according to your facility's protocol.

Equipment

Appropriate measuring container for each type of output being measured, marked in milliliters, such as urinal or graduated cylinder ■ appropriate devices for measuring input, such as syringe, medication cup, or water pitcher ■ intake and output form with volumes of specific containers listed ■ optional: gloves; intake and output worksheet; bedpan, urinal, or "hat"; commode.

Preparation of equipment

Label the measuring containers with patient's name. Inform the patient you'll be measuring intake and output. Provide a urinal, bedpan, or both for bedridden patients. For those patients who can use a commode, insert a bedpan or "hat" into the commode. For ambulatory patients, place a "hat" under the toilet seat. Label the intake and output record with all the sources of fluid intake and output *so that each source can be recorded separately.* For example, there should be a separate space for listing each of the following I.V. fluid sources: continuous I.V. fluid infusions, medications given by the I.V. route, and normal saline flushes.

Implementation

- Confirm the patient's identity using two patient identifiers according to your facility's policy.
- Explain to the patient and family that you'll be measuring intake and output *to elicit their support and cooperation.* Instruct the family to measure any fluids they give to the patient, to place any output in a urinal or bedpan in the bathroom, and to call the nurse to have it measured.
- Post an intake and output worksheet with the date and patient's name on the door or in the bathroom, according to your facility's policy, *to alert staff to measure intake and output and to have a convenient place to immediately record amounts.* The patient and family can also be taught to record fluid intake or output on this worksheet.

Measuring intake

- When a tube feeding or I.V. fluid is hung, note the type of solution, rate, and amount on the appropriate line of the intake section of the intake and output record. A separate flow sheet may be used for tube feedings or I.V. fluid administration. Shift totals may then be transferred to the intake and output record. (See *Intake and output record.*)
- Record the amount of oral fluids ingested. Include any food that's a fluid at room temperature, such as sherbet, ice cream, ice chips, and gelatin. Record ice chips at approximately one-half of their volume.
- Measure and record the type and amount of any instillations and how they were administered, such as bladder, nasogastric, and tube feeding irrigations.
- Include the amount of any medications in fluid or elixir form that are administered orally.
- Measure and record the amount of any medication given by the I.V. route, including normal saline and heparin flushes.
- Measure and record the amount of medications given through a GI tube, including any tap water flushes.

Measuring output

- Wash hands thoroughly and don gloves.
- Pour urine from bedpan or "hat" into a graduated measuring container, and record the amount on the worksheet or in the appropriate section of the intake and output record. If the patient is using a urinal, use the markings on the side of the container to obtain the amount.
- Record the color, clarity, and odor of the urine, if indicated. If the intake and output record doesn't provide space for this, include this information in a progress note.
- To empty a urinary drainage bag, open the clamp and allow the urine to flow into a calibrated measuring container. *A measuring container allows for a more accurate reading of urine output than using the markings on the side of the drainage bag.* Don't touch the drainage tube to the sides of the container *to reduce the risk of introducing microorganisms into the urinary drainage bag.* Close and secure the clamp after draining the urine. Record the urine output on the intake and output record.
- Measure and record all liquid stool and vomitus on the intake and output record. Describe the appearance of this output.

Intake and output record

As the sample shows, you can monitor your patient's fluid balance by using an intake and output record.

Name: Josephine Klein

Medical record #: 49731

Admission date: 2/13/08

INTAKE AND OUTPUT RECORD

	Intake						Output				
	Oral	*Tube feeding*	*Instilled*	*I.V. and IVPB*	*TPN*	*Total*	*Urine*	*Emesis*	*NG tubes*	*Other*	*Total*
DATE 2/15/08											
0700–1500	250	320	H_2O 50	1100		1720	1355				1355
1500–2300	200	320	H_2O 50	1100		1670	1200				1200
2300–0700		320	H_2O 50	1100		1470	1500				1500
24hr total	450	960	H_2O 150	3300		4860	4055				4055
DATE											
24hr total											
DATE											
24hr total											
DATE											
24hr total											

Key: IVPB = I.V. piggyback TPN = total parenteral nutrition NG = nasogastric

Standard measures

Styrofoam cup	240 ml	Water (large)	600 ml	Milk (large)	600 ml	Ice cream, sherbet, or gelatin	120 ml
Juice	120 ml	Water pitcher	750 ml	Coffee	240 ml		
Water (small)	120 ml	Milk (small)	120 ml	Soup	180 ml		

■ Empty drains into a graduated container, and record the amount in the appropriate space on the intake and output record. Label each drain and record the amount from each separately, *so that the source of any change in amount or characteristic can be identified.* A medication cup may be used to accurately measure amounts less than 30 ml. Record the color, consistency, odor, and other characteristics.
■ For systems that don't get emptied, such as a nasogastric suction container or chest tube drainage system, place a mark at the beginning of the shift at the appropriate height of drainage, and write the date, time and your initials next to it. Record hourly or shift totals, as indicated, in the appropriate place on the intake and output record. Record the color, consistency, odor, and other characteristics of the drainage.
■ In a progress note, describe insensible fluid losses, such as profuse diaphoresis.

Special considerations

■ Assess and record the patient's hydration status, such as vital signs, skin turgor, jugular vein distention, heart sounds, breath sounds, daily weight, thirst, edema, pulses, and mucous membranes. Notify the practitioner of abnormal findings.
■ Keep in mind normal intake and output values for a healthy adult when evaluating your patient's fluid status.
■ In addition to recording the amount of I.V. medication and liquid medication given orally or through a feeding tube on the intake and output record, be sure to record these medications on the medication administration record.

Documentation

Write the patient's name on the intake and output record. Record the date and time of your shift on the appropriate line. Record the total intake and output for each category of fluid for your shift, then total these categories and provide a shift total for intake and output. If hourly intake and output is needed, record these totals hourly and total them at the end of the shift. At the end of 24 hours, a daily total is calculated. Describe the characteristics of the output (such as urine, vomitus, and drainage) in a progress note if space isn't available on the intake and output record. Include the findings from your physical assessment. In a progress note, record the time and name of the practitioner notified of any abnormal findings, any orders given, nursing interventions performed, and the patient's response. Record any patient education performed.

Selected references

Craven, R.F. and Hirnle, C.J. *Fundamentals of Nursing: Human Health and Function,* 5th ed. Philadelphia: Lippincott Williams & Wilkins, 2007.
Fallis, W. M. "Indwelling Foley Catheters: Is the Current Design a Source of Erroneous Measurement of Urine Output?" *Critical Care Nurse* 25(2): 44-51, April 2005.
Hodgkinson, B., et. al. "Maintaining Oral Hydration in Older Adults: A Systematic Review," *International Journal of Nursing Practice* 9:S19-S28, 2003.
The Joanna Briggs Institute. "Maintaining Hydration in Older People. Evidence Based Practice Information Sheets For Health Professionals," 5(1), 2004. Available at *www.joannabriggs.edu.au/best_practice/BPIShyd.php.*

Feeding

Confusion, arm or hand immobility, injury, weakness, or restrictions on activities or positions may prevent a patient from feeding himself. Feeding the patient then becomes a key nursing responsibility. Injured or debilitated patients may experience depression and subsequent anorexia. Meeting such patients' nutritional needs requires determining food preferences; conducting the feeding in a friendly, unhurried manner; encouraging self-feeding to promote independence and dignity; and documenting intake and output.

Equipment

Meal tray ■ overbed table ■ linen-saver pad or towels ■ clean linens ■ flexible straws ■ basin of water ■ feeding syringe ■ assistive feeding devices if necessary.

Implementation

■ *Because many adults consider being fed demeaning,* allow the patient some control over mealtime, such as letting him set the pace of the meal or decide the order in which he eats various foods.
■ Raise the head of the bed if allowed. *Fowler's or semi-Fowler's position makes swallowing easier and reduces the risk of aspiration and choking.*
■ Before the meal tray arrives, give the patient soap, a basin of water or a wet washcloth, and a hand towel *to clean his hands.* If necessary, you may wash his hands for him.
■ Wipe the overbed table with soap and water or alcohol, especially if a urinal or bedpan was on it.
■ When the meal tray arrives, confirm the patient's identity using two patient identifiers according to your facility's policy; make sure they match the name on the tray. Check the tray to make sure it contains foods appropriate for the patient's condition.

■ Encourage the patient to feed himself if he can. If he's restricted to the prone or the supine position but can use his arms and hands, encourage him to try foods he can pick up such as sandwiches. If he can assume Fowler's or semi-Fowler's position but has limited use of his arms or hands, teach him how to use assistive feeding devices. (See *Using assistive feeding devices,* page 130.)
■ If necessary, tuck a napkin or towel under his chin *to protect his gown from spills.* Use a linen-saver pad or towel *to protect bed linens.*
■ Position a chair next to the patient's bed so you can sit comfortably if you need to feed him yourself.
■ Set up the patient's tray, remove the plate from the tray warmer, and discard all plastic wrappings. Then cut the food into bite-size pieces. Season the food per the patient's request as appropriate.
■ To help the blind or visually impaired patient feed himself, tell him that placement of various foods on his plate corresponds to the hours on a clock face. Maintain consistent placement for subsequent meals.
■ Ask the patient which food he prefers to eat first *to promote his sense of control over the meal.* Some patients prefer to eat one food at a time, while others prefer to alternate foods.
■ If the patient has difficulty swallowing, check the patient's plan of care for special instructions on swallowing techniques recommended by speech therapy. Offer liquids carefully with a spoon or feeding syringe *to help prevent aspiration.* Pureed or soft foods, such as custard or flavored gelatin, may be easier to swallow than liquids. If the patient doesn't have difficulty swallowing, use a flexible straw *to reduce the risk of spills.*
■ Ask the patient to indicate when he's ready for another mouthful. Pause between courses and whenever the patient wants to rest. During the meal, wipe the patient's mouth and chin as needed.
■ When the patient finishes eating, remove the tray. If necessary, clean up spills and change the bed linens. Provide mouth care.

Special considerations

■ Don't feed the patient too quickly *because this can upset him and impair digestion.*
■ If the patient is restricted to the supine position, provide foods that he can chew easily. If he's restricted to the supine position, feed him liquids carefully and only after he has swallowed his food *to reduce the risk of aspiration.*
■ If the patient won't eat, try to find out why. For example, confirm his food preferences. Also, make sure the patient isn't in pain at mealtimes or that he hasn't received any treatments immediately before a meal that could upset or nauseate him. Find out if any medications cause anorexia, nausea, or sedation. Of course, clear the bedside of emesis basins, urinals, bedpans, and similar distractions at mealtimes.
■ Establish a pattern for feeding the patient, and share this information with the rest of the staff *so the patient doesn't need to repeatedly instruct staff members about the best way to feed him.*
■ If the patient and his family are willing, suggest that family members assist with feeding. This will make the patient feel more comfortable at mealtimes and may ease discharge planning.
■ If the patient has a swallowing difficulty (such as in stroke or head injury), consult with speech therapy before feeding *to best determine the type of foods the patient requires (thickened, and so forth).*

Complications

Choking and aspiration of food can occur if the patient is fed too quickly or is given excessively large mouthfuls.

Documentation

Describe the feeding technique used in the nursing care plan to ensure continuity of care. In your notes, record the amount of food and fluid consumed; also note the fluids consumed on the intake and output record, if required. Note which foods the patient consistently fails to eat, then try to find the reason. Record the patient's level of independence. For the blind patient, record the pattern of feeding on the nursing care plan.

SELECTED REFERENCES

Bowman A., et al. "Implementation of an Evidence-Based Feeding Protocol and Aspiration Risk Reduction Algorithm," *Critical Care Nursing Quarterly* 28(4):324-333, October/December 2005.

Carlsson, E., et al. "Stroke and Eating Difficulties: Long-Term Experiences," *Journal of Clinical Nursing* 13(7):824-34, October 2004.

DiBartolo, M.C. "Careful Hand Feeding: A Reasonable Alternative to PEG Tube Placement in Individuals with Dementia," *Journal of Gerontologic Nursing* 3295:25-33, May 2006.

Hung, J.W., and Wu, Y.H. "Fitting a Bilateral Transhumeral Amputee with Utensil Prostheses and Their Functional Assessment 10 Years Later: A Case Report," *Archives of Physical Medicine and Rehabilitation* 86(11):2211-13, November 2005.

EQUIPMENT

Using assistive feeding devices

Various feeding devices, available through consulting occupational therapy, can help the patient who has limited arm mobility, grasp, range of motion (ROM), or coordination. Before introducing your patient to an assistive feeding device, assess his ability to master it. Don't introduce a device he can't manage. If his condition is progressively disabling, encourage him to use the device only until his mastery of it falters.

Introduce the assistive device before mealtime, with the patient seated in a natural position. Explain its purpose, show the patient how to use it, and encourage him to practice. After meals, wash the device thoroughly, and store it in the patient's bedside stand. Document the patient's progress, and share it with staff and family members to help reinforce the patient's independence. Specific devices include the following:

Plate guard

This device blocks food from spilling off the plate. Attach the guard to the side of the plate opposite the hand the patient uses to feed himself. Guiding the patient's hand, show him how to push food against the guard to secure it on the utensil. Then have him try again with food of a different consistency. When the patient tires, feed him the rest of the meal. At subsequent meals, encourage the patient to feed himself for progressively longer periods until he can feed himself an entire meal.

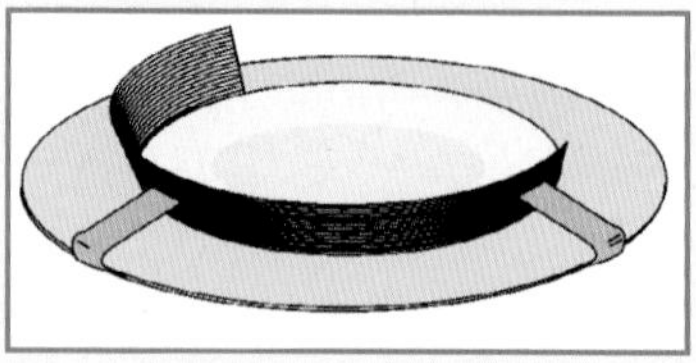

Swivel spoon

This utensil helps the patient with limited ROM in his forearm and will fit in universal cuffs.

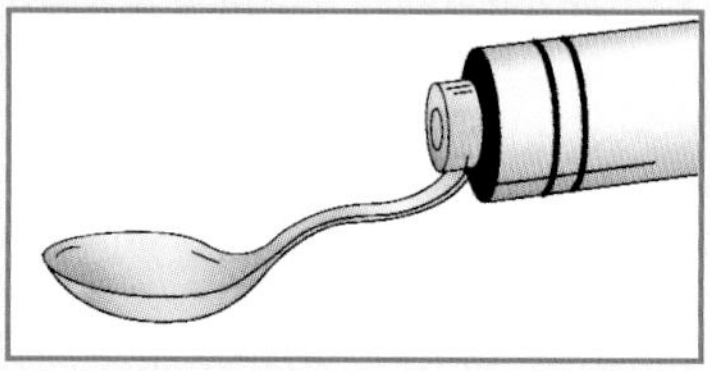

Universal cuffs

These flexible bands help the patient with flail hands or diminished grasp. Each cuff contains a slot that holds a fork or spoon. Attach the cuff to the hand the patient uses to feed himself. Then place the fork or spoon in the cuff slot. Bend the utensil to facilitate feeding.

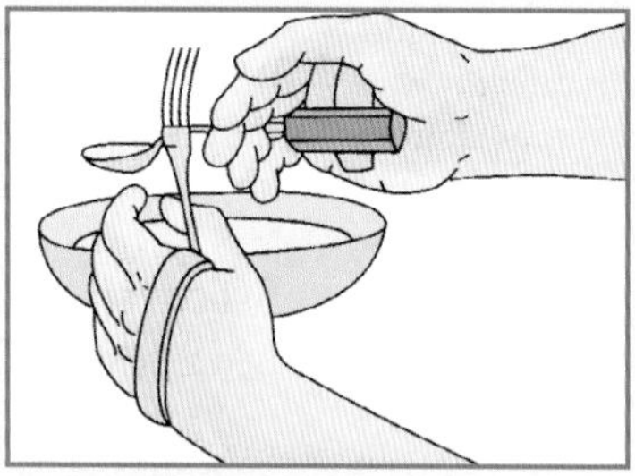

Long-handled utensils

These utensils have jointed stems to help the patient with limited ROM in his elbow and shoulder.

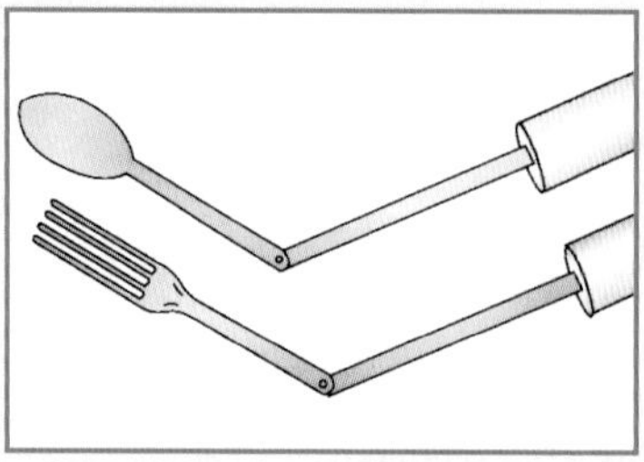

Utensils with built-up handles

These utensils can help the patient with diminished grasp. They can be purchased or can be improvised by wrapping tape around the handles.

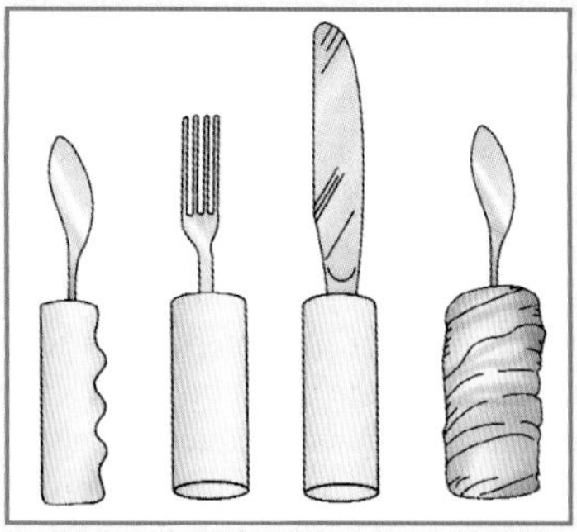

Spouted cups

These cups have a spout, which can prevent spills and burns in patients experiencing tremors or who have unsteady arms and hands.

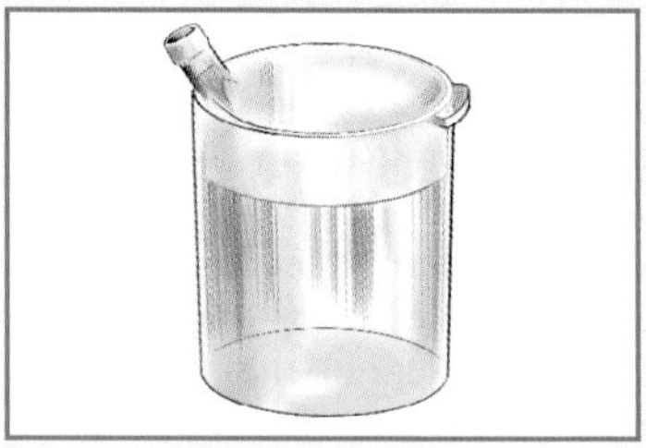

Slotted (Nosey) cups

These cups have a cut out for the nose to allow the patient to drink without bending his neck or tilting his head. Some have handles on both sides to ensure a firm grasp.

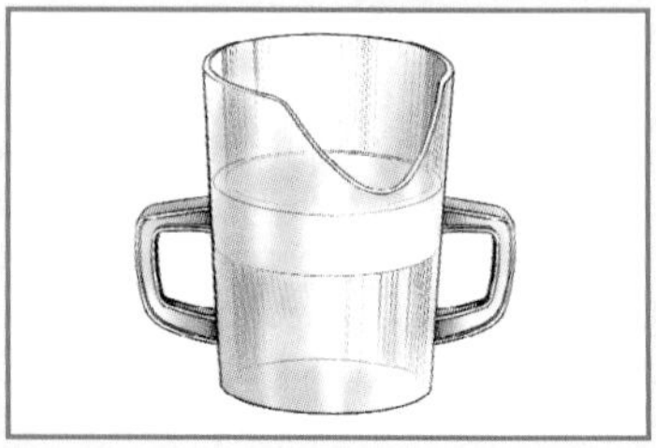

IMPAIRED SWALLOWING AND ASPIRATION PRECAUTIONS

Patients may experience impaired swallowing as a result of several specific problems. The first of these, oropharyngeal dysphagia, is impaired swallowing associated with deficits in oral and pharyngeal structure or function. These patients are at especially high risk for aspiration, and many of them experience silent aspiration. Patients at risk for oropharyngeal dysphagia include those with:

- nervous system damage such as stroke, head injury, or spinal cord injury
- neuromuscular diseases such as muscular dystrophy and cerebral palsy
- progressive neurologic disease such as Parkinson's disease, multiple sclerosis, amyotrophic lateral sclerosis, and dementia
- facial, oral, or neck surgery or trauma
- head and neck cancer.

Patients who were intubated for more than 3 days are also at risk for oropharyngeal dysphagia.

The second impaired swallowing problem is associated with esophageal dysphagia and aspiration risk due to:

- gastroesophageal reflux disease
- esophageal dysmotility or structural abnormality
- delayed gastric emptying
- nasogastric tubes.

Finally, impaired swallowing can be associated with tracheostomy or ventilation support due to:

- decreased sensation of the oral and pharyngeal cavities
- decreased sensation of food or fluids penetrating the laryngeal vestibule and aspirating (dropping below the level of the vocal cords)
- decreased ability to cough aspirated material off the vocal cords
- decreased laryngeal elevation and airway closure.

Equipment

Meal tray ■ call bell ■ wall suction or portable suction apparatus ■ suction kit ■ gloves ■ protective eyewear ■ pulse oximeter.

Implementation

- Confirm the patient's identity using two patient identifiers according to your facility's policy.
- Explain the procedure to the patient and his family.
- Wash your hands, and put on gloves and protective eyewear, if indicated, before suctioning the patient or providing mouth care.
- Set up the meal tray and position the patient for eating.
- If applicable, ensure that dentures are in place and fit well.

Managing impaired swallowing due to oropharyngeal dysphagia

- Assist with a bedside swallow evaluation (generally conducted by a speech-language pathologist).
- After completion of the swallowing evaluation, develop a management plan that includes common swallowing strategies, nutritional status, and supervision.

Using common swallowing strategies

- Have suction equipment available at the bedside.
- Position the patient at a 90-degree angle during meals *to decrease the risk of aspiration.*
- Provide for or perform oral care before and after meals, and be sure to check for food residue.
- If applicable, ensure that dentures are in place and that they fit well.
- Crush medications, as appropriate, and mix into applesauce.
- Minimize distractions when the patient is eating and drinking.
- If applicable, ensure that the temperature, consistency, and amount of foods and liquids are appropriate. Water should be chilled; avoid tepid liquids or food. Avoid mixed consistencies.
- Avoid straws. Encourage small sips.
- Encourage slow intake with adequate chewing.
- If one side of the patient's face is paralyzed, place food on the unaffected side. Check the affected side of the mouth for food that may lodge in the cheek during and after meals. If appropriate, teach the patient to perform a finger sweep.
- If fatigue impairs swallowing, provide rest periods before and during meals as needed.
- Assess swallowing between bites by feeling the rise and fall of the larynx (Adam's apple).
- Use cold or sour foods, and massage cheeks or throat *to stimulate the swallow trigger.*
- Have the patient remain sitting in an upright position for 30 minutes after meals.

Monitoring nutritional status

- Ask a dietitian to conduct a nutrition evaluation.
- Monitor the patient's hydration and nutrition.
- Implement calorie counts as needed.
- Weigh the patient daily or as ordered.
- Consult with the patient and family regarding food and fluid preferences.
- Provide small frequent meals and supplements.
- Praise the patient and family for achieving nutritional goals.

Using one-on-one supervision

- Monitor the patient for signs and symptoms of aspiration.
- Ensure that the patient has someone present throughout every meal.
- Provide feeding assistance or cueing for feeding and swallowing strategies during the entire meal, or ensure that a family member does this.
- *Because patients with dysphagia typically need to eat slowly,* allow these patients at least 30 to 45 minutes to eat.

Using close supervision

- Monitor the patient for signs and symptoms of aspiration.
- Check on the patient frequently during the meal, and spend 3 to 5 minutes each time recueing the patient to use swallowing strategies.
- Encourage the patient to increase intake, if needed, and provide other options *to maximize safety and nutritional intake.*
- Ensure that the call bell is within the patient's reach.

Using distant supervision

- Ensure that the call bell is within the patient's reach.
- Monitor the patient for signs and symptoms of aspiration.
- Provide initial cueing to initiate swallowing strategies.
- Check on the patient frequently.
- Assess the patient's progress at least two to three times during meals.

Managing impaired swallowing due to esophageal dysphagia

- Monitor for reflux and aspiration risks related to esophageal dysphagia.
- Initiate a bedside swallow evaluation to help differentiate oropharyngeal dysphagia from esophageal dysphagia.
- Consult with a speech-language pathologist to determine the need for alternative nutrition.
- Monitor respiratory rate, depth, and breath sounds for cough, dyspnea, cyanosis, crackles, or wheezes that may indicate aspiration and airway obstruction.
- Monitor bowel sounds and assess for abdominal distention.

NURSING ALERT *Absence of bowel sounds and increasing abdominal distention may indicate an ileus or bowel obstruction with resulting vomiting and risk of aspiration.*

- Monitor the patient's intake and output and daily weights.
- Weight loss can be an indicator of an esophageal problem.
- Implement strategies for oral intake.
- Position the patient at a 90-degree angle during oral feeding, and maintain the position for 45 to 60 minutes after the meal *to decrease the risk of reflux, regurgitation, and aspiration.*
- Offer thin liquids and pureed and moist foods that may be easier to swallow if the patient has esophageal dysmotility.
- Feed the patient slowly; allow adequate time for esophageal emptying.
- If the patient feels full quickly, offer small, frequent meals of foods high in caloric content.
- Alternate liquids and solids to improve esophageal emptying of the solids.
- Avoid spicy and acidic foods, and decrease caffeine intake *to decrease reflux.*
- Tell the patient to avoid eating before bedtime and to keep the head of his bed elevated above a 30-degree angle at night.

Managing impaired swallowing due to tracheostomy or endotracheal tube

- Request a referral to a speech-language pathologist for a bedside swallow evaluation before beginning feeding if aspiration risk is likely.
- Suction the patient every 2 hours or as needed *to maintain a patent airway.*
- Obtain a practitioner's order for speaking valve trials as appropriate.
- Follow speech therapy and practitioner recommendations on cuff inflation versus deflation for oral intake. The patient may still be able to aspirate around an inflated cuff.

Conducting speaking valve trials

- Have the speech-language pathologist assess the patient's tolerance of the speaking valve. In addition to hands-free speech, the speaking valve can also return oropharyngeal sensation and taste.
- Deflate the cuff before placing the valve. Monitor oxygen saturation at baseline, with the valve in place, and with the valve removed.
- Follow speaking valve recommendations for cleaning and wearing schedules.
- Place the speaking valve during meals (according to the speech-language pathologist's recommendations) because it's usually safer to eat with the valve in place; the valve increases the patient's ability to cough material off the vocal cords.

Managing a patient with a feeding tube

- Initiate a dietary consultation.
- Provide oral care for the patient who's on nothing-by-mouth status *to decrease colonization of bacteria in the mouth.*

■ Following feeding tube placement, use X-ray *to ensure its accurate placement.* X-ray verification of placement is the gold standard for safe placement, especially of small-bore feeding tubes.
■ Assess placement of the feeding tube before feeding and every 4 hours for patients with continuous feedings. Aspirate contents from the tube, and determine pH (less than 3.5 for stomach contents) and other characteristics of the aspirate. *Testing pH and noting the aspirate characteristics are the most reliable means of determining that the tube hasn't become dislodged.*

NURSING ALERT *Listening to stomach sounds as air is injected into the tube is no longer considered an accurate method to verify the placement of a feeding tube.*

■ If assessment indicates the possibility of feeding solution in mucus coughed or suctioned from the trachea, test the mucus for glucose. *A positive result may indicate tube displacement and aspiration of the feeding solution.*
■ Assess gastric residual amounts before feedings and at least every 4 hours for patients receiving continuous feeding. If the aspirate amount is greater than 100 ml, follow facility guidelines for withholding feeding. *Retained feeding solution can increase intragastric pressure, resulting in an increased risk of regurgitation and aspiration.*
■ Maintain the patient in semi-Fowler's position (at least 30 degrees) during feeding and for 30 to 45 minutes after feeding to facilitate movement of the feeding solution through the stomach and into the small intestine, thus decreasing the risk of regurgitation and aspiration.

Special considerations

Monitor the patient for signs and symptoms of swallowing problems and aspiration, including:
- coughing before, during, or after eating
- wet or "gurgling" voice
- increased chest congestion after eating
- multiple swallows on one mouthful or washing down food with liquids
- complaints of food getting "stuck" or painful swallowing
- unexplained changes in amount or rate of eating
- drooling or spitting food out of the mouth
- difficulty breathing during meals
- leakage from the tracheostomy site
- low-grade fevers shortly after meals
- weight loss and poor oral intake
- recurrent pneumonias
- increased white blood cell counts.

Patient teaching

■ Train the family to feed the patient, and supervise them as needed.
■ Teach family members the abdominal thrust maneuver.
■ Teach family members how to use suction equipment as needed.

Complications

Patients with impaired swallowing are more likely to experience airway obstruction and aspiration during meals. Aspiration may result in pneumonitis or pneumonia. Difficulty swallowing may result in decreased oral intake and eventually lead to dehydration and malnutrition.

Documentation

Record the amount of intake, the patient's food preferences, progress with meals, and any techniques effective in helping the swallowing process. Document the effectiveness of the family's assistance. Record any complications that arise and the interventions used to correct them.

SELECTED REFERENCES

Bowman, A., et al. "Implementation of an Evidence-Based Feeding Protocol and Aspiration Risk Reduction Algorithm," *Critical Care Nursing Quarterly* 28(4): 324-333, October-December 2005.

LeClerc, C., et al. "A Feeding Abilities Assessment for Persons with Dementia," *Alzheimer's Care Quarterly* 5(2):123-33, April-June 2004.

Serna, E.D., and McCarthy, M.S. "Doing It Better: Heads Up to Prevent Aspiration During Enteral Feeding," *Nursing* 36(1):76-77, January 2006.

Smith Hammond, C.A., and Goldstein, L. B. "Cough and Aspiration of Food and Liquids Due to Oral-Pharyngeal Dysphagia: ACCP Evidence-Based Clinical Practice Guidelines," *Chest* 129 (Suppl 1): 154S-168S, January 2006.

West, J., and Redstone, F. "Feeding the Adult with Neurogenic Disorders," *Topics in Geriatric Rehabilitation* 20(2): 131-134, April-June 2004.

Yoshikawa, M., et al. "Influence of Aging and Denture Use on Liquid Swallowing in Healthy Dentulous and Edentulous Older People," *Journal of the American Geriatrics Society* 54(3): 444-49, March 2006.

NUTRITIONAL SCREENING

A person's nutritional status is evaluated by examining information about the patient from several sources. A nutritional screening, along with the patient's medical history, physical assessment findings, and laboratory results, can be used to detect nutritional imbalances. If the nutritional screening determines the patient is at risk for a nutritional disorder, a comprehensive nutritional assessment may then be conducted to set goals and determine interventions to correct actual or potential imbalances.

Overcoming height measurement problems

A patient confined to a wheelchair or one who can't stand straight because of scoliosis poses a challenge in measuring accurate height. An approximate measurement of height can be obtained by measuring "wingspan."

Winging it

Have the patient hold his arms straight out from the sides of his body. Children may be told to hold their arms out "like bird wings." Measure from the tip of one middle finger to the tip of the other. That distance is the patient's approximate height.

Calculating BMI

Use one of the formulas below to calculate your patient's body mass index (BMI).

$$BMI = (\text{weight in pounds} \div \text{height in inches}^2) \times 703$$

or

$$BMI = (\text{weight in kilograms} \div \text{height in centimeters}^2) \times 10{,}000$$

or

$$BMI = \text{weight in kilograms} \div \text{height in meters}^2$$

Nutritional screening also examines certain variables to determine the risk of nutritional problems in specific populations. A screening may target pregnant women, the elderly, or those with certain disorders (such as cardiac disorders) to detect deficiencies or potential imbalances. Routine screening occurs during the initial history and physical assessment.

Equipment

Standing scale with measuring bars ■ nutritional screening form ■ optional: chair or bed scale, tape measure.

Preparation of equipment

Select the appropriate scale—usually, a standing scale for an ambulatory patient or a chair or bed scale for an acutely ill or debilitated patient. Then check to make sure the scale is balanced. *Standing scales and, to a lesser extent, bed scales may become unbalanced when transported.*

Implementation

- Confirm the patient's identity using two patient identifiers according to your facility's policy.
- Explain the purpose and procedure for nutritional screening to the patient.
- Ask the patient to remove his shoes, and obtain his weight using a scale. *Weight provides a rough estimate of body composition.*
- Ask about unplanned or unintentional weight loss. Determine how much weight the patient lost and over what period of time. A weight loss of more than 5% in 30 days or 10% in 180 days places the patient at nutritional risk.
- Measure the patient's height while standing erect without shoes, using the measuring bar on the scale. If the patient can't stand, approximate the height by measuring "wingspan." (See *Overcoming height measurement problems.*)
- Calculate or estimate body mass index (BMI) to evaluate weight in relation to height. A BMI of 18.5 to 24.9 defines healthy weight; a BMI of 25 to 29.9 defines overweight; a BMI of 30 or more defines obesity. (See *Calculating BMI.* See also *Determining BMI.*)
- Question the patient about his eating habits, living environment, and functional status to determine if he's at risk for nutritional problems. A problem in any of these areas places the patient at risk and requires further nutritional assessment.
- Examine the patient's laboratory values for information on nutritional status. A serum albumin level less than 3.5 mg/dl is a nonspecific indicator of poor nutrition. Prealbumin is the most accurate indicator because it reveals the most recent nutritional status (past 7 to 14 days). Serum transferrin reflects the patient's current protein status more accurately than albumin because of its shorter half-life. Elevated transferrin levels may indicate severe iron deficiency. Decreased hemoglobin and hematocrit levels suggest iron deficiency anemia. Decreased total lymphocyte count may indicate reduced protein stores.
- Review the medical record, and interview the patient *to determine if his present illness or medical history places him at nutritional risk.*
- Review physical assessment findings for signs of poor nutrition. (See *Evaluating nutritional disorders,* page 136.)
- Make a referral to a registered dietitian if a nutritional screening suggests the patient is at risk for nutritional problems. A registered dietitian will then perform a comprehensive nutritional assessment.

Special considerations

- The nutritional screening is typically performed during the initial nursing history and physical, but should be completed within 24 hours of admission.

Determining BMI

Body mass index (BMI) measures weight in relation to height. The BMI ranges shown here are for adults. They aren't exact ranges for healthy or unhealthy weights; however, they show that health risks increase at higher levels of overweight and obesity. To use the graph below, find your patient's weight along the bottom and then go straight up until you come to the line that matches his height. The shaded area indicates whether your patient is healthy, overweight, or obese.

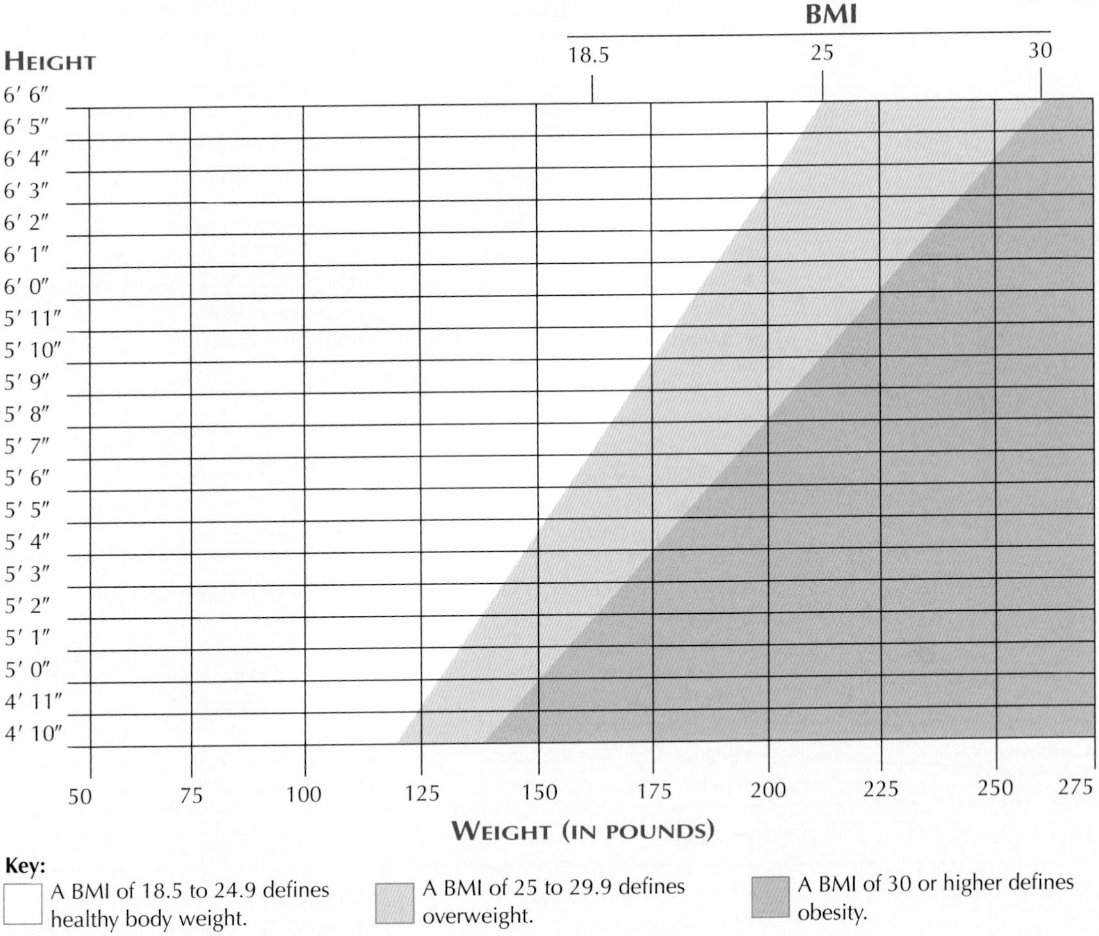

Adapted from *Nutrition and Your Health: Dietary Guidelines for Americans,* 5th ed. (Home and Garden Bulletin No. 232.) Washington, D.C.: U.S. Department of Agriculture, U.S. Department of Health and Human Services, 2000.

■ When measuring height, note the growth of children as well as diminishing height of older adults. Growth of children may be noted on standardized charts to assess growth patterns for possible abnormalities. Diminishing height of older adults may be related to osteoporotic changes and should be investigated.

■ The mini nutritional assessment may be used both for screening and assessing for malnutrition in the older adult.

Evaluating nutritional disorders

This table can help you interpret your nutritional assessment findings. Body systems are listed below with signs or symptoms and the implications for each.

BODY SYSTEM OR REGION	SIGN OR SYMPTOM	IMPLICATIONS
General	■ Weakness and fatigue ■ Weight loss	■ Anemia or electrolyte imbalance ■ Decreased calorie intake, increased calorie use, or inadequate nutrient intake or absorption
Skin, hair, and nails	■ Dry, flaky skin ■ Dry skin with poor turgor ■ Rough, scaly skin with bumps ■ Petechiae or ecchymoses ■ Sore that won't heal ■ Thinning, dry hair ■ Spoon-shaped, brittle, or ridged nails	■ Vitamin A, vitamin B-complex, or linoleic acid deficiency ■ Dehydration ■ Vitamin A deficiency ■ Vitamin C or K deficiency ■ Protein, vitamin C, or zinc deficiency ■ Protein deficiency ■ Iron deficiency
Eyes	■ Night blindness; corneal swelling, softening, or dryness; Bitot's spots (gray triangular patches on the conjunctiva) ■ Red conjunctiva	■ Vitamin A deficiency ■ Riboflavin deficiency
Throat and mouth	■ Cracks at the corner of the mouth ■ Magenta tongue ■ Beefy, red tongue ■ Soft, spongy, bleeding gums ■ Swollen neck (goiter)	■ Riboflavin or niacin deficiency ■ Riboflavin deficiency ■ Vitamin B_{12} deficiency ■ Vitamin C deficiency ■ Iodine deficiency
Cardiovascular	■ Edema ■ Tachycardia, hypotension	■ Protein deficiency ■ Fluid volume deficit
GI	■ Ascites	■ Protein deficiency
Musculoskeletal	■ Bone pain and bow leg ■ Muscle wasting	■ Vitamin D or calcium deficiency ■ Protein, carbohydrate, and fat deficiency
Neurologic	■ Altered mental status ■ Paresthesia	■ Dehydration and thiamine or vitamin B_{12} deficiency ■ Vitamin B_{12}, pyridoxine, or thiamine deficiency

Depending on the score on the screening portion of the tool, the second part of the tool is completed to provide a more detailed nutritional assessment.

Documentation

Record the date and time of the nutritional screening. Place the patient's height and weight on the screening form as well as the graphic sheet or patient care flow sheet, per your facility's policy. Note the type of scale used. Check off the appropriate patient responses on the screening tool for eating habits, living environment, and functional status. Calculate and record the BMI. Use a progress note to record information that doesn't have a space on the screening tool. Record whether the patient has experienced any weight loss, the period of time over which the loss has occurred, and how much weight was lost. Note the date and time of any blood samples obtained and the laboratory tests requested. Document laboratory results and the time and name of anyone you notified of abnormal results and whether orders were given. Note nutritional problems that were detected during the physical examination and review of the medical record. Include any patient teaching. For patients at nutritional risk, record the date, time, names of the people notified, whether they came to see the patient, orders given, nursing interventions, and patient response.

SELECTED REFERENCES

Ferguson, M., et al. "Development of a Valid and Reliable Malnutrition Screening Tool for Adult Acute Hospital Patients," *Nutrition* 15(6):458-464, June 1999.

Green, S.M., and Watson, R. "Nutritional Screening and Assessment Tools for Use by Nurses: Literature Review," *Journal of Advanced Nursing* 50(1):69-83, April 2005.

The Joint Commission. *Comprehensive Accreditation Manual for Hospitals. Update. The Official Handbook.* Chicago: 2007.

Kondrup, J., et al. "ESPEN Guidelines for Nutrition Screening 2002," *Clinical Nutrition* 22(4):415-421, August 2003.

U.S. Preventative Services Task Force. "Screening for Obesity in Adults: Recommendations and Rationale," *Annals of Internal Medicine 39*(11):930-32, December 2003.

BEDPAN AND URINAL

Bedpans and urinals permit elimination by the bedridden patient and accurate observation and measurement of urine and stool by the nurse. A bedpan is used by the female patient for defecation and urination and by the male patient for defecation; a urinal is used by the male patient for urination. Either device should be offered frequently—before meals, visiting hours, morning and evening care, and any treatments or procedures. Whenever possible, allow the patient privacy.

Equipment

Bedpan, fracture pan, or urinal with cover ▪ toilet tissue ▪ two washcloths ▪ soap ▪ gloves ▪ towel ▪ linen-saver pad ▪ bath blanket ▪ pillow ▪ optional: air freshener, talcum powder.

Available in adult and pediatric sizes, the bedpan may be disposable or reusable (the latter can be sterilized). The fracture pan, a type of bedpan, is used when spinal injuries, body or leg casts, or other conditions prohibit or restrict turning the patient. Like the bedpan, the urinal may be disposable or reusable.

Preparation of equipment

Obtain the appropriate bedpan or urinal. If necessary, sprinkle talcum powder on the edge of the bedpan *to reduce friction during placement and removal.* For a thin patient, place a linen-saver pad at the edge of the bedpan *to minimize pressure on the coccyx.*

Implementation

- If the patient's condition permits, provide privacy. Put on gloves *to prevent contact with body fluids, and comply with standard precautions.*

Placing a bedpan

- If allowed, elevate the head of the bed slightly *to prevent hyperextension of the spine when the patient raises the buttocks.*
- Rest the bedpan on the edge of the bed. Then, turn down the corner of the top linens, and draw up the patient's gown. Ask him to raise the buttocks by flexing his knees and pushing down on his heels. While supporting the patient's lower back with one hand, center the curved, smooth edge of the bedpan beneath the buttocks.
- If the patient can't raise his buttocks, lower the head of the bed to horizontal and help the patient roll onto one side, with buttocks toward you. Position the bedpan properly against the buttocks, and then help the patient roll back onto the bedpan. When the patient is positioned comfortably, raise the head of the bed as indicated.
- After positioning the bedpan, elevate the head of the bed to 30 degrees or higher, if allowed. *This position, like the normal elimination posture, aids in defecation and urination.* (See *Using a commode,* page 138.)
- If elevating the head of the bed is contraindicated, tuck a small pillow or folded bath blanket under the patient's back *to cushion the sacrum against the edge of the bedpan and support the lumbar region.*

Using a commode

An alternative to a bedpan, a commode is a portable chair made of plastic or metal, with a large opening in the center of the seat. It may have a bedpan or bucket that slides beneath the opening, or it may slide directly over the toilet, adding height to the standard toilet seat. Unlike a bedpan, a commode allows the patient to assume his normal elimination posture, *which aids in defecation.*

Before the patient uses it, inspect the commode's condition and make sure it's clean. Roll or carry the commode to the patient's room. Place it parallel and as close as possible to the patient's bed, and secure its brakes or wheel locks. If necessary, block its wheels with sandbags. Assist the patient onto the commode, provide toilet tissue, and place the call bell within his reach. Instruct the patient to push the call bell when finished.

If necessary, assist the patient with cleaning. Help him into bed and make him comfortable. Offer him soap, water, and a towel to wash his hands. Then close the lid of the commode or cover the bucket. Roll the commode or carry the bucket to the bathroom or utility room. If ordered, observe and measure the contents before disposal. Rinse and clean the bucket, and then spray or wipe the bucket and commode seat with disinfectant. Use an air freshener if appropriate.

- If the patient can be left alone, place the bed in a low position and raise the side rails *to ensure his safety.* Place toilet tissue and the call bell within the patient's reach, and instruct him to push the bell after elimination. If the patient is weak or disoriented, remain with him.
- Before removing the bedpan, lower the head of the bed slightly. Then ask the patient to raise his buttocks off the bed. Support the lower back with one hand, and gently remove the bedpan with the other *to avoid skin injury caused by friction.* If the patient can't raise his buttocks, ask him to roll away from you while you remove the bedpan. Hold the pan firmly with the other hand to avoid spills. Cover the bedpan and place it on the chair.
- Help clean the anal and perineal area, as necessary, *to prevent irritation and infection.* Turn the patient on his side, wipe carefully with toilet tissue, clean the area with a damp washcloth and soap, and dry well with a towel. Clean a female patient from front to back *to avoid introducing rectal contaminants into the vaginal or urethral openings.*

Placing a urinal

- Lift the corner of the top linens, hand the urinal to the patient, and allow him to position it.
- If the patient can't position the urinal himself, spread his legs slightly and hold the urinal in place *to prevent spills.*
- After the patient voids, carefully withdraw the urinal.

After use of a bedpan or urinal

- Give the patient a clean, damp, warm washcloth for his hands. Check the bed linens for wetness or soiling, and straighten or change them if needed. Make the patient comfortable. Place the bed in the low position, and raise the side rails.
- Take the bedpan or urinal to the bathroom or utility room. Observe the color, odor, amount, and consistency of its contents. If ordered, measure urine output or liquid stool, or obtain a specimen for laboratory analysis.
- Empty the bedpan or urinal into the toilet or designated waste area. Rinse with cold water and clean it thoroughly, using a disinfectant solution. (Some facilities use automatic bedpan washers as an alternative to hand washing these devices.) Dry the device and return it to the patient's bedside stand.
- Use an air freshener, if necessary, *to eliminate offensive odors and minimize embarrassment.*
- Remove gloves and wash your hands.

Special considerations

- Explain to the patient that drug treatment and changes in his environment, diet, and activities may disrupt his usual elimination schedule. Try to anticipate elimination needs, and offer the bedpan or urinal frequently *to help reduce embarrassment and minimize the risk of incontinence.*
- Avoid placing a bedpan or urinal on top of the bedside stand or overbed table *to avoid contamination of clean equipment and food trays.* Similarly, avoid placing it on the floor *to prevent the spread of microorganisms* from the floor to the patient's bed linens when the device is used.
- If the patient feels pain during turning or feels uncomfortable on a standard bedpan, use a fracture pan. Unlike the standard bedpan, the fracture pan is slipped under the buttocks from the front rather than the side. *Because it's shallower than the standard bedpan,* you need only lift the patient slightly to position it. If the patient is obese or otherwise difficult to lift, ask a coworker to help you.
- If the patient has an indwelling urinary catheter in place, carefully position and remove the bedpan *to avoid tension on the catheter, which could dislodge it or irritate the urethra.* After the patient defecates, wipe, clean, and dry the anal region, taking care to avoid catheter contamination. If necessary, clean the urinary meatus with antiseptic solution.

Documentation

Record the time, date, and type of elimination on the flowchart and the amount of urine output or liquid stool on the intake and output record, as needed. In your notes, document the amount, color, clarity, and odor of the urine or stool and the presence of blood, pus, or other abnormal characteristics in urine or stool. Document the condition of the perineum.

SELECTED REFERENCES

Craven, R.F., and Hirnle, C.J. *Fundamentals of Nursing: Human Health and Function,* 5th ed. Philadelphia: Lippincott Williams & Wilkins, 2007.

Holroyd-Leduc, J., et al. "Practical Management of Urinary Incontinence in the Long-Term Care Setting," *Annals of Long-Term Care* 14(2):30-37, February 2006.

National Guideline Clearinghouse. "Management of Urinary Incontinence in Primary Care: A National Clinical Guideline." Available at *www.guideline.gov/summary/summary.aspx?doc_id=6251&nbr=004011.*

National Institute for Occupational Safety and Health (NIOSH). Guidelines for Protecting the Safety and Health of Health Care Workers: *www.cdc.gov/niosh.*

INCONTINENCE MANAGEMENT

In elderly patients, incontinence commonly follows any loss or impairment of urinary or anal sphincter control. The incontinence may be transient or permanent. In all, about 10 million adults experience some form of urinary incontinence; this includes about 50% of the 1.5 million people in extended-care facilities. Fecal incontinence affects up to 10% of the patients in such facilities.

Contrary to popular opinion, urinary incontinence is neither a disease nor a part of normal aging. Incontinence may be caused by confusion, dehydration, fecal impaction, or restricted mobility. It's also a sign of various disorders, such as prostatic hyperplasia, bladder calculus, bladder cancer, urinary tract infection (UTI), stroke, diabetic neuropathy, Guillain-Barré syndrome, multiple sclerosis, prostatic cancer, prostatitis, spinal cord injury, and urethral stricture. It may also result from urethral sphincter damage after prostatectomy. In addition, certain drugs, including diuretics, hypnotics, sedatives, anticholinergics, antihypertensives, and alpha antagonists, may trigger urinary incontinence.

Urinary incontinence is classified as acute or chronic. Acute urinary incontinence results from disorders that are potentially reversible, such as delirium, dehydration, urine retention, restricted mobility, fecal impaction, infection or inflammation, drug reactions, and polyuria. Chronic urinary incontinence occurs as four distinct types: stress, overflow, urge, and functional incontinence.

In stress incontinence, leakage results from a sudden physical strain, such as a sneeze, cough, or quick movement. In overflow incontinence, urine retention causes dribbling because the distended bladder can't contract strongly enough to force a urine stream. In urge incontinence, the patient can't control the impulse to urinate. Finally, in functional (total) incontinence, urine leakage occurs despite the fact that the bladder and urethra are functioning normally. This condition is usually related to cognitive or mobility factors.

Fecal incontinence, the involuntary passage of feces, may occur gradually (as in dementia) or suddenly (as in spinal cord injury). It usually results from fecal stasis and impaction secondary to reduced activity, inappropriate diet, or untreated painful anal conditions. It can also result from chronic laxative use; reduced fluid intake; neurologic deficit; pelvic, prostatic, or rectal surgery; and the use of certain medications, including antihistamines, psychotropics, and iron preparations. Not usually a sign of serious illness, fecal incontinence can seriously impair an elderly patient's physical and psychological well-being.

Patients with urinary or fecal incontinence should be carefully assessed for underlying disorders. Most can be treated; some can even be cured. Treatment aims to control the condition through bladder or bowel retraining or other behavior management techniques, diet modification, drug therapy, pessaries, and, possibly, surgery. Corrective surgery for urinary incontinence includes transurethral resection of the prostate in men, urethral collagen injections for men or women, repair of the anterior vaginal wall or retropelvic suspension of the bladder in women, urethral sling, and bladder augmentation. (See *Correcting urinary incontinence with bladder retraining,* page 140.)

Equipment

Bladder retraining record sheet ■ gloves ■ stethoscope (to assess bowel sounds) ■ lubricant ■ moisture barrier cream ■ antidiarrheal or laxative suppository ■ incontinence pads ■ bedpan ■ specimen container ■ label ■ laboratory request form ■ optional: stool collection kit, urinary catheter.

Implementation

Whether the patient reports urinary or fecal incontinence or both, you'll need to perform initial and continuing assessments to plan effective interventions.

For urinary incontinence

■ Ask the patient when he first noticed urine leakage and whether it began suddenly or gradually. Have him describe his typical urinary pattern: Does he usually experience in-

HOME CARE

Correcting urinary incontinence with bladder retraining

The incontinent patient typically feels frustrated, embarrassed, and hopeless. Fortunately, his problem can usually be corrected by bladder retraining—a program that aims to establish a regular voiding pattern. Follow these guidelines.

Assess elimination patterns

First, assess the patient's intake and voiding patterns and reason for each accidental voiding (such as a coughing spell). Use an incontinence monitoring record.

Establish a voiding schedule

Encourage the patient to void regularly, for example, every 2 hours. When he can stay dry for 2 hours, increase the interval by 30 minutes every day until he achieves a 3- to 4-hour voiding schedule. Teach the patient to practice relaxation techniques such as deep breathing, *which help decrease the sense of urgency.*

Record results and remain positive

Keep a record of continence and incontinence for about 5 days *to help reinforce the patient's efforts to remain continent.* Remember, both your own and your patient's positive attitudes are crucial to his successful bladder retraining.

Take steps for success

Here are some additional tips to boost the patient's success:

- Be sure to locate the patient's bed near a bathroom or portable toilet. Leave a light on at night. If the patient needs assistance getting out of bed or a chair, promptly answer the call for help.
- Teach the patient measures to prevent urinary tract infections, such as adequate fluid intake (at least 2,000 ml/day unless contraindicated), drinking cranberry juice *to help acidify urine,* wearing cotton underpants, and bathing with nonirritating soaps. If the patient has urge incontinence, cranberry juice is contraindicated.
- Encourage the patient to empty his bladder completely before and after meals and at bedtime.
- Advise him to urinate whenever the urge arises and never to ignore it.
- Instruct the patient to take prescribed diuretics upon rising in the morning.
- Advise him to limit the use of sleeping aids, sedatives, and alcohol; *they decrease the urge to urinate and can increase incontinence, especially at night.*
- If the patient is overweight, encourage weight loss.
- Suggest exercises to strengthen pelvic muscles.
- Instruct the patient to increase dietary fiber *to decrease constipation and incontinence.*
- Monitor the patient for signs of anxiety and depression.
- Reassure the patient that periodic incontinent episodes don't mean that the program has failed. Encourage persistence, tolerance, and a positive attitude.

continence during the day or at night? Does he get the urge to go again immediately after emptying the bladder? Does he get strong urges to go? Ask him to rate his urinary control: Does he have moderate control, or is he completely incontinent? If he sometimes urinates with control, ask him to identify when and how much he usually urinates.

- Evaluate related problems, such as urinary hesitancy, frequency, urgency, nocturia, and decreased force or interrupted urine stream. Ask the patient to describe any previous treatment he has had for incontinence or measures he has performed by himself. Ask about medications, including nonprescription drugs.
- Assess the patient's environment. Is a toilet or commode readily available, and how long does the patient take to reach it? After the patient is in the bathroom, assess his manual dexterity; for example, how easily does he manipulate his clothes?
- Evaluate the patient's mental status and cognitive function.
- Quantify the patient's normal daily fluid intake.
- Review the patient's medication and diet history for drugs and foods that affect digestion and elimination.
- Review or obtain the patient's medical history, noting especially the number and route of births, hysterectomy (in women), and any incidence of UTI, prostate disorders, diabetes, spinal injury or tumor, stroke, and bladder, prostate, or pelvic surgery. Assess for such disorders as delirium, dehydration, urine retention, restricted mobility, fecal impaction, infection, inflammation, and polyuria.
- Inspect the urethral meatus for obvious inflammation or anatomic defects. Have the female patient bear down while

you note any urine leakage. Gently palpate the abdomen for bladder distention, which signals urine retention. Assess for costovertebral angle tenderness. If possible, have the patient examined by a urologist.

- Obtain specimens for appropriate laboratory tests as ordered. Label each specimen container, and send it to the laboratory with a request form.
- Begin incontinence management by implementing an appropriate bladder retraining program.

NURSING ALERT *Obtain a 24- to 48-hour bladder diary before implementing bladder retraining.*

- *To ensure healthful hydration and to prevent UTI,* make sure the patient maintains an adequate daily intake of fluids (six to eight 8-oz glasses). Restrict fluid intake after 6 p.m.
- *To manage stress incontinence,* begin an exercise program to help strengthen the pelvic floor muscles. (See *Strengthening pelvic floor muscles.*)
- *To manage functional incontinence,* frequently assess the patient's mental and functional status. Regularly remind him to void. Respond to his calls promptly, and help him get to the bathroom quickly. Provide positive reinforcement.

For fecal incontinence

- Ask the patient with fecal incontinence to identify its onset, duration, severity, and pattern (for instance, determine whether it occurs at night or with diarrhea). Focus the history on GI, neurologic, and psychological disorders.
- Note the frequency, consistency, and volume of stool passed in the past 24 hours. Obtain a stool specimen if ordered. Protect the patient's bed with an incontinence pad.
- Assess for chronic constipation, GI and neurologic disorders, and laxative abuse. Inspect the abdomen for distention, and auscultate for bowel sounds. If not contraindicated, check for fecal impaction (a factor in overflow incontinence).
- Assess the patient's medication regimen. Check for drugs that affect bowel activity, such as aspirin, some anticholinergic antiparkinsonian agents, aluminum hydroxide, calcium carbonate antacids, diuretics, iron preparations, opiates, tranquilizers, tricyclic antidepressants, and phenothiazines.
- For the neurologically capable patient with chronic incontinence, provide bowel retraining.
- Advise the patient to consume a fiber-rich diet that includes lots of raw, leafy vegetables (such as carrots and lettuce), unpeeled fruits (such as apples), and whole grains (such as wheat or rye breads and cereals). If the patient has a lactase deficiency, suggest that he take calcium supplements to replace calcium lost by eliminating dairy products from the diet.
- Encourage adequate fluid intake.

Strengthening pelvic floor muscles

Stress incontinence, the most common kind of urinary incontinence in women, usually results from weakening of the urethral sphincter. In men, it may sometimes occur after a radical prostatectomy.

You can help male and female patients prevent or minimize stress incontinence by teaching pelvic floor (Kegel) exercises to strengthen the pubococcygeal muscles. Here's how.

Learning Kegel exercises

First, explain how to locate the muscles of the pelvic floor. Instruct the patient to tense the muscles around the anus, as if to retain stool.

To identify this area initially, teach the patient to tighten the muscles of the pelvic floor to stop the flow of urine while urinating and then to release the muscles to restart the flow. Once learned, these exercises can be done anywhere. Although Kegel exercises shouldn't be done while urinating, they can be done at any other time.

Establishing a regimen

Explain to the patient that contraction and relaxation exercises are essential to muscle retraining. Suggest that the patient start out by contracting the pelvic floor muscles for 5 seconds, relax for 5 seconds, and then repeat the procedure as often as needed.

Typically, the patient starts with 10 contractions in the morning and 10 at night, gradually increasing the relaxation and contraction time.

Advise the patient not to use stomach, leg, or buttock muscles. Also discourage leg crossing or breath holding during these exercises.

- Teach the elderly patient to gradually eliminate laxative use. Point out that using laxatives to promote regular bowel movement may have the opposite effect, producing either constipation or incontinence over time. Suggest natural laxatives, such as prunes and prune juice, instead.
- Promote regular exercise by explaining how it helps to regulate bowel motility. Even a nonambulatory patient can perform some exercises while sitting or lying in bed.

Special considerations

- For fecal incontinence, maintain effective hygienic care *to increase the patient's comfort and prevent skin breakdown and infection.* Clean the perineal area frequently, and apply a moisture barrier cream. Control foul odors as well.
- Schedule extra time to provide encouragement and support for the patient, who may feel shame, embarrassment, and powerlessness from loss of control.

Complications

Skin breakdown and infection may result from incontinence. Psychological problems resulting from incontinence include social isolation, loss of independence, lowered self-esteem, and depression.

Documentation

Record all bladder and bowel retraining efforts, noting scheduled bathroom times, food and fluid intake, and elimination amounts, as appropriate. Document the duration of continent periods. Note any complications, including emotional problems and signs of skin breakdown and infection as well as the treatments given for them.

SELECTED REFERENCES

Ostaszkiewicz, J., et al. "Effects of Timed Voiding for the Management of Urinary Incontinence in Adults: Systematic Review," *Journal of Advanced Nursing* 52(4):420-31, November 2005.

Zarowitz, B.J., and Ouslander, J.G. "Management of Urinary Incontinence in Older Persons," *Geriatric Nursing* 27(5):265-70, September-October 2006.

MALE INCONTINENCE DEVICE

Many patients don't require an indwelling urinary catheter to manage their incontinence. For male patients, a male incontinence device reduces the risk of urinary tract infection from catheterization, promotes bladder retraining when possible, helps prevent skin breakdown, and improves the patient's self-image. The device consists of a condom catheter secured to the shaft of the penis and connected to a leg bag or drainage bag. It has no contraindications but can cause skin irritation and edema.

Equipment

Condom catheter ▪ drainage bag ▪ extension tubing ▪ hypoallergenic tape or incontinence sheath holder ▪ commercial adhesive strip or skin-bond cement ▪ elastic adhesive or Velcro, if needed ▪ gloves ▪ clippers if needed ▪ basin ▪ soap ▪ washcloth ▪ towel.

Preparation of equipment

Fill the basin with lukewarm water. Then bring the basin and the remaining equipment to the patient's bedside.

Implementation

- Confirm the patient's identity using two paitient identifiers according to your facility's policy.
- Explain the procedure to the patient, wash your hands thoroughly, put on gloves, and provide privacy.

Applying the device

- If the patient is circumcised, wash the penis with soap and water, rinse well, and pat dry with a towel. If the patient is uncircumcised, gently retract the foreskin and clean beneath it. Rinse well but don't dry *because moisture provides lubrication and prevents friction during foreskin replacement.* Replace the foreskin to avoid penile constriction. Then, if necessary, clip hair from the base and shaft of the penis *to prevent the adhesive strip or skin-bond cement from pulling pubic hair.*
- If you're using a precut commercial adhesive strip, insert the glans penis through its opening, and position the strip 1″ (2.5 cm) from the scrotal area. If you're using uncut adhesive, cut a strip to fit around the shaft of the penis. Remove the protective covering from one side of the adhesive strip, and press this side firmly to the penis to enhance adhesion. Then remove the covering from the other side of the strip. If a commercial adhesive strip isn't available, apply skin-bond cement, and let it dry for a few minutes.
- Position the rolled condom catheter at the tip of the penis, leaving ½″ (1.3 cm) between the condom end and the tip of the penis, with its drainage opening at the urinary meatus.
- Unroll the catheter upward, past the adhesive strip on the shaft of the penis. Then gently press the sheath against the strip until it adheres. (See *How to apply a condom catheter.*)
- After the condom catheter is in place, secure it with hypoallergenic tape or an incontinence sheath holder.
- Using extension tubing, connect the condom catheter to the leg bag or drainage bag. Remove and discard your gloves.

Removing the device

- After identifying the patient, wash your hands and put on gloves.
- Simultaneously roll the condom catheter and adhesive strip off the penis and discard them. If you've used skin-bond cement rather than an adhesive strip, remove it with solvent. Also remove and discard the hypoallergenic tape or incontinence sheath holder.
- Clean the penis with lukewarm water, rinse thoroughly, and dry. Check for swelling or signs of skin breakdown.

■ Remove the leg bag by closing the drain clamp, unlatching the leg straps, and disconnecting the extension tubing at the top of the bag. Discard your gloves.

Special considerations

■ If hypoallergenic tape or an incontinence sheath holder isn't available, secure the condom with a strip of elastic adhesive or Velcro. Apply the strip snugly—but not too tightly—*to prevent circulatory constriction.*

■ Inspect the condom catheter for twists and the extension tubing for kinks *to prevent obstruction of urine flow,* which could cause the condom to balloon, eventually dislodging it.

Documentation

Record the date and time of application and removal of the incontinence device. Also note skin condition and the patient's response to the device, including voiding pattern, *to assist with bladder retraining.*

SELECTED REFERENCES

Brodie, A. "A Guide to the Management of One-Piece Urinary Sheaths," *Nursing Times* 102(9):49, 51, February-March 2006.

Evans, D. "Lifestyle Solutions of Men with Continence Problems," *Nursing Times* 101(2):61-64, January 2005.

Milne, J.L., and Moore, K.N. "Factors Impacting Self-Care for Urinary Incontinence," *Urologic Nursing* 26(1):41-51, February 2006.

National Guideline Clearinghouse. "Management of Urinary Incontinence in Primary Care: A National Clinical Guideline."Available at *www.guideline.gov/summary/summary.aspx?doc_id=6251&nbr=004011.*

Newman, O.K. "Incontinence Products and Devices for the Elderly," *Urologic Nursing* 24(4):316-33, August 2004.

How to apply a condom catheter

Apply an adhesive strip to the shaft of the penis about 1" (2.5 cm) from the scrotal area.

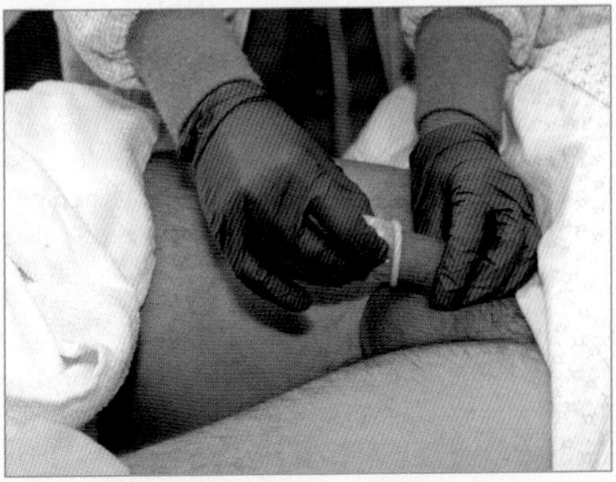

Then roll the condom catheter on to the penis past the adhesive strip, leaving about ½" (1.3 cm) clearance at the end. Press the sheath gently against the strip until it adheres.

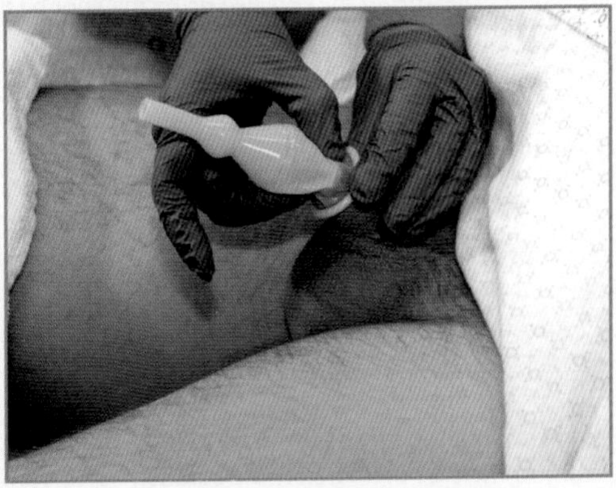

CREDÉ'S MANEUVER

When lower motor-neuron damage impairs the voiding reflex, the bladder may become flaccid or areflexic. Because the bladder fails to contract properly, urine collects inside it, causing distention. Credé's maneuver—application of manual pressure over the lower abdomen—promotes complete emptying of the bladder. After appropriate instruction, the patient can perform the maneuver himself, unless he can't reach his lower abdomen or lacks sufficient strength and dexterity. Even when performed properly, however, Credé's maneuver isn't always successful and doesn't always eliminate the need for catheterization.

Credé's maneuver can't be used after abdominal surgery if the incision isn't completely healed. When using Credé's maneuver, close monitoring of urine output is necessary to help detect possible infection from accumulation of residual urine.

Equipment

Bedpan, urinal, or bedside commode ■ gloves.

Implementation

- Confirm the patient's identity using two patient identifiers according to your facility's policy.
- Put on clean gloves.
- Explain the procedure to the patient, and wash your hands.
- If allowed, place the patient in Fowler's position, and position the bedpan or urinal. Alternatively, if the patient's condition permits, assist him onto the bedside commode.
- Place your hands flat on the patient's abdomen just below the umbilicus. Ask the female patient to bend forward from the hips. Then firmly stroke downward toward the bladder about six times to stimulate the voiding reflex.
- Place one hand on top of the other above the pubic arch. Press firmly inward and downward to compress the bladder and expel residual urine.

Special considerations

- Some facilities require a practitioner's order for performance of Credé's maneuver. This procedure shouldn't be performed on patients with normal bladder tone or bladder spasms.
- A bladder ultrasound scanner, if available, may be used to document residual urine volume after the Credé's maneuver is performed.
- After the patient has learned the procedure and can use it successfully, measuring the expelled urine may not be necessary. The patient may then use the maneuver to void directly into the toilet.

Patient teaching

- Explain to the patient that Credé's maneuver is a simple exercise that can be done at home. Tell the patient that he can start a stream of urine from his bladder by performing this easy-to-do maneuver. Tell the male patient to void directly into the toilet from a standing position if possible. The female patient should sit on the toilet as she normally would.
- Show the female patient how to lean forward, bending at the hips, to increase pressure on the bladder.
- Have the patient place one hand on top of the other in a return demonstration. Explain that the stroking movement compresses the bladder and expels urine.

Documentation

Record the date and time of the procedure, the amount of urine expelled, and the patient's tolerance of the procedure.

SELECTED REFERENCES

Almeida, E.G., et al. "Correlation between Urethral Sphincter Activity and Valsalva Leak Point Pressure at Different Bladder Distention: Revisiting the Urethral Pressure Profile," *Journal of Urology* 174(4 Pt1):1312-315, October 2005.

Fitzpatrick, J.M., and Kirby, R.S. "Management of Acute Urinary Retention," *BJU International* 97(Suppl2):16-20, April 2006.

National Diabetes Information Clearinghouse (NDIC). National Institute of Diabetes and Digestive and Kidney Diseases (NIDDK). "Diabetic Neuropathies: The Nerve Damage of Diabetes." Available at *www.diabteses.niddk.nih.gov/dm/pubs/neuropathies.*

Yerkes, A. "Diabetes and the Neurogenic Bladder," *Quality Care* 23(3):6, 3rd Quarter 2005.

DIGITAL REMOVAL OF FECAL IMPACTION

Fecal impaction—a large, hard, dry mass of stool in the folds of the rectum and, at times, in the sigmoid colon—results from prolonged retention and accumulation of stool. Common causes include poor bowel habits, inactivity, dehydration, improper diet (especially inadequate fluid intake), the use of constipation-inducing drugs, and incomplete bowel cleaning after a barium enema or barium swallow. Digital removal of fecal impaction is used when oil retention and cleansing enemas, suppositories, and laxatives fail to clear the impaction. It may require a practitioner's order.

This procedure is contraindicated during pregnancy; after rectal, genitourinary, abdominal, perineal, or gynecologic reconstructive surgery; in patients with myocardial infarction, coronary insufficiency, pulmonary embolus, heart failure, heart block, or Stokes-Adams syndrome (without pacemaker treatment); and in patients with GI or vaginal bleeding, hemorrhoids, rectal polyps, or blood dyscrasias.

Equipment

Gloves (two pairs) ▪ linen-saver pad ▪ bedpan plastic ▪ disposal bag ▪ soap ▪ water-filled basin ▪ towel ▪ water-soluble lubricant ▪ washcloth.

Implementation

- Confirm the patient's identity using two patient identifiers according to your facility's policy.
- Explain the procedure to the patient, and provide privacy.
- Position the patient on his left side, and flex his knees *to allow easier access to the sigmoid colon and rectum.*
- Drape the patient, and place a linen-saver pad beneath the buttocks *to prevent soiling the bed linens.*
- Put on gloves, and moisten an index finger with water-soluble lubricant *to reduce friction during insertion, thereby avoiding injury to sensitive tissue.*

■ Instruct the patient to breathe deeply *to promote relaxation.* Then gently insert your lubricated index finger beyond the anal sphincter until you touch the impaction. Rotate your finger gently around the stool to dislodge and break it into small fragments. Then work the fragments downward to the end of the rectum, and remove each one separately.
■ Before removing your finger, gently stimulate the anal sphincter with a circular motion two or three times *to increase peristalsis and encourage evacuation.*
■ Remove your finger and change your gloves. Then clean the anal area with soap and water, and lightly pat it dry with a towel.
■ Offer the patient the bedpan or commode *because digital manipulation stimulates the urge to defecate.*
■ Place disposable items in the plastic bag, and discard the bag properly. If necessary, clean the bedpan and return it to the bedside stand.
■ Wash your hands.

Special considerations

If the patient experiences pain, nausea, rectal bleeding, changes in pulse rate or skin color, diaphoresis, or syncope, stop the procedure immediately, and notify the practitioner.

Complications

Digital removal of fecal impaction can stimulate the vagus nerve and may decrease heart rate and cause syncope.

Documentation

Record the time and date of the procedure, the patient's response, and stool color, consistency, and odor.

Selected references

Craven, R.F., and Hirnle, C.J. *Fundamentals of Nursing: Human Health and Function,* 5th ed. Philadelphia: Lippincott Williams & Wilkins, 2007.
"Fecal Impaction." *Medical Encyclopedia, Medline Plus* U.S. National Library of Medicine and the National Institutes of Health. Ed by Jenifer K. Lehrer, MD, October 2006. Available at *www.nlm.nih.gove/medlineplus/ency/article/000230.htm.*
Taylor, C., et al. *Fundamentals of Nursing: The Art and Science of Nursing Care,* 6th ed. Philadelphia: Lippincott Williams & Wilkins, 2008.

CARE OF THE SURGICAL PATIENT

Preoperative care

Preoperative care begins when surgery is first planned and ends with the administration of anesthesia. This phase of care includes a preoperative interview and assessment to collect baseline subjective and objective data from the patient and his family; diagnostic tests such as urinalysis, electrocardiogram, and chest radiography; preoperative teaching; securing informed consent from the patient; and physical preparation.

Equipment

Gloves ■ thermometer ■ sphygmomanometer ■ stethoscope ■ watch with second hand ■ weight scale ■ tape measure.

Preparation of equipment

Assemble all equipment needed at the patient's bedside or in the admission area.

Implementation

■ If the patient is having same-day surgery, make sure he knows ahead of time not to eat or drink anything for 8 hours before surgery. Confirm with him what time he's scheduled to arrive at the facility, and tell him to leave all jewelry and valuables at home. Make sure the patient has arranged for someone to accompany him home after surgery.
■ Obtain a health history, and assess the patient's knowledge, perceptions, and expectations about his surgery. Ask about previous medical and surgical interventions. Also determine the patient's psychosocial needs; ask about occupational well-being, financial matters, support systems, mental status, and cultural beliefs. Use your facility's preoperative surgical assessment database, if available, to gather this information. Obtain a drug and anesthetic history. Ask about current prescriptions, over-the-counter medications, supplemental herbal preparations, and known allergies to foods and drugs.
■ Obtain the results of X-ray examinations and other preoperative tests.
■ Ask the patient if he has an advance directive. If he does, make a copy and place it in his chart. If he doesn't, ask him if he wants information about advance directives.
■ Measure the patient's height, weight, and vital signs.
■ Identify risk factors that may interfere with a positive expected outcome. Be sure to consider age, general health, medications, mobility, nutritional status, fluid and electrolyte disturbances, and lifestyle. Also consider the primary disor-

Obtaining informed consent

Informed consent means that the patient has consented to a procedure after receiving a full explanation of the procedure, its risks and complications, and the risk if the procedure isn't performed at this time. Although obtaining informed consent is the physician's responsibility, the nurse is responsible for verifying that this step has been taken.

You may be asked to witness the patient's signature. However, if you didn't hear the physician's explanation to the patient, you must sign that you're witnessing the patient's signature only.

Consent forms must be signed before the patient receives preoperative medication because forms signed after sedatives are given are legally invalid. Adults and emancipated minors can sign their own consent forms. Consent forms of children or of adults with impaired mental status must be signed by a parent or guardian.

der's duration, location, and nature and the extent of the surgical procedure.

- Explain preoperative procedures to the patient. Include typical events that the patient can expect. Discuss equipment that may be used postoperatively, such as nasogastric tubes and I.V. equipment. Explain the typical incision, dressings, and staples or sutures that will be used. Preoperative teaching can help reduce postoperative anxiety and pain, increase patient compliance, hasten recovery, and decrease length of stay.
- Discuss postoperative pain management. Teach the patient how to use your facility's pain scale. Find out his goals and expectations for pain relief.
- Talk the patient through the sequence of events from operating room, to postanesthesia care unit (PACU), and back to the patient's room. Some patients may be transferred from the PACU to an intensive care unit or surgical care unit. The patient may also benefit from a tour of the areas he'll see during the perioperative events.
- Tell the patient that when he goes to the operating room, he may have to wait a short time in the holding area. Explain that the physicians and nurses will wear surgical dress, and even though they'll be observing him closely, they'll refrain from talking to him very much. *Explain that minimal conversation will help the preoperative medication take effect.*
- When discussing transfer procedures and techniques, describe sensations that the patient will experience. Tell him that he'll be taken to the operating room on a stretcher and transferred from the stretcher to the operating room table. For his own safety, he'll be held securely to the table with soft restraints. The operating room nurses will check his vital signs frequently.
- Tell the patient that the operating room may feel cool. Electrodes may be put on his chest *to monitor his heart rate during surgery.* Describe the drowsy floating sensation he'll feel as the anesthetic takes effect. Tell him it's important that he relax at this time.
- Tell the patient about exercises that he may be expected to perform after surgery, such as deep-breathing, coughing (while splinting the incision if necessary), and extremity exercises, and movement and ambulation to minimize respiratory and circulatory complications. If the patient will undergo ophthalmic or neurologic surgery, he won't be asked to cough *because coughing increases intracranial pressure.*
- If the patient will have postoperative patient-controlled analgesia, explain how it works, and demonstrate the device *so he'll be able to use it immediately after surgery.*
- On the day of surgery, important interventions include giving morning care, verifying that the patient has signed an informed consent form, administering ordered preoperative medications, completing the preoperative checklist and chart, and providing support to the patient and his family. (See *Obtaining informed consent.*)
- Other immediate preoperative interventions may include preparing the GI tract (restricting food and fluids for about 8 hours before surgery) *to reduce vomiting and the risk of aspiration,* cleaning the lower GI tract of fecal material by enemas before abdominal or GI surgery, and giving antibiotics for 2 or 3 days preoperatively *to prevent contamination of the peritoneal cavity by GI bacteria.*
- Just before the patient is moved to the surgical area, make sure he's wearing a hospital gown, has his identification band in place, and has his vital signs recorded. Check to see that hairpins, nail polish, and jewelry have been removed. Note whether dentures, contact lenses, or prosthetic devices have been removed or left in place. Verify with the patient that the correct surgical site has been marked (see "Surgical site verification," page 147).

Special considerations

- Preoperative medications must be given on time *to enhance the effect of ordered anesthesia.* The patient should take nothing by mouth preoperatively. Don't give oral medications unless ordered. Be sure to raise the bed's side rails immediately after giving preoperative medications.
- If family members or others are present, direct them to the appropriate waiting area, and offer support as needed.

Documentation

Complete the preoperative checklist used by your facility. Record all nursing care measures and preoperative medications, results of diagnostic tests, and the time the patient is transferred to the surgical area. The chart and the surgical checklist must accompany the patient to surgery.

SELECTED REFERENCES

American Society of Peri-Anesthesia Nurses. "Clinical Evaluation of the ASPAN Pain and Comfort Clinical Guideline," *Journal of Perianesthesia Nursing* 19(3):150-59, June 2004.

AORN Guidance Statement: Preoperative Patient Care in the Ambulatory Surgery Setting. *AORN Journal:* April 2005.

Institute for Clinical Systems Improvement (ICSI). "Preoperative Evaluation," Bloomington: Minn.: ICSI, July 2006.

SURGICAL SITE VERIFICATION

Wrong-site surgery is a general term referring to a surgical procedure performed on the wrong body part or side of the body, or even the wrong patient. This error may occur in the operating room or in other settings, such as ambulatory care or interventional radiology.

Several factors may contribute to an increased risk of wrong-site surgery, including inadequate patient assessment, inadequate medical record review, inaccurate communication among health care team members, multiple surgeons involved in the procedure, failure to include the patient in the site-identification process, and relying solely on the physician for site identification.

Because serious consequences may result from wrong-site surgery, the nurse must confirm that the correct site has been identified before surgery begins.

Equipment

Surgical consent ■ medical record ■ procedure schedule ■ hypoallergenic, nonlatex permanent marker.

Implementation

■ Confirm the patient's identity using two patient identifiers according to your facility's policy.

■ Before the procedure, check the patient's chart for documentation, and compare the information using the history and physical examination form, nursing assessment, preprocedure checklist, signed informed consent with the exact procedure site identified, procedure schedule, and the patient's verbal confirmation of the correct site.

■ After verbally confirming the site with the patient, the person performing the procedure or another member of the surgical team who's fully informed about the patient and the intended procedure marks the site. The mark needs to be placed so that it's visible after the patient has been prepped and draped.

■ Make sure that the surgical team (surgeon, operating room or procedure staff, and anesthesia personnel) identifies the patient and verifies the correct procedure and correct site before beginning the surgery.

Special considerations

If the patient's condition prevents him from verifying the correct site, the surgeon will identify and mark the site using the history and physical examination forms, signed informed consent, preprocedure verification checklist, procedure schedule, X-rays, and other imaging studies.

Documentation

Complete the preprocedure checklist used by your facility, record that the correct site was verified, and note that the patient, family member, or surgeon has marked the correct site with a permanent marker. Verify that the procedure schedule coincides with the physician's order sheet.

SELECTED REFERENCES

AORN: Position Statement on Correct Site Surgery, February 2003.

The Joint Commission. 2008 Ambulatory Care and Office-Based National Patient Safety Goals, 2008.

The Joint Commission. National Patient Safety Goals, Critical Access Hospital, 2008.

The Joint Commission. Universal Protocol for Preventing Wrong Site, Wrong Procedure, Wrong Person Surgery, 2003.

Kwan, M.R., et al. "Incidence, Patterns, and Prevention of Wrong Site Surgery," *Archives of Surgery* 141(4):353-57, April 2006.

PREOPERATIVE SKIN PREPARATION

Proper preparation of the patient's skin for surgery renders it as free as possible from microorganisms, thereby reducing the risk of infection at the incision site. It doesn't duplicate or replace the full sterile preparation that immediately precedes surgery. Rather, it may involve a bath, shower, or local scrub with an antiseptic detergent solution, followed by hair removal. (See *Where to remove hair for surgery,* pages 148 and 149.)

Hair shouldn't be removed from the area surrounding the operative site unless it's thick enough to interfere with surgery because hair removal may increase the risk of infection. If hair needs to be removed, use clippers. Clipping hair should occur immediately before an opreation to decrease the risk of surgical site infection. Each facility has a hair removal policy.

The area of preparation always exceeds that of the expected incision to minimize the number of microorganisms

(Text continues on page 150.)

Where to remove hair for surgery

Shoulder and upper arm
On operative side, remove hair from fingertips to hairline and center chest to center spine, extending to iliac crest and including the axilla.

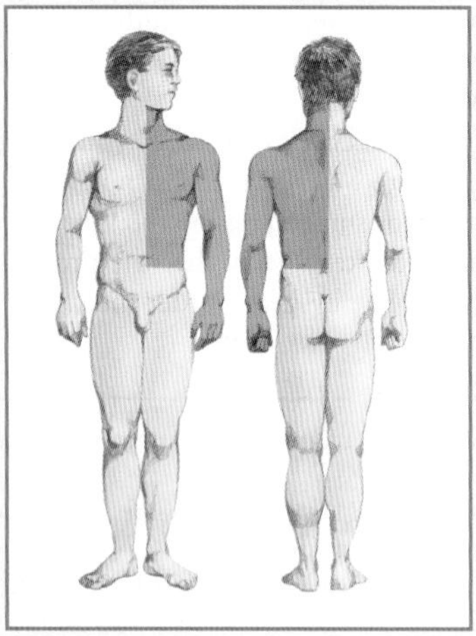

Forearm, elbow, and hand
On operative side, remove hair from fingertips to shoulder. Include the axilla unless surgery is for hand. Clean and trim fingernails.

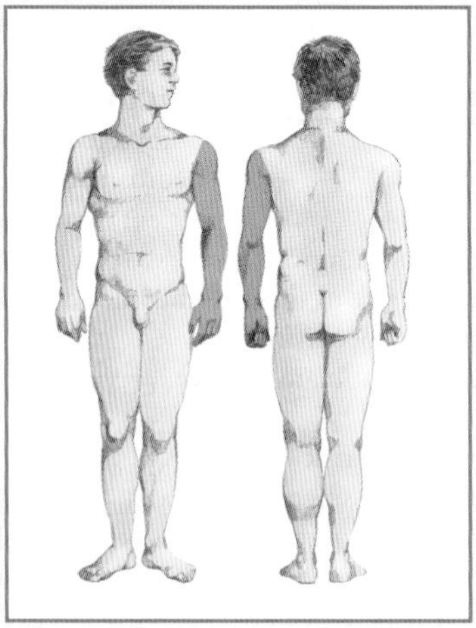

Thigh
On operative side, remove hair from toes to 3″ (7.6 cm) above umbilicus and from midline front to midline back, including pubis. Clean and trim toenails.

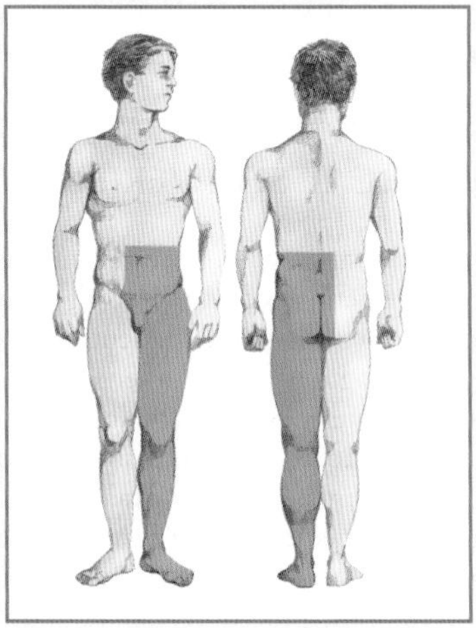

Chest
Remove hair from chin to iliac crests and nipple on unaffected side to midline of back on operative side (2″ [5 cm] beyond midline of back for thoracotomy). Include axilla and entire arm to elbow on operative side.

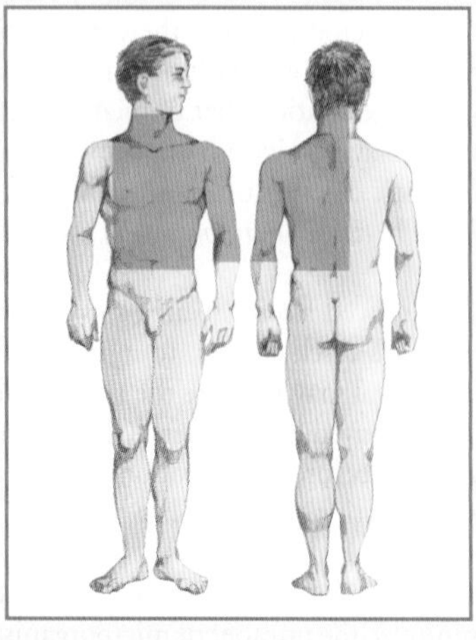

Abdomen
Remove hair from 3″ above nipples to upper thighs, including pubic area.

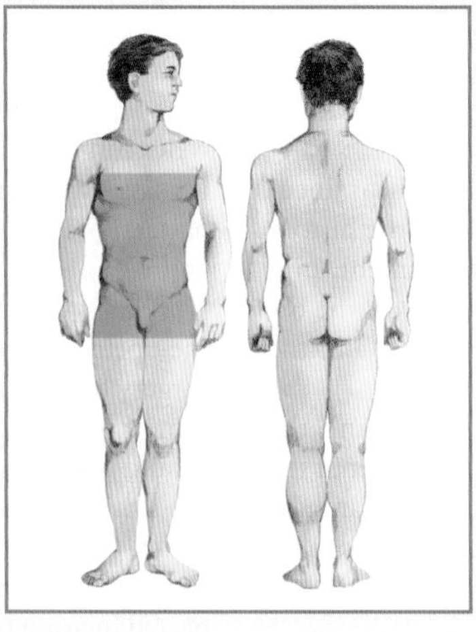

Lower abdomen
Remove hair from 2″ above umbilicus to midthigh, including pubic area; for femoral ligation, to midline of thigh in back; and for hernioplasty and embolectomy, to costal margin and down to knee.

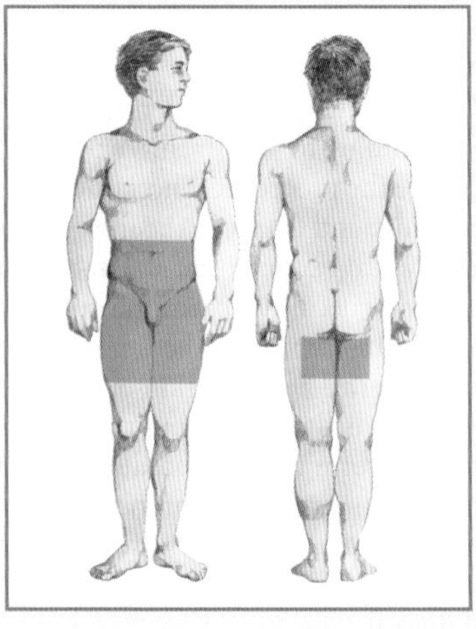

Where to remove hair for surgery *(continued)*

Hip

On operative side, remove hair from toes to nipples and at least 3″ (7.6 cm) beyond midline back and front, including the pubis. Clean and trim toenails.

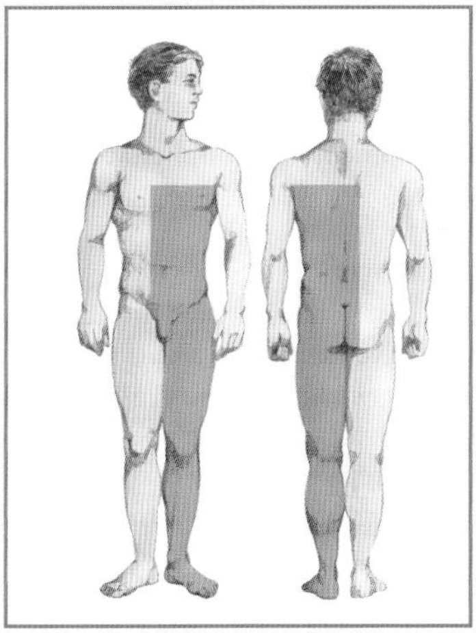

Knee and lower leg

On operative side, remove hair from toes to groin. Clean and trim toenails.

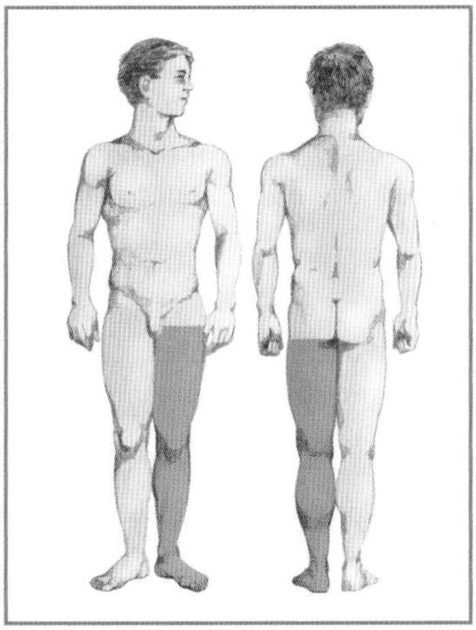

Ankle and foot

On operative side, remove hair from toes to 3″ above the knee. Clean and trim toenails.

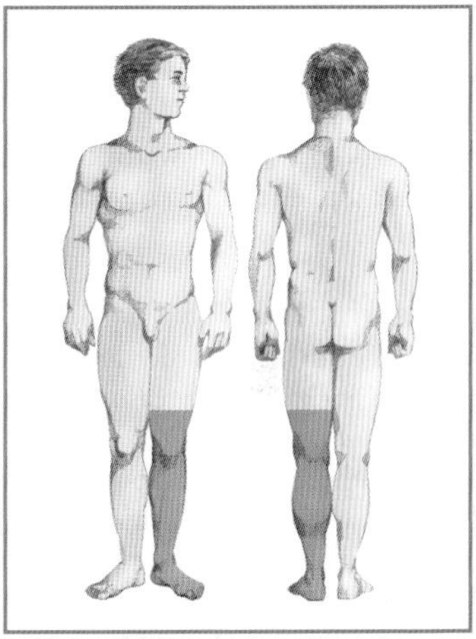

Flank

On operative side, remove hair from nipples to pubis, 3″ beyond midline in back, 2″ (5 cm) past abdominal midline. Include pubic area and, on affected side, upper thigh and axilla.

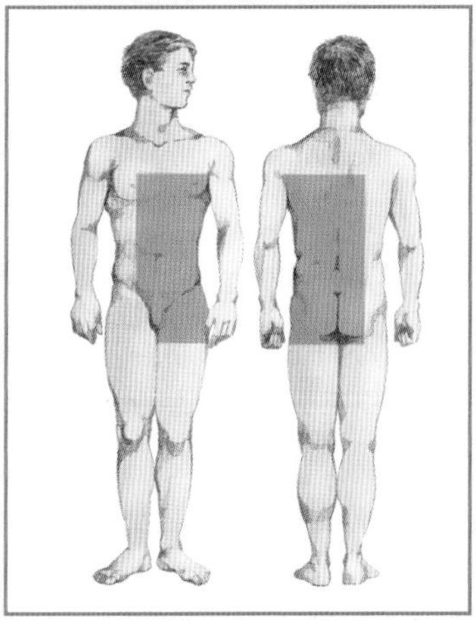

Perineum

Remove hair from pubis, perineum, and perianal area, and from the waist to at least 3″ below the groin in front and at least 3″ below the buttocks in back.

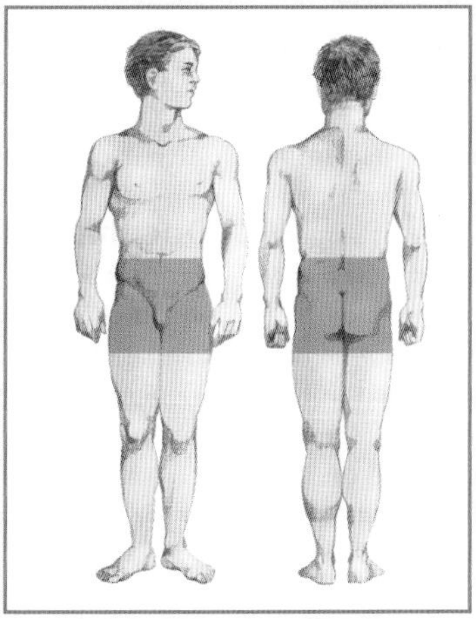

Spine

Remove hair from entire back, including shoulders and neck to hairline, and down to both knees. Include axillae.

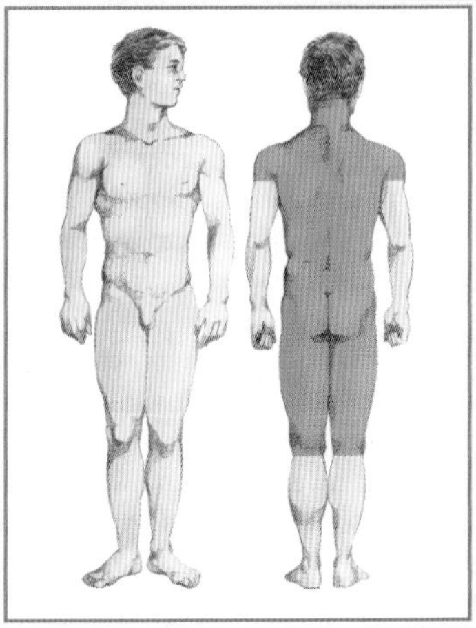

in the areas adjacent to the proposed incision and to allow surgical draping of the patient without contamination.

Equipment

Antiseptic soap solution ▪ tap water ▪ bath blanket ▪ two clean basins ▪ linen-saver pad ▪ adjustable light ▪ electric clippers ▪ scissors ▪ optional: 4″ × 4″ gauze pads, cotton-tipped applicators, acetone or nail polish remover, orangewood stick, trash bag, towel, gloves.

Preparation of equipment

Use warm tap water *because heat reduces the skin's surface tension and facilitates removal of soil and hair.* Dilute the antiseptic soap solution with warm tap water in one basin *for washing,* and pour plain warm water into the second basin *for rinsing.*

Implementation

- Check the physician's order, and explain the procedure to the patient, including the reason for the extensive preparations *to avoid causing undue anxiety.* Provide privacy, wash your hands thoroughly, and put on gloves.
- Place the patient in a comfortable position, drape him with the bath blanket, and expose the preparation area. For most surgeries, this area extends 12″ (30.5 cm) in each direction from the expected incision site. However, *to ensure privacy and avoid chilling the patient,* expose only one small area at a time while performing skin preparation.
- Position a linen-saver pad beneath the patient *to catch spills and avoid linen changes.* Adjust the light *to illuminate the preparation area.*
- Assess skin condition in the preparation area, and report any rash, abrasion, or laceration to the physician before beginning the procedure. *Any break in the skin increases the risk of infection and could cause cancellation of the planned surgery.*
- Have the patient remove all jewelry in or near the operative site.
- Put on gloves and, as ordered, begin removing hair from the preparation area by clipping any long hairs with clippers. Perform the procedure as near to the time of surgery as possible *so that microorganisms will have minimal time to proliferate.*
- Proceed with a 10-minute scrub *to ensure a clean preparation area.* Wash the area with a gauze pad dipped in the antiseptic soap solution. Using a circular motion, start at the expected incision site and work outward toward the periphery of the area *to avoid recontaminating the clean area.* Apply light friction while washing *to improve the antiseptic effect of the solution.* Replace the gauze pad as necessary.
- Carefully clean skin folds and crevices *because they harbor greater numbers of microorganisms.* Scrub the perineal area last, if it's part of the preparation area, for the same reason. Pull loose skin taut. If necessary, use cotton-tipped applicators to clean the umbilicus and an orangewood stick to clean under nails. Be sure to remove any nail polish *because the anesthetist uses nail bed color to determine adequate oxygenation and may place a probe on the nail to measure oxygen saturation.*
- Dry the area with a clean towel, and remove the linen-saver pad.
- Give the patient any special instructions for care of the prepared area, and remind him to keep the area clean for surgery. Make sure the patient is comfortable.
- Properly dispose of solutions and the trash bag, and clean or dispose of soiled equipment and supplies according to your facility's policy.

Special considerations

- Avoid shaving facial or neck hair on women and children unless ordered. Never shave eyebrows *because this disrupts normal hair growth and the new growth may prove unsightly.* Scalp shaving is usually performed in the operating room, but if you're required to prepare the patient's scalp, put all hair in a plastic or paper bag, and store it with the patient's possessions.
- Depilatory cream can also be used to remove hair. Although this method produces clean, intact skin without risking lacerations or abrasions, it can cause skin irritation or rash, especially in the groin area. If possible, cut long hairs with scissors before applying the cream *because removal of remaining hair then requires less cream.* Use a glove to apply the cream in a layer ½″ (1.3 cm) thick. After about 10 minutes, remove the cream with moist gauze pads. Next, wash the area with antiseptic soap solution, rinse, and pat dry.

Complications

Rashes, nicks, lacerations, and abrasions are the most common complications of skin preparation. They also increase the risk of postoperative infection.

Documentation

Record the date, time, and area of preparation; skin condition before and after preparation; any complications; and the patient's tolerance. If your facility requires it, complete an incident report if the patient suffers nicks, lacerations, or abrasions during skin preparation.

SELECTED REFERENCES

Bratzler D.W. "The Surgical Infection Prevention and Surgical Care Improvement Projects: Promises and Pitfalls," *The American Surgeon* 72(11):1010-16, November 2006.

Centers for Disease Control and Prevention. Guideline for Prevention of Surgical Site Infection, 1999. Available at *www.cdc.gov/ncidod/dhqp/gl_surgicalsite.html.*

Odom-Forren, J. "Preventing Surgical Site Infections," *Nursing* 36(6):59-64, June 2006.

Pyrek, K.M. "Preoperative Prep Should Safeguard Skin Integrity," *Infection Control Today* 2007. Available at *www.infectioncontroltoday.com/articles/406/406_23topics.html.*

Surgical Care Improvement Project Partnership. "Tips for Safer Surgery," *Oklahoma Foundation for Medical Quality,* 2007. Available at *www.medqlc.org/scip.*

POSTOPERATIVE CARE

This phase of care begins when the patient arrives in the postanesthesia care unit (PACU) and continues as he moves on to the short procedure unit, medical-surgical unit, or intensive care unit. Postoperative care aims to minimize postoperative complications by early detection and prompt treatment. After anesthesia, a patient may experience pain, inadequate oxygenation, or adverse physiologic effects of sudden movement.

Recovery from general anesthesia takes longer than induction because the anesthetic is retained in fat and muscle. Fat has a meager blood supply; thus, it releases the anesthetic slowly, providing enough anesthesia to maintain adequate blood and brain levels during surgery. The patient's recovery time varies with his amount of body fat, his overall condition, his premedication regimen, and the type, dosage, and duration of anesthesia.

Equipment

Thermometer ▪ watch with second hand ▪ stethoscope ▪ sphygmomanometer ▪ postoperative flowchart or other documentation tool.

Implementation

- Assemble the equipment at the patient's bedside.
- Obtain the patient's record from the PACU nurse. This should include:
  - a summary of operative procedures and pertinent findings
  - type of anesthesia
  - vital signs (preoperative, intraoperative, and postoperative)
  - medical history
  - medication history, including preoperative, intraoperative, and postoperative medications
  - fluid therapy, including estimated blood loss, type and number of drains and catheters, and amounts and characteristics of drainage
  - notes on the condition of the surgical wound. If the patient had vascular surgery, for example, knowing the location and duration of blood vessel clamping can prevent postoperative complications.
- Transfer the patient from the PACU stretcher to the bed, and position him properly. Get a coworker to help if necessary. When moving the patient, keep transfer movements smooth *to minimize pain and postoperative complications and avoid back strain among team members.* Use a transfer board *to facilitate moving the patient.*
- If the patient has had orthopedic surgery, always get a coworker to help transfer him. Ask the coworker to move only the affected extremity.
- If the patient is in skeletal traction, you may receive special orders for moving him. If you must move him, have a coworker move the weights as you and another coworker move the patient.
- Make the patient comfortable, and raise the bed's side rails *to ensure the patient's safety.*
- Assess the patient's level of consciousness, skin color, and mucous membranes.
- Monitor the patient's respiratory status by assessing his airway. Note breathing rate and depth, and auscultate for breath sounds. Administer oxygen and initiate oximetry *to monitor oxygen saturation if ordered.*
- Monitor the patient's pulse rate. It should be strong and easily palpable. The heart rate should be within 20% of the preoperative heart rate.
- Compare postoperative blood pressure to preoperative blood pressure. It should be within 20% of the preoperative level unless the patient suffered a hypotensive episode during surgery.
- Assess the patient's temperature *because anesthesia lowers body temperature.* Body temperature should be at least 95° F (35° C). If it's lower, apply blankets *to warm the patient* or use the Baer hugger patient-warming system.
- Assess the patient's infusion sites for redness, pain, swelling, or drainage. *This would indicate infiltration and requires discontinuing the I.V. and restarting it at another site.*
- Assess surgical wound dressings; they should be clean and dry. If they're soiled, assess the characteristics of the drainage and outline the soiled area. Note the date and time of assessment on the dressing. Assess the soiled area frequently; if it enlarges, reinforce the dressing and alert the physician. Don't remove the original dressing unless specified by the physician.
- Note the presence and condition of any drains and tubes. Note the color, type, odor, and amount of drainage and the patient's urine output. Make sure all drains are properly connected and free from obstructions.

■ If the patient has had vascular or orthopedic surgery, assess the appropriate extremity—or all extremities, depending on the surgical procedure. Perform neurovascular checks and assess color, temperature, sensation, movement, and presence and quality of pulses. Notify the physician of any abnormalities.
■ Assess the patient's pain intensity using your facility's pain scale. Assess pain type, location, frequency, and duration. Also assess other sources of discomfort, such as nausea and anxiety.
■ Provide pain medication as ordered.
■ As the patient recovers from anesthesia, monitor his respiratory and cardiovascular status closely. Be alert for signs of airway obstruction and hypoventilation caused by laryngospasm, or for sedation, which can lead to hypoxemia. *Cardiovascular complications—such as arrhythmias and hypotension—may result from the anesthetic agent or the operative procedure.*
■ Encourage coughing and deep-breathing exercises. Don't encourage them if the patient has just had nasal, ophthalmic, or neurologic surgery, *to avoid increasing intracranial pressure.*
■ Administer postoperative medications, such as antibiotics, analgesics, antiemetics, or reversal agents, as ordered and appropriate.
■ Remove all fluids from the patient's bedside until he's alert enough to eat and drink. Before giving him liquids, assess his gag reflex *to prevent aspiration.* To do this, lightly touch the back of his throat with a cotton swab—the patient will gag if the reflex has returned. Do this test quickly *to prevent a vagal reaction.*
■ Monitor the patient's intake and output.
■ Assess the presence of bowel sounds and passage of flatus before the patient can be allowed food.

Special considerations

■ Fear, pain, anxiety, hypothermia, confusion, and immobility can upset the patient and jeopardize his safety and postoperative status. Offer emotional support to the patient and his family. Keep in mind that the patient who has lost a body part or who has been diagnosed with an incurable disease will need ongoing emotional support. Refer him and his family for counseling as needed.
■ As the patient recovers from general anesthesia, reflexes appear in reverse order to that in which they disappeared. Hearing recovers first, so avoid holding inappropriate conversations.
■ Monitor the patient's blood pressure, heart rate, and oxygen saturation.
■ The patient under general anesthesia can't protect his own airway *because of muscle relaxation.* As he recovers, his cough and gag reflexes reappear. If he can lift his head without assistance, he usually can breathe on his own.
■ If the patient received spinal anesthesia, he may need to remain in a supine position with the bed adjusted to between 0 degrees and 20 degrees for at least 6 hours *to reduce the risk of spinal headache from leakage of cerebrospinal fluid.* Check your facility's policy and procedures for activity restriction after spinal anesthesia. The patient won't be able to move his legs, so be sure to reassure him that sensation and mobility will return.
■ If the patient has epidural analgesia infusion for postoperative pain control, monitor his respiratory status closely. *Respiratory arrest may result from the respiratory depressant effects of the opioid.* He may also suffer nausea, vomiting, or itching. Epidural analgesia may also include administering a local anesthetic with the opioid. Assess the patient's lower extremity motor strength every 2 to 4 hours. If sensorimotor loss occurs (numbness or weakness of the legs), notify the physician because the dosage may need to be decreased.
■ If the patient will be using a patient-controlled analgesia (PCA) unit, reinforce preoperative teaching and make sure he understands how to use it. Caution him to activate it only when he has pain, not when he feels sleepy or is pain-free. Review your facility's criteria for PCA use.

ELDER ALERT *If the patient is older, be aware of age-related changes that will alter your assessment. Cardiovascular status should be monitored carefully* **because it can be altered by blood loss, pain, bed rest, and fluid and electrolyte imbalances.** *Respiratory status should also be monitored carefully* **because ventilation and oxygenation can be altered by age-related changes, smoking, or chronic disease.** *Monitor level of consciousness and pain carefully because mental status changes can make pain control more difficult. Also,* **because drug metabolism slows with age,** *monitor the older adult for drug reactions, toxicity, and interactions. Monitor intake and output carefully, and watch for urinary tract infections* **due to decreased renal function and bladder capacity.**

Complications

Postoperative complications may include arrhythmias, hypotension, hypovolemia, septicemia, septic shock, atelectasis, pneumonia, thrombophlebitis, pulmonary embolism, urine retention, wound infection, wound dehiscence, evisceration, abdominal distention, paralytic ileus, constipation, altered body image, and postoperative psychosis.

Documentation

Document vital signs on the appropriate flowchart. Record the condition of dressings and drains and characteristics of drainage. Document all interventions taken to alleviate pain and anxiety and the patient's responses to them. Document any complications and interventions taken.

SELECTED REFERENCES

American Society of PeriAnesthesia Nurses. "Clinical Evaluation of the ASPAN Pain and Comfort Clinical Guideline," *Journal of Perianethseia Nursing* 19(3):150-59, June 2004.

Litusack, K. "Adjusting Postsurgical Care for Older Patients," *Nursing* 36(1): 66-67, January 2006.

Schwartz. A. "Learning the Essentials of Epidural Anesthesia," *Nursing* 36(1):44-49, January 2006.

SPIRITUAL AND TERMINAL CARE

SPIRITUAL CARE

Religious beliefs can profoundly influence a patient's recovery rate, attitude toward treatment, and overall response to hospitalization. In certain religious groups, beliefs can preclude diagnostic tests and therapeutic treatments, require dietary restrictions, and prohibit organ donation and artificial prolongation of life. (See *Beliefs and practices of selected religions,* pages 154 to 156.)

Consequently, effective patient care requires recognition of and respect for the patient's religious beliefs. Recognizing his beliefs and need for spiritual care may require close attention to his nonverbal cues or to seemingly casual remarks that express his spiritual concerns. Respecting his beliefs may require setting aside your own beliefs to help the patient follow his. Providing spiritual care may require contacting an appropriate member of the clergy in the facility or community, gathering any equipment that may be necessary to help the patient perform rites and administer sacraments, and preparing him for a pastoral visit.

Equipment

Clean towels (one or two) ■ teaspoon or 1-oz (30-ml) medicine cup (for baptism) ■ container of water (for emergency baptism).

Some facilities, particularly those with a religious affiliation, provide baptismal trays. The clergy member may bring holy water, holy oil, or other religious articles to minister to the patient.

Preparation of equipment

For baptism, cover a small table with a clean towel. Fold a second towel and place it on the table, along with the teaspoon or medicine cup. For communion and anointing, cover the bedside stand with a clean towel.

Implementation

■ Check the patient's admission record *to determine his religious affiliation.* Remember that even patients who claim to have no religious beliefs may desire spiritual or pastoral care. So watch and listen carefully for subtle expressions of this desire.

■ Evaluate the patient's behavior for signs of loneliness, anxiety, or fear—emotions that may signal his need for spiritual counsel. Also consider whether the patient is facing a health crisis, which may occur with chronic illness and before childbirth, surgery, or impending death. Remember that a patient may feel acutely distressed because of his inability to participate in religious observances. Help such a patient verbalize his beliefs *to relieve stress.* Listen to him and let him express his concerns, but carefully refrain from imposing your beliefs on him *to avoid conflict and further stress.* If the patient requests, arrange a visit by an appropriate member of the clergy. Consult this clergy member if you need more information about the patient's beliefs.

■ If the patient faces the possibility of abortion, amputation, transfusion, or other medical procedures with important religious implications, try to discover his or her spiritual attitude. Also try to determine the patient's attitude toward the importance of laying on of hands, confession, communion, observance of holy days (such as the Sabbath), and restrictions in diet or physical appearance. *Helping the patient continue his normal religious practices during hospitalization can help reduce stress.*

■ If the patient is pregnant, find out her beliefs concerning infant baptism and circumcision, and comply with them after delivery.

■ If a neonate is in critical condition, call an appropriate clergy member immediately. To perform an emergency baptism, the minister or priest pours a small amount of holy water into a teaspoon or a medicine cup and sprinkles a few drops of water over the infant's head while saying, "(Name of child), I baptize you in the name of the Father, the Son, and the Holy Spirit. Amen." In an extreme emergency, you can perform a Roman Catholic baptism, using a container of any available water. If you do so, be sure to notify the priest *because this sacrament must be administered only once.*

■ If a Jewish woman delivers a male infant prematurely or by cesarean birth, ask her whether she plans to observe the rite of circumcision, or bris, a significant ceremony per-

(Text continues on page 156.)

Beliefs and practices of selected religions

A patient's religious beliefs can affect his attitudes toward illness and traditional medicine. By trying to accommodate the patient's religious beliefs and practices in your care plan, you can increase his willingness to learn and comply with treatment regimens. Because religious beliefs may vary within particular sects, individual practices may differ from those described here.

Religion	Normal findings	Dietary restrictions	Practices in health crisis
Adventist	None (baptism of adults only)	Alcohol, coffee, tea, opioids, stimulants; in many groups, meat is also prohibited	Communion and baptism performed. Some members believe in divine healing, anointing with oil, and prayer. Some regard Saturday as the Sabbath.
Baptist	At birth, none (baptism of believers only); before death, counseling by clergy member and prayer	Alcohol; in some groups, coffee and tea is also prohibited	Some believe in healing by laying on of hands. Resistance to medical therapy occasionally approved.
Christian Scientist	At birth, none; before death, counseling by a Christian Science practitioner	Alcohol, coffee, and tobacco prohibited	Many members refuse all treatment, including drugs, biopsies, physical examination, and blood transfusions, and permit vaccination only when required by law. Alteration of thoughts is believed to cure illness. Hypnotism and psychotherapy are prohibited. (Christian Scientist nurses and nursing homes honor these beliefs.)
Church of Christ	None (baptism at age 8 or older)	Alcohol discouraged	Communion, anointing with oil, laying on of hands, and counseling by a minister.
Eastern Orthodox	At birth, baptism and confirmation; before death, last rites (For members of the Russian Orthodox Church, the arms are crossed after death, the fingers are set in a cross, and the unembalmed body is clothed in natural fiber.)	For members of the Russian Orthodox Church and usually the Greek Orthodox Church, no meat or dairy products on Wednesday, Friday, and during Lent	Anointing of the sick. For members of the Russian Orthodox Church, cross necklace is replaced immediately after surgery and shaving of male patients is prohibited, except in preparation for surgery. For members of the Greek Orthodox Church, communion and Sacrament of Holy Unction.
Episcopal	At birth, baptism; before death, occasional last rites	For some members, abstention from meat on Friday, fasting before communion (which may be daily)	Communion, prayer, and counseling performed by a minister.

Beliefs and practices of selected religions *(continued)*

Religion	Normal findings	Dietary restrictions	Practices in health crisis
Jehovah's Witnesses	None	Abstention from foods to which blood has been added	Typically, no blood transfusions are permitted; a court order may be required for an emergency transfusion.
Judaism	Ritual circumcision on eighth day after birth; burial of dead fetus; ritual washing of dead; burial (including organs and other body tissues) occurs as soon as possible; no autopsy or embalming	For Orthodox and Conservative Jews, kosher dietary laws (for example, pork and shellfish are prohibited); for Reform Jews, usually no restrictions	Donation or transplantation of organs requires rabbinical consultation. For Orthodox and Conservative Jews, medical procedures may be prohibited on the Sabbath—from sundown Friday to sundown Saturday—and special holidays.
Lutheran	Baptism usually performed 6 to 8 weeks after birth	None	Communion, prayer, and counseling performed by a minister.
Mormon	At birth, none (baptism at age 8 or older); before death, baptism, and gospel preaching	Alcohol, tobacco, tea, and coffee are prohibited; meat intake is limited	Belief in divine healing through the laying on of hands; communion on Sunday; some members may refuse medical treatment. Many wear a special undergarment.
Moslem	If spontaneous abortion occurs before 130 days, the fetus is treated as discarded tissue; after 130 days, it's treated as a human being. (Before death, confession of sins with family present; after death, only relatives or friends may touch the body.)	Pork is prohibited; daylight fasting during 9th month of Islamic calendar	Faith healing for the patient's morale only; conservative members reject medical therapy.
Orthodox Presbyterian	Infant baptism; scripture reading and prayer before death	None	Communion, prayer, and counseling performed by a minister.
Pentecostal Assembly of God, Foursquare Church	None (baptism only after age of accountability)	Abstention from alcohol, tobacco, meat slaughtered by strangling, any food to which blood has been added and, sometimes, pork	Belief in divine healing through prayer, anointing with oil, and laying on of hands.

(continued)

Beliefs and practices of selected religions *(continued)*

RELIGION	NORMAL FINDINGS	DIETARY RESTRICTIONS	PRACTICES IN HEALTH CRISIS
Roman Catholic	Infant baptism, including baptism of an aborted fetus without signs of clinical death (tissue necrosis); before death, anointing of the sick	Fasting or abstention from meat on Ash Wednesday and on Fridays during Lent; this practice is usually waived for the hospitalized	Burial of major amputated limb (sometimes) in consecrated ground; donation or transplantation of organs allowed if the benefit to recipient outweighs potential harm to donor. Sacraments of the Sick also performed when patients are ill, not just before death. Sometimes performed shortly after admission.
United Methodist	None (baptism of children and adults only)	None	Communion before surgery or similar crisis; donation of body parts encouraged.

formed on the eighth day after birth. (Because a patient who delivers a healthy, full-term baby vaginally is usually discharged quickly, this ceremony is normally performed outside the facility.) For a bris, ensure privacy and, if requested, sterilize the instruments. (For more information, see "Circumcision," page 905.)

- If the patient requests communion, prepare him for it before the clergy member arrives. First, place him in Fowler's or semi-Fowler's position if his condition permits. Otherwise, allow him to remain supine. Tuck a clean towel under his chin, and straighten the bed linens.
- If a terminally ill patient requests the Sacrament of the Sick (Last Rites) or special treatment of his body after death, call an appropriate clergy member. For the Roman Catholic patient, call a Roman Catholic priest to administer the sacrament, even if the patient is unresponsive or comatose. To prepare the patient for this sacrament, uncover his arms and fold back the top linens to expose his feet. After the clergy member anoints the patient's forehead, eyes, nose, mouth, hands, and feet, straighten and retuck the bed linens.

Special considerations

- Handle the patient's religious articles carefully to avoid damage or loss. Become familiar with religious resources in your facility. Some facilities employ one or more clergy members who counsel patients and staff and link patients to other pastoral resources.
- If the patient tries to convert you to his personal beliefs, tell him that you respect his beliefs but are content with your own. Likewise, avoid attempts to convert the patient to your personal beliefs.

Documentation

Complete a baptismal form and attach it to the patient's record; send a copy of the form to the appropriate clergy member. Record the rites of circumcision and last rites in your notes. Also, record last rites in red on the Kardex so it won't be repeated unnecessarily.

SELECTED REFERENCES

Gaskamp, C.D., et al. *Promoting Spirituality in the Older Adult.* Iowa City (IA): University of Iowa Gerontological Nursing Interventions Research Center, Research Dissemination Core, December 2004.

The Joint Commission. *Comprehensive Accreditation Manual for Hospitals: The Official Handbook.* Standard RI.2.10. 2007.

Meador. K.G. "Spiritual Care at the End of Life: What Is It and Who Does It?" *North Carolina Medical Journal* 65(4):226-28, July/August 2004.

Page, M. "How Well Do We Care for People's Spiritual Needs?" *The Australian and New Zealand Journal of Mental Health Nursing* 11(10):18-19, November 2005.

CARE OF THE DYING PATIENT

A patient needs intensive physical and emotional support as he approaches death. Signs and symptoms of impending death include reduced respiratory rate and depth, decreased or absent blood pressure, weak or erratic pulse rate, lowered skin temperature, decreased level of consciousness (LOC), diminished sensorium and neuromuscular control, diaphoresis, pallor, cyanosis, and mottling.

Five stages of dying

According to Elisabeth Kübler-Ross, author of *On Death and Dying*, the dying patient may progress through five psychological stages in preparation for death. Although each patient experiences these stages differently, and not necessarily in this order, understanding the stages will help you meet your patient's needs.

Denial

When the patient first learns of his terminal illness, he'll refuse to accept the diagnosis. He may experience physical symptoms similar to a stress reaction—shock, fainting, pallor, sweating, tachycardia, nausea, and GI disorders. During this stage, be honest with the patient but not blunt or callous. Maintain communication with him so he can discuss his feelings when he accepts the reality of death—but don't force him to confront this reality.

Anger

When the patient stops denying his impending death, he may show deep resentment toward those who will live on after he dies—including you, the hospital staff, and his own family. Although you may instinctively draw back from the patient or even resent this behavior, remember that he's dying and has a right to be angry. After you accept his anger, you can help him find different ways to express it and can help his family to understand it.

Bargaining

Although the patient acknowledges his impending death, he attempts to bargain with God or fate for more time. He'll probably strike this bargain secretly. If he does confide in you, don't urge him to keep his promises.

Depression

In this stage, the patient may first experience regrets about his past and then grieve about his current condition. He may withdraw from his friends, family, physician, and from you. He may suffer from anorexia, increased fatigue, or self-neglect. You may find him sitting alone, in tears. Accept the patient's sorrow, and if he talks to you, listen. Provide comfort by touch, as appropriate. Resist the temptation to make optimistic remarks or cheerful small talk.

Acceptance

In this last stage, the patient accepts the inevitability and imminence of his death, without emotion. The patient may simply desire the quiet company of a family member or friend. If, for some reason, a family member or friend can't be present, stay with the patient to satisfy his final need. Remember, however, that many patients die before reaching this stage.

Emotional support for the dying patient and his family usually means reassurance and the nurse's physical presence to help ease fear and loneliness. More intense emotional support is important at much earlier stages, especially for patients with long-term progressive illnesses, who can work through the stages of dying. (See *Five stages of dying*.)

Respect the patient's wishes about extraordinary means of supporting life. The patient may have signed a living will. This document, legally binding in most states, declares the patient's desire for a death unimpeded by the artificial support of defibrillators, respirators, life-sustaining drugs, auxiliary hearts, and other artificial means. If the patient has signed such a document, the nurse must respect his wishes and communicate the practitioner's "no code" order to all staff members.

Equipment

Clean bed linens ▪ clean gowns ▪ gloves ▪ water-filled basin ▪ soap ▪ washcloth ▪ towels ▪ lotion ▪ linen-saver pads ▪ petroleum jelly ▪ suction and resuscitation equipment, as necessary ▪ optional: indwelling urinary catheter.

Implementation

- Assemble equipment at the patient's bedside as needed.

Meeting physical needs

- Take vital signs often, and observe for pallor, diaphoresis, and decreased LOC.
- Reposition the patient in bed at least every 2 hours *because sensation, reflexes, and mobility diminish first in the legs and gradually in the arms.* Make sure the bed sheets cover him loosely *to reduce discomfort caused by pressure on arms and legs.*
- When the patient's vision and hearing start to fail, turn his head toward the light and speak to him from near the head of the bed. *Because hearing may be acute despite loss of consciousness,* avoid whispering or speaking inappropriately about the patient in his presence.

Understanding organ and tissue donation

A federal regulation was enacted in 1998 requiring facilities to report all deaths to the regional organ procurement organization. The regulation was enacted so that no potential donor is missed and ensures that the family of every potential donor will understand the option to donate. According to the American Medical Association, about 25 kinds of organs and tissues are being transplanted. Although donor organ requirements vary, the typical donor's age must be between a neonate and age 60 years and be free from transmissible disease. Tissue donations are less restrictive, and some tissue banks will accept skin from donors up to age 75.

Collection of most organs, such as the heart, liver, kidney, or pancreas, requires that the patient be pronounced brain dead and kept physically alive until the organs are harvested. Tissue such as eyes, skin, bone, and heart valves may be taken after death. Contact your regional organ procurement organization for specific organ donation criteria or to identify a potential donor. If you don't know the regional organ procurement organization in your area, call the United Network for Organ Sharing at (804) 782-4800.

- Change the bed linens and the patient's gown as needed. Provide skin care during gown changes, and adjust the room temperature for patient comfort if necessary.
- Observe for incontinence or anuria, the result of diminished neuromuscular control or decreased renal function. If necessary, obtain an order to catheterize the patient, or place linen-saver pads beneath the patient's buttocks. Put on gloves and provide perineal care with soap, a washcloth, and towels *to prevent irritation.*
- With suction equipment, suction the patient's mouth and upper airway *to remove secretions.* Elevate the head of the bed *to decrease respiratory resistance.* As the patient's condition deteriorates, he may breathe mostly through his mouth.
- Offer fluids frequently, and lubricate the patient's lips and mouth with petroleum jelly *to counteract dryness.*
- If the comatose patient's eyes are open, provide eye care to prevent corneal ulceration. *Such ulceration can cause blindness and prevent the use of these tissues for transplantation should the patient die.*
- Provide ordered pain medication as needed. Keep in mind that, as circulation diminishes, medications given I.M. will be poorly absorbed. Medications should be given I.V., if possible, *for optimum results.* Some medications can be given sublingually or rectally if the patient can't swallow or has no I.V. access.

Meeting emotional needs

- Fully explain all care and treatments to the patient even if he's unconscious *because he may still be able to hear.* Answer any questions as candidly as possible without sounding callous.
- Allow the patient to express his feelings, which may range from anger to loneliness. Take time to talk with the patient. Sit near the head of the bed, and avoid looking rushed or unconcerned.
- Notify family members, if they're absent, when the patient wishes to see them. Let the patient and his family discuss death at their own pace.
- Offer to contact a member of the clergy or social services department, if appropriate.

Special considerations

- If the patient has signed a living will, the practitioner will write a "do-not-resuscitate (DNR)" order on his progress notes and order sheets. Know your state's policy regarding the living will. If it's legal, transfer the DNR order to the patient's chart or Kardex and, at the end of your shift, inform the incoming staff of this order.
- If family members remain with the patient, show them the location of bathrooms, lounges, and cafeterias. Explain the patient's needs, treatments, and care plan to them. If appropriate, offer to teach them specific skills so they can take part in nursing care. Emphasize that their efforts are important and effective. As the patient's death approaches, give them emotional support.
- At an appropriate time, ask the family whether they have considered organ and tissue donation. Check the patient's records to determine whether he completed an organ donor card. (See *Understanding organ and tissue donation.*)

Documentation

Record changes in the patient's vital signs, intake and output, and LOC. Note the times of cardiac arrest and the end of respiration, and notify the practitioner when these occur.

SELECTED REFERENCES

Clinical Practice Guidelines for Quality Palliative Care. Brooklyn (NY): National Consensus Project for Quality Palliative Care; 2004.

Dobbins, E. "Helping Your Patient to a 'Good Death'," *Nursing* 35(20): 43-45, February 2005.

Hospice and Palliative Nurses Association and American Nurses Association. *Hospice and Palliative Nursing: Scope and Stan-*

dards of Practice, 2nd ed. Silver Spring, Md.: American Nurses Association, 2007.

Ramsey, G., and Motty, E. "Advance Directives: Protecting Patient's Rights," *Geriatric Nursing Protocols for Best Practice,* 2nd ed., New York: Springer Publishing Co., Inc., 2003.

POSTMORTEM CARE

After the patient dies, care includes preparing him for family viewing, arranging transportation to the morgue or funeral home, and determining the disposition of the patient's belongings. In addition, postmortem care entails comforting and supporting the patient's family and friends and providing for their privacy.

Postmortem care usually begins after a practitioner certifies the patient's death. If the death occurs within 24 hours of admission, or if the patient died violently or under suspicious circumstances (for example, an accident, a suicide, or a homicide), postmortem care may be postponed until the medical examiner completes an autopsy. Be aware that if an autopsy is necessary, it will influence the postmortem care.

Equipment

Gauze or soft string ties ▪ gloves ▪ chin straps ▪ abdominal pads ▪ cotton balls ▪ plastic shroud or body wrap ▪ three identification tags ▪ adhesive bandages to cover wounds or punctures ▪ plastic bag for patient's belongings ▪ water-filled basin ▪ soap ▪ towels ▪ washcloths ▪ stretcher.

A commercial morgue pack usually contains gauze or string ties, chin straps, a shroud, and identification tags.

Implementation

- Document any auxiliary equipment, such as a mechanical ventilator, still present. Put on gloves.
- Place the body in the supine position, arms at sides and head on a pillow. Then elevate the head of the bed 30 degrees *to prevent discoloration from blood settling in the face.*
- If the patient wore dentures, and your facility's policy permits, gently insert them; then close the mouth. Close the eyes by gently pressing on the lids with your fingertips. If they don't stay closed, place moist cotton balls on the eyelids for a few minutes, and then try again to close them. Place a folded towel under the chin *to keep the jaw closed.*
- Remove all indwelling urinary catheters, tubes, and tape, and apply adhesive bandages to puncture sites. Replace soiled dressings.
- Collect all the patient's valuables to prevent loss. If you're unable to remove a ring, cover it with gauze, tape it in place, and tie the gauze to the wrist *to prevent slippage and subsequent loss.*
- Clean the body thoroughly, using soap, a basin, and washcloths. Place one or more abdominal pads between the buttocks *to absorb rectal discharge or drainage.*
- Cover the body up to the chin with a clean sheet.
- Offer comfort and emotional support to the family and intimate friends. Ask if they wish to see the patient. If they do, allow them to do so in privacy. Ask if they would prefer to leave the patient's jewelry on the body.
- After the family leaves, remove the towel from under the chin of the deceased patient. Pad the chin, and wrap chin straps under the chin and tie them loosely on top of the head. Then pad the wrists and ankles *to prevent bruises,* and tie them together with gauze or soft string ties.
- Fill out the three identification tags. Each tag should include the deceased patient's name, room and bed numbers, date and time of death, and practitioner's name. Tie one tag to the deceased patient's hand or foot, but don't remove his identification bracelet *to ensure correct identification.*
- Place the shroud or body wrap on the morgue stretcher and, after obtaining assistance, transfer the body to the stretcher. Wrap the body, and tie the shroud or wrap with the string provided. Then attach another identification tag to the front of the shroud or wrap, and cover the shroud or wrap with a clean sheet. If a shroud or wrap isn't available, dress the deceased patient in a clean gown, and cover the body with a sheet.
- Place the deceased patient's personal belongings, including valuables, in a bag, and attach the third identification tag to it.
- If the patient died of an infectious disease, label the body according to your facility's policy.
- Close the doors of adjoining rooms if possible. Then take the body to the morgue. Use corridors that aren't crowded and, if possible, use a service elevator.

Special considerations

- If the patient is a trauma victim, the victim of a violent crime (such as a gunshot wound or stabbing), or has been in the hospital less than 24 hours, don't remove tubing or wash the patient until it's confirmed that an autopsy won't be done. If an autopsy is to be performed, keep all I.V. and other patient tubes intact and document as such.
- Give the deceased patient's personal belongings to his family, or bring them to the morgue. If you give the family jewelry or money, make sure a coworker is present as a witness. Obtain the signature of an adult family member *to verify receipt of valuables or to state their preference that jewelry remain on the patient.*
- Offer emotional support to the deceased patient's family and friends and to the patient's facility roommate, if appropriate.

Documentation

Although the extent of documentation varies among facilities, always record the disposition of the patient's possessions, especially jewelry and money. Also note the date and time the patient was transported to the morgue.

SELECTED REFERENCES

Harvey, J. "Debunking Myths about Postmortem Care," *Nursing* 31(7):44-45, July 2001.

Registered Nurses Association of Ontario (RNAO). *Supporting and Strengthening Families Through Expected and Unexpected Life Events Supplement.* Toronto (ON): Registered Nurses Association of Ontario, March 2006.

Research Dissemination Care. Family Bereavement Support before and after the Death of a Nursing Home Resident. Iowa City: University of Iowa Gerontological Nursing Interventions Research Center, October 2002.

2 ■ INFECTION CONTROL

INTRODUCTION

The mysteries of infection have been unfolding since Koch, Pasteur, and other microbiologists uncovered the link between bacteria and infection in the late 19th century. Despite our increased understanding of infectious diseases and the advent of programs to survey, prevent, identify, and control them, more than 2 million nosocomial infections occur each year. They raise health care costs by about $4.5 billion, lengthen hospital stays, and lead directly or indirectly to about 25,000 patient deaths annually.

Not all nosocomial infections can be prevented. Immunocompromised patients and those receiving immunosuppressive therapy, for example, may succumb to nosocomial infection despite all precautions. However, studies have shown that about one-third of all nosocomial infections could be prevented every year by faithful adherence to infection control principles. This chapter contains detailed instructions for using these principles effectively.

Causes and incidence

Infections result from aerobic and anaerobic bacteria, viruses, parasites, and fungi. The most common nosocomial infections involve the urinary tract, surgical wounds, the lower respiratory tract, and blood.

Urinary tract infections commonly result from catheter insertion or urogenital surgery or instrumentation. Surgical wound infections result from contamination during surgery, skin damage from preoperative hair removal, impaired blood supply, or coexisting medical problems. Lower respiratory tract infections can result from aspiration of oropharyngeal secretions, contaminated ventilation equipment, lung seeding by blood-borne pathogens, or airborne pathogens from other patients or caregivers. Bacteremia may arise as a complication of other infections, such as pneumonia and surgical wound infections, or from the presence of an intravascular device such as a central venous line.

The risk of nosocomial infection rises with the patient's age, underlying medical condition, use of invasive devices, and duration of hospitalization.

Infection control programs

According to recommendations issued in 1958 by the Joint Commission on Accreditation of Hospitals (now the Joint Commission) and the American Hospital Association, every accredited health care facility must have an infection control committee and a surveillance system as part of a formal infection control program. As health care delivery systems have changed since 1958, so has the challenge of adapting infection control programs for the surveillance, prevention, and control of infection. An effective infection control program can reduce the incidence of nosocomial infections by about one-third.

To guide health care facilities in their infection control efforts, in 1970, the Centers for Disease Control (now the Centers for Disease Control and Prevention [CDC]) published a manual that detailed seven categories of isolation techniques. The recommendations were revised in 1983 to reduce unnecessary procedures; to adapt to the increased use of intensive care units, invasive procedures, and immunosuppressive treatments; and to counter the spread of drug-resistant pathogens. In 1985, the CDC introduced its *universal precautions,* which recommended that health care workers wear gloves and other personal protective equipment (such as a mask, goggles, and a gown) to reduce exposure to blood and body fluids implicated in the transmission of blood-borne infections. In 1987, a new approach to infection control, known as *body substance isolation,* called for health care workers to wear gloves for contact with mucous membranes and broken skin, and anticipated contact with any moist body substances.

The CDC determined, however, that health care workers were confused about some aspects of universal precautions and body substance isolation; thus, in 1996, the CDC again revised the terminology used in its recommendations by introducing standard precautions as the basic unit of isolation precautions. *Standard precautions* call for health care workers to wear personal protective equipment appropriate for the task being performed and the risk of exposure to or contact with any moist body substance, mucous membrane, or broken skin. Three other transmission-based categories of isolation precautions were added to standard precautions as necessary to prevent the transmission of infection among patients, health care workers, and visitors. These categories are airborne precautions, droplet precautions, and contact precautions.

In most health care facilities, infection control practitioners are responsible for coordinating surveillance and other infection control activities. Although specific responsibilities may vary among facilities, typical activities include:

- teaching the staff the importance of correct hand hygiene between patient contacts (the most effective way to reduce infection risk)
- assessing patients for infection and recommending proper precautions against cross-contamination
- developing infection control guidelines, instructing the staff, and monitoring isolation procedures
- assisting staff in implementing procedures and using products to reduce the risk of nosocomial infection
- serving as a resource to the facility and the staff on the prevention and control of infection.

Isolation as prevention

Most isolation procedures aim at preventing transmission of disease from infected patients to other patients, health care workers, and visitors. In contrast, isolation may also aim at protecting immunocompromised patients from exogenous pathogens. Many factors contribute to the development of nosocomial infections. Strict adherence to your facility's infection control policies and the procedures outlined in this chapter can go a long way toward keeping infection at bay.

GENERAL PRINCIPLES

HAND HYGIENE

The hands are the conduits for almost every transfer of potential pathogens from one patient to another, from a contaminated object to the patient, or from a staff member to the patient. Thus, hand hygiene is the single most important procedure for preventing infection. To protect patients from nosocomial infections, hand hygiene must be performed routinely and thoroughly. In effect, clean and healthy hands with intact skin, short fingernails, and no rings minimize the risk of contamination. Artificial nails may serve as a reservoir for microorganisms, and microorganisms are more difficult to remove from rough or chapped hands.

In 2002, the CDC redefined hand washing when it published the *Guideline for Hand Hygiene in Health-Care Settings.* Hand hygiene is a general term that refers to hand washing, antiseptic hand wash, antiseptic hand rub, or surgical hand antisepsis. Hand washing refers to washing hands with plain (nonantimicrobial) soap and water. Use of an antiseptic agent (such as chlorhexidine, triclosan, or iodophor) to wash hands is an antiseptic hand wash. Whether a plain or an antiseptic agent is used, hand washing or hand hygiene is still the single most effective method to prevent the spread of infection. Washing with soap (plain or antimicrobial) and water is appropriate when hands are visibly soiled or contaminated with infectious material.

Equipment

Hand washing

Soap or detergent ▪ warm, running water ▪ paper towels ▪ optional: fingernail brush, antiseptic cleaning agent, disposable sponge brush, or plastic cuticle stick.

Hand sanitizing

Alcohol-based hand rub.

Implementation

Hand washing

- Remove rings as your facility's policy dictates *because they harbor dirt and skin microorganisms.* Remove your watch or wear it well above the wrist. *Note*: Artificial fingernails and nail polish must be kept in good repair *to minimize their potential to harbor microorganisms;* refer to your facility's policy pertaining to nail polish and artificial nails. Natural nails should be short (less than ¼"). The CDC Hand Hygiene Guideline recommends that artificial nails or extenders not be worn when having direct contact with patients at high risk such as those in intensive care units or the operating room areas.
- Wet your hands and wrists with warm water, and apply soap from a dispenser. Don't use bar soap *because it allows cross-contamination.* Hold your hands below elbow level *to prevent water from running up your arms and back down, thus contaminating clean areas.* (See *Proper hand-washing technique,* page 164.)
- Work up a generous lather by rubbing your hands together vigorously for about 10 seconds. *Soap and warm water reduce surface tension and this, aided by friction, loosens surface microorganisms, which wash away in the lather.*
- Pay special attention to the area under fingernails and around cuticles, and to the thumbs, knuckles, and sides of the fingers and hands *because microorganisms thrive in these protected or overlooked areas.* If you don't remove your wedding band, move it up and down your finger to clean beneath it.
- Avoid splashing water on yourself or the floor *because microorganisms spread more easily on wet surfaces and because slippery floors are dangerous.* Avoid touching the sink or faucets *because they're considered contaminated.*
- Rinse hands and wrists well *because running water flushes suds, soil, soap or detergent, and microorganisms away.*
- Pat hands and wrists dry with a paper towel. Avoid rubbing, *which can cause abrasion and chapping.*
- If the sink isn't equipped with knee or foot controls, turn off faucets by gripping them with a dry paper towel *to avoid recontaminating your hands.*

Hand sanitizing

- Apply a small amount of the alcohol-based hand rub to all surfaces of your hand.
- Rub your hands together.

Proper hand-washing technique

To minimize the spread of infection, follow these basic hand washing instructions. With your hands angled downward under the faucet, adjust the water temperature until it's comfortably warm.

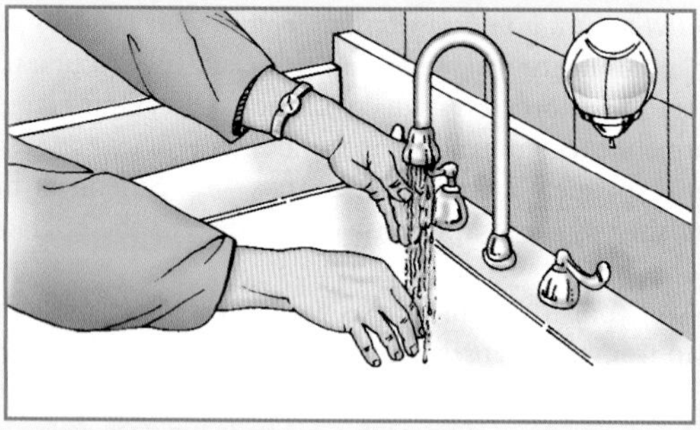

Add soap and work up a generous lather by scrubbing vigorously for 10 seconds. Be sure to clean beneath fingernails, around knuckles, and along the sides of fingers and hands.

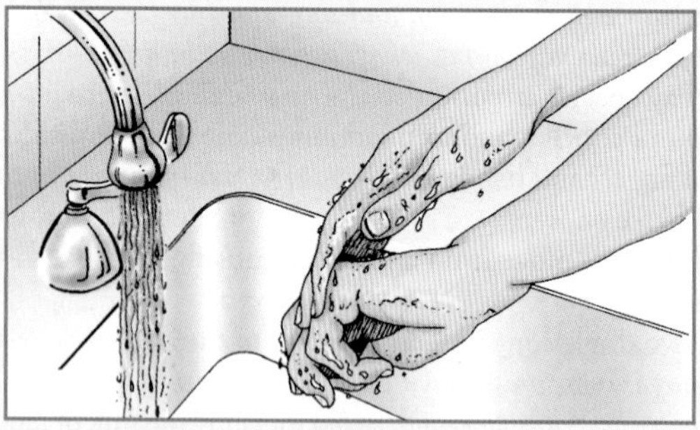

Rinse your hands completely *to wash away suds and microorganisms.* Pat dry with a paper towel. *To prevent recontaminating your hands on the faucet handles,* cover each one with a dry paper towel when turning off the water.

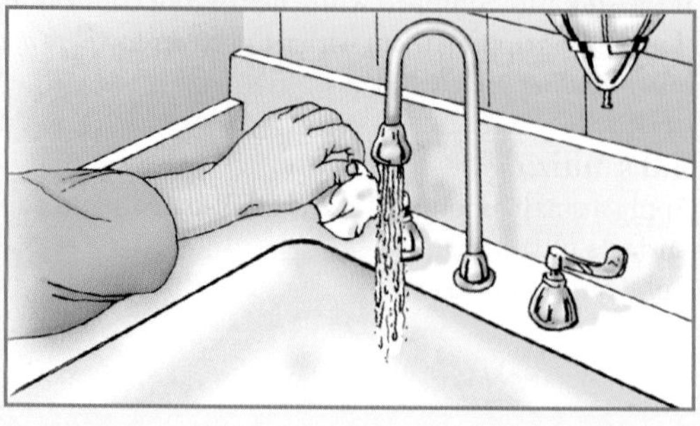

Special considerations

- Before participating in any sterile procedure or whenever your hands are grossly contaminated, wash your forearms also, and clean under the fingernails and in and around the cuticles with a fingernail brush, disposable sponge brush, or plastic cuticle stick. Use these softer implements *because brushes, metal files, or other hard objects may injure your skin and, if reused, may be a source of contamination.*
- Follow your facility's policy concerning when to wash with soap and when to use an antiseptic cleaning agent. Typically, you'll wash with soap before coming on duty; before and after direct or indirect patient contact; before and after performing any bodily functions, such as blowing your nose or using the bathroom; before preparing or serving food; before preparing or administering medications; after removing gloves or other personal protective equipment; and after completing your shift.
- Don't use an alcohol-based hand rub if contact with items contaminated with *Clostridium difficile* or *Bacillus anthracis* occurs. *These organisms can form spores, and alcohol won't kill the spores.* Wash your hands with soap and water instead.
- Use an antiseptic cleaning agent before performing invasive procedures, wound care, and dressing changes and after contamination. Antiseptics are also recommended for hand washing in isolation rooms, neonate and special care nurseries, and before caring for any highly susceptible patient.
- Wash your hands before and after performing patient care or procedures or having contact with contaminated objects, even though you may have worn gloves. Always wash your hands after removing gloves.
- Alcohol hand rubs usually contain *emollients to prevent drying and chapping of the skin.* Hand rubs and sanitizers are appropriate for decontaminating the hands after minimal contamination.

NURSING ALERT *If you're providing care in the patient's home, bring your own supply of soap and disposable paper towels. If running water isn't available, disinfect your hands with an alcohol-based hand sanitizer.*

Complications

Because it strips natural skin oils, frequent hand washing may result in dryness, cracking, and irritation. These effects are probably more common after repeated use of antiseptic cleaning agents, especially in people with sensitive skin. Be sure to rinse off any excess cleaning agents *to help minimize irritation.*

To prevent your hands from becoming dry or chapped, apply an emollient hand cream after each washing, or switch to a different cleaning agent. Make sure the hand cream or lotion you use won't cause the material in your gloves to deteriorate. If you develop dermatitis, you may need to be evaluated by your employee health provider to determine whether you should continue to work until the condition resolves.

SELECTED REFERENCES

Centers for Disease Control and Prevention. "Guidelines for Hand Hygiene in Health-Care Settings," *MMWR* 51(RR-16):1-144, October 2002.

Houghton, D. "HAI Prevention: The Power Is in Your Hands," *Nursing Management* 37(supplement):1-7, May 2006.

Hughes, N. "Handwashing: Going Back to Basics in Infection Control," *AJN* 107(7):96, July 2006.

Scalise, D. "Save Lives Now. 30 Things You Can Do to Eliminate Infections," *Hospital & Health Networks/AHA* 80(9):32-36, 38-40, September 2006.

BASIC STERILE TECHNIQUE

Sterile technique, also referred to as *aseptic technique,* is used for any procedure that requires the absence of microorganisms. Sterile technique should be followed any time the patient's skin is intentionally perforated, during procedures that involve entry into a sterile body cavity, or when coming into contact with nonintact skin resulting from trauma or surgery.

Sterile technique is used in conjunction with other procedures—it isn't a procedure in itself. Procedures requiring sterile technique include I.V. catheter insertion, any type of injection, inserting a urinary catheter, and dressing changes. Patients with a compromised immune system (such as those with burns, those following organ transplant, and those receiving chemotherapy or radiation therapy) also require sterile technique, even for some procedures that would normally only require clean technique.

Equipment

Sterile gloves ■ personal protective equipment ■ sterile supplies, as required by the procedure to be performed ■ optional: sterile bowl, sterile normal saline solution, sterile drape.

Many procedures have commercially prepared kits, which provide all of the necessary components.

Preparation of equipment

Assemble all the equipment in the patient's room. Check each package carefully, and discard any with a hole or tear or that's wet. Note the expiration date, and discard any package that's beyond the date. Make sure that the sterilization tape has turned the appropriate color (see your facility's policy; color will depend on the product used and sterilization method). Prepare a clean surface to set up the equipment for the sterile procedure.

Implementation

- Verify the practitioner's order *to ensure that the right procedure is being performed on the right patient at the right time.*
- Confirm the patient's identity using two patient identifiers according to your facility's policy.
- Explain the procedure to the patient and family *to relieve anxiety and ensure understanding and cooperation.*
- Assess the patient's level of pain, and administer analgesics 20 to 30 minutes before the procedure *to promote patient comfort.*
- Wash your hands thoroughly *to reduce the risk of transmission of microorganisms.* (See "Hand hygiene," page 163.)
- Follow standard precautions by putting on the necessary personal protective equipment for the procedure. (See "Standard precautions," page 177.)

Opening sterile kits

- Remove the plastic outer wrapper from the procedure kit, if one is present.
- Place the inner wrapped kit on a clean, dry, flat surface *because moisture on the table could be absorbed through the wrapper and contaminate the sterile supplies.*
- Position the kit so that the tip of the triangle-pointed wrapper is toward you—*this way you won't have to reach over the sterile contents once the other flaps are opened.*
- Grasp the outer portion of this outermost flap *to avoid contaminating the sterile field.*
- Open the flap away from the body (as shown below), keeping the arm outstretched to the side *so it doesn't cross over the sterile field.*

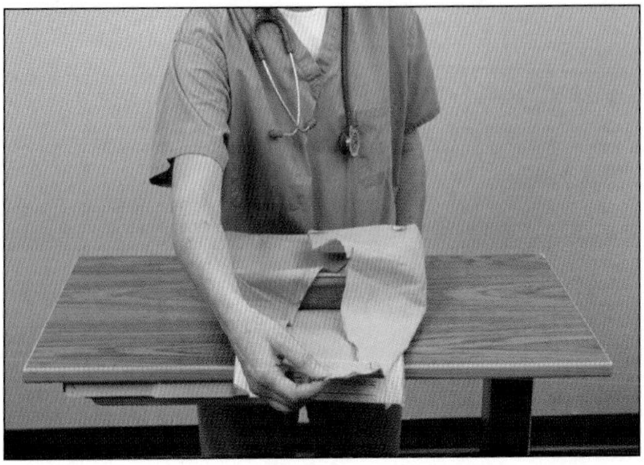

- Grasp the outer surface of the first side flap with the hand on the same side as the flap to avoid crossing over the sterile field (as shown below). Be sure to open the flap fully *to avoid allowing the wrapper to spring back.*

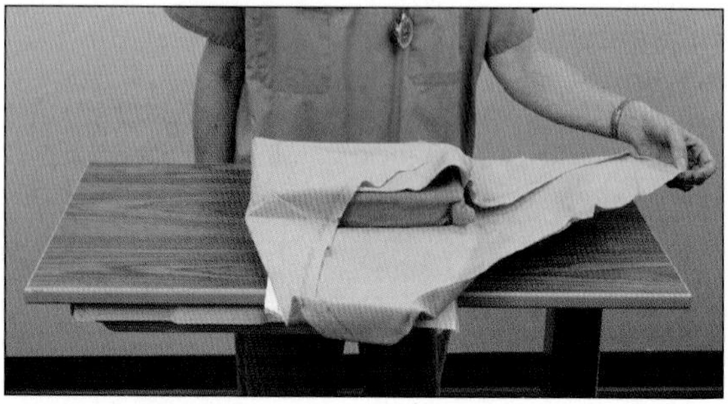

■ Grasp the outer surface of the second side flap, and open it with the hand on the same side (as shown below).

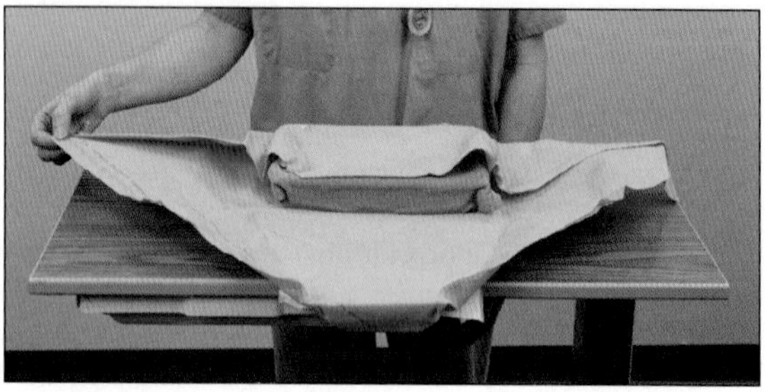

■ Grasp the outer surface of the innermost flap, and open it toward your body (as shown below).

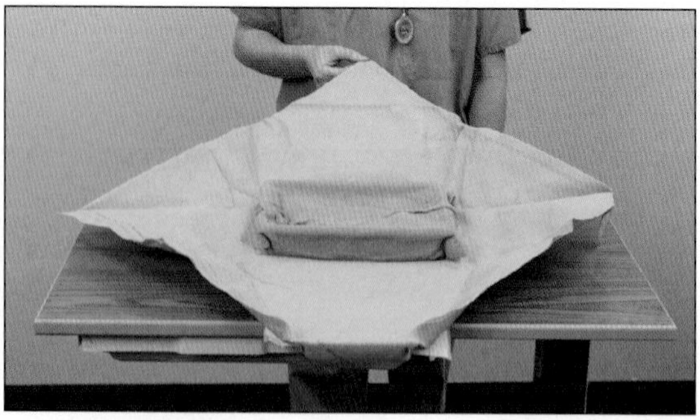

Opening wrapped sterile items

■ Grasp the sterile item wrapped in paper or linen in the nondominant hand.
■ Break the sterilization tape.
■ Use the dominant hand to grasp the outer surface of the top outermost flap *to avoid touching a sterile surface.*
■ Open the flap away from your body.
■ Grasp the outer surface of the first side flap, and open it fully to the side.
■ Repeat with the other side flap.
■ Secure all flaps in the nondominant hand *to avoid dangling and contaminating other items.*
■ Grasp the outer surface of the inner flap, and open it toward you.
■ Place the item on the sterile field, ensuring that only sterile surfaces touch other sterile surfaces *to avoid contamination.*
■ Be sure the item is at least 1″ (2.5 cm) from the edge of the sterile field *because any closer to the edge is considered unsterile.*

Opening peel pack containers or pouches

■ Grasp the unsealed corner of the wrapper, and pull it toward you.
■ If the item is light, it can be dropped onto the sterile field. Heavy items should be carefully set onto the sterile field.
■ Open a peel pack pouch (such as gloves and syringes) by grasping each side of the unsealed edge with the thumb side of each hand parallel to the seal, and pull it apart gently.
■ Hold the sides back so the wrap covers your hands and exposes the sterile item.
■ Don't allow the item to slide across the package side when dropping the item onto the sterile field.

Pouring sterile solutions

■ Open the wrapped package containing the sterile bowl, as described above, *to avoid contaminating the sterile field.*
■ Place the bowl on the edge of the sterile field but inside of the 1″ safety margin *so that solution can be poured without reaching across the sterile field.*
■ Unwrap the seal on the sterile normal saline solution bottle.
■ Unscrew the cap without touching the edges of the bottle.
■ Place the inverted cap on a nonsterile surface *to keep the inside of the cap from touching contaminated surfaces.*
■ Pour the solution into the bowl without reaching over the sterile field and from a distance of approximately 6″ (15 cm) above the bowl *to reduce the risk of touching sterile surfaces.*
■ Pour the solution slowly *to avoid splashing onto the drape and contaminating the sterile field.*
■ Discard unused solution or recap the container, and label the bottle with the date, time, and your initials to be used within 24 hours, depending on your facility's policy.

Opening and putting on sterile gloving

■ Open the package containing the sterile gloves following the above procedures. Some commercially prepared kits (such as the kit for inserting an indwelling urinary catheter) include a pair of sterile gloves. If gloves are included, they will be the uppermost item in the pack. Touch only the outer side of the glove wrapper.

■ Grasp the paper glove wrapper and place it on a clean, dry, flat surface.
■ Open the package, touching only the outer edges of the wrapper (as shown below).

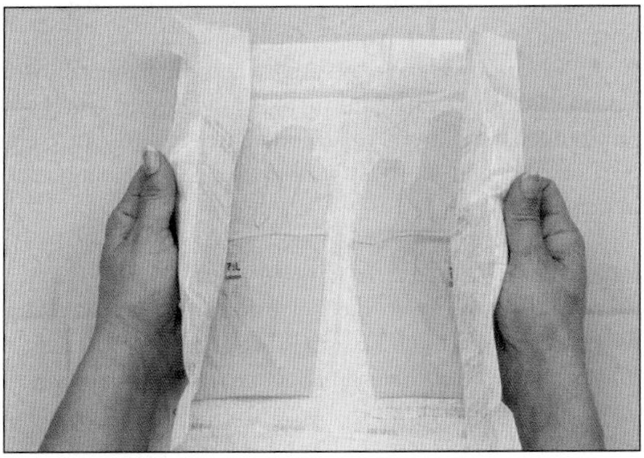

■ Use the thumb and fingers of the nondominant hand to grasp the folded inner surface portion of the glove for the dominant hand, touching only the inner portion of the glove (as shown below).

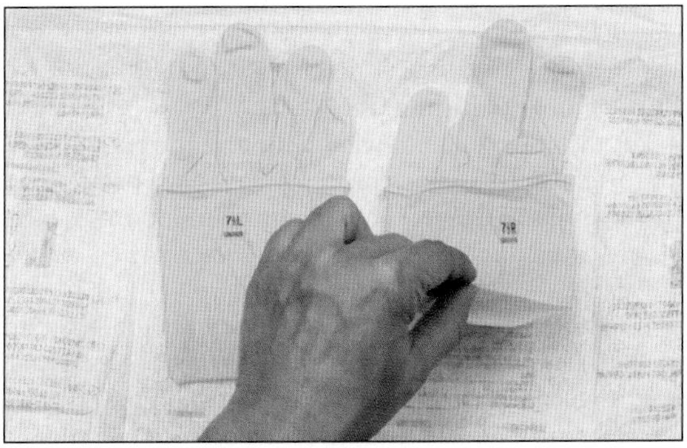

■ Lift the glove up, and insert the dominant hand into the glove, palm side up (as shown below).

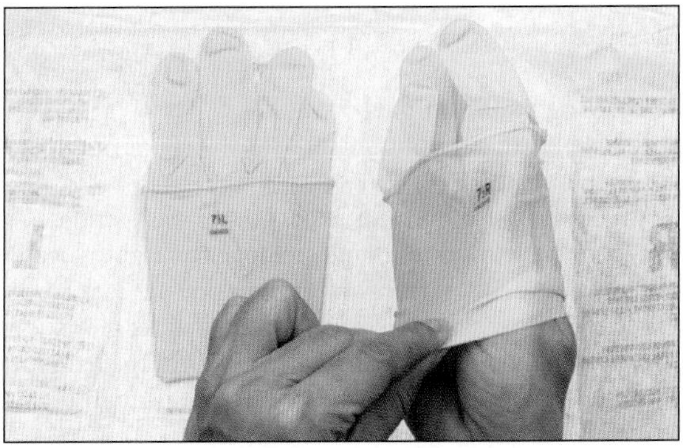

■ Pull the cuff down by touching only the inner surface of the glove.
■ Insert the four fingers of the dominant gloved hand into the sterile outer cuff of the other glove, keeping the thumb pulled back out of the way (as shown below).

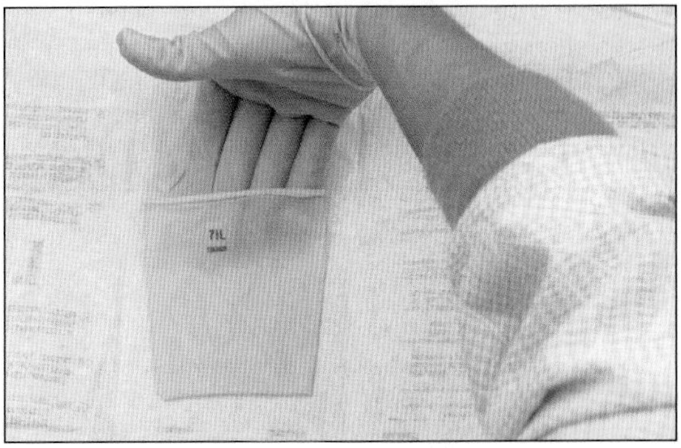

■ Lift the glove up, and insert the nondominant hand into the glove. Allow the cuff to come uncuffed as you finish putting it on, but don't touch the skin of the arm with the gloved hand.
■ Adjust fingers of the gloves once both hands are gloved.

Special considerations

■ If additional sterile supplies need to be added to a sterile field, open the sterile packages as described above. Be sure to open them away from the already set-up sterile field *to avoid contaminating the field.* Hold the opened additional supplies above the sterile field, and drop them onto the field.
■ Medical asepsis, also called *clean technique,* isn't the same as sterile technique. Medical asepsis is focused on the absence of pathogenic organisms and doesn't require items to be sterile. Sterile technique and surgical asepsis are focused on the elimination of all microorganisms.

Documentation

Document the procedure that was performed using guidelines for that procedure. Within this documentation, note the sterile supplies used and that sterile technique was followed. Note the date and time of the procedure.

SELECTED REFERENCES

Association of Perioperative Registered Nurses. *Standards, Recommended Practices, and Guidelines.* Denver: AORN, Inc., 2006.

Craven, R.F., and Hirnle, C.J. *Fundamentals of Nursing: Human Health and Function,* 5th ed. Philadelphia: Lippincott Williams & Wilkins, 2007.

Occupational Safety and Health Administration. Personal Protective Equipment Standard 1910.132.

Putting on a face mask

To avoid spreading airborne particles, wear a sterile or nonsterile face mask as indicated. Position the mask to cover your nose and mouth, and secure it high enough to ensure stability. Tie the top strings at the back of your head above the ears. Then tie the bottom strings at the base of your neck. If the mask has ear loops, place them securely around your ears.

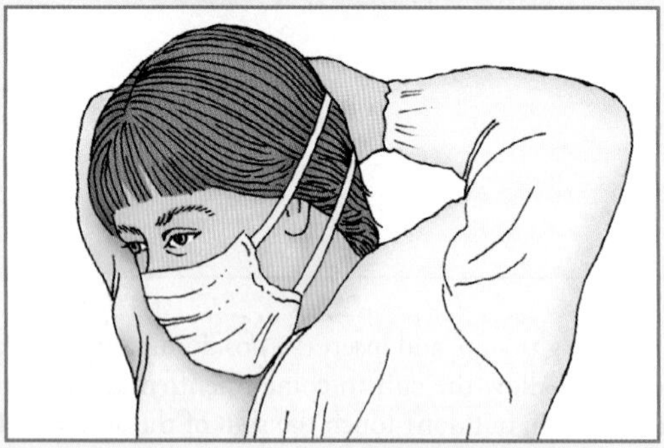

Adjust the metal nose strip if the mask has one.

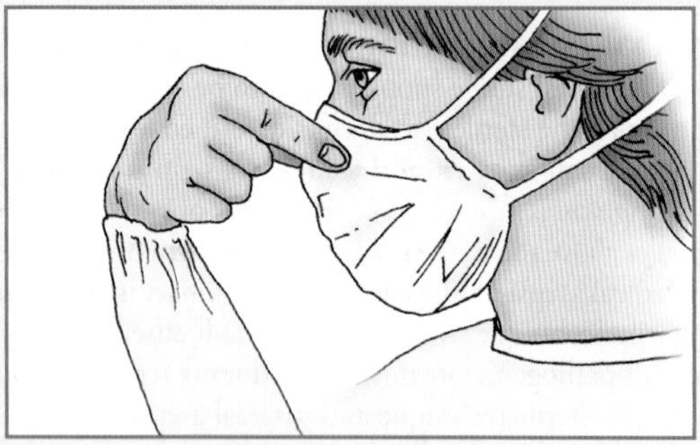

USE OF ISOLATION EQUIPMENT

Isolation procedures may be implemented to prevent the spread of infection from patient to patient, from the patient to health care workers, or from health care workers to the patient. They may also be used to reduce the risk of infection in immunocompromised patients. Central to the success of these procedures is the selection of the proper equipment and the adequate training of those who use it.

Equipment

Materials required for isolation typically include barrier clothing, an isolation cart or anteroom for storing equipment, and a door card announcing that isolation precautions are in effect.

***Barrier clothing*:** Gowns ▪ gloves ▪ goggles ▪ masks. Each staff member must be trained in their proper use.

Isolation supplies: Labels ▪ tape ▪ laundry bags (and water-soluble laundry bags, if used) ▪ plastic trash bags.

An isolation cart may be used when the patient's room has no anteroom. It should include a work area (such as a pull-out shelf), drawers or a cabinet area for holding isolation supplies and, possibly, a pole on which to hang coats or jackets.

Preparation of equipment

Remove the cover from the isolation cart if necessary, and set up the work area. Check the cart or anteroom *to ensure that correct and sufficient supplies are in place for the designated isolation category.*

Implementation

- Remove your watch (or push it well up your arm) and your rings according to your facility's policy. *These actions help to prevent the spread of microorganisms hidden under your watch or rings.*
- Wash your hands before putting on gloves *to prevent the growth of microorganisms under gloves.*

Putting on isolation garb

- Put the gown on, and wrap it around the back of your uniform. Tie the strings or fasten the snaps or pressure-sensitive tabs at the neck. Make sure your uniform is completely covered *to prevent contact with the patient or his environment.*
- Place the mask snugly over your nose and mouth. Secure ear loops around your ears or tie the strings behind your head high enough so the mask won't slip off. If the mask has a metal strip, squeeze it to fit your nose firmly but comfortably. (See *Putting on a face mask.*) If you wear eyeglasses, tuck the mask under their lower edge. If goggles are worn, put them on at this time.
- Put on the gloves. Pull the gloves over the cuffs to cover the edges of the gown's sleeves.

Removing isolation garb

- Remember that the outside surfaces of your barrier clothes are contaminated.
- While wearing gloves, untie the gown's waist strings.
- With your gloved left hand, remove the right glove by pulling on the cuff, turning the glove inside out as you pull. Don't touch any skin with the outside of either glove. (See *Removing contaminated gloves.*) Then remove the left glove by wedging one or two fingers of your right hand inside the

Removing contaminated gloves

Proper removal techniques are essential for preventing the spread of pathogens from gloves to your skin surface. Follow these steps carefully.

Using your left hand, pinch the right glove near the top. Avoid allowing the glove's outer surface to buckle inward against your wrist.

Pull downward, allowing the glove to turn inside out as it comes off. Keep the right glove in your left hand after removing it.

Now insert the first two fingers of your ungloved right hand under the edge of the left glove. Avoid touching the glove's outer surface or folding it against your left wrist.

Pull downward so that the glove turns inside out as it comes off. Continue pulling until the left glove completely encloses the right one and its uncontaminated inner surface is facing out.

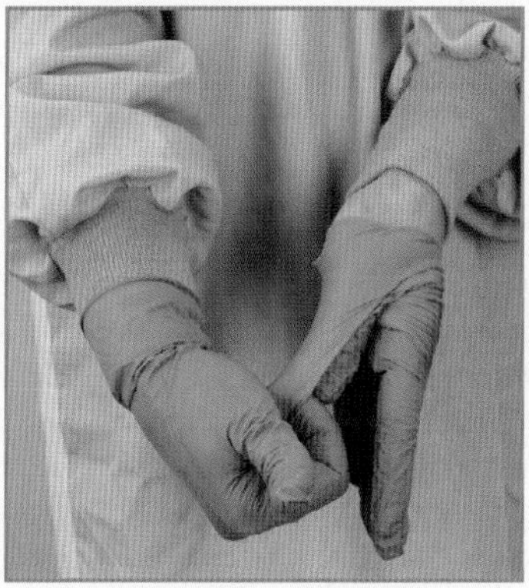

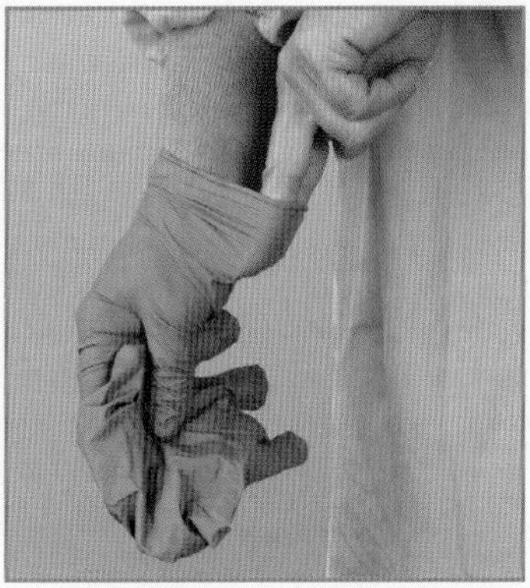

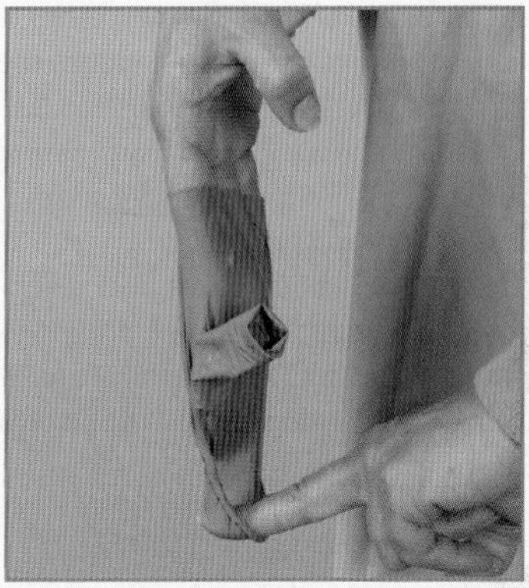

glove and pulling it off, turning it inside out as you remove it. Discard the gloves in the trash container.

- Untie the neck straps of your gown. Grasp the outside of the gown at the back of the shoulders, and pull the gown down over your arms, turning it inside out as you remove it *to ensure containment of the pathogens.*
- Holding the gown well away from your uniform, fold it inside out. Discard it in the laundry or trash container as necessary.
- If the sink is inside the patient's room, wash your hands and forearms with soap or antiseptic before leaving the room. Turn off the faucet using a paper towel, and discard the towel in the room. Grasp the door handle with a clean paper towel to open it, and discard the towel in a trash container inside the room. Close the door from the outside with your bare hand.
- Remove the mask last *to prevent contaminating your face or hair in the process.* Untie your mask, holding it only by the strings. Discard the mask in the trash container. Remove goggles.
- If the sink is in an anteroom, wash your hands and forearms with soap or antiseptic after leaving the room.

Special considerations

- If airborne precautions are required, a particulate respirator should be worn rather than a surgical mask.
- Use gowns, gloves, goggles, and masks only once, and discard them in the appropriate container before leaving a contaminated area. If your mask is reusable, retain it for further use unless it's damaged or damp. Be aware that isolation garb loses its effectiveness when wet *because moisture permits organisms to seep through the material.* Change masks and gowns as soon as moisture is noticeable or according to the manufacturer's recommendations or your facility's policy.
- At the end of your shift, restock used items for the next person. After patient transfer or discharge, return the isolation cart to the appropriate area for cleaning and restocking of supplies. An isolation room or other room prepared for isolation purposes must be thoroughly cleaned and disinfected before use by another patient.

SELECTED REFERENCES

Centers for Disease Control and Prevention. "Guideline for Isolation Precautions: Preventing Transmission of Infectious

Agents in Healthcare Settings 2007." Accessed August 2007 via the Web at *www.cdc.gov/ncidod/dhqp/g1_isolation.html.*
Perry, J., and Jagger, J. "Getting the Most from Your Personal Protective Gear," *Nursing* 34(12):72, December 2004.
Rushing, J. "Wearing Personal Protective Gear," *Nursing* 36(10): 56-57, October 2006.

SURGICAL ATTIRE

Surgical attire is worn in the semi-restricted and restricted areas of the surgical environment to reduce microbial contamination by surgical staff. The appropriate attire varies by restriction level. The *unrestricted* area is a central control point where the entrance of patients, personnel, and materials can be monitored. Street clothes are permitted in this area. The *semirestricted* area includes the peripheral support areas of the operating room, such as the corridors leading to the restricted areas of the operating room, scrub sink areas, clean and sterile supply storage rooms, and work areas for instrument processing. Surgical scrub attire is required, and all head and facial hair must be covered in this area. The *restricted* area includes the operating room suite, procedure rooms, and clean core. Surgical attire and hair coverings are required. Masks are required in the presence of open sterile items or scrubbed personnel.

Equipment

Two-piece scrub suit (pants and top) ■ head covering or hood ■ surgical mask ■ surgical gown ■ optional: cover gown or laboratory coat, protective eyewear or face shield, show covers.

Implementation

■ Put on a surgical head cover or hood and ensure that all hair and facial hair, including sideburns, are covered *to prevent hair, dandruff, and microoorganisms from falling onto the sterile field. Placing the head cover first reduces the risk of contaminants falling onto the scrub clothing.*

■ Put on scrub pants and top that are approved and laundered by the facility before entering semirestricted and restricted areas.

■ Place shoe covers over foot wear if splashing or spilling of body fluid is anticipated. However, studies suggest that shoe covers don't decrease the incidence of surgical wound infections. If worn, shoe covers should be removed when leaving the semirestricted area and new ones placed upon return.

■ Put on a surgical mask *to reduce the dispersal of microbial droplets from the mouth and nasopharynx.* Select a mask with microbial filtration of 95% or above *to protect yourself from aerosolized particles such as laser or electrosurgical plume.*

■ Ensure the mask covers the mouth and nose completely. Mold the malleable metal strip on the top of the mask to the nose.

■ Remove or confine all jewelry within scrub attire *to reduce the risk of transmission of microorganisms that may be on the jewelry as well as reducing the risk of the jewelry falling onto the sterile field or into the wound. Wearing rings interferes with proper hand antisepsis.*

■ Put on protective eyewear if splashing or splattering of body fluids is likely to occur.

Putting on a sterile gown and closed gloving technique

■ Open the sterile gown and gloves on a flat surface away from the sterile back table.

■ Grasp the sterile gown at the neckline, and lift up and away from the field. The exposed side of the folded gown is the inside of the gown.

■ Step back into an area where the gown can be unfolded without the risk of contamination.

■ Hold the gown with both hands on each side of the neckline, and allow the gown to unfold fully with the inside toward the wearer. Do not shake the gown open *as this causes air currents, which could lead to contamination.*

■ Keep your arms at shoulder level and away from the body as you slide both arms into the sleeves (as shown below), stopping when the hands reach the proximal edge of the cuff. Don't push the hands past the cuff, *or you won't be able to perform the closed gloving technique.*

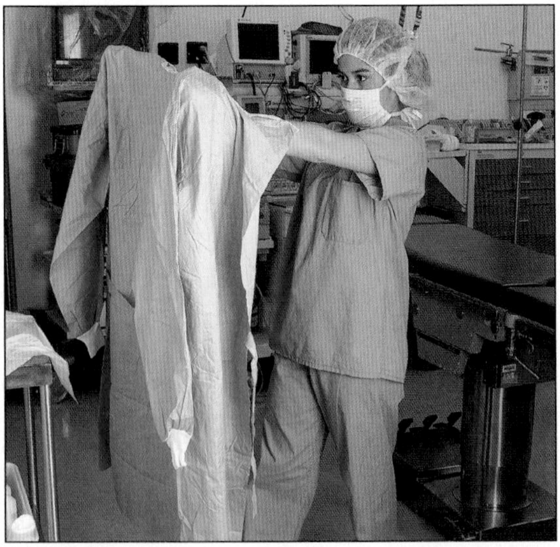

■ Have the circulating (unsterile) nurse touch the inside of the gown shoulders and sides to bring it over the scrub person's shoulders. The scrub nurse secures the neckline of the gown and the inner gown tie at the waist. This should be done before the scrub person puts on gloves *to keep the gown from flapping and becoming contaminated against a nonsterile surface.*

■ The scrub person returns to the sterile field created by the gown wrapper to put on sterile gloves.

Closed gloving technique

■ Keeping hands inside the gown sleeves, open the glove wrapper. Avoid getting too close to the sterile field *because the 1" (2.5 cm) margin of the gown wrapper is considered unsterile.*

■ Pick up the glove for the dominant hand with the nondominant hand still inside the gown sleeve. Extend the forearm of your dominant hand palm side up.

■ Place the glove for the dominant hand palm side down with the fingers facing toward the elbow. Grasp the glove cuff through the sleeve (as shown below).

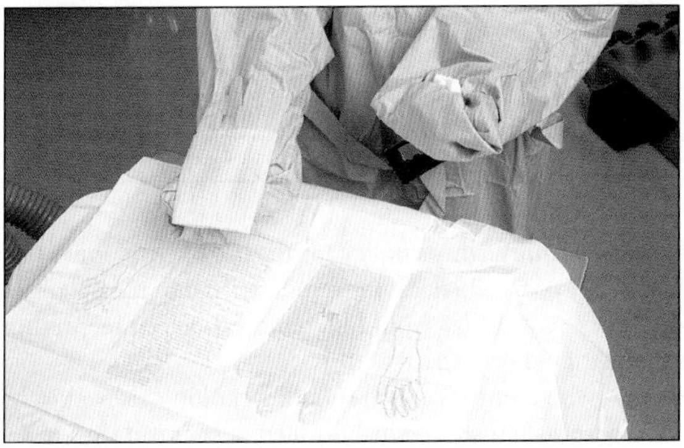

■ Use the nondominant hand to grasp the top side of the glove cuff and stretch it over the hand, covering the wrist entirely (as shown below).

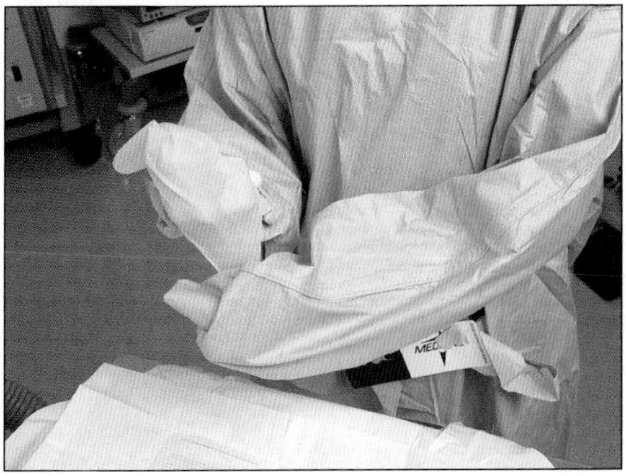

■ Advance the gown cuff down toward the wrist, direct fingers into the glove, and adjust glove on hand (as shown below).

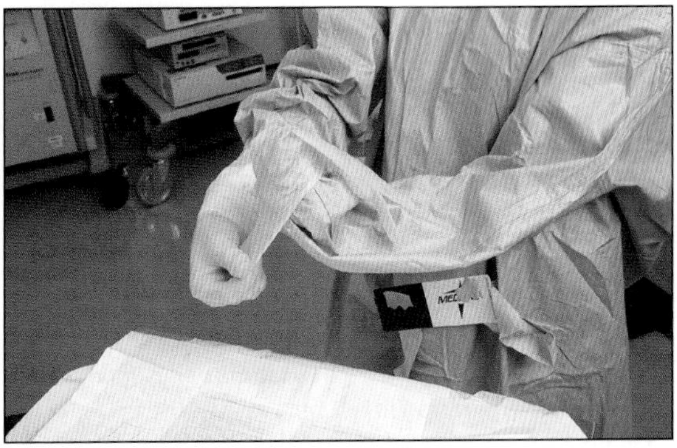

■ Repeat the procedure for the other hand.

■ Fold hands together and interlace fingers *to help the fingers fully extend into the gloves.*

■ Hold the short tie, attached to the card in front of the gown, in your left hand. Use your right hand to release the card from the front of the gown.

■ Hand the end of the card without the tie to another person. The person can be sterile or unsterile *because the person will keep the card but never touch the tie itself.*

■ Turn to the left to wrap the gown around your back (as shown below).

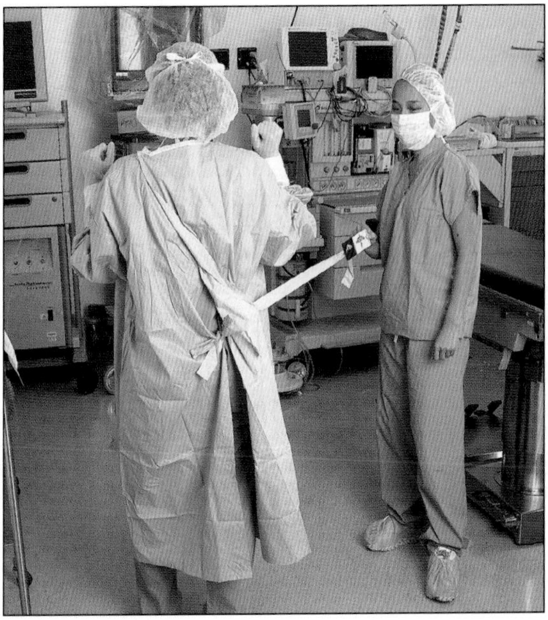

Reportable diseases checklist

Because reporting laws vary from state to state, this list isn't conclusive and may be changed periodically. Local agencies report certain diseases to their state health departments, which in turn determine which diseases are reported to the Centers for Disease Control and Prevention (CDC).

Acquired immunodeficiency syndrome (AIDS)
Anthrax
Botulism, food-borne
Botulism, infant
Botulism, other (wound and unspecified)
Brucellosis
California serogroup virus
Chancroid
Chlamydia trachomatis, genital infections
Cholera
Coccidioidomycosis
Cryptosporidiosis
Cyclosporiasis
Diphtheria
Eastern equine encephalitis
Ehrlichiosis
Escherichia coli, shiga toxin-producing
Giardiasis
Gonorrhea
Haemophilus influenza, invasive disease
Hansen's disease
Hantavirus pulmonary syndrome
Hemolytic uremic syndrome, postdiarrheal
Hepatitis A, acute
Hepatitis B, acute, chronic
Hepatitis B, perinatal infection
Hepatitis C, acute, chronic
Human immunodeficiency virus (HIV) infection
Influenza-associated pediatric mortality
Legionellosis
Listeriosis
Lyme disease
Malaria
Measles
Meningococcal infections
Mumps
Novel influenza A virus infections
Pertussis
Plague
Poliomyelitis, paralytic and nonparalytic
Powassan virus
Psittacosis
Q fever
Rabies, animal
Rabies, human
Rheumatic fever
Rocky Mountain spotted fever
Rubella
Salmonellosis
Severe acute respiratory syndrome

- While the other person holds the card securely, pull the tie out of the card without touching the card. Tie the gown in front of you.

Special considerations

- Sterile gowns are only sterile in front from the shoulders to the level of the sterile field. Sleeves are sterile from 2″ above the elbow to the cuff. The cuff itself collects moisture and is not an effective bacterial barrier and must be kept covered by sterile gloves. The neckline, shoulders, underarms, and back are not considered sterile *due to the surfaces rubbing together during head and neck movements, perspiration, and the inability to directly observe and protect these areas from contamination.* Hands must be kept in front of the body at or above the waist to be considered sterile.
- Choose a gown that is large enough to fully close in the back and whose cuffs do not extend beyond the glove. The cuffs of the gown are regarded as nonsterile once the hands pass through them.
- Surgical attire should only be worn once and then placed in the appropriate receptacle for laundering. They should not be hung in a locker or worn again. Surgical attire should not be laundered at home.
- Surgical attire that is clearly soiled or wet should be taken off and new attire put on *to reduce the risk of transmission of microorganisms.*
- Follow your facility's policy for the use of cover gowns or laboratory coats when leaving semirestricted or restricted areas. These coverings should be removed before reentering semirestricted or restricted areas.
- Staff who aren't scrubbed should wear long-sleeved jackets. These jackets should be buttoned or snapped shut *to reduce the risk of loose material contaminating sterile areas.* Arms should be covered *to decrease bacterial shedding from bare arms.*
- Avoid hanging a face mask around the neck after use. *Bacteria that's trapped in the mask can become dry and airborne.*
- Keep nails in good condition and, if worn, change nail polish every 4 days *because studies suggest that polish worn for longer time periods may support more bacteria.* Artificial nails should not be worn *because they may harbor microorganisms and prevent effective hand antisepsis.*

SELECTED REFERENCES

AORN Recommended Practices Committee. "Recommended Practices for Surgical Attire," *AORN Journal* 81(2):413-20, February 2005.

Association of Perioperative Registered Nurses. *Standards, Recommended Practices, and Guidelines.* Denver: AORN, Inc., 2007.

Shigellosis	Tetanus
St. Louis encephalitis	Toxic shock syndrome
Smallpox	Trichinosis
Streptococcal disease, invasive, Group A	Tuberculosis
	Tularemia
Streptococcal toxic-shock syndrome	Typhoid fever
	Vancomycin-intermediate *Staphylococcus aureus*
Streptococcus pneumonia, drug-resistant, invasive disease	Vancomycin-resistant *Staphylococcus aureus*
Streptococcus pneumonia, invasive in children over age 5	Varicella, morbidity and deaths only
	Vibriosis
Syphilis, all stages	West Nile virus
Syphilis, congenital	Western equine encephalitis
Syphilis, primary and secondary	Yellow

Reportable diseases

Certain contagious diseases must be reported to local and state public health officials and, ultimately, to the CDC. (See *Reportable diseases checklist.*) Typically, these diseases fit one of two categories: those reported individually based on a definitive or suspected diagnosis and those reported by the number of cases per week. The most commonly reported diseases include hepatitis, measles, salmonellosis, shigellosis, syphilis, and gonorrhea.

NURSING ALERT *Selected microorganisms are suspected as potential agents of biological warfare and are reportable immediately to the local or state health department. These agents include anthrax, botulinum toxin, plague, smallpox, and tularemia.*

In most states, the patient's practitioner must report communicable diseases to health officials. In hospitals, the infection control practitioner or epidemiologist reports them. The laboratory must also report organisms associated with reportable diseases. However, you should know the reporting requirements and procedures. Fast, accurate reporting helps identify and control infection sources, prevent epidemics, and guide public health planning and policy.

Equipment

Nursing procedure or infection control manual ▪ disease-reporting form, if available.

Implementation

- Make sure reportable diseases are listed and that the list is available to all shifts.
- Know your facility's protocol for reporting diseases. Typically, you'll contact the infection control practitioner or epidemiologist. If this person isn't available, contact your supervisor or the infectious disease physician on call.

Documentation

Document any diseases reported to the infection control practitioner, the practitioner's name, and the date and time of the report.

Selected references

Chorba, T.L., et al. "Mandatory Reporting of Infectious Diseases by Clinicians," *MMWR* 39(RR-9):1-17, June 1990.

Henning, K.J. "What is Syndromic Surveillance," *MMWR* 53:(Suppl):5-11, September 2004.

Nationally Notifiable Infectious Diseases, United States 2007, Revised. Available at *http://www.cdc.gov/EPO/DPHSI/phs/infdis2007r.htm.*

Immunization guidelines

Vaccines have reduced, and in some cases eliminated, numerous diseases that once injured or killed many infants, children, and adults. Although the United States has a low incidence of vaccine-preventable childhood diseases, not all such diseases have disappeared. That's why it's especially important that children, especially infants and young children, receive recommended immunizations on time. Catch-up schedules have been developed for those patients who did not receive their immunizations on time. (See *Childhood immunization schedule,* page 174. Also see *Adolescent immunization schedule,* page 175.)

Although immunization is common in the pediatric setting, it's unusual in the treatment of adults, despite the fact that morbidity and mortality from vaccine-preventable disease occur largely in adults. It's also important to assess the adult patient's immunization status and that they receive appropriate immunizations. (See *Adult immunization schedule,* page 176.)

Equipment

Patient history or immunization record form ▪ recommended immunization schedule, age-appropriate.

Childhood immunization schedule

This table shows the immunization schedule that the Centers for Disease Control and Prevention's Advisory Committee on Immunization Practices recommends for children.

VACCINE	SCHEDULE
Diphtheria-tetanus-acellular pertussis (DtaP)	Should be given at ages 2, 4, 6, and 15 to 18 months, and then at ages 4 to 6
Haemophilus influenzae type B (Hib)	Should be given at ages 2, 4, 6, and 12 and 15 months
Hepatitis A	Should be given in two doses at least 6 months apart starting at 1 year
Hepatitis B virus (HBV)	Should be given at birth, 1 to 2 months, and 6 to 18 months
Inactivated polio vaccine (IPV)	Should be given at ages 2, 4, and 6 to 18 months, and then at ages 4 to 6
Influenza	Should be given yearly from ages 6 months to 5 years
Measles-mumps-rubella (MMR)	Should receive two vaccinations, the first at age 2 months to 18 months and the second at ages 4 to 6
Varicella (chickenpox)	Should be given at 12 to 18 months and 4 to 6 years
Pneumococcal conjugate vaccine	Should be given at ages 2, 4, 6, and 12 to 15 months
Rotavirus	Should be given at ages 2, 4, and 6 months

Adapted from recommendations of the Advisory Committee on Immunization Practices, Centers for Disease Control and Prevention, published 2007. Available at *www.immunize.org/catg.d/p2010.pdf.*

Implementation

- As the patient's condition allows, review the importance of an up-to-date immunization status.
- Ask the patient or his family about his immunization history, and record where appropriate.
- Compare the patient's history to the recommended immunization schedule.
- Report deficiencies to the patient's medical provider.

Special considerations

Children ages 0 to 18

- The rotavirus vaccine (Rota) is recommended in a 3-dose series at 2, 4, and 6 months. The series shouldn't be started after age 12 weeks and shouldn't be administered after age 32 weeks *due to limited study results.*
- All children ages 6 to 59 months should receive the influenza vaccine.
- The second varicella vaccine is now recommended at ages 4 to 6 years.
- Human papillomavirus vaccine (HPV) has a recommended 3-dose schedule for females ages 11 or 12 with the second and third doses administered 2 and 6 months after the first dose. A catch-up schedule is recommended for unvaccinated females ages 13 to 26.

Adults ages 18 to 24

- A complete series of diphtheria and tetanus vaccinations is recommended for anyone who didn't receive these immunizations in infancy or childhood. In young adults, a primary series consists of three doses of preparations containing diphtheria and tetanus toxoids. The first two doses should be given at least 4 weeks apart and the third dose 6 to 12 months after the second dose. After the series is completed, a booster dose should be given every 10 years. If the person's

Adolescent immunization schedule

This table shows the immunization schedule that the Centers for Disease Control and Prevention's Advisory Committee on Immunization Practices recommends for children ages 7 to 18.

IMMUNIZATION	INDICATIONS	TIMING
Hepatitis A	Adolescents not vaccinated previously	Two doses: 6 to 18 months apart
Hepatitis B virus (HBV)	Adolescents not vaccinated previously for HBV	Three doses: second dose, 1 to 2 months after first dose; third dose, 4 months after first dose
Human papillomavirus (HPV)	Adolescents who are at increased risk for pneumococcal disease or its complications	First dose at ages 11 or 12; second dose, 2 months after the first; third dose, 6 months after the first
Influenza (flu)	Adolescents who are at risk for complications caused by influenza or who have contact with persons at increased risk for these complications	Annually
Measles-mumps-rubella (MMR)	Adolescents not vaccinated previously with two doses of MMR vaccine at age 12 months or older	Two doses at least 4 weeks apart
Meningococcal	All children	Ages 11 or 12
Pneumococcal	All females ages 11 to 13	One dose (may repeat dose 5 years later for those at highest risk)
Tetanus-diphtheria (Td)	At age 11 to 12, with no booster dose previously given	One dose at ages 11 or 12
Varicella (chickenpox)	Adolescents not vaccinated previously and who have no reliable history of chickenpox	Two doses at least 4 weeks apart

Adapted from recommendations of the Advisory Committee on Immunization Practices, Centers for Disease Control and Prevention, published 2007. Available at *www.immunize.org/catg.d/p2010.pdf.*

history is unknown or he's uncertain about having received diphtheria and tetanus toxoids, he should be considered unvaccinated and receive a full three-dose primary series. A one-time dose of tetanus, diphtheria, and acellular pertussis (Tdap) vaccine may be substituted for one Td dose.

■ Most young adults should be immune to measles, mumps, and rubella. However, as a result of the 1989 outbreak of measles in schools and colleges, recommendations were made to implement a routine two-dose schedule for the measles-mumps-rubella (MMR) vaccine. The first dose usually occurs in early childhood and the second before entry into middle or junior high school.

■ Young adults who are attending college or newly employed in an environment with a high risk of measles, mumps, or rubella transmission (a hospital or day care center, for example) should present documentation that they received two doses of live MMR or evidence of immunity, such as physician-diagnosed measles or laboratory evidence of immuni-

Adult immunization schedule

This table shows the immunizations that the Centers for Disease Control and Prevention's Advisory Committee on Immunization Practices recommends for individuals over age 18.

VACCINE	TIMING AND CONSIDERATIONS
Hepatitis A for those at risk	Two doses: 6 to 18 months apart for long-term protection; first dose, 4 weeks before departure to endemic countries
Hepatitis B virus (HBV) if never had initial series	Three doses: second dose, at least 1 month after first dose; third dose, 4 to 6 months after first dose
Influenza (flu)	Annually before flu season (September to December), especially for those age 50 or older, those with medical problems (heart or lung disease, diabetes, chronic conditions), and those who work or live with hish-risk individuals; now available in intranasal form
Measles-mumps-rubella (MMR)	Two doses: 1 month apart if born after 1957 or if immunity can't be proved* Ages 50 and older = 1 dose
Pneumococcal	One dose at age 65; also recommended for persons with chronic disease, kidney disorders, and sickle cell anemia; booster dose recommended 6 years after first dose
Tetanus-diphtheria (Td) if never had initial series	Three doses: second dose, after 1 month; third dose, 6 to 12 months after second; booster needed every 10 years, one tetanus booster every 10 years
Varicella (chickenpox)	Two doses for every patient who hasn't had chickenpox; second dose, 1 month after first dose**

*Shouldn't be given to pregnant patients or those considering pregnancy within 3 months of vaccination.
**Shouldn't be given to pregnant patients or those considering pregnancy within 1 month of vaccination.
All vaccines can be given simultaneously but not in the same syringe or site.
If patient is on pulse steroids, wait 1 month to immunize (inhaled or long-term steroids have no impact). For long-term steroid use, consult an infectious disease specialist.

Adapted from recommendations of the Advisory Committee on Immunization Practices, Centers for Disease Control and Prevention, published 2007. Available at *www.immunize.org/catg.d/p2011.pdf.*

ty. If the person was vaccinated with killed-measles-virus vaccine (available in the United States from 1963 until 1967) or with a measles vaccine of unknown type, he should receive two doses of live-measles-virus vaccine at least 1 month apart.

Adults ages 25 to 64

- Adults ages 25 to 64 should have completed a primary series of diphtheria and tetanus and should receive a booster dose every 10 years. If needed, a primary series should be given. A one-time does of tetanus, diphtheria, and acellular pertussis (Tdap) vaccine may be substituted for one Td booster.
- A person born in 1957 or later, who has no contraindications, should receive one dose of measles vaccine unless he has documented evidence of MMR vaccination, measles infection, or laboratory evidence of immunity.
- Unless proof of vaccination with rubella vaccine or laboratory evidence is available, rubella vaccine is recommended for adults, especially women of childbearing age. The vaccine of choice is MMR if recipients are likely to be susceptible to more than one of the three diseases.

Adults age 65 and older

■ Older adults should receive an influenza vaccine annually, in addition to a single dose of the pneumococcal polysaccharide vaccine. According to the Advisory Committee on Immunization Practices (ACIP), revaccination is suggested 6 years after the first dose for those at highest risk for fatal pneumococcal disease (such as asplenic patients), or a rapid decline in antibody levels (such as patients who have had a transplant or patients with chronic renal failure).

Special occupations

■ Persons in specific occupations with an increased risk of exposure to certain vaccine-preventable diseases need specific vaccines in addition to those recommended for their age-group. Health and public safety workers are particularly at risk for exposure to, and possible transmission of, vaccine-preventable diseases *because of their contact with patients or infectious materials from patients.*

■ *Because of the increased risk of exposure to hepatitis B,* all health care workers should receive the hepatitis B virus (HBV) vaccine. Serologic evidence of HBV infection is present in approximately 15% to 30% of health care personnel with frequent exposure to blood; the incidence in the public is 5%. The HBV vaccine provides protection against HBV for 7 years or more after vaccination; booster doses aren't needed during this interval.

■ An influenza vaccine is recommended yearly for physicians, nurses, and other personnel in hospitals and chronic-care and outpatient-care settings who have contact with high-risk patients in all age-groups.

Pregnancy

■ The ACIP recommends that any vaccine given during pregnancy should be delayed, when possible, until the second or third trimester. Pregnant women not previously vaccinated against tetanus and diphtheria should receive two doses of the vaccine. Those who received one or two doses of tetanus-diphtheria toxoid should complete their primary series during pregnancy. Pregnant women who have completed a primary series 10 years or more previously should receive a booster dose. *Because of a theoretical risk to the developing fetus,* pregnant women or those likely to become pregnant within 3 months shouldn't be given live virus vaccines.

■ The ACIP strongly recommends that an MMR and varicella vaccine be administered in the postpartum period to women not known to be immune, preferably before discharge from the hospital.

Documentation

Complete the patient history or immunization record, as required. Document the report of any immunization deficiencies to the health care practitioner, the practitioner's name, and the date and time of the report. Document any patient teaching provided.

SELECTED REFERENCES

"Immunization of Healthcare Workers: Recommendations of the Advisory Committee on Immunization Practices and the Hospital Infection Control Practices Advisory Committee (HICPAC)," *MMWR* 46(RR-18):1-42, December 1997.

"Recommended Adult Immunization Schedule—United States, October 2006-September 2007," *MMWR* 55:40, October 2006.

"Recommended Immunization Schedules for Persons Aged 0-18 years—United States," *MMWR* 55(51& 52):Q1-Q4, January 2007. Available at *http://www.cdc.gov/nip/publications/acip-list.htm.*

GUIDELINES

STANDARD PRECAUTIONS

Standard precautions were developed by the Centers for Disease Control and Prevention (CDC) to provide the widest possible protection against the transmission of infection. CDC officials recommend that health care workers handle all blood, body fluids (including secretions, excretions, and drainage), tissues, and contact with mucous membranes and broken skin as if they contain infectious agents, regardless of the patient's diagnosis.

Standard precautions encompass much of the isolation precautions previously recommended by the CDC for patients with known or suspected blood-borne pathogens as well as the precautions previously known as *body substance isolation.* They are to be used in conjunction with other transmission-based precautions: airborne, droplet, and contact precautions.

Standard precautions recommend wearing gloves for any known or anticipated contact with blood, body fluids, tissue, mucous membrane, and nonintact skin. (See *Choosing the right glove,* page 178.) If the task or procedure being performed may result in splashing or splattering of blood or body fluids to the face, a mask and goggles or face shield should be worn. If the task or procedure being performed may result in splashing or splattering of blood or body fluids to the body, a fluid-resistant gown or apron should be worn. Additional protective clothing, such as shoe covers,

EQUIPMENT

Choosing the right glove

Health care workers may develop allergic reactions as a result of their cumulative exposure to latex gloves and other products containing natural rubber latex. Patients also may have latex sensitivity. (See "Latex allergy protocol" in chapter 8.)

Take the following steps to protect yourself and your patient from allergic reactions to natural rubber latex:

- Use nonlatex (for example, vinyl or synthetic) gloves for activities that aren't likely to involve contact with infectious materials (such as food preparation and routine cleaning).
- Use appropriate barrier protection when handling infectious materials. If you choose latex gloves, use powder-free gloves with reduced protein content. *Powder in any glove is very drying to skin and may cause problems that may put health care workers at greater risk for exposure to infection if skin is dry and cracked.*
- After wearing and removing gloves, wash your hands with soap and dry them thoroughly.
- When wearing latex gloves, don't use oil-based hand creams or lotions *(which can cause gloves to deteriorate)* unless they've been shown to maintain glove barrier protection.
- Refer to the material safety data sheet for the appropriate glove to wear when handling chemicals.
- Learn procedures for preventing latex allergy, and learn how to recognize the following symptoms of latex allergy: skin rashes, hives, flushing, itching, asthma, shock, and nasal, eye, or sinus symptoms.
- If you have (or suspect you have) a latex sensitivity, use nonlatex gloves, avoid contact with latex gloves and other latex-containing products, and consult a practitioner experienced in treating latex allergy. Report problems to your supervisor, and follow your facility's policy for evaluation.

For known latex allergy

If you're allergic to latex, consider the following precautions:

- Avoid contact with latex gloves and other products that contain latex.
- Avoid areas where you might inhale the powder from latex gloves worn by other workers.
- Inform your employers and your health care providers (physicians, nurses, dentists, and others).
- Wear a medical identification bracelet.
- Follow your practitioner's instructions for dealing with allergic reactions to latex.
- Check packages, trays, and kits for items containing latex. *Products containing natural rubber latex must be labeled clearly on the exterior.*

may be appropriate to protect the caregiver's feet in situations that may expose him to large amounts of blood or body fluids (or both), such as care of a trauma patient in the operating room or emergency department.

Airborne precautions are initiated in situations of suspected or known infections spread by the airborne route. The causative organisms are coughed, talked, or sneezed into the air by the infected person in droplets of moisture. The moisture evaporates, leaving the microorganisms suspended in the air to be breathed in by susceptible persons who enter the shared air space. Airborne precautions recommend placing the infected patient in a negative-pressure isolation room and the wearing of respiratory protection by all persons entering the patient's room.

Droplet precautions are used to protect health care workers and visitors from mucous membrane contact with oral and nasal secretions of the infected individual.

Contact precautions use barrier precautions to interrupt the transmission of specific epidemiologically important organisms by direct or indirect contact. Each institution must establish an infection control policy that lists specific barrier precautions.

Equipment

Gloves ▪ masks ▪ goggles, glasses with side pieces, or face shields ▪ gowns or aprons ▪ resuscitation bag ▪ bags for specimens ▪ Environmental Protection Agency (EPA)–registered tuberculocidal disinfectant or diluted bleach solution (diluted between 1:10 and 1:100, mixed fresh daily), or both, or EPA-registered disinfectant labeled effective against hepatitis B virus (HBV), and human immunodeficiency virus (HIV).

Implementation

- Wash your hands immediately if they become contaminated with blood or body fluids, excretions, secretions, or drainage; also wash your hands before and after patient care and after removing gloves. *Hand washing removes microorganisms from your skin.* If your hands aren't visibly soiled, an alcohol-based hand rub can be used for routine decontamination.
- Wear gloves if you will or could come in contact with blood, specimens, tissue, body fluids, secretions or excretions, mucous membrane, broken skin, or contaminated surfaces or objects.
- Change your gloves and wash your hands between patient contacts *to avoid cross-contamination.*
- Wear a fluid-resistant gown, face shield, or goggles and a mask during procedures likely to generate splashing or splattering of blood or body fluids, such as surgery, endoscopic procedures, dialysis, assisting with intubation or manipulation of arterial lines, or any other procedure with potential for splashing or splattering of body fluids.
- Handle used needles and other sharp instruments carefully. Don't bend, break, reinsert them into their original sheaths, remove needles from syringes, or unnecessarily handle them. Discard them intact immediately after use into a puncture-resistant disposal box. Use tools to pick up broken glass or other sharp objects. Use safety devices according to the instructions provided by the manufacturer. Activate all safety mechanisms on sharp devices immediately after use, even if the sharps disposal container is very close. Evaluate your work practices to make sure you're working safely, both for your own protection and for the protection of your patients and coworkers. *These measures reduce the risk of accidental injury or infection.* When available, use a needleless I.V. system.
- Immediately notify your employee health provider of all needle-stick or other sharp object injuries, mucosal splashes, or contamination of open wounds or nonintact skin with blood or body fluids *to allow investigation of the incident and appropriate care and documentation.* Be sure to complete all follow-up screening and care as recommended by your employee health care provider.
- Properly label all specimens collected from patients, and place them in plastic bags at the collection site. Attach requisition slips to the outside of the bag.
- Place all items that have come in direct contact with the patient's secretions, excretions, blood, drainage, or body fluids—such as nondisposable utensils or instruments—in a single impervious bag or container before removal from the room. Carry soiled linens in outstretched arms *to avoid contaminating your uniform.* Place linens and trash in single bags of sufficient thickness to contain the contents.
- While wearing the appropriate personal protective equipment, promptly clean all blood and body fluid spills with detergent and water followed by an EPA-registered tuberculocidal disinfectant or diluted bleach solution (diluted between 1:10 and 1:100, mixed daily), or both, or an EPA-registered disinfectant labeled effective against HBV and HIV, provided that the surface hasn't been contaminated with agents or volumes of or concentrations of agents for which higher-level disinfection is recommended.
- Disposable food trays and dishes aren't necessary.
- If you have an exudative lesion, avoid all direct patient contact until the condition has resolved, and you've been cleared by the employee health provider.
- If you have dermatitis or other conditions resulting in broken skin on your hands, avoid situations where you may have contact with blood and body fluids (even though gloves could be worn) until the condition has resolved, and you've been cleared by the employee health provider.

Special considerations

- Standard precautions, such as hand hygiene and appropriate use of personal protective equipment, should be routine infection control practices.
- Keep mouthpieces, resuscitation bags, and other ventilation devices nearby *to eliminate the need for emergency mouth-to-mouth resuscitation, thus reducing the risk of exposure to body fluids.*

NURSING ALERT Because you may not always know what organisms may be present in every clinical situation, *you must use standard precautions for every contact with blood, body fluids, secretions, excretions, drainage, mucous membranes, and nonintact skin. Use your judgment in individual cases about whether to implement additional isolation precautions, such as airborne, droplet, or contact precautions or a combination of them. What's more, if your work requires you to be exposed to blood, you should receive the HBV vaccine series.*

Complications

Failure to follow standard precautions may lead to exposure to blood-borne diseases or other infections and to all the complications they may cause.

Documentation

Record any special needs for isolation precautions on the nursing care plan and as otherwise indicated by your facility. Document patient and family teaching about isolation precautions.

Diseases requiring airborne precautions

The following table lists the diseases that require airborne precautions and the length of the precautionary period.

DISEASE	PRECAUTIONARY PERIOD
Avian influenza	For 14 days after onset of symptoms or until alternate diagnosis is confirmed
Chickenpox (varicella)	Until lesions are crusted and no new lesions appear
Herpes zoster (disseminated)	Duration of illness
Herpes zoster (localized in immunocompromised patients)	Duration of illness
Measles (rubeola)	Duration of illness
Monkey pox	Until lesions are crusted
Severe acute respiratory syndrome	Duration of illness
Smallpox	Duration of illness until all scabs fall off
Tuberculosis (pulmonary or laryngeal, suspected or confirmed)	Depends on clinical response; patient must be on effective therapy, be improving clinically (decreased cough and fever and improved findings on chest radiograph), and have three consecutive negative sputum smears collected on different days, or TB must be ruled out
Viral hemorrhagic fevers (Ebola, Lassa, Marburg)	Duration of illness with severe pulmonary involvement or when patient is undergoing aerolized treatment or procedures that induce cough

SELECTED REFERENCES

Centers for Disease Control and Prevention. "Guideline for Isolation Precautions: Preventing Transmission of Infectious Agents in Healthcare Settings 2007." Accessed August 2007 via the Web at *www.cdc.gov/ncidod/dhqp/g1_isolation.html.*

Centers for Disease Control and Prevention. "Guidelines for Hand Hygiene in Health-Care Settings," *MMWR* 51(RR-16):1-144, October 2002.

Department of Labor Occupational Safety and Health Administration. "29 C.F.R. Part 1920 Occupational Exposure to Bloodborne Pathogens; Needlesticks and Other Sharps Injuries; Final Rule," *Federal Register* 66(12):5318-325, January 2001.

Gardner, J.S. "Hospital Infection Control Practices Advisory Committee Guidelines for Isolation Precautions in Hospitals," *Infection Control and Hospital Epidemiology* 17:53-80, January 1996.

Houghton, D. "HAI Prevention: The Power Is in Your Hands," *Nursing Management* 37(supplement):1-7, May 2006.

Rushing, J. "Wearing Personal Protective Gear," *Nursing* 36(10):56-57, October 2006.

AIRBORNE PRECAUTIONS

Airborne precautions, used in addition to standard precautions, prevents the spread of infectious diseases transmitted by airborne pathogens that are breathed, sneezed, or coughed into the environment. (See *Diseases requiring airborne precautions.*) This precaution category includes the former categories of acid-fast bacillus isolation and respiratory isolation.

Effective airborne precautions require a negative-pressure room with the door kept closed to maintain the proper air pressure balance between the isolation room and the adjoining hallway or corridor. An anteroom is preferred. The negative air pressure must be monitored, and the air is either vented directly to the outside of the building or filtered through high-efficiency particulate air (HEPA) filtration before recirculation.

Respiratory protection must be worn by all persons who enter the room. Such protection is provided by a disposable respirator (such as an N95 respirator or HEPA respirator) or a reusable respirator (such as a HEPA respirator or a powered air-purifying respirator [PAPR]). Regardless of the type of respirator used, the health care worker must ensure proper fit to the face each time she wears the respirator. If the patient must leave the room for an essential procedure, he should wear a surgical mask covering his nose and mouth while out of the room.

Equipment

Respirators (either disposable N95 or HEPA respirators or reusable HEPA respirators or PAPRs) ▪ surgical masks ▪ isolation door card ■ other personal protective equipment, as needed, for standard precautions.

Gather any additional supplies, such as a thermometer, stethoscope, and blood pressure cuff.

Preparation of equipment

Keep all airborne precaution supplies outside the patient's room in a cart or anteroom.

Implementation

■ Situate the patient in a negative-pressure room with the door closed. If possible, the room should have an anteroom. The negative pressure should be monitored. If necessary, two patients with the same infection may share a room. Explain isolation precautions to the patient and his family *to ease patient anxiety and promote cooperation.*

■ Keep the patient's door (and the anteroom door) closed at all times *to maintain the negative pressure and contain the airborne pathogens.* Put the airborne precautions sign on the door to notify anyone entering the room.

■ Pick up your respirator, and put it on according to the manufacturer's directions. Adjust the straps for a firm but comfortable fit. Check the respiratory seal. (See *Respirator seal check.*)

■ Instruct the patient to cover his nose and mouth with a facial tissue while coughing or sneezing.

■ Tape an impervious bag to the patient's bedside *so the patient can dispose of facial tissues correctly.*

■ Make sure all visitors wear respiratory protection while in the patient's room.

■ Limit the patient's movement from the room. If he must leave the room for essential procedures, make sure he wears a surgical mask over his nose and mouth. Notify the receiving department or area of the patient's isolation precautions *so that the precautions will be maintained, and the patient can be returned to the room promptly.*

Special considerations

■ Before leaving the room, remove gloves (if worn) and wash your hands. Remove your respirator outside the patient's room after closing the door.

■ Depending on the type of respirator and recommendations from the manufacturer, follow your facility's policy and either discard your respirator or store it until the next use. If your respirator is to be stored until the next use, store it in a dry, well-ventilated place (not a plastic bag) *to prevent microbial growth.* Nondisposable respirators must be cleaned according to the manufacturer's recommendations.

Respirator seal check

Always check the respirator seal before using a respirator. To do this, place both of your hands over the respirator and exhale. If air leaks around your nose, adjust the nosepiece. If air leaks at the respirator's edges, adjust the straps along the side of your head. Recheck respirator fit after making any adjustments.

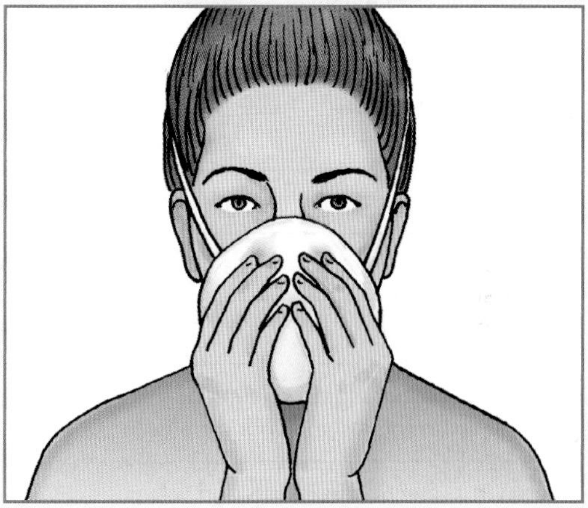

Documentation

Record the need for airborne precautions on the nursing care plan and as otherwise indicated by your facility. Document initiation and maintenance of the precautions, the patient's tolerance of the procedure, and any patient or family teaching. Also document the date airborne precautions were discontinued.

SELECTED REFERENCES

Centers for Disease Control and Prevention. "Guideline for Isolation Precautions: Preventing Transmission of Infectious Agents in Healthcare Settings 2007." Accessed August 2007 via the Web at *www.cdc.gov/ncidod/dhqp/g1_isolation.html.*

"Guidelines for Environmental Infection Control in Health Care Facilities: Recommendations of the CDC and the Health Care Infection Control Practices Advisory Committee (HICPAC)," *MMWR* 52(RR-10):1-42, June 2003.

Hughes, N. "Respiratory Protection, Part 1," *AJN* 106(1):96, January 2006.

Hughes, N. "Respiratory Protection, Part 2," *AJN* 106(2):88, February 2006.

Rushing, J. "Wearing Personal Protective Gear," *Nursing* 36(10):56-57, October 2006.

Diseases requiring droplet precautions

DISEASE	PRECAUTIONARY PERIOD
Invasive *Haemophilus influenzae* type b disease, including meningitis, pneumonia, sepsis, and epiglottitis	Until 24 hours after initiation of effective therapy
Invasive *Neisseria meningitidis* disease, including meningitis, pneumonia, and sepsis	Until 24 hours after initiation of effective therapy
Diphtheria (pharyngeal)	Until off antibiotics and two cultures taken at least 24 hours apart are negative
Mycoplasma pneumoniae infection	Duration of illness
Pertussis	Until 5 days after initiation of effective therapy
Pneumonic plague	Until 72 hours after initiation of effective therapy
Streptococcal pharyngitis, pneumonia, or scarlet fever in infants and young children	Until 24 hours after initiation of effective therapy
Adenovirus infection in infants and young children	Duration of illness
Influenza	Duration of illness
Mumps	For 9 days after onset of swelling
Parvovirus B19	Maintain precautions for duration of hospitalization when chronic disease occurs in an immunocompromised patient. For patients with transient aplastic crisis or red-cell crisis, maintain precautions for 7 days.
Rubella (German measles)	Until 7 days after onset of rash
Avian influenza	For 14 days after onset of symptoms or until an alternate diagnosis is confirmed; airborne precautions preferred but droplet precautions may be used if a negative pressure room isn't available
Severe acute respiratory syndrome	Duration of illness; airborne precautions preferred
Viral hemorrhagic infection	Duration of illness

DROPLET PRECAUTIONS

Droplet precautions prevent the spread of infectious diseases transmitted by contact of nasal or oral secretions (droplets arising from coughing or sneezing) from the infected patient with the mucous membranes of the susceptible host. This category includes some diseases formerly included in respiratory isolation. The droplets of moisture are heavy and generally fall to the ground within 3′ (1 m); the organisms contained in the droplets don't become airborne or suspended in the air. (See *Diseases requiring droplet precautions.*)

Effective droplet precautions require a single room (not necessarily a negative-pressure room), and the door doesn't need to be closed. Persons having direct contact with, or who will be within 3′ (1 m) of the patient, should wear a surgical mask covering the nose and mouth.

When handling infants or young children who require droplet precautions, you may also need to wear gloves and a gown to prevent soiling of clothing with nasal and oral secretions.

Equipment

Masks ▪ gowns, if necessary ▪ gloves ▪ plastic bags ▪ droplet precautions door card.

Gather any additional supplies, such as a thermometer, stethoscope, and blood pressure cuff.

Preparation of equipment

Keep all droplet precaution supplies outside the patient's room in a cart or anteroom.

Implementation

- Place the patient in a single room with private toilet facilities and an anteroom if possible. If necessary, two patients with the same infection may share a room. Explain isolation procedures to the patient and his family *to ease patient anxiety and promote cooperation.*
- Put a droplet precautions card on the door *to notify anyone entering the room.*
- Wash your hands before entering and after leaving the room and during patient care as indicated.
- Pick up your mask by the top strings, adjust it around your nose and mouth, and tie the strings or adjust the ear loops around your ears for a comfortable fit. If the mask has a flexible metal nose strip, adjust it to fit firmly but comfortably.
- Instruct the patient to cover his nose and mouth with a facial tissue while coughing or sneezing.
- Tape an impervious bag to the patient's bedside *so that the patient can dispose of facial tissues correctly.*
- Make sure all visitors wear masks when in close proximity with the patient (within 3′) and, if necessary, gowns and gloves.
- If the patient must leave the room for essential procedures, make sure he wears a surgical mask over his nose and mouth. Notify the receiving department or area of the patient's isolation precautions *so that the precautions will be maintained and the patient can be returned to the room promptly.*

Special considerations

- Before removing your mask, remove your gloves (if worn) and wash your hands.
- Untie the strings and dispose of the mask, handling it by the strings only.

Documentation

Record the need for droplet precautions on the nursing care plan and as otherwise indicated by your facility. Document initiation and maintenance of the precautions, the patient's tolerance of the procedure, and any patient or family teaching. Also document the date droplet precautions were discontinued.

SELECTED REFERENCES

Centers for Disease Control and Prevention. "Guideline for Isolation Precautions: Preventing Transmission of Infectious Agents in Healthcare Settings 2007." Accessed August 2007 via the Web at *www.cdc.gov/ncidod/dhqp/gl_isolation.html.*

"Guidelines for Environmental Infection Control in Health-Care Facilities: Recommendations of CDC and the Healthcare Infection Control Practices Advisory Committee (HICPAC)," *MMWR* 52(RR-10):1-42, June 2003.

Rushing, J. "Wearing Personal Protective Gear," *Nursing* 36(10):56-57, October 2006.

CONTACT PRECAUTIONS

Contact precautions prevent the spread of infectious diseases transmitted by contact with body substances containing the infectious agent or items contaminated with the body substances containing the infectious agent. Contact precautions apply to patients who are infected or colonized (presence of microorganism without clinical signs and symptoms of infection) with epidemiologically important organisms that can be transmitted by direct or indirect contact. (See *Diseases requiring contact precautions,* page 184.)

Effective contact precautions require a single room and the use of gloves and gowns by anyone having contact with the patient, the patient's support equipment, or items soiled with body substances containing the infectious agent. Thorough hand washing and proper handling and disposal of articles contaminated by the body substance containing the infectious agent are also essential.

Equipment

Gloves ▪ gowns or aprons ▪ masks, if necessary ▪ isolation door card ▪ plastic bags.

Gather any additional supplies, such as a thermometer, stethoscope, and blood pressure cuff.

Diseases requiring contact precautions

DISEASE	PRECAUTIONARY PERIOD
Infection or colonization with multidrug-resistant bacteria	Until off antibiotics and culture negative
Clostridium difficile enteric infection	Duration of illness
Escherichia coli disease, in diapered or incontinent patient	Duration of illness
Shigellosis, in diapered or incontinent patient	Duration of illness
Hepatitis A, in diapered or incontinent patient	Duration of illness
Rotavirus infection, in diapered or incontinent patient	Duration of illness
Respiratory syncytial virus infection, in infants and young children	Duration of illness
Parainfluenza virus infection, in diapered or incontinent patient	Duration of illness
Enteroviral infection, in diapered or incontinent patient	Duration of illness
Scabies	Until 24 hours after initiation of effective therapy
Diphtheria (cutaneous)	Duration of illness
Herpes simplex virus infection (neonatal or mucocutaneous)	Duration of illness
Impetigo	Until 24 hours after initiation of effective therapy
Major abscesses, cellulitis, or pressure ulcer	Until 24 hours after initiation of effective therapy
Pediculosis (lice)	Until 24 hours after initiation of effective therapy
Rubella, congenital syndrome	Place infant on precautions during any admission until age 1, unless nasopharyngeal and urine culture are negative for virus after age 3 months
Staphylococcal furunculosis in infants and young children	Duration of illness
Acute viral (acute hemorrhagic) conjunctivitis	Duration of illness
Viral hemorrhagic infections (Ebola, Lassa, Marburg)	Duration of illness
Zoster (chickenpox, disseminated zoster, or localized zoster in immunocompromised patient)	Until all lesions are crusted; requires airborne precautions
Smallpox	Duration of illness; requires airborne precautions
Avian influenza	For 14 days after onset of symptoms or until an alternate diagnosis is confirmed
Monkey pox	Until all lesions are crusted; requires airborne precautions
Severe acute respiratory syndrome	Duration of illness; requires airborne precautions

Preparation of equipment

Keep all contact precaution supplies outside the patient's room in a cart or anteroom.

Implementation

- Situate the patient in a single room with private toilet facilities and an anteroom if possible. If necessary, two patients with the same infection may share a room. Explain isolation procedures to the patient and his family *to ease his anxiety and promote cooperation.*
- Place a contact precautions card on the door *to notify anyone entering the room.*
- Wash your hands before entering and after leaving the patient's room and after removing gloves.
- Place any laboratory specimens in impervious, labeled containers, and send them to the laboratory at once. Attach requisition slips to the outside of the container.
- Instruct visitors to wear gloves and a gown while visiting the patient and to wash their hands after removing the gown and gloves.
- Place all items that have come in contact with the patient in a single impervious bag, and arrange for their disposal or disinfection and sterilization.
- Limit the patient's movement from the room. If the patient must be moved, cover any draining wounds with clean dressings. Notify the receiving department or area of the patient's isolation precautions *so that the precautions will be maintained and the patient can be returned to the room promptly.*

Special considerations

- Cleaning and disinfection of equipment between patients is essential.
- Try to dedicate certain reusable equipment (thermometer, stethoscope, blood pressure cuff) for the patient in contact precautions *to reduce the risk of transmitting infection to other patients.*
- Remember to change gloves during patient care as indicated by the procedure or task. Wash your hands after removing gloves and before putting on new gloves.

Documentation

Record the need for contact precautions on the nursing care plan and as otherwise indicated by your facility. Document initiation and maintenance of the precautions, the patient's tolerance of the procedure, and any patient or family teaching. Also document the date contact precautions were discontinued.

SELECTED REFERENCES

Centers for Disease Control and Prevention. "Guideline for Isolation Precautions: Preventing Transmission of Infectious Agents in Healthcare Settings 2007." Accessed August 2007 via the Web at *www.cdc.gov/ncidod/dhqp/gl_isolation.html.*

"Guidelines for Environmental Infection Control in Health-Care Facilities: Recommendations of CDC and the Healthcare Infection Control Practices Advisory Committee (HICPAC)," *MMWR* 52(RR-10):1-42, June 2003.

Rushing, J. "Wearing Personal Protective Gear," *Nursing* 36(10):56-57, October 2006.

NEUTROPENIC PRECAUTIONS

Unlike other types of precaution procedures, neutropenic precautions (also known as protective precautions and reverse isolation) guard the patient who is at increased risk for infection against contact with potential pathogens. These precautions are used primarily for patients with extensive noninfected burns, those who have leukopenia or a depressed immune system, and those receiving immunosuppressive treatments. (See *Conditions and treatments requiring neutropenic precautions,* page 186.)

Neutropenic precautions require a single room equipped with positive air pressure, if possible, to force suspended particles down and out of the room. The degree of precautions may range from using a single room, thorough hand-hygiene technique, and limitation of traffic into the room to more extensive precautions requiring the use of gowns, gloves, and masks by facility staff and visitors. The extent of neutropenic precautions may vary from facility to facility, depending on the reason for and the degree of the patient's immunosuppression.

To care for patients who have temporarily increased susceptibility, such as those who have undergone bone marrow transplantation, neutropenic precautions may also require a patient isolator unit and the use of sterile linens, gowns, gloves, and head and shoe coverings. In such cases, all other items taken into the room should be sterilized or disinfected. The patient's diet also may be modified to eliminate raw fruits and vegetables and to allow only cooked foods and possibly only sterile beverages.

Equipment

Gloves ▪ gowns ▪ masks ▪ neutropenic precautions door card.

Gather any additional supplies, such as a thermometer, stethoscope, and blood pressure cuff, *so you don't have to leave the isolation room unnecessarily.*

Conditions and treatments requiring neutropenic precautions

CONDITION OR TREATMENT	PRECAUTIONARY PERIOD
Acquired immunodeficiency syndrome	Until white blood cell count reaches 1,000/ml or more, or according to facility guidelines
Agranulocytosis	Until remission
Burns, extensive noninfected	Until skin surface heals substantially
Dermatitis, noninfected vesicular, bullous, or eczematous disease (when severe and extensive)	Until skin surface heals substantially
Immunosuppressive therapy	Until patient's immunity is adequate
Lymphomas and leukemia, especially late stages of Hodgkin's disease or acute leukemia	Until clinical improvement is substantial

Preparation of equipment

Keep supplies in a clean enclosed cart or in an anteroom outside the room.

Implementation

- After placing the patient in a single room, explain isolation precautions to the patient and his family *to ease patient anxiety and promote cooperation.*
- Place a neutropenic precautions card on the door *to caution those entering the room.*
- Wash your hands with an antiseptic agent before putting on gloves, after removing gloves, and as indicated during patient care.
- Wear gloves and gown according to standard precautions, unless the patient's condition warrants a sterile gown, gloves, and a mask.
- Avoid transporting the patient out of the room; if he must be moved, make sure he wears a gown and mask. Notify the receiving department or area *so that the precautions will be maintained and the patient will be returned to the room promptly.*
- Don't allow visits by anyone known to be ill or infected.

Special considerations

- Don't perform invasive procedures, such as urethral catheterization, unless absolutely necessary *because these procedures risk serious infection in the patient with impaired resistance.*
- Instruct the housekeeping staff to put on gowns, gloves, and masks before entering the room; no ill or infected person should enter. They should follow the same requirements as the staff, depending on the patient's condition and your facility's policy.
- Make sure the room is cleaned with freshly prepared cleaning solutions. *Because the patient doesn't have a contagious disease,* materials leaving the room need no special precautions beyond standard precautions.
- All equipment and supplies entering the room should be cleaned or disinfected before entry.

Documentation

Document the need for neutropenic precautions on the nursing care plan and as otherwise indicated by your facility. Document initiation and maintenance of the precautions and any patient or family teaching provided.

SELECTED REFERENCES

Centers for Disease Control and Prevention. "Guideline for Isolation Precautions: Preventing Transmission of Infectious Agents in Healthcare Settings 2007." Accessed August 2007 via the Web at *www.cdc.gov/ncidod/dhqp/g1_isolation.html.*

"Guidelines for Environmental Infection Control in Health-Care Facilities: Recommendations of CDC and the Healthcare Infection Control Practices Advisory Committee (HICPAC)," *MMWR* 52(RR-10):1-42, June 2003.

Larson, E., and Nirenburg, A. "Evidence-Based Nursing Practice to Prevent Infection in Hospitalized Neutropenic Patients with Cancer," *Oncology Nurse Forum* 31(4):717-25, July 2004.

3 ■ Specimen collection and testing

INTRODUCTION

Collecting specimens promptly and correctly can directly affect a patient's diagnosis, treatment, and recovery. In many cases, the nurse is solely responsible for collecting appropriate specimens. Even for tests that aren't a nurse's hands-on responsibility, you may have to schedule the test, prepare the patient, assist the physician or other caregiver in performing the test, and care for the patient afterward. For some tests, for example, you may have to teach the patient how to perform the procedure at home, as with blood glucose tests and fecal occult blood tests. In every case, your nursing responsibilities depend on the clinical setting and your facility's policies as well as the guidelines provided in your state's or province's nurse practice act.

Patient preparation

A thorough working knowledge of diagnostic tests will help you prepare patients for them. If you can explain a test with clarity and compassion, you'll help put the patient at ease, gain his trust and cooperation, and thus ensure more accurate results. Helping him understand a procedure based on the practitioner's explanations also paves the way for consent that's truly informed.

When preparing a patient, your explanations should be clear, straightforward, and complete. For example, before a difficult or painful procedure, such as a bone marrow biopsy, warn the patient about the type of discomfort he'll probably feel. Letting him know exactly what to expect helps him tolerate such a procedure. Preparation should include telling the patient how long the procedure takes and how soon the results will be available.

If you're assisting the practitioner with a test, talk to the patient throughout to comfort and encourage him. Prepare him for upcoming sensations, if necessary. Afterward, watch for adverse reactions or complications, and be prepared to implement appropriate care.

Some tests require more detailed instructions to promote cooperation and ensure accurate specimen collection, especially when the patient must modify his behavior before the test and when he'll be collecting the specimen himself. For example, you may have to instruct him to observe a special diet, suspend taking certain medications, or learn a special collection technique.

Whenever possible, reinforce your verbal explanations with appropriate information. Make sure the patient has time to read the information before physical preparation for the test or procedure begins. Many facilities also have videocassettes, telelectures, and films available to augment the patient-teaching process.

Informed consent

Fundamental requirements have been established to protect a patient's rights while he's receiving care. One of the most important rights is informed consent, which states that the patient (or a responsible family member if the patient is legally incompetent) must fully understand what will be done during a test, surgery, or any medical procedure and must understand its risks and implications *before* he can legally consent to it.

Explaining a procedure, its purpose, how it will be performed, and its potential risks is primarily the physician's responsibility. The nurse typically reinforces the physician's explanation, confirms that the patient comprehends it, and verifies that written consent has been given when necessary. Written consent isn't always necessary for individual tests; informed consent may be adequate. The patient retains the legal right to withdraw consent—oral or written—at any time and for any reason and to refuse care or treatment.

Safety measures

Proper specimen collection not only helps to ensure accurate test results but also protects you and the patient. The use of gloves and other barriers, as necessary, is mandated by the Occupational Safety and Health Administration standard, better known as standard precautions. Before you're exposed to a patient's body fluids, make sure you observe the appropriate precautions.

BLOOD SAMPLES

VENIPUNCTURE

Performed to obtain a venous blood sample, venipuncture involves piercing a vein with a needle and collecting blood in a syringe or evacuated tube. Typically, venipuncture is performed using the antecubital fossa. If necessary, however, it can be performed on a vein in the dorsal forearm, the dorsum of the hand or foot, or another accessible location. The inner wrist shouldn't be used because of the high risk of damage to underlying structures. Although laboratory personnel usually perform this procedure in the hospital setting, you may perform it. You should also determine if special conditions exist before venipuncture, such as anticoagulant therapy, low platelet count, bleeding disorders, and other abnormalities that increase the risk of bleeding and hematoma formation.

EQUIPMENT

Guide to color-top collection tubes

TUBE COLOR	DRAW VOLUME	ADDITIVE	PURPOSE
Red	2 to 20 ml	None	Serum studies
Lavender	2 to 10 ml	EDTA	Whole-blood studies
Green	2 to 15 ml	Heparin (sodium, lithium, or ammonium)	Plasma studies
Blue	2.7 or 4.5 ml	Sodium citrate and citric acid	Coagulation studies on plasma
Black	2.7 or 4.5 ml	Sodium oxalate	Coagulation studies on plasma
Gray	3 to 10 ml	Glycolytic inhibitor, such as sodium fluoride, powdered oxalate, or glycolytic-microbial inhibitor	Glucose determinations on serum or plasma
Yellowm	12 ml	Acid-citrate-dextrose	Whole-blood studies

Equipment

Tourniquet ▪ gloves ▪ syringe or evacuated tubes and needle holder ▪ alcohol or antiseptic pads ▪ 20G or 21G needle for the forearm or 25G needle for the wrist, hand, and ankle, and for children ▪ color-coded collection tubes containing appropriate additives ▪ labels ▪ laboratory request form and laboratory biohazard transportation bag ▪ 2″ × 2″ gauze pads ▪ adhesive bandage. (See *Guide to color-top collection tubes.*)

Preparation of equipment

If you're using evacuated tubes, open the needle packet, attach the needle to its holder, and select the appropriate tubes. If you're using a syringe, attach the appropriate needle to it. Be sure to choose a syringe large enough to hold all the blood required for the test. Label all collection tubes clearly with the patient's name and room number, the practitioner's name, the date and time of collection, and initials of the person performing the venipuncture.

Implementation

- Wash your hands thoroughly and put on gloves.
- Confirm the patient's identity using two patient identifiers according to your facility's policy.
- Tell him that you're about to collect a blood sample, and explain the procedure *to ease his anxiety and ensure his cooperation.* Ask him if he has ever felt faint, sweaty, or nauseated when having blood drawn.

PEDIATRIC ALERT *If the patient is a child, try distracting him with a toy or game* to reduce anxiety.

- If the patient is on bed rest, ask him to lie in a supine position, with his head slightly elevated and his arms at his sides. Ask the ambulatory patient to sit in a chair and support his arm securely on an armrest or a table.
- Assess the patient's veins *to determine the best puncture site.* (See *Common venipuncture sites,* page 190.) Observe the skin for the vein's blue color, or palpate the vein for a firm rebound sensation.
- Tie a tourniquet 2″ (5 cm) proximal to the area chosen. *By impeding venous return to the heart while still allowing arterial flow, a tourniquet produces venous dilation.* If arterial perfusion remains adequate, you'll be able to feel the radial pulse. (If the tourniquet fails to dilate the vein, have the patient open and close his fist a few times. Then ask him to close his fist as you insert the needle and to open it again when the needle is in place.)
- Clean the venipuncture site with an alcohol or antiseptic pad. Don't wipe off the antiseptic with alcohol *because alcohol cancels the effect of the antiseptic.* Wipe in a circular motion, spiraling outward from the site *to avoid introducing potentially infectious skin flora into the vessel during the procedure.* If you use alcohol, apply it with friction for 30 seconds

Common venipuncture sites

These illustrations show the anatomic locations of veins commonly used for venipuncture. The most commonly used sites are on the forearm, followed by those on the hand.

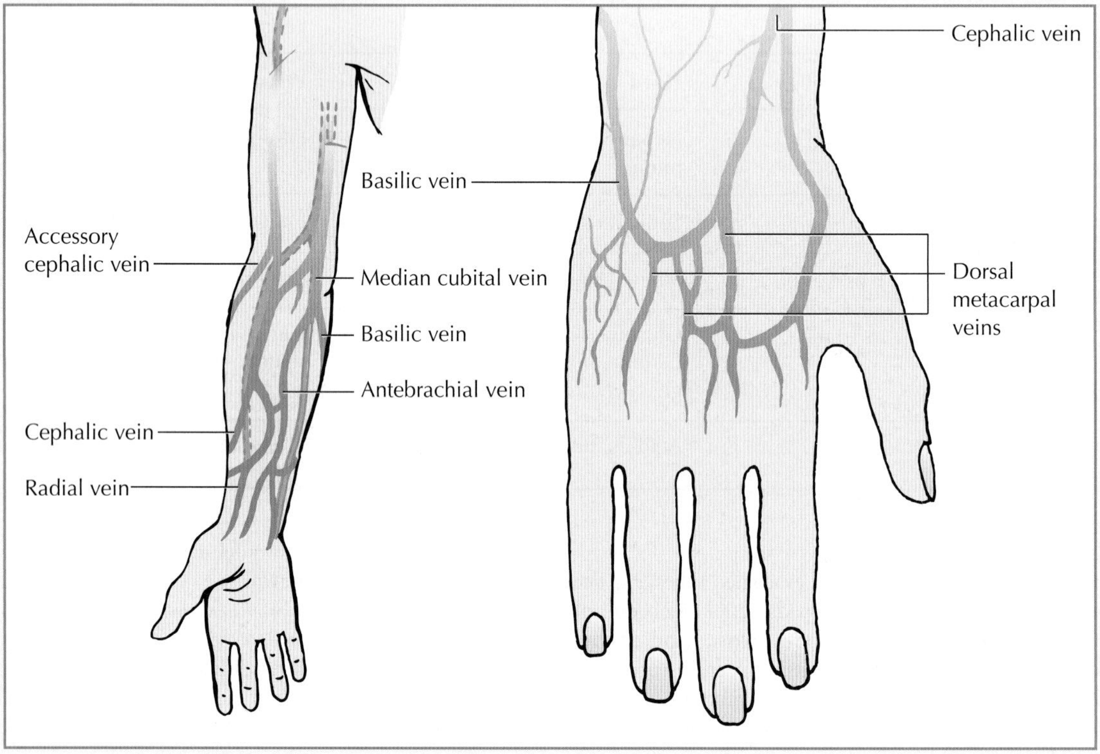

or until the final pad comes away clean. Allow the skin to dry before performing venipuncture.

- Immobilize the vein by pressing just below the venipuncture site with your thumb and drawing the skin taut.
- Position the needle holder or syringe with the needle bevel up and the shaft parallel to the path of the vein and at a 30-degree angle to the arm. Insert the needle into the vein. If you're using a syringe, venous blood will appear in the hub; withdraw the blood slowly, pulling the plunger of the syringe gently *to create steady suction* until you obtain the required sample. *Pulling the plunger too forcibly may collapse the vein.* If you're using a needle holder and an evacuated tube, grasp the holder securely to stabilize it in the vein, and push down on the collection tube until the needle punctures the rubber stopper. Blood will flow into the tube automatically.
- Remove the tourniquet as soon as blood flows adequately *to prevent stasis and hemoconcentration, which can impair test results.* If the flow is sluggish, leave the tourniquet in place longer, but always remove it before withdrawing the needle. Don't leave the tourniquet on for more than 3 minutes.
- Continue to fill the required tubes, removing one and inserting another. Gently rotate each tube as you remove it *to help mix the additive with the sample.*
- After you've drawn the sample, place a gauze pad over the puncture site, and slowly and gently remove the needle from the vein. When using an evacuated tube, remove it from the needle holder *to release the vacuum* before withdrawing the needle from the vein.
- Apply gentle pressure to the puncture site for 2 to 3 minutes or until bleeding stops. *This prevents extravasation into the surrounding tissue, which can cause a hematoma.*

■ After bleeding stops, apply an adhesive bandage.
■ If you've used a syringe, transfer the sample to a collection tube. Place the specimen tubes inside the biohazard transport bag, being careful to avoid foaming, *which can cause hemolysis.*
■ Finally, check the venipuncture site *to see if a hematoma has developed.* If it has, apply pressure until you're sure bleeding has stopped (about 5 minutes), after which you may apply warm soaks to the site.
■ Discard syringes, needles, and used gloves in the appropriate containers.

Special considerations

■ Many manufacturers make safety-engineered blood collection sets; their use is recommended *to prevent needle sticks.*
■ Never collect a venous sample from an arm or a leg that's already being used for I.V. therapy or blood administration *because this may affect test results.* Don't collect a venous sample from an infection site *because this may introduce pathogens into the vascular system.* Likewise, avoid collecting blood from edematous areas, arteriovenous shunts, an upper extremity on the same side as a previous lymph node dissection, and sites of previous hematomas or vascular injury.
■ If the patient has large, distended, highly visible veins, perform venipuncture without a tourniquet *to minimize the risk of hematoma formation.* If the patient has a clotting disorder or is receiving anticoagulant therapy, maintain firm pressure on the venipuncture site for at least 5 minutes after withdrawing the needle *to prevent hematoma formation.*
■ Avoid using veins in the patient's legs for venipuncture, if possible, *because this increases the risk of thrombophlebitis.* Some facilities require a practitioner's order to collect blood from a leg or foot vein. Check your facility's policy and procedure.

Complications

A hematoma at the needle insertion site is the most common complication of venipuncture. Infection may result from poor technique.

Documentation

Record the date, time, and site of the venipuncture; the name of the test; the time the sample was sent to the laboratory; the amount of blood collected; the patient's temperature; and any adverse reactions to the procedure.

SELECTED REFERENCES

Centers for Disease Control and Prevention. Hospital Infection Control Practices Advisory Committee. "Guideline for Prevention of Intravascular Device-Related Infections." Accessed August 2007 via the Web at *www.cdc.gov/ncidod/dhqp/g1_intravascular.html.*

Occupational Safety and Health Administration. "Bloodborne Pathogens," 1910.1030. Accessed August 2007 via the Web at *www.osha.gov/pls/oshaweb/owadisp.show_document?p_table=STANDARDS&p_id=10051.*

Rosenthal, K., "Tips for Venipuncture in Children," Nursing 35(12):31, December 2005.

Standard 71. Phlebotomy. "Infusion Nursing Standards of Practice," *Journal of Infusion Nursing* 29(15):571-72, January-February 2006.

BLOOD CULTURE

Normally bacteria-free, blood is susceptible to infection through infusion lines as well as from thrombophlebitis, infected shunts, and bacterial endocarditis due to prosthetic heart valve replacements. Bacteria may also invade the vascular system from local tissue infections through the lymphatic system and the thoracic duct.

Blood cultures are performed to detect bacterial invasion (bacteremia) and the systemic spread of such an infection (septicemia) through the bloodstream. In this procedure, a venous blood sample is collected by venipuncture at the patient's bedside and then transfered it into two bottles, one containing an anaerobic medium and the other, an aerobic medium. The bottles are incubated, encouraging any organisms that are present in the sample to grow in the media. Blood cultures allow identification of about 67% of pathogens within 24 hours and up to 90% within 72 hours.

Although some authorities consider the timing of culture collections debatable and possibly irrelevant, others advocate drawing three blood samples at least 1 hour apart. The first of these should be collected at the earliest sign of suspected bacteremia or septicemia. To check for suspected bacterial endocarditis, three or four samples may be collected at 5- to 30-minute intervals before starting antibiotic therapy.

Equipment

Tourniquet ■ gloves ■ alcohol ■ povidone-iodine pads ■ 10-ml syringe for an adult; 6-ml syringe for a child ■ three or four 20G 1″ needles ■ two or three blood culture bottles (50-ml bottles for adults; 20-ml bottles for infants and children) with sodium polyethanol sulfonate added (one aerobic bottle containing a suitable medium, such as Trypticase soy broth with 10% carbon dioxide atmosphere; one anaerobic bottle with prereduced medium; and, possibly, one hyperosmotic bottle with 10% sucrose medium) ■ laboratory request form and laboratory biohazard transport bags ■ 2″ × 2″ gauze pads ■ small adhesive bandages ■ labels.

Preparation of equipment

Check the expiration dates on the culture bottles and replace outdated bottles.

Implementation

- Confirm the patient's identity using two patient identifiers according to your facility's policy. Tell the patient that you need to collect a series of blood samples to check for infection. Explain the procedure *to ease his anxiety and promote cooperation.* Explain that the procedure usually requires three blood samples collected at different times.
- Wash your hands and put on gloves.
- Tie a tourniquet 2″ (5 cm) proximal to the area chosen. (See "Venipuncture," page 188.)
- Clean the venipuncture site with an alcohol pad.
- Then clean the area with a povidone-iodine pad. Don't wipe off the povidone-iodine with alcohol *because alcohol cancels the effect of povidone-iodine.* Start at the site and work outward in a circular motion. Wait 30 to 60 seconds for the skin to dry.
- Perform a venipuncture, drawing 10 ml of blood from an adult.

PEDIATRIC ALERT *Draw only 2 to 6 ml of blood from a child.*

- Wipe the diaphragm tops of the culture bottles with a povidone-iodine pad, and change the needle on the syringe used to draw the blood.
- Inject 5 ml of blood into each 50-ml bottle or 2 ml into each 20-ml pediatric culture bottle. (Bottle size may vary according to your facility's policy, but the sample dilution should always be 1:10.)
- Remove the tourniquet. Apply pressure to the venipuncture site using a 2″ × 2″ dressing. Then cover the site with a small adhesive bandage.
- Label the culture bottles with the patient's name and identification number, practitioner's name, and date and time of collection. Indicate the suspected diagnosis and the patient's temperature, and note on the laboratory request form any recent antibiotic therapy. Place the samples in the laboratory biohazard transport bag. Send the samples to the laboratory immediately.
- Discard syringes, needles, and gloves in the appropriate containers.

Special considerations

- Obtain each set of cultures from a different site.
- Avoid using existing blood lines for cultures unless sample is drawn when line is inserted or catheter sepsis is suspected.

Complications

The most common complication of venipuncture is formation of a hematoma. If a hematoma develops, apply warm soaks to the site.

Documentation

Record the date and time of blood sample collection, name of the test, amount of blood collected, number of bottles used, patient's temperature, and adverse reactions to the procedure.

SELECTED REFERENCES

Bekeris, B., et al. "Trends in Blood Culture Contamination: A College of American Pathologists Q-Tracks Study of 356 Institutions," *Archives of Pathology and Laboratory Medicine* 129(10):1222-225, October 2005.

Clinical Laboratory Standards. "Principles and Procedures for Blood Cultures." Approved Guidelines MH7-A, 2007.

College of American Pathologists. "Drawing Blood for a Valid Culture." Accessed August 2007 at *www.cap.org/apps/docs/newspath/spring_2004/0404_Laboratory_Report_Drawing_Blood_for_a_Valid_Culture.doc.*

Craven, R.F., and Hirnle, C.J. *Fundamentals of Nursing: Human Health and Function,* 5th ed. Philadelphia: Lippincott Williams & Wilkins, 2007.

Fischbach, F.T. *A Manual of Laboratory and Diagnostic Tests,* 7th ed. Philadelphia: Lippincott Williams & Wilkins, 2003.

Rushing, J. "Drawing Blood Culture Specimens for Reliable Results," *Nursing* 34(12):20, December 2004.

BLOOD GLUCOSE TESTS

Reagent strip tests (such as Glucostix and Multistix) use a drop of capillary blood obtained by fingerstick, heelstick, or earlobe puncture as a sample. A reagent patch on the tip of a handheld plastic strip changes color in response to the amount of glucose in the blood sample. Comparing the color change with a standardized color chart provides a semiquantitative measurement of blood glucose levels. These tests can be performed in the hospital, practitioner's office, or patient's home.

Blood glucose monitors measure blood glucose concentrations. A drop of whole blood is placed on a blood glucose test strip before or after the strip is inserted into the monitor. A portable blood glucose meter (such as Glucometer, Accu-Chek, and One Touch) provides quantitative measurements that compare in accuracy with other laboratory tests. Some meters store successive test results electronically to help determine glucose patterns.

Equipment

For reagent strip testing: Reagent strips ■ alcohol pads ■ gauze pads ■ disposable lancets or mechanical blood-letting devices ■ watch or clock with a second hand ■ optional: small adhesive bandage.

For blood glucose monitor testing: Portable blood glucose meter ■ alcohol pads ■ gauze pads ■ disposable lancets or mechanical blood-letting devices ■ blood glucose test strips ■ optional: small adhesive bandage.

Preparation of equipment

When using a blood glucose meter, calibrate it and run it with a quality control test *to ensure accurate test results.* Follow the manufacturer's instructions for calibration. If appropriate, ensure that the code strip number on the test strip matches the code number on the meter.

Implementation

■ Confirm the patient's identity using two patient identifiers according to your facility's policy.
■ Explain the procedure to the patient or child's parents.
■ Next, select the puncture site—usually the fingertip or earlobe for an adult or a child.

PEDIATRIC ALERT *Select the heel or great toe for infant.*

■ Wash your hands and put on gloves.
■ If necessary, dilate the capillaries by applying warm, moist compresses to the area for about 10 minutes.
■ Wipe the puncture site with an alcohol pad, and allow to dry completely.
■ To collect a sample from the fingertip with a disposable lancet (smaller than 2 mm), position the lancet on the side of the patient's fingertip, perpendicular to the lines of the fingerprints. Pierce the skin sharply and quickly *to minimize the patient's anxiety and pain and to increase blood flow.* Alternatively, you can use a mechanical blood-letting device, such as an Autolet, which uses a spring-loaded lancet.
■ After puncturing the fingertip, don't squeeze the puncture site *to avoid diluting the sample with tissue fluid.*

For reagent strip testing

■ Touch a drop of blood to the reagent patch on the strip; make sure you cover the entire patch.
■ After collecting the blood sample, briefly apply pressure to the puncture site *to prevent painful extravasation of blood into subcutaneous tissues.* Ask the adult patient to hold a gauze pad firmly over the puncture site until bleeding stops.
■ Make sure you leave the blood on the strip for exactly 60 seconds.
■ After waiting the recommended time, compare the color change on the strip with the standardized color chart on the product container. If you're using a blood glucose meter, follow the manufacturer's instructions.
■ After bleeding has stopped, you may apply a small adhesive bandage to the puncture site.

For blood glucose monitor testing

■ Turn on the monitor.
■ Touch a drop of blood to the test area of the test strip.
■ After collecting the blood sample, briefly apply pressure to the puncture site *to prevent painful extravasation of blood into subcutaneous tissues.* Ask the adult patient to hold a gauze pad firmly over the puncture site until bleeding stops.
■ Insert the test strip into the blood glucose meter according to the manufacturer's instructions.
■ Read the digital display when the alarm sounds.
■ Remove the test strip and dispose of it according to your facility's policy.
■ After bleeding has stopped, you may apply a small adhesive bandage to the puncture site.
■ Remove your gloves and wash your hands.

NURSING ALERT *If you obtain an extremely low or high blood glucose monitor result obtain a serum blood glucose level immediately to confirm the result.*

■ Clean the blood glucose monitor when it becomes contaminated with blood, at intervals recommended by the manufacturer, or according to your facility's policy.

Special considerations

■ Before using reagent strips, check the expiration date on the package, and replace outdated strips. Check for special instructions related to the specific reagent. The reagent area of a fresh strip should match the color of the "0" block on the color chart. Protect the strips from light, heat, and moisture.
■ Before using a blood glucose meter, calibrate it and run it with a control sample *to ensure accurate test results.* Follow the manufacturer's instructions for calibration.
■ Follow your facility's policy for bedside point-of-care testing.
■ Avoid selecting cold, cyanotic, or swollen puncture sites *to ensure an adequate blood sample.* If you can't obtain a capillary sample, perform venipuncture, and place a large drop of venous blood on the reagent strip. If you want to test blood from a refrigerated sample, allow the blood to return to room temperature before testing it.
■ *To help detect abnormal glucose metabolism and diagnose diabetes mellitus,* the practitioner may order other blood glucose tests. (See *Oral and I.V. glucose tolerance tests,* page 194.)
■ Some blood glucose meters, such as the One Touch Ultra, require smaller amounts of blood; the puncture may be done on the patient's arm instead of his finger.

Oral and I.V. glucose tolerance tests

For monitoring trends in glucose metabolism, the two tests described here may offer benefits over blood testing with reagent strips.

Oral glucose tolerance test

The most sensitive test for detecting borderline diabetes mellitus, the oral glucose tolerance test (OGTT) measures carbohydrate metabolism after ingestion of a challenge dose of glucose. The body absorbs this dose rapidly, causing plasma glucose levels to rise and peak within 30 minutes to 1 hour. The pancreas responds by secreting insulin, causing glucose levels to return to normal within 2 to 3 hours. During this period, plasma and urine glucose levels are monitored to assess insulin secretion and the body's ability to metabolize glucose.

Although you may not collect the blood and urine specimens (usually five of each) required for this test, you're responsible for preparing the patient for the test and monitoring his physical condition during the test.

Begin by explaining the OGTT to the patient. Then tell him to maintain a high-carbohydrate diet for 3 days and to fast for 10 to 16 hours before the test, as ordered. The patient must not smoke, drink coffee or alcohol, or exercise strenuously for 8 hours before or during the test. Inform him that he'll then receive a challenge dose of 100 g of carbohydrate (usually a sweetened carbonated beverage or gelatin).

Tell the patient who will perform the venipunctures, when they'll be performed, and that he may feel slight discomfort from the needle punctures and the pressure of the tourniquet. Reassure him that collecting each blood sample usually takes less than 3 minutes. As ordered, withhold drugs that may affect test results. Remind him not to discard the first urine specimen voided after waking.

During the test period, watch for signs and symptoms of hypoglycemia—weakness, restlessness, nervousness, hunger, and sweating—and report them to the practitioner immediately. Encourage the patient to drink plenty of water to promote adequate urine excretion. Provide a bedpan, urinal, or specimen container when necessary.

I.V. glucose tolerance test

The I.V. glucose tolerance test may be chosen for patients who are unable to absorb an oral dose of glucose; for example, those with malabsorption disorders and short-bowel syndrome or those who have had a gastrectomy. The test measures blood glucose after an I.V. infusion of 50% glucose over 3 to 4 minutes. Blood samples are then collected after 30 minutes, 1 hour, 2 hours, and 3 hours. After an immediate glucose peak of 300 to 400 mg/dl (accompanied by glycosuria), the normal glucose curve falls steadily, reaching fasting levels within 1 to $1\frac{1}{4}$ hours. Failure to achieve fasting glucose levels within 2 to 3 hours typically confirms diabetes.

Home care

If the patient will be using the reagent strip system at home, teach him the proper use of the lancet or Autolet, reagent strips and color chart, and portable blood glucose meter, as necessary. Also provide written guidelines.

Documentation

Record reading from reagent strip (using a portable blood glucose meter or a color chart) in your notes or on a special flowchart, if available. Also record time and date of the test.

SELECTED REFERENCES

Clinical Laboratories Standards Institute. "Point-of-care Blood Glucose Testing in Acute and Chronic Care Facilities," Approved guideline, 2nd ed. C30-A2, 2002.

Dale, L. "Make a Point about Alternate Site Blood Glucose Sampling," *Nursing* 36(2):52-53, February 2006.

Miller, C. "Using Standards of Care to Drive Evidence-Based Clinical Practice and Outcomes for Diabetes Mellitus," *Home Healthcare Nurse* 24(5):307-12, May 2006.

Rizvi, A.A., and Sanders, M.B. "Assessment and Monitoring of Glycemic Control in Primary Diabetes Care: Monitoring Techniques, Record Keeping, Meter Downloads, Tests of Average Glycemia, and Point-of-Care Evaluation," *Journal of American Academy of Nurse Practitioners* 18(1):11-21, January 2006.

Scovell, C. "Using Audit to Change Practice for Routine Glucochecks," *Nursing Times* 102(39):33-34, September-October 2006.

Seley, J.J., and Zaldivar, A. "Read That Meter! Getting the Most Out of Blood Glucose Monitoring," *Advance for Nurse Practitioners* 14(4):55-56, April 2006.

BEDSIDE HEMOGLOBIN TESTING

Nurses monitor hemoglobin levels at the patient's bedside because the fast, accurate results obtained this way allow immediate intervention, if necessary. In contrast, with traditional monitoring methods, blood samples must be sent to the laboratory for interpretation. Numerous testing systems are available for bedside monitoring. Bedside systems are also convenient for the patient's home use.

HemoCue, one system available, gives accurate results without having to pipette, dispense, or mix blood and reagents to obtain readings. Thus, it eliminates the risk of leakage, broken tubes, and splattered blood. A plastic, disposable microcuvette functions as a combination pipette, test tube, and measuring vessel. It contains a reagent that produces a precise chemical reaction as soon as it contacts blood. The photometer is a handheld device that recharges its battery and downloads its data at a docking station. (See *Using a bedside hemoglobin monitor.*)

Normal hemoglobin values range from 12.5 to 15 g/dl. A below-normal hemoglobin value may indicate anemia, recent hemorrhage, or fluid retention, causing hemodilution. An elevated hemoglobin value suggests hemoconcentration from polycythemia or dehydration.

Equipment

Lancet ▪ microcuvette ▪ photometer ▪ gloves ▪ alcohol pads ▪ gauze pads.

Implementation

- Confirm the patient's identity using two patient identifiers according to your facility's policy.
- Take the equipment to the patient's bedside, and explain the purpose of the test to him. Tell him that he'll feel a pinprick in his finger during blood sampling.
- Turn the photometer on. If it hasn't been used recently, insert the control cuvette *to make sure that the photometer is working properly.*
- Wash your hands and put on gloves.
- Select an appropriate puncture site. You'll usually use a fingertip for an adult. The middle and fourth fingers are the best choices. *The second finger is usually the most sensitive, and the thumb may have thickened skin or calluses. Blood should circulate freely in the finger from which you're collecting blood,* so avoid using a ring-bearing finger.

PEDIATRIC ALERT *For an infant, use the heel or great toe.*

- Keep the patient's finger straight, and ask him to relax it. Holding his finger between the thumb and index finger of your nondominant hand, gently rock the patient's finger as you move your fingers from his top knuckle to his fingertip. *This causes blood to flow to the sampling point.*

EQUIPMENT

Using a bedside hemoglobin monitor

Monitoring hemoglobin levels at the patient's bedside is a straightforward procedure. A photometer, such as the HemoCue analyzer featured here, relies on capillary action to draw blood into a disposable microcuvette.

This method of obtaining blood minimizes a health care worker's exposure to the patient's blood and decreases the risk of cross-contamination. Follow the steps shown here when using the HemoCue system.

After you pierce the skin, the microcuvette draws blood automatically.

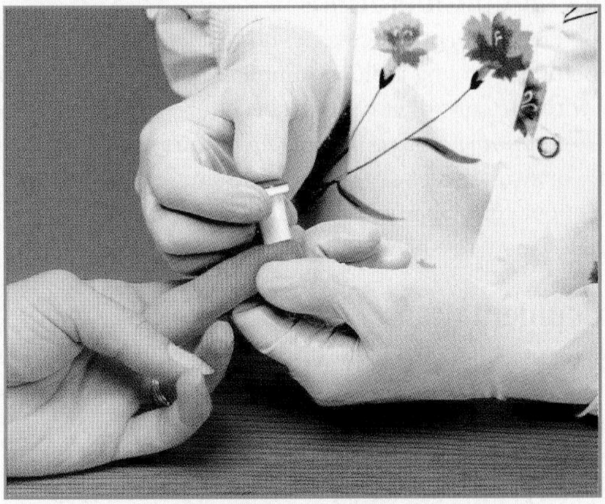

Next, place the microcuvette in the photometer. The photometer screen displays the hemoglobin levels.

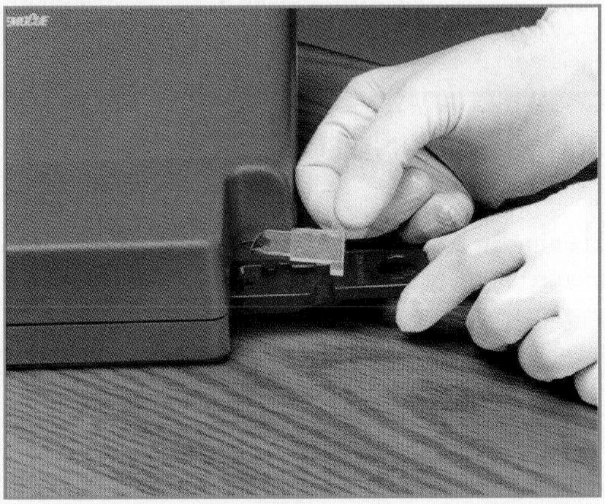

- Use an alcohol pad to clean the puncture site, wiping in a circular motion from the center of the site outward. Dry the site thoroughly with a gauze pad.
- Pierce the skin quickly and sharply with the lancet, and apply the microcuvette, which automatically collects a precise amount of blood (about 5 µl).
- Wipe any excessive blood from the sides of the microcuvette *to obtain the most accurate reading.*
- Place the microcuvette into the photometer. Results will appear on the photometer screen within 1 minute.
- Place a gauze pad over the puncture site until the bleeding stops.
- Dispose of the lancet and microcuvette according to your facility's policy. Remove your gloves and wash your hands. Notify the practitioner if the test result is outside the expected parameters.

Special considerations

- Before using a microcuvette, note its expiration date.
- Before collecting a blood sample, operate the photometer with the control cuvette to check for proper function.
- *To ensure an adequate blood sample,* don't use a cold, cyanotic, or swollen area as the puncture site.
- Follow your facility's policy and procedure for point-of-care testing when performing bedside hemoglobin testing.

Documentation

Document the values obtained from the photometer as well as the date and time of the test and any interventions performed.

SELECTED REFERENCES

Diesel, D., et al. "Point-of-care Testing (POCT): Key Factors to Ensure Efficiency and High Quality," *International Journal of Clinical Chemistry,* May 2004. Available at *www.cli-online.com/uploads/tx_itproducts/datasheet/point-of-care-testing-(poct)-key-factors-to-ensure-efficiency-and-high-quality.pdf.*

ARTERIAL PUNCTURE FOR BLOOD GAS ANALYSIS

Obtaining an arterial blood sample requires percutaneous puncture of the brachial, radial, or femoral artery or withdrawal of a sample from an arterial line. Once collected, the sample can be analyzed to determine arterial blood gas (ABG) values.

ABG analysis evaluates ventilation by measuring blood pH and the partial pressures of arterial oxygen ($Pa{O_2}$) and carbon dioxide ($Pa{CO_2}$). Blood pH measurement reveals the blood's acid-base balance. $Pa{O_2}$ indicates the amount of oxygen that the lungs deliver to the blood, and $Pa{CO_2}$ indicates the lungs' capacity to eliminate carbon dioxide. ABG samples can also be analyzed for oxygen content and saturation and for bicarbonate values.

Typically, ABG analysis is ordered for patients who have chronic obstructive pulmonary disease, pulmonary edema, acute respiratory distress syndrome, myocardial infarction, or pneumonia. It's also performed during episodes of shock and after coronary artery bypass surgery, resuscitation from cardiac arrest, changes in respiratory therapy or status, and prolonged anesthesia.

Most ABG samples can be collected by a respiratory technician or specially trained nurse. Collection from the femoral artery, however, is usually performed by a physician or as your facility's policy indicates. Before attempting a radial puncture, Allen's test should be performed. (See *Performing Allen's test.*)

Equipment

10-ml syringe specially made for drawing blood for ABG analysis ▪ 20G 1¼" needle ▪ 22G 1" needle ▪ glove ▪ alcohol pad ▪ two 2" × 2" gauze pads ▪ rubber cap for syringe hub or rubber stopper for needle ▪ ice-filled plastic bag ▪ label ▪ laboratory request form ▪ adhesive bandage ▪ optional: 1% lidocaine solution.

Many health care facilities use a commercial ABG kit that contains all the equipment listed above (except the adhesive bandage and ice). If your facility doesn't use such a kit, obtain a sterile syringe made for drawing blood for ABG values.

Preparation of equipment

Prepare the collection equipment before entering the patient's room. Wash your hands thoroughly; then open the ABG kit and remove the sample label and the plastic bag. Record on the label the patient's name, room number, body temperature, date and collection time, the flow rate and delivery method of oxygen if present, and the practitioner's name. Fill the plastic bag with ice and set it aside.

Implementation

- Confirm the patient's identity using two patient identifiers according to your facility's policy.
- Tell the patient you need to collect an arterial blood sample, and explain the procedure *to help ease anxiety and promote cooperation.* Tell him that the needle stick will cause some discomfort but that he must remain still during the procedure.
- Wash your hands, and put on gloves
- Place a rolled towel under the patient's wrist *for support.* Locate the artery, and palpate it for a strong pulse.

- Clean the puncture site with an alcohol pad, starting in the center of the site and spiraling outward in a circular motion for 30 seconds or until the pad comes away clean. Allow the skin to dry.
- Palpate the artery with the index and middle fingers of one hand while holding the syringe over the puncture site with the other hand. The puncture site should be between your index and middle fingers as they palpate the pulse.
- Hold the needle bevel up at a 30- to 45-degree angle. When puncturing the brachial artery, hold the needle at a 60-degree angle. (See *Arterial puncture technique,* page 198.)
- Puncture the skin and arterial wall in one motion, following the path of the artery.
- Watch for blood backflow in the syringe. Don't pull back on the plunger *because arterial blood should enter the syringe automatically.* Fill the syringe to the 5-ml mark.
- After collecting the sample, press a gauze pad firmly over the puncture site until the bleeding stops—at least 5 minutes. If the patient is receiving anticoagulant therapy or has a blood dyscrasia, apply pressure for 10 to 15 minutes; if necessary, ask a coworker to hold the gauze pad in place while you prepare the sample for transport to the laboratory. Don't ask the patient to hold the pad. *If he fails to apply sufficient pressure, a large, painful hematoma may form, hindering future arterial punctures at that site.*
- Check the syringe for air bubbles. If any appear, remove them by holding the syringe upright and slowly ejecting some of the blood onto a 2″ × 2″ gauze pad.
- Insert the needle into a rubber stopper, or remove the needle and place a rubber cap directly on the syringe tip *to prevent the sample from leaking and to keep air out of the syringe.*
- Put the labeled sample into the ice-filled plastic bag basin. Attach a properly completed laboratory request form, and send the sample to the laboratory immediately.
- When bleeding stops, apply a small adhesive bandage to the site.
- Monitor the patient's vital signs, and observe for signs of circulatory impairment, such as swelling, discoloration, pain, numbness, or tingling in the bandaged arm or leg. Watch for bleeding at the puncture site.

Special considerations

- If the patient is receiving oxygen, make sure that his therapy has been under way for at least 15 minutes before collecting an arterial blood sample.
- Unless ordered, don't turn off existing oxygen therapy before collecting arterial blood samples. Be sure to indicate on the laboratory request form the amount and type of oxygen therapy the patient is receiving.
- If the patient isn't receiving oxygen, indicate that he's breathing room air.

Performing Allen's test

Rest the patient's arm on the mattress or bedside stand, and support his wrist with a rolled towel. Have him clench his fist. Then, using your index and middle fingers, press on the radial and ulnar arteries. Hold this position for a few seconds.

Without removing your fingers from the patient's arteries, ask him to unclench his first and hold his hand in a relaxed position. The palm will be blanched *because pressure from your fingers has impaired the normal blood flow.*

Blanched palm

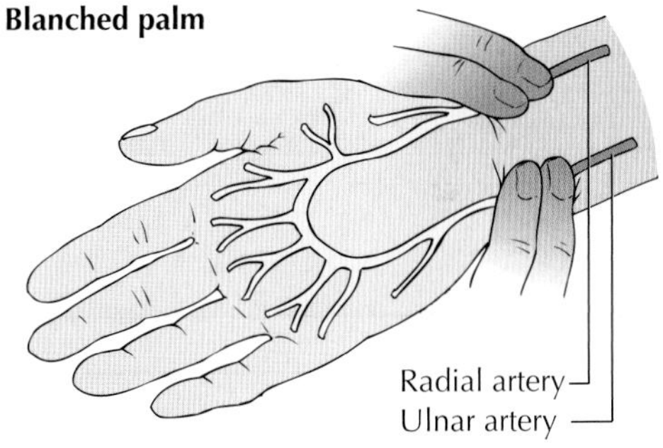

Release pressure on the patient's ulnar artery. If the hand becomes flushed, which indicates blood filling the vessels, you can safely proceed with the radial artery puncture. If the hand doesn't flush, perform the test on the other arm.

Flushed palm

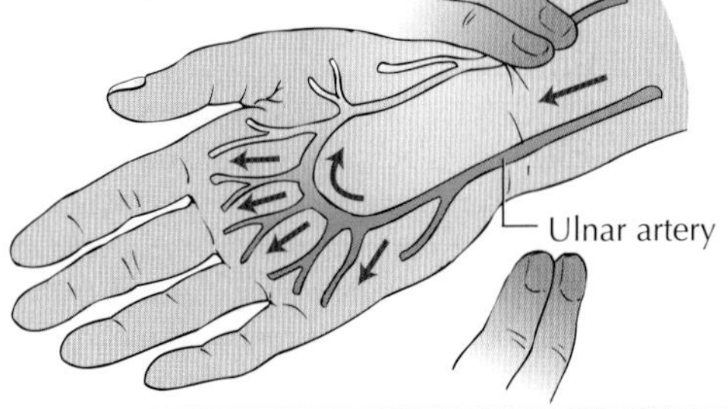

- If the patient has just received a nebulizer treatment, wait about 20 minutes before collecting the sample.
- If necessary, you can anesthetize the puncture site with 1% lidocaine solution or 0.9% benzyl alcohol according to your facility's policy. Consider such use of lidocaine carefully *because it delays the procedure, the patient may be aller-*

Arterial puncture technique

The angle of needle penetration in arterial blood gas sampling depends on which artery will be sampled. For the radial artery, which is used most often, the needle should enter bevel-up at a 30- to 45-degree angle over the radial artery.

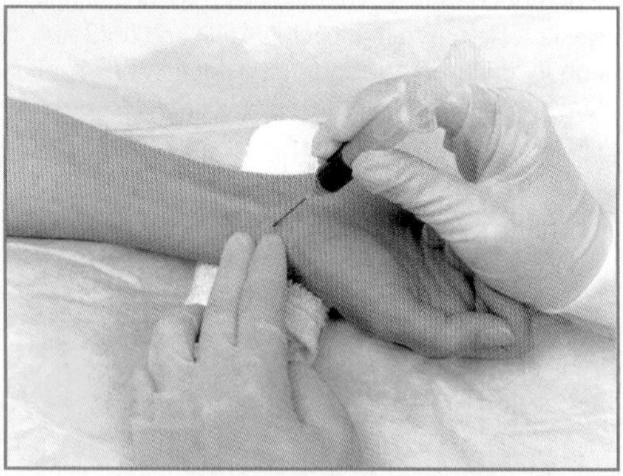

gic to the drug, or the resulting vasoconstriction may prevent successful puncture.

- When filling out a laboratory request form for ABG analysis, include the following information *to help the laboratory staff calibrate the equipment and evaluate results correctly:* the patient's current temperature, most recent hemoglobin level, current respiratory rate and, if the patient is on a ventilator, fraction of inspired oxygen, tidal volume, and ventilatory frequency.

Complications

If you use too much force when attempting to puncture the artery, the needle may touch the periosteum of the bone, causing the patient considerable pain, or you may advance the needle through the opposite wall of the artery. If this happens, slowly pull the needle back a short distance, and check to see if you obtain a blood return. If blood still fails to enter the syringe, withdraw the needle completely, and start with a fresh heparinized needle. Don't make more than two attempts to withdraw blood from the same site. *Probing the artery may injure it and the radial nerve. Also, hemolysis will alter test results.*

If arterial spasm occurs, blood won't flow into the syringe, and you won't be able to collect the sample. If this happens, replace the needle with a smaller one, and try the puncture again. *A smaller-bore needle is less likely to cause arterial spasm.*

Documentation

Record the results of Allen's test, the time the sample was drawn, the patient's temperature, the site of the arterial puncture, the amount of time that pressure was applied to the site to control bleeding, and the type and amount of oxygen therapy the patient was receiving.

SELECTED REFERENCES

American Association for Respiratory Care. "AARC Clinical Guidelines: Blood Gas Analysis and Hemoximetry. 2001 Revision and Update," *Respiratory Care* 46(5):498-505, May 2001.

Crawford, A. "An Audit of the Patient's Experience of Arterial Blood Gas Testing," *British Journal of Nursing* 13(9):529-32, May 2004.

Hudson, T.L., et al. "Use of Local Anesthesia for Arterial Punctures," *American Journal of Critical Care* 15(6):595-66, November 2006.

Lynn-McHale Wiegand, D.J., and Carlson, K.K., eds. *AACN Procedure Manual for Critical Care,* 5th ed. Philadelphia: W.B. Saunders Co., 2005.

National Committee for Clinical Laboratory Standards. *Procedures for the Collection of Arterial Blood Specimens,* 4th ed. Approved Standard H11-A4, 2004.

URINE SPECIMENS

URINE COLLECTION

A random urine specimen, usually collected as part of the physical examination or at various times during hospitalization, permits laboratory screening for urinary and systemic disorders as well as for drug screening. A clean-catch midstream specimen is replacing random collection because it provides a virtually uncontaminated specimen without the need for catheterization.

An indwelling catheter specimen—obtained either by clamping the drainage tube and emptying the accumulated urine into a container or by aspirating a specimen with a syringe—requires sterile collection technique to prevent catheter contamination and urinary tract infection. This method is contraindicated after genitourinary surgery.

Equipment

For a random specimen: Bedpan or urinal with cover, if necessary ▪ gloves ▪ graduated container ▪ specimen container with lid ▪ label ▪ laboratory request form and laboratory biohazard transport bag.

For a clean-catch midstream specimen: Soap and water ▪ gloves ▪ graduated container ▪ three sterile 2″ × 2″

gauze pads ■ antiseptic solution ■ sterile specimen container with lid ■ label ■ bedpan or urinal, if necessary ■ laboratory request form and laboratory biohazard transport bag. (Commercial clean-catch kits containing antiseptic towelettes, sterile specimen container with lid and label, and instructions for use in several languages are widely used.)

For an indwelling catheter specimen: Gloves ■ antiseptic pad ■ 10-ml syringe ■ 21G or 22G ½" ■ needle ■ tube clamp ■ sterile specimen container with lid ■ label ■ laboratory request form and laboratory biohazard transport bag.

Implementation

■ Verify the order for the urine specimen.
■ Confirm the patient's identity using two patient identifiers according to your facility's policy.
■ Tell the patient that you need a urine specimen for laboratory analysis. Explain the procedure to him and his family, if necessary, *to promote cooperation and prevent accidental disposal of specimens.*

Collecting a random specimen

■ Provide privacy. Instruct the patient on bed rest to void into a clean bedpan or urinal, or ask the ambulatory patient to void into either one in the bathroom.
■ Put on gloves. Then pour at least 120 ml of urine into the specimen container, and cap the container securely. If the patient's urine output must be measured and recorded, pour the remaining urine into the graduated container. Otherwise, discard the remaining urine. If you inadvertently spill urine on the outside of the container, clean and dry it *to prevent cross-contamination.*
■ After you label the specimen container with the patient's name and identification number and the date and time of collection, attach the laboratory request form, place it in the laboratory biohazard transport bag, and send it the laboratory immediately. *Delayed transport of the specimen may alter test results.*
■ Clean the graduated container and urinal or bedpan, and return them to their proper storage area. Discard disposable items.
■ Wash your hands thoroughly *to prevent cross-contamination.* Offer the patient a washcloth and soap and water to wash his hands.

Collecting a clean-catch midstream specimen

■ *Because the goal is a virtually uncontaminated specimen,* explain the procedure to the patient carefully. Provide illustrations *to emphasize the correct collection technique,* if possible.
■ Tell the male patient to remove all clothing from the waist down and to stand in front of the toilet as for urination or, if female, to sit far back on the toilet seat and spread her legs. Then have the patient clean the periurethral area (tip of the penis or labial folds, vulva, and urinary meatus) with soap and water and wipe the area three times, each time with a fresh 2" × 2" gauze pad soaked in antiseptic solution or with the wipes provided in a commercial kit. Instruct the female patient to separate her labial folds with the thumb and forefinger. Tell her to wipe down one side with the first pad and discard it, to wipe the other side with the second pad and discard it and, finally, to wipe down the center over the urinary meatus with the third pad and discard it. Stress the importance of cleaning from front to back *to avoid contaminating the genital area with fecal matter.* For the uncircumcised male patient, emphasize the need to retract his foreskin *to effectively clean the meatus* and to keep it retracted during voiding.
■ Tell the female patient to straddle the bedpan or toilet to allow labial spreading and to keep her labia separated while voiding.
■ Instruct the patient to begin voiding into the bedpan, urinal, or toilet. Then, without stopping the urine stream, the patient should move the collection container into the stream, collecting 30 to 50 ml at the midstream portion of the voiding. He can then finish voiding into the bedpan, urinal, or toilet.
■ Put on gloves before discarding the first and last portions of the voiding, and measure the remaining urine in a graduated container for intake and output records, if necessary. Be sure to include the amount in the specimen container when recording the total amount voided.
■ Take the sterile container from the patient, and cap it securely. Avoid touching the inside of the container or the lid. If the outside of the container is soiled, clean it and wipe it dry. Remove gloves and discard them properly.
■ Wash your hands thoroughly. Tell the patient to wash his hands also.
■ Label the container with the patient's name and identification number, name of test, type of specimen, collection time, and suspected diagnosis, if known. If a urine culture has been ordered, note any current antibiotic therapy on the laboratory request form. Place the specimen in a laboratory biohazard transport bag, and send the container to the laboratory immediately or place it on ice *to prevent specimen deterioration and altered test results.*

Collecting an indwelling catheter specimen

■ About 30 minutes before collecting the specimen, clamp the drainage tube *to allow urine to accumulate.*
■ Put on gloves. If the drainage tube has a built-in sampling port, wipe the port with an antiseptic pad. Uncap the needle on the syringe, and insert the needle into the sampling

Aspirating a urine specimen

If the patient has an indwelling urinary catheter in place, clamp the tube distal to the aspiration port for about 30 minutes. Wipe the port with an alcohol pad, and insert a needle and a 10-ml or 20-ml syringe into the port perpendicular to the tube. Aspirate the required amount of urine, and expel it into the specimen container. Remove the clamp on the drainage tube.

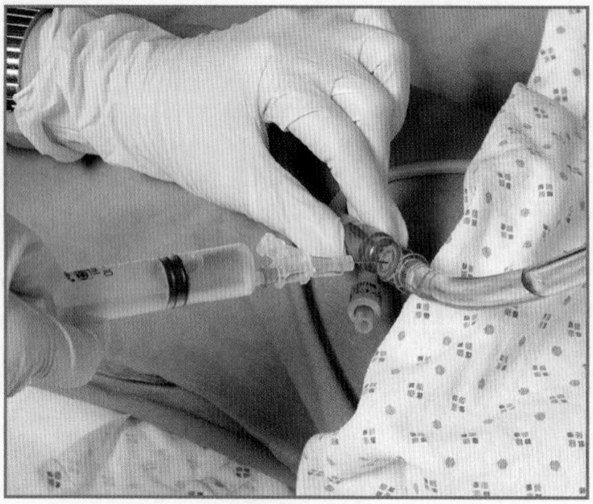

port at a 90-degree angle to the tubing. Aspirate the specimen into the syringe. (See *Aspirating a urine specimen.*)

- If the drainage tube doesn't have a sampling port, and the catheter is made of rubber, obtain the specimen from the catheter. *Other types of catheters will leak after you withdraw the needle.* To withdraw the specimen from a rubber catheter, wipe it with an antiseptic pad just above where it connects to the drainage tube. Insert the needle into the rubber catheter at a 45-degree angle and withdraw the specimen. Never insert the needle into the shaft of the catheter *because this may puncture the lumen leading to the catheter balloon.*
- Transfer the specimen to a sterile container, label it, and send it to the laboratory immediately in a laboratory biohazard transport bag, or place it on ice. If a urine culture is to be performed, be sure to list any current antibiotic therapy on the laboratory request form.
- If the catheter isn't made of rubber or has no sampling port, wipe the area where the catheter joins the drainage tube with an antiseptic pad. Disconnect the catheter, and allow urine to drain into the sterile specimen container. Avoid touching the inside of the sterile container with the catheter, and don't touch anything with the catheter drainage tube *to avoid contamination.* When you've collected the specimen, wipe both connection sites with an antiseptic pad, and join them. Cap the specimen container, label it, and send it to the laboratory immediately, or place it on ice.

NURSING ALERT *Make sure you unclamp the drainage tube after collecting the specimen to prevent urine backflow, which may cause bladder distention and infection.*

Home care

Instruct the patient to collect the specimen in a clean container with a tight-fitting lid and to keep it on ice or in the refrigerator (separate from food items) for up to 24 hours.

Documentation

Record the times of specimen collection and transport to the laboratory. Specify the test as well as the appearance, odor, and color and any unusual characteristics of the specimen. If necessary, record the urine volume in the intake and output record.

SELECTED REFERENCES

Craven, R.F., and Hirnle, C.J. *Fundamentals of Nursing: Human Health and Function,* 5th ed. Philadelphia: Lippincott Williams & Wilkins, 2007.

Davis, K. "Need Urine from a Catheter System? Forget the Needle," *Nursing* 34(12):64, December 2004.

Fernandez, R.S., et al. "Clamping Short-Term Indwelling Catheters: A Systematic Review of the Evidence," *Journal of Wound, Ostomy, and Continence Nursing* 32(5):329-36, September-October, 2005.

Fischbach, F. *A Manual of Laboratory and Diagnostic Tests,* 7th ed. Philadelphia: Lippincott Williams & Wilkins, 2004.

Occupational Safety and Health Administration. "Bloodborne Pathogens," 1910.1030. Accessed August 2007 via the Web at *www.osha.gov/pls/oshaweb/owadisp.show_document?p_table=STANDARDS&p_id=10051.*

"Preferred Medical Devices Announces New Urine Collection and Containment System for Patients with Limited Mobility" *Journal of Hospice and Palliative Nursing* 8(3):131, May-June 2006.

Ribby, K.J. "Decreasing Urinary Tract Infections through Staff Development, Outcomes, and Nursing Process," *Journal of Nursing Quality Care* 21(2):194-98, April-June, 2006.

U.S. Department of Health and Human Services Division of Workplace Program. "Drug Testing Specimen Collection." Available at *http://www.workplace.samhsa.gov/DrugTesting/SpecimenCollection/index.html.*

Wilson, L.A. "Urinalysis," *Nursing Standard* 19(35):51-54, May 2005.

TIMED URINE COLLECTION

Because hormones, proteins, and electrolytes are excreted in small, variable amounts in urine, specimens for measuring these substances must typically be collected over an extended period to yield quantities of diagnostic value.

A 24-hour specimen is used most commonly because it provides an average excretion rate for substances eliminated during this period. Timed specimens may also be collected for shorter periods, such as 2 or 12 hours, depending on the specific information needed.

A timed urine specimen may also be collected after administering a challenge dose of a chemical—insulin, for example—to detect various renal disorders.

Equipment

Large collection bottle with a cap or stopper, or a commercial plastic container ▪ preservative, if necessary ▪ gloves ▪ bedpan or urinal if patient doesn't have an indwelling catheter ▪ graduated container if patient is on intake and output measurement ▪ ice-filled container if a refrigerator isn't available ▪ label ▪ laboratory request form and laboratory biohazard transport container ▪ four patient-care reminders.

Check with the laboratory to find out which preservatives may need to be added to the specimen or whether a dark collection bottle is required.

Implementation

- Confirm the patient's identity using two patient identifiers according to your facility's policy.
- Explain the procedure to the patient and his family, as necessary, *to enlist their cooperation and prevent accidental disposal of urine during the collection period.* Emphasize that failure to collect even one specimen during the collection period invalidates the test and requires that it begin again.
- Place patient-care reminders over the patient's bed, in his bathroom, and on the urinal or indwelling catheter collection bag. Include the date and the collection interval.
- Instruct the patient to save all urine during the collection period, to notify you after each voiding, and to avoid contaminating the urine with stool or toilet tissue. Explain any dietary or drug restrictions, and make sure he understands and is willing to comply with them.

For 2-hour collection

- If possible, instruct the patient to drink two to four 8-oz (480 to 960 ml) glasses of water about 30 minutes before collection begins. After 30 minutes, tell him to void. Put on gloves, and discard this specimen *so the patient starts the collection period with an empty bladder.* Note this time as the beginning time for collection.
- If ordered, administer a challenge dose of medication (such as glucose solution or corticotropin), and record the time.
- If possible, offer the patient a glass of water at least every hour during the collection period *to stimulate urine production.* After each voiding, put on gloves, and add the specimen to the collection bottle.
- Instruct the patient to void about 15 minutes before the end of the collection period, if possible, and add this specimen to the collection bottle.
- At the end of the collection period, remove and discard your gloves, and send the appropriately labeled collection bottle to the laboratory immediately in an approved laboratory biohazard transport container, along with a properly completed laboratory request form.

For 12- and 24-hour collection

- Put on gloves, and ask the patient to void. Then discard this urine *so the patient starts the collection period with an empty bladder.* Record the time.
- After putting on gloves and pouring the first urine specimen into the collection bottle, add the required preservative. Then refrigerate the bottle or keep it on ice until the next voiding, as appropriate.
- Collect all urine voided during the prescribed period. Just before the collection period ends, ask the patient to void again, if possible. Add this last specimen to the collection bottle, pack it in ice *to inhibit deterioration of the specimen,* and remove and discard your gloves. Label the collection bottle, place it in an approved laboratory biohazard transport container, and send it to the laboratory with a properly completed laboratory request form.

Special considerations

- Keep the patient well hydrated before and during the test *to ensure adequate urine flow.*
- Before collection of a timed specimen, make sure the laboratory will be open when the collection period ends *to help ensure prompt, accurate results.*
- Never store a specimen in a refrigerator that contains food or medication *to avoid contamination.* If the patient has an indwelling catheter in place, put the collection bag in an ice-filled container at his bedside.
- Instruct the patient to avoid exercise and ingestion of coffee, tea, or any drugs (unless directed otherwise by the physician) before the test *to avoid altering test results.*
- If you accidentally discard a specimen during the collection period, you'll need to restart the collection. This may result in an additional day of hospitalization, which may cause the patient personal and financial hardship. Therefore, emphasize the need to save all the patient's urine during the

collection period to everyone involved in his care as well as to his family and other visitors.

Home care

If the patient must continue collecting urine at home, provide written instructions for the appropriate method. Tell him that he can keep the collection bottle in a brown bag in his refrigerator at home, separate from other refrigerator contents.

Documentation

Record the date and intervals of specimen collection and when the collection bottle was sent to the laboratory.

SELECTED REFERENCES

Craven, R.F., and Hirnle, C.J. *Fundamentals of Nursing: Human Health and Function,* 5th ed. Philadelphia: Lippincott Williams & Wilkins, 2007.

Fischbach, F. *A Manual of Laboratory and Diagnostic Tests,* 7th ed. Philadelphia: Lippincott Williams & Wilkins, 2004.

Hellerstein, S., et al. "Timed-Urine Collections for Renal Clearance Studies," *Pediatric Nephrology* 21(1):96-101, January 2006.

National Kidney Foundation. Kidney Disease Outcome Quality Initiative (K/DOQI) Clinical Practice Guidelines for Chronic Kidney Disease. Available at *www.kidney.org/PROFESSIONALS/kdoqi/guidelines/.*

Occupational Safety and Health Administration. "Bloodborne Pathogens," 1910.1030. Accessed August 2007 via the Web at *www.osha.gov/pls/oshaweb/owadisp.show_document?p_table=STANDARDS&p_id=10051.*

URINE GLUCOSE AND KETONE TESTS

Reagent strip tests are used to monitor urine glucose and ketone levels and to screen for diabetes. Urine glucose tests are less accurate than blood glucose tests and are used less frequently because of the increasing convenience of blood self-testing. Urine ketone tests monitor fat metabolism, help diagnose carbohydrate deprivation and diabetic ketoacidosis, and help distinguish between diabetic and nondiabetic coma.

Glucose oxidase tests (such as Diastix, Tes-Tape, and Clinistix strips) produce color changes when patches of reagents implanted in handheld plastic strips react with glucose in the patient's urine; urine ketone strip tests (such as Keto-Diastix and Ketostix) are similar. All test results are read by comparing color changes with a standardized reference chart.

Equipment

Specimen container ▪ gloves ▪ glucose or ketone test strip ▪ reference color chart.

NURSING ALERT *Wear gloves as barrier protection when performing all urine tests.*

Implementation

- Confirm the patient's identity using two patient identifiers according to your facility's policy.
- Explain the test to the patient, and if he's a newly diagnosed diabetic, teach him how to perform the test himself. Check his history for medications that may interfere with test results.
- Before each test, instruct the patient not to contaminate the urine specimen with stool or toilet tissue.
- Test urine specimen immediately after the patient voids.
- Instruct the patient to void. Ask him to drink a glass of water, if possible, and collect a second-voided specimen after 30 to 45 minutes.

Glucose oxidase strip tests

- Put on gloves before collecting a specimen for the test, and remove them to record test results.
- If you're using a Clinistix strip, dip the reagent end of the strip into the urine for 2 seconds. Remove excess urine by tapping the strip against the specimen container's rim, wait for exactly 10 seconds, and then compare its color with the color chart on the test strip container. Ignore color changes that occur after 10 seconds.
- If you're using a Diastix strip, dip the reagent end of the strip into the urine for 2 seconds. Tap off excess urine from the strip, wait for exactly 30 seconds, and then compare the strip's color with the color chart on the test strip container. Ignore color changes that occur after 30 seconds.
- If you're using a Tes-Tape strip, pull about 1½" (3.8 cm) of the reagent strip from the dispenser, and dip one end about ¼" (0.6 cm) into the specimen for 2 seconds. Tap off excess urine from the strip, wait exactly 60 seconds, and then compare the darkest part of the tape with the color chart on the dispenser. If the test result exceeds 0.5%, wait an additional 60 seconds, and make a final comparison.
- Discard the specimen and your gloves.
- Record the results.

Ketone strip test

- Put on gloves, and collect a second-voided midstream specimen.
- If you're using a Ketostix strip, dip the reagent end of the strip into the specimen, and remove it immediately. Wait exactly 15 seconds, and then compare the color of the strip with the color chart on the test strip container. Ignore col-

or changes that occur after 15 seconds. Remove and discard your gloves, and record the test result.

- If you're using a Keto-Diastix strip, dip the reagent end of the strip into the specimen, and remove it immediately. Tap off excess urine from the strip, and hold the strip horizontally *to prevent mixing of chemicals between the two reagent squares.* Wait exactly 15 seconds, and then compare the color of the ketone part of the strip with the color chart on the test strip container. After 30 seconds, compare the color of the glucose part of the strip with the color chart.
- Remove and discard your gloves, and record the test result.

Special considerations

Keep reagent strips in a cool, dry place at a temperature below 86° F (30° C), but don't refrigerate them. Keep the container tightly closed. Don't use discolored or outdated tablets or strips.

Documentation

Record test results according to the information on the reagent containers, or use a flowchart designed to record this information. If you're teaching a patient how to perform the test, keep a record of his progress.

SELECTED REFERENCES

Department of Health and Human Services, U.S. Food and drug Administration. "Glucose Meters and Diabetes Management." Accessed August 2007 via the Web at *www.fda.gov/diabetes/glucose.html.*

Emery, S.P., et al. "Twenty-four-hour Urine Insulin as a Measure of Hyperinsulinemia/Insulin Resistance before Onset of Pre-Eclampsia and Gestational Hypertension," *BJOG* 112(11):1479-85, November 2005.

International Diabetes Federation. Position Statement: "The Role of Urine Glucose Monitoring in Diabetes," March 2005. Available at *http://www.idf.org/home/index.cfm?node=183.*

Wei, O.Y., and Teece, S. "Best Evidence Topic Report. Urine Dipsticks in Screening for Diabetes Mellitus," *Emergency Medicine Journal* 23(2):138, February 2006.

Wilson, L.A. "Urinalysis," *Nursing Standard* 19(35):51-54, May 2005.

URINE SPECIFIC GRAVITY

The kidneys maintain homeostasis by varying urine output and urine concentration of dissolved salts. Urine specific gravity measures the concentration of urine solutes, which reflects the kidneys' capacity to concentrate urine. The capacity to concentrate urine is among the first functions lost when renal tubular damage occurs.

Urine specific gravity is determined by comparing the weight of a urine specimen with that of an equivalent volume of distilled water, which is 1.000. Because urine contains dissolved salts and other substances, it's heavier than 1.000. Urine specific gravity ranges from 1.003 (very dilute) to 1.035 (highly concentrated); normal values range from 1.010 to 1.025. Specific gravity is commonly measured with a urinometer (a specially calibrated hydrometer designed to float in a cylinder of urine). The more concentrated the urine, the higher the urinometer floats—and the higher the specific gravity. Specific gravity may also be measured by a refractometer, which measures the refraction of light as it passes through a urine specimen, or a reagent strip test.

Elevated specific gravity reflects an increased concentration of urine solutes, which occurs in conditions that cause renal hypoperfusion, and may indicate heart failure, dehydration, hepatic disorders, or nephrosis. Low specific gravity reflects failure to reabsorb water and concentrate urine; it may indicate hypercalcemia, hypokalemia, alkalosis, acute renal failure, pyelonephritis, glomerulonephritis, or diabetes insipidus.

Although urine specific gravity is commonly measured with a random urine specimen, more accurate measurement is possible with a controlled specimen collected after fluids are withheld for 12 to 24 hours.

Equipment

Calibrated urinometer and cylinder, refractometer, or reagent strips (Multistix) ■ gloves ■ graduated specimen container.

Implementation

- Confirm the patient's identity using two patient identifiers according to your facility's policy.
- Check the patient's history for drugs that may increase specific gravity, such as dextran, sucrose, or radiographic contrast medium within the past 3 days.
- Explain the procedure to the patient, and tell him when you'll need the specimen. Explain why you're withholding fluids and for how long *to ensure his cooperation.*

Measuring with a urinometer

- Put on gloves and collect a random urine specimen. Let the specimen reach room temperature (71.6° F [22° C]) before testing *because this is the temperature at which most urinometers are calibrated.*
- Fill the cylinder about three-quarters full of urine. Then gently spin the urinometer, and drop it into the cylinder.
- When the urinometer stops bobbing, read the specific gravity from the calibrated scale marked directly on the stem of the urinometer. Make sure the instrument floats freely and doesn't touch the sides of the cylinder. Read the scale at

EQUIPMENT

Using a urinometer

With the urinometer floating in a cylinder of urine, position your eye at a level even with the bottom of the meniscus, and read the specific gravity from the scale printed on the urinometer.

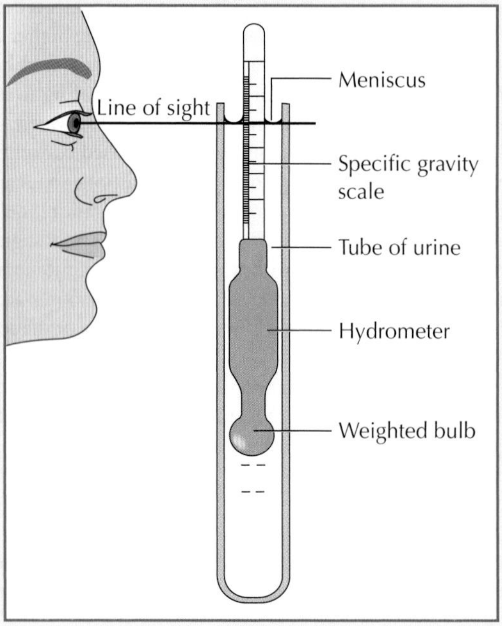

the lowest point of the meniscus *to ensure an accurate reading.* (See *Using a urinometer.*)

- Discard the urine, and rinse the cylinder and urinometer in cool water. *Warm water coagulates proteins in urine, making them stick to the instrument.*
- Remove your gloves and wash your hands thoroughly *to prevent cross-contamination.*

Measuring with a refractometer

- Put on gloves, and collect a random or controlled urine specimen.
- Place a single drop of urine on the refractometer slide.
- Turn on the light and look through the eyepiece to see the specific gravity indicated on a scale. (Some instruments have a digital display.)
- Discard the urine, and clean the equipment according to the manufacturer's guidelines.
- Discard your gloves and wash your hands.

Measuring with a reagent strip

- Put on gloves, and obtain a random or controlled urine specimen.
- Dip the reagent end of the test strip into the specimen for 2 seconds.
- Tap the strip on the rim of the specimen container *to remove excess urine,* and compare the resultant color change with the color chart supplied with the kit.
- Discard the urine and specimen container
- Discard your gloves and wash your hands.

Special considerations

Test the urinometer in distilled water at room temperature *to ensure that its calibration is 1.000.* If necessary, correct the urinometer reading for temperature effects; add 0.001 to your observed reading for every 5.4° F (3° C) above the calibration temperature of 71.6° F (22° C); subtract 0.001 for every 5.4° F below 71.6° F.

Documentation

Record the specific gravity, volume, color, odor, and appearance of the collected urine specimen.

SELECTED REFERENCES

Mentes, J.C., et al. "Use of a Urine Color Chart to Monitor Hydration Status in Nursing Home Residents," *Biological Research for Nursing* 7(3):197-203, January 2006.

National Institute of Diabetes and Digestive and Kidney Diseases. Accessed August 2007 at *www.niddk.nih.gov.*

Opplinger, R.A., et al. "Accuracy of Urine Specific Gravity and Osmolality as Indicators of Hydration Status," *International Journal of Sport Nutrition and Exercise Metabolism* 15(3):236-51, June 2005.

URINE PH

The pH of urine—its alkalinity or acidity—reflects the kidneys' ability to maintain a normal hydrogen ion concentration in plasma and extracellular fluids. The normal hydrogen ion concentration in urine varies, ranging from pH 4.6 to 8.0, but it usually averages around pH 6.0.

The simplest procedure for testing the pH of urine consists of dipping a reagent strip (such as Combistix) into a fresh specimen of the patient's urine and comparing the resultant color change with a standardized color chart.

An alkaline pH (above 7.0), resulting from a diet low in meat but high in vegetables, dairy products, and citrus fruits, causes turbidity and the formation of phosphate, carbonate, and amorphous crystals. Alkaline urine may also result from urinary tract infection and from metabolic or respiratory alkalosis.

An acid pH (below 7.0), resulting from a high-protein diet, also causes turbidity as well as the formation of oxalate, cystine, amorphous urate, and uric acid crystals. Acid urine may also result from renal tuberculosis, phenylketonuria, alkaptonuria, pyrexia, diarrhea, starvation, renal failure, and all forms of acidosis.

Measuring urine pH can also help monitor some medications, such as methenamine, that are active only at certain pH levels.

Equipment

Clean-catch kit ▪ urine specimen container ▪ gloves ▪ reagent strips. (The reagent strip has a pH indicator as part of a battery of indicators.)

Implementation

■ Confirm the patient's identity using two patient identifiers according to your facility's policy.

■ Wash your hands thoroughly and put on gloves.

■ Provide patient with a specimen container, and instruct him to collect a clean-catch midstream specimen. (See "Urine collection," page 198.) Dip the reagent strip into the urine, remove it, and tap off the excess urine from the strip.

■ Hold the strip horizontally *to avoid mixing reagents from adjacent test areas on the strip*. Then compare the color on the strip with the standardized color chart on the strip package. This comparison can be made up to 60 seconds after immersing the strip. Note the results promptly *as the reagent strip may continue to change color.*

■ Discard the urine specimen. If you're monitoring the patient's intake and output, measure the amount of urine discarded.

■ Remove and discard your gloves, and wash your hands thoroughly *to prevent cross-contamination*.

Special considerations

■ Use only a fresh urine specimen *because bacterial growth at room temperature changes urine pH.*

■ Avoid letting a drop of urine run off the reagent strip onto adjacent reagent spots on the strip *because the other reagents can change the pH result.*

■ Be aware that urine collected at night is usually more acidic than urine collected during the day.

Documentation

Record test results, time of voiding, and amount voided.

SELECTED REFERENCES

Kamel, K.S., et al. "Studies to Identify the Basis for an Alkaline Urine pH in Patients with Calcium Hydrogen Phosphate Kidney Stones," *Nephrology Dialysis Transplantation* 22(2):424-31, November 2006.

Midthun, S., et al. "A Protocol for the Urine Dipstick/Pad Method," *Journal of Wound, Ostomy, and Continence Nursing* 33(4):396-400, July-August 2006.

Midthun, S., et al. "Are True-Negative Nitrite Results Affected by a Two-Hour Delay in Dipstick/Pad Analysis of Urine in Incontinence Pads?" *Journal of Wound, Ostomy, and Continence Nursing* 33(3):292-95, May-June 2006.

STRAINING URINE FOR CALCULI

Renal calculi, or *kidney stones*, may develop anywhere in the urinary tract. They may be excreted with the urine or become lodged in the urinary tract, causing hematuria, urine retention, renal colic and, possibly, hydronephrosis.

Ranging in size from microscopic to several centimeters, calculi form in the kidneys when mineral salts—principally calcium oxalate or calcium phosphate—collect around a nucleus of bacterial cells, blood clots, or other particles. Other substances involved in calculus formation include uric acid, xanthine, and ammonia.

Renal calculi result from many causes, including hypercalcemia, which may occur with hyperparathyroidism, excessive dietary intake of calcium, prolonged immobility, abnormal urine pH levels, dehydration, hyperuricemia associated with gout, and some hereditary disorders. Most commonly, calculi form as a result of urine stasis stemming from dehydration (which concentrates urine), benign prostatic hyperplasia, neurologic disorders, or urethral strictures.

Testing for the presence of calculi requires careful straining of all the patient's urine through a gauze pad or fine-mesh sieve and, at times, quantitative laboratory analysis of questionable specimens. Such testing typically continues until the patient passes the calculi or until surgery, as ordered.

Equipment

Fine-mesh sieve or 2″ × 2″ gauze pad ▪ graduated container ▪ urinal or bedpan ▪ gloves ▪ laboratory request form and laboratory biohazard transport bag ▪ three patient-care reminders ▪ specimen container (for use if calculi are found).

Implementation

■ Confirm the patient's identity using two patient identifiers according to your facility's policy.

■ Explain the procedure to the patient and his family, if possible, *to ensure cooperation and to stress the importance of straining all the patient's urine.*

■ Post a patient-care reminder stating STRAIN ALL URINE over the patient's bed, in his bathroom, and on the collection container.

- Tell the patient to notify you after each voiding.
- If a commercial strainer isn't available, unfold a 4" × 4" gauze pad, place it over the top of a graduated measuring container, and secure it with a rubber band.
- Put on gloves. With the strainer secured over the mouth of the collection container, pour the specimen from the urinal or bedpan into the container. If the patient has an indwelling catheter in place, strain all urine from the collection bag before discarding it.
- Examine the strainer for calculi. If you detect calculi or if the filter looks questionable, notify the practitioner, place the filtrate in a specimen container, and send it to the laboratory in a laboratory biohazard transport bag with a laboratory request form.
- If the strainer is intact, rinse it carefully and reuse it. If it has become damaged, discard it, and replace it with a new strainer. Remove and discard your gloves.

Special considerations

- Save and send to the laboratory any small or suspicious-looking residue in the specimen container *because even tiny calculi can cause hematuria and pain.*
- Be aware that calculi may appear in various colors, each of which has diagnostic value.
- Don't leave the stone in contact with urine or other fluids *because this may alter the results of the analysis.*

Home care

If the patient will be straining his urine at home, teach him how to use a strainer and the importance of straining all his urine for the prescribed period.

Documentation

Chart the time of the specimen collection and transport to the laboratory, if necessary. Describe any filtrate passed, and note any pain or hematuria that occurred during the voiding.

SELECTED REFERENCES

Colella, J., et al. "Urolithiasis/Nephrolithiasis: What's It All About?" *Urologic Nursing* 25(6):427-48, 449, 475, December 2005.

Krieg, C. "The Role of Diet in Prevention of Common Kidney Stones," *Urologic Nursing* 25(6):451-57, December 2005.

Matlaga, B.R., et al. "Changing Composition of Renal Calculi in Patients with Neurogenic Bladder," *Journal of Urology* 175(5):1716-719, May 2006.

Ringold, S., et al. "Kidney Stones," *JAMA* 293(9):1158, March 2005.

STOOL SPECIMENS

STOOL COLLECTION

Stool is collected to determine the presence of blood, ova and parasites, bile, fat, pathogens, or substances such such as ingested drugs. Gross examination of stool characteristics, such as color, consistency, and odor, can reveal such conditions as GI bleeding and steatorrhea.

Stool specimens are collected randomly or for specific periods, such as 72 hours. Because stool specimens can't be obtained on demand, proper collection requires careful instructions to the patient to ensure an uncontaminated specimen.

Equipment

Specimen container with lid ▪ gloves ▪ two tongue blades ▪ paper towel or paper bag ▪ bedpan or portable commode ▪ two patient-care reminders (for timed specimens) ▪ laboratory request form and laboratory biohazard transport bag.

Implementation

- Explain the procedure to the patient and his family, if possible, to ensure their cooperation and prevent inadvertent disposal of timed stool specimens.

Collecting a random specimen

- Tell the patient to notify you when he has the urge to defecate. Have him defecate into a clean, dry bedpan or commode. Instruct him not to contaminate the specimen with urine or toilet tissue *because urine inhibits fecal bacterial growth and toilet tissue contains bismuth, which interferes with test results.*
- Put on gloves.
- Using a tongue blade, transfer the most representative stool specimen from the bedpan to the container, and cap the container. If the patient passes blood, mucus, or pus with the stool, be sure to include this with the specimen.
- Wrap the tongue blade in a paper towel, and discard it. Remove and discard your gloves, and wash your hands thoroughly *to prevent cross-contamination.*

Collecting a timed specimen

- Place a patient-care reminder stating SAVE ALL STOOL over the patient's bed and in his bathroom.
- After putting on gloves, collect the first specimen, and include this in the total specimen.
- Obtain the timed specimen as you would a random specimen, but remember to transfer all stool to the specimen container.

■ If stool must be obtained with an enema, use only tap water or normal saline solution.
■ As ordered, send each specimen to the laboratory immediately with a laboratory request form or, if permitted, refrigerate the specimens collected during the test period, and send them when collection is complete. All specimens must be stored and transported in an approved laboratory biohazard container. Remove and discard gloves.
■ Make sure the patient is comfortable after the procedure and that he has the opportunity to thoroughly clean his hands and perianal area. Perineal care may be necessary for some patients.

Special considerations

■ Never place a stool specimen in a refrigerator that contains food or medication *to prevent contamination.*
■ Notify the practitioner if the stool specimen looks unusual.

Home care

If the patient is to collect a specimen at home, instruct him to collect it in a clean container with a tight-fitting lid, to wrap the container in a brown paper bag, and to keep it in the refrigerator (separate from any food items) until it can be transported.

Documentation

Record the time of specimen collection and transport to the laboratory. Note stool color, odor, and consistency, and unusual characteristics; also note whether the patient had difficulty passing the stool.

Selected references

Centers for Disease Control and Prevention. "Guidelines for Specimen Collection." Available at *http://www.cdc.gov/foodborneoutbreaks/guide_sc.htm.*

Fischbach, F. *A Manual of Laboratory and Diagnostic Tests,* 7th ed. Philadelphia: Lippincott Williams & Wilkins, 2004.

Mai, V., et al. "Timing in Collection of Stool Samples," *Science* 310(5751):1118, November 2005.

Occupational Safety and Health Administration. "Bloodborne Pathogens," 1910.1030. Accessed August 2007 via the Web at *www.osha.gov/pls/oshaweb/owadisp.show_document?p_table=STANDARDS&p_id=10051.*

Fecal occult blood test

Fecal occult blood tests are valuable for determining the presence of occult blood (hidden GI bleeding) and for distinguishing between true melena and melena-like stools. Certain medications, such as iron supplements and bismuth compounds, can darken stools so that they resemble melena.

Two common occult blood screening tests are Hematest (an orthotolidine reagent tablet) and the Hemoccult slide (filter paper impregnated with guaiac). Both tests produce a blue reaction in a fecal smear if occult blood loss exceeds 5 ml in 24 hours. One test, ColoCARE, doesn't require the patient to handle the stool.

Occult blood tests are particularly important for early detection of colorectal cancer because 80% of patients with this disorder test positive. However, a single positive test result doesn't necessarily confirm GI bleeding or indicate colorectal cancer. To confirm a positive result, the test must be repeated at least three times while the patient follows a special diet according to the manufacturers' recommendations for the occult blood test being used. Even then, a confirmed positive test doesn't necessarily indicate colorectal cancer. It does indicate the need for further diagnostic studies because GI bleeding can result from many causes other than cancer, such as ulcers and diverticula. These tests are easily performed on collected specimens or smears from a digital rectal examination.

Equipment

Test kit ■ gloves ■ glass or porcelain plate ■ tongue blade or other wooden applicator.

Implementation

■ Confirm the patient's identity using two patient identifiers according to your facility's policy.
■ Explain the procedure to the patient, and check the patient's history for medications that may interfere with the test.
■ Put on gloves and collect a stool specimen.

Hematest reagent tablet test

■ Use a wooden applicator to smear a bit of the stool specimen on the filter paper supplied with the test kit. Or, after performing a digital rectal examination, wipe the finger you used for the examination on a square of the filter paper.
■ Place the filter paper with the stool smear on a glass plate.
■ Remove a reagent tablet from the bottle, and immediately replace the cap tightly. Then place the tablet in the center of the stool smear on the filter paper.
■ Add one drop of water to the tablet, and allow it to soak in for 5 to 10 seconds. Add a second drop, letting it run from the tablet onto the specimen and filter paper. If necessary, tap the plate gently *to dislodge any water from the top of the tablet.*
■ After 2 minutes, the filter paper will turn blue if the test is positive. Don't read the color that appears on the tablet

HOME CARE

Home tests for fecal occult blood

Most fecal occult blood tests require the patient to collect a specimen of his stool and smear some of it on a slide. In contrast, some new tests don't require the patient to handle stool, making the procedure safer and simpler. One example is a test called Colocare.

If the patient will be performing the Colocare test at home, tell him to avoid red meat and vitamin C supplements for 2 days before the test. He should check with his practitioner about discontinuing any medications before the test. Some drugs that may interfere with test results are aspirin, indomethacin, corticosteroids, phenylbutazone, reserpine, dietary supplements, anticancer drugs, and anticoagulants.

Tell the patient to flush the toilet twice just before performing the test *to remove any toilet-cleaning chemicals from the tank.* Tell him to defecate into the toilet but to throw no toilet paper into the bowl. Within 5 minutes, he should remove the test pad from its pouch and float it printed side up on the surface of the water. Tell him to watch the pad for 15 to 30 seconds for any evidence of blue or green color changes, and have him record the result on the reply card.

Emphasize that he should perform this test with three consecutive bowel movements and then send the completed card to his practitioner. However, he should call his practitioner immediately if he notes a positive color change in the first test.

itself or that develops on the filter paper after the 2-minute period.

- Note the results and discard the filter paper.
- Remove and discard your gloves, and wash your hands thoroughly.

Hemoccult slide test

- Open the flap on the slide packet, and use a wooden applicator to apply a thin smear of the stool specimen to the guaiac-impregnated filter paper exposed in box A. Or, after performing a digital rectal examination, wipe the finger you used for the examination on a square of the filter paper.
- Apply a second smear from another part of the specimen to the filter paper exposed in box B *because some parts of the specimen may not contain blood.*
- Allow the specimens to dry for 3 to 5 minutes.
- Open the flap on the reverse side of the slide package, and place two drops of Hemoccult developing solution on the paper over each smear. A blue reaction will appear in 30 to 60 seconds if the test is positive.
- Record the results and discard the slide package.
- Remove and discard your gloves, and wash your hands thoroughly.

Special considerations

- Make sure stool specimens aren't contaminated with urine, soap solution, or toilet tissue, and test them as soon as possible after collection.
- Test samples from several portions of the same specimen because occult blood from the upper GI tract isn't always evenly dispersed throughout the formed stool; likewise, blood from colorectal bleeding may occur mostly on the outer stool surface.
- Check the condition of the reagent tablets, and note their expiration date. Use only fresh tablets and discard outdated ones. Protect Hematest tablets from moisture, heat, and light.
- Check the expiration date on the hemoccult slides and developer, and protect the unused slides from heat, moisture, light, and chemicals.
- Don't collect samples during or until 3 days after a female's menstrual period *to avoid a false-positive test from contamination of the specimen.*
- Ingestion of 2 to 5 ml of blood, such as from bleeding gums or active bleeding from hemorrhoids, may produce a false positive.
- If repeat testing is necessary after a positive screening test, explain the test to the patient. Instruct him to maintain a high-fiber diet and to refrain from eating red meat, poultry, fish, turnips, and horseradish for 48 to 72 hours before the test as well as throughout the collection period *because these substances may alter test results.*
- As ordered, have the patient discontinue use of iron preparations, bromides, iodides, rauwolfia derivatives, indomethacin, colchicine, salicylates, potassium, phenylbutazone, bismuth compounds, steroids, and ascorbic acid for 48 to 72 hours before the test and during it *to ensure accurate test results and avoid possible bleeding, which some of these compounds may cause.*

Home care

If the patient will be using the Hemoccult slide packet at home, advise him to complete the label on the slide packet before specimen collection. If he'll be using a ColoCARE test packet, inform him that this test is a preliminary screen for occult blood in his stool. Tell him that he won't have to obtain a stool specimen to perform the test but that he should follow your instructions carefully. (See *Home tests for fecal occult blood.*)

Documentation

Record the time and date of the test, the result, and any unusual characteristics of the stool tested. Report positive results to the practitioner.

SELECTED REFERENCES

Fischbach, F. *A Manual of Laboratory and Diagnostic Tests,* 7th ed. Philadelphia: Lippincott Williams & Wilkins, 2004.

Greenwald, B. "A Comparison of Three Stool Tests for Colorectal Cancer Screening," *MedSurg Nursing* 14(5):292-300, October 2005.

Greenwald, B. "A Pilot Study Evaluating Two Alternate Methods of Stool Collection for the Fecal Occult Blood Test,"*MedSurg Nursing* 15(2):89-94, April 2006.

Lastella, V.P. "Fecal Occult Blood Test," *Gastroenterology* 130(1):285, January 2006.

National Cancer Institute. "Screening for Colorectal Cancer." Accessed August 2007 via the Web at *http://cis.nci.nih.gov/fact/5_31.htm.*

"Review Criteria for Assessment of Qualitative Fecal Occult Blood In Vitro Diagnostic Devices," U.S. Department of Health and Human Services, Food and Drug Administration, August 8, 2007.

OTHER SPECIMENS

SPUTUM COLLECTION

Secreted by mucous membranes lining the bronchioles, bronchi, and trachea, sputum helps protect the respiratory tract from infection. When expelled from the respiratory tract, sputum carries saliva, nasal and sinus secretions, dead cells, and normal oral bacteria from the respiratory tract. Sputum specimens may be cultured for identification of respiratory pathogens.

The usual method of sputum specimen collection, expectoration, may require ultrasonic nebulization, hydration, or chest percussion and postural drainage. Less common methods include tracheal suctioning and, rarely, bronchoscopy. Tracheal suctioning is contraindicated within 1 hour of eating and in patients with esophageal varices, nausea, facial or basilar skull fractures, laryngospasm, or bronchospasm. It should be performed cautiously in patients with heart disease because it may precipitate arrhythmias.

Equipment

For expectoration: Sterile specimen container with tight-fitting cap ▪ gloves ▪ label ▪ laboratory request form and laboratory biohazard transport bag ▪ aerosol (10% sodium chloride, propylene glycol, acetylcysteine, or sterile or distilled water), as ordered ▪ facial tissues ▪ emesis basin.

For tracheal suctioning: #12 to #14 French sterile suction catheter ▪ water-soluble lubricant ▪ laboratory request form and laboratory biohazard transport bag ▪ sterile gloves ▪ mask ▪ goggles ▪ sterile in-line specimen trap (Lukens trap) ▪ normal saline solution ▪ portable suction machine, if wall unit is unavailable ▪ oxygen therapy equipment ▪ optional: nasal airway, to obtain a nasotracheal specimen with suctioning, if needed. Commercial suction kits are available that contain the suction catheter, lubricant, sterile gloves, and specimen trap.

Preparation of equipment

Equipment and preparation depend on the method of collection. Gather the appropriate equipment for the task.

Implementation

- Confirm the patient's identity using two patient identifiers according to your facility's policy.
- Tell the patient that you'll collect a specimen of sputum (not saliva), and explain the procedure *to promote cooperation.* If possible, collect the specimen early in the morning, before breakfast, *to obtain an overnight accumulation of secretions.*

Collection by expectoration

- Instruct the patient to sit in a chair or at the edge of the bed. If he can't sit up, place him in high Fowler's position.
- Ask the patient to rinse his mouth with water *to reduce specimen contamination.* (Avoid mouthwash or toothpaste *because they may affect the mobility of organisms in the sputum sample.*) Then tell him to cough deeply and expectorate directly into the specimen container. Ask him to produce at least 15 ml of sputum, if possible.
- Put on gloves.
- Cap the container and, if necessary, clean its exterior. Remove and discard your gloves, and wash your hands thoroughly.
- Label the container with the patient's name and room number, practitioner's name, date and time of collection, and initial diagnosis. Also include on the laboratory request form whether the patient was febrile or taking antibiotics and whether sputum was induced *(because such specimens commonly appear watery and may resemble saliva).* Send the specimen to the laboratory immediately in a laboratory biohazard transport bag.

EQUIPMENT

Attaching a specimen trap to a suction catheter

Wearing gloves, push the suction tubing onto the male adapter of the in-line trap.

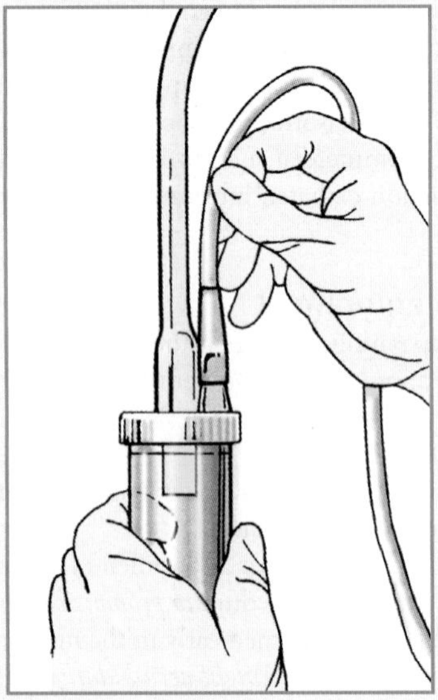

Insert the suction catheter into the rubber tubing of the trap.

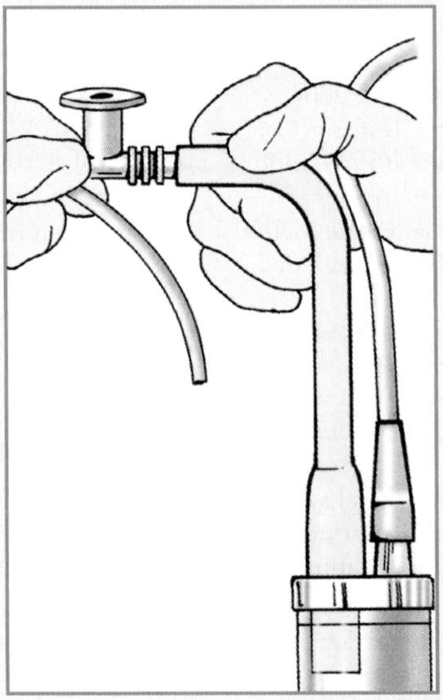

After suctioning, disconnect the in-line trap from the suction tubing and catheter. To seal the container, connect the rubber tubing to the male adapter of the trap

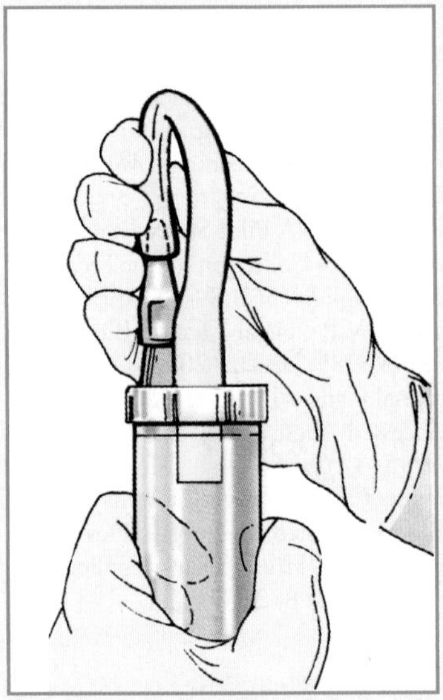

Collection by tracheal suctioning

■ If the patient can't produce an adequate specimen by coughing, prepare to suction him to obtain the specimen. Explain the suctioning procedure to him, and tell him that he may cough, gag, or feel short of breath during the procedure.

■ Check the suction machine *to make sure it's functioning properly*. Then place the patient in high Fowler's or semi-Fowler's position.

■ Administer oxygen to the patient before beginning the procedure.

■ Wash your hands thoroughly.

■ Put on sterile gloves. Consider one hand sterile and the other hand clean *to prevent cross-contamination.*

■ Connect the suction tubing to the male adapter of the in-line specimen trap. Attach the sterile suction catheter to the rubber tubing of the trap. (See *Attaching a specimen trap to a suction catheter.*)

■ Position a mask and goggles over your face. Tell the patient to tilt his head back slightly. Then lubricate the catheter with normal saline solution, and gently pass it through the patient's nostril without suction.

■ When the catheter reaches the larynx, the patient will cough. As he does, quickly advance the catheter into the trachea. Tell him to take several deep breaths through his mouth *to ease insertion.*

■ To obtain the specimen, apply suction for 5 to 10 seconds but never longer than 15 seconds *because prolonged suction can cause hypoxia.* If the procedure must be repeated, let the patient rest for four to six breaths. When collection is completed, discontinue the suction, gently remove the catheter, and administer oxygen.

■ Detach the catheter from the in-line trap, gather it up in your dominant hand, and pull the glove cuff inside out and down around the used catheter to enclose it for disposal. Remove and discard the other glove and your mask and goggles.

■ Detach the trap from the tubing connected to the suction machine. Seal the trap tightly by connecting the rubber tubing to the male adapter of the trap. Examine the specimen *to make sure it's actually sputum, not saliva.*

■ Label the trap's container as an expectorated specimen, place in a laboratory biohazard transport bag, and send it to the laboratory immediately with a completed laboratory request form.

■ Offer the patient a glass of water or mouthwash.

Special considerations

■ If you can't obtain a sputum specimen through tracheal suctioning, perform chest percussion *to loosen and mobilize secretions,* and position the patient for optimal drainage. After 20 to 30 minutes, repeat the tracheal suctioning procedure.

■ Before sending the specimen to the laboratory, examine it to make sure it's actually sputum, not saliva, *because saliva will produce inaccurate test results.*

■ *Because expectorated sputum is contaminated by normal mouth flora,* tracheal suctioning provides a more reliable specimen for diagnosis.

■ If the patient becomes hypoxic or cyanotic during suctioning, remove the catheter immediately and administer oxygen.

■ If the patient has asthma or chronic bronchitis, watch for aggravated bronchospasms with the use of more than a 10% concentration of sodium chloride or acetylcysteine in an aerosol. If he's suspected of having tuberculosis, don't use more than 20% propylene glycol with water when inducing a sputum specimen *because a higher concentration inhibits growth of the pathogen and causes erroneous test results.* If propylene glycol isn't available, use 10% to 20% acetylcysteine with water or sodium chloride.

Complications

Patients with cardiac disease may develop arrhythmias during the procedure as a result of coughing, especially when the specimen is obtained by suctioning. Other potential complications include tracheal trauma or bleeding, vomiting, aspiration, and hypoxemia.

Documentation

In your notes, record the collection method used, time and date of collection, how the patient tolerated the procedure, color and consistency of the specimen, and its proper disposition.

SELECTED REFERENCES

Agnes,K., and Condon, M. "Tuberculosis Guidelines and Update," *AJN* 106(6):104, June 2006.

Lynn, P. *Taylor's Clinical Nursing Skills,* 2nd ed. Philadelphia: Lippincott Williams & Wilkins, 2007.

Villarino, M., and Mazurek, G. "Tuberculosis Contact, Concerns, and Controls: What Matters for Healthcare Workers," *Infection Control and Hospital Epidemiology* 27(5):433-35, May 2006.

LUMBAR PUNCTURE

Lumbar puncture involves the insertion of a sterile needle into the subarachnoid space of the spinal canal, usually between the third and fourth lumbar vertebrae. This procedure is used to determine the presence of blood in cerebrospinal fluid (CSF), to obtain CSF specimens for laboratory analysis, and to inject dyes for contrast in radiologic studies. The pressure of the CSF, which flows freely between the brain and the spinal column, may be measured during the procedure. It's also used to administer drugs or anesthetics and to relieve intracranial pressure (ICP) by removing CSF.

Performed by a physician or advanced practice nurse, lumbar puncture requires sterile technique and careful patient positioning. This procedure is contraindicated in patients with ICP, lumbar deformity, or infection at the puncture site. It isn't recommended in patients with increased ICP because the rapid reduction in pressure that follows withdrawal of CSF can cause tonsillar herniation and medullary compression.

Equipment

Overbed table ■ one or two pairs of sterile gloves for the physician ■ sterile gloves for the nurse ■ face masks ■ antiseptic solution ■ sterile gauze pads ■ alcohol pads ■ sterile fenestrated drape ■ 3-ml syringe for local anesthetic ■ 25G ¾″ sterile needle for injecting anesthetic ■ local anesthetic (usually 1% lidocaine) ■ 18G or 20G 3½″ spinal needle with stylet (22G needle for children) ■ three-way stopcock ■ manometer ■ small adhesive bandage ■ three sterile collection tubes with stoppers ■ laboratory request forms and laboratory biohazard transport bag ■ labels ■ light source such as a gooseneck lamp ■ sterile marker ■ sterile labels ■ optional: patient-care reminder.

Disposable lumbar puncture trays contain most of the needed sterile equipment.

Preparation of equipment

Gather the equipment, and take it to the patient's bedside.

Implementation

■ Confirm the patient's identity using two patient identifiers according to your facility's policy.

■ Explain the procedure to the patient *to ease his anxiety and ensure his cooperation.* Make sure a consent form has been signed.

Positioning for lumbar puncture

Have the patient lie on his side at the edge of the bed, with his chin tucked to his chest and his knees drawn up to his abdomen. Make sure the patient's spine is curved and his back is at the edge of the bed (as shown below). *This position widens the spaces between the vertebrae, easing insertion of the needle.*

To help the patient maintain this position, place one of your hands behind his neck and the other hand behind his knees, and pull gently. Hold the patient firmly in this position throughout the procedure *to prevent accidental needle displacement.*

Patient positioning

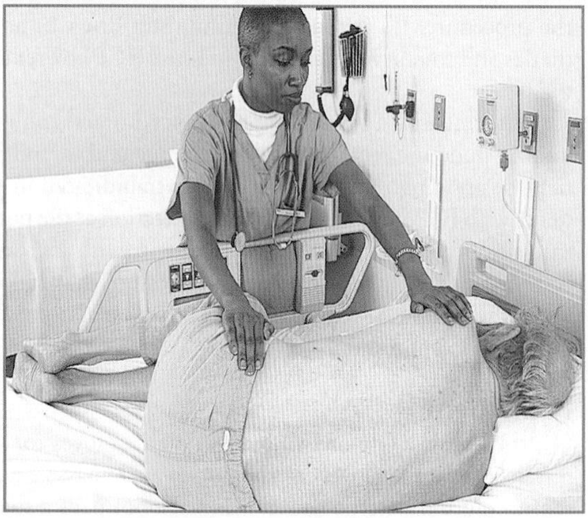

Typically, the physician inserts the needle between the third and fourth lumbar vertebrae (as shown below).

Needle insertion

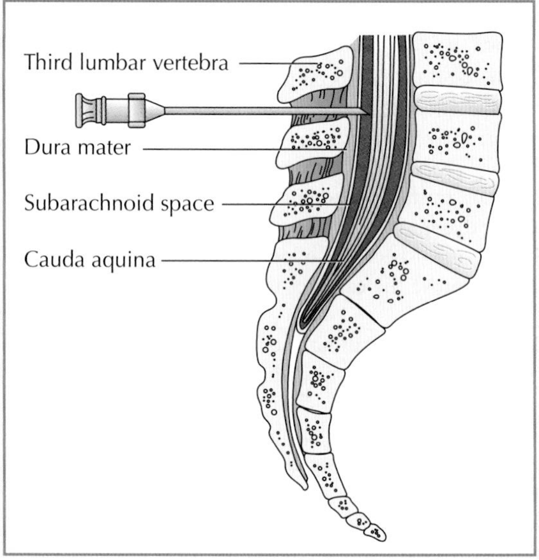

■ Inform the patient that he may experience headache after lumbar puncture, but reassure him that his cooperation during the procedure minimizes such an effect. (*Note:* Sedatives and analgesics are usually withheld before this test if there's evidence of a central nervous system disorder *because they may mask important symptoms.*)
■ Immediately before the procedure, provide privacy, and instruct the patient to void.
■ Wash your hands thoroughly.
■ Open the equipment tray on an overbed table, being careful not to contaminate the sterile field when you open the wrapper. Label all medications, medication containers, and other solutions on and off the sterile field.
■ Provide adequate lighting at the puncture site, and adjust the height of the patient's bed *to allow the physician to perform the procedure comfortably.*
■ Position the patient and reemphasize the importance of remaining as still as possible *to minimize discomfort and trauma.* (See *Positioning for lumbar puncture.*)
■ The physician cleans the puncture site with sterile gauze pads soaked in antiseptic solution, wiping in a circular motion away from the puncture site; he uses three different pads *to prevent contamination of spinal tissues by the body's normal skin flora.* Next, he drapes the area with the fenestrated drape *to provide a sterile field.* (If the physician uses povidone-iodine pads instead of sterile gauze pads, he may remove his sterile gloves and put on another pair *to avoid introducing povidone-iodine into the subarachnoid space with the lumbar puncture needle.*)
■ If no ampule of anesthetic is included on the equipment tray, clean the injection port of a multidose vial of anesthetic with an alcohol pad. Then invert the vial 45 degrees so that the physician can insert a 25G needle and syringe and withdraw the anesthetic for injection.

■ Before the physician injects the anesthetic, tell the patient he'll experience a transient burning sensation and local pain. Ask him to report any other persistent pain or sensations *because they may indicate irritation or puncture of a nerve root, requiring repositioning of the needle.*
■ When the physician inserts the sterile spinal needle into the subarachnoid space between the third and fourth lumbar vertebrae, instruct the patient to remain still and breathe normally. If necessary, hold the patient firmly in position *to prevent sudden movement that may displace the needle.*
■ If the lumbar puncture is being performed to administer contrast media for radiologic studies or spinal anesthetic, the physician injects the dye or anesthetic at this time.
■ When the needle is in place, the physician attaches a manometer with a three-way stopcock to the needle hub *to read CSF pressure.* If ordered, help the patient extend his legs *to provide a more accurate pressure reading.*
■ The physician then detaches the manometer and allows CSF to drain from the needle hub into the collection tubes. When he has collected 2 to 3 ml in each tube, mark the tubes in sequence, insert a stopper to secure them, and label them.
■ If the physician suspects an obstruction in the spinal subarachnoid space, he may check for Queckenstedt's sign. After he takes an initial CSF pressure reading, compress the patient's jugular vein for 10 seconds as ordered. *This increases ICP and—if no subarachnoid block exists—causes CSF pressure to rise as well.* The physician then takes pressure readings every 10 seconds until the pressure stabilizes.
■ After the physician collects the specimens and removes the spinal needle, clean the puncture site with povidone-iodine, and apply a small adhesive bandage.
■ Send the CSF specimens to the laboratory immediately, with completed laboratory request forms in a laboratory biohazard transport bag.

Special considerations

■ During lumbar puncture, watch closely for signs of adverse reaction: elevated pulse rate, pallor, and clammy skin. Alert the physician immediately to any significant changes.
■ The patient may be ordered to lie flat for 8 to 12 hours after the procedure *to allow the restoration of spinal fluid to prevent postspinal headache.* If necessary, place a patient-care reminder on his bed to this effect.
■ Collected CSF specimens must be sent to the laboratory immediately; they can't be refrigerated for later transport.
■ Encourage the patient to drink fluids after the procedure *to reduce the risk of spinal headache.*
■ Check the puncture site for redness, swelling, and drainage every hour for the first 4 hours and then every 4 hours for the next 24 hours.

Complications

Headache is the most common adverse effect of lumbar puncture. Others include a reaction to the anesthetic, meningitis, epidural or subdural abscess, bleeding into the spinal canal, CSF leakage through the dural defect remaining after needle withdrawal, local pain caused by nerve root irritation, edema or hematoma at the puncture site, transient difficulty voiding, and fever. The most serious complications of lumbar puncture, although rare, are tonsillar herniation and medullary compression.

Documentation

Record the initiation and completion times of the procedure, the patient's response, administration of drugs, number of specimen tubes collected, time of transport to the laboratory, and color, consistency, and any other characteristics of the collected specimens.

SELECTED REFERENCES

Lenfeldt, N., et al. "CSF Pressure Assessed by Lumbar Punture Agrees with Intracranial Pressure," *Neurology* 68(2):155-58, January 2007.
Rushing, J. "Assisting with Lumbar Puncture," *Nursing* 37(1):23, January 2007.
Straus, S.E., et al. "How Do I Perform a Lumbar Puncture and Analyze the Results to Diagnose Bacterial Meningitis?" *JAMA* 296(16):2012-2022, October 2006.
Strout, T.D., et al. "Reducing Pain in ED Patients during Lumbar Puncture: The Efficacy and Feasibility of Iontophoresis, Collaborative Approach," *Journal of Emergency Nursing* 30(5):423-30, October 2004.

PAPANICOLAOU TEST

Also known as the *Pap test* or *Pap smear,* this cytologic test developed in the 1920s by George N. Papanicolaou allows early detection of cervical cancer. The test involves scraping secretions from the cervix, spreading them on a slide, and immediately coating the slide with fixative spray or solution to preserve specimen cells for nuclear staining. Alternately, the collection device may be rinsed in a vial of fluid transport medium for slide preparation in the laboratory. Cytologic evaluation then outlines cell maturity, morphology, and metabolic activity. Although cervical scrapings are the most common test specimen, the Pap test also permits cytologic evaluation of the vaginal pool, prostatic secretions, urine, gastric secretions, cavity fluids, bronchial aspirations, and sputum.

Using a vaginal speculum

The following three steps show you how to insert a vaginal speculum.

1. Insert the speculum into the vagina holding the blades obliquely.

2. As the blades pass the introitus, rotate the blades to a horizontal position.

3. Separate the blades by depressing the thumbscrew and elevating the handle. The blades maintain their position by adjustment of the thumbscrew.

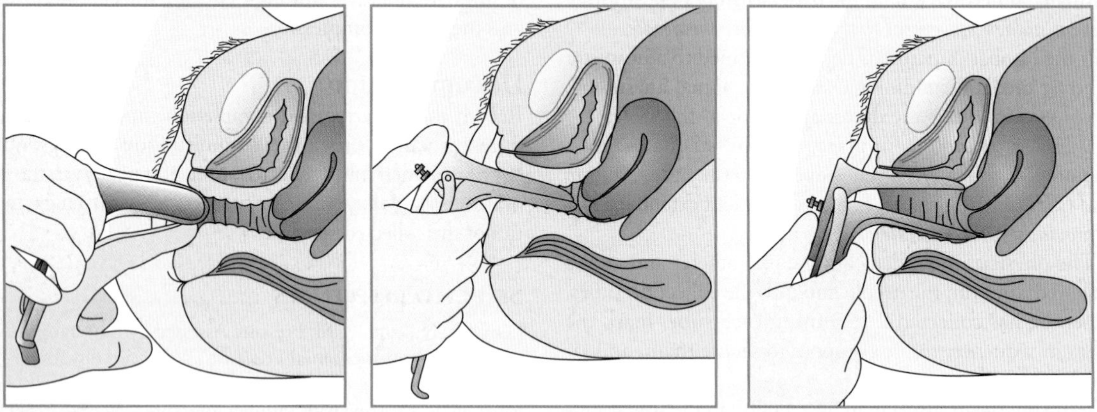

Equipment

Bivalve vaginal speculum ▪ gloves ▪ cervical sampling device (wooden spatula or broom collection device such as Cytobrush or Cervexbrush) ▪ long cotton-tipped applicator ▪ three glass microscope slides and fixative (a commercial spray or 95% ethyl alcohol solution) or vial of preservative (such as ThinPrep) ▪ adjustable lamp ▪ drape ▪ laboratory request forms and laboratory biohazard transport bag.

Preparation of equipment

Select a speculum of the appropriate size, and gather the equipment in the examining room. Label each glass slide with the patient's name and the letter "E," "C," or "V" *to differentiate endocervical, cervical, and vaginal specimens.* If using a liquid-based Pap test, label the vial of preservative and open it.

Implementation

- Confirm the patient's identity using two patient identifiers according to your facility's policy.
- Explain the procedure to the patient, and wash your hands.
- Instruct the patient to void *to relax the perineal muscles and facilitate bimanual examination of the uterus.*
- Provide privacy, and instruct the patient to undress below the waist but to wear her shoes, if desired, *to cushion her feet against the stirrups.* Then instruct her to sit on the examination table and to drape her genital region.
- Place the patient in the lithotomy position, with her feet in the stirrups and her buttocks extended slightly beyond the edge of the table. Adjust the drape.
- Adjust the lamp so that it fully illuminates the genital area. Then fold back the corner of the drape to expose the perineum.
- If you're performing the procedure, first put on gloves. Then take the speculum in your dominant hand and moisten it with warm water *to ease insertion.* Avoid using water-soluble lubricants, *which can interfere with accurate laboratory testing.*
- Warn the patient that you're about to touch her *to avoid startling her.* Then gently separate the labia with the thumb and forefinger of your nondominant hand.
- Instruct the patient to take several deep breaths, and insert the speculum into the vagina. Once it's in place, slowly open the blades to expose the cervix. Then lock the blades in place. (See *Using a vaginal speculum.*)
- Insert a cotton-tipped applicator through the speculum 5 mm into the cervical os. Rotate the applicator 360 degrees to obtain an endocervical specimen. Then remove the applicator, and gently roll it in a circle across the slide marked "E." Refrain from rubbing the applicator on the slide *to prevent cell destruction.* Immediately place the slide in a fixative

solution, or spray it with a fixative *to prevent drying of the cells, which interferes with nuclear staining and cytologic interpretation.*

- Insert the small curved end of the Pap stick through the speculum, and place it directly over the cervical os. Rotate the stick gently but firmly *to scrape cells loose.* Remove the stick, spread the specimen across the slide marked "C," and fix it immediately, as before.
- Insert the opposite end of the Pap stick or a cotton-tipped applicator through the speculum, and scrape the posterior fornix or vaginal pool, an area that collects cells from the endometrium, vagina, and cervix. Remove the stick or applicator, spread the specimen across the slide marked "V," and fix it immediately.
- If you're using the liquid-based Pap test, collect the sample from the patient by rotating the broom-like device 360 degrees on the cervix five times. Rinse the collection device in the vial of preservative solution, and seal the container.
- Unlock the speculum *to ease removal and avoid accidentally pinching the vaginal wall.* Withdraw the speculum.
- Remove the glove from your nondominant hand to perform the bimanual examination, which usually follows the Pap test. Remove your other glove and discard both gloves.
- Gently remove the patient's feet from the stirrups, and assist her to a sitting position. Provide privacy for her to dress.
- Fill out the appropriate laboratory request forms, including the date of the patient's last menses. Place the specimen in a laboratory biohazard transport bag, and send it to the laboratory.

Special considerations

- Many preventable factors can interfere with the Pap test's accuracy, so provide appropriate patient teaching beforehand. For example, use of a vaginal douche in the 48-hour period before specimen collection washes away cellular deposits and prevents adequate sampling. Instillation of vaginal medications in the same period makes cytologic interpretation difficult. Collection of a specimen during menstruation prevents adequate sampling because menstrual flow washes away cells; ideally, such collection should take place 5 to 6 days before menses or 1 week after it. Application of topical antibiotics promotes rapid, heavy shedding of cells and requires postponement of the Pap test for at least 1 month.
- If the patient has had a complete hysterectomy, collect test specimens from the vaginal pool and cuff.
- The American College of Obstetricians and Gynecologists recommends annual Pap tests starting within 3 years of vaginal intercourse or by age 21 until age 30. After age 30, and if a healthy woman has had three consecutive normal Pap tests, she may be able to increase the test intervals to every 2 to 3 years while still having routine gynecologic exams. Women who have human immunodeficiency virus infection, multiple partners, or other risk factors should continue testing on a yearly basis.

Complications

Failure to unlock the speculum blades before removal can pinch vaginal tissue. Slight cramping normally accompanies this examination, but rough handling of the speculum can cause severe cramping. Scraping an inflamed cervix with the Pap stick can cause slight bleeding.

Documentation

On the patient's chart, record the date and time of specimen collection, any complications, and the nursing action taken.

SELECTED REFERENCES

Buechler, E.J. "Pap Tests and HPV Infection. Advances in Screening and Interpretation," *Postgraduate Medicine* 118(2):37-40, 43-46, August 2005.

Rosenthal, D.L., et al. "The PapSpin: A Reasonable Alternative to Other, More Expensive Liquid-Based Papanicolaou Tests," *Cancer* 108(3):137-43, June 2006.

Schan, M. "What are the Current Pap Test Guidelines," *Nursing* 34(12):26, December 2004.

Sperling, R. "American College of Obstetricians and Gynecologists Releases New Guidelines for Papanicolaou (Pap) Tests," *Home Healthcare Nurse* 22(3):163, March 2004.

Tiffen, J., and Mahon, S. "Cerival Cancer Screening: What Should We Tell Women about Screening?" *Clinical Journal of Oncology Nursing* 10(4):527-31, August 2006.

SWAB SPECIMENS

Correct collection and handling of swab specimens helps the laboratory staff identify pathogens accurately with a minimum of contamination from normal bacterial flora. Collection normally involves sampling inflamed tissues and exudates from the throat, nasopharynx, wounds, eye, ear, or rectum with sterile swabs of cotton or other absorbent material. The type of swab used depends on the part of the body affected. For example, collection of a nasopharyngeal specimen requires a cotton-tipped swab.

After the specimen has been collected, the swab is immediately placed in a sterile tube containing a transport medium and, in the case of sampling for anaerobes, an inert gas. Swab specimens are usually collected to identify pathogens and sometimes to identify asymptomatic carriers of certain easily transmitted disease organisms.

Equipment

For a throat specimen: Gloves ▪ tongue blade ▪ penlight ▪ sterile cotton-tipped swab ▪ sterile culture tube with transport medium (or commercial collection kit) ▪ label ▪ laboratory request form and laboratory biohazard transport bag.

For a nasopharyngeal specimen: Gloves ▪ penlight ▪ sterile, flexible cotton-tipped swab ▪ tongue blade ▪ sterile culture tube with transport medium ▪ label ▪ laboratory request form and laboratory biohazard transport bag ▪ optional: small open-ended Pyrex tube or nasal speculum.

For a wound specimen: Sterile gloves ▪ sterile forceps ▪ alcohol or povidone-iodine pads ▪ sterile swabs ▪ sterile 10-ml syringe ▪ 21G needle ▪ sterile culture tube with transport medium (or commercial collection kit for aerobic culture) ▪ labels ▪ special anaerobic culture tube containing carbon dioxide or nitrogen ▪ fresh dressings for the wound ▪ laboratory request form and laboratory biohazard transport bag ▪ optional: rubber stopper for needle.

For an ear specimen: Gloves ▪ normal saline solution ▪ two 2″ × 2″ gauze pads ▪ sterile swabs ▪ sterile culture tube with transport medium ▪ label ▪ 10-ml syringe and 22G 1″ needle (for tympanocentesis) ▪ label ▪ laboratory request form and laboratory biohazard transport bag.

For an eye specimen: Sterile gloves ▪ sterile normal saline solution ▪ two 2″ × 2″ gauze pads ▪ sterile swabs ▪ sterile wire culture loop (for corneal scraping) ▪ sterile culture tube with transport medium ▪ label ▪ laboratory request form and laboratory biohazard transport bag.

For a rectal specimen: Gloves ▪ soap and water ▪ washcloth ▪ sterile swab ▪ normal saline solution ▪ sterile culture tube with transport medium ▪ label ▪ laboratory request form and laboratory biohazard transport bag.

Implementation

▪ Confirm the patient's identity using two patient identifiers according to your facility's policy. Explain the procedure to the patient *to ease his anxiety and ensure cooperation.*

Collecting a throat specimen

▪ Tell the patient that he may gag during the swabbing but that the procedure will probably take less than 1 minute.
▪ Instruct the patient to sit erect at the edge of the bed or in a chair, facing you. Then wash your hands and put on gloves.
▪ Ask the patient to tilt his head back. Depress his tongue with the tongue blade, and illuminate his throat with the penlight *to check for inflamed areas.*
▪ If the patient starts to gag, withdraw the tongue blade and tell him to breathe deeply. Once he's relaxed, reinsert the tongue blade but not as deeply as before.
▪ Using the cotton-tipped swab, wipe the tonsillar areas from side to side, including any inflamed or purulent sites. Make sure you don't touch the tongue, cheeks, or teeth with the swab *to avoid contaminating it with oral bacteria.*
▪ Withdraw the swab and immediately place it in the culture tube. If you're using a commercial kit, crush the ampule of culture medium at the bottom of the tube, and then push the swab, into the medium *to keep the swab moist.*
▪ Remove and discard your gloves, and wash your hands.
▪ Label the specimen with the patient's name and identification number, the practitioner's name, and the date, time, and site of collection.
▪ On the laboratory request form, indicate whether any organism is strongly suspected, especially *Corynebacterium diphtheriae* (requires two swabs and special growth medium), *Bordetella pertussis* (requires a nasopharyngeal culture and special growth medium), and *Neisseria meningitidis* (requires enriched selective media).
▪ Place in a laboratory biohazard transport bag, and send the specimen to the laboratory immediately *to prevent growth or deterioration of microbes.*

Collecting a nasopharyngeal specimen

▪ Tell the patient that he may gag or feel the urge to sneeze during the swabbing but that the procedure takes less than 1 minute.
▪ Have the patient sit erect at the edge of the bed or in a chair, facing you. Then wash your hands and put on gloves.
▪ Ask the patient to blow his nose *to clear his nasal passages.* Then check his nostrils for patency with a penlight.
▪ Tell the patient to occlude one nostril first and then the other as he exhales. Listen for the more patent nostril *because you'll insert the swab through it.*
▪ Ask the patient to cough *to bring organisms to the nasopharynx for a better specimen.*
▪ While it's still in the package, bend the sterile swab in a curve, and then open the package without contaminating the swab.
▪ Ask the patient to tilt his head back, and gently pass the swab through the more patent nostril about 3″ to 4″ (7.5 to 10 cm) into the nasopharynx, keeping the swab near the septum and floor of the nose. Rotate the swab quickly and remove it. (See *Obtaining a nasopharyngeal specimen.*)
▪ Alternatively, depress the patient's tongue with a tongue blade, and pass the bent swab up behind the uvula. Rotate the swab and withdraw it.
▪ Remove the cap from the culture tube, insert the swab, and break off the contaminated end. Then close the tube tightly.
▪ Remove and discard your gloves, and wash your hands.

■ Label the specimen for culture, complete a laboratory request form, and send the specimen to the laboratory immediately in a laboratory biohazard transport bag. If you're collecting a specimen to isolate a possible virus, check with the laboratory for the recommended collection technique.

Collecting a wound specimen
■ Wash your hands, prepare a sterile field, and put on sterile gloves. With sterile forceps, remove the dressing to expose the wound. Dispose of the soiled dressings properly.
■ Clean the area around the wound with an alcohol or a povidone-iodine pad *to reduce the risk of contaminating the specimen with skin bacteria.* Then allow the area to dry.
■ For an aerobic culture, use a sterile cotton-tipped swab to collect as much exudate as possible, or insert the swab deeply into the wound, and gently rotate it. Remove the swab from the wound, and immediately place it in the aerobic culture tube. Send the tube to the laboratory immediately with a completed laboratory request form. Never collect exudate from the skin and then insert the same swab into the wound; *this could contaminate the wound with skin bacteria.*
■ For an anaerobic culture, insert the sterile cotton-tipped swab deeply into the wound, rotate it gently, remove it, and immediately place it in the anaerobic culture tube. (See *Obtaning an anaerobic specimen,* page 218.) Or insert a sterile 10-ml syringe, without a needle, into the wound, and aspirate 1 to 5 ml of exudate into the syringe. Then attach the 21G needle to the syringe, and immediately inject the aspirate into the anaerobic culture tube. If an anaerobic culture tube is unavailable, obtain a rubber stopper, attach the needle to the syringe, and gently push all the air out of the syringe by pressing on the plunger. Stick the needle tip into the rubber stopper, remove and discard your gloves, and send the syringe of aspirate to the laboratory immediately with a completed laboratory request form in a laboratory biohazard transport bag.
■ Put on sterile gloves.
■ Apply a new dressing to the wound. (See chapter 4, Physical treatments.)

Collecting an external ear specimen
■ Wash your hands and put on gloves.
■ Gently clean excess debris from the patient's ear with normal saline solution and gauze pads.
■ Insert the sterile swab into the ear canal, and rotate it gently along the walls of the canal *to avoid damaging the eardrum.*
■ Withdraw the swab, being careful not to touch other surfaces *to avoid contaminating the specimen.*
■ Place the swab in the sterile culture tube with transport medium.
■ Remove and discard your gloves, and wash your hands.

Obtaining a nasopharyngeal specimen

After you've passed the swab into the nasopharynx, quickly but gently rotate the swab to collect the specimen. Then remove the swab, taking care not to injure the nasal mucous membrane.

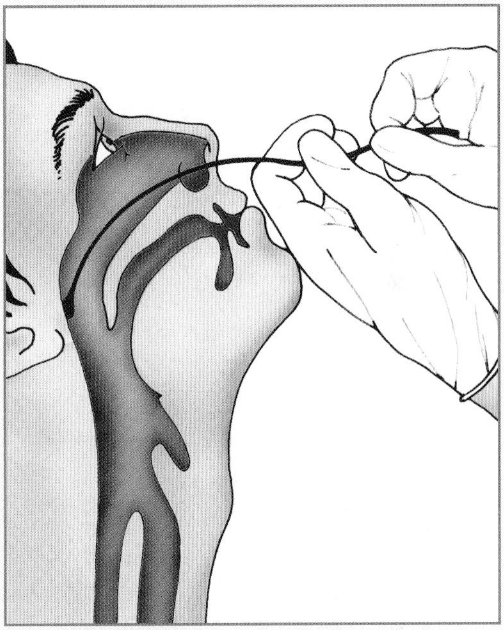

■ Label the specimen for culture, complete a laboratory request form, and send the specimen to the laboratory immediately in a laboratory biohazard transport bag.

Collecting a middle ear specimen
■ Put on gloves and clean the outer ear with normal saline solution and gauze pads. Remove and discard your gloves. After the physician punctures the eardrum with a needle and aspirates fluid into the syringe, label the container, complete a laboratory request form, and send the specimen to the laboratory immediately in a laboratory biohazard transport bag.

Collecting an eye specimen
■ Wash your hands and put on sterile gloves.
■ Gently clean excess debris from the outside of the eye with normal saline solution and gauze pads, wiping from the inner to the outer canthus.

EQUIPMENT

Obtaining an anaerobic specimen

Because most anaerobes die when exposed to oxygen, they must be transported in tubes filled with carbon dioxide or nitrogen. The anaerobic specimen collector shown here includes a rubber-stoppered tube filled with carbon dioxide, a small inner tube, and a swab attached to a plastic plunger.

Before specimen collection, the small inner tube containing the swab is held in place with the rubber stopper (as shown below left). After collecting the specimen, quickly replace the swab in the inner tube and depress the plunger to separate the inner tube from the stopper (as shown below right), forcing it into the larger tube and exposing the specimen to a carbon dioxide-rich environment.

Before

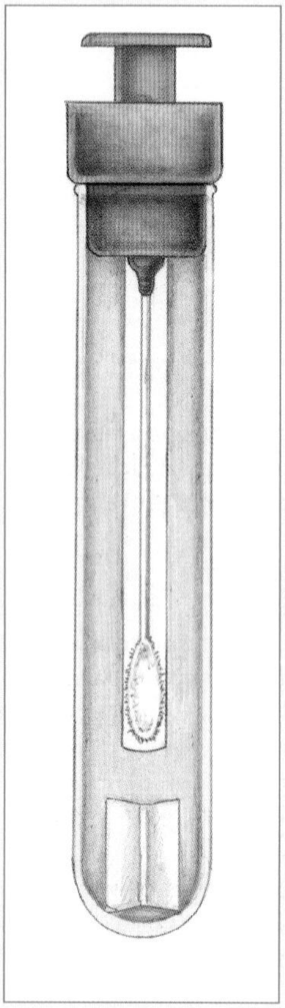

After

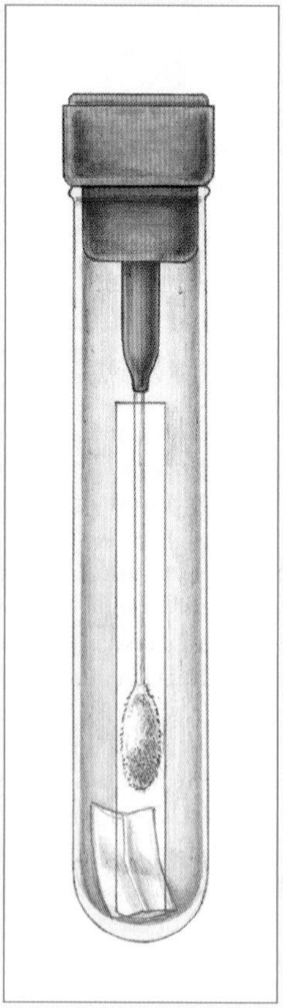

■ Retract the lower eyelid to expose the conjunctival sac. Gently rub the sterile swab over the conjunctiva, being careful not to touch other surfaces. Hold the swab parallel to the eye, rather than pointed directly at it, *to prevent corneal irritation or trauma due to sudden movement.* (If a corneal scraping is required, this procedure is performed by a physician, using a wire culture loop.)
■ Immediately place the swab or wire loop in the culture tube with transport medium.
■ Remove and discard your gloves, and wash your hands.
■ Label the specimen for culture, complete a laboratory request form, and send the specimen to the laboratory immediately in a laboratory biohazard transport bag.

Collecting a rectal specimen

■ Wash your hands and put on gloves.
■ Clean the area around the patient's anus using a washcloth and soap and water.
■ Insert the swab, moistened with normal saline solution or sterile broth medium, through the anus, and advance it about 3⁄8″ (1 cm) for infants or 1½″ (4 cm) for adults. While withdrawing the swab, gently rotate it against the walls of the lower rectum *to sample a large area of the rectal mucosa.*
■ Place the swab in a culture tube with transport medium.
■ Remove and discard your gloves, and wash your hands.
■ Label the specimen for culture, complete a laboratory request form, and send the specimen to the laboratory immediately in a laboratory biohazard transport bag.

Special considerations

■ Note recent antibiotic therapy on the laboratory request form.
■ *For a wound specimen:* Although you would normally clean the area around a wound to prevent contamination by normal skin flora, don't clean a perineal wound with alcohol *because this could irritate sensitive tissues.* Also, make sure that antiseptic doesn't enter the wound.
■ *For an eye specimen:* Don't use an antiseptic before culturing *to avoid irritating the eye and inhibiting growth of organisms in the culture.* If the patient is a child or an uncooperative adult, ask a coworker to restrain the patient's head *to prevent eye trauma resulting from sudden movement.*

Documentation

Record the time, date, and site of specimen collection and any recent or current antibiotic therapy. Also note whether the specimen has an unusual appearance or odor.

SELECTED REFERENCES

Brook, I., and Gober, A.E. "Recovery of Potential Pathogens and Interfering Bacteria in the Nasopharynx of Smokers and Nonsmokers," *Chest* 127(6):2072-2075, June 2005.

Centers for Disease Control and Prevention. "Public Health Guidance for Community-level Preparedness and Response to Severe Acute Respiratory Syndrome (SARS)," Version 2, Supplement F: Laboratory Guidance. Accessed August 2007 via the Web at *www.cdc.gov/ncidod/sars/guidance/f/word/app4.doc.*

Clinical and Laboratory Standards Institute. "Quality Control of Microbiological Transport Systems," Approved Standard, M40, 2003.

Fischbach, F. *A Manual of Laboratory and Diagnostic Tests,* 7th ed. Philadelphia: Lippincott Williams & Wilkins, 2004.

Macfarlane, P., et al. "RSV Testing in Bronchiolitis: Which Nasal Sampling Method is Best?" *Archives of Diseases in Childhood* 90(6):634-35, June 2005.

Rushing, J. "Obtaining a Throat Culture," *Nursing* 37(3):20, March 2007.

BONE MARROW ASPIRATION AND BIOPSY

A specimen of bone marrow—the major site of blood cell formation—may be obtained by aspiration or needle biopsy. The procedure allows evaluation of overall blood composition by studying blood elements and precursor cells as well as abnormal or malignant cells. Aspiration removes cells through a needle inserted into the marrow cavity of the bone; a biopsy removes a small, solid core of marrow tissue through the needle. Both procedures are usually performed by a physician, but some facilities authorize specially trained chemotherapy nurses or nurse clinicians to perform them with an assistant.

Aspirates aid in diagnosing various disorders and cancers, such as oat cell carcinoma, leukemia, and lymphomas such as Hodgkin's disease. Biopsies are often performed simultaneously to stage the disease and monitor response to treatment. Bone marrow biopsy is contraindicated in patients with severe bleeding disorder.

Equipment

For aspiration: Mask ▪ gown ▪ nonsterile gloves ▪ prepackaged bone marrow set, which includes antiseptic pads ▪ two sterile drapes (one fenestrated, one plain) ▪ ten 4″ × 4″ gauze pads ▪ ten 2″ × 2″ gauze pads ▪ two 12-ml syringes ▪ 22G 1″ or 2″ ▪ scalpel ▪ sedative ▪ specimen containers ▪ bone marrow needle ▪ 70% isopropyl alcohol ▪ 1% lidocaine (unopened bottle) ▪ 26G or 27G ½″ to ⅝″needle ▪ adhesive tape ▪ sterile gloves ▪ glass slides and coverglass ▪ labels and laboratory biohazard transport bags.

For biopsy: All equipment listed above ▪ biopsy needle, such as Vim-Silverman, Jamshidi, Illinois sternal, or Westerman-Jensen needle ▪ Zenker's fixative.

Implementation

- Confirm the patient's identity using two patient identifiers according to your facility's policy.
- Tell the patient that the physician will collect a bone marrow specimen, and explain the procedure *to ease his anxiety and ensure cooperation.* Make sure the patient or a responsible family member understands the procedure and signs a consent form obtained by the physician.
- Inform the patient that the procedure normally takes about 20 minutes, that test results usually are available in 1 to 3 days, and that more than one marrow specimen may be required.
- Check the patient's history for hypersensitivity to the local anesthetic. Tell him which bone—sternum or posterior superior or anterior iliac crest—will be sampled. Inform him that he will receive a local anesthetic and will feel heavy pressure from insertion of the biopsy or aspiration needle as well as a brief, pulling sensation.
- If the patient has osteoporosis, tell him that the needle pressure may be minimal; if he has osteopetrosis, inform him that a drill may be needed.
- Provide a sedative, as ordered, before the test.
- Position the patient according to the selected puncture site. (See *Common sites for bone marrow aspiration and biopsy,* page 220.)
- Label all medications, medication containers, and other solutions on and off the sterile field.
- Using sterile technique, the puncture site is cleaned with antiseptic pads and allowed to dry; then the area is draped.
- To anesthetize the site, the physician infiltrates it with 1% lidocaine, using a 26G or 27G ½″ to ⅝″ needle to inject a small amount intradermally and then a larger 22G 1″ to 2″ needle to anesthetize the tissue down to the bone.
- When the needle tip reaches the bone, the physician anesthetizes the periosteum by injecting a small amount of lidocaine in a circular area about ¾″ (2 cm) in diameter. The needle should be withdrawn from the periosteum after each injection.
- After allowing about 1 minute for the lidocaine to take effect, a scalpel may be used to make a small stab incision in the patient's skin to accommodate the bone marrow needle. *This technique avoids pushing skin into the bone marrow and also helps avoid unnecessary skin tearing to help reduce the risk of infection.*

Common sites for bone marrow aspiration and biopsy

The posterior superior iliac crest is the preferred site for bone marrow aspiration *because no vital organs or vessels are nearby*. The patient is placed either in the lateral position with one leg flexed or in the prone position. The anterior iliac crest may be used with patients who can't lie in a prone position.

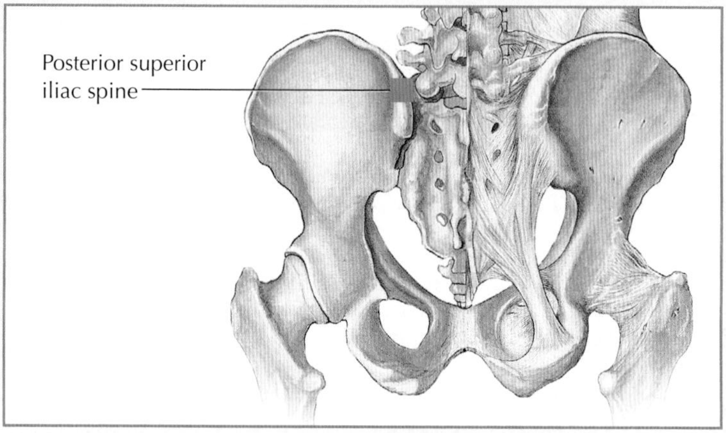

The spinous process of the third or fourth lumbar vertebra is the preferred site if multiple punctures are necessary or if marrow is absent at other sites. The patient sits on the edge of the bed, leaning over the bedside stand.

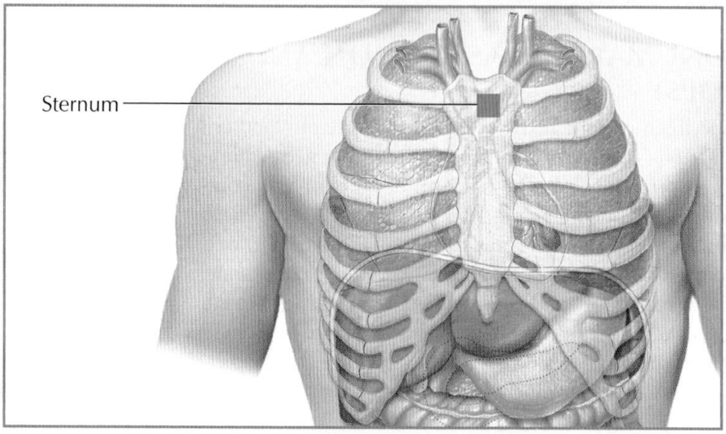

Aspiration from the sternum involves the greatest risk but may be used because the site is near the surface, the cortical bone is thin, and the marrow cavity contains numerous cells and relatively little fat or supporting bone. The patient is placed in a supine position. This site is seldom used for biopsy.

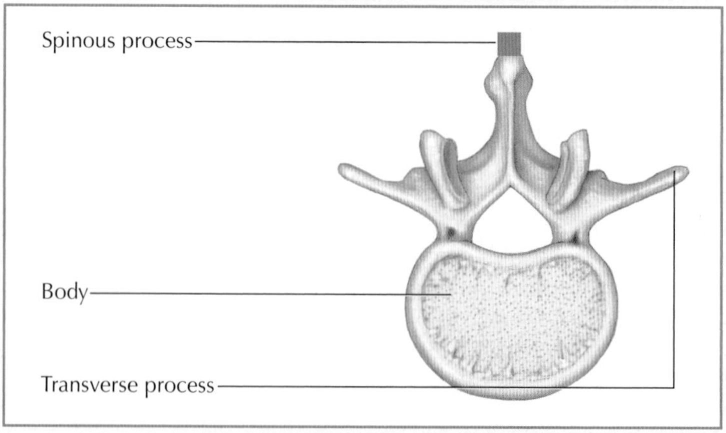

Bone marrow aspiration

- The physician inserts the bone marrow needle and lodges it firmly in the bone cortex. If the patient feels sharp pain instead of pressure when the needle first touches bone, the needle was probably inserted outside the anesthetized area. If this happens, the needle should be withdrawn slightly and moved to the anesthetized area.
- The needle is advanced by applying an even, downward force with the heel of the hand or the palm, while twisting it back and forth slightly. A crackling sensation means that the needle has entered the marrow cavity.
- Next, the physician removes the inner cannula, attaches the syringe to the needle, aspirates the required specimen, and withdraws the needle.
- The nurse puts on gloves and applies pressure to the aspiration site with a gauze pad for 5 minutes to control bleeding while an assistant prepares the marrow slides. The area is then cleaned with alcohol to remove the povidone-iodine, the skin is dried thoroughly with a 4″ × 4″ gauze pad, and a sterile pressure dressing is applied. Specimens are labeled appropriately, placed in laboratory biohazard transport bags, and sent to the laboratory.

Bone marrow biopsy

- The physician inserts the biopsy needle into the periosteum and advances it steadily until the outer needle passes into the marrow cavity.
- The biopsy needle is directed into the marrow cavity by alternately rotating the inner needle clockwise and counterclockwise. Then a plug of tissue is removed, the needle assembly is withdrawn, and the marrow specimen is expelled into a properly labeled specimen bottle containing Zenker's fixative or formaldehyde. It's then placed in the laboratory biohazard transport bag and sent to the laboratory.
- The nurse puts on gloves, cleans the area around the biopsy site with alcohol to remove the povidone-iodine solution, firmly presses a sterile 2″ × 2″ gauze pad against the incision *to control bleeding,* and applies a sterile pressure dressing.

Special considerations

- Faulty needle placement may yield too little aspirate. If no specimen is produced, the needle must be withdrawn from the bone (but not from the overlying soft tissue), the stylet replaced, and the needle inserted into a second site within the anesthetized field.
- Bone marrow specimens shouldn't be collected from irradiated areas *because radiation may have altered or destroyed the marrow.*

Complications

Bleeding and infection are potentially life-threatening complications of aspiration or biopsy at any site. Complications of sternal needle puncture are uncommon but include puncture of the heart and major vessels, causing severe hemorrhage; puncture of the mediastinum, causing mediastinitis or pneumomediastinum; and puncture of the lung, causing pneumothorax.

If a hematoma occurs around the puncture site, apply warm soaks. Give analgesics for site pain or tenderness.

Documentation

Chart the time, date, location, and patient's tolerance of the procedure. Note the amount and color of marrow aspirate, laboratory tests ordered, and time the specimen was sent. Document patient's vital signs, pain level, and complications, and the type of dressing applied.

SELECTED REFERENCES

Christensen, J., and Fatchett, D. "Promoting Parental Use of Distraction and Relaxation in Pediatric Oncology Patients During Invasive Procedures," *Journal of Pediatric Oncology Nursing* 19(4):127-32, July-August 2002.

Islam, A. "Bone Marrow Aspiration Before Bone Marrow Core Biopsy Using the Same Bone Marrow Biopsy Needle: A Good or Bad Practice?" *Journal of Clinical Pathology* 60(2):212-15, February 2007.

Rushing, J. "Assisting with Bone Marrow Aspiration and Biopsy," *Nursing* 36(3):68, March 2006.

SKIN BIOPSY

Skin biopsy is a diagnostic test in which a small piece of tissue is removed, under local anesthesia, from a lesion that is suspected of being malignant or from another dermatosis.

One of three techniques may be used: shave biopsy, punch biopsy, or excisional biopsy. *Shave biopsy* cuts the lesion above the skin line, which allows further biopsy of the site. *Punch biopsy* removes an oval core from the center of the lesion. *Excisional biopsy* removes the entire lesion and is indicated for rapidly expanding lesions; for sclerotic, bullous, or atrophic lesions; and for examination of the border of a lesion surrounding normal skin.

Lesions suspected of being malignant usually have changed color, size, or appearance or have failed to heal properly after injury. Fully developed lesions should be selected for biopsy whenever possible because they provide more diagnostic information than lesions that are resolving or in early stages of development. For example, if the skin shows blisters, the biopsy should include the most mature ones.

Normal skin consists of squamous epithelium (epidermis) and fibrous connective tissue (dermis). Histologic examination of the tissue specimen obtained during biopsy may reveal a benign or malignant lesion. Benign growths include cysts, seborrheic keratoses, warts, pigmented nevi (moles), keloids, dermatofibromas, and neurofibromas. Malignant tumors include basal cell carcinoma, squamous cell carcinoma, and malignant melanoma.

Equipment

Gloves (sterile and clean) ▪ #15 scalpel for shave or excisional biopsy ▪ punch for punch biopsy ▪ local anesthetic ▪ specimen bottle containing 10% formaldehyde solution ▪ 4-0 sutures for punch or excisional biopsy ▪ adhesive bandage ▪ forceps ▪ laboratory specimen labels and laboratory biohazard transport bags.

Implementation

- Confirm the patient's identity using two patient identifiers according to your facility's policy.
- Describe the procedure, and tell him who will perform it. Answer any questions he may have *to ease anxiety and ensure cooperation.*
- Inform the patient that he need not restrict food or fluids.
- Tell him that he'll receive a local anesthetic for pain.
- Inform him that the biopsy will take about 15 minutes and that the test results are usually available within 7 days.
- Have the patient or an appropriate family member sign a consent form.
- Check the patient's history for hypersensitivity to the local anesthetic.
- Label all medications, medication containers, and other solutions on and off the sterile field.
- Position the patient comfortably, and clean the biopsy site before the local anesthetic is administered.
- For a *shave biopsy,* the protruding growth is cut off at the skin line with a #15 scalpel. The tissue is placed immediately in a properly labeled specimen bottle containing 10% formaldehyde solution. Apply pressure to the area *to stop the bleeding.* Apply an adhesive bandage.
- For a *punch biopsy,* the skin surrounding the lesion is pulled taut, and the punch is firmly introduced into the lesion and rotated to obtain a tissue specimen. The plug is lifted with forceps or a needle and is severed as deeply into the fat layer as possible. The specimen is placed in a properly labeled specimen bottle containing 10% formaldehyde solution or in a sterile container if indicated. Closing the wound depends on the size of the punch: A 3-mm punch requires only an adhesive bandage, a 4-mm punch requires one suture, and a 6-mm punch requires two sutures.
- For an *excisional biopsy,* a #15 scalpel is used to excise the lesion; the incision is made as wide and as deep as necessary. The tissue specimen is removed and placed immediately in a properly labeled specimen bottle containing 10% formaldehyde solution. Apply pressure to the site *to stop the bleeding.* The wound is closed using a 4-0 suture. If the incision is large, a skin graft may be required.
- Check the biopsy site for bleeding.
- Label the specimen, and send it to the laboratory immediately in a laboratory biohazard transport bag.
- If the patient experiences pain, administer analgesics.

Special considerations

- Advise the patient going home with sutures to keep the area clean and as dry as possible. Tell him that facial sutures will be removed in 3 to 5 days and trunk sutures, in 7 to 14 days.
- Instruct the patient with adhesive strips to leave them in place for 14 to 21 days or until they fall off.

Complications

Possible complications include bleeding and infection of the surrounding tissue.

Documentation

Document the time and location where the specimen was obtained, the appearance of the specimen and site, and whether bleeding occurred at the biopsy site.

SELECTED REFERENCES

Baron, J.M., and Abazahra, F. "Evidenced-based Staging System for Malignant Melanoma: Is Now Necessarily Better?" *Lancet* 364(9432):395-96, July-August 2004.

Maguire-Eisen, M. "Risk Assessment and Early Detection of Skin Cancers," *Seminars in Oncology Nursing* 19(1):43-51, February 2003.

Trent, J.T., et al. "Skin and Wound Biopsy: When, Why and How," *Advances in Skin and Wound Care* 16(7):372-75, December 2003.

4 ■ Physical Treatments

INTRODUCTION

Used effectively for centuries, many physical treatments have become fundamental nursing procedures. The principles behind such treatments as application of heat and cold—and often the techniques for performing them—remain essentially unchanged. However, that doesn't make them any less important than more-involved or specialized procedures created by new, high-technology medical treatments. In fact, physical treatments that many nurses might consider routine are those most responsible for maintaining patient comfort, decreasing anxiety, and reducing the risk of infection.

Proven effectiveness

Most physical treatments have endured procedurally intact because of their effectiveness. Some treatments stimulate or support normal physiologic processes. For example, the application of heat enhances healing because the warmth causes vasodilation, thereby increasing blood supply to the affected area and making more nutrients available for tissue growth. Antiembolism stockings support blood vessels, increasing venous return and thereby reducing the risk of deep vein thrombosis. Drains allow wound secretions to escape to the surface from underlying tissue, thus assisting the healing process.

Other physical treatments prevent a pathologic response or inhibit a full-blown response. For example, cold application produces vasoconstriction and increases blood viscosity, thereby reducing inflammation, bleeding, and localized tissue edema. Medicated baths relieve itching and reduce the irritation caused by various skin disorders. Wound irrigation performed with an antiseptic solution inhibits bacterial growth. Also, radiation therapy inhibits or destroys cancerous cells, offering patients palliation, control, or cure. In all these instances, nursing assessment and interventions are essential to the success of physical treatments.

Advances in equipment

Improvements in physical treatments have resulted in part from equipment advances. For example, single-use or single-patient disposable products have heightened efficiency and safety. Hot-water bottles and ice collars, sterile gauze dressings, presaturated sterile swabs, and aquathermia pads are all available for single use. The number and types of disposable items and the variety of prepackaged procedure setup trays available continue to expand. One of the latest such products is the single-patient hyperthermia-hypothermia blanket. This disposable, lightweight vinyl blanket connects to a conventional module for use both under and over the patient.

A portable Fiberglas tub makes it possible to bathe rather than sponge patients on bed rest. The full-sized tub stands as high as the bed, rolls easily on casters, and fills and empties at the bedside through a hose that attaches to any faucet.

Vinyl pressure cuffs improve on the well-known and effective antiembolism stockings. This portable system stimulates the normal pumping action of leg muscles by inflating progressively from the ankle to the thigh, assisting venous return and preventing blood backflow.

Hypoallergenic adhesive gauze dressings cover an entire wound site with a single sheet of air- and exudate-permeable adhesive gauze. This type of occlusive dressing is particularly well suited for large or curved body areas and holds dressings securely without tapes or straps. The gauze can be lifted off easily and painlessly for examination of the wound—even on sensitive or hairy skin—and then can be pressed back into place.

The silicone-foam dressing has improved the care of open, granulating wounds. Poured into the wound in liquid form, this new packing quickly congeals into an absorbent rubber pad with the exact contour of the wound, but it permits air circulation and doesn't cause irritation.

The new portable and disposable equipment saves nursing time because it's easier to use than the equipment it replaces. And nursing time saved means fewer delays in delivering patient care. What's more, disposables reduce the spread of healthcare-acquired infection and enhance patient comfort.

HEAT AND COLD

DIRECT HEAT APPLICATION

Heat applied directly to the patient's body raises tissue temperature and enhances the inflammatory process by causing vasodilation and increasing local circulation. This promotes leukocytosis, suppuration, drainage, and healing. Heat also increases tissue metabolism, reduces pain caused by muscle spasm, and decreases congestion in deep visceral organs.

Direct heat may be dry or moist. Dry heat can be delivered at a higher temperature and for a longer time. Devices for applying dry heat include the hot-water bottle, electric heating pad, aquathermia pad, and chemical hot pack.

Moist heat softens crusts and exudates, penetrates deeper than dry heat, doesn't dry the skin, produces less perspiration, and usually is more comfortable for the patient. Devices for applying moist heat include warm compresses for small body areas and warm packs for large areas.

Direct heat treatment can't be used on a patient at risk for hemorrhage. It also is contraindicated if the patient has a sprained limb in the acute stage (because vasodilation would increase pain and swelling) or if he has a condition associated with acute inflammation such as appendicitis. Direct heat should be applied cautiously to pediatric and elderly patients and to patients with impaired renal, cardiac, or respiratory function; arteriosclerosis or atherosclerosis; or impaired sensation. It should be applied with extreme caution to heat-sensitive areas, such as scar tissue and stomas.

Equipment

Patient thermometer ▪ towel ▪ adhesive tape or roller gauze ▪ absorbent, protective cloth covering ▪ gloves, if the patient has an open lesion.

For a hot-water bottle: Hot tap water ▪ pitcher ▪ bath (utility) thermometer ▪ absorbent, protective cloth covering.

For an electric heating pad: Absorbent, protective cloth covering.

For an aquathermia pad: Distilled water ▪ temperature-adjustment key ▪ absorbent, protective cloth covering.

For a chemical hot pack (disposable): Absorbent, protective cloth covering.

For a warm compress or pack (sterile or nonsterile): Basin of hot tap water or container of sterile water, normal saline, or other solution, as ordered ▪ hot-water bottle, aquathermia pad, or chemical hot pack ▪ linen-saver pad ▪ bath thermometer ▪ optional: forceps.

The following items may be sterile or nonsterile, as needed: compress material (flannel, 4″ × 4″ gauze pads) or pack material (absorbent towels, large absorbent pads) ▪ cotton-tipped applicators ▪ forceps ▪ bowl or basin ▪ bath (utility) thermometer ▪ waterproof covering ▪ towel ▪ dressing.

Preparation of equipment

Hot-water bottle: Fill the bottle with hot tap water *to detect leaks and warm the bottle*; then empty it. Run hot tap water into a pitcher, and measure the water temperature with the bath thermometer. Adjust the temperature as ordered, usually to 115° to 125° F (46.1° to 51.7° C) for adults.

PEDIATRIC ALERT *Adjust the water temperature to 105° to 115° F (40.6° to 46.1° C) for children under age 2.*

ELDER ALERT ***Adjust the water temperature to 105° to 115° F for elderly patients.***

Next, pour hot water into the bottle, filling it one-half to two-thirds full. *Partially filling the bottle keeps it lightweight and flexible to mold to the treatment area.* Squeeze the bottle until the water reaches the neck *to expel any air that would make the bottle inflexible and reduce heat conduction.* Fasten the top, and cover the bag with an absorbent cloth. Secure the cover with tape or roller gauze.

Electric heating pad: Check the cord for frayed or damaged insulation. Then plug in the pad, and adjust the control switch to the desired setting. Wrap the pad in a protective cloth covering, and secure the cover with tape or roller gauze.

Aquathermia pad: Check the cord for safety, as above, and fill the control unit two-thirds full with distilled water. Don't use tap water *because it leaves mineral deposits in the unit.* Check for leaks, and then tilt the unit in several directions *to clear the pad's tubing of air.* Tighten the cap, and then loosen it a quarter turn *to allow heat expansion within the unit.* After making sure the hoses between the control unit and the pad are free of tangles, place the unit on the bedside table, slightly above the patient *so that gravity can assist water flow.* If the central supply department hasn't preset the temperature, use the temperature-adjustment key provided to set the temperature on the control unit. The usual temperature is 105° F (40.6° C). Then place the pad in a protective cloth covering, and secure the cover with tape or roller gauze. Plug in the unit, turn it on, and allow the pad to warm for 2 minutes.

Chemical hot pack: Select a pack of the correct size. Then follow the manufacturer's directions (strike, squeeze, or knead) to activate the heat-producing chemicals. Place the pack in a protective cloth covering, and secure the cover with tape or roller gauze.

Sterile warm compress or pack: Warm the container of sterile water or solution by setting it in a sink or basin of hot water. Measure its temperature with a sterile bath thermometer. If a sterile thermometer is unavailable, pour some heated sterile solution into a clean container, check the temperature with a regular bath thermometer, and then discard the tested solution. Adjust the temperature by adding hot or cold water to the sink or basin until the solution reaches 131° F (55° C) for adults.

PEDIATRIC ALERT *Adjust the water temperature to 105° F (40.6° C) for children or for an eye compress.*

ELDER ALERT ***Adjust the water temperature to 105° F for elderly patients or for an eye compress.***

Pour the heated solution into a sterile bowl or basin. Then, using sterile technique, soak the compress or pack in the heated solution. If necessary, prepare a hot-water bottle, aquathermia pad, or chemical hot pack to keep the compress or pack warm.

Nonsterile warm compress or pack: Fill a bowl or basin with hot tap water or other solution, and measure the temperature of the fluid with a bath thermometer. Adjust the temperature as ordered, usually to 131° F (55° C) for adults.

PEDIATRIC ALERT *Adjust the water temperature to 105° F for children or for an eye compress.*

HOME CARE

Using moist heat to relieve muscle spasm

Tell patients to choose moist heat rather than dry heat when attempting to ease muscle tension or spasm. Moist heat is less drying to the skin, less apt to cause burns, less likely to cause excessive fluid and salt loss through sweating, and more likely to penetrate deeper tissues. Instruct the patient to apply heat for 20 to 30 minutes, as follows:

- Place a moist towel over the painful area.
- Cover the towel with a hot-water bottle properly filled and at the correct temperature.
- Remove the hot-water bottle and wet pack after 20 to 30 minutes. Don't continue application for longer than 30 minutes *because vasoconstriction begins to occur, and the therapeutic value decreases after that time.*

ELDER ALERT *Adjust the water temperature to 105° F (40.6° C) for elderly patients or for an eye compress.* Then soak the compress or pack in the hot liquid. If necessary, prepare a hot-water bottle, aquathermia pad, or chemical hot pack *to keep the compress or pack warm.*

Implementation

- Check the practitioner's order.
- Assess the patient's condition.
- Confirm the patient's identity using two patient identifiers according to your facility's policy.
- Explain the procedure to the patient, and tell him not to lean or lie directly on the heating device *because this reduces air space and increases the risk of burns.* Warn him against adjusting the temperature of the heating device or adding hot water to a hot-water bottle. Advise him to report pain immediately and to remove the device if necessary.
- Provide privacy, and make sure the room is warm and free from drafts. Wash your hands.
- Take the patient's temperature, pulse, and respiration *to serve as a baseline.* If heat treatment is being applied to raise the patient's body temperature, monitor temperature, pulse, and respirations throughout the application.
- Expose only the treatment area *because vasodilation will make the patient feel chilly.*

Applying a hot-water bottle, an electric heating pad, an aquathermia pad, or a chemical hot pack

- Before applying the heating device, press it against your inner forearm *to test its temperature and heat distribution.* If it heats unevenly, obtain a new device.
- Apply the device to the treatment area and, if necessary, secure it with tape or roller gauze. Begin timing the application.
- Assess the patient's skin condition frequently, and remove the device if you observe increased swelling or excessive redness, blistering, maceration, or pallor or if the patient reports discomfort. Refill the hot-water bottle as necessary *to maintain the correct temperature.*
- Remove the device after 20 to 30 minutes, or as ordered.

NURSING ALERT *Tissue exposed to heat for more than 30 minutes begins to develop vasoconstriction.*

- Dry the patient's skin with a towel and re-dress the site, if necessary. Take the patient's temperature, pulse, and respiration *for comparison with the baseline.* Position him comfortably in bed.
- If the treatment is to be repeated, store the equipment in the patient's room, out of his reach; otherwise, return it to its proper place.

Applying a warm compress or pack

- Place a linen-saver pad under the site.
- Remove the warm compress or pack from the bowl or basin. (Use sterile forceps throughout the procedure if necessary.)
- Wring excess solution from the compress or pack (using sterile forceps if needed). *Excess moisture increases the risk of burns.*
- Apply the compress gently to the affected site (using forceps, if warranted). After a few seconds, lift the compress (with forceps, if needed) and check the skin for excessive redness, maceration, or blistering. When you're sure the compress isn't causing a burn, mold it firmly to the skin *to keep air out, which reduces the temperature and effectiveness of the compress.* Work quickly *so the compress retains its heat.*
- Apply a waterproof covering (sterile, if necessary) to the compress. Secure it with tape or roller gauze *to prevent it from slipping.*
- Place a hot-water bottle, aquathermia pad, or chemical hot pack over the compress and waterproof covering *to maintain the correct temperature.* Begin timing the application.
- Check the patient's skin every 5 minutes for tissue tolerance. Remove the device if the skin shows excessive redness, maceration, or blistering or if the patient experiences pain or discomfort. Change the compress as needed to maintain the correct temperature.

■ After 15 to 20 minutes or as ordered, remove the compress. (Use forceps, if warranted.) Discard the compress into a waterproof trash bag.
■ Dry the patient's skin with a towel (sterile, if necessary). Note the condition of the skin and re-dress the area, if necessary. Take the patient's temperature, pulse, and respiration *for comparison with baseline.* Then make sure the patient is comfortable.

Special considerations

■ If the patient is unconscious, anesthetized, irrational, neurologically impaired, or insensitive to heat, stay with him throughout the treatment.
■ When direct heat is ordered to decrease congestion within internal organs, the application must cover a large enough area *to increase blood volume at the skin's surface.* For relief of pelvic organ congestion, for example, apply heat over the patient's lower abdomen, hips, and thighs. To achieve local relief, you may concentrate heat only over the specified area. (See *Using moist heat to relieve muscle spasm.*)
■ As an alternative method of applying sterile moist compresses, use a bedside sterilizer to sterilize the compresses. Saturate the compress with tap water or another solution and wring it dry. Then place it in the bedside sterilizer at 275° F (135° C) for 15 minutes. Remove the compress with sterile forceps or sterile gloves, and wring out the excess solution. Then place the compress in a sterile bowl, and measure its temperature with a sterile thermometer.
■ Be sure to follow manufacturer's instructions for heating compresses, and avoid over-heating.

Complications

Because tissue damage may result from direct heat application, monitor the temperature of the compress carefully. Frequently assess the condition of the patient's skin under the heat application device.

Documentation

Record the time and date of heat application; type, temperature or heat setting, duration, and site of application; patient's temperature, pulse, respirations, and skin condition before, during, and after treatment; signs of complications; and the patient's tolerance of treatment.

SELECTED REFERENCES

Cosqray, N.A., et al. "Effect of Heat Modalities on Hamstring Length: A Comparison of Pneumatherm, Moist Heat Pack, and a Control," *Journal of Orthopedic Sports and Physical Therapy* 34(7):377-84, July 2004.

Craven, R.F., and Hirnle, C.J. *Fundamentals of Nursing: Human Health and Function,* 5th ed. Philadelphia: Lippincott Williams & Wilkins, 2007.

Mayer, J.M., et al. "Treating Acute Low Back Pain with Continuous Low-level Heat Wrap Therapy and/or Exercises: A Randomized Controlled Trial," *The Spine Journal* 5(4):395-403, July-August 2005.

Taylor, C., et al. *Fundamentals of Nursing: The Art and Science of Nursing Care,* 6th ed. Philadelphia: Lippincott Williams & Wilkins, 2008.

COLD APPLICATION

The application of cold constricts blood vessels; inhibits local circulation, suppuration, and tissue metabolism; relieves vascular congestion; slows bacterial activity in infections; reduces body temperature; and may act as a temporary anesthetic during brief, painful procedures. (See *Reducing pain with ice massage,* page 228.) Because treatment with cold also relieves inflammation, reduces edema, and slows bleeding, it may provide effective initial treatment after eye injuries, strains, sprains, bruises, muscle spasms, and burns. Cold doesn't reduce existing edema, however, because it inhibits reabsorption of excess fluid.

Cold may be applied in dry or moist forms, but ice shouldn't be placed directly on a patient's skin because it may further damage tissue. Moist application is more penetrating than dry because moisture facilitates conduction. Devices for applying cold include an ice bag or collar, aquathermia pad (which can produce cold or heat), and chemical cold packs and ice packs. Devices for applying moist cold include cold compresses for small body areas and cold packs for large areas.

Apply cold treatments cautiously on patients with impaired circulation, on children, and on elderly or arthritic patients because of the risk of ischemic tissue damage.

Equipment

Patient thermometer ■ towel ■ adhesive tape or roller gauze ■ gloves, if necessary.

For an ice bag or collar: Tap water ■ ice chips ■ absorbent, protective cloth covering.

For an aquathermia pad: Distilled water ■ temperature-adjustment key ■ absorbent, protective cloth covering.

For a chemical cold pack: Single-use packs are available for applying dry cold. These lightweight plastic packs contain a chemical that turns cold when activated. Reusable, sealed cold packs, filled with an alcohol-based solution, are also available. These packs may be stored frozen until use and, after exterior disinfection, may be refrozen and used again. Other chemical packs are activated by striking, squeezing, or kneading them.

For a cold compress or pack: Basin of ice chips ■ container of tap water ■ bath thermometer ■ compress mater-

Reducing pain with ice massage

Normally, ice shouldn't be applied directly to a patient's skin *because it can damage the skin surface and underlying tissues.* However, when carefully performed, ice massage may help patients tolerate brief, painful procedures, such as bone-marrow aspiration, catheterization, chest-tube removal, injection into joints, lumbar puncture, and suture removal.

Prepare for ice massage by gathering the ice, a porous covering to hold it (if desired), and a cloth for wiping water from the patient as the ice melts. Water may be frozen in a cup ahead of time. The paper is removed from half of the cup exposing the ice to be used for the procedure.

Just before the procedure begins, rub the ice over the appropriate area *to numb it.* Assess the site frequently; stop rubbing immediately if you detect signs of tissue intolerance.

As the procedure begins, rub the ice over a point near but not at the site *to distract the patient from the procedure itself and give him another stimulus on which to concentrate.*

If the procedure lasts longer than 10 minutes or if you think tissue damage may occur, move the ice to a different site and continue massage.

If you know in advance that the procedure will probably last longer than 10 minutes, massage the site intermittently—2 minutes of massage alternating with a rest period until the skin regains its normal color. Alternatively, you can divide the area into several sites, and apply ice to each one for several minutes at a time.

ial (4″ × 4″ gauze pads or washcloths) or pack material (towels or flannel) ▪ linen-saver pad ▪ waterproof covering.

Preparation of equipment

Ice bag or collar: Select a device of the correct size, fill it with cold tap water, and check for leaks. Then empty the device and fill it about halfway with crushed ice. *Using small pieces of ice helps the device mold to the patient's body.* Squeeze the device *to expel air that might reduce conduction.* Fasten the cap, and wipe any moisture from the outside of the device. Wrap the bag or collar in a cloth covering, and secure the cover with tape or roller gauze. *The protective cover prevents tissue trauma and absorbs condensation.*

Aquathermia pad: Check the cord for frayed or damaged insulation. Then fill the control unit two-thirds full with distilled water. Don't use tap water *because it leaves mineral deposits in the unit.* Check for leaks, and then tilt the unit several times *to clear the pad's tubing of air.* Tighten the cap. After ensuring that the hoses between the control unit and pad are free of tangles, place the unit on the bedside table, slightly above the patient *so that gravity can assist water flow.* If the central supply department hasn't preset the temperature, use the temperature-adjustment key to adjust the control unit setting to the lowest temperature. Cover the pad with an absorbent, protective cloth, and secure the cover with tape or roller gauze. Plug in the unit and turn it on. Allow the pad to cool for 2 minutes before placing it on the patient.

Chemical cold pack: Select a pack of the appropriate size, and follow the manufacturer's directions (strike, squeeze, or knead) *to activate the cold-producing chemicals.* Make certain that the container hasn't been broken during activation. Wrap the pack in a cloth cover, and secure the cover with tape or roller gauze.

Cold compress or pack: Cool a container of tap water by placing it in a basin of ice or by adding ice to the water. Using a bath thermometer for guidance, adjust the water temperature to 59° F (15° C) or as ordered. Immerse the compress or pack material in the water.

Implementation

- Confirm the patient's identity using two patient identifiers according to your facility's policy.
- Check the practitioner's order, and assess the patient's condition.
- Explain the procedure to the patient, provide privacy, and make sure the room is warm and free of drafts. Wash your hands thoroughly.
- Record the patient's temperature, pulse, and respirations *to serve as a baseline.*
- Expose only the treatment site *to avoid chilling the patient.*

Applying an ice bag or collar, an aquathermia pad, or a chemical cold pack

- Place the covered cold device on the treatment site, and begin timing the application.
- Observe the site frequently for signs of tissue intolerance, such as blanching, mottling, cyanosis, maceration, and blisters. Also be alert for shivering and complaints of burning or numbness. If these signs or symptoms develop, discontinue treatment and notify the practitioner.
- Refill or replace the cold device as necessary *to maintain the correct temperature.* Change the protective cover if it becomes wet.

HOME CARE

Using cold for a muscle sprain

Cold can help relieve pain and reduce edema during the first 24 to 72 hours after a sprain occurs. Tell the patient to apply cold to the area four times daily for 20 to 30 minutes each time.

For each application, instruct the patient to obtain enough crushed ice to cover the painful area, place it in a plastic bag, and place the bag inside a pillowcase or large piece of cloth (as shown at right).

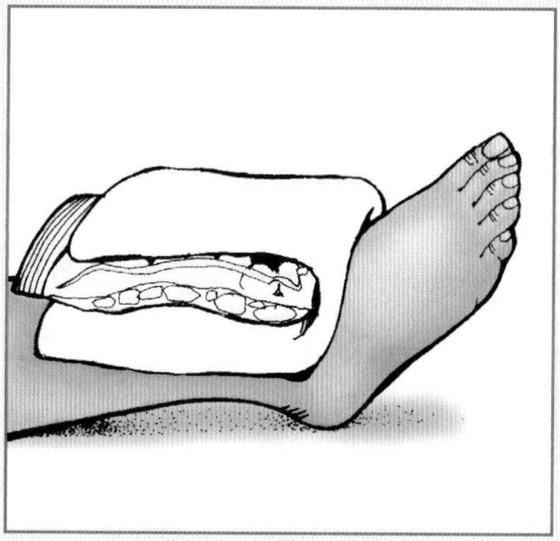

For later applications, the patient may want to fill a paper cup with water, stand a tongue blade in the cup, and place it in the freezer. After the water freezes, he can peel the paper off the ice and hold it with the protruding handle. If he chooses this method, tell him to first cover the area with a cloth. *Applying ice directly to the skin can cause frostbite or cold shock.*

Instruct the patient to rub the ice over the painful area for the specified treatment time. Warn him that although ice eases pain in a joint that has begun to stiffen, he shouldn't let the analgesic effect encourage overuse of the joint.

After 24 to 72 hours, when heat and swelling have subsided or when cold no longer helps, the patient should switch to heat application.

- Remove the device after the prescribed treatment period (usually 30 minutes *because reflex vasodilation begins to occur after that time*).

Applying a cold compress or pack

- Place a linen-saver pad under the site.
- Remove the compress or pack from the water, and wring it out *to prevent dripping.* Apply it to the treatment site, and begin timing the application.
- Cover the compress or pack with a waterproof covering *to provide insulation and to keep the surrounding area dry.* Secure the covering with tape or roller gauze *to prevent it from slipping.*
- Check the application site frequently for signs of tissue intolerance, and note complaints of burning or numbness. If these symptoms develop, discontinue treatment and notify the practitioner.
- Change the compress or pack as needed *to maintain the correct temperature.* Remove it after the prescribed treatment period (usually 20 minutes).

Concluding all cold applications

- Dry the patient's skin, and re-dress the treatment site according to the practitioner's orders. Then position the patient comfortably, and take his temperature, pulse, and respirations *for comparison with baseline.*
- Dispose of liquids and soiled materials properly. If the cold treatment will be repeated, clean and store the equipment in the patient's room, out of his reach; otherwise, return it to storage.

Special considerations

- Apply cold immediately after an injury *to minimize edema.* (See *Using cold for a muscle sprain.*) Although colder temperatures can be tolerated for a longer time when the treatment site is small, don't continue any application for longer than 1 hour *to avoid reflex vasodilation.* The application of temperatures below 59° F (15° C) also causes local reflex vasodilation.
- Use sterile technique when applying cold to an open wound or to a lesion that may open during treatment. Also maintain sterile technique during eye treatment, with separate sterile equipment for each eye *to prevent cross-contamination.*
- Avoid securing cooling devices with pins *because an accidental puncture could allow extremely cold fluids to leak out and burn the patient's skin.*
- If the patient is unconscious, anesthetized, neurologically impaired, irrational, or otherwise insensitive to cold, stay with him throughout the treatment, and check the application site frequently for complications.

■ Warn the patient against placing ice directly on his skin *because the extreme cold can cause burns.*

Complications

Hemoconcentration may cause thrombi. Intense cold may cause pain, burning, or numbness.

Documentation

Record the time, date, and duration of cold application; type of device used (ice bag or collar, aquathermia pad, or chemical cold pack); site of application; temperature or temperature setting; patient's temperature, pulse, and respirations before and after application; skin appearance before, during, and after application; signs of complications; and the patient's tolerance of treatment.

SELECTED REFERENCES

Craven, R.F., and Hirnle, C.J. *Fundamentals of Nursing: Human Health and Function,* 5th ed. Philadelphia: Lippincott Williams & Wilkins, 2007.

Kanlayanaphotoporn, R., et al. "Comparison of Skin Surface Temperature during the Application of Various Cryotherapy Modalities," *Archives of Physical Medicine and Rehabilitation* 86(7):1411-415, July 2005.

Laureanofilho, J.R., et al. "The Influence of Cryotherapy on Reduction of Swelling, Pain, and Trimus after Third Molar Extraction: A Preliminary Study," *Journal of the American Dental Association* 136(6):774-78, June 2005.

Ownby, K.K. "Effects of Ice Massage on Neuropathic Pain in Persons with AIDS," *The Journal of the Association of Nurses in AIDS Care* 17(5):15-22, September-October 2006.

Taylor, C., et al. *Fundamentals of Nursing: The Art and Science of Nursing Care,* 6th ed. Philadelphia: Lippincott Williams & Wilkins, 2008.

HYPERTHERMIA-HYPOTHERMIA BLANKET

A blanket-sized aquathermia pad, the hyperthermia-hypothermia blanket raises, lowers, or maintains body temperature through conductive heat or cold transfer between the blanket and the patient. It can be operated manually or automatically.

In manual operation, the nurse or physician sets the temperature on the unit. The blanket reaches and maintains this temperature regardless of the patient's temperature. The temperature control must be adjusted manually to reach a different setting. The nurse monitors the patient's body temperature with a conventional thermometer.

In automatic operation, the unit directly and continually monitors the patient's temperature by means of a thermistor probe (rectal, skin, or esophageal) and alternates heating and cooling cycles as necessary to achieve and maintain the desired body temperature. The thermistor probe also may be used in conjunction with manual operation but isn't essential. The unit is equipped with an alarm to warn of abnormal temperature fluctuations and a circuit breaker that protects against current overload.

The blanket is most commonly used to reduce high fever when more conservative measures—such as baths, ice packs, and antipyretics—are unsuccessful. Its other uses include maintaining normal temperature during surgery or shock; inducing hypothermia during surgery to decrease metabolic activity and thereby reduce oxygen requirements; reducing intracranial pressure; controlling bleeding and intractable pain in patients with amputations, burns, or cancer; and providing warmth in cases of severe hypothermia.

Equipment

Hyperthermia-hypothermia control unit ■ fluid for the control unit (distilled water or distilled water and 20% ethyl alcohol) ■ thermistor probe (rectal, skin, or esophageal) ■ patient thermometer ■ one or two hyperthermia-hypothermia blankets ■ one or two disposable blanket covers (or one or two sheets or bath blankets) ■ lanolin or a mixture of lanolin and cold cream ■ adhesive tape ■ towel ■ sphygmomanometer ■ gloves, if necessary ■ optional: protective wraps for the patient's hands and feet.

Disposable hyperthermia-hypothermia blankets are available for single-patient use.

Preparation of equipment

Inspect the control unit and each blanket for leaks and the plugs and connecting wires for broken prongs, kinks, and fraying. If you detect or suspect malfunction, don't use the equipment.

Review the practitioner's order, and prepare one or two blankets by covering them with disposable covers (or use a sheet or bath blanket when positioning the blanket on the patient). *The cover absorbs perspiration and condensation, which could cause tissue breakdown if left on the skin.* Connect the blanket to the control unit, and set the controls for manual or automatic operation and for the desired blanket or body temperature. Make sure the machine is properly grounded before plugging it in.

Turn on the machine, and add liquid to the unit reservoir, if necessary, as fluid fills the blanket. Allow the blanket to preheat or precool *so that the patient receives immediate thermal benefit.* Place the control unit at the foot of the bed.

Implementation

■ Confirm the patient's identity using two patient identifiers according to your facility's policy.
■ Assess the patient's condition, and explain the procedure to him. Provide privacy, and make sure the room is warm and free of drafts.
■ Check your facility's policy and, if necessary, make sure the patient or a responsible family member has signed a consent form.
■ Wash your hands thoroughly. If the patient isn't already wearing a patient gown, ask him to put one on. Use a gown with cloth ties rather than metal snaps or pins *to prevent heat or cold injury.*
■ Take the patient's temperature, pulse, respirations, and blood pressure *to serve as a baseline,* and assess his level of consciousness, pupil reaction, limb strength, and skin condition.
■ Keeping the bottom sheet in place and the patient recumbent, roll the patient to one side and slide the rolled blanket halfway underneath him, so that its top edge aligns with his neck. Then roll the patient back, and pull and flatten the blanket across the bed. Place a pillow under the patient's head. Make sure his head doesn't lie directly on the blanket *because the blanket's rigid surface may be uncomfortable, and the heat or cold may lead to tissue breakdown.* Use a sheet or bath blanket as insulation between the patient and the blanket. (See *Using a cooling system.*)
■ Apply lanolin or a mixture of lanolin and cold cream to the patient's skin where it touches the blanket *to help protect the skin from heat or cold sensation.*
■ In automatic operation, insert the thermistor probe in the patient's rectum, and tape it in place *to prevent accidental dislodgment.* If rectal insertion is contraindicated, tuck a skin probe deep into the axilla, and secure it with tape. If the patient is comatose or anesthetized, insert an esophageal probe. Plug the other end of the probe into the correct jack on the unit's control panel.
■ Place a sheet or, if ordered, the second hyperthermia-hypothermia blanket over the patient. *This increases the thermal benefit by trapping cooled or heated air.*
■ Wrap the patient's hands and feet if he wishes *to minimize chilling and promote comfort.* Monitor vital signs and perform a neurologic assessment every 5 minutes until the desired body temperature is reached and then every 15 minutes until temperature is stable or as ordered.
■ Check fluid intake and output hourly or as ordered. Observe the patient regularly for color changes in skin, lips, and nail beds and for edema, induration, inflammation, pain, and sensory impairment. If they occur, discontinue the procedure, and notify the practitioner.

EQUIPMENT

Using a cooling system

A hypothermia or cooling blanket is used to lower a patient's body temperature. The pad has coils that circulate a chilled solution. While the blanket is in use, you must monitor the patient's temperature, which can be adjusted to help keep the patient's temperature in his ordered range.

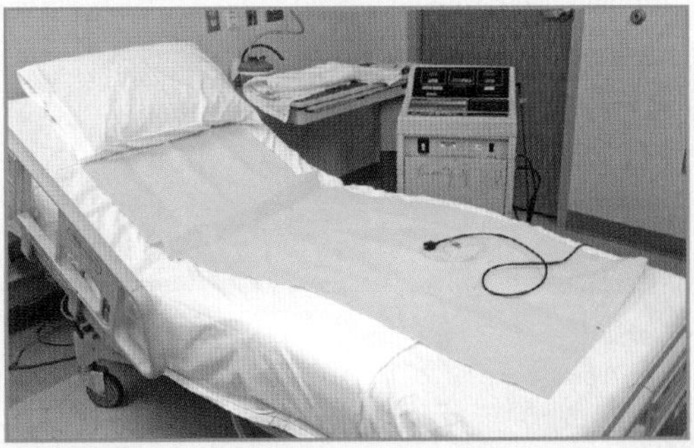

■ Reposition the patient every 30 minutes to 1 hour, unless contraindicated, *to prevent skin breakdown.* Keep the patient's skin, bedclothes, and blanket cover free of perspiration and condensation, and reapply cream to exposed body parts as needed.
■ After turning off the machine, follow the manufacturer's directions. *Some units must remain plugged in for at least 30 minutes to allow the condenser fan to remove water vapor from the mechanism.* Continue to monitor the patient's temperature until it stabilizes *because body temperature can fall as much as 5° F (2.8° C) after this procedure.*
■ Remove all equipment from the bed. Dry the patient and make him comfortable. Supply a fresh patient gown, if necessary. Cover him lightly.
■ Continue to perform neurologic checks and monitor vital signs, fluid intake and output, and general condition every 30 minutes for 2 hours and then hourly or as ordered.
■ Return the equipment to the central supply department for cleaning, servicing, and storage.

Special considerations

■ If the patient shivers excessively during hypothermia treatment, discontinue the procedure, and notify the practitioner immediately. *By increasing metabolism, shivering elevates body temperature.*

EQUIPMENT

Using a warming system

Shivering, the compensatory response to falling body temperature, may use more oxygen than the body can supply—especially in a surgical patient. In the past, patients were covered with blankets to warm their bodies. Now, health care facilities may supply a warming system such as the Bair Hugger patient-warming system (shown below).

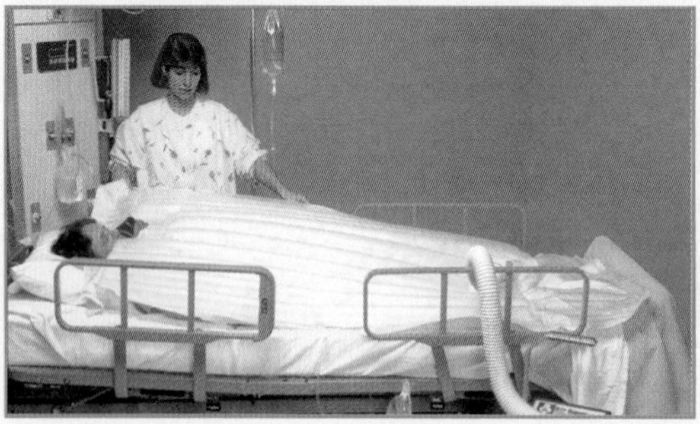

This system helps to gradually increase body temperature by drawing air through a filter, warming the air to the desired temperature, and circulating it through a hose to a warming blanket placed over the patient.

When using the warming system, follow these guidelines:

- Use a bath blanket in a single layer over the warming blanket *to minmize heat loss.*
- Place the warming blanket directly over the patient with the paper side facing down and the clear tubular side facing up.
- Make sure the connection hose is at the foot of the bed.
- Take the patient's temperature during the first 15 to 30 minutes and at least every 30 minutes while the warming blanket is in use.
- Obtain guidelines from the patient's practitioner for discontinuing use of the warming blanket.

- Avoid lowering the temperature more than 1 degree every 15 minutes *to prevent premature ventricular contractions.*
- Don't use pins to secure catheters, tubes, or blanket covers *because an accidental puncture of the blanket can result in fluid leakage and burns.*
- With hyperthermia or hypothermia therapy, the patient may experience a secondary defense reaction (vasoconstriction or vasodilation, respectively) that causes body temperature to rebound and thus defeat the treatment's purpose.
- If the patient requires isolation, place the blanket, blanket cover, and probe in a plastic bag clearly marked with the type of isolation *so that the central supply department can give it special handling.* If the blanket is disposable, discard it, using appropriate precautions.
- *To avoid bacterial growth in the reservoir or blankets,* always use sterile distilled water and change it monthly. Check to see if your facility's policy calls for adding a bacteriostatic agent to the water. Avoid using deionized water *because it may corrode the system.*
- *To gradually increase body temperature,* especially in postoperative patients, the practitioner may order a disposable warming system. (See *Using a warming system.*)

Complications

Use of a hyperthermia-hypothermia blanket can cause shivering, marked changes in vital signs, increased intracranial pressure, respiratory distress or arrest, cardiac arrest, oliguria, and anuria.

Documentation

Record the patient's pulse, respirations, blood pressure, neurologic signs, fluid intake and output, skin condition, and position change. Record the patient's temperature and that of the blanket every 30 minutes while the blanket is in use. Also document the type of hyperthermia-hypothermia unit used; control settings (manual or automatic and temperature settings); date, time, duration, and the patient's tolerance of treatment; and signs of complications.

Selected references

Loke, A.Y., et al. "Comparing the Effectiveness of Two Types of Cooling Blankets for Febrile Patients," *Nursing in Critical Care* 10(5):247-43, September-October 2005.

Mayer, S.A., et al. "Clinical Trial of a Novel Surface Cooling System for Fever Control in Neurocritical Care Patients," *Critical Care Medicine* 32(12):2508-515, December 2004.

Singer, A.J., et al. "The Effects of a Commercially Available Burn-Cooling Blanket on Core Body Temperatures in Volunteers," *Academy of Emergency Medicine* 13(6):58-64, June 2006.

Tepid water sponge bath

A tepid water sponge bath reduces fever by dilating superficial blood vessels, thus releasing heat and lowering body temperature. A tepid water sponge bath may lower systemic temperature when routine fever treatments fail, particularly for infants and children, whose temperatures tend to rise very high, very quickly.

Equipment

Basin of tepid water, about 80° to 93° F (27° to 34° C) ▪ bath (utility) thermometer ▪ bath blanket ▪ linen-saver pad ▪ washcloths ▪ patient thermometer ▪ hot-water bottle and cover ▪ ice bag and cover ▪ towel ▪ clean patient gown ▪ gloves, if the patient has open lesions or has been incontinent.

Preparation of equipment

Prepare a hot-water bottle and an ice bag. Then place the bath thermometer in a basin, and run water over it until the temperature reaches the high end of the tepid range (93° F [34° C]) *because the water will cool during the bath.* Immerse the washcloths in the tepid solution until saturated.

Implementation

- Check the practitioner's order and assess the patient's condition.
- Check the medication Kardex for recent administration of an antipyretic *because this can affect patient response to the bath.*
- Explain the procedure to the patient, provide privacy, and make sure the room is warm and free of drafts. Wash your hands thoroughly and put on gloves, if necessary.
- Place a linen-saver pad under the patient *to catch any spills* and a bath blanket over him *for privacy.* Then remove his pajamas. Also remove the top bed linen *to avoid wetting it.*
- Take the patient's temperature, pulse, and respirations *to serve as a baseline.*
- Place the hot-water bottle with protective covering on the patient's feet *to reduce the sensation of chilliness.* Place the covered ice bag on his head *to prevent headache and nasal congestion that occur as the rest of the body cools.*
- Wring out each washcloth before sponging the patient *so they don't drip and cause discomfort.*
- Place moist washcloths over the major superficial blood vessels in the axillae, groin, and popliteal areas *to accelerate cooling.* Change the washcloths as they warm.
- Bathe each extremity separately for about 5 minutes; then sponge the chest and abdomen for 5 minutes. Turn the patient, and bathe his back and buttocks for 5 to 10 minutes. Keep the patient covered except for the body part you're sponging.
- Add warm water to the basin as necessary *to maintain the desired water temperature.*
- Check the patient's temperature, pulse, and respirations every 10 minutes. Notify the practitioner if the patient's temperature doesn't fall within 30 minutes. Stop the bath when the patient's temperature reaches 1° to 2° F (0.6° to 1° C) above the desired level *because his temperature will continue to fall naturally.* Continue to monitor his temperature until it stabilizes.
- Observe the patient for chills, shivering, pallor, mottling, cyanosis of the lips or nail beds, and vital sign changes—especially a rapid, weak, or irregular pulse—*because such signs may indicate an emergency.* If any of these signs occur, discontinue the bath, cover the patient lightly, and notify the practitioner.
- If no adverse effects occur, bathe the patient for at least 30 minutes *to reduce his temperature.*
- Pat each area dry after sponging, but avoid rubbing with the towel *because rubbing increases cell metabolism and produces heat.*
- After the bath, make sure the patient is dry and comfortable. Dress him in a fresh gown, and cover him lightly.
- Dispose of liquids and soiled materials properly. If the treatment will be repeated, clean and store the equipment in the patient's room, out of his reach; otherwise, return the items to storage.
- Check the patient's temperature, pulse, and respirations after the bath and again in 30 minutes *to determine the treatment's effectiveness.*

Special considerations

- If ordered, administer an antipyretic 15 to 20 minutes before the sponge bath *to achieve more rapid fever reduction.* Consider covering the patient's trunk with a wet towel for 15 minutes *to speed cooling.* Resaturate the towel as necessary.
- Refrain from bathing the breasts of a postpartum patient *because they could become overly dry or fissures could develop on the nipples.*
- Take a rectal or tympanic temperature, unless contraindicated, *for accuracy.* Axillary temperatures are unreliable *because the cool compresses applied to these areas alter the readings.* If you must take an oral temperature, use an electronic thermometer *because it gives the temperature reading quickly.*
- Sponge baths to reduce fever are used most commonly in nonhospital settings; febrile hospitalized patients usually receive antibiotics or antipyretics and, if needed, treatment with hypothermia blankets, which can lower and maintain body temperature more effectively than sponge baths.

Complications

Accelerated temperature reduction can provoke seizure activity.

Documentation

Record the date, time, and duration of the bath; the temperature of the solution; the patient's temperature, pulse, and respirations before, during, and after the procedure; any complications that arise; and the patient's tolerance for treatment.

SELECTED REFERENCES

Craven, R.F., and Hirnle, C.J. *Fundamentals of Nursing: Human Health and Function,* 5th ed. Philadelphia: Lippincott Williams & Wilkins, 2007.

Taylor, C. "Managing Infants with Pyrexia," *Nursing Times* 102(39):42-43, September-October 2006.

Taylor, C., et al. *Fundamentals of Nursing: The Art and Science of Nursing Care,* 6th ed. Philadelphia: Lippincott Williams & Wilkins, 2008.

BATHS AND SOAKS

SITZ BATH

A sitz bath involves immersion of the pelvic area in warm or hot water. It's used to relieve discomfort, especially after perineal or rectal surgery or childbirth. The bath promotes wound healing by cleaning the perineum and anus, increasing circulation, and reducing inflammation. It also helps relax local muscles.

To be performed correctly, the sitz bath requires frequent checks of water temperature to ensure therapeutic effects as well as correct draping of the patient during the bath and prompt dressing afterward to prevent vasoconstriction.

Equipment

Sitz tub, portable sitz bath, or regular bathtub ▪ bath mat ▪ rubber mat ▪ bath (utility) thermometer ▪ two bath blankets ▪ towels ▪ patient gown ▪ gloves, if the patient has an open lesion or has been incontinent ▪ optional: rubber ring, footstool, overbed table, I.V. pole (to hold irrigation bag), wheelchair or cart, dressing supplies.

A disposable sitz bath kit is available for single-patient use. It includes a plastic basin that fits over a commode and an irrigation bag with tubing and clamp.

Preparation of equipment

Make sure the sitz tub, portable sitz bath, or regular bathtub is clean and disinfected. Or, obtain a disposable sitz bath kit from the central supply department.

Position the bath mat next to the bathtub, sitz tub, or commode. If you're using a tub, place a rubber mat on its surface *to prevent falls.* Place the rubber ring on the bottom of the tub *to serve as a seat for the patient,* and cover the ring with a towel *for comfort. Keeping the patient elevated improves water flow over the wound site and avoids unnecessary pressure on tender tissues.* If you're using a commercial kit, open the package, and familiarize yourself with the equipment.

Fill the sitz tub or bathtub one-third to one-half full, so that the water will reach the seated patient's umbilicus. Use warm water (94° to 98° F [34° to 37° C]) for relaxation or wound cleaning and healing and hot water (110° to 115° F [43° to 46° C]) for heat application. Run the water slightly warmer than desired *because it will cool while the patient prepares for the bath.* Measure the water temperature using the bath thermometer.

If you're using a commercial kit, fill the basin to the specified line with water at the prescribed temperature. Place the basin under the commode seat, clamp the irrigation tubing to block water flow, and fill the irrigation bag with water of the same temperature as that in the basin. *To create flow pressure,* hang the bag above the patient's head on a hook, towel rack, or I.V. pole.

Implementation

- Confirm the patient's identity using two patient identifiers according to your facility's policy.
- Check the practitioner's order and assess the patient's condition.
- Explain the procedure to the patient. Wash your hands thoroughly and put on gloves.
- Have the patient void.
- Assist the patient to the bath area, provide privacy, and make sure the area is warm and free of drafts. Help the patient undress as needed.
- Remove and dispose of any soiled dressings. If a dressing adheres to a wound, allow it to soak off in the tub.
- Assist the patient into the tub or onto the commode as needed. Instruct him to use the safety rail for balance. Explain that the sensation may be unpleasant initially *because the wound area is already tender.* Assure him that this discomfort will soon be relieved by the warm water.
- For any apparatus except a regular bathtub, if the patient's feet don't reach the floor and the weight of his legs presses against the edge of the equipment, place a small stool under the patient's feet. *This decreases pressure on local blood vessels.* Also place a folded towel against the patient's lower back *to prevent discomfort and promote correct body alignment.*
- Drape the patient's shoulders and knees with bath blankets *to avoid chills that cause vasoconstriction.*
- If you're using the sitz bath kit, open the clamp on the irrigation tubing *to allow a stream of water to flow continuously over the wound site.* Refill the bag with water of the correct

temperature as needed, and encourage the patient to regulate the flow himself. Place the patient's overbed table in front of him *to provide support and comfort.*

- If you're using a tub, check the water temperature frequently with the bath thermometer. If the temperature drops significantly, add warm water. For maximum safety, first help the patient stand up slowly *to prevent dizziness and loss of balance.* Then, with the patient holding the safety rail *for support,* run warm water into the tub. Check the water temperature. When the water reaches the correct temperature, help the patient sit down again to resume the bath.
- If necessary, stay with the patient during the bath. If you must leave, show him how to use the call button, and ensure his privacy.
- Check the patient's color and general condition frequently. If he complains of feeling weak, faint, or nauseated or shows signs of cardiovascular distress, discontinue the bath, check the patient's pulse and blood pressure, and assist him back to bed. Use a wheelchair or cart to transport the patient to his room if necessary. Notify the practitioner.
- When the prescribed bath time has elapsed—usually 15 to 20 minutes—tell the patient to use the safety rail *for balance,* and help him to a standing position slowly *to prevent dizziness and to allow him to regain his equilibrium.*
- If necessary, help the patient to dry himself. Put on clean gloves, and re-dress the wound, as needed, and assist the patient to dress and return to bed or back to his room.
- Dispose of soiled materials properly. Empty, clean, and disinfect the sitz tub, bathtub, or portable sitz bath. Return the commercial kit to the patient's bedside for later use.

Special considerations

- Use a regular bathtub only if a special sitz tub, portable sitz bath, or commercial sitz bath kit is unavailable. *Because the application of heat to the extremities causes vasodilation and draws blood away from the perineal area,* a regular bathtub is less effective for local treatment than a sitz device.
- If the patient will be sitting in a bathtub with his extremities immersed in the hot water, check his pulse before, during, and after the bath *to help detect vasodilation that could make him feel faint when he stands up.*
- Tell the patient never to touch an open wound *because of the risk of infection.*

Home care

Instruct the patient to adhere to the manufacturer's guidelines for disposable equipment.

Complications

Weakness or faintness can result from heat or the exertion of changing position. Irregular or accelerated pulse may indicate cardiovascular distress.

Documentation

Record the date, time, duration, and temperature of the bath; wound condition before and after treatment, including color, odor, and amount of drainage; any complications; and the patient's response to treatment.

SELECTED REFERENCES

Albers, L.L., and Borders, N. "Minimizing Genital Tract Trauma and Related Pain Following Spontaneous Vaginal Birth," *Journal of Midwifery and Women's Health* 52(3):246-53, May-June 2007.

Craven, R.F., and Hirnle, C.J. *Fundamentals of Nursing: Human Health and Function,* 5th ed. Philadelphia: Lippincott Williams & Wilkins, 2007.

Guta, P. "Randomized, Controlled Study Comparing Sitz-Bath and No Sitz-Bath Treatments in Patients with Anal Fissures," *ANZ Journal of Surgery* 76(8):718-21, August 2006.

Taylor, C., et al. *Fundamentals of Nursing: The Art and Science of Nursing Care,* 6th ed. Philadelphia: Lippincott Williams & Wilkins, 2008.

THERAPEUTIC BATH

Also referred to as balneotherapy, a therapeutic bath combines water and additives to soothe and relax the patient, clean the skin, relieve inflammation and pruritus, and soften and remove crusts, scales, debris, and old medications. Used primarily for their antipruritic and emollient actions, these baths coat irritated skin with a soothing, protective film. Because they constrict surface blood vessels, they also have an anti-inflammatory effect.

The addition of oatmeal powder, soluble cornstarch, or soybean complex to water creates a colloid bath, which has a soothing effect and is used to treat generalized itching. Oil baths are useful for lubricating dry skin and easing eczematous eruptions. Sodium bicarbonate added to water produces an alkaline bath that has a cooling effect and helps relieve pruritus. A medicated tar bath may be used to treat psoriasis. The film of tar left on the skin works in combination with ultraviolet light to inhibit the rapid cell turnover characteristic of psoriasis. (See *Comparing therapeutic baths,* page 236.)

A bedridden patient may benefit from a local soak with the therapeutic additive instead of a therapeutic tub bath.

Comparing therapeutic baths

TYPE	AGENTS	PURPOSE
Antibacterial	■ Acetic acid ■ Potassium permanganate ■ Povidone-iodine	Used to treat infected eczema, dirty ulcerations, furunculosis, and pemphigus
Colloidal	■ Aveeno colloidal oatmeal ■ Aveeno colloidal oatmeal, oilated ■ Starch and baking soda	Used to relieve pruritus and to soothe irritated skin; indicated for any irritated or oozing condition, such as atopic eczema
Emollient	■ Bath oils ■ Mineral oil	Used to clean and hydrate the skin, indicated for any dry skin condition
Tar	■ Bath oils with tar ■ Coal tar concentrate	Used to treat scaly dermatoses, sometimes in combination with ultraviolet light therapy; loosens scales and relieves pruritus

Equipment

Bathtub ■ bath mat ■ rubber mat ■ bath (utility) thermometer ■ therapeutic additive ■ measuring device ■ colander or sieve for oatmeal powder ■ two washcloths ■ two towels ■ patient gown or loose-fitting cotton pajamas ■ lubricating cream or ointment, if ordered.

Preparation of equipment

Assemble supplies and draw the bath before bringing the patient to the bath area *to prevent chilling him.* Make sure the tub is clean and disinfected *because a patient with skin breakdown is particularly vulnerable to infection.* Place the bath mat next to the tub and the rubber mat on the bottom of the tub *to prevent falls; the therapeutic additive may make the tub exceptionally slippery.* Fill the tub with 6″ to 8″ (15 to 20 cm) of water.

The treatment's purpose and the type of additive used determine the water temperature. Cool to lukewarm water is used for relieving pruritus and when adding tar or starch. Warm baths soothe, but water warmer than 100° F causes vasodilation, which could aggravate pruritus. Use the bath thermometer to check the water temperature.

Measure the correct amount of therapeutic additive, according to the practitioner's order or package instructions. As the tub is filling, thoroughly mix the additive in the water. Add most substances directly to the water, but place oatmeal powder in a sieve or colander under the tub faucet *to help it dissolve.* Begin with 2 tbs of oatmeal powder; then add more powder or water as needed to regulate the thickness of the oatmeal bath.

When giving a tar bath, wear a plastic apron or protective gown *because tar preparations stain clothing.*

Implementation

- Confirm the patient's identity using two patient identifiers according to your facility's policy.
- Check the practitioner's order.
- Assess the patient's condition.
- Explain the procedure to the patient, and have him void. Wash your hands thoroughly, and then escort the patient to the bath area. Close the door *to provide privacy and eliminate drafts.*
- Check the water temperature. Assist the patient to undress, and help him into the tub, if necessary. Advise him to use the safety rails *to prevent falls.*
- Tell him that the bath may feel unpleasant at first *because his skin is irritated,* but assure him that the medication will soon coat and soothe his skin.
- Ask the patient to stretch out in the tub and submerge his body up to the chin. If he's capable, give him a washcloth to apply the bath solution gently to his face and other body areas not immersed if these areas require treatment.

NURSING ALERT ***If the patient is taking a tar bath, tell him not to get the bath solution in his eyes*** **because tar is an eye irritant.**

- Warn the patient against scrubbing his skin *to prevent further irritation.*
- Add warm water to the bath as needed *to maintain a comfortable temperature.*

■ Allow the patient to soak for 15 to 30 minutes. If you must stay with him, pull the bath curtain; *this gives him some privacy and protects him from drafts.* If you must leave the room, show the patient how to use the call button, and ensure his privacy.
■ After the bath, assist the patient from the tub. Have him use the safety rails *to prevent falls.*
■ Help the patient pat his skin dry with towels. Don't rub the skin *because rubbing removes some solutes and oils clinging to the skin and produces friction, thereby worsening pruritus.*
■ Apply lubricating cream or ointment, if ordered, *to help hold water in the newly hydrated skin.*
■ Provide a fresh patient gown or loose-fitting cotton pajamas. Advise the patient to avoid wearing pajamas, underwear, or other clothing that isn't cotton and loose-fitting. *Tight clothing and scratchy or synthetic materials can aggravate skin conditions by causing friction and increasing perspiration.*
■ Escort the patient to his room, and make sure he's comfortable.
■ Drain the bath water, clean and disinfect the tub, and dispose of soiled materials properly. If you've given an oatmeal powder bath, drain and rinse the tub immediately, or the powder will cake, making later removal difficult.

Special considerations

■ *Because pruritus seems worse at night,* give a therapeutic bath before bedtime, unless ordered otherwise, *to promote restful sleep. Because the patient with a skin disorder may be self-conscious,* maintain eye contact during conversation and avoid staring at his skin. Also avoid nonverbal expressions and gestures that show revulsion. If the patient wishes, allow him to talk about his condition and how it affects his self-esteem.
■ Refrain from using soap during a therapeutic bath *because its drying effect counteracts the bath emollient.*
■ *A patient with skin breakdown chills easily,* so protect him from drafts. However, after the bath, avoid covering or dressing him too warmly *because perspiration aggravates pruritus.* Instruct the patient not to scratch his skin *to prevent excoriation and infection.*
■ If the patient is confined to bed, you can place the therapeutic additive in a basin of water at 95° to 100° F (35° to 37.8° C) and apply it with a washcloth, using light, gentle strokes.

Home care

Instruct the patient to bathe only as often as prescribed. Excessive bathing can dry the skin. Advise him to purchase commercial bath oil. Salad or cooking oils may give clothes an unpleasant odor, and mineral oil mixes poorly with water. Tell the patient to follow the manufacturer's instructions for commercially prepared colloid preparations. Colloid for an oatmeal bath can be made at home by putting one-half cup of raw oatmeal into a blender and blending at medium-high speed until the material has the consistency of flour, then sifting it to remove unground pieces.

Documentation

Record the date, time, and duration of the bath. Note the water temperature, type and amount of additive, skin appearance before and after the bath, the patient's tolerance of the treatment, and the bath's effectiveness.

SELECTED REFERENCES

Bender, T., et al. "Hydrotherapy, Balneotherapy, and Spa Treatment in Pain Management," *Rheumatology International* 25(3):2204, April 2005.

SOAKS

A soak involves immersion of a body part in warm water or a medicated solution. This treatment helps to soften exudates, facilitate debridement, enhance suppuration, clean wounds or burns, rehydrate wounds, apply medication to infected areas, and increase local blood supply and circulation.

Most soaks are applied with clean tap water and clean technique. Sterile solution and sterile equipment are required for treating wounds, burns, and other breaks in the skin.

Equipment

Basin or arm or foot tub ■ bath (utility) thermometer ■ hot tap water or prescribed solution ■ cup ■ pitcher ■ linen-saver pad ■ overbed table ■ footstool ■ pillows ■ towels ■ gauze pads and other dressing materials ■ clean and sterile gloves, if necessary.

Preparation of equipment

Clean and disinfect the basin or tub. Run hot tap water into a pitcher, or heat the prescribed solution, as applicable. Measure the water or solution temperature with a bath thermometer. If the temperature isn't within the prescribed range (usually 105° to 110° F [40.6° to 43.3° C]), add hot or cold water or reheat or cool the solution, as needed.

If you're preparing the soak outside the patient's room, heat the liquid slightly above the correct temperature *to allow for cooling during transport.* If the solution for a medicated soak isn't premixed, prepare the solution and heat it.

Implementation

- Confirm the patient's identity using two patient identifiers according to your facility's policy.
- Check the practitioner's order.
- Assess the patient's condition, and check for an allergy to the medicated solution.
- Explain the procedure to the patient. Provide privacy. Wash your hands thoroughly.
- If the soak basin or tub will be placed in bed, make sure the bed is flat beneath it *to prevent spills.* For an arm soak, have the patient sit erect. For a leg or foot soak, ask him to lie down and bend the appropriate knee. For a foot soak in the sitting position, let him sit on the edge of the bed or transfer him to a chair.
- Place a linen-saver pad under the treatment site and, if necessary, cover the pad with a towel *to absorb spillage.*
- Expose the treatment site. Put on gloves before removing any dressing; dispose of the soiled dressing properly. If the dressing is encrusted and stuck to the wound, leave it in place and proceed with the soak. Remove the dressing several minutes later when it has begun to soak free.
- Position the soak basin under the treatment site on the bed, overbed table, footstool, or floor, as appropriate. Pour the heated liquid into the soak basin or tub. Then lower the arm or leg into the basin gradually *to allow adjustment to the temperature change.* Make sure the soak solution covers the treatment site.
- Support other body parts with pillows or towels as needed *to prevent discomfort and muscle strain.* Make the patient comfortable and ensure proper body alignment.
- Check the temperature of the soak solution with the bath thermometer every 5 minutes. If the temperature drops below the prescribed range, remove some of the cooled solution with a cup. Then lift the patient's arm or leg from the basin *to avoid burns,* and add hot water or solution to the basin. Mix the liquid thoroughly, and then check its temperature. If the temperature is within the prescribed range, lower the patient's affected part back into the basin.
- Observe the patient for signs of tissue intolerance: extreme redness at the treatment site, excessive drainage, bleeding, or maceration. If such signs develop or the patient complains of pain, discontinue the treatment and notify the practitioner.
- After 15 to 20 minutes or as ordered, lift the patient's arm or leg from the basin, and remove the basin.
- Dry the arm or leg thoroughly with a towel. If the patient has a wound, dry the skin around it without touching the wound.
- While the skin is hydrated from the soak, use gauze pads to remove loose scales or crusts.
- Observe the treatment area for general appearance, degree of swelling, debridement, suppuration, and healing. Put on sterile gloves and re-dress the wound, if appropriate.
- Remove the towel and linen-saver pad, and make the patient comfortable in bed.
- Discard the soak solution, dispose of soiled materials properly, and clean and disinfect the basin. Remove and discard your gloves. If the treatment is to be repeated, store the equipment in the patient's room, out of his reach; otherwise, return it to the central supply department.

Special considerations

- To treat large areas, particularly burns, a soak may be administered in a whirlpool or Hubbard tank.

Documentation

Record the date, time, and duration of the soak; treatment site; solution and its temperature; skin and wound appearance before, during, and after treatment; and the patient's tolerance for the treatment.

SELECTED REFERENCES

Craven, R.F., and Hirnle, C.J. *Fundamentals of Nursing: Human Health and Function,* 5th ed. Philadelphia: Lippincott Williams & Wilkins, 2007.

Gutman, A.B., et al. "Soak and Smear: A Standard Technique Revisited," *Archives of Dermatology* 141(12):1556-59, December 2005.

Taylor, C., et al. *Fundamentals of Nursing: The Art and Science of Nursing Care,* 6th ed. Philadelphia: Lippincott Williams & Wilkins, 2008.

SUPPORT DEVICES

ANTIEMBOLISM STOCKING APPLICATION

Elastic antiembolism stockings help prevent deep vein thrombosis (DVT) and pulmonary embolism by compressing superficial leg veins. This compression increases venous return by forcing blood into the deep venous system rather than allowing it to pool in the legs and form clots.

Antiembolism stockings can provide equal pressure over the entire leg or a graded pressure that is greatest at the ankle and decreases over the length of the leg. Usually indicated for postoperative, bedridden, elderly, or other patients at risk for DVT, these stockings shouldn't be used on patients with dermatoses or open skin lesions, gangrene, severe arteriosclerosis or other ischemic vascular diseases, pul-

Measuring for antiembolism stockings

Measure the patient carefully to ensure that his antiembolism stockings provide enough compression for adequate venous return.

To choose the correct *knee-length* stocking, measure the circumference of the calf at its widest point (top left) and the leg length from the bottom of the heel to the back of the knee (bottom left).

To choose a *thigh-length* stocking, measure the calf as for a knee-length stocking and the thigh at its widest point (top right). Then measure leg length from the bottom of the heel to the gluteal fold (bottom right).

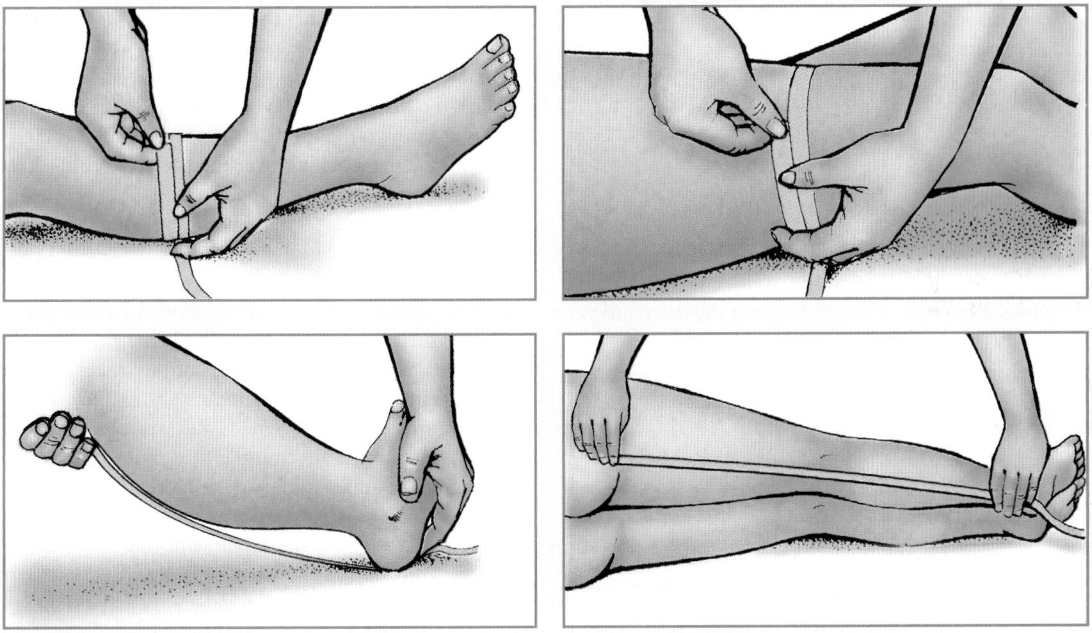

monary or any massive edema, recent vein ligation, or vascular or skin grafts. For patients with chronic venous problems, intermittent pneumatic compression stockings may be ordered during surgery and postoperatively.

Equipment

Tape measure ▪ antiembolism stockings of correct size and length ▪ talcum powder.

Preparation of equipment

Before applying a knee-length stocking: Measure the circumference of the patient's calf at its widest point and leg length from the bottom of the heel to the back of the knee. (See *Measuring for antiembolism stockings.*)

Before applying a thigh-length stocking: Measure the circumference of the calf and thigh at their widest points and the leg length from the bottom of the heel to the gluteal fold.

Before applying a waist-length stocking: Measure the circumference of the calf and thigh at their widest points and the leg length from the bottom of the heel along the side to the waist.

Obtain the correct size stocking according to the manufacturer's specifications. If the patient's measurements are outside the range indicated by the manufacturer, or if his legs are deformed or edematous, ask the practitioner if he wants to order custom-made stockings.

Implementation

- Confirm the patient's identity using two patient identifiers according to your facility's policy.
- Check the practitioner's order.

Applying antiembolism stockings: Three key steps

Gather the loose part of the stocking at the toes, and pull this portion toward the heel.

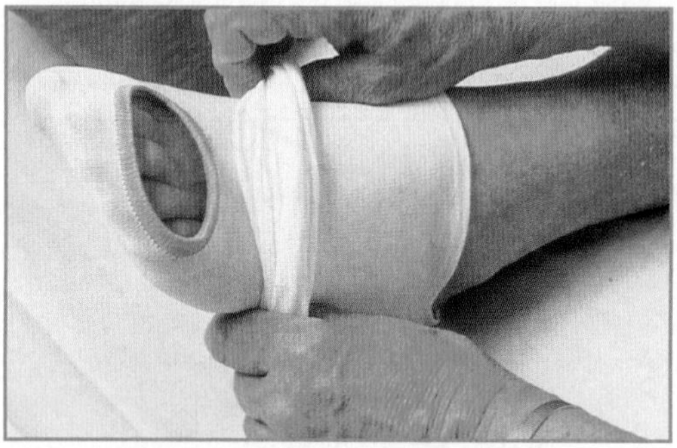

Then gather the loose part of the stocking and bring it over the heel with short alternating front and back pulls.

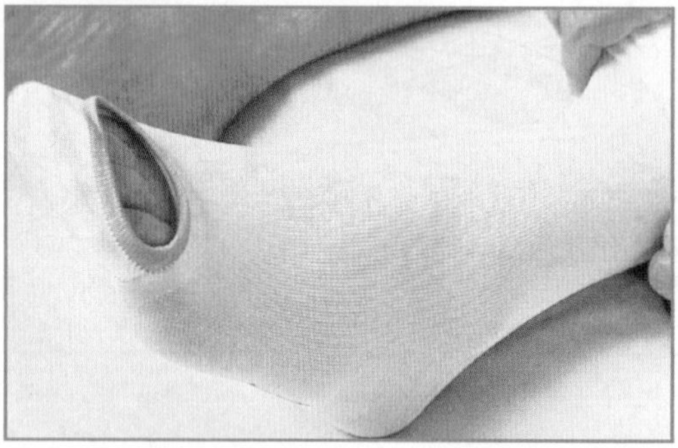

Insert the index and middle fingers into the gathered part of the stocking at the ankle, and ease it upward by rocking it slightly up and down.

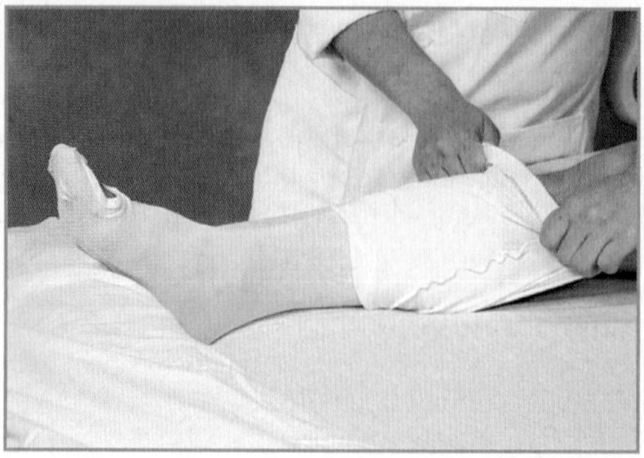

- Assess the patient's condition. If his legs are cold or cyanotic, notify the practitioner before proceeding.
- Explain the procedure to the patient, provide privacy, and wash your hands thoroughly.
- Have the patient lie down. Then dust his ankle with talcum powder *to ease application.*

Applying a knee-length stocking

- Insert your hand into the stocking from the top, and grasp the heel pocket from the inside. Holding the heel, turn the stocking inside out so that the foot is inside the stocking leg. *This method allows easier application than gathering the entire stocking and working it up over the foot and ankle.*
- With the heel pocket down, hook the index and middle fingers of both your hands into the foot section. Facing the patient, ease the stocking over the toes, stretching it sideways as you move it up the foot.
- Support the patient's ankle with one hand, and use the other hand to pull the heel pocket under the heel. Then center the heel in the pocket.
- Gather the loose portion of the stocking at the toe, and pull only this section over the heel. Gather the loose material at the ankle, and slide the rest of the stocking up over the heel with short pulls, alternating front and back. (See *Applying antiembolism stockings: Three key steps.*)
- Insert your index and middle fingers into the gathered stocking at the ankle, and ease the fabric up the leg to the knee.
- Supporting the patient's ankle with one hand, use your other hand to stretch the stocking toward the knee, front and back, *to distribute the material evenly.* The stocking top should be 1″ to 2″ (2.5 to 5 cm) below the bottom of the patella.
- Gently snap the fabric around the ankle *to ensure a tight fit and eliminate gaps that could reduce pressure.*
- Adjust the foot section for fabric smoothness and toe comfort by tugging on the toe section. Properly position the toe window, if any.
- Repeat the procedure for the second stocking, if ordered.

Applying a thigh-length stocking

- Follow the procedure for applying a knee-length stocking, taking care to distribute the fabric evenly below the knee before continuing the procedure.
- With the patient's leg extended, stretch the rest of the stocking over the knee.
- Flex the patient's knee, and pull the stocking over the thigh until the top is 1″ to 3″ (2.5 to 7.5 cm) below the gluteal fold.
- Stretch the stocking from the top, front and back, *to distribute the fabric evenly over the thigh.*

■ Gently snap the fabric behind the knee *to eliminate gaps that could reduce pressure.*

Applying a waist-length stocking

■ Follow the procedure for applying knee-length and thigh-length stockings, and extend the stocking top to the gluteal fold.

■ Fit the patient with the adjustable belt that accompanies the stockings. Make sure the waistband and the fabric don't interfere with any incision, drainage tube, catheter, or other device.

Special considerations

■ Apply the stockings in the morning, if possible, *before edema develops.* If the patient has been ambulating, ask him to lie down and elevate his legs for 15 to 30 minutes before applying the stockings *to facilitate venous return.*

■ Don't allow the stockings to roll or turn down at the top or toe *because the excess pressure could cause venous strangulation.* Have the patient wear the stockings in bed and during ambulation *to provide continuous protection against thrombosis.*

■ Check the patient's toes at least once every 4 hours—more often in the patient with a faint pulse or edema. Note skin color and temperature, sensation, swelling, and ability to move. If complications occur, remove the stockings, and notify the practitioner immediately.

■ Be alert for an allergic reaction *because some patients can't tolerate the sizing in new stockings.* Laundering the stockings before applying them reduces the risk of an allergic reaction to sizing. Remove the stockings at least once daily *to bathe the skin and observe for irritation and breakdown.*

■ Using warm water and mild soap, wash the stockings when soiled. Keep a second pair handy *for the patient to wear while the other pair is being laundered.*

Home care

If the patient will require antiembolism stockings after discharge, teach him or a family member how to apply them correctly, and explain why he needs to wear them. Instruct the patient or family member to care for the stockings properly and to replace them when they lose elasticity.

Complications

Obstruction of arterial blood flow—characterized by cold and bluish toes, dusky toenail beds, decreased or absent pedal pulses, and leg pain or cramps—can result from application of antiembolism stockings. Less serious complications, such as an allergic reaction and skin irritation, can also occur.

Documentation

Record the date and time of stocking application and removal, stocking length and size, condition of the leg before and after treatment, condition of the toes during treatment, any complications, and the patient's tolerance of the treatment.

SELECTED REFERENCES

Howard, A., et al. "Randomized Clinical Trial of Low Molecular Weight Heparin with Thigh-Length or Knee-Length Antiembolism Stockings for Patients Undergoing Surgery," *British Journal of Surgery* 91(7): 842-47, July 2004.

Ingram, J.E., et al. "A Review of Thigh-Length vs. Knee-Length Antiembolism Stockings," *British Journal of Nursing* 12(14):845-51, July-August 2003.

Segal, J.E., et al. "Management of Venous Thromboembolism: A Systemic Review for a Practice Guideline," *Annals of Internal Medicine* 146(3):I43, February 2007.

SEQUENTIAL COMPRESSION THERAPY

Safe, effective, and noninvasive, sequential compression therapy helps prevent deep vein thrombosis (DVT) in surgical patients. This therapy massages the legs in a wavelike, milking motion that promotes blood flow and deters thrombosis.

Typically, sequential compression therapy complements other preventive measures, such as antiembolism stockings and anticoagulant medications. Although patients at low risk for DVT may require only antiembolism stockings, those at moderate to high risk may require both antiembolism stockings and sequential compression therapy. These preventive measures are continued for as long as the patient remains at risk.

Both antiembolism stockings and sequential compression sleeves are commonly used preoperatively because blood clots tend to form during surgery. About 20% of blood clots form in the femoral vein. Sequential compression therapy counteracts blood stasis and coagulation changes, two of the three major factors that promote DVT. It reduces stasis by increasing peak blood flow velocity, helping to empty the femoral vein's valve cusps of pooled or static blood. Also, the compressions cause an anticlotting effect by increasing fibrinolytic activity, which stimulates the release of a plasminogen activator.

Equipment

Measuring tape and sizing chart for the brand of sleeves you're using ■ pair of compression sleeves in correct size ■ connecting tubing ■ compression controller.

Implementation

■ Confirm the patient's identity using two patient identifiers according to your facility's policy.
■ Explain the procedure to the patient *to ensure his cooperation.*
■ Wash your hands.

Determining proper sleeve size

■ Before applying the compression sleeve, determine the proper size of sleeve that you need.
■ Measure the circumference of the upper thigh while the patient rests in bed. Do this by placing the measuring tape under the thigh at the gluteal furrow (as shown below).

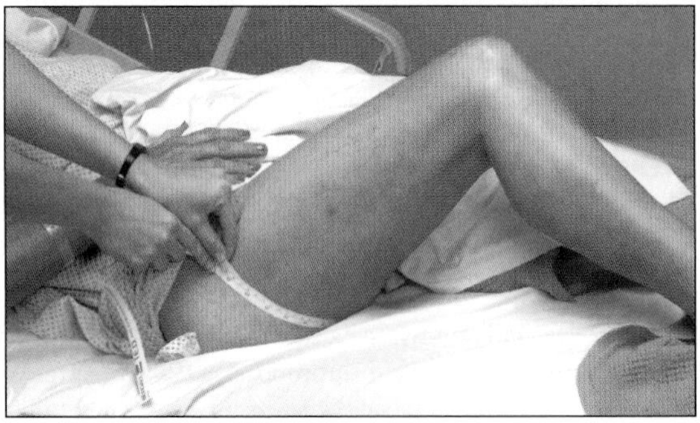

■ Hold the tape snugly, but not tightly, around the patient's leg. Note the exact circumference.
■ Find the patient's thigh measurement on the sizing chart, and locate the corresponding size of the compression sleeve.
■ Remove the compression sleeves from the package, and unfold them.
■ Lay the unfolded sleeves on a flat surface with the cotton lining facing up (as shown below).

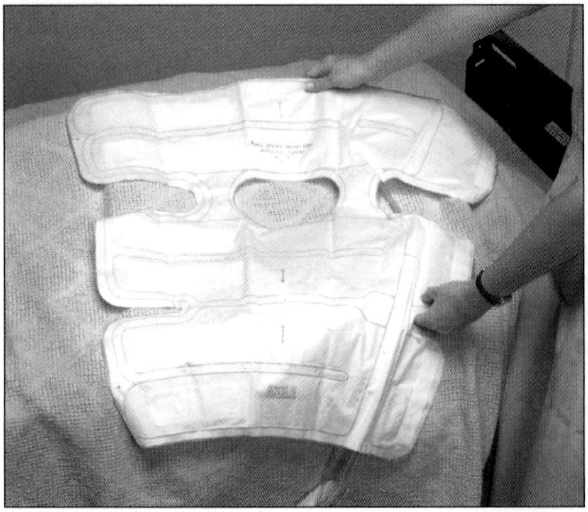

■ Notice the markings on the lining denoting the ankle and the area behind the knee at the popliteal pulse point. *Use these markings to position the sleeve at the appropriate landmarks.*

Applying the sleeves

■ Place the patient's leg on the sleeve lining. Position the back of the knee over the popliteal opening.
■ Make sure the back of the ankle is over the ankle marking.
■ Starting at the side opposite the clear plastic tubing, wrap the sleeve snugly around the patient's leg.
■ Fasten the sleeve securely with the Velcro fasteners. For the best fit, first secure the ankle and calf sections and then the thigh.
■ The sleeve should fit snugly but not tightly. Check the fit by inserting two fingers between the sleeve and the patient's leg at the knee opening. Loosen or tighten the sleeve by readjusting the Velcro fastener.
■ Using the same procedure, apply the second sleeve (as shown below).

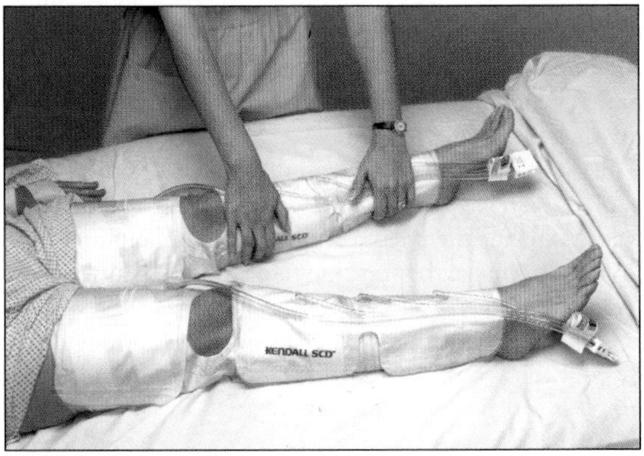

Operating the system

■ Connect each sleeve to the tubing leading to the controller. Both sleeves must be connected to the compression controller for the system to operate. Line up the blue arrows on the sleeve connector with the arrows on the tubing connectors, and push the ends together firmly. Listen for a click, *signaling a firm connection.* Make sure the tubing isn't kinked.
■ Plug the compression controller into the proper wall outlet. Turn on the power.
■ The controller automatically sets the compression sleeve pressure at 45 mm Hg, which is the midpoint of the normal range (35 to 55 mm Hg).
■ Observe the patient to see how well he tolerates the therapy and the controller as the system completes its first cy-

cle. With the instrument shown here, each cycle lasts 71 seconds—11 seconds of compression and 60 seconds of decompression.

■ Check the AUDIBLE ALARM key. The green light should be lit, indicating that the alarm is working.

■ The compression sleeves should function continuously (24 hours daily) until the patient is fully ambulatory. Be sure to check the sleeves at least once each shift *to ensure proper fit and inflation.*

Removing the sleeves

■ You may remove the sleeves when the patient is walking, bathing, or leaving the room for tests or other procedures. Reapply them immediately after any of these activities. To disconnect the sleeves from the tubing, press the latches on each side of the connectors, and pull the connectors apart.

■ Store the tubing and compression controller according to facility protocol. This equipment isn't disposable.

Special considerations

■ Remove the sleeves and assess and document skin integrity every 8 hours *to avoid skin breakdown,* especially in patients with decreased sensation or who are unresponsive.

■ The compression controller also has a mechanism to help cool the patient.

■ If you're applying only one sleeve—for example, if the patient has a cast—leave the unused sleeve folded in the plastic bag. Cut a small hole in the bag's sealed bottom edge, and pull the sleeve connector (the part that holds the connecting tubing) through the hole. Then you can join both sleeves to the compression controller.

■ If a malfunction triggers the instrument's alarm, you'll hear beeping. The system shuts off whenever the alarm is activated.

■ To respond to the alarm, remove the operator's card from the slot on the top of the compression controller. Follow the instructions printed on the card next to the matching code.

Complications

Don't use this therapy in patients with any of the following conditions:

■ acute DVT (or DVT diagnosed within the past 6 months)

■ severe arteriosclerosis or any other ischemic vascular disease

■ massive edema of the legs resulting from pulmonary edema or heart failure

■ any local condition that the compression sleeves would aggravate, such as dermatitis, vein ligation, gangrene, and recent skin grafting. A patient with a pronounced leg deformity also would be unlikely to benefit from the compression sleeves.

Documentation

Document the procedure, the patient's response to and understanding of the procedure, and the status of the alarm and cooling settings.

SELECTED REFERENCES

Bartley, M. "Keep Venous Thromboembolism at Bay," *Nursing* 36(10):36-41, October 2006.

Beck, D. "Venous Thromboembolism (VTE) Prophylaxis: Implications for Medical-Surgical Nurses," *Medsurg Nursing* 15(5):282-87, October 2006.

"Graduate Compression Stockings: Prevention of Postoperative Venous Thromboembolism Is Crucial," *AJN* 106(2):72AA-DD, February 2006.

Lachiewicz, P.F., et al. "Two Mechanical Devices for Prophylaxis of Thromboembolism after Total Knee Arthroplasty: A Prospective, Randomized Study," *Journal of Bone and Joint Surgery* 86(8):1137-141, November 2004.

ELASTIC BANDAGE APPLICATION

Elastic bandages exert gentle, even pressure on a body part. By supporting blood vessels, these rolled bandages promote venous return and prevent pooling of blood in the legs. They're typically used in place of antiembolism stockings to prevent thrombophlebitis and pulmonary embolism in postoperative or bedridden patients who can't stimulate venous return by muscle activity.

Elastic bandages also minimize joint swelling after trauma to the musculoskeletal system. Used with a splint, they immobilize a fracture during healing. They can provide hemostatic pressure and anchor dressings over a fresh wound or after surgical procedures, such as vein stripping.

Equipment

Elastic bandage of appropriate width ■ tape, pins, or self-closures ■ gauze pads or absorbent cotton.

Bandages usually come in 2″to 6″ widths and 4′ and 6′ (1.2- and 1.8-m) lengths. The 3″ width is adaptable to most applications. An elastic bandage with self-closures is also available.

Preparation of equipment

Select a bandage that wraps the affected body part completely but isn't excessively long. In most cases, use a narrower bandage for wrapping the foot, lower leg, hand, or arm, and a wider bandage for the thigh or trunk. The bandage should be clean and rolled before application.

Implementation

- Confirm the patient's identity using two patient identifiers according to your facility's policy.
- Check the practitioner's order.
- Examine the area to be wrapped for lesions or skin breakdown. If these conditions are present, consult the practitioner before applying the elastic bandage.
- Explain the procedure to the patient, provide privacy, and wash your hands thoroughly. Position him comfortably, with the body part to be bandaged in normal functioning position *to promote circulation and prevent deformity and discomfort.*
- Avoid applying a bandage to a dependent extremity. If you're wrapping an extremity, elevate it for 15 to 30 minutes before application *to facilitate venous return.*
- Apply the bandage so that two skin surfaces don't remain in contact when wrapped. Place gauze or absorbent cotton as needed between skin surfaces, such as between toes and fingers and under breasts and arms, *to prevent skin irritation.*
- Hold the bandage with the roll facing upward in one hand and the free end of the bandage in the other hand. Hold the bandage roll close to the part being bandaged *to ensure even tension and pressure.*
- Unroll the bandage as you wrap the body part in a spiral or spiral-reverse method. Never unroll the entire bandage before wrapping *because this could produce uneven pressure, which interferes with blood circulation and cell perfusion.*
- Overlap each layer of bandage by one-half to two-thirds the width of the strip. (See *Bandaging techniques.*)
- Wrap firmly but not too tightly. As you wrap, ask the patient to tell you if the bandage feels comfortable. If he complains of tingling, itching, numbness, or pain, loosen the bandage.
- Begin wrapping an extremity at the most distal part and work proximally *to promote venous return.*
- When wrapping an extremity, anchor the bandage initially by circling the body part twice. *To prevent the bandage from slipping out of place on the foot,* wrap it in a figure eight around the foot, the ankle, and then the foot again before continuing. The same technique works on any joint, such as the knee, wrist, or elbow. Include the heel when wrapping the foot, but never wrap the toes (or fingers) unless absolutely necessary *because the distal extremities are used to detect impaired circulation.*
- When you're finished wrapping, secure the end of the bandage with tape, pins, or self-closures, being careful not to scratch or pinch the patient. Avoid using metal clips *because they typically come loose when the patient moves and may get lost in the bed linens and injure him.*
- Check distal circulation after the bandage is in place *because the elastic may tighten as you wrap.*
- Elevate a wrapped extremity for 15 to 30 minutes *to facilitate venous return.*
- Check distal circulation once or twice every 8 hours *because an elastic bandage that is too tight may result in neurovascular damage.* Lift the distal end of the bandage, and assess the skin underneath for color, temperature, and integrity.
- Remove the bandage every 8 hours or whenever it's loose and wrinkled. Roll it up as you unwrap *to ready it for reuse.* Observe the area and provide skin care before rewrapping the bandage.
- Change the bandage at least once daily. Bathe the skin, dry it thoroughly, and observe for irritation and breakdown before applying a fresh bandage.

Special considerations

- Avoid leaving gaps in bandage layers or exposed skin surfaces *because this may result in uneven pressure on the body part.*
- Observe the patient for an allergic reaction *because some patients can't tolerate the sizing in a new bandage.* Laundering it reduces this risk.
- Launder the bandage daily or whenever it becomes limp; *laundering restores its elasticity.* Always keep two bandages handy *so one can be applied while the other bandage is being laundered.*
- When using an elastic bandage after a surgical procedure on an extremity (such as vein stripping) or with a splint to immobilize a fracture, remove it only as ordered rather than every 8 hours.

Home care

If the patient will be using an elastic bandage at home, teach him or a family member how to apply it correctly and how to assess for restricted circulation. Tell him to keep two bandages available so he'll have one while the other is being laundered.

Complications

Arterial obstruction—characterized by a decreased or an absent distal pulse, blanching or bluish discoloration of skin, dusky nail beds, numbness and tingling or pain and cramping, and cold skin—can result from elastic bandage application. Edema can occur from obstruction of venous return. Less serious complications include allergic reaction and skin irritation.

Documentation

Record the date and time of bandage application and removal; the application site, bandage size, skin condition before application, skin care provided after removal, and com-

Bandaging techniques

Circular
Each turn encircles the previous one, covering it completely. Use this technique to anchor a bandage.

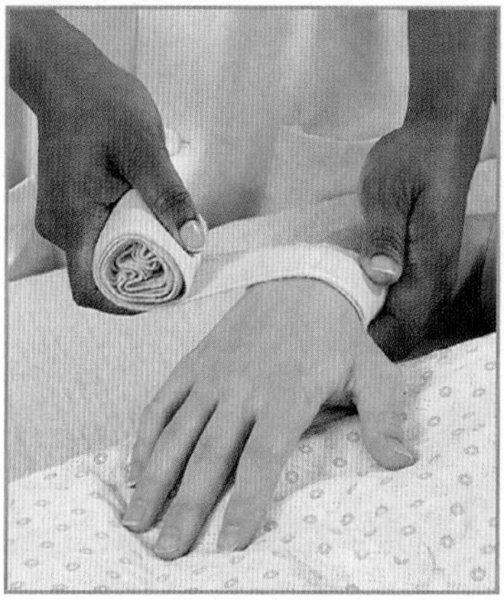

Spiral
Each turn partially overlaps the previous one. Use this technique to wrap a long, straight body part or one of increasing circumference.

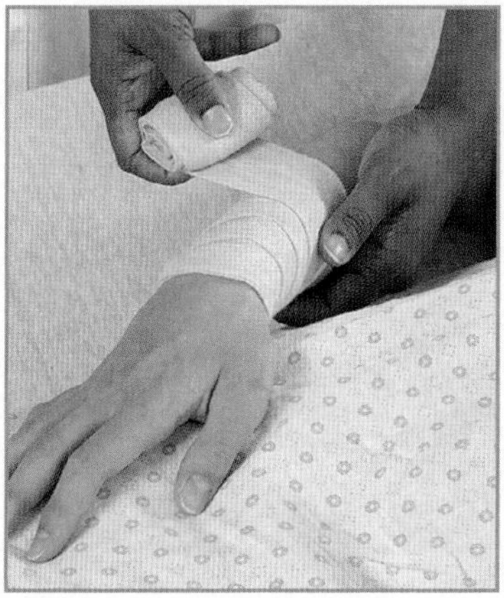

Spiral-reverse
Anchor the bandage, and then reverse direction halfway through each spiral turn. Use this technique to accommodate the increasing circumference of a body part.

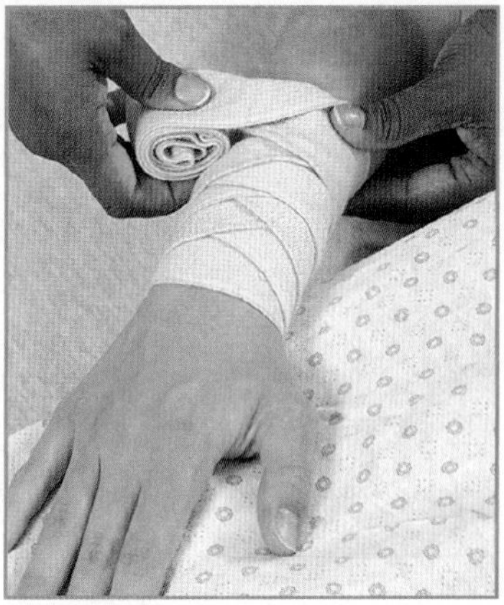

Figure eight
Anchor below the joint, and then use alternating ascending and descending turns to form a figure eight. Use this technique around joints.

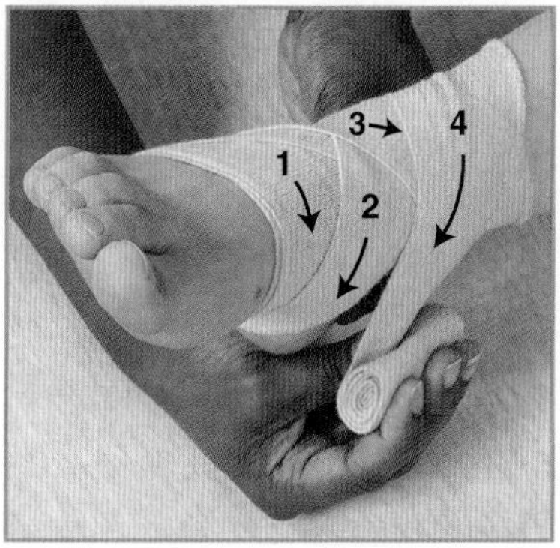

Recurrent
This technique includes a combination of recurrent and circular turns. Hold the bandage as you make each recurrent turn, and then use the circular turns as a final anchor. Use this technique for a stump, a hand, or the scalp.

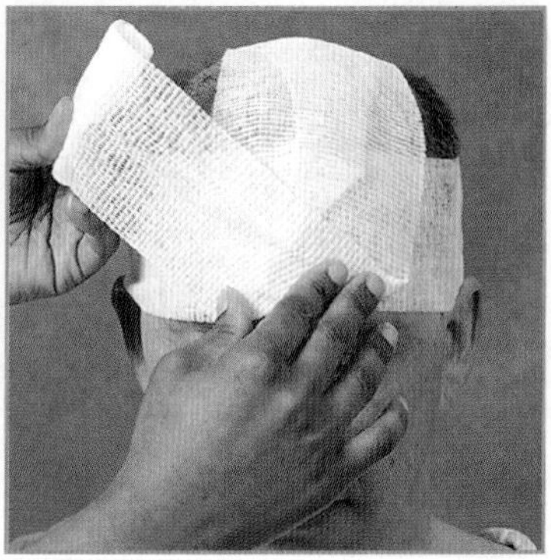

plications; the patient's tolerance of the treatment; and any patient teaching.

SELECTED REFERENCES

Coull, A., et al. "Class 3C Compression Bandaging for Venous Ulcers: Comparison of Spiral and Figure-Eight Techniques," *Journal of Advanced Nursing* 54(3):274-83, May 2006.

Types of binders

Straight abdominal
Keeps suture line intact after abdominal surgery so patient can move more freely and provides abdominal support after delivery or paracentesis

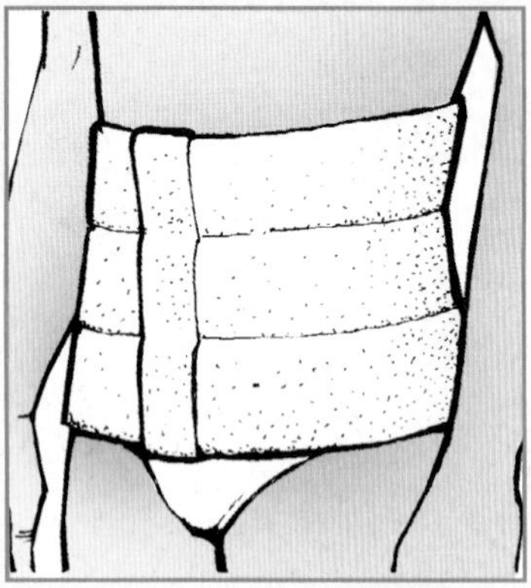

Scultetus
Keeps suture line intact after abdominal surgery so patient can move more freely and provides abdominal support after delivery or paracentesis

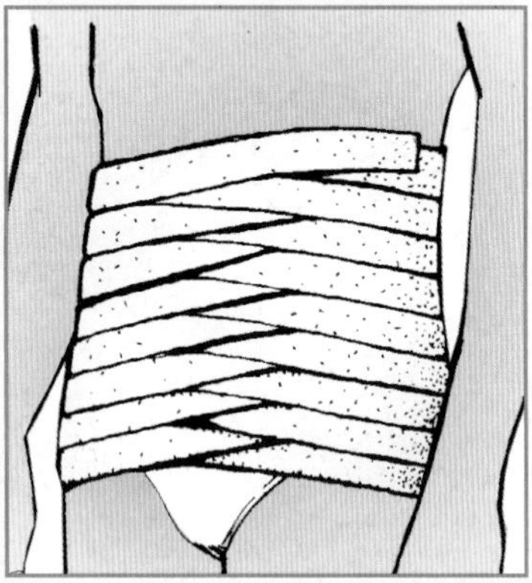

Breast
Reduces breast engorgement in the non–breast-feeding mother

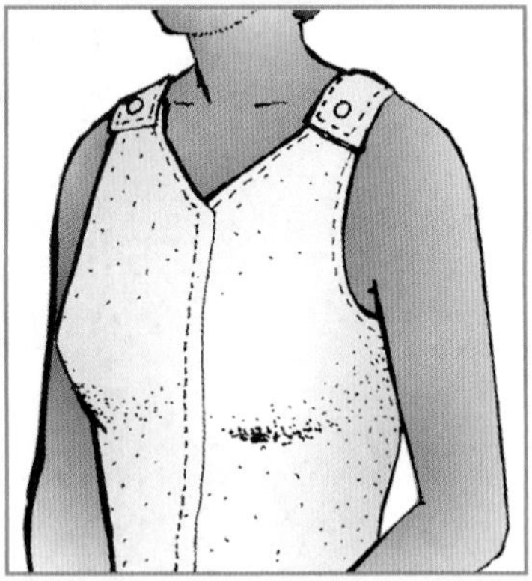

Single T
Keeps perineal dressings in place for the female patient

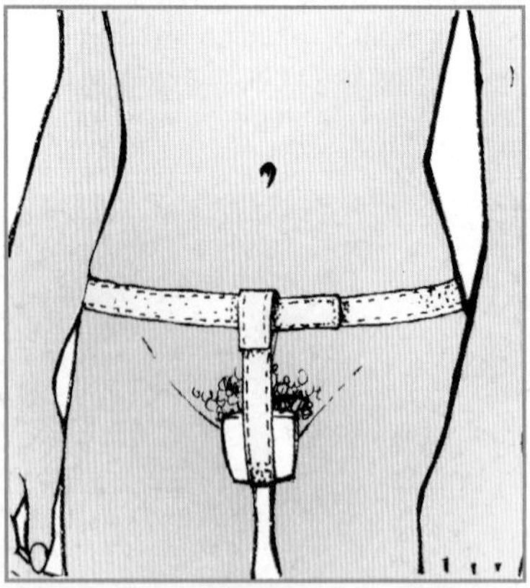

Double T
Secures perineal dressings for the male patient or for the female patient requiring a bulky dressing

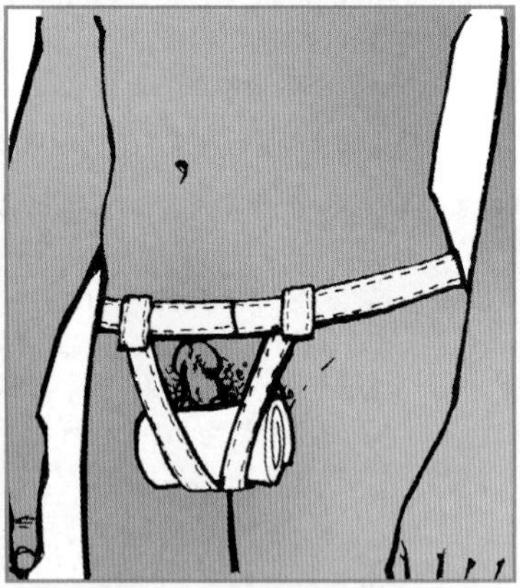

Fletcher, J. "The Importance of Correctly Choosing a Bandage and Bandaging Technique," *Nursing Times* 100(32):52-53, August 2004.

Lynn, P. *Taylor's Clinical Nursing Skills,* 2nd ed. Philadelphia: Lippincott Williams & Wilkins, 2008.

BINDER APPLICATION

Also known as self-closures, binders are lengths of cloth or elasticized material that encircle the chest, abdomen, or groin to provide support, keep dressings in place (especially for patients allergic to tape), reduce tension on wounds and suture lines, and reduce breast engorgement in the non–breast-feeding mother (although a snug-fitting support bra is usually recommended instead). Typically, cloth binders are fastened with safety pins, and elasticized binders are fastened with Velcro.

Equipment

Tape measure ■ binder of appropriate size and type ■ safety pins ■ gloves, if necessary. Commercial elastic binders with Velcro closings are now commonly used instead of standard cotton straight and scultetus binders that require pins. Disposable T-binders are available, and scrotal supports typically replace binders for male patients, except after abdominal-perineal resection. (See *Types of binders.*)

Preparation of equipment

Measure the area that the binder must fit, and obtain the proper size and type of binder from the central supply department.

Implementation

■ Confirm the patient's identity using two patient identifiers according to your facility's policy.
■ Check the practitioner's order.
■ Assess the patient's condition.
■ Explain the procedure to the patient, provide privacy, wash your hands thoroughly, and put on gloves, if needed.
■ Raise the patient's bed to its highest position *to avoid muscle strain when applying the binder.*
■ Change the dressing, and inspect the wound or suture line if appropriate.

Applying a straight abdominal binder

■ Accordion-fold half of the binder, slip it under the patient, and pull it through from the other side. Make sure the binder is straight, free of wrinkles, and evenly distributed under the patient. Its lower edge should extend well below the hips.
■ Overlap one side snugly onto the other. Then insert one finger under the binder's edge *to ensure a snug fit that's still loose enough to avoid impaired circulation and patient discomfort.*
■ Starting at the lower edge, close the Velcro closure.
■ Make darts in the binder as needed. Avoid making the binder too tight around the diaphragm *because it may interfere with breathing.*

Applying a scultetus binder

■ Slide the binder under the patient's hips and buttocks so that its top aligns with the waist and its lowest tail crosses the extreme lower abdomen.

Applying a scultetus binder

After centering the binder's solid portion under the patient, with tails distributed evenly on each side, bring the lowest tail straight across the patient's abdomen, hold it snugly, and bring the next higher tail across to overlap it. Alternate tails in this manner, with the next higher tail overlapping the one below it by about half its width.

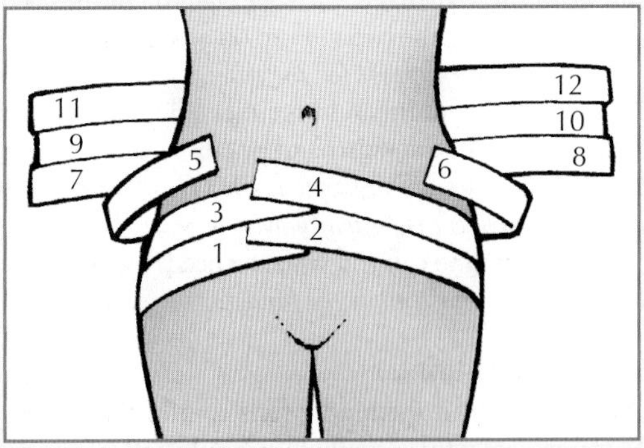

■ Adjust the binder so that its solid part is centered under the patient and its tails are evenly distributed on either side. Spread the tails out flat *so you can pick them up easily.*
■ Beginning at the lower edge of the binder, bring one tail straight across the patient's abdomen. If the tail is too long, fold it over flat at the end. Hold this tail snugly in place as you bring the opposite tail across on top of it, overlapping the first tail's upper half and continuing with succeeding tail pieces. (See *Applying a scultetus binder.*)
■ Secure the top strap, using two safety pins placed horizontally *so they won't interfere with body movement.*

Applying a breast binder

■ Slip the binder under the patient's chest so that its lower edge aligns with the waist. Straighten the binder to distribute it evenly on either side.
■ Place the binder so that the patient's nipples are centered in the breast tissue. *This ensures proper breast alignment and support and produces faster tissue involution.*
■ Pull the binder's edges snugly together, and begin closing the Velcro closures upward from the waist.
■ Adjust the shoulder straps to fit properly and secure them with the Velcro fasteners.

Applying a T-binder

■ Slip the T-binder under the patient's waist, with its tails extending below the buttocks. Smooth the waistband and tails *to remove twists, which can chafe the patient's skin.*

■ Pull the waistband snugly into position at the patient's waistline or lower across the abdomen. Then fasten the Velcro closure. Next, bring the free tail up between the patient's legs over the dressing or perineal pad.

■ For a female patient, bring the single tail up to the center of the waist, loop it behind and over the waistband, and secure it to the waistband with the Velcro closures. For a male patient, bring the two tails up on either side of the penis *to provide even support for the testes.* Loop the ends behind and over the waistband on either side of the midline, and fasten them to the waistband by closing the Velcro closures. *Pinning through multiple layers keeps the straps from slipping sideways as the patient moves.*

■ Tell the patient to call you when he needs to void or defecate *to unfasten and reapply the binder.*

Applying any binder

■ Ask the patient if the binder feels comfortable. Tell him that it may feel tight initially but should feel comfortable shortly. Instruct the patient to notify you immediately if the binder feels too tight or too loose or comes apart.

■ If the patient can ambulate, ask him to do so *to evaluate the fit of the binder.*

Special considerations

■ *For maximum support,* wrap the binder so that it applies even pressure across the body section. Eliminate all wrinkles, and avoid placing pressure over bony prominences.

■ In surgical applications, fasten straight and scultetus binders from the bottom upward *to relieve gravitational pull on the wound.* In obstetric applications, fasten from the top downward *to direct the uterus into the pelvis. Because this places extra pressure on weak abdominal muscles,* observe the patient closely for precipitate delivery.

■ Be careful not to compress any tubes, drains, or catheters and not to position them so that they are working against gravity. Also, don't allow binder placement to interfere with elimination.

■ Use a double T-binder on a female patient after extensive surgery that requires a large dressing. Use a straight or scultetus binder as a breast binder, if necessary.

■ Observe the patient and check binder placement every 8 hours. Check the skin for color, palpate it for warmth, check pulses, and assess for tingling or numbness.

■ Reapply the binder when a dressing needs changing, when the binder becomes loose or too tight, and at other times according to the practitioner's orders. When changing the binder, observe the skin for signs of irritation. Provide appropriate skin care before reapplying the binder.

Home care

If the patient will need a binder after discharge, teach him and a family member how to remove it, inspect the skin, bathe the area, and reapply it. Tell the patient and family member where binders can be purchased and how to care for them. For a patient with cancer, the American Cancer Society may provide assistance in obtaining binders. If commercially manufactured binders are unavailable, advise the patient and family that a clean towel or sheeting material can be used instead. Periodically reinforce prior teaching and instructions.

Complications

Irritation of the underlying skin can result from perspiration or friction.

Documentation

Record the date and time of binder application, reapplication, and removal; binder type and location; purpose of application; skin condition before and after application; dressing changes or skin care; complications; and the patient's tolerance of the treatment.

SELECTED REFERENCES

Doughty, D. "Preventing and Managing Surgical Wound Dehiscence," *Advances in Skin & Wound Care* 18(6):319-22, July-August 2005.

Hahler, B. "Surgical Wound Dehiscence," *Medsurg Nursing* 15(5):296-300, October 2006.

Meloni, R., et al. "Evaluation of the Complexity of Post-Operative Care Following Breast and Gynecologic Cancer Surgery," *Cancer Nursing* 29(6):499-505, November-December 2006.

Taylor, C., et al. *Fundamentals of Nursing: The Art and Science of Nursing Care,* 6th ed. Philadelphia: Lippincott Williams & Wilkins, 2008.

Wilson, J., and Clark, J. "Obesity: Impediment to Postsurgical Wound Healing," *Advances in Skin & Wound Care* 17(8):426-35, October 2004.

PRESSURE DRESSING APPLICATION

For effective control of capillary or small-vein bleeding, temporary application of pressure directly over a wound may be achieved with a bulk dressing held by a glove-protected hand, bound into place with a pressure bandage, or held under pressure by an inflated air splint. A pressure dressing requires frequent checks for wound drainage to determine its effectiveness in controlling bleeding.

Equipment

Two or more sterile gauze pads ▪ roller gauze ▪ adhesive tape ▪ clean disposable gloves ▪ metric ruler.

Preparation of equipment

Obtain the pressure dressing quickly *to avoid excessive blood loss.* Use clean cloth for the dressing if sterile gauze pads are unavailable.

Implementation

- Quickly explain the procedure to the patient *to help decrease his anxiety,* and put on gloves.
- Elevate the injured body part *to help reduce bleeding.*
- Place enough gauze pads over the wound to cover it. Don't clean the wound until the bleeding stops.
- For an extremity or a trunk wound, hold the dressing firmly over the wound and wrap the roller gauze tightly across it and around the body part *to provide pressure on the wound.* Secure the bandage with adhesive tape.
- To apply a dressing to the neck, the shoulder, or another location that can't be tightly wrapped, don't use roller gauze. Instead, apply tape directly over the dressings *to provide the necessary pressure at the wound site.*
- Check pulse, temperature, and skin condition distal to the wound site *because excessive pressure can obstruct normal circulation.*
- Check the dressing frequently *to monitor wound drainage.* Use the metric standard of measurement to determine the amount of drainage, and document these serial measurements for later reference. Don't circle a potentially wet dressing with ink *because this provides no permanent documentation in the medical record and also runs the risk of contaminating the dressing.*
- If the dressing becomes saturated, don't remove it *because this will interfere with the pressure.* Instead, apply an additional dressing over the saturated one and continue to monitor and record drainage.
- Obtain additional medical care as soon as possible.

Special considerations

- Apply pressure directly to the wound with your gloved hand if sterile gauze pads and clean cloth are unavailable.
- Avoid using an elastic bandage to bind the dressing *because it can't be wrapped tightly enough to create pressure on the wound site.*

Complications

A pressure dressing that is applied too tightly can impair circulation.

Documentation

When the bleeding is controlled, record the date and time of dressing application, presence or absence of distal pulses, integrity of distal skin, amount of wound drainage, and complications.

SELECTED REFERENCES

Dean, R. "Emergency First Aid for Nurses," *Nursing Standard* 20(6):57-65, October 2005.
Karabagli, Y., et al. "Industrial Foam Rubber as a Pressure Dressing," *Plastic and Reconstructive Surgery* 114(3):826, September 2004.
Kauvar, D., et al. "Impact of Hemorrhage on Trauma Outcome: An Overview of Epidemiology, Clinical Presentation, and Therapeutic Considerations," *The Journal of Trauma* 60(6suppl):53-61, June 2006.
Laskowski-Jones, L. "First Aid for Bleeding Wounds," *Nursing* 36(9):50-51, September 2006.

WOUND CARE

SURGICAL WOUND MANAGEMENT

When caring for a surgical wound, you carry out procedures that help prevent infection by stopping pathogens from entering the wound. Besides promoting patient comfort, such procedures protect the skin surface from maceration and excoriation caused by contact with irritating drainage. They also allow you to measure wound drainage to monitor fluid and electrolyte balance.

The two primary methods used to manage a draining surgical wound are dressing and pouching. Dressing is preferred unless caustic or excessive drainage is compromising your patient's skin integrity. Usually, lightly seeping wounds with drains and wounds with minimal purulent drainage can be managed with packing and gauze dressings. Some wounds, such as those that become chronic, may require an occlusive dressing.

A wound with copious, excoriating drainage calls for pouching to protect the surrounding skin. If your patient has a surgical wound, you must monitor him and choose the appropriate dressing.

Dressing a wound calls for sterile technique and sterile supplies to prevent contamination. You may use the color of the wound to help determine which type of dressing to

Tailoring wound care to wound color

Promote healing in any wound by keeping it moist, clean, and free of debris. For open wounds, use wound color to guide the specific management approach and assess how well the wound is healing.

Red wounds

Red, the color of healthy granulation tissue, indicates normal healing. When a wound begins to heal, a layer of pale pink granulation tissue covers the wound bed. As this layer thickens, it becomes beefy red. Cover a red wound, keep it moist and clean, and protect it from trauma. Use a transparent dressing (such as Tegaderm or Op-site), a hydrocolloidal dressing (such as Duo-Derm), or a gauze dressing moistened with sterile normal saline solution or impregnated with petroleum jelly or an antibiotic.

Yellow wounds

Yellow is the color of exudate produced by microorganisms in an open wound. When a wound heals without complications, the immune system removes microorganisms. However, if there are too many microorganisms to remove, exudate accumulates and becomes visible. Exudate usually appears whitish yellow, creamy yellow, yellowish green, or beige. Dry exudate appears darker.

If your patient has a yellow wound, clean it and remove exudate, using irrigation; then cover it with a moist dressing. Use absorptive products (for example, Debrisan beads and paste) or a moist gauze dressing with or without an antibiotic. You may also use hydrotherapy with whirlpool or high-pressure irrigation.

Black wounds

Black, the least healthy color, signals necrosis. Dead, avascular tissue slows healing and provides a site for microorganisms to proliferate.

You should debride a black wound. After removing dead tissue, apply a dressing to keep the wound moist and guard against external contamination. As ordered, use enzyme products, surgical debridement, hydrotherapy with whirlpool or irrigation, or a moist gauze dressing.

Multicolored wounds

You may note two or even all three colors in a wound. In this case, classify the wound according to the least healthy color present. For example, if your patient's wound is both red and yellow, classify it as a yellow wound.

apply. (See *Tailoring wound care to wound color.*) Be sure to change the dressing often enough to keep the skin dry. Always follow standard precautions set by the Centers for Disease Control and Prevention (CDC).

Equipment

Waterproof trash bag ▪ clean gloves ▪ sterile gloves ▪ gown and face shield or goggles, if indicated ▪ sterile 4″ × 4″ gauze pads ▪ large absorbent dressings, if indicated ▪ sterile cotton-tipped applicators ▪ sterile dressing set ▪ antiseptic swabs ▪ topical medication, if ordered ▪ adhesive or other tape ▪ soap and water ▪ optional: forceps; skin protectant; nonadherent pads; acetone-free adhesive remover; sterile normal saline solution; graduated container; and Montgomery straps, a fishnet tube elasticized dressing support, or a T-binder.

For a wound with a drain: Sterile scissors ▪ sterile 4″ × 4″ gauze pads without cotton lining ▪ sump drain ▪ ostomy pouch or another collection bag ▪ sterile precut tracheostomy pads or drain dressings ▪ adhesive tape (paper or silk tape if the patient is hypersensitive) ▪ surgical mask.

For pouching a wound: Collection pouch with drainage port ▪ sterile gloves ▪ skin protectant ▪ sterile gauze pads.

Preparation of equipment

Ask the patient about allergies to tapes and dressings. Assemble all equipment in the patient's room. Check the expiration date on each sterile package, and inspect for tears.

Open the waterproof trash bag, and place it near the patient's bed. Position the bag to avoid reaching across the sterile field or the wound when disposing of soiled articles. Form a cuff by turning down the top of the trash bag *to provide a wide opening and to prevent contamination of instruments or gloves by touching the bag's edge.*

Implementation

- Confirm the patient's identity using two patient identifiers according to your facility's policy.
- Explain the procedure to the patient *to allay his fears and ensure his cooperation.*

Removing the old dressing

■ Check the practitioner's order for specific wound care and medication instructions. Note the location of surgical drains *to avoid dislodging them during the procedure.*

■ Assess the patient's condition.

■ Identify the patient's allergies, especially to adhesive tape, povidone-iodine or other topical solutions, or medications.

■ Provide privacy, and position the patient as necessary. *To avoid chilling him,* expose only the wound site.

■ Wash your hands thoroughly. Put on a gown and a face shield, if necessary. Then put on clean gloves.

■ Loosen the soiled dressing by holding the patient's skin and pulling the tape or dressing toward the wound. *This protects the newly formed tissue and prevents stress on the incision.* Moisten the tape with acetone-free adhesive remover, if necessary, *to make the tape removal less painful (particularly if the skin is hairy).* Don't apply solvents to the incision *because they could contaminate the wound.*

■ Slowly remove the soiled dressing. If the gauze adheres to the wound, loosen the gauze by moistening it with sterile normal saline solution.

■ Observe the dressing for the amount, type, color, and odor of drainage.

■ Discard the dressing and gloves in the waterproof trash bag.

Caring for the wound

■ Wash your hands. Establish a sterile field with all the equipment and supplies you'll need for suture-line care and the dressing change, including a sterile dressing set and antiseptic swabs. If the practitioner has ordered ointment, squeeze the needed amount onto the sterile field. If you're using an antiseptic from an unsterile bottle, pour the antiseptic cleaning agent into a sterile container *so you won't contaminate your gloves.* Then put on sterile gloves.

■ Saturate the sterile gauze pads with the prescribed cleaning agent. Avoid using cotton balls *because they may shed fibers in the wound, causing irritation, infection, or adhesion.*

■ If ordered, obtain a wound culture; then proceed to clean the wound.

■ Irrigate the wound, if ordered, using the specified solution.

■ Pick up the moistened gauze pad or swab, and squeeze out the excess solution.

■ For an open wound, clean the wound in a full or half circle, beginning in the center and working outward (as shown top of next column). Use a new swab or pad for each circle. Clean to at least1″ (3.5 cm) beyond the end of the new dressing or 2″ (5 cm) beyond the wound margins if you aren't applying a new dressing.

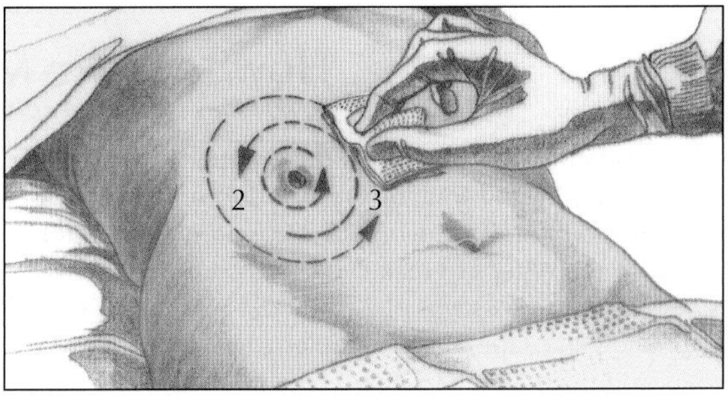

■ For a linear incision, work from the top of the incision, wipe once to the bottom, and then discard the gauze pad. With a second moistened pad, wipe from top to bottom in a vertical path next to the incision (as shown below).

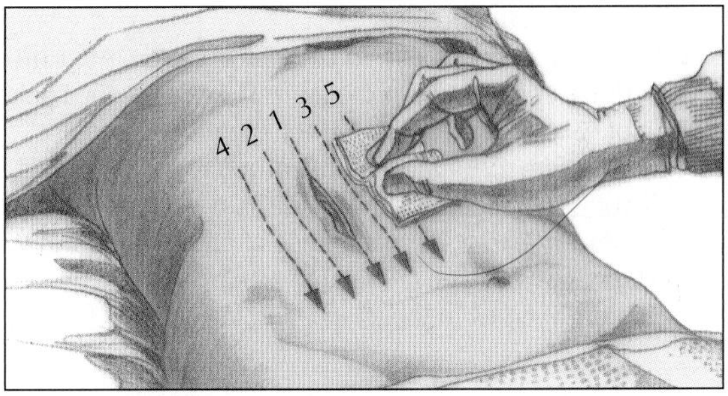

■ Continue to work outward from the incision in lines running parallel to it. Always wipe from the clean area toward the less clean area (usually from top to bottom). Use each gauze pad or swab for only one stroke *to avoid tracking wound exudate and normal body flora from surrounding skin to the clean areas.* Remember that the suture line is cleaner than the adjacent skin and the top of the suture line is usually cleaner than the bottom *because more drainage collects at the bottom of the wound.*

■ Use sterile, cotton-tipped applicators for efficient cleaning of tight-fitting wire sutures, deep and narrow wounds, and wounds with pockets. *Because the cotton on the swab is tightly wrapped,* it's less likely than a cotton ball to leave fibers in the wound. Remember to wipe only once with each applicator.

■ If the patient has a surgical drain, clean the drain's surface last. *Because moist drainage promotes bacterial growth,* the drain is considered the most contaminated area. Clean the skin around the drain by wiping in half or full circles from the drain site outward.

■ Clean all areas of the wound to wash away debris, pus, blood, and necrotic material. Try not to disturb sutures or irritate the incision. Clean to at least 1″ beyond the end of the new dressing. If you aren't applying a new dressing, clean to at least 2″ beyond the incision.

How to make Montgomery straps

An abdominal dressing requiring frequent changes can be secured with Montgomery straps *to promote the patient's comfort.* If ready-made straps aren't available, follow these steps to make your own:

- Cut four to six strips of 2″ to 3″ (5 to 7.5 cm) wide hypoallergenic tape of sufficient length to allow the tape to extend about 6″ (15.2 cm) beyond the wound on each side. (The length of the tape will vary according to the patient's size and the type and amount of dressing.)
- Fold one of each strip 2″ to 3″ back on itself (sticky sides together) to form a nonadhesive tab. Then cut a small hole in the folded tab's center, close to its top edge. Make as many pairs of straps as you'll need to snugly secure the dressing.
- Clean the patient's skin *to prevent irritation.* After his skin dries, apply a skin protectant. Then apply the sticky side of each tape to a skin barrier sheet composed of opaque hydrocolloidal or nonhydrocolloidal materials, and apply the sheet directly to the skin near the dressing. Next, thread a separate piece of gauze tie, umbilical tape, or twill tape (about 12″ [30.5 cm]) through each pair of holes in the straps, and fasten each tie as you would a shoelace. Don't stress the surrounding skin by securing the ties too tightly.
- Repeat this procedure according to the number of Montgomery straps needed.
- Replace Montgomery straps every 2 or 3 days or whenever they become soiled. If skin maceration occurs, place new tapes about 1″ (2.5 cm) away from any irritation.

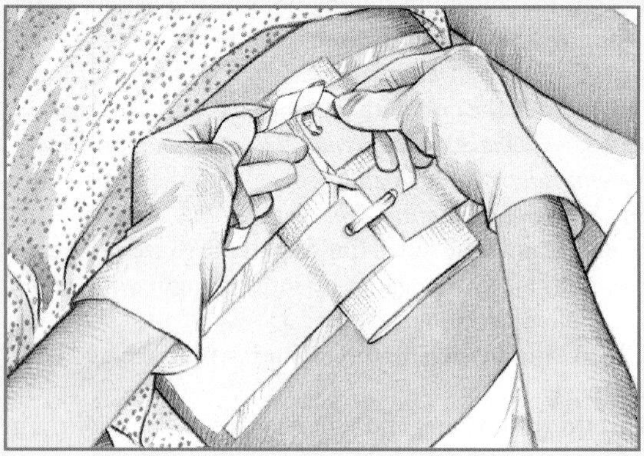

- Check to make sure the edges of the incision are lined up properly, and check for signs of infection (heat, redness, swelling, induration, and odor), dehiscence, and evisceration. If you observe such signs or if the patient reports pain at the wound site, notify the practitioner.
- Wash skin surrounding the wound with soap and water, and pat dry using a sterile 4″ × 4″ gauze pad. Avoid oil-based soap *because it may interfere with pouch adherence.* Apply any prescribed topical medication.
- Apply a skin protectant, if needed.
- If ordered, pack the wound with gauze pads or strips folded to fit, using a sterile forceps. Avoid using cotton-lined gauze pads *because cotton fibers can adhere to the wound surface and cause complications.* Pack the wound, using the wet-to-damp method. Soaking the packing material in solution and wringing it out so that it's slightly moist provides a moist wound environment that absorbs debris and drainage. However, removing the packing won't disrupt new tissue. Don't pack the wound tightly; *doing so will exert pressure and may damage the wound.*

Applying a fresh gauze dressing

- Gently place sterile 4″ × 4″ gauze pads at the center of the wound, and move progressively outward to the edges of the wound site. Extend the gauze at least 1″ beyond the incision in each direction, and cover the wound evenly with enough sterile dressings (usually two or three layers) to absorb all drainage until the next dressing change. Use large absorbent dressings to form outer layers, if needed, *to provide greater absorbency.*
- Secure the dressing's edges to the patient's skin with strips of tape *to maintain the sterility of the wound site* (as shown below). Or secure the dressing with a T-binder or Montgomery straps *to prevent skin excoriation,* which may occur with repeated tape removal necessitated by frequent dressing changes. (See *How to make Montgomery straps.*)

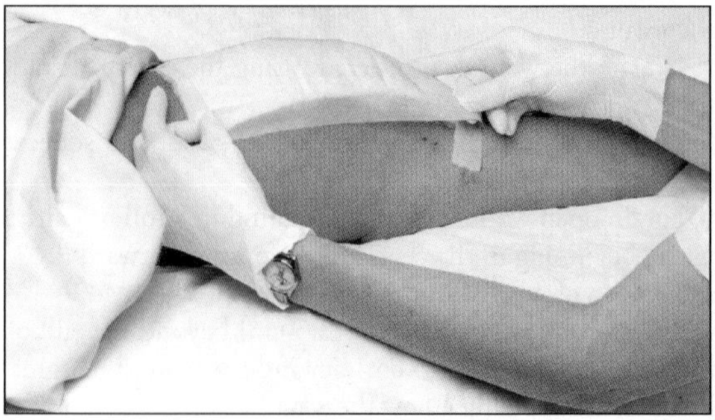

- Make sure the patient is comfortable.

■ Properly dispose of the solutions and trash bag, and clean or discard soiled equipment and supplies according to your facility's policy. If your patient's wound has purulent drainage, don't return unopened sterile supplies to the sterile supply cabinet *because this could cause cross-contamination of other equipment.*

Dressing a wound with a drain

■ Use commercially precut gauze drain dressings or prepare a drain dressing by using sterile scissors to cut a slit in a sterile 4″ × 4″ gauze pad. Fold the pad in half; then cut inward from the center of the folded edge. Don't use a cotton-lined gauze pad *because cutting the gauze opens the lining and releases cotton fibers into the wound.* Prepare a second pad the same way.

■ Gently press one drain dressing close to the skin around the drain so that the tubing fits into the slit. Press the second drain dressing around the drain from the opposite direction so that the two dressings encircle the tubing.

■ Layer as many uncut sterile 4″ × 4″ gauze pads or large absorbent dressings around the tubing as needed *to absorb expected drainage.* Tape the dressing in place, or use a T-binder or Montgomery straps.

Pouching a wound

■ If your patient's wound is draining heavily or if drainage may damage surrounding skin, you'll need to apply a pouch.

■ Measure the wound. Cut an opening ¼″ (1 cm) larger than the wound in the facing of the collection pouch (as shown below).

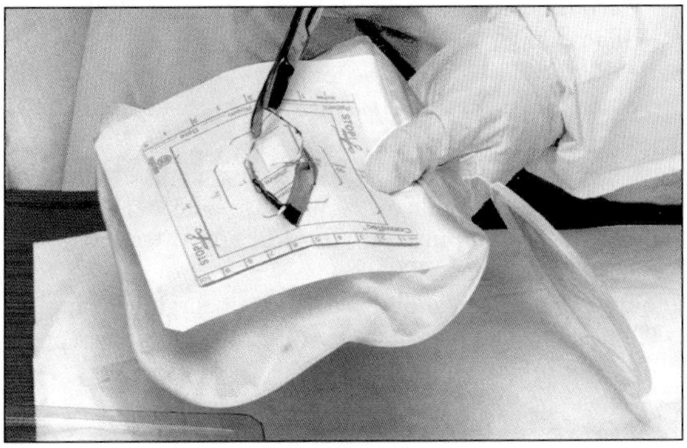

■ Apply a skin protectant as needed. (Some protectants are incorporated within the collection pouch and also provide adhesion.)

■ Make sure the drainage port at the bottom of the pouch is closed firmly *to prevent leaks.* Then gently press the contoured pouch opening around the wound, starting at its lower edge, *to catch any drainage* (as shown top of next column).

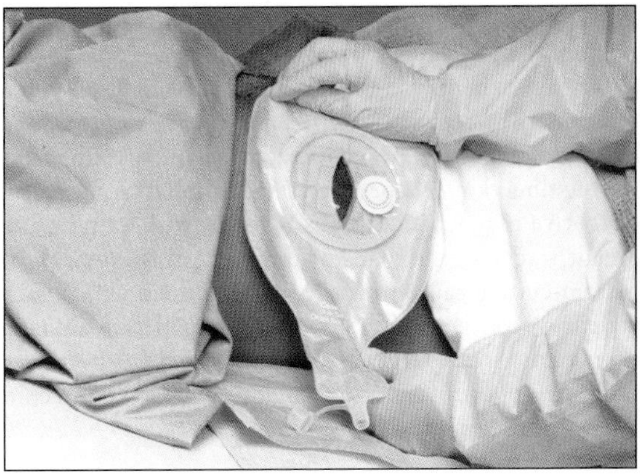

■ To empty the pouch, put on gloves and a face shield or mask and goggles to avoid any splashing. Then insert the pouch's bottom half into a graduated biohazard container, and open the drainage port (as shown below). Note the color, consistency, odor, and amount of fluid. If ordered, obtain a culture specimen, and send it to the laboratory immediately. Remember to follow the CDC's standard precautions when handling infectious drainage.

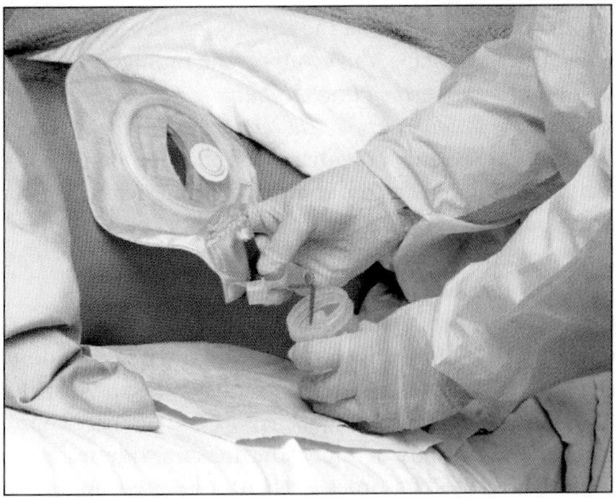

■ Wipe the bottom of the pouch and the drainage port with a gauze pad *to remove any drainage that could irritate the patient's skin or cause an odor.* Then reseal the port. Change the pouch only if it leaks or fails to adhere. *More frequent changes are unnecessary and only irritate the patient's skin.*

Special considerations

■ If the patient has two wounds in the same area, cover each wound separately with layers of sterile 4″ × 4″ gauze pads. Then cover each site with a large absorbent dressing secured to the patient's skin with tape. Don't use a single large absorbent dressing to cover both sites *because drainage quickly saturates a pad, promoting cross-contamination.*

- When packing a wound, don't pack it too tightly *because this compresses adjacent capillaries and may prevent the wound edges from contracting.* Avoid overlapping damp packing onto surrounding skin *because it macerates the intact tissue.*
- To save time when dressing a wound with a drain, use precut tracheostomy pads or drain dressings instead of custom-cutting gauze pads to fit around the drain. If your patient is sensitive to adhesive tape, use paper or silk tape *because it is less likely to cause a skin reaction and peels off more easily than adhesive tape.* Use a surgical mask to cradle a chin or jawline dressing; *this provides a secure dressing and avoids the need to shave the patient's hair.*
- If ordered, use a collodion spray or similar topical protectant instead of a gauze dressing. Moisture- and contaminant-proof, this covering dries in a clear, impermeable film that leaves the wound visible for observation and avoids the friction caused by a dressing.
- If a sump drain isn't adequately collecting wound secretions, reinforce it with an ostomy pouch or another collection bag. Use waterproof tape to strengthen a spot on the front of the pouch near the adhesive opening; then cut a small "X" in the tape. Feed the drain catheter into the pouch through the "X" cut. Seal the cut around the tubing with more waterproof tape; then connect the tubing to the suction pump. *This method frees the drainage port at the bottom of the pouch so you don't have to remove the tubing to empty the pouch.* If you use more than one collection pouch for a wound or wounds, record drainage volume separately for each pouch. Avoid using waterproof material over the dressing *because it reduces air circulation and promotes infection from accumulated heat and moisture.*
- Because many practitioners prefer to change the first postoperative dressing themselves to check the incision, don't change the first dressing unless you have specific instructions to do so. If you have no such order and drainage comes through the dressings, reinforce the dressing with fresh sterile gauze. Request an order to change the dressing, or ask the practitioner to change it as soon as possible. A reinforced dressing shouldn't remain in place longer than 24 hours *because it's an excellent medium for bacterial growth.*
- For the recent postoperative patient or a patient with complications, check the dressing every 15 to 30 minutes or as ordered. For the patient with a properly healing wound, check the dressing at least once every 8 hours.
- If the dressing becomes wet from the outside (for example, from spilled drinking water), replace it as soon as possible *to prevent wound contamination.*
- If your patient will need wound care after discharge, provide appropriate teaching. If he'll be caring for the wound himself, stress the importance of using sterile technique, and teach him how to examine the wound for signs of infection and other complications. Also show him how to change dressings, and give him written instructions for all procedures to be performed at home.

Complications

A major complication of a dressing change is an allergic reaction to an antiseptic cleaning agent, a prescribed topical medication, or adhesive tape. This reaction may lead to skin redness, rash, excoriation, or infection.

NURSING ALERT *Take care when removing adhesive tape to prevent skin tears, especially in elderly patients.*

Documentation

Document the date, time, and type of wound management procedure; amount of soiled dressing and packing removed; wound appearance (size, condition of margins, presence of necrotic tissue) and odor (if present); type, color, consistency, and amount of drainage (for each wound); presence and location of drains; additional procedures, such as irrigation, packing, or application of a topical medication; type and amount of new dressing or pouch applied; and the patient's tolerance of the procedure.

Document special or detailed wound care instructions and pain management steps on the care plan. Record the color and amount of drainage on the intake and output sheet.

SELECTED REFERENCES

Baranoski, S., and Ayello, E. *Wound Care Essentials: Practice Principles,* 2nd ed. Philadelphia: Lippincott Williams & Wilkins, 2008.

Barie, P., and Eachempati, S. "Surgical Site Infections," *The Surgical Clinics of North America* 85(6):1115-135, viii-ix, December 2005.

Hess, C. *Clinical Guide: Skin & Wound Care,* 6th ed. Philadelphia: Lippincott Williams & Wilkins, 2008.

Schweon, S. "Stamping Out Surgical Site Infections," *RN* 69(10):12, October 2006.

Vuolo, J. "Assessment and Management of Surgical Wounds in Clinical Practice," *Nursing Standard* 20(52):46-56, September 2006.

SUTURE REMOVAL

The goal of this procedure is to remove skin sutures from a healed wound without damaging newly formed tissue. The timing of suture removal depends on the shape, size, and location of the sutured incision; the absence of inflammation, drainage, and infection; and the patient's general condition. Usually, for a sufficiently healed wound, sutures are removed

7 to 10 days after insertion. Techniques for removal depend on the method of suturing, but all require sterile procedure to prevent contamination. Although sutures usually are removed by a physician, in many facilities, a nurse may remove them on the physician's order.

Equipment

Waterproof trash bag ▪ adjustable light ▪ clean gloves, if the wound is dressed ▪ sterile gloves ▪ sterile forceps or sterile hemostat ▪ normal saline solution ▪ sterile gauze pads ▪ antiseptic cleaning agent ▪ sterile curve-tipped suture scissors ▪ povidone-iodine pads ▪ optional: adhesive butterfly strips or Steri-Strips and compound benzoin tincture or other skin protectant.

Prepackaged, sterile suture-removal trays are available.

Preparation of equipment

Assemble all equipment in the patient's room. Check the expiration date on each sterile package, and inspect for tears. Open the waterproof trash bag, and place it near the patient's bed. Position the bag properly *to avoid reaching across the sterile field or the suture line when disposing of soiled articles.* Form a cuff by turning down the top of the trash bag *to provide a wide opening and prevent contamination of instruments or gloves by touching the bag's edge.*

Implementation

- If your facility allows you to remove sutures, check the practitioner's order *to confirm the details for this procedure.*
- Check for patient allergies, especially to adhesive tape and povidone-iodine or other topical solutions or medications.
- Tell the patient that you're going to remove the stitches from his wound. Assure him that this procedure typically is painless, but that he may feel a tickling sensation as the stitches come out. Reassure him that because his wound is healing properly, removing the stitches won't weaken the incision.
- Provide privacy, and position the patient so he's comfortable without placing undue tension on the suture line. *Because some patients experience nausea or dizziness during the procedure,* have the patient recline if possible. Adjust the light to have it shine directly on the suture line.
- Wash your hands thoroughly. If the patient's wound has a dressing, put on clean gloves and carefully remove the dressing. Discard the dressing and the gloves in the waterproof trash bag.
- Observe the patient's wound for possible gaping, drainage, inflammation, signs of infection, and embedded sutures. Notify the practitioner if the wound has failed to heal properly. The absence of a healing ridge under the suture line 5 to 7 days after insertion indicates that the line needs continued support and protection during the healing process.
- Establish a sterile work area with all the equipment and supplies you'll need for suture removal and wound care. Open the sterile suture-removal tray, maintaining sterility of the contents, and put on sterile gloves.
- Using sterile technique, clean the suture line *to decrease the number of microorganisms present and reduce the risk of infection.* The cleaning process should also moisten the sutures sufficiently *to ease removal.* Soften them further, if needed, with normal saline solution.
- Proceed according to the type of suture you're removing. (See *Methods for removing sutures,* pages 256 and 257.) *Because the visible part of a suture is exposed to skin bacteria and considered contaminated,* be sure to cut sutures at the skin surface on one side of the visible part of the suture. Remove the suture by lifting and pulling the visible end off the skin *to avoid drawing this contaminated portion back through subcutaneous tissue.*
- If ordered, remove every other suture *to maintain some support for the incision.* Then go back and remove the remaining sutures.
- After removing sutures, wipe the incision gently with gauze pads soaked in an antiseptic cleaning agent or with a povidone-iodine pad. Apply a light sterile gauze dressing, if needed, *to prevent infection and irritation from clothing.* Then discard your gloves.
- Make sure the patient is comfortable. According to the practitioner's preference, inform the patient that he may shower in 1 or 2 days if the incision is dry and heals well.
- Properly dispose of the solutions and trash bag, and clean or dispose of soiled equipment and supplies according to your facility's policy.

Special considerations

- Be sure to check the practitioner's order for the time of suture removal. Usually, you'll remove sutures on the head and neck 3 to 5 days after insertion; on the chest and abdomen, 5 to 7 days after insertion; and on the lower extremities, 7 to 10 days after insertion.
- If the patient has interrupted sutures or an incompletely healed suture line, remove only those sutures specified by the practitioner. He may want to leave some sutures in place for an additional day or two *to support the suture line.*
- If the patient has both retention and regular sutures in place, check the practitioner's order for the sequence in which they are to be removed. *Because retention sutures link underlying fat and muscle tissue and give added support to the obese or slow-healing patient,* they usually remain in place for 14 to 21 days.

Methods for removing sutures

Removal techniques depend on the type of sutures to be removed. The illustrations below show removal steps for four common suture types. Keep in mind that for all suture types, it's important to grasp and cut sutures in the correct place to avoid pulling the exposed (thus contaminated) suture material through subcutaneous tissue.

Plain interrupted sutures

Using sterile forceps, grasp the knot of the first suture and raise it off the skin. This will expose a small portion of the suture that was below skin level. Place the rounded tip of sterile curved-tip suture scissors against the skin, and cut through the exposed portion of the suture. Then, still holding the knot with the forceps, pull the cut suture up and out of the skin in a smooth continuous motion *to avoid causing the patient pain.* Discard the suture. Repeat the process for every other suture, initially; if the wound doesn't gape, you can then remove the remaining sutures as ordered.

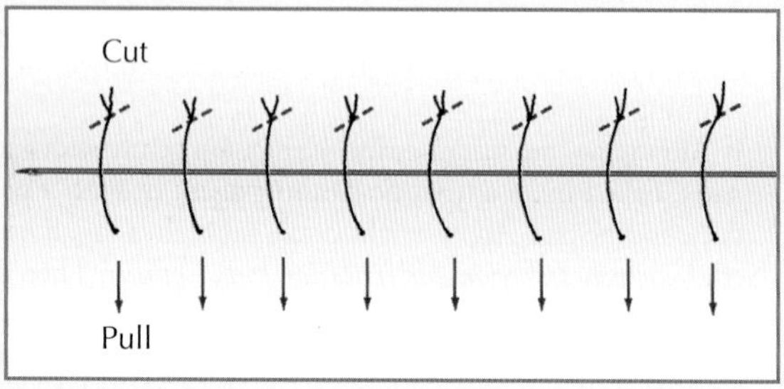

Plain continuous sutures

Cut the first suture on the side opposite the knot. Next, cut the same side of the next suture in line. Then lift the first suture out in the direction of the knot. Proceed along the suture line, grasping each suture where you grasped the knot on the first one.

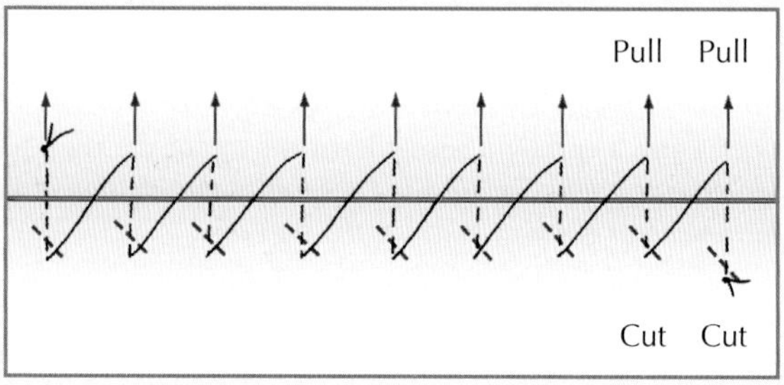

■ Be particularly careful to clean the suture line before attempting to remove mattress sutures. This decreases the risk of infection when the visible, contaminated part of the stitch is too small to cut twice for sterile removal and must be pulled through tissue. After you have removed mattress sutures this way, monitor the suture line carefully for subsequent infection.

■ If the wound dehisces during suture removal, apply butterfly adhesive strips or Steri-Strips to support and approximate the edges, and call the practitioner immediately to repair the wound.

■ Apply butterfly adhesive strips or Steri-Strips after any suture removal, if desired, *to give added support to the incision line and prevent lateral tension on the wound from forming a wide scar.* Use a small amount of compound benzoin tincture or other skin protectant *to ensure adherence.* Leave the strips in place for 3 to 5 days as ordered.

Home care

If the patient is being discharged, teach him how to remove the dressing and care for the wound. Instruct him to call the practitioner immediately if he observes wound discharge or any other abnormal change. Tell him that the redness surrounding the incision should gradually disappear and only a thin line should show after a few weeks.

Documentation

Record the date and time of suture removal, type and number of sutures, appearance of the suture line, signs of wound complications, dressings or butterfly strips applied, and the patient's tolerance of the procedure.

SELECTED REFERENCES

Taylor, C., et al. *Fundamentals of Nursing: The Art and Science of Nursing Care,* 6th ed. Philadelphia: Lippincott Williams & Wilkins, 2008.

Mattress interrupted sutures

If possible, remove the small, visible portion of the suture opposite the knot by cutting it at each visible end and lifting the small piece away from the skin to prevent pulling it through and contaminating subcutaneous tissue. Then remove the rest of the suture by pulling it out in the direction of the knot. If the visible portion is too small to cut twice, cut it once, and pull the entire suture out in the opposite direction. Repeat these steps for the remaining sutures, and monitor the incision carefully for infection.

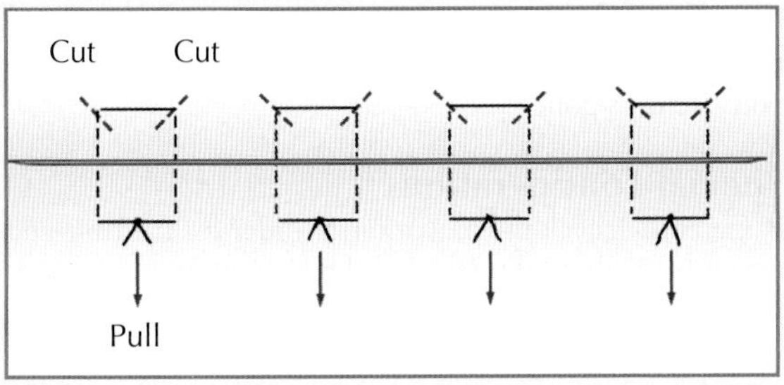

Mattress continuous sutures

Follow the procedure for removing mattress interrupted sutures, first removing the small visible portion of the suture, if possible, *to prevent pulling it through and contaminating subcutaneous tissue*. Then extract the rest of the suture in the direction of the knot.

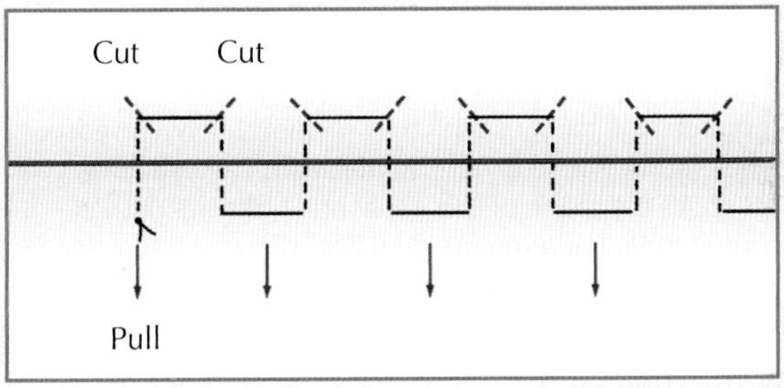

SKIN STAPLE AND CLIP REMOVAL

Skin staples or clips may be used instead of standard sutures to close lacerations or surgical wounds. Because they can secure a wound more quickly than sutures, they may substitute for surface sutures when cosmetic results aren't a prime consideration, such as in abdominal closure. When properly placed, staples and clips distribute tension evenly along the suture line with minimal tissue trauma and compression, facilitating healing and minimizing scarring. Because staples and clips are made from surgical stainless steel, tissue reaction to them is minimal. Usually, physicians remove skin staples and clips, but some facilities permit qualified nurses to perform this procedure.

Skin staples and clips are contraindicated when wound location requires cosmetically superior results or when the incision site makes it impossible to maintain at least a 5-mm distance between the staple and underlying bone, vessels, or internal organs.

Equipment

Waterproof trash bag ▪ adjustable light ▪ clean gloves, if needed ▪ sterile gloves ▪ sterile gauze pads ▪ sterile staple or clip extractor ▪ antiseptic cleaning agent ▪ sterile cotton-tipped applicators ▪ optional: butterfly adhesive strips or Steri-Strips, compound benzoin tincture or other skin protectant.

Prepackaged, sterile, disposable staple or clip extractors are available.

Preparation of equipment

Assemble all equipment in the patient's room. Check the expiration date on each sterile package, and inspect for tears. Open the waterproof trash bag, and place it near the patient's bed. Position the bag *to avoid reaching across the sterile field or the wound when disposing of soiled articles.* Form a cuff by turning down the top of the bag *to provide a wide opening, then preventing contamination of instruments or gloves by touching the bag's edge.*

Removing a staple

Position the extractor's lower jaws beneath the span of the first staple (as shown below).

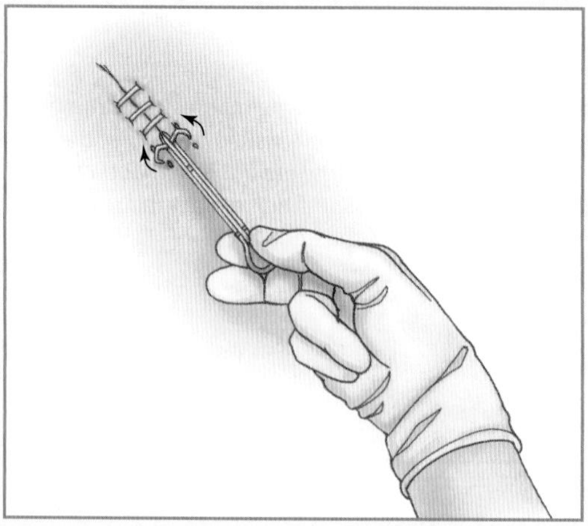

Squeeze the handles until they're completely closed; then lift the staple away from the skin. The extractor changes the shape of the staple and pulls the prongs out of the intradermal tissue.

Implementation

- If your facility allows you to remove skin staples and clips, check the practitioner's order *to confirm the exact timing and details for this procedure.*
- Check for patient allergies, especially to adhesive tape and povidone-iodine or other topical solutions or medications.
- Explain the procedure to the patient. Tell him that he may feel a slight pulling or tickling sensation but little discomfort during staple removal. Reassure him that because his incision is healing properly, removing the supporting staples or clips won't weaken the incision line.
- Provide privacy, and place the patient in a comfortable position that doesn't place undue tension on the incision. *Because some patients experience nausea or dizziness during the procedure,* have the patient recline if possible. Adjust the light to shine directly on the incision.
- Wash your hands thoroughly.
- If the patient's wound has a dressing, put on clean gloves and carefully remove it. Discard the dressing and the gloves in the waterproof trash bag.
- Assess the patient's incision. Notify the practitioner of gaping, drainage, inflammation, and other signs of infection.
- Establish a sterile work area with all the equipment and supplies you'll need for removing staples or clips and for cleaning and dressing the incision. Open the package containing the sterile staple or clip extractor, maintaining asepsis. Put on sterile gloves.
- Wipe the incision gently with sterile gauze pads soaked in an antiseptic cleaning agent or with sterile cotton-tipped applicators *to remove surface encrustations.*
- Pick up the sterile staple or clip extractor. Then, starting at one end of the incision, remove the staple or clip. (See *Removing a staple.*) Hold the extractor over the trash bag, and release the handle to discard the staple or clip.
- Repeat the procedure for each staple or clip until all are removed.
- Apply a sterile gauze dressing, if needed, *to prevent infection and irritation from clothing.* Then discard your gloves.
- Make sure the patient is comfortable. According to the practitioner's preference, inform the patient that he may shower in 1 or 2 days if the incision is dry and healing well.
- Properly dispose of solutions and the trash bag, and clean or dispose of soiled equipment and supplies according to your facility's policy .

Special considerations

- Carefully check the practitioner's order for the time and extent of staple or clip removal. The practitioner may want you to remove only alternate staples or clips initially and to leave the others in place for an additional day or two *to support the incision.*
- When removing a staple or clip, place the extractor's jaws carefully between the patient's skin and the staple or clip *to avoid patient discomfort.* If extraction is difficult, notify the practitioner; *staples or clips placed too deeply within the skin or left in place too long may resist removal.*
- If the wound dehisces after staples or clips are removed, apply butterfly adhesive strips or Steri-Strips *to approximate and support the edges,* and call the practitioner immediately to repair the wound. (See *Types of adhesive skin closures.*)
- You may also apply butterfly adhesive strips or Steri-Strips after removing staples or clips even if the wound is healing normally *to give added support to the incision and prevent lateral tension from forming a wide scar.* Use a small amount of compound benzoin tincture or other skin protectant *to ensure adherence.* Leave the strips in place for 3 to 5 days.

Home care

If the patient is being discharged, teach him how to remove the dressing and care for the wound. Instruct him to call the practitioner immediately if he observes wound discharge or any other abnormal change. Tell him that the redness surrounding the incision should gradually disappear and that after a few weeks, only a thin line will be visible.

Documentation

Record the date and time of staple or clip removal, number of staples or clips removed, appearance of the incision, dressings or butterfly strips applied, signs of wound complications, and the patient's tolerance of the procedure.

SELECTED REFERENCES

Taylor, C., et al. *Fundamentals of Nursing: The Art and Science of Nursing Care,* 6th ed. Philadelphia: Lippincott Williams & Wilkins, 2008.

Vuolo, J. "Assessment and Management of Surgical Wounds in Clinical Practice," *Nursing Standard* 20(52):46-56, September 2006.

WOUND DEHISCENCE AND EVISCERATION MANAGEMENT

Although surgical wounds typically heal without incident, occasionally the edges of a wound may fail to join or may separate even after they seem to be healing normally. This development, called wound dehiscence, may lead to an even more serious complication: evisceration, in which a portion of the viscera (usually a bowel loop) protrudes through the incision. Evisceration, in turn, can lead to peritonitis and septic shock. (See *Recognizing dehiscence and evisceration,* page 260.) Dehiscence and evisceration are most likely to occur 6 to 7 days after surgery. By then, sutures may have been removed and the patient can cough easily and breathe deeply—both of which strain the incision. Some wound dehiscence may be managed conservatively using a medical approach, such as sterile dressing application and wound monitoring.

NURSING ALERT ***Wound evisceration requires quick intervention to prevent potentially fatal shock; the wound is usually closed in the operating room.***

Several factors can contribute to these complications. Poor nutrition—either from inadequate intake or a condition such as diabetes mellitus—may hinder wound healing. Chronic pulmonary or cardiac disease can also slow healing because the injured tissue doesn't get needed nutrients and oxygen. Localized wound infection may limit closure, delay healing, and weaken the incision. Also, stress on the incision from coughing or vomiting may cause abdominal distention or severe stretching. A midline abdominal incision, for instance, poses a high risk of wound dehiscence.

Types of adhesive skin closures

Steri-Strips are used as a primary means of keeping a wound closed after suture removal. They're made of thin strips of sterile, nonwoven, porous fabric tape.

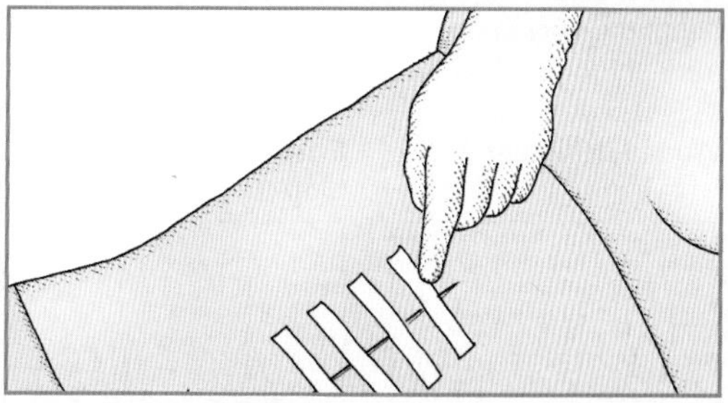

Butterfly closures consist of sterile, waterproof adhesive strips. A narrow, nonadhesive "bridge" connects the two expanded adhesive portions. These strips are used to close small wounds and assist healing after suture removal.

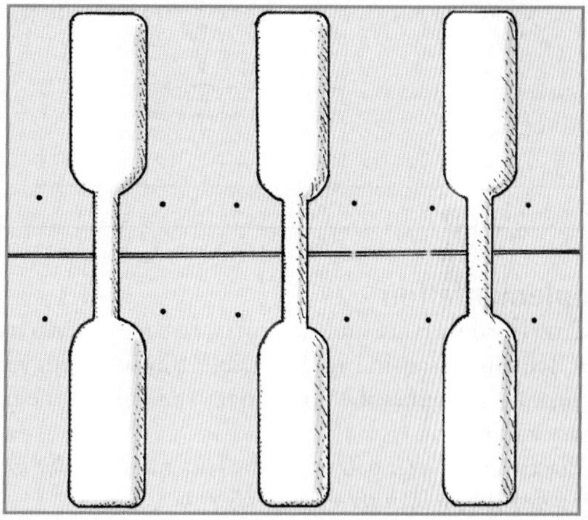

Equipment

Two sterile towels ▪ 1 L of sterile normal saline solution ▪ sterile irrigation set, including a basin, solution container, and 50-ml catheter-tip syringe ▪ several large abdominal dressings ▪ sterile, waterproof drape ▪ linen-saver pads ▪ sterile gloves.

If the patient will return to the operating room, also gather the following equipment: I.V. administration set and I.V. fluids ▪ equipment for nasogastric (NG) intubation ▪ sedative, as ordered ▪ suction apparatus.

Recognizing dehiscence and evisceration

In wound dehiscence (below left), the layers of the surgical wound separate. In evisceration (below right), the viscera (in this case, a bowel loop) protrude through the surgical incision.

Wound dehiscence **Evisceration of bowel loop**

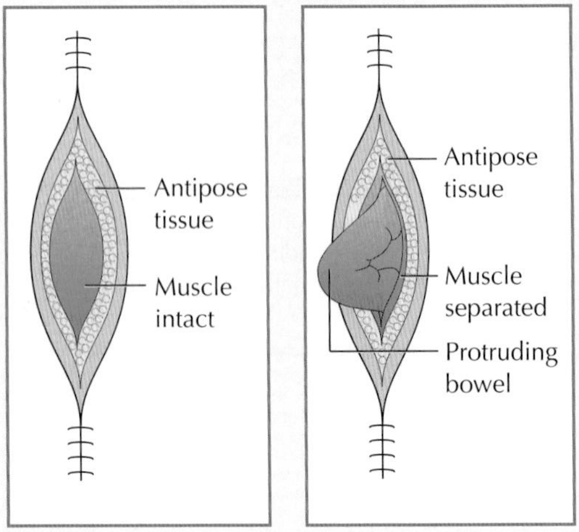

Implementation

- Provide reassurance and support *to ease the patient's anxiety.* Tell him to stay in bed. If possible, stay with him while someone else notifies the practitioner and collects the necessary equipment.
- Place a linen-saver pad under the patient *to keep the sheets dry when you moisten the exposed viscera.*
- Using sterile technique, unfold a sterile towel *to create a sterile field.* Open the package containing the irrigation set, and place the basin, solution container, and 50-ml syringe on the sterile field.
- Open the bottle of normal saline solution, and pour about 400 ml into the solution container. Also pour about 200 ml into the sterile basin.
- Open several large abdominal dressings, and place them on the sterile field.
- Put on the sterile gloves, and place one or two of the large abdominal dressings into the basin *to saturate them with saline solution.*
- Place the moistened dressings over the exposed viscera. Then place a sterile, waterproof drape over the dressings *to prevent the sheets from getting wet.*
- Moisten the dressings every hour by withdrawing saline solution from the container through the syringe and then gently squirting the solution on the dressings.
- When you moisten the dressings, inspect the color of the viscera. If it appears dusky or black, notify the practitioner immediately. *With its blood supply interrupted, a protruding organ may become ischemic and necrotic.*
- Keep the patient on absolute bed rest in low Fowler's position (no more than 20 degrees' elevation) with his knees flexed. *This prevents injury and reduces stress on an abdominal incision.*
- Don't allow the patient to have anything by mouth *to decrease the risk of aspiration during surgery.*
- Monitor the patient's pulse, respirations, blood pressure, and temperature every 15 minutes *to detect shock.*
- If necessary, prepare the patient to return to the operating room. After gathering the appropriate equipment, start an I.V. infusion as ordered.
- Insert an NG tube, and connect it to continuous or intermittent low suction, as ordered.
- Continue to reassure the patient while you prepare him for surgery. Make sure he has signed a consent form and that the operating room staff has been informed about the procedure.
- Administer preoperative medications to the patient as ordered.

Special considerations

- Depending on the circumstances, some of these procedures may not be done at the bedside. For instance, NG intubation may make the patient gag or vomit, causing further evisceration. For this reason, the physician may choose to have the NG tube inserted in the operating room with the patient under anesthesia.
- The best treatment is prevention. If you're caring for a postoperative patient who's at risk for poor healing, make sure he receives an adequate supply of protein, vitamins, and calories. Monitor his dietary deficiencies, and discuss any problems with the practitioner and the dietitian.
- When changing wound dressings, always use sterile technique. Inspect the incision with each dressing change, and if you recognize the early signs of infection, start treatment before dehiscence or evisceration can occur. If local infection develops, clean the wound as necessary *to eliminate a buildup of purulent drainage.* Make sure bandages aren't so tight that they limit blood supply to the wound.

Complications

Infection, which can lead to peritonitis and, possibly, septic shock, is the most severe and most common complication of wound dehiscence and evisceration. Caused by bacterial contamination or by drying of normally moist abdominal contents, infection can impair circulation and lead to necrosis of the affected organ.

Documentation

Note when the problem occurred, the patient's activity preceding the problem, his condition, and the time the practitioner was notified. Describe the appearance of the wound or eviscerated organ; amount, color, consistency, and odor of any drainage; and nursing actions taken. Record the patient's vital signs, his response to the incident, and the practitioner's actions.

Finally, make sure you change the patient care plan to reflect nursing actions needed to promote proper healing.

SELECTED REFERENCES

Banwell, P.E., et al. "Treatment of Dehisced and Infected Wounds," *Journal of Wound Care* 14(3):110, March 2005.

Doughty, D.B. "Preventing and Managing Surgical Wound Dehiscence," *Home Healthcare Nurse* 22(6):364-7, June 2004.

Hahler, B. "Surgical Wound Dehiscence," *Medsurg Nursing* 15(5):296-300, October 2006.

Wilson, J.A., and Clark, J.J. "Obesity: Impediment to Postsurgical Wound Healing," *Advances in Skin & Wound Care* 17(8):426-35, October 2004.

TRAUMATIC WOUND MANAGEMENT

Traumatic wounds include abrasions, lacerations, puncture wounds, and amputations. In an abrasion, the skin is scraped, with partial loss of the skin surface. In a laceration, the skin is torn, causing jagged, irregular edges; the severity of a laceration depends on its size, depth, and location. A puncture wound occurs when a pointed object, such as a knife or glass fragment, penetrates the skin. Traumatic amputation refers to the removal of part of the body, a limb, or part of a limb.

When caring for a patient with a traumatic wound, first assess his ABCs—airway, breathing, and circulation. It may seem natural to focus on a gruesome injury, but a patent airway and pumping heart take first priority. Once the patient's ABCs are stabilized, you can turn your attention to the traumatic wound. Initial management concentrates on controlling bleeding, usually by applying firm, direct pressure and elevating the extremity. If bleeding continues, you may need to compress a pressure point. Assess the condition of the wound. Management and cleaning technique usually depend on the specific type of wound and degree of contamination.

Equipment

Sterile basin ■ normal saline solution ■ sterile 4″ × 4″ gauze pads ■ sterile gloves ■ clean gloves ■ sterile cotton-tipped applicators ■ dry sterile dressing, nonadherent pad, or petroleum gauze ■ linen-saver pad ■ optional: clippers, towel, goggles, mask, gown, 50-ml catheter-tip syringe, surgical scrub brush, antibacterial ointment, porous tape, sterile forceps, sutures and suture set, hydrogen peroxide.

Preparation of equipment

Place a linen-saver pad under the area to be cleaned. Remove any clothing covering the wound. If necessary, clip hair around the wound with scissors *to promote cleaning and treatment.*

Assemble needed equipment at the patient's bedside. Fill a sterile basin with normal saline solution. Make sure the treatment area has enough light to allow close observation of the wound. Depending on the nature and location of the wound, wear sterile or clean gloves *to avoid spreading infection.*

Implementation

- Check the patient's medical history for previous tetanus immunization and, if needed and ordered, arrange for immunization.
- Administer pain medication if ordered.
- Wash your hands.
- Use appropriate protective equipment, such as a gown, a mask, and goggles, if spraying or splashing of body fluids is possible.

For an abrasion

- Flush the scraped skin with normal saline solution.
- Remove dirt or gravel with a sterile 4″ × 4″ gauze pad moistened with normal saline solution. Rub in the opposite direction from which the dirt or gravel became embedded.
- If the wound is extremely dirty, you may use a surgical brush to scrub it.
- With a small wound, allow it to dry and form a scab. With a larger wound, you may need to cover it with a nonadherent pad or petroleum gauze and a light dressing. Apply antibacterial ointment if ordered.

For a laceration

- Moisten a sterile 4″ × 4″ gauze pad with normal saline solution. Clean the wound gently, working outward from its center to about 2″ (5 cm) beyond its edges. Discard the

Caring for a severed body part

After traumatic amputation, a surgeon may be able to reimplant the severed body part through microsurgery. The chance of successful reimplantation is much greater if the amputated part has received proper care.

If a patient arrives at the hospital with a severed body part, first make sure that bleeding at the amputation site has been controlled. Then follow these guidelines for preserving the body part.

- Put on sterile gloves. Place several sterile gauze pads and an appropriate amount of sterile roller gauze in a sterile basin, and pour sterile normal saline or sterile lactated Ringer's solution over them. *Never* use another solution, and don't try to scrub or debride the part.
- Holding the body part in one gloved hand, carefully pat it dry with sterile gauze. Place saline-soaked gauze pads over the stump, and then wrap the whole body part with saline-soaked roller gauze. Wrap the gauze with a sterile towel, if available. Then put this package in a watertight container or bag and seal it.
- Fill another plastic bag with ice, and place the part, still in its watertight container, inside (as shown at right). Seal the outer bag. (Always protect the part from direct contact with ice and—*never* use dry ice—*to prevent irreversible tissue damage, which would make the part unsuitable for reimplantation.*) Keep this bag ice-cold until the surgeon is ready to do the reimplantation surgery.
- Label the bag with the patient's name, identification number, identification of the amputated part, the hospital identification number, and the date and time when cooling began.

Note: The body part must be wrapped and cooled quickly. *Irreversible tissue damage occurs after only 6 hours at ambient temperature.* However, hypothermic management seldom preserves tissues for more than 24 hours.

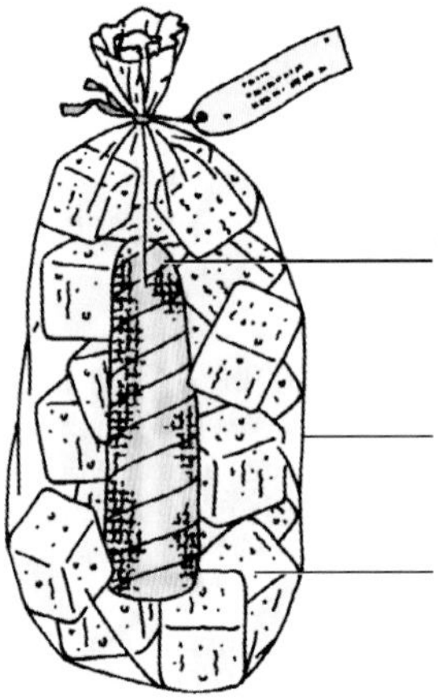

soiled gauze pad, and use a fresh one as necessary. Continue until the wound appears clean.

- If the wound is dirty, you may irrigate it with a 50-ml catheter-tip syringe and normal saline solution.
- Assist the practitioner in suturing the wound edges using the suture kit, or apply sterile strips of porous tape.
- Apply the prescribed antibacterial ointment *to help prevent infection.*
- Apply a dry sterile dressing over the wound *to absorb drainage and help prevent bacterial contamination.*

For a puncture wound

- If the wound is minor, allow it to bleed for a few minutes before cleaning it.
- For a larger puncture wound, you may need to irrigate it before applying a dry dressing.
- Stabilize any embedded foreign object until the practitioner can remove it. After he removes the object and bleeding is stabilized, clean the wound as you'd clean a laceration or deep puncture wound.

For an amputation

- Apply a gauze pad moistened with normal saline solution to the amputation site. Elevate the affected part, and immobilize it for surgery.
- Recover the amputated part, and prepare it for transport to a facility where microvascular surgery is performed. (See *Caring for a severed body part.*)

Special considerations

- When irrigating a traumatic wound, avoid using more than 8 psi of pressure. *High-pressure irrigation can seriously interfere with healing, kill cells, and allow bacteria to infiltrate the tissue.*
- To clean the wound, you may use normal saline or hydrogen peroxide (its foaming action facilitates debris removal). However, peroxide should *never* be instilled into a

deep wound *because of the risk of embolism from the evolving gases.* Be sure to rinse your hands well after using hydrogen peroxide.

■ Avoid cleaning a traumatic wound with alcohol *because alcohol causes pain and tissue dehydration.* Also, avoid using antiseptics for wound cleaning *because they can impede healing.* In addition, never use a cotton ball or cotton-filled gauze pad to clean a wound *because cotton fibers left in the wound can cause contamination.*

■ After a wound has been cleaned, the practitioner may want to debride it *to remove dead tissue and reduce the risk of infection and scarring.* If this is necessary, pack the wound with gauze pads soaked in normal saline solution until debridement.

■ Observe for signs and symptoms of infection, such as warm red skin at the site or purulent discharge. Be aware that infection of a traumatic wound can delay healing, increase scar formation, and trigger systemic infection such as septicemia.

■ Observe all dressings. If edema is present, adjust the dressing *to avoid impairing circulation to the area.*

Complications

Cleaning and care of traumatic wounds may temporarily increase the patient's pain. Excessive, vigorous cleaning may further disrupt tissue integrity.

Documentation

Document the date and time of the procedure, wound size and condition, medication administration, specific wound care measures, and patient teaching.

SELECTED REFERENCES

Adriansson, C., et al. "The Use of Topical Anaesthesia at Children's Minor Lacerations: An Experimental Study," *Accident and Emergency Nursing* 12(2):74-84, April 2004.

Day, M.W. "Traumatic Amputation," *Nursing* 36(10):88, October 2006.

Gustafsson, M., and Ahlstrom, G. "Problems Experienced During the First Year of an Acute Traumatic Hand Injury: A Prospective Study," *Journal of Clinical Nursing* 13(8):986-95, November 2004.

Khan, M.N., and Naqvi, A.H. "Antiseptics, Iodine, Povidone-Iodine and Traumatic Wound Cleansing," *Journal of Tissue Viability* 16(4):6-10, November 2006.

Laskowski-Jones, L. "First Aid for Amputation," *Nursing* 36(4):50-52, April 2006.

Pereira, C. "Policy for the Handling of Amputation Parts in Accident and Emergency Departments," *Plastic and Reconstructive Surgery* 116(1):346-47, July 2005.

Venkatramani, H., and Sabapathy, S.R. "A Simple Technique for Stabilizing Subtotal Digital Amputation During Transport," *Plastic and Reconstructive Surgery* 113(5):1527-528, April 2004.

WOUND IRRIGATION

Irrigation cleans tissues and flushes cell debris and drainage from an open wound. Irrigation with a commercial wound cleaner helps the wound heal properly from the inside tissue layers outward to the skin surface; it also helps prevent premature surface healing over an abscess pocket or infected tract. Performed properly, wound irrigation requires strict sterile technique. After irrigation, open wounds usually are packed to absorb additional drainage. Always follow the standard precaution guidelines of the Centers for Disease Control and Prevention (CDC).

Equipment

Waterproof trash bag ■ linen-saver pad ■ emesis basin ■ clean gloves ■ sterile gloves ■ goggles, if indicated ■ gown, if indicated ■ prescribed irrigant such as sterile normal saline solution ■ sterile water or normal saline solution ■ sterile irrigating syringe ■ sterile container ■ materials as needed for wound care ■ sterile dressing ■ commercial wound cleaner ■ 35-ml piston syringe with 19G catheter ■ skin protectant wipe ■ gauze pad.

Preparation of equipment

Assemble all equipment in the patient's room. Check the expiration date on each sterile package and inspect for tears. Check the sterilization date and the date that each bottle of irrigating solution was opened; don't use any solution that's been open longer than 24 hours.

Using aseptic technique, dilute the prescribed irrigant to the correct proportions with sterile water or normal saline solution, if necessary. Let the solution stand until it reaches room temperature, or warm it to 90° to 95° F (32.2° to 35° C).

Open the waterproof trash bag, and place it near the patient's bed. Position the bag *to avoid reaching across the sterile field or the wound when disposing of soiled articles.* Form a cuff by turning down the top of the trash bag *to provide a wide opening, which will keep instruments or gloves from touching the bag's edge, thus preventing contamination.*

Implementation

■ Confirm the patient's identity using two patient identifiers according to your facility's policy.

■ Check the practitioner's order.

■ Assess the patient's condition. Identify the patient's allergies, especially to povidone-iodine or other topical solutions or medications.

Irrigating a deep wound

When preparing to irrigate a wound, attach a 19G needle or catheter to a 30-ml piston syringe. This setup delivers an irrigation pressure of 8 psi, which is effective in cleaning the wound and reducing the risk of trauma and wound infection. *To prevent tissue damage or, in an abdominal wound, intestinal perforation,* avoid forcing the needle or catheter into the wound.

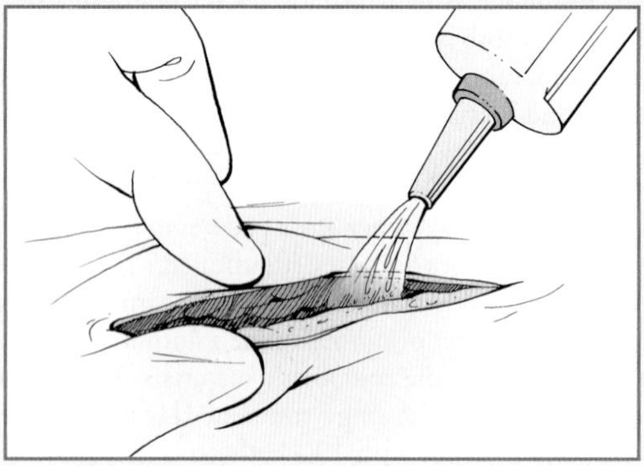

Irrigate the wound with gentle pressure until the solution returns clean. Then position the emesis basin under the wound to collect any remaining

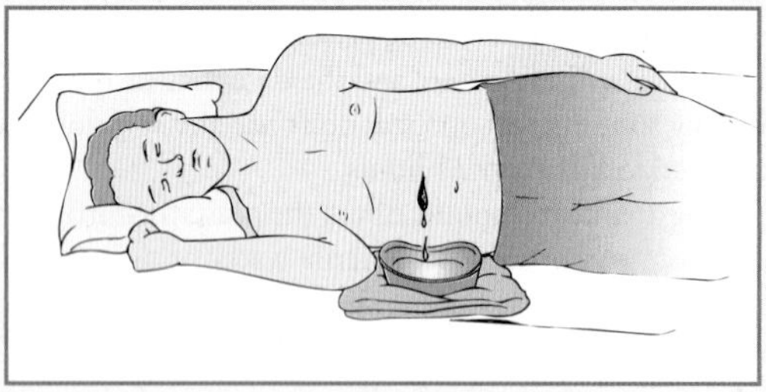

- Explain the procedure to the patient, provide privacy, and position the patient correctly for the procedure.
- Place the linen-saver pad under the patient to catch any spills and avoid linen changes. Place the emesis basin below the wound so that the irrigating solution flows from the wound into the basin and so that the irrigating solution will drain from the clean to the dirty end of the wound.
- Wash your hands thoroughly. If necessary, put on a gown and goggles *to protect your clothing from wound drainage and contamination.* Put on clean gloves.
- Remove the soiled dressing; then discard the dressing and gloves in the trash bag.
- Assess the wound and surrounding tissue for information about the healing process or presence of infection.
- Establish a sterile field with all the equipment and supplies you'll need for irrigation and wound care. Pour the prescribed amount of irrigating solution into a sterile container *so you won't contaminate your sterile gloves later by picking up unsterile containers.*
- Put on sterile gloves, gown, and goggles, if indicated.
- Fill the syringe with the irrigating solution. Gently instill a slow, steady stream of irrigating solution into the wound until the syringe empties. (See *Irrigating a deep wound.*) Make sure the solution flows from the clean to the dirty area of the wound *to prevent contamination of clean tissue by exudate.* Also make sure the solution reaches all areas of the wound.
- Refill the syringe and repeat the irrigation.
- Continue to irrigate the wound until you've administered the prescribed amount of solution or until the solution returns clear. Note the amount of solution administered. Then discard the syringe in the waterproof trash bag.
- Keep the patient positioned to allow further wound drainage into the basin.
- Dry intact skin with a sterile gauze pad, apply with a skin protectant wipe, and allow it to dry well *to help prevent skin breakdown and infection.*
- Pack the wound, if ordered, and apply a sterile dressing. Remove and discard your gloves and gown.
- Make sure the patient is comfortable.
- Properly dispose of drainage, solutions, and trash bag, and clean or dispose of soiled equipment and supplies according to your facility's policy and CDC guidelines. *To prevent contamination of other equipment,* don't return unopened sterile supplies to the sterile supply cabinet.

Special considerations

- Try to coordinate wound irrigation with the practitioner's visit *so that he can inspect the wound.*
- Use only the irrigant specified by the practitioner *because others may be erosive or otherwise harmful.*
- Remember to follow your facility's policy and CDC guidelines concerning wound and skin precautions.
- Irrigate with a bulb syringe if the wound is small or not particularly deep or if a piston syringe is unavailable. However, use a bulb syringe cautiously *because this type of syringe doesn't deliver enough pressure to adequately clean the wound.*
- If the procedure is likely to cause the patient pain, premedicate him before beginning irrigation as ordered.

Home care

If the wound must be irrigated at home, teach the patient or a family member how to perform this procedure using strict sterile technique. Ask for a return demonstration of the proper technique. Provide written instructions. Arrange for home health supplies and nursing visits as appropriate. Urge the patient to call the practitioner if he detects signs of infection.

Complications

Wound irrigation increases the risk of infection and may cause excoriation and increased pain. Pressure over 15 psi causes trauma to the wound and directs bacteria back into the tissue.

Documentation

Record the date and time of irrigation, amount and type of irrigant, appearance of the wound, sloughing tissue or exudate, amount of solution returned, skin care performed around the wound, dressings applied, and the patient's tolerance of the treatment.

SELECTED REFERENCES

Hassinger, H.M., et al. "High-Pressure Pulsatile Lavage Propagates Bacteria into Soft Tissue," *Clinical Orthopaedics and Related Research* 439:27-31, October 2005.

Svoboda, S.J., et al. "Comparison of Bulb Syringe and Pulsed Lavage Irrigation with Use of a Bioluminescent Musculoskeletal Wound Model," *The Journal of Bone and Joint Surgery* 88(10):2167-174, October 2006.

Willcox, M. "Cleaning Simple Wounds: Healing by Secondary Intention," *Nursing Times* 100(46):57, November 2004.

CLOSED-WOUND DRAIN MANAGEMENT

Typically inserted during surgery in anticipation of substantial postoperative drainage, a closed-wound drain promotes healing and prevents swelling by suctioning the exudate that accumulates at the wound site. By removing this fluid, the closed-wound drain helps reduce the risk of infection and skin breakdown as well as the number of dressing changes. The drain is usually emptied every 4 to 8 hours. Hemovac and Jackson-Pratt closed drainage systems are used most commonly. (See *Types of closed drainage systems.*)

A closed-wound drain consists of perforated tubing connected to a portable vacuum unit. The distal end of the tubing lies within the wound and usually leaves the body from a site other than the primary suture line to preserve the integrity of the surgical wound. The tubing exit site is treated as an additional surgical wound; the drain is usually sutured to the skin.

EQUIPMENT

Types of closed drainage systems

There are two common types of closed drainage systems. The Jackson-Pratt drain collects exudate in a bulblike device that's typically used with breast and abdominal surgery.

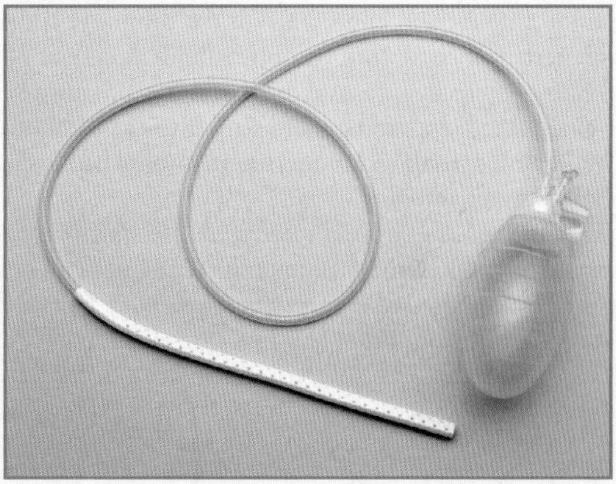

The Hemovac drain is used when blood drainage is expected after surgery, such as in abdominal and orthopedic surgeries.

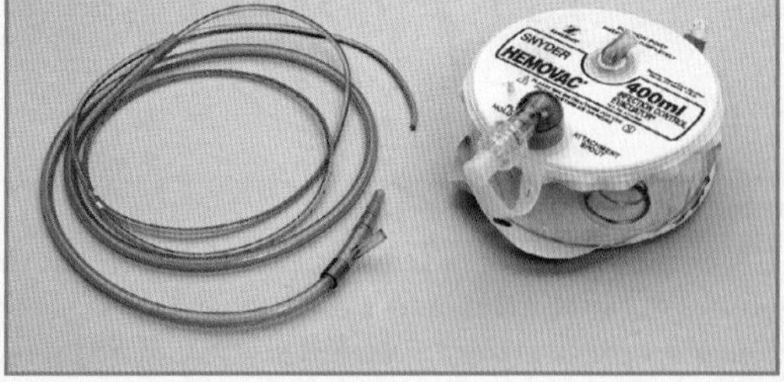

If the wound produces heavy drainage, the closed-wound drain may be left in place for longer than 1 week. Drainage must be emptied and measured frequently to maintain maximum suction and prevent strain on the suture line.

Equipment

Graduated cylinder ▪ sterile laboratory container, if needed ▪ alcohol pads ▪ gloves ▪ gown ▪ face shield ▪ sterile gauze pads ▪ antiseptic cleaning agent ▪ antiseptic swabs ▪ optional: label.

Implementation

■ Check the practitioner's order and assess the patient's condition.
■ Explain the procedure to the patient, provide privacy, and wash your hands.
■ Unclip the vacuum unit from the patient's bed or gown.
■ Using sterile technique, release the vacuum by removing the spout plug on the collection chamber. The container expands completely as it draws in air.
■ Empty the unit's contents into a graduated cylinder, and note the amount and appearance of the drainage. If diagnostic tests will be performed on the fluid specimen, pour the drainage directly into a sterile laboratory container, note the amount and appearance, and send it to the laboratory.
■ Maintaining sterile technique, use an alcohol pad to clean the unit's spout and plug.
■ *To reestablish the vacuum that creates the drain's suction power,* fully compress the vacuum unit. With one hand holding the unit compressed *to maintain the vacuum,* replace the spout plug with your other hand (as shown below).

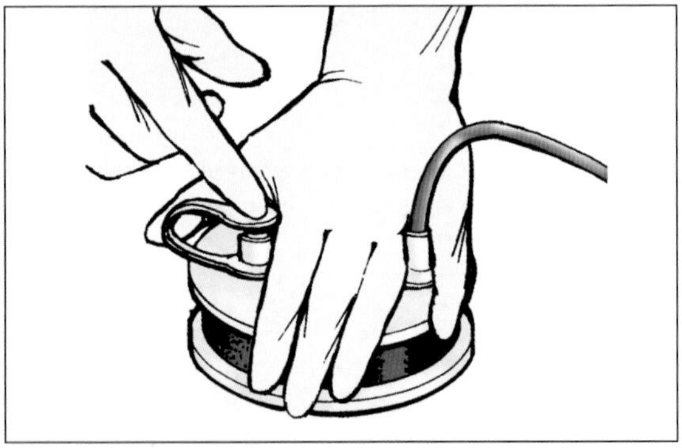

■ Check the patency of the equipment. Make sure the tubing is free of twists, kinks, and leaks *because the drainage system must be airtight to work properly.* The vacuum unit should remain compressed when you release manual pressure; rapid reinflation indicates an air leak. If this occurs, recompress the unit and make sure the spout plug is secure.
■ Secure the vacuum unit to the patient's gown. Fasten it below wound level *to promote drainage.* Don't apply tension on drainage tubing when fastening the unit *to prevent possible dislodgment.*
■ Remove and discard your gloves, and wash your hands thoroughly.
■ Observe the sutures that secure the drain to the patient's skin; look for signs of pulling or tearing and for swelling or infection of surrounding skin. Gently clean the sutures with sterile gauze pads soaked in an antiseptic cleaning agent or with an antiseptic swab.
■ Properly dispose of drainage, solutions, and clean or dispose of soiled equipment and supplies according to your facility's policy.

Special considerations

■ Empty the drain and measure its contents once during each shift if drainage has accumulated, more often if drainage is excessive. *Removing excess drainage maintains maximum suction and avoids straining the drain's suture line.*
■ If the patient has more than one closed drain, number the drains *so you can record drainage from each site.*

NURSING ALERT *Be careful not to mistake chest tubes with water seal drainage devices for closed-wound drains* because the care of these devices differs from closed-wound drainage systems, and the vacuum of a chest tube should never be released.

Complications

Occlusion of the tubing by fibrin, clots, or other particles can reduce or obstruct drainage. Infection may develop at the tubing exit site.

Documentation

Record the date and time you empty the drain, appearance of the drain site and presence of swelling or signs of infection, equipment malfunction and consequent nursing action, and the patient's tolerance of the treatment. On the intake and output sheet, record drainage color, consistency, type, and amount. If the patient has more than one closed-wound drain, number the drains, and record the information above separately for each drainage site.

SELECTED REFERENCES

Jeter, K. "Closed Suction Wound Drainage System," *Journal of Wound, Ostomy, and Continence Nursing* 31(2):51, March-April 2004.
Patel, V.P., et al. "Factors Associated with Prolonged Wound Drainage after Primary Total Hip and Knee Arthroplasty," *Journal of Bone and Joint Surgery* 89(1):33-38, January 2007.

VACUUM-ASSISTED CLOSURE THERAPY

Vacuum-assisted closure (VAC) therapy, also known as negative pressure wound therapy, is used to enhance delayed or impaired wound healing. The VAC device applies localized subatmospheric pressure to draw the edges of the wound toward the center. It's applied after a special dressing is placed in the wound or over a graft or flap; this wound packing removes fluids from the wound and stimulates growth of

Understanding vacuum-assisted closure therapy

Vacuum-assisted closure (VAC) therapy, also called negative pressure wound therapy, is an option to consider when a wound fails to heal in a timely manner. VAC therapy encourages healing by applying localized subatmospheric pressure at the site of the wound. This reduces edema and bacterial colonization and stimulates the formation of granulation tissue.

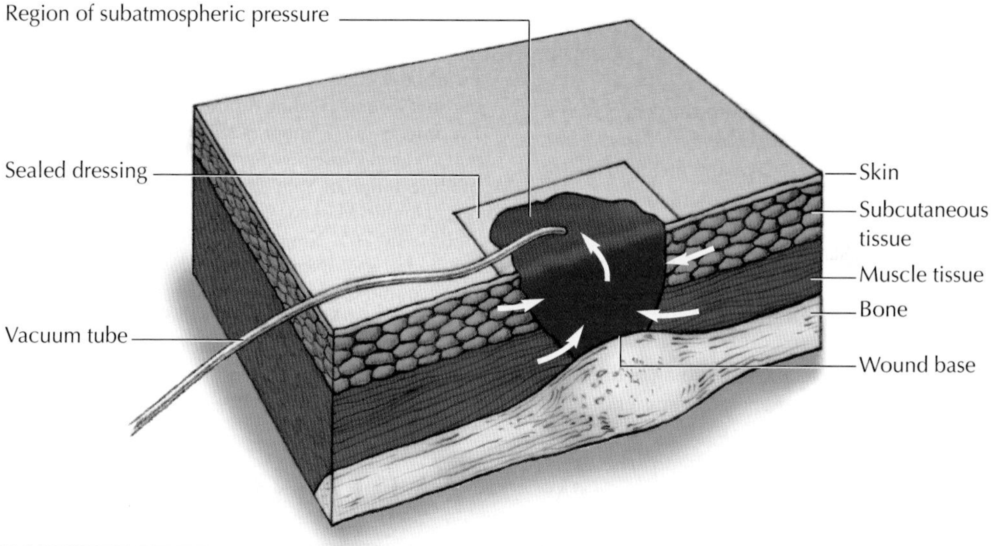

healthy granulation tissue. (See *Understanding vacuum-assisted closure therapy*.)

VAC therapy is indicated for acute and traumatic wounds, pressure ulcers, and chronic open wounds, such as diabetic ulcers, meshed grafts, and skin flaps. It's contraindicated for fistulas that involve organs or body cavities, necrotic tissue with eschar, untreated osteomyelitis, malignant wounds, and wounds with exposed arteries and veins. This therapy should be used cautiously in patients with active bleeding, in those taking anticoagulants, and when achieving wound hemostasis has been difficult.

Equipment

Waterproof trash bag ▪ goggles ▪ gown, if indicated ▪ emesis basin ▪ sterile irrigating solution ▪ normal saline solution ▪ clean gloves ▪ sterile gloves ▪ sterile scissors ▪ linen-saver pad ▪ irrigating syringe ▪ reticulated foam ▪ fenestrated tubing ▪ evacuation tubing ▪ skin protectant wipe ▪ transparent occlusive air-permeable drape ▪ evacuation canister ▪ vacuum unit.

Preparation of equipment

Assemble the VAC device at the bedside per manufacturer's instructions. Set negative pressure according to the practitioner's order (25 to 200 mm Hg). Warm the irrigating solution to 90° to 95° F *to reduce discomfort.*

Implementation

- Confirm the patient's identity using two patient identifiers according to your facility's policy.
- Assess the patient's condition.
- Explain the procedure to the patient, provide privacy, and wash your hands. Put on goggles—and a gown, if necessary—*to protect yourself from wound drainage and contamination.*
- Place a linen-saver pad under the patient *to catch any spills and avoid linen changes.* Position the patient to allow maximum wound exposure. Place the emesis basin under the wound *to collect any drainage.*
- Use sterile technique, and prepare a sterile field with all your supplies.

- Put on clean gloves. Remove the soiled dressing, and discard it in the waterproof trash bag. Remove your gloves.
- Put on sterile gloves, and irrigate the wound thoroughly using the normal saline solution and the irrigating syringe.
- Clean the area around the wound with normal saline solution; wipe intact skin with a skin protectant wipe and allow it to dry well. Remove and discard your gloves.
- If your sterile gloves are contaminated, remove them and put on a new pair. Using sterile scissors, cut the foam to the shape and measurement of the wound. More than one piece of foam may be necessary if the first piece is cut too small.

  Carefully place the foam in the wound.
- Next, place the fenestrated tubing into the center of the foam. *The fenestrated tubing, embedded into the foam, delivers negative pressure to the wound.* Make sure there's foam between the tubing and the base of the wound and over the top of the tubing.
- Place the transparent occlusive air permeable drape over the foam, enclosing both the foam and the tubing. Leave at least a 2″ (5 cm) margin around the wound of intact skin covered by the dressing.
- Connect the free end of the fenestrated tubing to the evacuation tubing connected to the evacuation canister.
- Remove and discard your gloves.
- Turn on the vacuum unit. Make sure the transparent dressing shrinks to the foam and the skin. *This confirms a good seal is present.*
- Make sure the patient is comfortable.
- Properly dispose of drainage, solution, linen-saver pad, and trash bag, and clean or dispose of soiled equipment and supplies according to your facility's policy and Centers for Disease Control and Prevention guidelines.

Special considerations

- Change the dressing every 48 to 72 hours. Try to coordinate dressing change with the practitioner's visit *so he can inspect the wound.*
- Measure the amount of drainage every shift.
- Adjust the negative pressure setting according to the practitioner's orders.
- Audible and visual alarms alert you if the unit is tipped greater than 45 degrees, the canister is full, the dressing has an air leak, or the canister becomes dislodged.
- Change the canister once a week or according to your facility's policy.
- *To obtain optimal therapy,* the unit must be applied at least 22 out of 24 hours.

Complications

Care and cleaning of wounds may temporarily increase the patient's pain. They also increase the risk for infection.

Documentation

Document the frequency and duration of therapy, the amount of negative pressure applied, the size and condition of the wound, and the patient's response to treatment.

SELECTED REFERENCES

Andros, G., et al. "Consensus Statement on Negative Pressure Wound Therapy (V.A.C. Therapy) for the Management of Diabetic Foot Wounds," *Ostomy/Wound Management* Suppl:1-32, June 2006.

Attinger, C.E., et al. "Clinical Approach to Wounds: Debridement and Wound Bed Preparation Including the Use of Dressing and Wound-Healing Adjuvants," *Plastic and Reconstructive Surgery* 117(7 Suppl):72S-109S, June 2006.

Llanos, S., et al. "Effectiveness of Negative Pressure Closure in the Integration of Split Thickness Skin Grafts: A Randomized, Double-Masked, Controlled Trial," *Annals of Surgery* 244(5):700-705, November 2006.

Morris, G.H., et al. "Negative Pressure Wound Therapy Achieved By Vacuum-Assisted Closure: Evaluating the Assumption," *Ostomy/Wound Management* 53(1):52-57, January 2007.

Pham, C.T., et al. "The Safety and Efficacy of Topical Negative Pressure in Non-Healing Wounds: A Systematic Review," *Journal of Wound Care* 15(6):240-50, June 2006.

RADIATION THERAPY

EXTERNAL RADIATION THERAPY

About 60% of all cancer patients are treated with some form of external radiation therapy. Also called radiotherapy, this treatment delivers X-rays or gamma rays directly to the cancer site. Its effects are local because only the area being treated experiences direct effects.

Radiation doses are based on the type, stage, and location of the tumor as well as on the patient's size, condition, and overall treatment goals. Doses are given in increments, usually three to five times a week, until the total dose is reached.

The goals of radiation therapy include *cure,* in which the cancer is completely destroyed and not expected to recur; *control,* in which the cancer doesn't progress or regress but is expected to progress at some later time; or *palliation,* in which radiation is given to relieve symptoms caused by the cancer (such as bone pain, bleeding, and headache).

External beam radiation therapy is delivered by machines that aim a concentrated beam of high-energy particles (photons and gamma rays) at the target site. Two types of machines are commonly used: units containing cobalt or cesium as radioactive sources for gamma rays, and linear accelerators that use electricity to produce X-rays. Linear accelerators produce high energy with great penetrating ability.

Radiation therapy may be augmented by chemotherapy, brachytherapy (radiation implant therapy), or surgery, as needed. (For information on chemotherapy, see chapter 5, Drug administration.)

Equipment

Radiation therapy machine ■ film badge or pocket dosimeter.

Implementation

- Confirm the patient's identity using two patient identifiers according to your facility's policy.
- Explain the treatment to the patient and his family. Review the treatment goals, and discuss the range of potential adverse effects as well as interventions to minimize them. Also discuss possible long-term complications and treatment issues. Educate the patient and his family about local cancer services.
- Make sure the radiation oncology department has obtained informed consent.
- Review the patient's clinical record for recent laboratory and imaging results, and alert the radiation oncology staff to any abnormalities or other pertinent results (such as myelosuppression, paraneoplastic syndromes, oncologic emergencies, and tumor progression).
- Transport the patient to the radiation oncology department.
- The patient begins by undergoing simulation (treatment planning), in which the target area is mapped out on his body using a machine similar to the radiation therapy machine. Then the target area is tattooed or marked in ink on his body *to ensure accurate treatments.*
- The physician and radiation oncologist determine the duration and frequency of treatments, depending on the patient's body size, size of portal, extent and location of cancer, and treatment goals.
- The patient is positioned on the treatment table beneath the machine. Treatments last from a few seconds to a few minutes. Reassure the patient that he won't feel anything and won't be radioactive. After treatment is complete, the patient may return home or to his room.

Special considerations

- Explain to the patient that the full benefit of radiation treatments may not occur until several weeks or months after treatments begin. Instruct him to report long-term adverse effects.
- Emphasize the importance of keeping follow-up appointments with the physician.
- Refer the patient to a support group, such as a local chapter of the American Cancer Society.

Home care

Instruct the patient and his family about proper skin care and management of possible adverse effects.

Complications

Adverse effects arise gradually and diminish gradually after treatments. They may be acute, subacute (accumulating as treatment progresses), chronic (following treatment), or long-term (arising months to years after treatment). Adverse effects are localized to the area of treatment, and their severity depends on the total radiation dose, underlying organ sensitivity, and the patient's overall condition.

Common acute and subacute adverse effects can include altered skin integrity, altered GI and genitourinary function, altered fertility and sexual function, altered bone marrow production, fatigue, and alopecia.

Chronic and long-term complications or adverse effects may include radiation pneumonitis, neuropathy, skin and muscle atrophy, telangiectasia, fistulas, altered endocrine function, and secondary cancers. Other complications of treatment include headache, alopecia, xerostomia, dysphagia, stomatitis, altered skin integrity (wet or dry desquamation), nausea, vomiting, heartburn, diarrhea, cystitis, and fatigue.

Documentation

Record radiation precautions taken during treatment; interventions used and their effectiveness; grading of adverse effects; teaching given to the patient and his family and their responses to it; the patient's tolerance of isolation procedures and the family's compliance with procedures; discharge plans and teaching; and referrals to local cancer services, if any.

SELECTED REFERENCES

Ahlberg, K., et al. "Fatigue, Psychological Distress, Coping Resources, and Functional Status during Radiotherapy for Uterine Cancer," *Oncology Nursing Forum* 32(3):633-40, May 2005.

Aistars, J. "The Validity of Skin Care Protocols Followed by Women with Breast Cancer Receiving External Radiation," *Clinical Journal of Oncology Nursing* 10(4):487-92, August 2006.

Delaney, G., et al. "The Role of Radiotherapy in Cancer Treatment: Estimating Optimal Utilization from a Review of Evidence-Based Clinical Guidelines," *Cancer* 104(6):1129-137, September 2005.

Recht, A., et al. "Post-Mastectomy Radiotherapy: Clinical Practice Guidelines of the American Society of Clinical Oncology," *Journal of Clinical Oncology* 19(5):1539-569, March 2001.

RADIATION IMPLANT THERAPY

In this treatment, also called *brachytherapy,* the physician uses implants of radioactive isotopes (encapsulated in seeds, needles, or sutures) to deliver ionizing radiation within a body cavity or interstitially to a tumor site. Implants can deliver a continuous radiation dose over several hours or days to a specific site while minimizing exposure to adjacent tissues. The implants may be permanent or temporary. Isotopes such as cesium 131, cesium 137, gold 198, iodine 125, iridium 192, palladium 103, and phosphorus 32 are used to treat cancers. (See *Radioisotopes and their uses.*)

Common implant sites include the brain, breast, cervix, endometrium, lung, neck, oral cavity, prostate, and vagina. Radiation implant therapy is commonly combined with external radiation therapy (teletherapy) for increased effectiveness.

For treatment, the patient is usually placed in a private room (with its own bathroom) located as far away from high-traffic areas as practical. If monitoring shows an increased radiation hazard, adjacent rooms and hallways may also need to be restricted. Consult your facility's radiation safety policy for specific guidelines.

Equipment

Film badge or pocket dosimeter ■ RADIATION PRECAUTION sign for door ■ RADIATION PRECAUTION warning labels ■ masking tape ■ lead-lined container ■ long-handled forceps ■ male T-binder and two sanitary napkins with safety pin (if Burnett applicator is being used) ■ optional: lead shield and lead strip.

Preparation of equipment

Place the lead-lined container and long-handled forceps in a corner of the patient's room. Mark a "safe line" on the floor with masking tape 6′ (1.8 m) from the patient's bed *to warn visitors to keep clear of the patient to minimize their radiation exposure.* If desired, place a portable lead shield in the back of the room *to use when providing care.*

Place an emergency tracheotomy tray in the room if an implant will be inserted in the oral cavity or neck.

Implementation

- Confirm the patient's identity using two patient identifiers according to your facility's policy.
- Explain the treatment and its goals to the patient. Before treatment begins, review radiation safety procedures, visitation policies, potential adverse effects, and interventions for those effects. Also review long-term concerns and home care issues.
- Place the RADIATION PRECAUTION sign on the door.
- Check to see that informed consent has been obtained.
- Ensure that all laboratory tests are performed before beginning treatment. If laboratory work is required during treatment, the badged technician obtains the specimen, labels the collection tube with a RADIOACTIVE PRECAUTION label, and alerts the laboratory personnel before bringing it. If urine tests are needed for phosphorus 32 therapy, ask the radiation oncology department or laboratory technician how to transport the specimens safely.
- Affix a RADIATION PRECAUTION warning label to the patient's identification wristband.
- Affix warning labels to the patient's chart and Kardex *to ensure staff awareness of the patient's radioactive status.*
- Wear a film badge or dosimeter at waist level during the entire shift. Turn in the radiation badge monthly or according to your facility's protocol. Pocket dosimeters measure immediate exposures. In many centers, these measurements aren't part of the permanent exposure record but are used to ensure that nurses receive the lowest possible exposure.
- Each nurse must have a personal, nontransferable film badge or ring badge. *Badges document each person's cumulative lifetime radiation exposure.* Only primary caregivers are badged and allowed into the patient's room.
- To minimize exposure to radiation, use the three principles of time, distance, and shielding: Time—plan to give care in the shortest time possible. *Less time equals less exposure.* Distance—work as far away from the radiation source as possible. Give care from the side opposite the implant or from a position allowing the greatest working distance possible. *The intensity of radiation exposure varies inversely as the square of the distance from the source.* Shielding—use a portable shield, if needed and desired.
- Provide essential nursing care only; omit bed baths. If ordered, provide perineal care, making sure that wipes, sanitary pads, and similar items are bagged correctly and monitored. (Refer to your facility's radiation policy.)
- Dressing changes over an implanted area must be supervised by the radiation technician or another designated caregiver.
- Before discharge, a patient's temporary implant must be removed and properly stored by the radiation oncology department. A patient with a permanent implant may not be released until his radioactivity level is less than 5 millirems/hour at 1 m.

Radioisotopes and their uses

Radioisotopes are unstable elements that emit three kinds of energy particles as they "decay" to a stable state. These particles are ranked by their penetrating power.

Alpha particles possess the lowest energy level and are easily stopped by a sheet of paper. More powerful *beta particles* can be stopped by the skin's surface. *Gamma rays,* the most powerful, can be stopped only by dense shielding such as lead. Some isotopes commonly used in cancer treatments are described below.

ISOTOPE AND INDICATIONS	DESCRIPTION	NURSING CONSIDERATIONS
Cesium 137 (^{137}Cs) Gynecologic cancers	▪ 30-year half-life ▪ Emits gamma particles ▪ Encased in steel capsules that are placed in the patient temporarily in the operating room	▪ Elevate the head of the bed no more than 45 degrees. ▪ Encourage fluids and implement a low-residue diet. ▪ Encourage quiet activities; enforce strict bed rest, as ordered.
Gold 198 (^{198}Au) Localized male genitourinary tumors	▪ 3-day half-life ▪ Emits gamma particles ▪ Permanently implanted as tiny seeds directly into the tumor or tumor bed	▪ If a seed is dislodged and found, call the radiation oncology department for disposal.
Iodine 125 (^{125}I) Localized or unresectable tumors; slow-growing tumors; recurrent disease	▪ 60-day half-life ▪ Emits gamma particles ▪ Permanently implanted as tiny seeds or sutures directly into the tumor or tumor bed	▪ Because a seed may become dislodged, no linens, body fluids, instruments, or utensils may leave the patient's room until they're monitored. ▪ If a seed is dislodged and found, call the radiation oncology department; use long-handled forceps to put it in a lead-lined container in the room. ▪ Monitor body fluids to detect displaced seeds. Give the patient a 24-hour urine container that can be closed.
Iridium 192 (^{192}Ir) Gynecologic cancers; tumors of the prostate, brain, and breast	▪ 74-day half-life ▪ Emits gamma particles ▪ Temporarily implanted as seeds strung inside special catheters that are implanted around the tumor	▪ If a catheter is dislodged, call the radiation oncology department; use long-handled forceps to put the implant in a lead-lined container in the room.
Palladium 103 (^{103}Pd) Prostate cancer	▪ 17-day half-life ▪ Emits gamma particles ▪ Permanently implanted as seeds in the tumor or tumor bed	▪ See Iodine 125.
Phosphorus 32 (^{32}P) Polycythemia, leukemia, bone metastasis, and malignant ascites	▪ 14-day half-life ▪ Emits beta particles ▪ Used as an I.V. solution rather than an implant because of its low energy level	▪ Patients receiving ^{32}P are placed in a private room with a separate bathroom.
Cesium 131 (^{131}Cs) Prostate, liver, and head and neck tumors	▪ 10-day half-life ▪ Permanently implanted as tiny seeds directly into the tumor bed ▪ Emits gamma particles	▪ See Gold 198.

Special considerations

- Nurses and visitors who are pregnant or trying to conceive or father a child must not attend patients receiving radiation implant therapy *because the gonads and developing embryo and fetus are highly susceptible to the damaging effects of ionizing radiation.*
- If the patient must be moved out of his room, notify the appropriate department of the patient's status *to give receiving personnel time to make appropriate preparations to receive the patient.* When moving the patient, ensure that the route is clear of equipment and other people and that the elevator, if there is one, is keyed and ready to receive the patient. Move the patient in a bed or wheelchair, accompanied by two badged caregivers. If the patient is delayed along the way, stand as far away from the bed as possible until you can continue.
- The patient's room must be monitored daily by the radiation oncology department, and disposables must be monitored and removed according to facility guidelines.
- If a code is called on a patient with an implant, follow your facility's code procedures as well as these steps: Notify the code team of the patient's radioactive status *to exclude any team member who is pregnant or trying to conceive or father a child.* Also notify the radiation oncology department. Cover the implant site with a strip of lead shielding if possible. Don't allow anything to leave the patient's room until it's monitored for radiation. The primary care nurse must remain in the room (as far from the patient as possible) *to act as a resource person for the patient and to provide film badges or dosimeters to code team members.*
- If an implant becomes dislodged, notify the radiation oncology department staff, and follow their instructions. Typically, the dislodged implant is collected with long-handled forceps and placed in a lead-shielded canister.
- Tell the patient who has had a cervical implant to expect slight to moderate vaginal bleeding after being discharged. This flow normally changes color from pink to brown to white. Instruct her to notify the physician if bleeding increases, persists for more than 48 hours, or has a foul odor. Explain to the patient that she may resume most normal activities but should avoid sexual intercourse and the use of tampons until after her follow-up visit to the physician (about 6 weeks after discharge). Instruct her to take showers rather than baths for 2 weeks, to avoid douching unless allowed by the physician, and to avoid activities that cause abdominal strain for 6 weeks.
- Refer the patient for sexual or psychological counseling if needed.
- If a patient with an implant dies on the unit, notify the radiation oncology department *so they can remove a temporary implant and store it properly.* If the implant was permanent, radiation oncology staff members will determine which precautions to follow before postmortem care can be provided and before the body can be moved to the morgue.

Complications

Depending on the implant site and total radiation dose, complications of implant therapy may include dislodgment of the radiation source or applicator, tissue fibrosis, xerostomia, radiation pneumonitis, muscle atrophy, sterility, vaginal dryness or stenosis, fistulas, hypothyroidism, altered bowel habits, infection, airway obstruction, diarrhea, cystitis, myelosuppression, neurotoxicity, and secondary cancers. Encourage the patient and family members to keep in contact with the radiation oncology department and to call them if concerns or physical changes occur.

Documentation

Record radiation precautions taken during treatment, adverse effects of therapy, teaching given to the patient and his family and their responses to it, the patient's tolerance of isolation procedures and the family's compliance with procedures, and referrals to local cancer services.

Selected references

Phan, T.P., et al. "High Dose Rate Brachytherapy as a Boost for the Treatment of Localized Prostate Cancer," *The Journal of Urology* 177(1):123-27, January 2007.

Stipetich, R., et al. "Nursing Considerations in Brachytherapy-Related Erectile Dysfunction," *Urology Nursing* 25(4):249-54, August 2005.

Thompson, S., et al. "Estimation of the Optimal Brachytherapy Utilization Rate in the Treatment of the Uterine Cervix: Review of Clinical Practice Guidelines and Primary Evidence," *Cancer* 107(12):2932-941, December 2006.

Radioactive iodine therapy

Because the thyroid gland concentrates iodine, radioactive iodine 131 (^{131}I) can be used to treat thyroid cancer. Usually administered orally, this isotope is used to treat postoperative residual cancer, recurrent disease, inoperable primary thyroid tumors, invasion of the thyroid capsule, and thyroid ablation as well as cancers that have metastasized to cervical or mediastinal lymph nodes or other distant sites.

Because ^{131}I is absorbed systemically, all body secretions, especially urine, must be considered radioactive. For ^{131}I treatments, the patient usually is placed in a private room (with its own bathroom) located as far away from high-traffic areas as practical. Adjacent rooms and hallways may also need to be restricted. Consult your facility's radiation safety policy for specific guidelines.

In lower doses, ^{131}I also may be used to treat hyperthyroidism. Most patients receive this treatment on an outpatient basis and are sent home with appropriate home care instructions.

Equipment

Film badges, pocket dosimeters, or ring badges ■ RADIATION PRECAUTION sign for door ■ RADIATION PRECAUTION warning labels ■ waterproof gowns ■ clear and red plastic bags for contaminated articles ■ plastic wrap ■ absorbent plastic-lined pads ■ masking tape ■ radioresistant gloves ■ trash cans ■ optional: portable lead shield.

Preparation of equipment

Assemble all necessary equipment in the patient's room. Keep an emergency tracheotomy tray just outside the room or in a handy place at the nurses' station. Place the RADIATION PRECAUTION sign on the door. Affix warning labels to the patient's chart and Kardex *to ensure staff awareness of the patient's radioactive status.*

Place an absorbent plastic-lined pad on the bathroom floor and under the sink; if the patient's room is carpeted, cover it with such a pad as well. Place an additional pad over the bedside table. Secure plastic wrap over the telephone, television controls, bed controls, mattress, call button, and toilet. *These measures prevent radioactive contamination of working surfaces.*

Keep large trash cans in the room lined with plastic bags (two clear bags inserted inside an outer red bag). Monitor all objects before they leave the room.

Notify the dietitian to supply foods and beverages only in disposable containers and with disposable utensils.

Implementation

■ Explain the procedure and review treatment goals with the patient and his family. Before treatment begins, review the facility's radiation safety procedures and visitation policies, potential adverse effects, interventions, and home care procedures. (See *What to do after ^{131}I treatment.*)

■ Verify that the physician has obtained informed consent.

■ Check for allergies to iodine-containing substances, such as contrast media and shellfish. Review the medication history for thyroid-containing or thyroid-altering drugs and for lithium carbonate, *which may increase ^{131}I uptake.*

■ Review the patient's health history for vomiting, diarrhea, productive cough, and sinus drainage, *which could increase the risk of radioactive secretions.*

■ If necessary, remove the patient's dentures *to avoid contaminating them and to reduce radioactive secretions.* Tell him that they'll be returned 48 hours after treatment.

HOME CARE

What to do after ^{131}I treatment

■ Instruct the patient to report long-term adverse reactions. In particular, review signs and symptoms of hypothyroidism and hyperthyroidism. Also ask him to report signs and symptoms of thyroid cancer, such as enlarged lymph nodes, dyspnea, bone pain, nausea, vomiting, and abdominal discomfort.

■ Although the patient's radiation level at discharge will be safe, suggest that he take extra precautions during the first week, such as using separate eating utensils, sleeping in a separate bedroom, and avoiding body contact.

■ Sexual intercourse may be resumed 1 week after ^{131}I treatment. However, urge a female patient to avoid pregnancy for 6 months after treatment, and tell a male patient to avoid impregnating his partner for 3 months after treatment.

■ Affix a RADIATION PRECAUTION warning label to the patient's identification wristband.

■ Encourage the patient to use the toilet rather than a bedpan or urinal and to flush it three times after each use *to reduce radiation levels.*

■ Tell the patient to remain in his room except for tests or procedures. Allow him to ambulate in the room.

■ Unless contraindicated, instruct the patient to increase his fluid intake to 3 qt (3 L) daily.

■ Encourage the patient to chew or suck on hard candy *to keep salivary glands stimulated and prevent them from becoming inflamed (which may develop in the first 24 hours).*

■ Ensure that all laboratory tests are performed before beginning treatment. If laboratory work is required, the badged laboratory technician obtains the specimen, labels the collection tube with a RADIATION PRECAUTION warning label, and alerts the laboratory personnel before transporting it. If urine tests are needed, ask the radiation oncology department or laboratory technician how to transport the specimens safely.

■ Wear a film badge or dosimeter at waist level during the entire shift. Turn in the radiation badge monthly or according to your facility's protocol, and be sure to record your exposures accurately. *Pocket dosimeters measure immediate exposures. These measurements may not be part of the permanent exposure record but help to ensure that nurses receive the lowest possible exposure.*

■ Each nurse must have a personal, nontransferable film badge or ring badge. *Badges document each person's cumulative lifetime radiation exposure.* Only primary caregivers are badged and allowed into the patient's room.
■ Wear gloves to touch the patient or objects in his room.
■ Allow visitors to stay no longer than 30 minutes every 24 hours with the patient. Stress that no visitors will be allowed who are pregnant or trying to conceive or father a child.
PEDIATRIC ALERT *Visitors younger than age 18 aren't allowed.*
■ Restrict direct contact to no longer than 30 minutes or 20 millirems per day. If the patient is receiving 200 millicuries of ^{131}I , remain with him only 2 to 4 minutes and stand no closer than 1′ (30 cm) away. If standing 3′ (1 m) away, the time limit is 20 minutes; if standing 5′ (1.5 m) away, the limit is 30 minutes.
■ Give essential nursing care only; omit bed baths. If ordered, provide perineal care, making sure that wipes, sanitary pads, and similar items are bagged correctly.
■ If the patient vomits or urinates on the floor, notify the nuclear medicine department, and use nondisposable radioresistant gloves when cleaning the floor. After cleanup, wash your gloved hands, remove the gloves and leave them in the room, and then rewash your hands.
■ If the patient must be moved from his room, notify the appropriate department of his status *so that receiving personnel can make appropriate arrangements to receive him.* When moving the patient, ensure that the route is clear of equipment and other people and that the elevator, if there is one, is keyed and ready to receive the patient. Move the patient in a bed or wheelchair, accompanied by two badged caregivers. If delayed, stand as far away from him as possible until you can continue.
■ The patient's room must be cleaned by the radiation oncology department, not by housekeeping. The room must be monitored daily, and disposables must be monitored and removed according to facility guidelines.
■ At discharge, schedule the patient for a follow-up examination. Also arrange for a whole-body scan about 7 to 10 days after ^{131}I treatment.
■ Inform the patient and his family of community support services for cancer patients.

Special considerations

■ Nurses and visitors who are pregnant or trying to conceive or father a child must not attend or visit patients receiving ^{131}I therapy *because the gonads and developing embryo and fetus are highly susceptible to the damaging effects of ionizing radiation.*
■ If a code is called on a patient undergoing ^{131}I therapy, follow your facility's code procedures as well as these steps: Notify the code team of the patient's radioactive status *to exclude any team member who is pregnant or trying to conceive or father a child.* Also notify the radiation oncology department. Don't allow anything out of the patient's room until it's monitored. The primary care nurse must remain in the room (as far as possible from the patient) *to act as a resource person and to provide film badges or dosimeters to code team members.*
■ If the patient dies on the unit, notify the radiology safety officer, who will determine which precautions to follow before postmortem care is provided and before the body can be removed to the morgue.

Complications

Myelosuppression is common in patients who undergo repeated ^{131}I treatments. Radiation pulmonary fibrosis may develop if extensive lung metastasis was present when ^{131}I was administered.

Other complications may include nausea, vomiting, headache, radiation thyroiditis, fever, sialadenitis, and pain and swelling at metastatic sites.

Documentation

Record radiation precautions taken during treatment, teaching given to the patient and his family, the patient's tolerance of (and the family's compliance with) isolation procedures, and referrals to local cancer counseling services.

SELECTED REFERENCES

American Association of Clinical Endocrinologists. "AACE Medical Guidelines for Clinical Practice for the Evaluation and Treatment of Hyperthyroidism and Hypothyroidism," *Endocrine Practice* 81(6):457-469, November-December 2002.

Podnos, Y.D., et al. "Radioactive Iodine Offers Survival Improvement in Patients with Follicular Carcinoma of the Thyroid," *Surgery* 138(6):1072-1076, December 2005.

5 ■ DRUG ADMINISTRATION

INTRODUCTION

Administering drugs is one of your most crucial nursing responsibilities. To ensure safe and effective drug therapy for your patients, you need to be familiar with the indications, customary dosages, and intended effects of prescribed drugs. And you need to assess each patient before administering a drug, delaying or withholding it if necessary. Just as important, you need the skills to be able to administer a drug capably, minimizing your patient's anxiety and maximizing the drug's effectiveness. This chapter will help you perform this task by providing the information you need to give drugs by injection, instillation, inhalation, topical application, and the intravascular route. You'll also learn how to give I.V. bolus injections, and prepare and administer chemotherapeutic drugs.

SELECTING THE APPROPRIATE ROUTE

Drugs may be administered by many routes. The *topical,* or *dermatomucosal, route* includes aural, ocular, nasal, and vaginal administration; oropharyngeal inhalation; and transdermal absorption. The *enteral route,* the most commonly used one, involves drug absorption through the GI tract. The *parenteral route* includes intradermal, subcutaneous, I.M., I.V., intrathecal, and intraosseous infusions or injections. The *endotracheal route* involves administering a drug into the respiratory system through an endotracheal tube. The *epidural route* involves giving a drug (usually an anesthetic or an opioid analgesic) through a catheter inserted near the spinal cord by a lumbar puncture. The *intrapleural route* involves injecting a drug through the chest wall into the pleural space.

More than any other factor, the administration route determines the onset of a drug's effect. For example, drugs administered I.V. act almost instantly because they're immediately available in the bloodstream. Antibiotics, for instance, are commonly given I.V. to provoke a quick, continuous response. Other drugs must be given I.V. because they're ineffective, or even dangerous, when given by other routes.

Conversely, some drugs, such as NPH insulin and penicillin G, can't be given I.V. because they obstruct blood flow. Drugs administered intrathecally, such as spinal anesthetics, also act rapidly. Drugs administered orally must be absorbed into the bloodstream before they can take effect.

AVOIDING MEDICATION ERRORS

Before you administer any medication, always compare the practitioner's order with the order on the patient's medication record. Then mentally check off the first five "rights" of drug administration: *right patient, right drug, right dose, right route,* and *right time.* If the practitioner's order and the patient's medication record match, then compare the label on the medication with the medication record. If you find any discrepancies, withhold the drug and verify the order with the practitioner or pharmacist. If a patient questions any of his drugs, double-check the orders and the dose before administration. Also check the drug's expiration date.

Before giving any drug, you need to be aware of two more "rights": the patient's right to know why he's getting the drug and what adverse effects to expect, if any, and his right to refuse medication.

Some drugs, such as opioids, barbiturates, and other controlled substances, have automatic stop dates mandated by law. Other medications, such as antibiotics, have stop dates set by facility policy. Check your facility's policy on how to handle outdated orders. Also learn your facility's policies on acceptance and documentation of verbal orders and correct use of p.r.n. (as needed) orders.

Many facilities are implementing high-alert medication infusion policies to ensure the safe administration of certain medications. Medications that possess a narrow margin of safety are deemed high-alert medications. The following I.V. infusion medications are some examples of high-alert medications:

- Antiarrhythmics
- Anticoagulants
- Benzodiazepines
- Chemotherapy
- Dopamine
- Dobutamine
- Electrolytes
- Insulin
- Lidocaine
- Opioids (morphine)
- Neuromuscular blocking agents
- Thrombolytics.

To facilitate safe medication administration practices, many facilities are designing and implementing specific error-reduction strategies targeting these and other high-alert medications. For example, high-alert medications should be mixed by a pharmacist or purchased as a premixed infusion whenever possible. Prior to initiating high-alert medication infusion, two nurses may be required to independently double-check all medication-related calculations and verify the rate of infusion. Many facilities require the initials or signature of both nurses who performed the calculated rate of administration on the medication record. It's also recommended that subsequent adjustments to the infusion rate of a high-alert medication be reverified by two nurses. Refer to your facility's specific policies pertaining to high-alert medications prior to administering these medications.

The U.S. Pharmacopeia's (USP) Center for the Advancement of Patient Safety suggests the following practices to prevent medication errors:

- Encourage the reporting of medication errors.
- Improve staff communication and leadership.
- Recruit qualified staff by establishing partnerships with academic institutions and clinical practices.
- Educate staff about safe medication practices.
- Increase the number of pharmacists available in patient-care areas.
- Use standardized protocols for high-alert medications.
- Use premixed I.V. solutions and unit-dose medications.
- Automate the medication process through bar-coding systems, wristband-scanning devices, identification wristbands with patient photos, and computerized records.

Understanding patient response and drug interactions

Assessing a patient's response to medication requires a thorough understanding of his condition and the drug's desired or expected effect. If a patient is receiving an antiarrhythmic, for example, but continues to have premature ventricular contractions, you should tell the practitioner that the drug isn't producing the desired effect.

When assessing the patient's response to therapy, also consider the results of laboratory tests, which can indicate a therapeutic effect, an adverse effect, or a toxic level. For example, prothrombin times help to evaluate the therapeutic effect of warfarin, and low serum potassium levels may signal an adverse effect of certain diuretics. Be aware that some drugs may affect diagnostic test results, causing "false positives." For example, codeine may elevate cerebrospinal fluid pressure.

Monitor the patient's condition carefully; changes such as weight loss or gain can affect the action of some drugs. Other factors, such as the patient's age, body build, gender, and emotional state, may also affect the patient's response to drug therapy.

Because many patients receive more than one drug, you should also understand drug interactions. A drug interaction is a change in drug absorption, distribution, metabolism, and excretion that may occur with or shortly after administration of another drug. A desirable interaction is the basis for combination therapy, which may be used for additive effect, for helping to maintain an effective blood level, or for minimizing or preventing adverse effects. Some interactions, however, can have undesirable results, such as weakening a drug's desired effects or exaggerating its toxic ones. For example, patients who smoke require larger doses of theophylline than do nonsmokers because cigarette smoke activates oxidative enzymes in the liver, increasing drug metabolism.

Watching for adverse effects

When you administer drugs, you need to recognize and identify adverse effects, toxic reactions, and drug allergies. Some adverse effects are transient and subside as the patient develops a tolerance for the drug; others may require a change in therapy.

A *toxic reaction* to a drug can be acute, resulting from excessive doses, as in acetaminophen overdose, or chronic, resulting from progressive accumulation of the drug in the body. It can also result from impaired metabolism or excretion that can cause elevated blood levels of a drug.

A *drug allergy* (hypersensitivity) results from an antigen-antibody reaction in susceptible patients. Such a reaction can range from mild urticaria to potentially fatal anaphylaxis. Therefore, always check for allergies before administering medications. In some instances, sensitivity tests may be done before giving the first dose. Be aware that a negative history doesn't rule out a future allergic reaction.

Other undesirable effects to watch for when administering drugs include idiosyncratic reactions and dependence.

Documenting carefully

Documentation aims to preserve an accurate record of patient assessment and interventions as well as your reasons for giving the care specified. Documenting a patient's medications provides a legal record of drugs he received during his stay in the facility. Medication administration involves documenting on a medication administration record (MAR) as well as in the nurses' notes. Many facilities also require documentation of opioid administration in a central record.

After administering a drug, document the following on the patient's Kardex or computer file: drug name, dosage, route and time of administration, and your signature and title. In the nurses' notes, include any assessment data that refer to the patient's response to the medication or any adverse effects of the medication.

If your facility documents medications by computer, be sure to enter each drug immediately after you give it. This gives all health care team members access to current medication information and is especially important if the system has no hard-copy backup. If a patient refuses or is unable to take medication or if, in your judgment, the patient shouldn't receive the medication, document this on the MAR and in the nurses' notes.

Many facilities use an MAR to document medication orders and administration. Usually contained in a Kardex file, the MAR serves as the central source for recording the practitioner's medication orders and documenting administration. It becomes part of the patient's permanent medical record. When using the MAR, know and follow your facility's policy and procedure for recording medication orders and charting medication administration. Make sure medication orders include the patient's full name, date ordered, drug dose, administration route or method, frequency, and time ordered for the first dose. Some drugs may be ordered with a specific number of doses or a stop date. If that's so, be sure to note this on the MAR.

Always write legibly. Use only acceptable abbreviations, and use them correctly. When in doubt as to how to abbreviate a term, spell it out. When documenting parenteral medications, be sure to include the injection site and the route you used. After administering the first dose, sign your full name, licensure status, and identifying initials in the appropriate place on the MAR.

If all medications have been given according to the plan of care, no further documentation is needed. However, if your facility's MAR doesn't include a place to document parenteral administration sites, the patient's response to p.r.n. medications, or any deviation from the medication order, further narrative documentation is necessary. Document any patient teaching given as well as the patient's response and knowledge level.

TOPICAL ADMINISTRATION

SKIN MEDICATIONS

Topical drugs are applied directly to the skin surface. They include lotions, pastes, ointments, creams, powders, shampoos, patches, and aerosol sprays. Topical medications are absorbed through the epidermal layer into the dermis. The extent of absorption depends on the vascularity of the region.

Nitroglycerin, fentanyl, nicotine, and certain supplemental hormone replacements are used for systemic effects. Most other topical medications are used for local effects. Ointments have a fatty base, which is an ideal vehicle for drugs such as antimicrobials and antiseptics. Typically, topical medications should be applied two or three times per day to achieve their therapeutic effect.

Equipment

Patient's medication record and chart ▪ prescribed medication ▪ gloves ▪ 4″ × 4″ sterile gauze pads ▪ transparent semipermeable dressing ▪ adhesive tape ▪ solvent (such as cottonseed oil).

Implementation

- Verify the order on the patient's medication record by checking it against the practitioner's order on the chart. Also check the patient's medication record for allergies.
- Make sure the label on the medication agrees with the medication order. Read the label again before you open the container and as you remove the medication from the container. Check the expiration date.
- Confirm the patient's identity using two patient identifiers according to your facility's policy.
- If your facility uses a bar code scanning system, be sure to scan your ID badge, the patient's ID bracelet, and the medication's bar code.
- Provide privacy.
- Explain the procedure thoroughly to the patient *because he may have to apply the medication by himself after discharge.*
- Wash your hands *to prevent cross-contamination,* and put on gloves.
- Help the patient assume a comfortable position that provides access to the area to be treated.
- Expose the area to be treated. Make sure the skin or mucous membrane is intact (unless the medication has been ordered to treat a skin lesion such as an ulcer). *Applying medication to broken or abraded skin may cause unwanted systemic absorption and result in further irritation.*
- If necessary, clean the skin of debris, including crusts, epidermal scales, and old medication. You may have to change your gloves if they become soiled.

Applying paste, cream, or ointment

- Open the container. Place the lid or cap upside down *to prevent contamination of the inside surface.*
- Apply the medication to the affected area with long, smooth strokes that follow the direction of hair growth using your gloved hands. *This technique avoids forcing medication into hair follicles, which can cause irritation and lead to folliculitis.* Avoid excessive pressure when applying the medication *because it could abrade the skin.*

Removing ointment

- Wash your hands and apply gloves. Then rub solvent on them, and apply it liberally to the ointment-treated area in the direction of hair growth. Alternatively, saturate a sterile gauze pad with the solvent, and use the pad to gently remove the ointment. Remove excess oil by gently wiping the area with a sterile gauze pad. Don't rub too hard to remove the medication *because you could irritate the skin.*

Applying other topical medications

- To apply shampoos, follow package directions. (See *Using medicated shampoos.*)

■ To apply aerosol sprays, shake the container, if indicated, *to completely mix the medication.* Hold the container 6" to 12" (15 to 30 cm) from the skin, or follow the manufacturer's recommendation. Spray a thin film of the medication evenly over the treatment area.
■ To apply powders, dry the skin surface, making sure to spread skin folds where moisture collects. Then apply a thin layer of powder over the treatment area.
■ *To protect applied medications and prevent them from soiling the patient's clothes,* tape an appropriate amount of sterile gauze pad or a transparent semipermeable dressing over the treated area. With certain medications (such as topical steroids), semipermeable dressings may be contraindicated. Check medication information and cautions. If you're applying a topical medication to the patient's hands or feet, cover the site with white cotton gloves for the hands or terry cloth scuffs for the feet.

PEDIATRIC ALERT *In children, topical medications (such as steroids) should be covered only loosely with a diaper. Don't use plastic pants.*

■ Assess the patient's skin for signs of irritation, allergic reaction, or breakdown.

Special considerations

■ Never apply medication without first removing previous applications *to prevent skin irritation from an accumulation of medication.*
■ Be sure to wear gloves *to prevent absorption by your own skin.* If the patient has an infectious skin condition, use sterile gloves and dispose of old dressings according to your facility's policy.
■ Don't apply ointments to mucous membranes as liberally as you would to skin *because mucous membranes are usually moist and absorb ointment more quickly than skin does.* Also, don't apply too much ointment to any skin area *because it might cause irritation and discomfort, stain clothing and bedding, and make removal difficult.*
■ Never apply ointment to the eyelids or ear canal unless ordered. *The ointment might congeal and occlude the tear duct or ear canal.*
■ Inspect the treated area frequently for adverse effects such as signs of an allergic reaction.
■ When applying an aerosol spray or powder, make sure to protect the patient from direct inhalation of the medication.

Complications

Skin irritation, a rash, or an allergic reaction may occur.

Documentation

Record the medication applied; time, date, and site of application; and condition of the patient's skin at the time of application. Note the patient's tolerance and subsequent effects of the medication, if any.

Using medicated shampoos

Medicated shampoos include keratolytic and cytostatic agents, coal tar preparations, and lindane (gamma benzene hexachloride) solutions. They can be used to treat conditions such as dandruff, psoriasis, and head lice. However, they're contraindicated in patients with broken or abraded skin.

Because application instructions may vary among brands, check the label on the shampoo before starting the procedure *to ensure use of the correct amount.* Keep the shampoo away from the patient's eyes. If any shampoo should accidentally get in his eyes, irrigate them promptly with water. Likewise, keep the shampoo from running into the patient's mouth. Selenium sulfide, used in cytostatic agents, is extremely toxic if ingested.

To apply a medicated shampoo, follow these steps:
■ Prepare the patient for shampoo treatment.
■ Shake the bottle of shampoo well *to mix the solution evenly.*
■ Wet the patient's hair thoroughly, and wring out excess water.
■ Apply the proper amount of shampoo as directed on the label.
■ Work the shampoo into a lather, adding water as necessary. Part the hair, and work the shampoo into the scalp, taking care not to use your fingernails.
■ Leave the shampoo on the scalp and hair for as long as instructed (usually 5 to 10 minutes). Then rinse the hair thoroughly.
■ Towel-dry the patient's hair.
■ After the hair is dry, comb or brush it. Use a fine-tooth comb *to remove nits* if necessary.

SELECTED REFERENCES

Craven, R.F., and Hirnle, C.J. *Fundamentals of Nursing: Human Health and Function,* 5th ed. Philadelphia: Lippincott Williams & Wilkins, 2006.
McCleane, G. "Topical Analgesics," *The Medical Clinics of North America* 91(1):125-39, January 2007.
McIntyre, L.J., and Courey, T.J. "Safe Medication Administration," *Journal of Nursing Care Quality* 22(1):40-42, January-March 2007.

TRANSDERMAL DRUGS

Through an adhesive patch or a measured dose of ointment applied to the skin, transdermal drugs deliver constant, controlled medication directly into the bloodstream for a prolonged systemic effect.

Medications available in transdermal form include nitroglycerin, used to control angina; scopolamine, used to treat motion sickness; estradiol, used for postmenopausal hormone replacement; clonidine, used to treat hypertension; nicotine, used for smoking cessation; fentanyl, an opioid analgesic used to control chronic pain; and hormonal birth control. Nitroglycerin ointment dilates coronary vessels for up to 4 hours; a nitroglycerin disk or pad can produce the same effect for as long as 24 hours. A scopolamine patch can relieve motion sickness for as long as 72 hours, transdermal estradiol and hormonal birth control last for up to 1 week, clonidine and nicotine patches last for 24 hours, and a fentanyl patch can last for up to 72 hours.

Contraindications for transdermal drug application include skin allergies or skin reactions to the drug. Transdermal drugs shouldn't be applied to broken or irritated skin because they would increase irritation, or to scarred or callused skin, which might impair absorption.

Equipment

Patient's medication record and chart ▪ gloves ▪ prescribed medication (patch or ointment) ▪ application strip or measuring paper (for nitroglycerin ointment) ▪ adhesive tape ▪ plastic wrap (optional for nitroglycerin ointment) or semipermeable dressing.

Applying nitroglycerin ointment

Unlike most topical medications, nitroglycerin ointment is used for its transdermal *systemic* effect. It's used to dilate the veins and arteries, thus improving cardiac perfusion in a patient with cardiac ischemia or angina pectoris.

To apply nitroglycerin ointment, start by taking the patient's baseline blood pressure *so that you can compare it with later readings.* Remove any previously applied nitroglycerin ointment. Gather your equipment. Nitroglycerin ointment, which is prescribed by the inch, comes with a rectangular piece of ruled paper to be used in applying the medication. Squeeze the prescribed amount of ointment onto the ruled paper (as shown below). Put on gloves, if desired, *to avoid contact with the medication.*

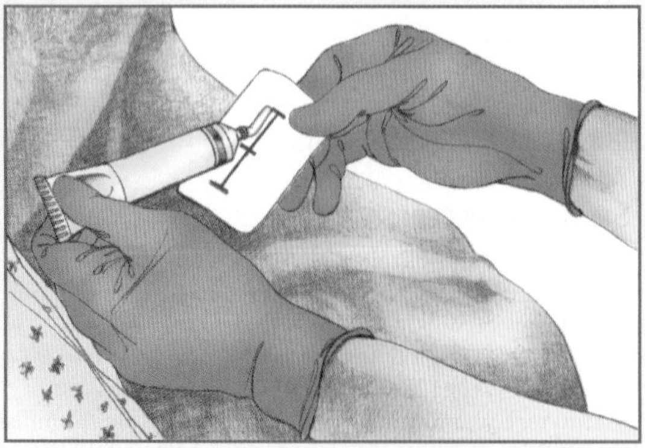

After measuring the correct amount of ointment, tape the paper—drug side down—directly to the skin (as shown below). *For increased absorption,* the practitioner may request that you cover the site with plastic wrap or a transparent semipermeable dressing.

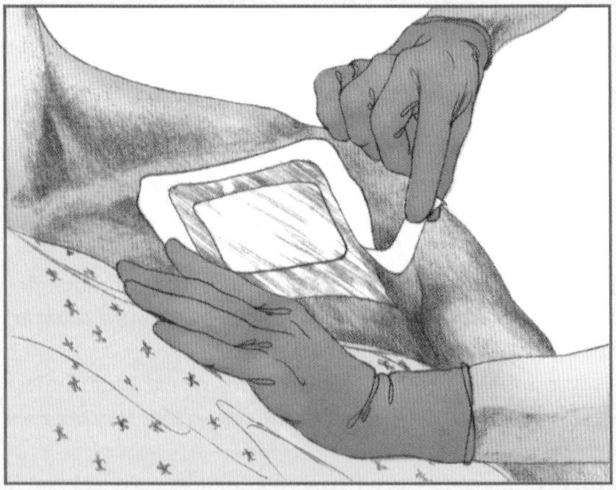

After 5 minutes, record the patient's blood pressure. If it has dropped significantly and he has a headache (from vasodilation of blood vessels in his head), notify the practitioner immediately. He may reduce the dose. If the patient's blood pressure has dropped but he's asymptomatic, instruct him to lie still until it returns to normal.

Implementation

- Verify the order on the patient's medication record by checking it against the practitioner's order.
- Wash your hands and, if necessary, put on gloves.
- Check the label on the medication *to make sure you'll be giving the correct drug in the correct dose.* Note the expiration date.
- Confirm the patient's identity using two patient identifiers according to your facility's policy.
- If your facility uses a bar code scanning system, be sure to scan your ID badge, the patient's ID bracelet, and the medication's bar code.
- Explain the procedure to the patient, and provide privacy.
- Remove any previously applied medication.

Applying transdermal ointment

- Place the prescribed amount of ointment on the application strip or measuring paper, taking care not to get any on your skin. (See *Applying nitroglycerin ointment.*)
- Apply the strip to any dry, hairless area of the body. Don't rub the ointment into the skin.
- Tape the strip and ointment to the skin.
- If desired, cover the application strip with plastic wrap, and tape the wrap in place.

Applying a transdermal patch

- Open the package and remove the patch.
- Without touching the adhesive surface, remove the clear plastic backing.
- Apply the patch to a dry, hairless area—behind the ear, for example, as with scopolamine. (See *Applying a transdermal medication patch.*)
- Write the date, time, and your initials on the dressing.

After applying transdermal medications

- Store the medication as ordered.
- Instruct the patient to keep the area around the patch or ointment as dry as possible.
- If you didn't wear gloves, wash your hands immediately after applying the patch or ointment *to avoid absorbing the drug yourself.*

Special considerations

- Reapply daily transdermal medications at the same time every day *to ensure a continuous effect,* but alternate the application sites *to avoid skin irritation.* Before reapplying nitroglycerin ointment, remove the plastic wrap, application strip, and any remaining ointment from the patient's skin at the previous site.

HOME CARE

Applying a transdermal medication patch

If the patient will be receiving medication by transdermal patch, instruct him in its proper use, as described below:

- Explain to the patient that the patch consists of several layers. The layer closest to his skin contains a small amount of the drug and allows prompt introduction of the drug into the bloodstream. The next layer controls release of the drug from the main portion of the patch. The third layer contains the main dose of the drug. The outermost layer consists of an aluminized polyester barrier.
- Teach the patient to apply the patch to appropriate skin areas, such as the upper arm or chest and behind the ear. Warn him to avoid touching the gel or surrounding tape. Tell him to use a different site for each application *to avoid skin irritation.* If necessary, he can clip the hair at the site. Caution him to avoid any area that may cause uneven absorption, such as skin folds, scars, and calluses, or any irritated or damaged skin areas. Also, tell him not to apply the patch below the elbow or knee.
- Instruct the patient to wash his hands after application *to remove any medication that may have rubbed off.*
- Warn the patient not to get the patch wet. Tell him to discard it if it leaks or falls off and then to clean the site and apply a new patch at a different site.
- Instruct the patient to apply the patch at the same time at the prescribed interval *to ensure continuous drug delivery.* Bedtime application is ideal *because body movement is reduced during the night.* Finally, tell him to apply a new patch about 30 minutes before removing the old one.

- When applying a scopolamine or fentanyl patch, instruct the patient not to drive or operate machinery until his response to the drug has been determined.
- Warn a patient using a clonidine patch to check with his practitioner before taking an over-the-counter cough preparation *because such drugs may counteract clonidine's effects.*

Complications

Topical medications may cause skin irritation, such as pruritus and a rash. The patient may also suffer adverse effects of the specific drug administered. For example, transdermal nitroglycerin medications may cause headaches and, in elderly patients, orthostatic hypotension. Scopolamine has various adverse effects; dry mouth and drowsiness are the most common. Transdermal estradiol carries an increased risk of endometrial cancer, thromboembolic disease, and birth defects. Clonidine may cause severe rebound hypertension, especially if withdrawn suddenly.

Documentation

Record the type of medication; date, time, and site of application; and dose. Also note any adverse effects and the patient's response.

SELECTED REFERENCES

The Joint Commission. *Comprehensive Accreditation Manual for Hospitals: The Official Handbook.* Standard MM.1.10. 2007.

The Joint Commission. *Comprehensive Accreditation Manual for Hospitals: The Official Handbook.* Standard MM.2.10. 2007.

The Joint Commission. *Comprehensive Accreditation Manual for Hospitals: The Official Handbook.* Standard MM.3.10. 2007.

The Joint Commission. *Comprehensive Accreditation Manual for Hospitals: The Official Handbook.* Standard MM.4.10. 2007.

The Joint Commission. *Comprehensive Accreditation Manual for Hospitals: The Official Handbook.* Standard MM.4.20. 2007.

The Joint Commission. *Comprehensive Accreditation Manual for Hospitals: The Official Handbook.* Standard MM.5.10. 2007.

The Joint Commission. *Comprehensive Accreditation Manual for Hospitals: The Official Handbook.* Standard MM.6.10. 2007.

The Joint Commission. *Comprehensive Accreditation Manual for Hospitals: The Official Handbook.* Standard MM.6.20. 2007.

McErlane, K. "Keeping Track of the Patch: Transdermal Delivery in Obese Patients," *AJN* 105(6):36-37, June 2005.

Taylor, C., et al. *Fundamentals of Nursing: The Art and Science of Nursing Care,* 6th ed. Philadelphia: Lippincott Williams & Wilkins, 2008.

EYE MEDICATIONS

Eye medications — drops, ointments, and disks — serve diagnostic and therapeutic purposes. During an eye examination, eyedrops can be used to anesthetize the eye, dilate the pupil to facilitate examination, and stain the cornea to identify corneal abrasions, scars, and other anomalies. Eye medications can also be used to lubricate the eye, treat certain eye conditions (such as glaucoma and infections), protect the vision of neonates, and lubricate the eye socket for insertion of a prosthetic eye.

Understanding the ocular effects of medications is important because certain drugs may cause eye disorders or have serious ocular effects. For example, anticholinergics, which are commonly used during eye examinations, can precipitate acute glaucoma in patients with a predisposition to the disorder.

Equipment

Prescribed eye medication ■ patient's medication record and chart ■ gloves ■ warm water or normal saline solution ■ sterile gauze pads ■ facial tissues ■ optional: ocular dressing.

Preparation of equipment

Make sure the medication is labeled for ophthalmic use. Then check the expiration date. Remember to date the container the first time you use the medication. After it's opened, an eye medication may be used for a maximum of 2 weeks to avoid contamination.

Inspect ocular solutions for cloudiness, discoloration, and precipitation, but remember that some eye medications are suspensions and normally appear cloudy. Don't use any solution that appears abnormal. If the tip of an eye ointment tube has crusted, turn the tip on a sterile gauze pad *to remove the crust.*

Implementation

- Verify the order on the patient's medication record by checking it against the practitioner's order on his chart.
- Wash your hands.
- Check the medication label against the patient's medication record.

NURSING ALERT *Make sure you know which eye to treat* because different medications or doses may be ordered for each eye.

- Confirm the patient's identity using two patient identifiers according to your facility's policy.
- If your facility uses a bar code scanning system, be sure to scan your ID badge, the patient's ID bracelet, and the medication's bar code.
- Explain the procedure to the patient, and provide privacy. Put on gloves.
- If the patient is wearing an eye dressing, remove it by gently pulling it down and away from his forehead. Take care not to contaminate your hands.
- Remove any discharge by cleaning around the eye with sterile gauze pads moistened with warm water or normal saline solution. With the patient's eye closed, clean from the inner to the outer canthus, using a fresh sterile gauze pad for each stroke.

■ *To remove crusted secretions around the eye,* moisten a gauze pad with warm water or normal saline solution. Ask the patient to close the eye, and then place the gauze pad over it for 1 or 2 minutes. Remove the pad, and then reapply moist sterile gauze pads, as necessary, until the secretions are soft enough to be removed without traumatizing the mucosa.
■ Have the patient sit or lie in the supine position. Instruct him to tilt his head back and toward the side of the affected eye *so that excess medication can flow away from the tear duct, minimizing systemic absorption through the nasal mucosa.*

Instilling eyedrops

■ Remove the dropper cap from the medication container, if necessary, and draw the medication into it. Be careful to avoid contaminating the dropper tip or bottle top.
■ Before instilling the eyedrops, instruct the patient to look up and away. *This moves the cornea away from the lower lid and minimizes the risk of touching the cornea with the dropper if the patient blinks.*
■ You can steady the hand holding the dropper by resting it against the patient's forehead. Then, with your other hand, gently pull down the lower lid of the affected eye and instill the drops in the conjunctival sac. Try to avoid placing the drops directly on the eyeball *to prevent the patient from experiencing discomfort.* (See *Instilling eye medications.*) If you're instilling more than one drop agent, you should wait 5 or more minutes between agents.

Applying eye ointment

■ Squeeze a small ribbon of medication on the edge of the conjunctival sac from the inner to the outer canthus. Cut off the ribbon by turning the tube. You can steady the hand holding the medication tube by bracing it against the patient's forehead or cheek. If you're applying more than one ribbon of medication, wait 10 minutes before applying the second medication.

Using a medication disk

■ A medication disk can release medication in the eye for up to 1 week before needing to be replaced. Pilocarpine, for example, can be administered this way to treat glaucoma. (See *How to insert and remove an eye medication disk,* page 284.)

After instilling eyedrops or eye ointment

■ Instruct the patient to close his eyes gently, without squeezing the lids shut. If you instilled drops, tell the patient to blink. If you applied ointment, tell him to roll his eyes behind closed lids *to help distribute the medication over the surface of the eyeball.*

Instilling eye medications

To instill eyedrops, pull the lower lid down to expose the conjunctival sac. Have the patient look up and away, then squeeze the prescribed number of drops into the sac, as shown below. Release the patient's eyelid, and have him blink to distribute the medication.

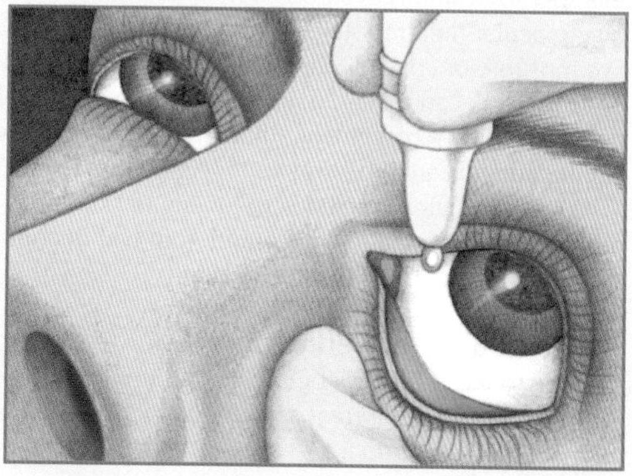

To apply an ointment, gently lay a thin strip of the medication along the conjunctival sac from the inner canthus to the outer canthus, as shown below. Avoid touching the tip of the tube to the patient's eye. Then release the eyelid, and have the patient roll his eye behind closed lids to distribute the medication.

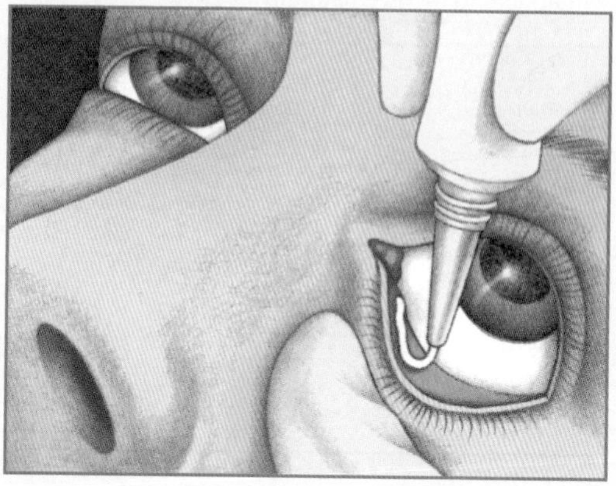

■ Use a clean tissue to remove any excess solution or ointment leaking from the eye. Remember to use a fresh tissue for each eye *to prevent cross-contamination.*
■ Apply a new eye dressing if necessary. (See "Hot and cold eye compresses," page 814.)

How to insert and remove an eye medication disk

Small and flexible, an oval eye medication disk consists of three layers: two soft outer layers and a middle layer that contains the medication. Floating between the eyelids and the sclera, the disk stays in the eye while the patient sleeps and even during swimming and athletic activities. The disk frees the patient from having to remember to instill his eyedrops. When the disk is in place, ocular fluid moistens it, releasing the medication. Eye moisture or contact lenses don't adversely affect the disk. The disk can release medication for up to 1 week before needing replacement. Pilocarpine, for example, can be administered this way to treat glaucoma.

Contraindications include conjunctivitis, keratitis, retinal detachment, and any condition in which constriction of the pupil should be avoided.

To insert an eye medication disk

Arrange to insert the disk before the patient goes to bed. *This minimizes the blurring that usually occurs immediately after disk insertion.*

- Wash your hands and put on gloves.
- Press your fingertip against the oval disk so that it lies lengthwise across your fingertip. It should stick to your finger. Lift the disk out of its packet.
- Gently pull the patient's lower eyelid away from the eye, and place the disk in the conjunctival sac. It should lie horizontally, as shown below, not vertically. The disk will adhere to the eye naturally.

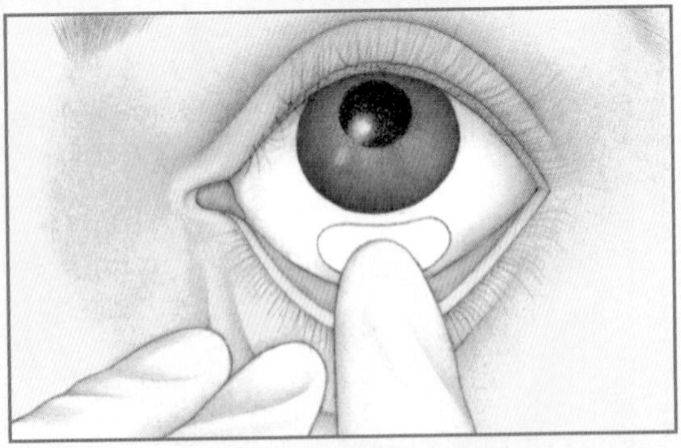

- Pull the lower eyelid out, up, and over the disk. Tell the patient to blink several times. If the disk is still visible, pull the lower lid out and over the disk again. Tell the patient that when the disk is in place, he can adjust its position by *gently* pressing his finger against his closed lid. Caution him against rubbing his eye or moving the disk across the cornea.
- If the disk falls out, wash your hands, rinse the disk in cool water, and reinsert it. If the disk appears bent, replace it.
- If both of the patient's eyes are being treated with medication disks, replace both disks at the same time *so that both eyes receive medication at the same rate.*
- If the disk repeatedly slips out of position, reinsert it under the upper eyelid. To do this, gently lift and evert the upper eyelid, and insert the disk in the conjunctival sac. Then gently pull the lid back into position, and tell the patient to blink several times. Again, the patient may press gently on the closed eyelid to reposition the disk. The more the patient uses the disk, the easier it should be for him to retain it. If he can't retain it, notify the practitioner.
- If the patient will continue therapy with an eye medication disk after discharge, teach him how to insert and remove it himself. To check his mastery of these skills, have him demonstrate insertion and removal for you.
- Also teach the patient about possible adverse reactions. Foreign-body sensation in the eye, mild tearing or redness, increased mucous discharge, eyelid redness, and itchiness can occur with the use of disks. Blurred vision, stinging, swelling, and headaches can occur with pilocarpine, specifically. Mild symptoms are common but should subside within the first 6 weeks of use. Tell the patient to report persistent or severe symptoms to his practitioner.

To remove an eye medication disk

- You can remove an eye medication disk with one or two fingers. To use one finger, put on gloves, and evert the lower eyelid to expose the disk. Then use the forefinger of your other hand to slide the disk onto the lid and out of the patient's eye. To use two fingers, evert the lower lid with one hand to expose the disk. Then pinch the disk with the thumb and forefinger of your other hand, and remove it from the eye.
- If the disk is located in the upper eyelid, apply long circular strokes to the patient's closed eyelid with your finger until you can see the disk in the corner of the patient's eye. When the disk is visible, you can place your finger directly on the disk and move it to the lower sclera. Then remove it as you would a disk located in the lower lid.

■ Return the medication to the storage area. Make sure you store it according to the label's instructions.
■ Wash your hands.

Special considerations

■ When administering an eye medication that may be absorbed systemically (such as atropine), gently press your thumb on the inner canthus for 1 to 2 minutes after instilling drops while the patient closes his eyes. *This helps prevent medication from flowing into the tear duct.*
■ *To maintain the drug container's sterility,* never touch the tip of the bottle or dropper to the patient's eyeball, lids, or lashes. Discard any solution remaining in the dropper before returning the dropper to the bottle. If the dropper or bottle tip has become contaminated, discard it and obtain another sterile dropper. *To prevent cross-contamination,* never use a container of eye medication for more than one patient.
■ Teach the patient to instill eye medications *so that he can continue treatment at home, if necessary.* Review the procedure, and ask for a return demonstration.
■ If an ointment and drops have been ordered, the drops should be instilled first.

Complications

Instillation of some eye medications may cause transient burning, itching, and redness. Rarely, systemic effects may also occur.

Documentation

Record the medication instilled or applied, eye or eyes treated, and date, time, and dose. Note any adverse effects and the patient's response.

SELECTED REFERENCES

Joanna Briggs Institute. "Strategies to Reduce Medication Errors with Reference to Older Adults," *Nursing Standards* 20(41):53-57, June 2006.
The Joint Commission. *Comprehensive Accreditation Manual for Hospitals: The Official Handbook.* Standard MM.4.30. 2007.
The Joint Commission. *Comprehensive Accreditation Manual for Hospitals: The Official Handbook.* Standard MM.5.10. 2007.
The Joint Commission. *Comprehensive Accreditation Manual for Hospitals: The Official Handbook.* Standard MM.5.20. 2007.
The Joint Commission. *Comprehensive Accreditation Manual for Hospitals: The Official Handbook.* Standard MM.6.20. 2007.
McIntyre, L.J., and Courey, T.J. "Safe Medication Administration," *Journal of Nursing Care Quality* 22(1):40-42, January-March 2007.
Taylor, C., et al. *Fundamentals of Nursing: The Art and Science of Nursing Care,* 6th ed. Philadelphia: Lippincott Williams & Wilkins, 2008.

EARDROPS

Eardrops may be instilled to treat infection and inflammation, soften cerumen for later removal, produce local anesthesia, or facilitate removal of an insect trapped in the ear by immobilizing and smothering it.

Instillation of eardrops is usually contraindicated if the patient has a perforated eardrum, but it may be permitted with certain medications and adherence to sterile technique. Other conditions may also prohibit instillation of certain medications into the ear. For instance, instillation of drops containing hydrocortisone is contraindicated if the patient has herpes, another viral infection, or a fungal infection.

Equipment

Prescribed eardrops ■ patient's medication record and chart ■ light source ■ facial tissue or cotton-tipped applicator ■ optional: cotton ball, bowl of warm water.

Preparation of equipment

To avoid adverse effects (such as vertigo, nausea, and pain) resulting from instillation of eardrops that are too cold, warm the medication to body temperature in the bowl of warm water, or carry it in your pocket for 30 minutes before administration. If necessary, test the temperature of the medication by placing a drop on your wrist. *(If the medication is too hot, it may burn the patient's eardrum.)*

Implementation

■ Verify the order on the patient's medication record by checking it against the practitioner's order.
■ Wash your hands.
■ Confirm the patient's identity using two patient identifiers according to your facility's policy.
■ If your facility uses a bar code scanning system, be sure to scan your ID badge, the patient's ID bracelet, and the medication's bar code.
■ Provide privacy if possible. Explain the procedure to the patient.
■ Have the patient lie on the side opposite the affected ear.
■ Straighten the patient's ear canal. For an adult, pull the auricle of the ear up and back. (See *Positioning the patient for eardrop instillation,* page 286.)

PEDIATRIC ALERT *For an infant or a child younger than age 3, gently pull the auricle down and back* because the ear canal is straighter at this age.

Positioning the patient for eardrop instillation

Before instilling eardrops, have the patient lie on his side. Then straighten the patient's ear canal to help the medication reach the eardrum. For an adult, gently pull the auricle *up and back;* for an infant or a young child, gently pull *down and back.*

Adult

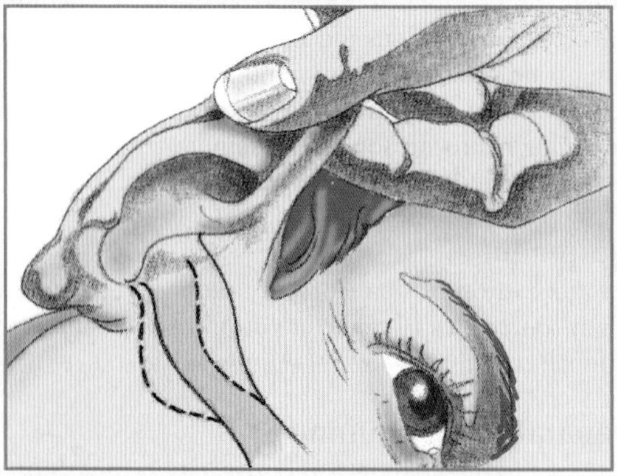

Child

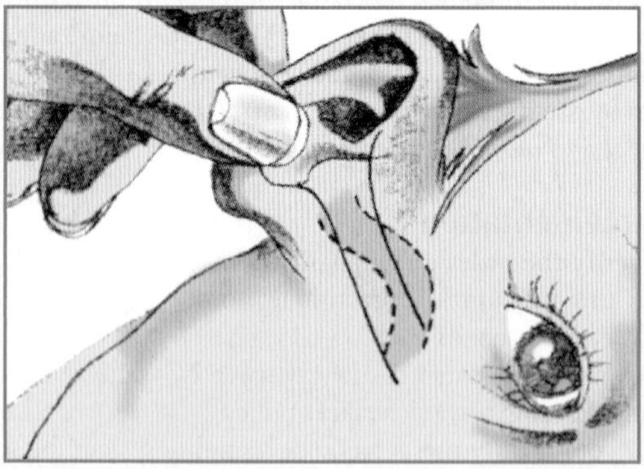

■ Using a light source, examine the ear canal for drainage. If you find any, clean the canal with a tissue or cotton-tipped applicator *because drainage can reduce the medication's effectiveness.*

■ Compare the label on the eardrops with the order on the patient's medication record. Check the label again while drawing the medication into the dropper. Check the label for the final time before returning the eardrops to the shelf or drawer.

■ *To avoid damaging the ear canal with the dropper,* gently support the hand holding the dropper against the patient's head. Straighten the patient's ear canal once again, and instill the ordered number of drops. *To avoid patient discomfort,* aim the dropper so that the drops fall against the sides of the ear canal, not on the eardrum. Hold the ear canal in position until you see the medication disappear down the canal. Then release the ear.

■ Instruct the patient to remain on his side for 5 to 10 minutes *to let the medication run down into the ear canal.*

■ If ordered, tuck the cotton ball loosely into the opening of the ear canal *to prevent the medication from leaking out.* Be careful not to insert it too deeply into the canal *because this would prevent drainage of secretions and increase pressure on the eardrum.*

■ Clean and dry the outer ear.

■ If ordered, repeat the procedure in the other ear after 5 to 10 minutes.

■ Assist the patient into a comfortable position.

■ Wash your hands.

Special considerations

■ *Remember that some conditions make the normally tender ear canal even more sensitive,* so be especially gentle when performing this procedure.

■ Wash your hands before and after caring for the patient's ear and between caring for each ear.

■ *To prevent injury to the eardrum,* never insert a cotton-tipped applicator into the ear canal past the point where you can see the tip. After applying eardrops to soften the cerumen, irrigate the ear as ordered *to facilitate its removal.*

■ If the patient has vertigo, keep the side rails of his bed up, and help him during the procedure as needed. Also, move slowly and unhurriedly *to avoid exacerbating his vertigo.*

■ Teach the patient to instill the eardrops correctly *so that he can continue treatment at home,* if necessary. Review the procedure, and let the patient try it himself while you observe.

Documentation

Record the medication used, the ear treated, and the date, time, and number of eardrops instilled. Also document any signs or symptoms that the patient experienced during the procedure, such as drainage, redness, vertigo, nausea, and pain.

SELECTED REFERENCES

The Joint Commission. *Comprehensive Accreditation Manual for Hospitals: The Official Handbook.* Standard MM.1.10. 2007.

The Joint Commission. *Comprehensive Accreditation Manual for Hospitals: The Official Handbook.* Standard MM.3.10. 2007.
The Joint Commission. *Comprehensive Accreditation Manual for Hospitals: The Official Handbook.* Standard MM.4.10. 2007.
The Joint Commission. *Comprehensive Accreditation Manual for Hospitals: The Official Handbook.* Standard MM.4.20. 2007.
The Joint Commission. *Comprehensive Accreditation Manual for Hospitals: The Official Handbook.* Standard MM.4.30. 2007.
The Joint Commission. *Comprehensive Accreditation Manual for Hospitals: The Official Handbook.* Standard MM.5.10. 2007.
The Joint Commission. *Comprehensive Accreditation Manual for Hospitals: The Official Handbook.* Standard MM.6.10. 2007.
The Joint Commission. *Comprehensive Accreditation Manual for Hospitals: The Official Handbook.* Standard MM.6.20. 2007.
Taylor, C., et al. *Fundamentals of Nursing: The Art and Science of Nursing Care,* 6th ed. Philadelphia: Lippincott Williams & Wilkins, 2008.

HANDHELD OROPHARYNGEAL INHALERS

Handheld inhalers include the metered dose inhaler (or nebulizer), the turbo-inhaler, and the nasal inhaler. These devices deliver topical medications to the respiratory tract, producing local and systemic effects. The mucosal lining of the respiratory tract absorbs the inhalant almost immediately. Examples of common inhalants are bronchodilators, used to improve airway patency and facilitate mucous drainage; mucolytics, which attain a high local concentration to liquefy tenacious bronchial secretions; and corticosteroids, used to decrease inflammation.

The use of these inhalers may be contraindicated in patients who can't form an airtight seal around the device and in patients who lack the coordination or clear vision necessary to assemble a turbo-inhaler. Specific inhalant drugs may also be contraindicated. For example, bronchodilators are contraindicated if the patient has tachycardia or a history of cardiac arrhythmias associated with tachycardia.

Equipment

Patient's medication record and chart ■ metered dose inhaler, turbo-inhaler, or nasal inhaler ■ prescribed medication ■ normal saline solution (or another appropriate solution) for gargling ■ optional: emesis basin. (See *Types of handheld inhalers,* page 288.)

Implementation

- Verify the order on the patient's medication record by checking it against the practitioner's order.
- Wash your hands.
- Check the label on the inhaler against the order on the medication record. Verify the expiration date.
- Confirm the patient's identity using two patient identifiers according to your facility's policy.
- If your facility uses a bar code scanning system, be sure to scan your ID badge, the patient's ID bracelet, and the medication's bar code.
- Explain the procedure to the patient.

Using a metered dose inhaler

- Shake the inhaler bottle *to mix the medication and aerosol propellant.*
- Remove the mouthpiece and cap. *Note:* Some metered dose inhalers have a spacer built into the inhaler. Pull the spacer away from the section holding the medication canister until it clicks into place.
- Insert the metal stem on the bottle into the small hole on the flattened portion of the mouthpiece. Then turn the bottle upside down.
- Have the patient exhale; then place the mouthpiece in his mouth, and close his lips around it.
- As you firmly push the bottle down against the mouthpiece, ask the patient to inhale slowly and to continue inhaling until his lungs feel full. *This action draws the medication into his lungs.* Compress the bottle against the mouthpiece only once.
- Remove the mouthpiece from the patient's mouth, and tell him to hold his breath for several seconds *to allow the medication to reach the alveoli.* Then instruct him to exhale slowly through pursed lips *to keep the distal bronchioles open, allowing increased absorption and diffusion of the drug and better gas exchange.*
- Have the patient gargle with normal saline solution, if desired, *to remove medication from the mouth and back of the throat.* (The lungs retain only about 10% of the inhalant; most of the remainder is exhaled, but substantial amounts may remain in the oropharynx.)
- Rinse the mouthpiece thoroughly with warm water *to prevent accumulation of residue.*

Using a turbo-inhaler

- Hold the mouthpiece in one hand, and with the other hand, slide the sleeve away from the mouthpiece as far as possible.
- Unscrew the tip of the mouthpiece by turning it counterclockwise.
- Firmly press the colored portion of the medication capsule into the propeller stem of the mouthpiece.

EQUIPMENT

Types of handheld inhalers

Handheld inhalers use air under pressure to produce a mist containing tiny droplets of medication. Drugs delivered in this form (such as mucolytics and bronchodilators) can travel deep into the lungs.

Metered dose inhaler

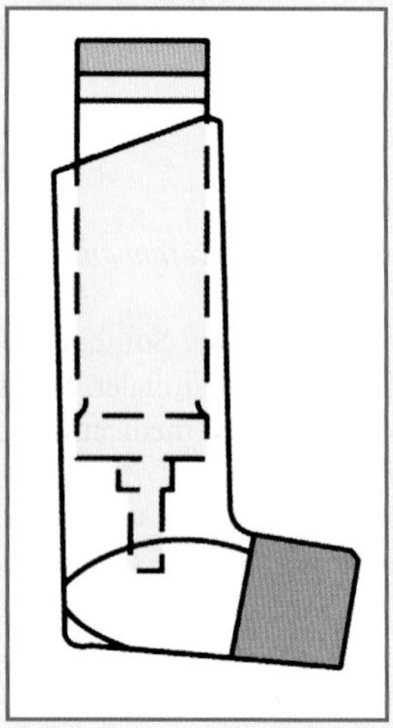

Nasal inhaler

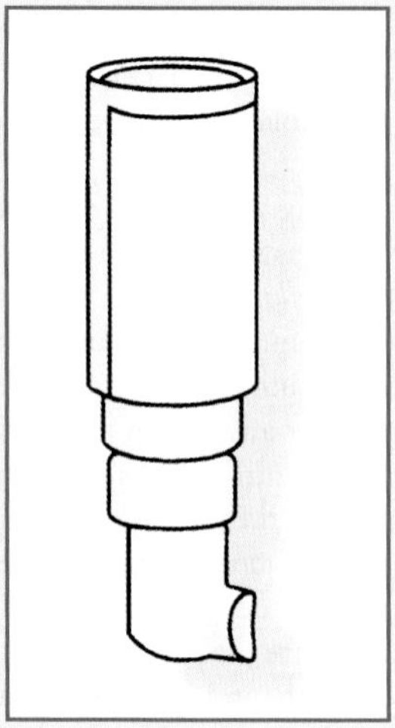

Inhaler with built-in spacer

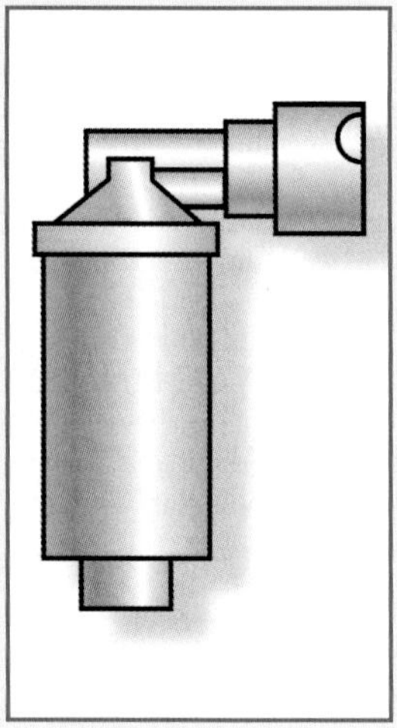

Turbo inhaler

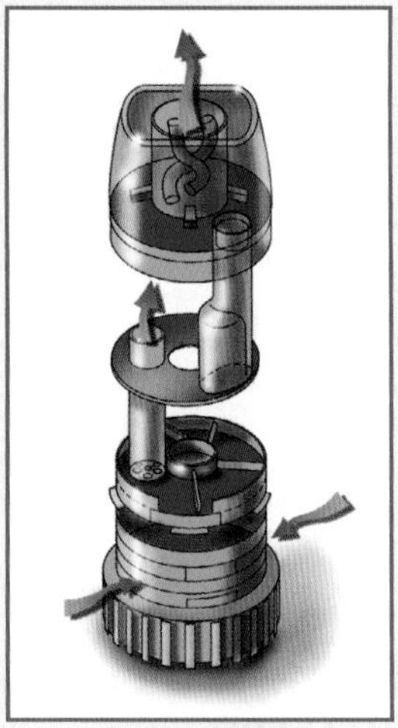

- Screw the inhaler together again securely.
- Holding the inhaler with the mouthpiece at the bottom, slide the sleeve all the way down and then up again *to puncture the capsule and release the medication.* Do this only once.
- Have the patient exhale and tilt his head back. Tell him to place the mouthpiece in his mouth, close his lips around it, and inhale once — quickly and deeply — through the mouthpiece.
- Tell the patient to hold his breath for several seconds *to allow the medication to reach the alveoli.* (Instruct him not to exhale through the mouthpiece.)
- Remove the inhaler from the patient's mouth, and tell him to exhale as much air as possible.
- Repeat the procedure until all the medication in the device is inhaled.
- Have the patient gargle with normal saline solution, if desired, *to remove medication from the mouth and back of the throat.* Be sure to provide an emesis basin if the patient needs one.
- Discard the empty medication capsule, put the inhaler in its can, and secure the lid. Rinse the inhaler with warm water at least once per week.

Using a nasal inhaler

- Have the patient blow his nose *to clear his nostrils.*
- Shake the medication cartridge, and then insert it in the adapter. (Before inserting a refill cartridge, remove the protective cap from the stem.)
- Remove the protective cap from the adapter tip.
- Hold the inhaler with your index finger on top of the cartridge and your thumb under the nasal adapter. The adapter tip should be pointing toward the patient.
- Have the patient tilt his head back. Then tell him to place the adapter tip into one nostril while occluding the other nostril with his finger.
- Instruct the patient to inhale gently as he presses the adapter and the cartridge together firmly *to release a measured dose of medication.* Be sure to follow the manufacturer's instructions. With some medications, such as dexamethasone sodium phosphate (Turbinaire), inhaling during administration isn't desirable.
- Tell the patient to remove the inhaler from his nostril and to hold his breath for a few seconds.
- Have the patient exhale through his mouth.
- Shake the inhaler, and have the patient repeat the procedure in the other nostril.

■ Have the patient gargle with normal saline solution *to remove medication from his mouth and throat.*
■ Remove the medication cartridge from the nasal inhaler, and wash the nasal adapter in lukewarm water. Let the adapter dry thoroughly before reinserting the cartridge.

Special considerations

■ When using a turbo-inhaler or nasal inhaler, make sure the pressurized cartridge isn't punctured or incinerated. Store the medication cartridge below 120° F (48.9° C).
■ If you're using a turbo-inhaler, keep the medication capsules wrapped until needed *to keep them from deteriorating.*
■ Spacer inhalers may be recommended to provide greater therapeutic benefit for children and for patients who have difficulty with coordination. A spacer attachment is an extension to the inhaler's mouthpiece that provides more dead-air space for mixing the medication. Some inhalers have built-in spacers.
■ Teach the patient how to use the inhaler *so that he can continue treatments himself after discharge,* if necessary. Explain that overdosage — which is common — can cause the medication to lose its effectiveness. Tell him to record the date and time of each inhalation as well as his response *to prevent overdosage and to help the practitioner determine the drug's effectiveness.* Also, note whether the patient uses an unusual amount of medication — for example, more than one cartridge for a metered-dose nebulizer every 3 weeks. Inform the patient of possible adverse reactions.
■ If more than one inhalation is ordered, advise the patient to wait at least 2 minutes before repeating the procedure.
■ If the patient is also using a steroid inhaler, instruct him to use the bronchodilator first and then wait 5 minutes before using the steroid. *This allows the bronchodilator to open the air passages for maximum effectiveness.*

Documentation

Record the inhalant administered as well as the dose and time. Note any significant change in the patient's heart rate and any other adverse reactions.

SELECTED REFERENCES

The Joint Commission. *Comprehensive Accreditation Manual for Hospitals: The Official Handbook.* Standard MM.1.10. 2007.

The Joint Commission. *Comprehensive Accreditation Manual for Hospitals: The Official Handbook.* Standard MM.2.10. 2007.

The Joint Commission. *Comprehensive Accreditation Manual for Hospitals: The Official Handbook.* Standard MM.3.10. 2007.

The Joint Commission. *Comprehensive Accreditation Manual for Hospitals: The Official Handbook.* Standard MM.4.10. 2007.

The Joint Commission. *Comprehensive Accreditation Manual for Hospitals: The Official Handbook.* Standard MM.4.20. 2007.

The Joint Commission. *Comprehensive Accreditation Manual for Hospitals: The Official Handbook.* Standard MM.5.10. 2007.

The Joint Commission. *Comprehensive Accreditation Manual for Hospitals: The Official Handbook.* Standard MM.6.10. 2007.

The Joint Commission. *Comprehensive Accreditation Manual for Hospitals: The Official Handbook.* Standard MM.6.20. 2007.

Leach, C.L. "Inhalation Aspects of Therapeutic Aerosols," *Toxicologic Pathology* 35(1):23-26, January 2007.

Maggio, E.T. "Intraval: Highly Effective Intranasal Delivery of Peptide and Protein Drugs," *Expert Opinions in Drug Delivery* 3(4):529-39, June 2006.

Newell, K., and Hume, S. "Choosing the Right Inhaler for Patients with Asthma," *Nursing Standard* 21(5):46-48, October 2006.

Taylor, C., et al. *Fundamentals of Nursing: The Art and Science of Nursing Care,* 6th ed. Philadelphia: Lippincott Williams & Wilkins, 2008.

NASAL MEDICATIONS

Nasal medications may be instilled by means of drops, a spray (using an atomizer), or an aerosol (using a nebulizer). Most drugs instilled by these methods produce local rather than systemic effects. Drops can be directed at a specific area; sprays and aerosols diffuse medication throughout the nasal passages.

Most nasal medications, such as phenylephrine, are vasoconstrictors, which relieve nasal congestion by coating and shrinking swollen mucous membranes. Because vasoconstrictors may be absorbed systemically, they are usually contraindicated in hypersensitive patients. Other types of nasal medications include antiseptics, anesthetics, and corticosteroids. Local anesthetics may be administered to promote patient comfort during rhinolaryngologic examination, laryngoscopy, bronchoscopy, and endotracheal intubation. Corticosteroids reduce inflammation in allergic or inflammatory conditions and nasal polyps.

Equipment

Prescribed medication ■ patient's medication record and chart ■ emesis basin (with nose drops only) ■ facial tissues ■ optional: pillow, small piece of soft rubber or plastic tubing, gloves.

Implementation

- Verify the order on the patient's medication record by checking it against the practitioner's order. Note the concentration of the medication. Phenylephrine, for example, is available in various concentrations from 0.125% to 1%. Verify the expiration date.
- Confirm the patient's identity using two patient identifiers according to your facility's policy.
- If your facility uses a bar code scanning system, be sure to scan your ID badge, the patient's ID bracelet, and the medication's bar code.
- Explain the procedure and provide privacy.
- Wash your hands. Put on gloves if you notice drainage from the nostrils.

Instilling nose drops

- When possible, position the patient so that the drops flow back into the nostrils, toward the affected area. (See *Positioning the patient for nose drop instillation.*)
- Draw up some medication into the dropper.
- Push up the tip of the patient's nose slightly. Position the dropper just above the nostril, and direct its tip toward the midline of the nose *so that the drops flow toward the back of the nasal cavity rather than down the throat.*
- Insert the dropper about 3/8" (1 cm) into the nostril. Don't let the dropper touch the sides of the nostril *because this would contaminate the dropper or could cause the patient to sneeze.*
- Instill the prescribed number of drops, observing the patient carefully for signs of discomfort.
- *To prevent the drops from leaking out of the nostrils,* ask the patient to keep his head tilted back for at least 5 minutes and to breathe through his mouth. *This also allows sufficient time for the medication to constrict mucous membranes.*
- Keep an emesis basin handy *so that the patient can expectorate any medication that flows into the oropharynx and mouth.* Use a facial tissue to wipe any excess medication from the patient's nostrils and face.
- Clean the dropper by separating the plunger and pipette and flushing them with warm water. Allow them to air-dry.

Using a nasal spray

- Have the patient sit upright with his head tilted back slightly. Alternatively, have the patient lie on his back with his shoulders elevated, neck hyperextended, and head tilted back over the edge of the bed. Support his head with one hand *to prevent neck strain.*
- Remove the protective cap from the atomizer.
- *To prevent air from entering the nasal cavity and to allow the medication to flow properly,* occlude one of the patient's nostrils with your finger. Insert the atomizer tip into the open nostril.
- Instruct the patient to inhale, and as he does so, squeeze the atomizer once, quickly and firmly. Use just enough force to coat the inside of the patient's nose with medication. Then tell the patient to exhale through his mouth.
- If ordered, spray the nostril again. Then repeat the procedure in the other nostril.
- Instruct the patient to keep his head tilted back for several minutes and to breathe slowly through his nose *so that the medication has time to work.* Tell him not to blow his nose for several minutes.

Using a nasal aerosol

- Instruct the patient to blow his nose gently *to clear his nostrils.*
- Insert the medication cartridge according to the manufacturer's directions. With some models, you'll fit the medication cartridge over a small hole in the adapter. When inserting a refill cartridge, first remove the protective cap from the stem. Spacer inhalers may be recommended. (See "Handheld oropharyngeal inhalers," page 287.)
- Shake the aerosol well before each use, and remove the protective cap from the adapter tip.
- Hold the aerosol between your thumb and index finger, with your index finger positioned on top of the medication cartridge.
- Tilt the patient's head back, and carefully insert the adapter tip in one nostril while sealing the other nostril with your finger.
- Press the adapter and cartridge together firmly *to release one measured dose of medication.*
- Shake the aerosol, and repeat the procedure to instill medication into the other nostril.
- Remove the medication cartridge, and wash the nasal adapter in lukewarm water daily. Allow the adapter to dry before reinserting the cartridge.

Special considerations

PEDIATRIC ALERT *Before instilling nose drops in a young child, attach a small piece of tubing to the end of the dropper. Do the same for an uncooperative patient.*

- If using a metered-dose pump spray system, prime the delivery system with four sprays or until a fine mist appears. Reprime the system with two sprays or until a fine mist appears if 3 or more days have lapsed since the last use.
- When using an aerosol, be careful not to puncture or incinerate the pressurized cartridge. Store it at temperatures below 120° F (48.9° C).
- *To prevent the spread of infection,* label the medication bottle so that it will be used only for that patient.

Positioning the patient for nose drop instillation

To reach the ethmoid and sphenoid sinuses, have the patient lie on her back with her neck hyperextended and her head tilted back over the edge of the bed. Support her head with one hand *to prevent neck strain.*

To reach the maxillary and frontal sinuses, have the patient lie on her back with her head toward the affected side and hanging slightly over the edge of the bed. Ask her to rotate her head laterally after hyperextension, and support her head with one hand *to prevent neck strain.*

To administer drops for relief of ordinary nasal congestion, help the patient to a reclining or supine position with her head tilted slightly toward the affected side. Aim the dropper upward, toward the patient's eye, rather than downward, toward her ear.

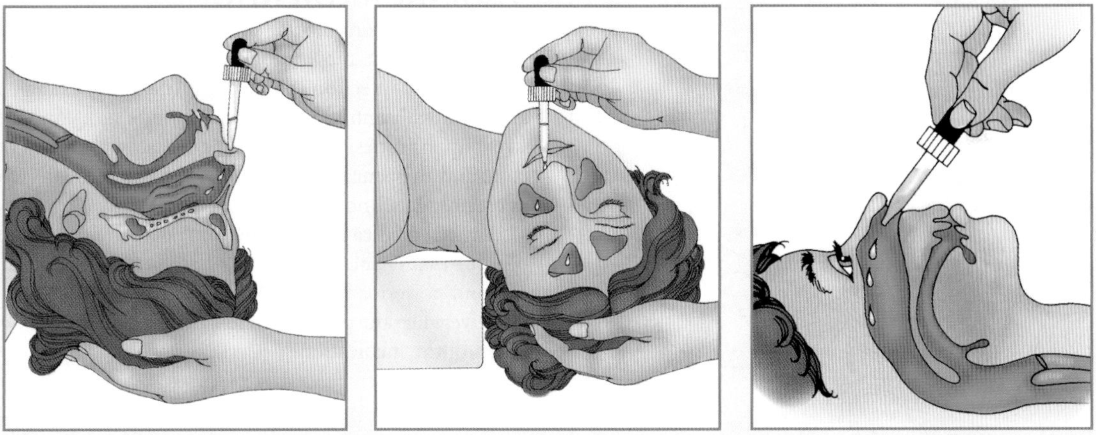

- Teach the patient how to instill nasal medications correctly *so that he can continue treatment after discharge if necessary.* Caution him against using nasal medications longer than prescribed *because they may cause a rebound effect that worsens the condition.* A rebound effect occurs when the medication loses its effectiveness and relaxes the vessels in the nasal turbinates, producing a stuffiness that can be relieved only by discontinuing the medication.
- Inform the patient of possible adverse reactions. In addition, explain that when corticosteroids are given by nasal aerosol, therapeutic effects may not appear for 2 days to 2 weeks.
- Teach the patient good oral and nasal hygiene.

Complications

Some nasal medications may cause restlessness, palpitations, nervousness, and other systemic effects. For example, excessive use of corticosteroid aerosols may cause hyperadrenocorticism and adrenal suppression.

Documentation

Record the medication instilled and its concentration, number of drops or instillations administered, and whether the medication was instilled in one or both nostrils. Also note the time and date of instillation and any resulting adverse effects.

SELECTED REFERENCES

DelGaudio, J.M., and Wise, S.K. "Topical Steroid Drops for the Treatment of Sinus Ostia Stenosis in the Postoperative Period," *American Journal of Rhinology* 20(6):563-67, November-December 2006.

Farkas, A., et al. "Characterization of Regional and Local Deposition of Inhaled Aerosol Drugs in the Respiratory System by Computational Fluid and Particle Dynamics Methods," *Journal of Aerosol Medications* 19(3):329-43, 2006.

The Joint Commission. *Comprehensive Accreditation Manual for Hospitals: The Official Handbook.* Standard MM.1.10. 2007.

The Joint Commission. *Comprehensive Accreditation Manual for Hospitals: The Official Handbook.* Standard MM.2.10. 2007.

How to insert a vaginal cream

Fill the applicator with the prescribed amount of medication. Then lubricate the applicator, hold it by the cylinder, and insert it into the vagina. *To ensure the patient's comfort,* direct the applicator down initially, toward the spine, and then up and back, toward the cervix (as shown below).

Administer the medication by depressing the plunger. Remove the applicator while the plunger is still depressed.

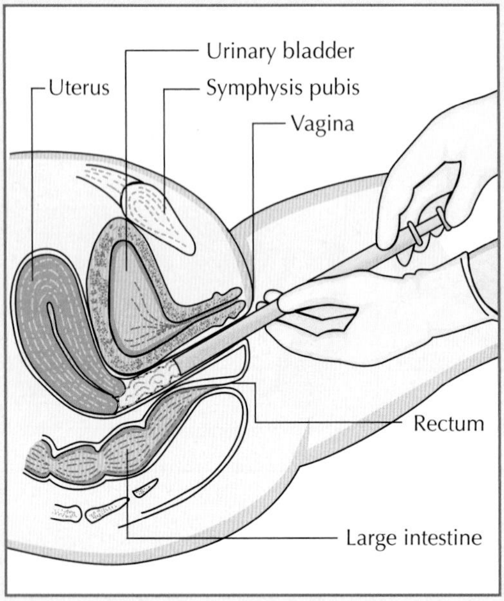

The Joint Commission. *Comprehensive Accreditation Manual for Hospitals: The Official Handbook.* Standard MM.3.10. 2007.

The Joint Commission. *Comprehensive Accreditation Manual for Hospitals: The Official Handbook.* Standard MM.4.10. 2007.

The Joint Commission. *Comprehensive Accreditation Manual for Hospitals: The Official Handbook.* Standard MM.4.20. 2007.

The Joint Commission. *Comprehensive Accreditation Manual for Hospitals: The Official Handbook.* Standard MM.5.10. 2007.

The Joint Commission. *Comprehensive Accreditation Manual for Hospitals: The Official Handbook.* Standard MM.6.10. 2007.

The Joint Commission. *Comprehensive Accreditation Manual for Hospitals: The Official Handbook.* Standard MM.6.20. 2007.

Merkus, P., et al. "The 'Best Method' of Topical Nasal Drugs Delivery: Comparison of Seven Techniques," *Rhinology* 44(2):102-107, June 2006.

Raghavan, U., and Jones, N.S. "A Prospective Randomized Blinded Cross-Over Trial Using Nasal Drops in Patients with Nasal Polyposis: An Evaluation of Effectiveness and Comfort Level if Two Head Positions," *American Journal of Rhinology* 20(4):397-400, July-August 2006.

Taylor, C., et al. *Fundamentals of Nursing: The Art and Science of Nursing Care,* 6th ed. Philadelphia: Lippincott Williams & Wilkins, 2008.

VAGINAL MEDICATIONS

Vaginal medications include suppositories, creams, gels, and ointments. These medications can be inserted as a topical treatment for infection (particularly Trichomonas vaginalis and monilial vaginitis) or inflammation or as a contraceptive. Suppositories melt when they contact the vaginal mucosa, and their medication diffuses topically (as effectively as creams, gels, and ointments).

Vaginal medications usually come with a disposable applicator that enables placement of medication in the anterior and posterior fornices. Vaginal administration is most effective when the patient can remain lying down afterward to retain the medication.

Equipment

Patient's medication record and chart ▪ prescribed medication and applicator, if necessary ▪ water-soluble lubricant ▪ gloves ▪ small sanitary pad.

Implementation

- If possible, plan to insert vaginal medications at bedtime, when the patient is recumbent.
- Verify the order on the patient's medication record by checking it against the practitioner's order.
- Confirm the patient's identity using two patient identifiers according to your facility's policy.
- If your facility uses a bar code scanning system, be sure to scan your ID badge, the patient's ID bracelet, and the medication's bar code.
- Wash your hands, explain the procedure to the patient, and provide privacy.
- Ask the patient to void.
- Ask the patient if she would rather insert the medication herself. If so, provide appropriate instructions. If not, proceed with the following steps.
- Help the patient into the lithotomy position.
- Expose only the perineum.

Inserting a suppository
- Remove the suppository from the wrapper, and lubricate it with water-soluble lubricant.
- Put on gloves, and expose the vagina by spreading the labia.
- With an applicator or the forefinger of your free hand, insert the suppository about 2″ (5 cm) into the vagina.

Inserting ointments, creams, or gels
- Insert the plunger into the applicator. Then attach the applicator to the tube of medication.
- Gently squeeze the tube to fill the applicator with the prescribed amount of medication. Detach the applicator from the tube, and lubricate the applicator.
- Put on gloves, and expose the vagina by spreding the labia.
- Insert the applicator as you would a small suppository, and administer the medication by depressing the plunger on the applicator. (See *How to insert a vaginal cream.*)

After vaginal insertion
- Remove and discard your gloves.
- Wash the applicator with soap and warm water and store it, unless it's disposable. If the applicator can be used again, label it *so that it will be used only for the same patient.*
- *To prevent the medication from soiling the patient's clothing and bedding,* provide a sanitary pad.
- Help the patient return to a comfortable position, and advise her to remain in bed as much as possible for the next several hours.
- Wash your hands thoroughly.

Special considerations
- Refrigerate vaginal suppositories that melt at room temperature.
- If possible, teach the patient how to insert the vaginal medication *because she may have to administer it herself after discharge.* Give her a patient-teaching sheet if one is available.
- Instruct the patient not to wear a tampon after inserting vaginal medication *because it would absorb the medication and decrease its effectiveness.*
- Instruct the patient to avoid sexual intercourse during treatment.

Complications
Vaginal medications may cause local irritation.

Documentation
Record the medication administered as well as time and date. Note adverse effects and any other pertinent information.

Selected references

The Joint Commission. *Comprehensive Accreditation Manual for Hospitals: The Official Handbook.* Standard MM.1.10. 2007.

The Joint Commission. *Comprehensive Accreditation Manual for Hospitals: The Official Handbook.* Standard MM.2.10. 2007.

The Joint Commission. *Comprehensive Accreditation Manual for Hospitals: The Official Handbook.* Standard MM.3.10. 2007.

The Joint Commission. *Comprehensive Accreditation Manual for Hospitals: The Official Handbook.* Standard MM.4.10. 2007.

The Joint Commission. *Comprehensive Accreditation Manual for Hospitals: : The Official Handbook.* Standard MM.4.20. 2007.

The Joint Commission. *Comprehensive Accreditation Manual for Hospitals: The Official Handbook.* Standard MM.5.10. 2007.

The Joint Commission. *Comprehensive Accreditation Manual for Hospitals: The Official Handbook.* Standard MM.6.10. 2007.

The Joint Commission. *Comprehensive Accreditation Manual for Hospitals: The Official Handbook.* Standard MM.6.20. 2007.

Taylor, C., et al. *Fundamentals of Nursing: The Art and Science of Nursing Care,* 6th ed. Philadelphia: Lippincott Williams & Wilkins, 2008.

ENTERAL ADMINISTRATION

Oral drugs
Because oral administration is usually the safest, most convenient, and least expensive method, most drugs are administered by this route. Drugs for oral administration are available in many forms: tablets, enteric-coated tablets, capsules, syrups, elixirs, oils, liquids, suspensions, powders, and granules. Some require special preparation before administration, such as mixing with juice to make them more palatable; oils, powders, and granules most often require such preparation.

Sometimes oral drugs are prescribed in higher dosages than their parenteral equivalents because after absorption through the GI system, they are immediately broken down by the liver before they reach the systemic circulation.

ELDER ALERT *Oral dosages normally prescribed for adults may be dangerous for elderly patients.*

Oral administration is contraindicated for unconscious patients; it may also be contraindicated in patients with nausea and vomiting and in those unable to swallow.

Measuring liquid medications

To pour liquid medications, hold the medication cup at eye level. Use your thumb to mark off the correct level on the cup. Then set the cup down and read the bottom of the meniscus at eye level *to ensure accuracy.* If you've poured too much medication into the cup, discard the excess. Don't return it to the bottle.

Here are a few additional tips:

- Hold the container so that the medication flows from the side opposite the label *so it won't run down the container and stain or obscure the label.* Remove drips from the lip of the bottle first and then from the sides, using a clean, damp paper towel.
- For a liquid measured in drops, use only the dropper supplied with the medication.

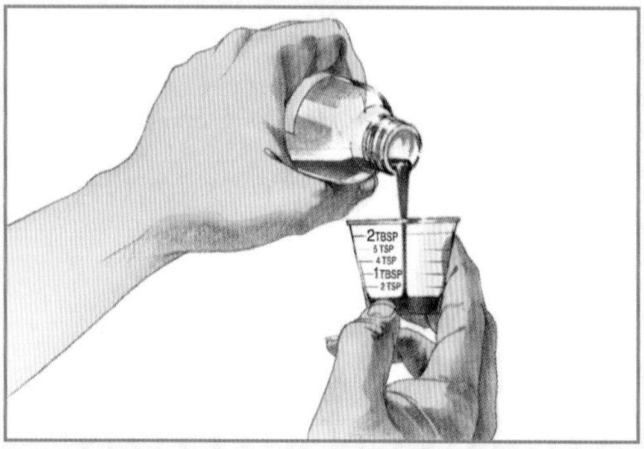

Equipment

Patient's medication record and chart ■ prescribed medication ■ medication cup ■ optional: appropriate vehicle, such as jelly or applesauce, for crushed pills commonly used with children or elderly patients, and juice, water, or milk for liquid medications; drinking straw; mortar and pestle for crushing pills; pill-cutting device for scored tablets.

Implementation

- Verify the order on the patient's medication record by checking it against the practitioner's order.
- Wash your hands.
- Check the label on the medication three times before administering it *to make sure you'll be giving the prescribed medication.* Check when you take the container from the shelf or drawer, again before you pour the medication into the medication cup, and again before returning the container to the shelf or drawer. If you're administering a unit-dose medication, check the label for the final time at the patient's bedside immediately after pouring the medication and before discarding the wrapper.
- Confirm the patient's identity using two patient identifiers according to your facility's policy.
- If your facility uses a bar code scanning system, be sure to scan your ID badge, the patient's ID bracelet, and the medication's bar code.
- Assess the patient's condition, including level of consciousness and vital signs, as needed. *Changes in the patient's condition may warrant withholding medication.* For example, you may need to withhold a medication that will slow the patient's heart rate if his apical pulse rate is less than 60 beats/minute.
- Give the patient his medication and an appropriate vehicle or liquid, as needed, *to aid swallowing, minimize adverse effects, or promote absorption.* For example, cyclophosphamide is given with fluids to minimize adverse effects; antitussive cough syrup is given without a fluid to avoid diluting its soothing effect on the throat. If appropriate, crush the medication *to facilitate swallowing.*
- Stay with the patient until he has swallowed the drug. If he seems confused or disoriented, check his mouth *to make sure he has swallowed it.* Return and reassess the patient's response within 1 hour after giving the medication.

Special considerations

- Make sure you have a written order for every medication given. Verbal orders should be signed by the practitioner within the specified time period. (Hospitals usually require a signature within 24 hours; long-term-care facilities, within 48 hours.)
- Notify the practitioner about any medication withheld, unless instructions to withhold are already written.
- Use care in measuring out the prescribed dose of liquid oral medication. (See *Measuring liquid medications.*)
- Don't give medication from a poorly labeled or unlabeled container. Don't attempt to label or reinforce drug labels yourself. *This must be done by a pharmacist.*
- Never give a medication poured by someone else. Never allow your medication cart or tray out of your sight. *This prevents anyone from rearranging the medications or taking one without your knowledge.* Never return unwrapped or prepared medications to stock containers. Instead, dispose of them and notify the pharmacy. Keep in mind that the disposal of any controlled substance must be cosigned by another nurse, as mandated by law.
- If the patient questions you about his medication or the dosage, check his medication record again. If the medication is correct, reassure him. Make sure you tell him about any changes in his medication or dosage. Instruct him, as appropriate, about possible adverse effects. Ask him to report anything he thinks may be an adverse effect.

- *To avoid damaging or staining the patient's teeth,* administer iron preparations through a straw. An unpleasant-tasting liquid can usually be made more palatable if taken through a straw *because the liquid contacts fewer taste buds.*
- If the patient can't swallow a whole tablet or capsule, ask the pharmacist if the drug is available in liquid form or if it can be administered by another route. If not, ask him if you can crush the tablet or open the capsule and mix it with food. Keep in mind that many enteric-coated or time-release medications and gelatin capsules shouldn't be crushed. Remember to contact the practitioner for an order to change the administration route when necessary.

PEDIATRIC ALERT *Oral medications are relatively easy to give to infants* because of infants' natural sucking instinct and, in infants under 4 months old, their undeveloped sense of taste.

Documentation

Note the drug administered, dose, date and time, and patient's reaction, if any. If the patient refuses a drug, document the refusal, and notify the charge nurse and the patient's practitioner as needed. Also note if a drug was omitted or withheld for other reasons, such as radiology or laboratory tests, or if, in your judgment, the drug was contraindicated at the ordered time. Sign out all opioids given on the appropriate opioids central record.

SELECTED REFERENCES

Craven, R.F., and Hirnle, C.J. *Fundamentals of Nursing: Human Health and Function*, 5th ed. Philadelphia: Lippincott Williams & Wilkins, 2006.

Hohenhaus, S.M. "Giving Liquid Medications to Pediatric Patients," *Journal of Emergency Nursing* 32(1):69-70, February 2006.

Joanna Briggs Institute. "Strategies to Reduce Medication Errors with Reference to Older Adults," *Nursing Standard* 209(1):53-57, June 2006.

NASOGASTRIC TUBE DRUG ADMINISTRATION

Besides providing an alternate means of nourishment, a nasogastric (NG) tube or gastrostomy tube allows direct instillation of medication into the GI system of patients who can't ingest the drug orally. Before instillation, the patency and positioning of the tube must be carefully checked because the procedure is contraindicated if the tube is obstructed or improperly positioned; if the patient is vomiting around the tube; or if his bowel sounds are absent.

Oily medications and enteric-coated or sustained-release tablets or capsules are contraindicated for instillation through an NG tube. Oily medications cling to the sides of the tube and resist mixing with the irrigating solution, and crushing enteric-coated or sustained-release tablets to facilitate transport through the tube destroys their intended properties.

Equipment

Patient's medication record and chart ▪ prescribed medication ▪ towel or linen-saver pad ▪ 50- or 60-ml piston-type catheter-tip syringe ▪ two 4″ × 4″ gauze pads ▪ pH test strip ▪ gloves ▪ diluent ▪ cup for mixing medication and fluid ▪ spoon ▪ 50 ml of water ▪ rubber band ▪ gastrostomy tube and funnel, if needed (for gastrostomy tube) ▪ optional: mortar and pestle, clamp.

For maximum control of suction, use a piston syringe instead of a bulb syringe. The liquid for diluting the medication can be juice, water, or a nutritional supplement.

Preparation of equipment

Gather equipment for use at the bedside. Liquids should be at room temperature. *Administering cold liquids through an NG tube can cause abdominal cramping.* Although this isn't a sterile procedure, make sure the cup, syringe, spoon, and gauze are clean.

Implementation

- Verify the order on the patient's medication record by checking it against the practitioner's order.
- Wash your hands and put on gloves.
- Check the label on the medication three times before preparing it for administration *to make sure you'll be giving the medication correctly.*
- If the prescribed medication is in tablet form, crush the tablets *to ready them for mixing in a cup with the diluting liquid.* Request liquid forms of medications, if available. Bring the medication and equipment to the patient's bedside.
- Confirm the patient's identity using two patient identifiers according to your facility's policy.
- If your facility uses a bar code scanning system, be sure to scan your ID badge, the patient's ID bracelet, and the medication's bar code.
- Explain the procedure to the patient; provide privacy.
- Unpin the tube from the patient's gown. *To avoid soiling the sheets,* fold back the bed linens to the patient's waist, and drape his chest with a towel or linen-saver pad.
- Elevate the head of the bed so that the patient is in Fowler's position, as tolerated.
- After unclamping the tube, take the 50- or 60-ml syringe and attach it to the end of the tube.
- Aspirate stomach contents, and place a small amount on a pH test strip. Probability of gastric placement is increased if aspirate has a typical gastric fluid appearance (grassy-green, clear and colorless with mucus shreds, or brown) and pH is

Giving medications through an NG tube

Holding the nasogastric (NG) tube at a level somewhat above the patient's nose, pour up to 30 ml of diluted medication into the syringe barrel. *To prevent air from entering the patient's stomach,* hold the tube at a slight angle, and add more medication before the syringe empties. If necessary, raise the tube slightly higher to increase the flow rate.

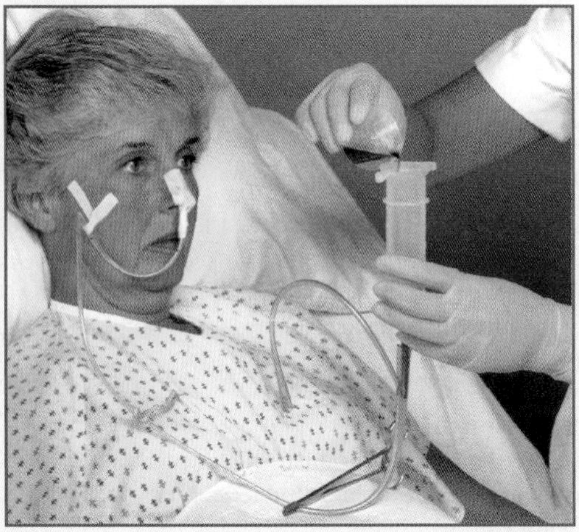

After you've delivered the whole dose, position the patient on her right side, head slightly elevated, *to minimize esophageal reflux.*

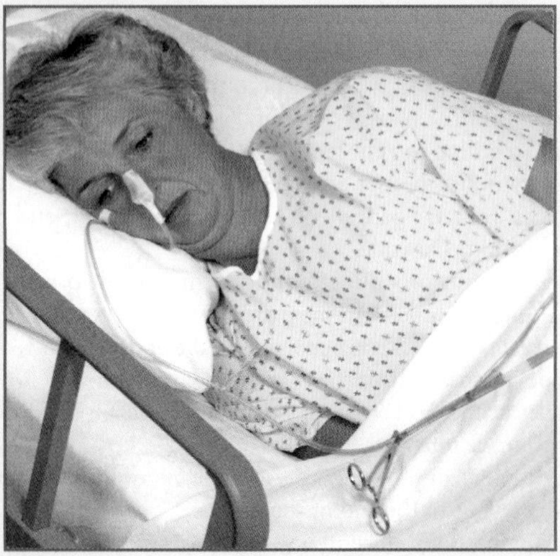

5.0. If no gastric contents appear when you draw back on the syringe, the tube may have risen into the esophagus, and you'll have to advance it and confirm placement before proceeding.

- If you meet resistance when aspirating for gastric contents, stop the procedure. *Resistance may indicate a nonpatent tube or improper tube placement.* (Keep in mind that some smaller NG tubes may collapse when aspiration is attempted.) If the tube seems to be in the stomach, resistance probably means that the tube is lying against the stomach wall. *To relieve resistance,* withdraw the tube slightly or turn the patient.
- After you have established that the tube is patent and in the correct position, clamp the tube, detach the syringe, and lay the end of the tube on the 4″ × 4″ gauze pad.
- Mix the crushed tablets or liquid medication with the diluent. If the medication is in capsule form, open the capsules and empty their contents into the liquid. Pour liquid medications directly into the diluent. Stir well. (If the medication was in tablet form, make sure the particles are small enough to pass through the eyes at the distal end of the tube.)
- Reattach the syringe, without the piston, to the end of the tube and open the clamp.
- Deliver the medication slowly and steadily. (See *Giving medications through an NG tube*.)
- If the medication flows smoothly, slowly add more until the entire dose has been given.
- If the medication doesn't flow properly, don't force it. If it's too thick, dilute it with water. If you suspect that tube placement is inhibiting the flow, stop the procedure and reevaluate tube placement.
- Watch the patient's reaction throughout the instillation. If he shows any sign of discomfort, stop the procedure immediately.
- As the last of the medication flows out of the syringe, start to irrigate the tube by adding 30 to 50 ml of water. *Irrigation clears medication from the sides of the tube and from the distal end, reducing the risk of clogging.*

PEDIATRIC ALERT *For a child, irrigate the tube using only 15 to 30 ml of water.*

- When the water stops flowing, quickly clamp the tube. Detach the syringe and dispose of it.
- Fasten the NG tube to the patient's gown.
- Remove the towel or linen-saver pad, and replace bed linens.
- Leave the patient in Fowler's position, or have him lie on his right side with the head of the bed partially elevated. Tell him to maintain this position for at least 30 minutes after the procedure. *This position facilitates the downward flow of medication into his stomach and prevents esophageal reflux.*

■ If medication is prescribed for a patient with a gastrostomy tube, follow the steps outlined in *Giving medications through a gastrostomy tube.*
■ If medication is prescribed for a patient with a gastrostomy feeding button, ask the practitioner to order the liquid form of the drug if possible. If not, you may give a tablet or capsule dissolved in 30 to 50 ml of warm water (15 to 30 ml for children). To administer medication this way, use the same procedure as for feeding the patient through the button. (See "Gastrostomy feeding button care," page 693.) Then draw up the dissolved medication into a syringe, and inject it into the feeding tube.
■ Withdraw the medication syringe, and flush the tube with 50 ml of warm water.

PEDIATRIC ALERT *Flush the tube with 30 ml of water for a child.*

■ Then replace the safety plug, and keep the patient upright at a 30-degree angle for 30 minutes after giving the medication.

Special considerations

■ *To prevent instillation of too much fluid* (for an adult, more than 400 ml of liquid at one time), don't schedule the drug instillation with the patient's regular tube feeding, if possible.
■ If you must schedule a tube feeding and medication instillation simultaneously, give the medication first *to ensure that the patient receives the prescribed drug therapy even if he can't tolerate an entire feeding.* Remember to avoid giving foods that interact adversely with the drug. Tube feedings must be held 2 hours before and 2 hours after phenytoin or warfarin administration.
■ If the patient receives continuous tube feedings, stop the feeding, and check the quantity of residual stomach contents. If it's more than 50% of the previous hour's intake, withhold the medication and feeding, and notify the practitioner. *An excessive amount of residual contents may indicate intestinal obstruction or paralytic ileus.*
■ If the NG tube is attached to suction, be sure to turn off the suction for 20 to 30 minutes after administering medication.
■ If possible, teach the patient who requires long-term treatment to instill his medication himself through the NG tube. Have him observe the procedure several times before trying it himself.
■ Remain with the patient when he performs the procedure for the first few times *so that you can provide assistance and answer any questions.* Encourage him, and correct any errors in technique as necessary.

Giving medications through a gastrostomy tube

Surgically inserted into the stomach, a gastrostomy tube reduces the risk of fluid aspiration—a constant danger with a nasogastric (NG) tube. To administer medication by this route, prepare the patient and medication as for an NG tube. Then gently lift the dressing around the tube to assess the skin for irritation. Report any irritation to the practitioner. If none appears, follow these steps:
■ Remove the dressing that covers the tube. Then remove the dressing or plug at the tip of the tube, and attach the syringe or funnel to the tip.
■ Release the clamp and instill about 10 ml of water into the tube through the syringe *to check for patency.* If the water flows in easily, the tube is patent. If it flows in slowly, raise the funnel to increase pressure. If the water still doesn't flow properly, stop the procedure and notify the practitioner.

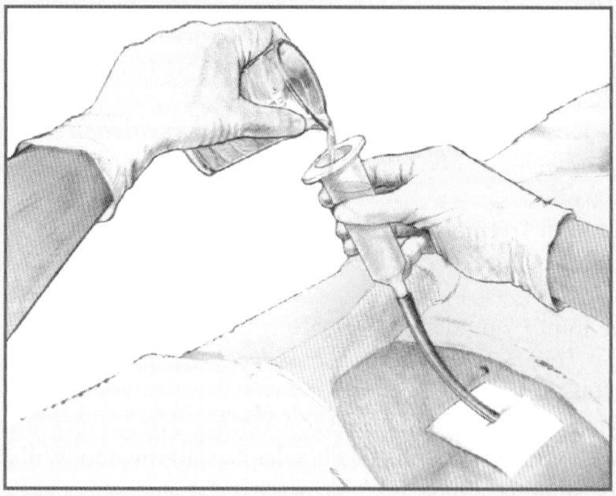

■ Pour up to 30 ml of medication into the syringe or funnel. Tilt the tube *to allow air to escape as the fluid flows downward.* Just before the syringe empties, add medication as needed.
■ After giving the medication, pour in about 30 ml of water to *irrigate the tube.*
■ Tighten the clamp, place a 4″ × 4″ gauze pad on the end of the tube, and secure it with a rubber band.
■ Cover the tube with two more 4″ × 4″ gauze pads, and secure them firmly with tape.
■ Keep the head of the bed elevated for at least 30 minutes after the procedure *to aid digestion.*

Documentation

Record the instillation of medication, date and time of instillation, dose, and patient's tolerance of the procedure. On his intake and output sheet, note the amount of fluid instilled.

SELECTED REFERENCES

Dansereau, R.J., and Crail, D.J. "Extemporaneous Procedures for Dissolving Tablets for Oral Administration and for Feeding Tubes," Annals of Pharmacotherapy 39(1):63-66, January 2005.

The Joint Commission. *Comprehensive Accreditation Manual for Hospitals: The Official Handbook.* Standard MM.1.10. 2007.

The Joint Commission. *Comprehensive Accreditation Manual for Hospitals: The Official Handbook.* Standard MM.2.10. 2007.

The Joint Commission. *Comprehensive Accreditation Manual for Hospitals: The Official Handbook.* Standard MM.3.10. 2007.

The Joint Commission. *Comprehensive Accreditation Manual for Hospitals: The Official Handbook.* Standard MM.4.10. 2007.

The Joint Commission. *Comprehensive Accreditation Manual for Hospitals: The Official Handbook.* Standard MM.4.20. 2007.

The Joint Commission. *Comprehensive Accreditation Manual for Hospitals: The Official Handbook.* Standard MM.5.10. 2007.

The Joint Commission. *Comprehensive Accreditation Manual for Hospitals: The Official Handbook.* Standard MM.6.10. 2007.

The Joint Commission. *Comprehensive Accreditation Manual for Hospitals: The Official Handbook.* Standard MM.6.20. 2007.

Taylor, C., et al. *Fundamentals of Nursing: The Art and Science of Nursing Care,* 6th ed. Philadelphia: Lippincott Williams & Wilkins, 2008.

BUCCAL, SUBLINGUAL, AND TRANSLINGUAL DRUGS

Certain drugs are given buccally, sublingually, or translingually to prevent their destruction or transformation in the stomach or small intestine. These drugs act quickly because the oral mucosa's thin epithelium and abundant vasculature allow direct absorption into the bloodstream.

Drugs given buccally include nitroglycerin and methyltestosterone; drugs given sublingually include ergotamine tartrate, isosorbide dinitrate, and nitroglycerin. Translingual drugs, which are sprayed onto the tongue, include nitrate preparations for patients with chronic angina.

Equipment

Patient's medication record and chart ■ prescribed medication ■ medication cup.

Implementation

- Verify the order on the patient's medication record by checking it against the practitioner's order on his chart.
- Wash your hands with warm water and soap. Explain the procedure to the patient if he's never taken a drug buccally, sublingually, or translingually before.
- Check the label on the medication before administering it *to make sure you'll be giving the prescribed medication.* Verify the expiration date of all medications, especially nitroglycerin.
- Confirm the patient's identity using two patient identifiers according to your facility's policy.
- If your facility uses a bar code scanning system, be sure to scan your ID badge, the patient's ID bracelet, and the medication's bar code.

Buccal and sublingual administration

- For buccal administration, place the tablet in the buccal pouch, between the cheek and gum. For sublingual administration, place the tablet under the patient's tongue. (See *Placing drugs in the oral mucosa.*)
- Instruct the patient to keep the medication in place until it dissolves completely *to ensure absorption.*
- Caution him against chewing the tablet or touching it with his tongue *to prevent accidental swallowing.*
- Tell him not to smoke before the drug has dissolved *because nicotine's vasoconstrictive effects slow absorption.*

Translingual administration

- To administer a translingual drug, tell the patient to hold the medication canister vertically, with the valve head at the top and the spray orifice as close to his mouth as possible.
- Instruct him to spray the dose onto his tongue by pressing the button firmly.
- Remind the patient using a translingual aerosol form that he shouldn't inhale the spray but should release it under his tongue. Also tell him to wait 10 seconds or so before swallowing.

Special considerations

- Don't give liquids to a patient who is receiving buccal medication *because some buccal tablets can take up to 1 hour to be absorbed.* Tell the patient not to rinse his mouth until the tablet has been absorbed.
- Tell the patient with angina to moisten the nitroglycerin tablet with saliva and to keep it under his tongue until it has been fully absorbed.

Complications

Some buccal medications may irritate the mucosa. Alternate sides of the mouth for repeat doses *to prevent continuous irritation of the same site.* Sublingual medications — such as nitroglycerin — may cause a tingling sensation under the tongue. If the patient finds this annoying, try placing the drug in the buccal pouch instead.

Documentation

Record the medication administered, dose, date and time, and patient's reaction, if any.

SELECTED REFERENCES

Ferguson, A. "Administration of Oral Medication," *Nursing Times* 101(45):24-25, November 2005.

Finn, A., et al. "Bioavailability and Metabolism of Prochlorperazine Administered via the Buccal or Oral Delivery Route," *Journal of Clinical Pharmacology* 45(12):1383-390, December 2005.

The Joint Commission. *Comprehensive Accreditation Manual for Hospitals: The Official Handbook.* Standard MM.1.10. 2007.

The Joint Commission. *Comprehensive Accreditation Manual for Hospitals: The Official Handbook.* Standard MM.2.10. 2007.

The Joint Commission. *Comprehensive Accreditation Manual for Hospitals: The Official Handbook.* Standard MM.3.10. 2007.

The Joint Commission. *Comprehensive Accreditation Manual for Hospitals: The Official Handbook.* Standard MM.4.10. 2007.

The Joint Commission. *Comprehensive Accreditation Manual for Hospitals: The Official Handbook.* Standard MM.4.20. 2007.

The Joint Commission. *Comprehensive Accreditation Manual for Hospitals: The Official Handbook.* Standard MM.5.10. 2007.

The Joint Commission. *Comprehensive Accreditation Manual for Hospitals: The Official Handbook.* Standard MM.6.10. 2007.

The Joint Commission. *Comprehensive Accreditation Manual for Hospitals: The Official Handbook.* Standard MM.6.20. 2007.

Smart, J.D. "Buccal Drug Delivery," *Expert Opinion on Drug Delivery* 2(3):507-17, May 2005.

Taylor, C., et al. *Fundamentals of Nursing: The Art and Science of Nursing Care,* 6th ed. Philadelphia: Lippincott Williams & Wilkins, 2008.

Placing drugs in the oral mucosa

Buccal and sublingual administration routes allow some drugs, such as nitroglycerin and methyltestosterone, to enter the bloodstream rapidly without being degraded in the GI tract. To give a drug buccally, insert it between the patient's cheek and teeth (as shown below). Ask him to close his mouth and hold the tablet against his cheek until the tablet is absorbed.

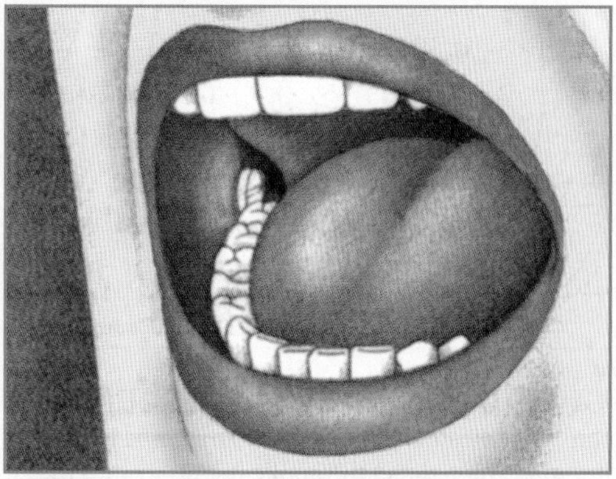

To give a drug sublingually, place it under the patient's tongue (as shown below), and ask him to leave it there until it's dissolved.

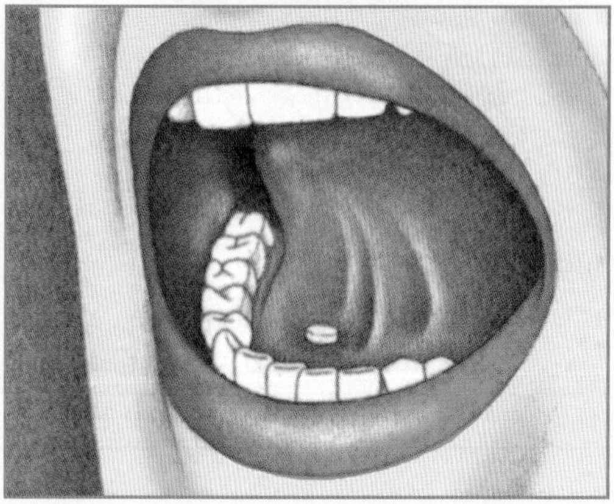

RECTAL SUPPOSITORIES AND OINTMENTS

A rectal suppository is a small, solid, medicated mass, usually cone-shaped, with a cocoa butter or glycerin base. It may be inserted to stimulate peristalsis and defecation or to relieve pain, vomiting, and local irritation. Rectal suppositories commonly contain drugs that reduce fever, induce relaxation, interact poorly with digestive enzymes, or have a

How to administer a rectal suppository or ointment

When inserting a suppository, direct its tapered end toward the side of the rectum so that it contacts the membranes *to encourage absorption of the medication.*

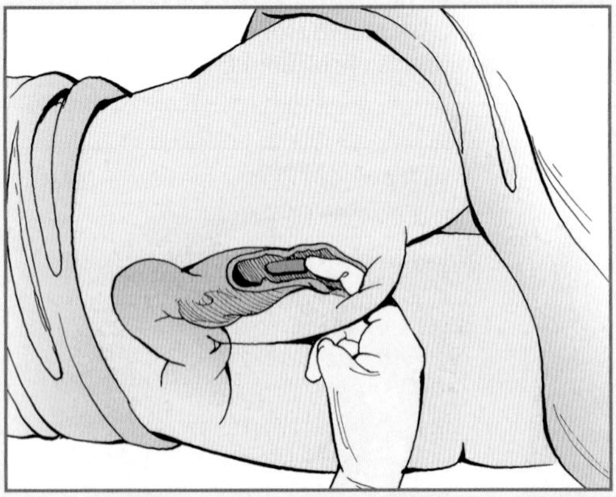

When applying a rectal ointment internally, be sure to lubricate the applicator *to minimize pain on insertion.* Then direct the applicator tip toward the patient's umbilicus.

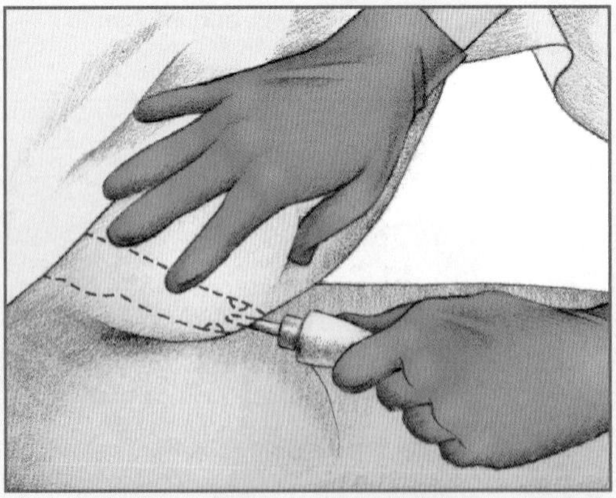

taste too offensive for oral use. Rectal suppositories melt at body temperature and are absorbed slowly.

Because insertion of a rectal suppository may stimulate the vagus nerve, this procedure is contraindicated in patients with potential cardiac arrhythmias. It may have to be avoided in patients with recent rectal or prostate surgery because of the risk of local trauma or discomfort during insertion. An ointment is a semisolid medication used to produce local effects. It may be applied externally to the anus or internally to the rectum. Rectal ointments commonly contain drugs that reduce inflammation or relieve pain and itching.

Equipment

Rectal suppository or tube of ointment and applicator ▪ patient's medication record and chart ▪ gloves ▪ water-soluble lubricant ▪ 4″ × 4″ gauze pads ▪ optional: bedpan.

Preparation of equipment

Store rectal suppositories in the refrigerator until needed *to prevent softening and, possibly, decreased effectiveness of the medication.* A softened suppository is also difficult to handle and insert. To harden it again, hold the suppository (in its wrapper) under cold running water.

Implementation

- Verify the order on the patient's medication record by checking it against the practitioner's order.
- Make sure the label on the medication package agrees with the medication order. Read the label again before you open the wrapper and again as you remove the medication. Check the expiration date.
- Wash your hands with warm water and soap.
- Confirm the patient's identity using two patient identifiers according to your facility's policy.
- If your facility uses a bar code scanning system, be sure to scan your ID badge, the patient's ID bracelet, and the medication's bar code.
- Explain the procedure and the purpose of the medication to the patient.
- Provide privacy.

Inserting a rectal suppository

- Place the patient on his left side in Sims' position. Drape him with the bedcovers to expose only the buttocks.
- Put on gloves. Remove the suppository from its wrapper, and lubricate it with water-soluble lubricant.
- Lift the patient's upper buttock with your nondominant hand *to expose the anus.*
- Instruct the patient to take several deep breaths through his mouth *to help relax the anal sphincters and reduce anxiety or discomfort during insertion.*
- Using the index finger of your dominant hand, insert the suppository—tapered end first—about 3″ (7.6 cm), until you feel it pass the internal anal sphincter. Try to direct the tapered end toward the side of the rectum *so that it contacts*

the membranes. (See *How to administer a rectal suppository or ointment.*)
- Ensure the patient's comfort. Encourage him to lie quietly and, if applicable, to retain the suppository for the appropriate length of time. A suppository administered to relieve constipation should be retained as long as possible (at least 20 minutes) to be effective. Press on the anus with a gauze pad if necessary until the urge to defecate passes.
- Remove and discard your gloves.

Applying rectal ointment
- Put on gloves.
- Place the patient on his left side in Sims' position; then drape him to expose only the buttocks.
- *To apply externally,* use gloves or a gauze pad to spread medication over the anal area.
- *To apply internally,* attach the applicator to the tube of ointment, and coat the applicator with water-soluble lubricant.
- Expect to use about 1″ (2.5 cm) of ointment. *To gauge how much pressure to use during application,* squeeze a small amount from the tube before you attach the applicator.
- Lift the patient's upper buttock with your nondominant hand *to expose the anus.*
- Instruct the patient to take several deep breaths through his mouth *to relax the anal sphincters and reduce anxiety or discomfort during insertion.*
- Gently insert the applicator, directing it toward the umbilicus.
- Slowly squeeze the tube *to eject the medication.*
- Remove the applicator, and place a folded 4″ × 4″ gauze pad between the patient's buttocks *to absorb excess ointment.*
- Detach the applicator from the tube, and recap the tube. Then clean the applicator thoroughly with soap and warm water.

Special considerations
- *Because the intake of food and fluid stimulates peristalsis,* a suppository for relieving constipation should be inserted about 30 minutes before mealtime *to help soften the feces in the rectum and facilitate defecation.* A medicated retention suppository should be inserted between meals.
- Instruct the patient to avoid expelling the suppository. If he has difficulty retaining it, place him on a bedpan.
- Make sure the patient's call button is handy, and watch for his signal *because he may be unable to suppress the urge to defecate.* For example, a patient with proctitis has a highly sensitive rectum and may not be able to retain a suppository for long.
- Be sure to inform the patient that the suppository may discolor his next bowel movement. Anusol suppositories, for example, can give feces a silver-gray pasty appearance.

Documentation
Record the administration time, dose, and patient's response.

SELECTED REFERENCES

The Joint Commission. *Comprehensive Accreditation Manual for Hospitals: The Official Handbook.* Standard MM.1.10. 2007.

The Joint Commission. *Comprehensive Accreditation Manual for Hospitals: The Official Handbook.* Standard MM.2.10. 2007.

The Joint Commission. *Comprehensive Accreditation Manual for Hospitals: The Official Handbook.* Standard MM.3.10. 2007.

The Joint Commission. *Comprehensive Accreditation Manual for Hospitals: The Official Handbook.* Standard MM.4.10. 2007.

The Joint Commission. *Comprehensive Accreditation Manual for Hospitals: The Official Handbook.* Standard MM.4.20. 2007.

The Joint Commission. *Comprehensive Accreditation Manual for Hospitals: The Official Handbook.* Standard MM.5.10. 2007.

The Joint Commission. *Comprehensive Accreditation Manual for Hospitals: The Official Handbook.* Standard MM.6.10. 2007.

The Joint Commission. *Comprehensive Accreditation Manual for Hospitals: The Official Handbook.* Standard MM.6.20. 2007.

Taylor, C., et al. *Fundamentals of Nursing: The Art and Science of Nursing Care,* 6th ed. Philadelphia: Lippincott Williams & Wilkins, 2008.

PARENTERAL ADMINISTRATION

ADMIXTURE OF DRUGS IN A SYRINGE

Combining two drugs in one syringe avoids the discomfort of two injections. Usually, drugs can be mixed in a syringe in one of four ways. They may be combined from two multidose vials (for example, regular and long-acting insulin), from one multidose vial and one ampule, from two ampules, or from a cartridge-injection system combined with either a multidose vial or an ampule.

Such combinations are contraindicated when the drugs aren't compatible and when the combined doses exceed the amount of solution that can be absorbed from a single injection site.

Cartridge-injection system

A cartridge-injection system, such as Tubex or Carpuject, is a convenient, easy-to-use method of injection that facilitates accuracy and sterility. The device consists of a plastic cartridge-holder syringe and a prefilled medication cartridge with needle attached, as shown below.

The medication in the cartridge is premixed and premeasured, *which saves time and helps ensure an exact dose*. The medication remains sealed in the cartridge and sterile until the injection is administered to the patient.

The disadvantage of this system is that not all drugs are available in cartridge form. However, compatible drugs can be added to partially filled cartridges.

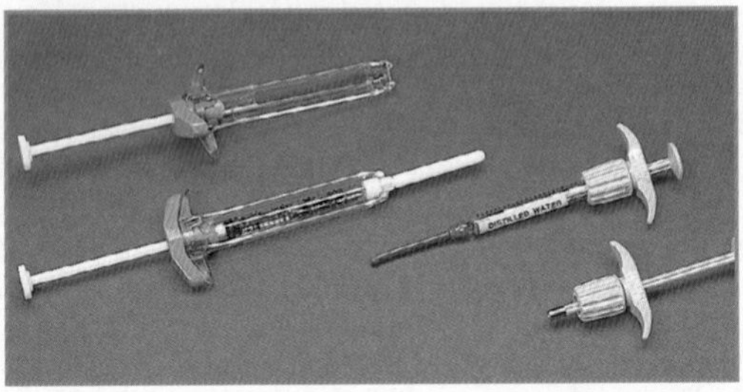

Equipment

Prescribed medications ▪ patient's medication record and chart ▪ alcohol pads ▪ syringe and needle ▪ optional: cartridge-injection system and filter needle.

The type and size of the syringe and needle depend on the prescribed medications, patient's body build, and route of administration. Medications that come in prefilled cartridges require a cartridge-injection system. (See *Cartridge-injection system*.)

Implementation

- Verify that the drugs to be administered agree with the patient's medication record and the practitioner's orders.
- Calculate the dose to be given.
- Wash your hands.

Mixing drugs from two multidose vials

- Using an alcohol pad, wipe the rubber stopper on the first vial. *This reduces the risk of contaminating the medication as you insert the needle into the vial.*
- Pull back the syringe plunger until the volume of air drawn into the syringe equals the volume to be withdrawn from the drug vial.
- Without inverting the vial, insert the needle into the top of the vial, making sure that the needle's bevel tip doesn't touch the solution. Inject the air into the vial, and withdraw the needle. *This replaces air in the vial, thus preventing creation of a partial vacuum on withdrawal of the drug.*
- Repeat the steps above for the second vial. Then, after injecting the air into the second vial, invert the vial, withdraw the prescribed dose, and then withdraw the needle.
- Wipe the rubber stopper of the first vial again, and insert the needle, taking care not to depress the plunger. Invert the vial, withdraw the prescribed dose, and then withdraw the needle.

Mixing drugs from a multidose vial and an ampule

- Using an alcohol pad, clean the vial's rubber stopper.
- Pull back on the syringe plunger until the volume of air drawn into the syringe equals the volume to be withdrawn from the drug vial.
- Insert the needle into the top of the vial, and inject the air. Then invert the vial, and keep the needle's bevel tip below the level of the solution as you withdraw the prescribed dose. Put the sterile needle cover over the needle.
- Tap the stem of the ampule *to move any medication from the stem into the body of the ampule.*
- Wrap a sterile gauze pad or an alcohol pad around the ampule's neck *to protect yourself from injury in case the glass splinters.* Break open the ampule, directing the force away from you.
- Switch to the filter needle at this point *to filter out any glass splinters.*
- Insert the needle into the ampule. Be careful not to touch the outside of the ampule with the needle. Draw the correct dose into the syringe.
- Change back to a regular needle to administer the injection.

Mixing drugs from two ampules

- Tap the stem of the ampule *to move any medication from the stem into the body of the ampule.*
- Open both ampules; wrap a small gauze pad or alcohol pad around the neck of the ampule, and quickly snap off the top along the scored line at the neck. Snap the neck away from your body.
- Insert a syringe—with the needle attached—into the ampule without allowing the needle to come in contact with the rim of the ampule. Use a filter needle, as appropriate.
- Withdraw the amount ordered from the first ampule, and remove the needle from the solution.

■ Change the needle, if necessary, and repeat with the second ampule.
■ Discard the used equipment appropriately.

Special considerations

■ Insert a needle through the vial's rubber stopper at a slight angle, bevel up, and exert slight lateral pressure. *This way you won't cut a piece of rubber out of the stopper, which can then be pushed into the vial.*
■ When withdrawing the medication from an ampule, place the ampule upright on a flat surface, and insert the needle into the solution. Then withdraw the ordered amount. Alternatively, once the needle is in the solution, you can invert the ampule, keeping the needle centered and in the solution to withdraw the ordered amount. *Fluid is held in place in the inverted ampule by surface tension.*
■ When mixing drugs from multidose vials, be careful not to contaminate one drug with the other. Ideally, the needle should be changed after drawing the first medication into the syringe. This isn't always possible *because many disposable syringes don't have removable needles.*

NURSING ALERT ***Never combine drugs if you're unsure of their compatibility, and never combine more than two drugs. Although drug incompatibility usually causes a visible reaction, such as clouding, bubbling, or precipitation, some incompatible combinations produce no visible reaction even though they alter the chemical nature and action of the drugs. Check appropriate references, and consult a pharmacist when you're unsure about specific compatibility. When in doubt, administer two separate injections.***

■ Some medications are compatible for only a brief time after being combined and should be administered within 10 minutes after mixing. *After this time, environmental factors, such as temperature, exposure to light, and humidity, may alter compatibility.*
■ *To reduce the risk of contamination,* most facilities dispense parenteral medications in single-dose vials. Insulin is one of the few drugs still packaged in multidose vials. Be careful when mixing regular and long-acting insulin. Draw up the regular insulin first *to avoid contamination by the long-acting suspension.* (If a minute amount of the regular insulin is accidentally mixed with the long-acting insulin, it won't appreciably change the effect of the long-acting insulin.) Check your facility's policy before mixing insulins.
■ When you combine a cartridge-injection system and a multidose vial, use a separate needle and syringe to inject air into the multidose vial. *This prevents contamination of the multidose vial by the cartridge-injection system.*

Documentation

Record the drugs administered, injection site, and time of administration. Document adverse drug effects or other pertinent information.

SELECTED REFERENCES

The Joint Commission. *Comprehensive Accreditation Manual for Hospitals: The Official Handbook.* Standard MM.1.10. 2007.

The Joint Commission. *Comprehensive Accreditation Manual for Hospitals: The Official Handbook.* Standard MM.2.10. 2007.

The Joint Commission. *Comprehensive Accreditation Manual for Hospitals: The Official Handbook.* Standard MM.3.10. 2007.

The Joint Commission. *Comprehensive Accreditation Manual for Hospitals: The Official Handbook.* Standard MM.4.10. 2007.

The Joint Commission. *Comprehensive Accreditation Manual for Hospitals: The Official Handbook.* Standard MM.4.20. 2007.

The Joint Commission. *Comprehensive Accreditation Manual for Hospitals: The Official Handbook.* Standard MM.5.10. 2007.

The Joint Commission. *Comprehensive Accreditation Manual for Hospitals: The Official Handbook.* Standard MM.6.10. 2007.

The Joint Commission. *Comprehensive Accreditation Manual for Hospitals: The Official Handbook.* Standard MM.6.20. 2007.

The Joint Commission. *Comprehensive Accreditation Manual for Hospitals: The Official Handbook.* Standard MM.7.10. 2007.

Preston, S.T., and Hegadoren, K. "Glass Contamination in Parenterally Administered Medication," *Journal of Advanced Nursing* 48(3):266-70, November 2004.

"Standard 32. Filters. Infusion Nursing Standards of Practice," *Journal of Infusion Nursing* 29(15):533-34, January-February 2006.

Taylor, C., et al. *Fundamentals of Nursing: The Art and Science of Nursing Care,* 6th ed. Philadelphia: Lippincott Williams & Wilkins, 2008.

SUBCUTANEOUS INJECTION

When injected into the adipose (fatty) tissues beneath the skin, a drug moves into the bloodstream more rapidly than if given by mouth. Subcutaneous (subQ) injection allows slower, more sustained drug administration than I.M. injection; it also causes minimal tissue trauma and carries little risk of striking large blood vessels and nerves.

Absorbed mainly through the capillaries, drugs recommended for subQ injection include nonirritating aqueous

EQUIPMENT

Types of insulin infusion pumps

A subcutaneous insulin infusion pump provides continuous, long-term insulin therapy for patients with type 1 diabetes mellitus. Complications include infection at the injection site, catheter clogging, and insulin loss from loose reservoir-catheter connections. Insulin pumps work on either an open-loop or a closed-loop system.

Open-loop system

The open-loop pump is used most commonly. It infuses insulin but can't respond to changes in the patient's serum glucose levels. These portable, self-contained, programmable insulin pumps are smaller and less obtrusive than ever—about the size of a credit card—and have fewer buttons.

The pump delivers insulin in small (basal) doses every few minutes and large (bolus) doses that the patient sets manually. The system consists of a reservoir containing the insulin syringe, a small pump, an infusion-rate selector that allows insulin release adjustments, a battery, and a plastic catheter with an attached needle leading from the syringe to the subcutaneous injection site. The needle is typically held in place with waterproof tape. The patient can wear the pump on his belt or in his pocket—practically anywhere as long as the infusion line has a clear path to the injection site.

The infusion-rate selector automatically releases about one-half the total daily insulin requirement. The patient releases the remainder in bolus doses before meals and snacks. He must change the syringe daily, and the needle, catheter, and injection site every other day.

Closed-loop system

The self-contained closed-loop system detects and responds to changing serum glucose levels. The typical closed-loop system includes a glucose sensor, a programmable computer, a power supply, a pump, and an insulin reservoir. The computer triggers continuous insulin delivery in appropriate amounts from the reservoir.

Nonneedle catheter system

In the nonneedle delivery system, a tiny plastic catheter is inserted into the skin over a needle using a special insertion device (below). The needle is then withdrawn, leaving the catheter in place. This catheter can be placed in the abdomen, thigh, or flank and should be changed every 2 to 3 days.

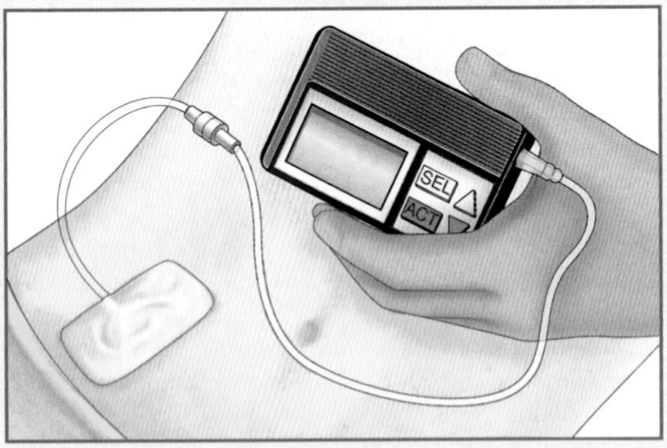

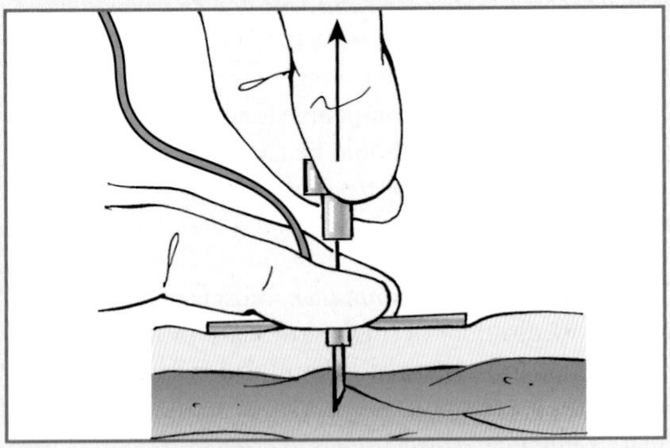

solutions and suspensions contained in 0.5 to 2 ml of fluid. Heparin and insulin, for example, are usually administered subQ. (Some diabetic patients, however, may benefit from an insulin infusion pump. See *Types of insulin infusion pumps.*)

Drugs and solutions for subQ injection are injected through a relatively short needle, using meticulous sterile technique. The most common subQ injection sites are the outer aspect of the upper arm, anterior thigh, loose tissue of the lower abdomen, upper hips, buttocks, and upper back. (See *Locating subcutaneous injection sites.*) Injection is contraindicated in sites that are inflamed, edematous, scarred, or covered by a mole, birthmark, or other lesion. It may also be contraindicated in patients with impaired coagulation mechanisms.

Equipment

Prescribed medication ▪ patient's medication record and chart ▪ 25G to 27G ⅝" or ½" needle or insulin syringe ▪

gloves ▪ 1- or 3-ml syringe ▪ alcohol pads ▪ 2″ × 2″ gauze pad ▪ optional: antiseptic cleaning agent, filter needle.

Preparation of equipment

Verify the order on the patient's medication record by checking it against the practitioner's order. Also note whether the patient has any allergies, especially before the first dose.

Inspect the medication to make sure it isn't abnormally discolored or cloudy and doesn't contain precipitates (unless the manufacturer's instructions allow it).

Wash your hands. Choose equipment appropriate to the prescribed medication and injection site, and make sure it works properly.

Check the medication label against the patient's medication record. Read the label again as you draw up the medication for injection.

For single-dose ampules: Wrap an alcohol pad around the ampule's neck, and snap off the top, directing the force away from your body. Attach a filter needle to the needle and withdraw the medication, keeping the needle's bevel tip below the level of the solution. Tap the syringe *to clear air from it.* Cover the needle with the needle sheath.

Before discarding the ampule, check the medication label against the patient's medication record. Discard the filter needle and the ampule. Attach the appropriate needle to the syringe.

For single-dose or multidose vials: Reconstitute powdered drugs according to instructions. Make sure all crystals have dissolved in the solution. Warm the vial by rolling it between your palms *to help the drug dissolve faster.*

Clean the vial's rubber stopper with an alcohol pad. Pull the syringe plunger back until the volume of air in the syringe equals the volume of drug to be withdrawn from the vial.

Without inverting the vial, insert the needle into the vial. Inject the air, invert the vial, and keep the needle's bevel tip below the level of the solution as you withdraw the prescribed amount of medication. Cover the needle with the needle sheath. Tap the syringe to clear any air from it. Check the medication label against the patient's medication record before discarding the single-dose vial or returning the multidose vial to the shelf.

Locating subcutaneous injection sites

Subcutaneous (subQ) injection sites (as indicated by the colored areas in the illustration below) include the fat pads on the abdomen, upper hips, upper back, and lateral upper arms and thighs. For subQ injections administered repeatedly, such as insulin, rotate sites. Choose one injection site in one area, move to a corresponding injection site in the next area, and so on.

When returning to an area, choose a new site in that area. Preferred injection sites for insulin are the arms, abdomen, thighs, and buttocks. The preferred injection site for heparin is the lower abdominal fat pad, just below the umbilicus.

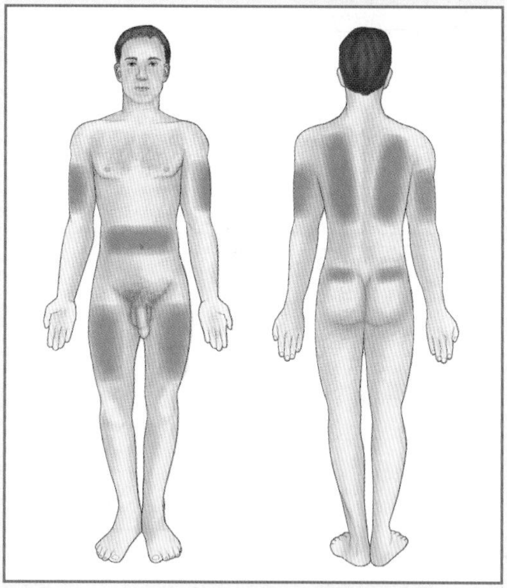

Implementation

▪ Confirm the patient's identity using two patient identifiers according to your facility's policy.

▪ If your facility uses a bar code scanning system, be sure to scan your ID badge, the patient's ID bracelet, and the medication's bar code.

▪ Explain the procedure to the patient, and provide privacy.

▪ Select an appropriate injection site. Rotate sites according to a schedule for repeated injections, using different areas of the body unless contraindicated. (Heparin, for example, should be injected only in the abdomen if possible.)

▪ Put on gloves.

▪ Position and drape the patient if necessary.

▪ Clean the injection site with an alcohol pad, beginning at the center of the site and moving outward in a circular motion. Allow the skin to dry before injecting the drug *to avoid a stinging sensation from introducing alcohol into subcutaneous tissues.*

▪ Loosen the protective needle sheath.

Technique for subcutaneous injection

Before giving the injection, elevate the subcutaneous tissue at the site by grasping it firmly.

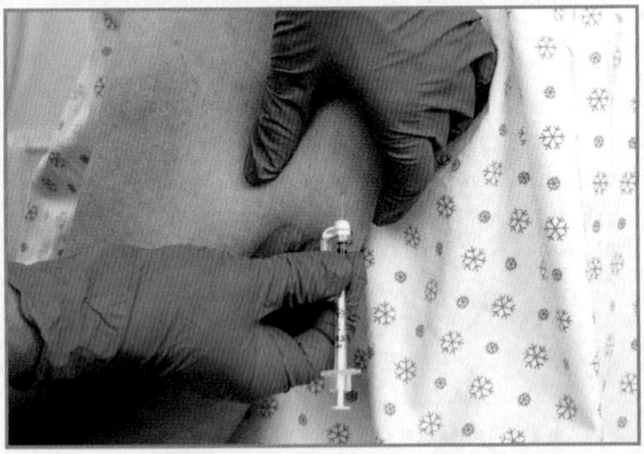

Insert the needle at a 45- or 90-degree angle to the skin surface, depending on needle length and the amount of subcutaneous tissue at the site. Some medications, such as heparin, should always be injected at a 90-degree angle.

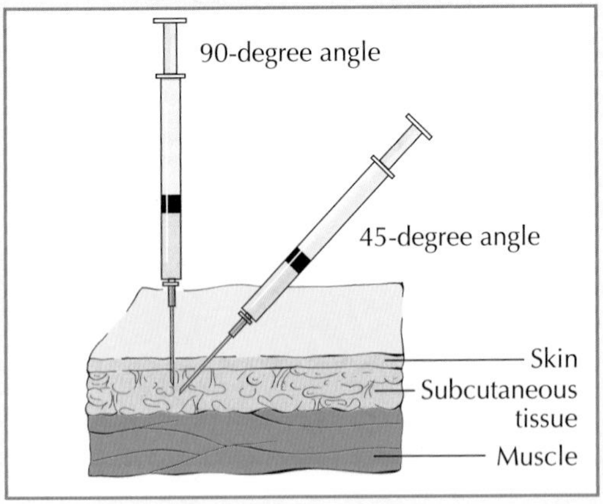

- With your nondominant hand, grasp the skin around the injection site firmly to elevate the subcutaneous tissue, forming a 1″ (2.5-cm) fat fold.
- Holding the syringe in your dominant hand, insert the loosened needle sheath between the fourth and fifth fingers of your other hand while still pinching the skin around the injection site. Pull back the syringe with your dominant hand *to uncover the needle by grasping the syringe like a pencil.* Don't touch the needle.
- Position the needle with its bevel up.
- Tell the patient he'll feel a needle prick.
- Insert the needle quickly in one motion at a 45- or 90-degree angle. (See *Technique for subcutaneous injection.*) Release the patient's skin *to avoid injecting the drug into compressed tissue and irritating nerve fibers.*
- Pull back the plunger slightly *to check for blood return.* If none appears, begin injecting the drug slowly. If blood appears on aspiration, withdraw the needle, prepare another syringe, and repeat the procedure.
- Don't aspirate for blood return when giving insulin or heparin. *It isn't necessary with insulin and may cause a hematoma with heparin.*
- After injection, remove the needle gently but quickly at the same angle used for insertion.
- Cover the site with an alcohol pad or a 2″ × 2″ gauze pad, and massage the site gently (unless contraindicated, as with heparin and insulin) *to distribute the drug and facilitate absorption.*
- Remove the alcohol pad, and check the injection site for bleeding and bruising.
- Dispose of injection equipment according to your facility's policy. *To avoid needle-stick injuries,* don't resheath the needle.

Special considerations

- When using prefilled syringes, adjust the angle and depth of insertion according to needle length.

For insulin injections

- *To establish more consistent blood insulin levels,* rotate insulin injection sites within anatomic regions. Preferred insulin injection sites are the arms, abdomen, thighs, and buttocks.
- Make sure the type of insulin, unit dosage, and syringe are correct.
- When combining insulins in a syringe, make sure they're compatible. Regular insulin can be mixed with all other types. Prompt insulin zinc suspension (Semilente insulin) can't be mixed with NPH insulin. Follow your facility's policy regarding which insulin to draw up first.
- Before drawing up insulin suspension, gently roll and invert the bottle. Don't shake the bottle *because this can cause foam or bubbles to develop in the syringe.*

For heparin injections

- The preferred site for a heparin injection is the lower abdominal fat pad, 2″ (5 cm) beneath the umbilicus, between the right and left iliac crests. *Injecting heparin into this area, which isn't involved in muscle activity, reduces the risk of local capillary bleeding.* Always rotate the sites from one side to the other.

- Inject the drug slowly into the fat pad. Leave the needle in place for 10 seconds after injection; then withdraw it.
- Don't administer an injection within 2″ of a scar, a bruise, or the umbilicus.
- Don't aspirate to check for blood return *because this can cause bleeding into the tissues at the site.*
- Don't rub or massage the site after the injection. *Rubbing can cause localized minute hemorrhages or bruises.*
- If the patient bruises easily, apply ice to the site for the first 5 minutes after the injection *to minimize local hemorrhage,* and then apply pressure.

Complications

Concentrated or irritating solutions may cause sterile abscesses to form. Repeated injections in the same site can cause lipodystrophy. A natural immune response, lipodystrophy can be minimized by rotating injection sites.

Documentation

Record the time and date of the injection, medication and dose administered, injection site and route, and patient's reaction.

SELECTED REFERENCES

Annersten, M., and Willman, A. "Performing Subcutaneous Injections: A Literature Review," *Worldviews on Evidence-Based Nursing* 2(3):122-30, 2005.

The Joint Commission. *Comprehensive Accreditation Manual for Hospitals: The Official Handbook.* Standard MM.1.10. 2007.

The Joint Commission. *Comprehensive Accreditation Manual for Hospitals: The Official Handbook.* Standard MM.2.10. 2007.

The Joint Commission. *Comprehensive Accreditation Manual for Hospitals: The Official Handbook.* Standard MM.3.10. 2007.

The Joint Commission. *Comprehensive Accreditation Manual for Hospitals: The Official Handbook.* Standard MM.4.10. 2007.

The Joint Commission. *Comprehensive Accreditation Manual for Hospitals: The Official Handbook.* Standard MM.4.20. 2007.

The Joint Commission. *Comprehensive Accreditation Manual for Hospitals: The Official Handbook.* Standard MM.5.10. 2007.

The Joint Commission. *Comprehensive Accreditation Manual for Hospitals: The Official Handbook.* Standard MM.6.10. 2007.

The Joint Commission. *Comprehensive Accreditation Manual for Hospitals: The Official Handbook.* Standard MM.6.20. 2007.

The Joint Commission. *Comprehensive Accreditation Manual for Hospitals: The Official Handbook.* Standard MM.7.10. 2007.

Rushing, J. "How to Administer a Subcutaneous Injection," *Nursing* 34(6):32, June 2004.

Taylor, C., et al. *Fundamentals of Nursing: The Art and Science of Nursing Care,* 6th ed. Philadelphia: Lippincott Williams & Wilkins, 2008.

Locating intradermal injection sites

The most common intradermal injection site is the ventral forearm. Other sites (indicated by dotted areas) include the upper chest, upper arm, and shoulder blades. Skin in these areas is usually lightly pigmented, thinly keratinized, and relatively hairless, facilitating detection of adverse reactions.

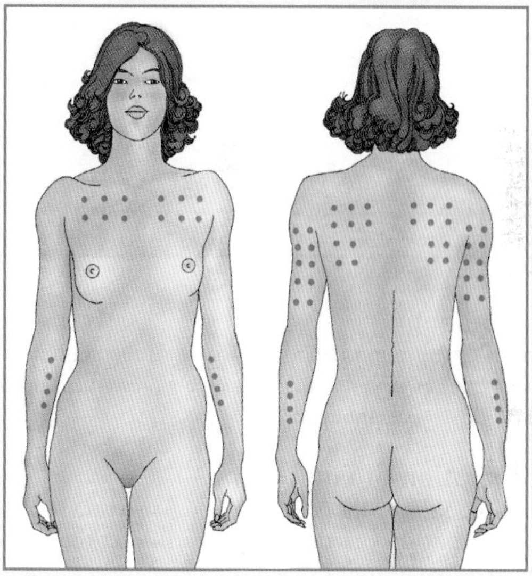

INTRADERMAL INJECTION

Because little systemic absorption of intradermally injected agents takes place, this type of injection is used primarily to produce a local effect, as in allergy or tuberculin testing. Intradermal injections are administered in small volumes (usually 0.5 ml or less) into the outer layers of the skin.

The ventral forearm is the most commonly used site for intradermal injection because of its easy accessibility and lack of hair. In extensive allergy testing, the outer aspect of the upper arms may be used as well as the area of the back located between the scapulae. (See *Locating intradermal injection sites.*)

Giving an intradermal injection

Secure the patient's forearm. Insert the needle at a 10- to 15-degree angle so that it just punctures the skin's surface. The antigen should raise a small wheal as it's injected.

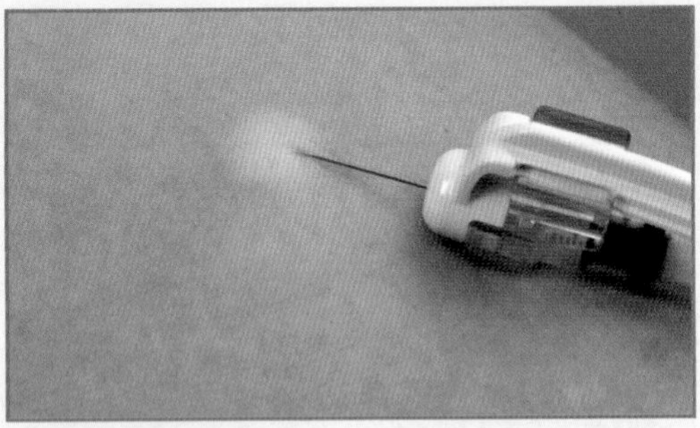

Equipment

Patient's medication record and chart ■ tuberculin syringe with a 26G or 27G ½″ to ⅜″ needle ■ prescribed medication ■ gloves ■ alcohol pads.

Preparation of equipment

Verify the order on the patient's medication record by checking it against the practitioner's order. Inspect the medication *to make sure it isn't abnormally discolored or cloudy and doesn't contain precipitates.* Wash your hands.

Choose equipment appropriate to the prescribed medication and injection site, and make sure it works properly. Check the medication label against the patient's medication record. Read the label again as you draw up the medication for injection.

Implementation

- Confirm the patient's identity using two patient identifiers according to your facility's policy.
- If your facility uses a bar code scanning system, be sure to scan your ID badge, the patient's ID bracelet, and the medication's bar code.
- Tell the patient where you'll be giving the injection.
- Instruct the patient to sit up and to extend his arm and support it on a flat surface, with the ventral forearm exposed.
- Put on gloves.
- With an alcohol pad, clean the surface of the ventral forearm about two or three fingerbreadths distal to the antecubital space. Make sure the test site you have chosen is free from hair or blemishes. Allow the skin to dry completely before administering the injection.
- While holding the patient's forearm in your hand, stretch the skin taut with your thumb.
- With your free hand, hold the needle at a 10- to 15-degree angle to the patient's arm, with its bevel up.
- Insert the needle about ⅛″ (0.3 cm) below the epidermis at sites 2″ (5 cm) apart. Stop when the needle's bevel tip is under the skin, and inject the antigen slowly. You should feel some resistance as you do this, and a wheal should form as you inject the antigen. (See *Giving an intradermal injection.*) If no wheal forms, you have injected the antigen too deeply; withdraw the needle, and administer another test dose at least 2″ from the first site.
- Withdraw the needle at the same angle at which it was inserted. Don't rub the site. *This could irritate the underlying tissue, which may affect test results.*
- Circle each test site with a marking pen, and label each site according to the recall antigen given. Instruct the patient to refrain from washing off the circles until the test is completed.
- Dispose of needles and syringes according to your facility's policy.
- Remove and discard your gloves.
- Assess the patient's response to the skin testing in 24 to 48 hours.

Special considerations

In patients who are hypersensitive to the test antigens, a severe anaphylactic response can result. This requires immediate epinephrine injection and other emergency resuscitation procedures. Be especially alert after giving a test dose of penicillin or tetanus antitoxin.

Documentation

On the patient's medication record, document the type and amount of medication given, the time it was given, and the injection site. Note skin reactions and other adverse reactions.

SELECTED REFERENCES

The Joint Commission. *Comprehensive Accreditation Manual for Hospitals: The Official Handbook.* Standard MM.1.10. 2007.

The Joint Commission. *Comprehensive Accreditation Manual for Hospitals: The Official Handbook.* Standard MM.2.10. 2007.

The Joint Commission. *Comprehensive Accreditation Manual for Hospitals: The Official Handbook.* Standard MM.3.10. 2007.

The Joint Commission. *Comprehensive Accreditation Manual for Hospitals: The Official Handbook.* Standard MM.4.10. 2007.

The Joint Commission. *Comprehensive Accreditation Manual for Hospitals: The Official Handbook.* Standard MM.4.20. 2007.

The Joint Commission. *Comprehensive Accreditation Manual for Hospitals: The Official Handbook.* Standard MM.5.10. 2007.

The Joint Commission. *Comprehensive Accreditation Manual for Hospitals: The Official Handbook.* Standard MM.6.10. 2007.

The Joint Commission. *Comprehensive Accreditation Manual for Hospitals: The Official Handbook.* Standard MM.6.20. 2007.

The Joint Commission. *Comprehensive Accreditation Manual for Hospitals: The Official Handbook.* Standard MM.7.10. 2007.

La Montagne, J.R., and Fauci, A.S. "Intradermal Influenza Vaccination—Can Less Be More?" *New England Journal of Medicine* 351(2):2330-332, November 2004.

Love, G.H. "Administering an Intradermal Injection," *Nursing* 36(6):20, June 2006.

Taylor, C., et al. *Fundamentals of Nursing: The Art and Science of Nursing Care,* 6th ed. Philadelphia: Lippincott Williams & Wilkins, 2008.

I.M. INJECTION

I.M. injections deposit medication deep into muscle tissue. This route of administration provides rapid systemic action and absorption of relatively large doses (up to 5 ml in appropriate sites). I.M. injections are recommended for patients who are uncooperative or can't take medication orally and for drugs that are altered by digestive juices. Because muscle tissue has few sensory nerves, I.M. injection allows less painful administration of irritating drugs.

The site for an I.M. injection must be chosen carefully, taking into account the patient's general physical status and the purpose of the injection. I.M. injections shouldn't be administered at inflamed, edematous, or irritated sites or at sites that contain moles, birthmarks, scar tissue, or other lesions. I.M. injections may also be contraindicated in patients with impaired coagulation mechanisms, occlusive peripheral vascular disease, edema, and shock; after thrombolytic therapy; and during an acute myocardial infarction because these conditions impair peripheral absorption. I.M. injections require sterile technique to maintain the integrity of muscle tissue.

Oral or I.V. routes are preferred for administration of drugs that are poorly absorbed by muscle tissue, such as phenytoin, digoxin, chlordiazepoxide, and diazepam.

Equipment

Patient's medication record and chart ▪ prescribed medication ▪ diluent or filter needle, if needed ▪ 3- or 5-ml syringe ▪ 20G to 25G 1″ to 3″ needle ▪ gloves ▪ alcohol pads ▪ 2″ × 2″ gauze pad.

The prescribed medication must be sterile. The needle may be packaged separately or already attached to the syringe. Needles used for I.M. injections are longer than subcutaneous needles *because they must reach deep into the muscle.* Needle length also depends on the injection site, patient's size, and amount of subcutaneous fat covering the muscle. The needle gauge for I.M. injections should be larger *to accommodate viscous solutions and suspensions.*

Preparation of equipment

Verify the order on the patient's medication record by checking it against the practitioner's order. Also note whether the patient has any allergies, especially before the first dose. Wash your hands.

Check the prescribed medication for color and clarity. Also note the expiration date. Never use medication that's cloudy or discolored or contains a precipitate unless the manufacturer's instructions allow it. Remember that for some drugs (such as suspensions), the presence of drug particles is normal. Observe for abnormal changes. If in doubt, check with the pharmacist.

Choose equipment appropriate to the prescribed medication and injection site, and make sure it works properly. The needle should be straight, smooth, and free of burrs.

For single-dose ampules: Wrap an alcohol pad around the ampule's neck, and snap off the top, directing the force away from your body. Attach a filter needle and withdraw the medication, keeping the needle's bevel tip below the level of the solution. Tap the syringe *to clear air from it.* Cover the needle with the needle sheath.

Before discarding the ampule, check the medication label against the patient's medication record. Discard the filter needle and the ampule. Attach the appropriate needle to the syringe.

For single-dose or multidose vials: Reconstitute powdered drugs according to instructions. Make sure all crystals have dissolved in the solution. Warm the vial by rolling it between your palms *to help the drug dissolve faster.*

Wipe the stopper of the medication vial with an alcohol pad, and then draw up the prescribed amount of medication. Read the medication label as you select the medication, as you draw it up, and after you've drawn it up *to verify the correct dosage.*

Don't use an air bubble in the syringe. *Syringes are calibrated to administer the correct dose without an air bubble.* Gather all necessary equipment, and proceed to the patient's room.

Implementation

- Confirm the patient's identity using two patient identifiers according to your facility's policy.
- If your facility uses a bar code scanning system, be sure to scan your ID badge, the patient's ID bracelet, and the medication's bar code.
- Provide privacy, and explain the procedure to the patient.
- Select an appropriate injection site. The ventrogluteal site is used most commonly for healthy adults, although the deltoid muscle may be used for a small-volume injection (2 ml or less). Remember to rotate injection sites for patients who require repeated injections. (See *Locating I.M. injection sites.*)

PEDIATRIC ALERT *For infants and children, the vastus lateralis muscle of the thigh is used most commonly* because it's usually the best developed and contains no large nerves or blood vessels, minimizing the risk of serious injury. *The rectus femoris muscle may also be used in infants but is usually contraindicated in adults.*

- Position and drape the patient appropriately, making sure the site is well exposed and that lighting is adequate.
- Loosen the protective needle sheath, but don't remove it.
- After selecting the injection site, gently tap it *to stimulate the nerve endings and minimize pain when the needle is inserted.* Clean the skin at the site with an alcohol pad. Move the pad outward in a circular motion to a circumference of about 2″ (5 cm) from the injection site, and allow the skin to dry. Keep the alcohol pad for later use.
- Put on gloves. With the thumb and index finger of your nondominant hand, gently stretch the skin of the injection site taut.
- While you hold the syringe in your dominant hand, remove the needle sheath by slipping it between the free fingers of your nondominant hand and then drawing back the syringe.
- Position the syringe at a 90-degree angle to the skin surface, with the needle a couple of inches from the skin. Tell the patient that he'll feel a prick as you insert the needle. Then quickly and firmly thrust the needle through the skin and subcutaneous tissue, deep into the muscle.
- Support the syringe with your nondominant hand, if desired. Pull back slightly on the plunger with your dominant hand to aspirate for blood. If no blood appears, *slowly* inject the medication into the muscle. *A slow, steady injection rate allows the muscle to distend gradually and accept the medication under minimal pressure.* You should feel little or no resistance against the force of the injection.

NURSING ALERT ***If blood appears in the syringe on aspiration, the needle is in a blood vessel. If this occurs, stop the injection, withdraw the needle, prepare another injection with new equipment, and inject another site. Don't inject the bloody solution.***

- After the injection, gently but quickly remove the needle at a 90-degree angle.
- Using a gloved hand, cover the injection site immediately with the used alcohol pad or 2″ × 2″ gauze pad, apply gentle pressure, and unless contraindicated, massage the relaxed muscle *to help distribute the drug.*
- Remove the alcohol pad, and inspect the injection site for signs of active bleeding or bruising. If bleeding continues, apply pressure to the site; if bruising occurs, you may apply ice.
- Watch for adverse reactions at the site for 10 to 30 minutes after the injection.

ELDER ALERT ***An older patient will probably bleed or ooze from the site after the injection*** **because of decreased tissue elasticity.** ***Applying a small pressure bandage may be helpful.***

- Discard all equipment according to standard precautions and your facility's policy. Don't recap needles; dispose of them in an appropriate sharps container to avoid needlestick injuries.

Special considerations

- *To slow their absorption*, some drugs for I.M. administration are dissolved in oil or other special solutions. Mix these preparations well before drawing them into the syringe.

PEDIATRIC ALERT *The gluteal muscles can be used as the injection site only after a toddler has been walking for about 1 year.*

- Never inject into sensitive muscles, especially those that twitch or tremble when you assess site landmarks and tissue depth. *Injections into these trigger areas may cause sharp or referred pain such as the pain caused by nerve trauma.*
- Keep a rotation record that lists all available injection sites, divided into various body areas, for patients who require repeated injections. Rotate from a site in the first area to a site in each of the other areas. Then return to a site in the first area that is at least 1″ (2.5 cm) away from the previous injection site in that area.
- If the patient has experienced pain or emotional trauma from repeated injections, consider numbing the area before cleaning it by holding ice on it for several seconds, or consider the use of an eulectic mixture of local anesthetics (EMLA) cream applied 60 to 90 minutes prior to the procedure. If you must inject more than 5 ml of solution, divide the solution, and inject it at two separate sites.
- Always encourage the patient to relax the muscle you'll be injecting *because injections into tense muscles are more painful than usual and may bleed more readily.*
- I.M. injections can damage local muscle cells, causing elevations in serum enzyme levels (creatine kinase [CK]) that can be confused with elevations resulting from cardiac muscle damage, as in myocardial infarction. *To distinguish be-*

Locating I.M. injection sites

Deltoid

Find the lower edge of the acromial process and the point on the lateral arm in line with the axilla. Insert the needle 1″ to 2″ (2.5 to 5 cm) below the acromial process, usually two or three fingerbreadths, at a 90-degree angle or angled slightly toward the process. Typical injection: 0.5 ml (range: 0.5 to 2 ml).

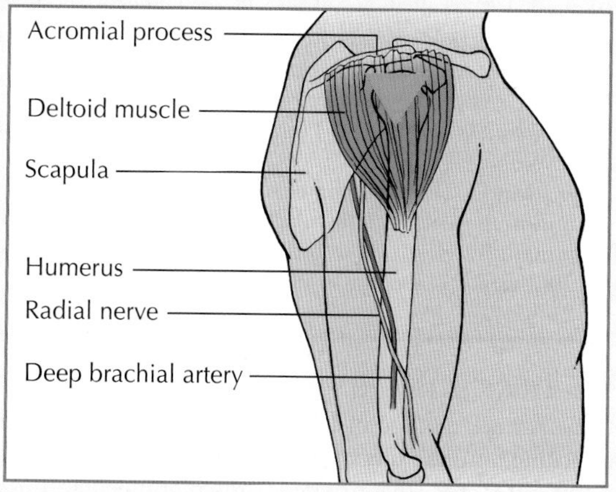

Dorsogluteal

Inject above and outside a line drawn from the posterior superior iliac spine to the greater trochanter of the femur. Or, divide the buttock into quadrants, and inject in the upper outer quadrant, about 2″ to 3″ (5 to 7.6 cm) below the iliac crest. Insert the needle at a 90-degree angle. Typical injection: 1 to 4 ml (range: 1 to 5 ml).

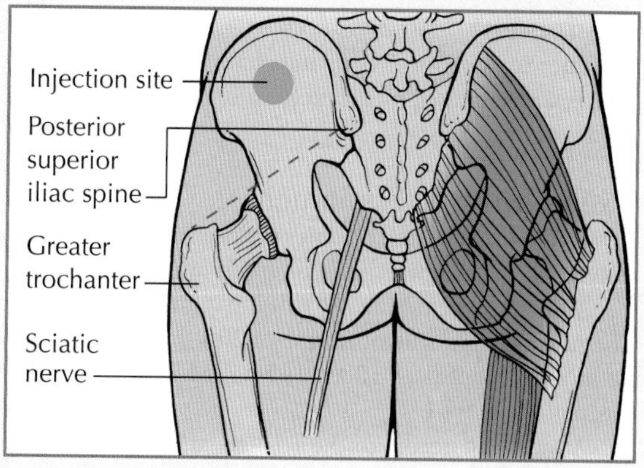

Ventrogluteal

Locate the greater trochanter of the femur with the heel of your hand. Then spread your index and middle fingers from the anterior superior iliac spine to as far along the iliac crest as you can reach. Insert the needle between the two fingers at a 90-degree angle to the muscle. (Remove your fingers before inserting the needle.) Typical injection: 1 to 4 ml (range: 1 to 5 ml).

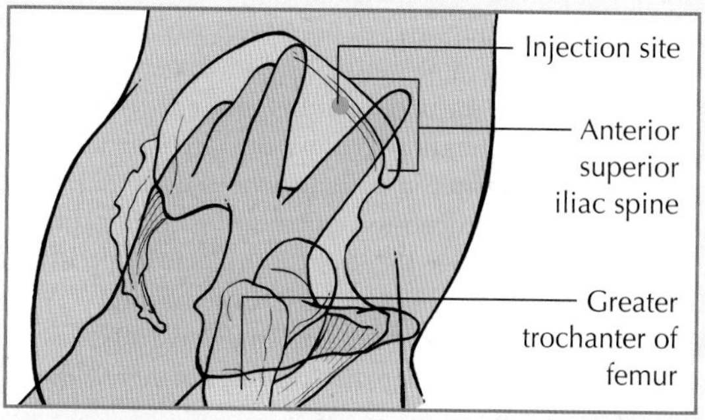

Vastus lateralis

Use the lateral muscle of the quadriceps group, from a handbreadth below the greater trochanter to a handbreadth above the knee. Insert the needle into the middle third of the muscle parallel to the surface on which the patient is lying. You may have to bunch the muscle before insertion. Typical injection: 1 to 4 ml (range: 1 to 5 ml; 1 to 3 ml for infants).

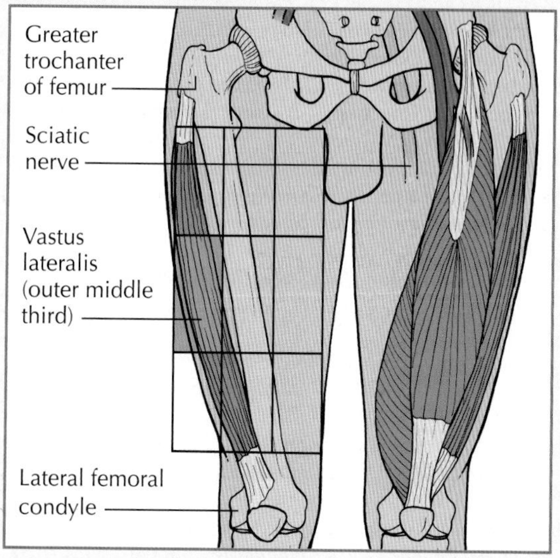

tween skeletal and cardiac muscle damage, diagnostic tests for suspected myocardial infarction must identify the isoenzyme of CK specific to cardiac muscle (CK-MB) and include tests to determine lactate dehydrogenase and aspartate aminotransferase levels. If it's important to measure these enzyme levels, suggest that the practitioner switch to I.V. administration and adjust dosages accordingly.

- Dosage adjustments are usually necessary when changing from the I.M. route to the oral route.

Complications

Accidental injection of concentrated or irritating medications into subcutaneous tissue or other areas where they can't be fully absorbed can cause sterile abscesses to develop. Such abscesses result from the body's natural immune response in which phagocytes attempt to remove the foreign matter.

Failure to rotate sites in patients who require repeated injections can lead to deposits of unabsorbed medications. Such deposits can reduce the desired pharmacologic effect and may lead to abscess formation or tissue fibrosis.

ELDER ALERT Because older patients have decreased muscle mass, *I.M. medications can be absorbed more quickly than expected.*

Documentation

Chart the drug administered, dose, date, time, route of administration, and injection site. Also, note the patient's tolerance of the injection and the injection's effects, including any adverse effects.

SELECTED REFERENCES

Craven, R.F., and Hirnle, C.J. *Fundamentals of Nursing: Human Health and Function,* 5th ed. Philadelphia: Lippincott Williams & Wilkins, 2007.

Donaldson, D., and Green, J. "Using the Ventrogluteal Site for Intramuscular Injections," *Nursing Times* 101(16):36-38, April 2005.

"I.M. Injections: Pick Your Site," Nursing 36(6):34, June 2006.

The Joint Commission. *Comprehensive Accreditation Manual for Hospitals: The Official Handbook.* Standard MM.1.10. 2007.

The Joint Commission. *Comprehensive Accreditation Manual for Hospitals: The Official Handbook.* Standard MM.2.10. 2007.

The Joint Commission. *Comprehensive Accreditation Manual for Hospitals: The Official Handbook.* Standard MM.3.10. 2007.

The Joint Commission. *Comprehensive Accreditation Manual for Hospitals: The Official Handbook.* Standard MM.4.10. 2007.

The Joint Commission. *Comprehensive Accreditation Manual for Hospitals: The Official Handbook.* Standard MM.4.20. 2007.

The Joint Commission. *Comprehensive Accreditation Manual for Hospitals: The Official Handbook.* Standard MM.5.10. 2007.

The Joint Commission. *Comprehensive Accreditation Manual for Hospitals: The Official Handbook.* Standard MM.6.10. 2007.

The Joint Commission. *Comprehensive Accreditation Manual for Hospitals: The Official Handbook.* Standard MM.6.20. 2007.

Prettyman, J. "Subcutaneous or Intramuscular? Confronting a Parenteral Administration Dilemma," *Medsurg Nursing* 14(2):93-98, April 2005.

Ramtahal, J., et al. "Sciatic Nerve Injury Following Intramuscular Injection: A Case Report and Review of Literature," *Journal of Neuroscience Nursing* 38(4):238-40, August 2006.

Taylor, C., et al. *Fundamentals of Nursing: The Art and Science of Nursing Care,* 6th ed. Philadelphia: Lippincott Williams & Wilkins, 2008.

Wynaden, D. "Establishing Best Practice Guidelines for Administration of Intramuscular Injections in the Adult: A Systematic Review of the Literature," *Contemporary Nurse* 20(2):267-77, December 2005.

Z-TRACK INJECTION

The Z-track method of I.M. injection prevents leakage, or tracking, into the subcutaneous tissue. It's typically used to administer drugs that irritate and discolor subcutaneous tissue, primarily iron preparations such as iron dextran. It may also be used in elderly patients who have decreased muscle mass. Lateral displacement of the skin during the injection helps to seal the drug in the muscle.

This procedure requires careful attention to technique because leakage into subcutaneous tissue can cause patient discomfort and may permanently stain some tissues.

Equipment

Patient's medication record and chart ■ two 20G 1¼″ to 2″ needles ■ prescribed medication ■ gloves ■ 3- or 5-ml syringe ■ two alcohol pads.

Preparation of equipment

Verify the order on the patient's medication record by checking it against the practitioner's order. Wash your hands.

Make sure the needle you're using is long enough to reach the muscle. As a rule of thumb, a 200-lb (90.7-kg) patient requires a 2″ needle; a 100-lb (45-kg) patient, a 1¼″ to 1½″ needle.

Attach one needle to the syringe, and draw up the prescribed medication. Then draw 0.2 to 0.5 cc of air (depending on your facility's policy) into the syringe. Remove the first needle and attach the second *to prevent tracking the medication through the subcutaneous tissue as the needle is inserted.*

Displacing the skin for Z-track injection

By blocking the needle pathway after an injection, the Z-track technique allows I.M. injection while minimizing the risk of subcutaneous irritation and staining from such drugs as iron dextran. The illustrations here show you how to perform a Z-track injection.

Before the procedure begins, the skin, subcutaneous fat, and muscle lie in their normal positions.

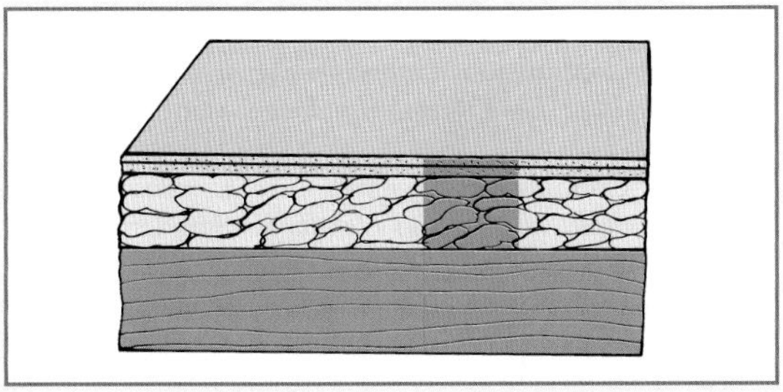

To begin, place your finger on the skin surface, and pull the skin and subcutaneous layers out of alignment with the underlying muscle. You should move the skin about ½″ (1 cm).

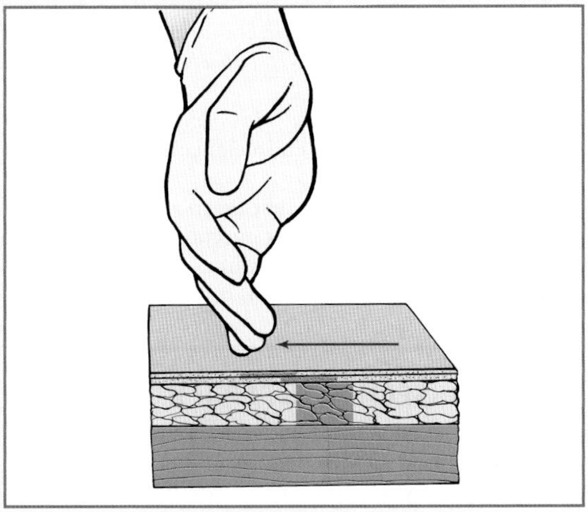

Insert the needle at a 90-degree angle at the site where you initially placed your finger. Inject the drug and withdraw the needle.

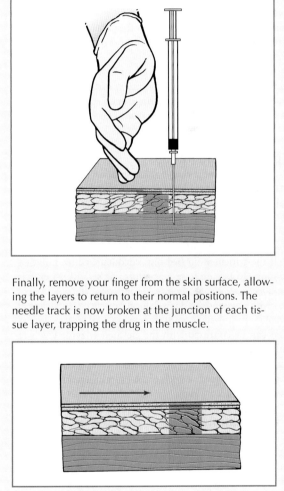

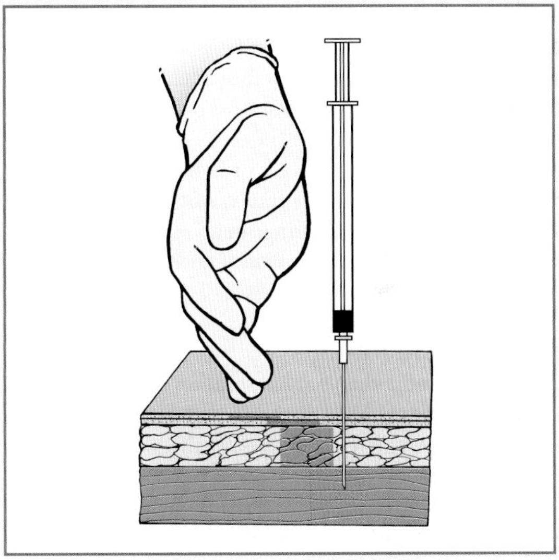

Finally, remove your finger from the skin surface, allowing the layers to return to their normal positions. The needle track is now broken at the junction of each tissue layer, trapping the drug in the muscle.

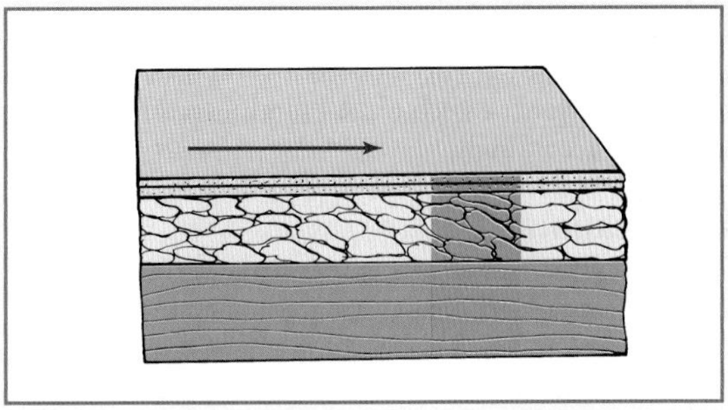

Implementation

- Confirm the patient's identity using two patient identifiers according to your facility's policy.
- If your facility uses a bar code scanning system, be sure to scan your ID badge, the patient's ID bracelet, and the medication's bar code.
- Explain the procedure and provide privacy.
- Place the patient in the lateral position, exposing the gluteal muscle to be used as the injection site. The patient may also be placed in the prone position.
- Clean an area on the upper outer quadrant of the patient's buttock with an alcohol pad.
- Put on gloves. Then displace the skin laterally by pulling it away from the injection site. (See *Displacing the skin for Z-track injection.*)

- Insert the needle into the muscle at a 90-degree angle.
- Aspirate for blood return; if none appears, inject the drug slowly, followed by the air. *Injecting air after the drug helps clear the needle and prevents tracking the medication through subcutaneous tissues as the needle is withdrawn.*
- Wait 10 seconds before withdrawing the needle *to ensure dispersion of the medication.*
- Withdraw the needle slowly. Then release the displaced skin and subcutaneous tissue *to seal the needle track.* Don't massage the injection site or allow the patient to wear a tight-fitting garment over the site *because it could force the medication into subcutaneous tissue.*
- Encourage the patient to walk or move about in bed *to facilitate absorption of the drug from the injection site.*
- Discard the needles and syringe in an appropriate sharps container. Don't recap needles *to avoid needle-stick injuries.*
- Remove and discard your gloves.

Special considerations

- Never inject more than 5 ml of solution into a single site using the Z-track method. Alternate gluteal sites for repeat injections.
- Always encourage the patient to relax the muscle you'll be injecting *because injections into tense muscle are more painful than usual and may bleed more readily.*
- If the patient is on bed rest, encourage active range-of-motion (ROM) exercises or perform passive ROM exercises *to facilitate absorption from the injection site.*
- I.M. injections can damage local muscle cells, causing elevated serum enzyme levels (for example, of creatine kinase) that can be confused with the elevated enzyme levels resulting from damage to cardiac muscle, as in myocardial infarction. If measuring enzyme levels is important, suggest that the practitioner switch to I.V. administration, and adjust dosages accordingly.

Complications

Discomfort and tissue irritation may result from drug leakage into subcutaneous tissue. Failure to rotate sites in patients who require repeated injections can interfere with the absorption of medication. Unabsorbed medications may build up in deposits. Such deposits can reduce the desired pharmacologic effect and may lead to abscess formation or tissue fibrosis.

Documentation

Record the medication, dosage, date, time, and site of injection on the patient's medication record. Include the patient's response to the injected drug.

Selected references

"Administering Medication by the Z-track Method," *Nursing* 35(7):24, July 2005.

Donaldson, D., and Green, J. "Using the Ventrogluteal Site for Intramuscular Injections," *Nursing Times* 101(16):36-38, April 2005.

"I.M. Injections: Pick Your Site," *Nursing* 36(6):34, June 2006.

The Joint Commission. *Comprehensive Accreditation Manual for Hospitals: The Official Handbook.* Standard MM.1.10. 2007.

The Joint Commission. *Comprehensive Accreditation Manual for Hospitals: The Official Handbook.* Standard MM.2.10. 2007.

The Joint Commission. *Comprehensive Accreditation Manual for Hospitals: The Official Handbook.* Standard MM.3.10. 2007.

The Joint Commission. *Comprehensive Accreditation Manual for Hospitals: The Official Handbook.* Standard MM.4.10. 2007.

The Joint Commission. *Comprehensive Accreditation Manual for Hospitals: The Official Handbook.* Standard MM.4.20. 2007.

The Joint Commission. *Comprehensive Accreditation Manual for Hospitals: The Official Handbook.* Standard MM.5.10. 2007.

The Joint Commission. *Comprehensive Accreditation Manual for Hospitals: The Official Handbook.* Standard MM.6.10. 2007.

The Joint Commission. *Comprehensive Accreditation Manual for Hospitals: The Official Handbook.* Standard MM.6.20. 2007.

Taylor, C., et al. *Fundamentals of Nursing: The Art and Science of Nursing Care,* 6th ed. Philadelphia: Lippincott Williams & Wilkins, 2008.

Wynaden, D. "Establishing Best Practice Guidelines for Administration of Intramuscular Injections in the Adult: A Systematic Review of the Literature," *Contemporary Nurse* 20(2):267-77, December 2005.

Intraosseous infusion

When rapid venous infusion is difficult or impossible, intraosseous infusion allows delivery of fluids, medications, or whole blood into the bone marrow. Most commonly performed on infants and children, this technique is used in such emergencies as cardiopulmonary arrest, circulatory collapse, hypokalemia from traumatic injury or dehydration, status epilepticus, status asthmaticus, burns, near-drowning, and overwhelming sepsis.

Any drug that can be given I.V. can be given by intraosseous infusion with comparable absorption and effectiveness. Intraosseous infusion has been used as an acceptable alternative for infants and children.

Intraosseous infusion is commonly undertaken at the anterior surface of the tibia. Alternative sites include the iliac crest, spinous process and, rarely, the upper anterior portion of the sternum. Intraosseous infusion can only be performed by trained personnel. This is usually a physician, but may be a specially trained nurse. (See *Understanding intraosseous infusion.*)

This procedure is contraindicated in patients with osteogenesis imperfecta, osteopetrosis, and ipsilateral fracture because of the potential for subcutaneous extravasation. Infusion through an area with cellulitis or an infected burn increases the risk of infection.

Understanding intraosseous infusion

During intraosseous infusion, the bone marrow serves as a noncollapsible vein; thus, fluid infused into the marrow cavity rapidly enters the circulation by way of an extensive network of venous sinusoids. Here, the needle is shown positioned in the patient's tibia.

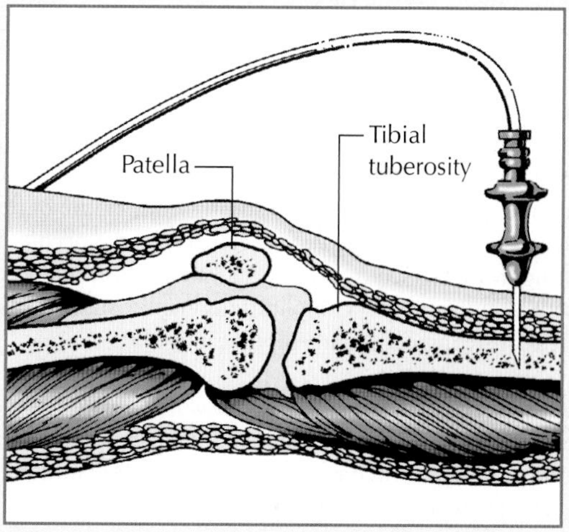

Equipment

Bone marrow biopsy needle or specially designed intraosseous infusion needle (cannula and obturator) ▪ antiseptic skin pads ▪ sterile gauze pads ▪ sterile gloves ▪ sterile drape ▪ bone marrow set ▪ heparin flush solution ▪ I.V. fluids and tubing ▪ 1% lidocaine ▪ 3- or 5-ml syringe ▪ tape ▪ two 5-ml syringes.

Preparation of equipment

Prepare I.V. fluids and tubing as ordered. Label all medications, medication containers, and other solutions on and off the sterile field.

Implementation

- Confirm the patient's identity using two patient identifiers according to your facility's policy.
- If the patient is conscious, explain the procedure *to allay his fears and promote his cooperation.* Make sure that patient or responsible family member understands procedure and signs a consent form.
- If your facility uses a bar code scanning system, be sure to scan your ID badge, the patient's ID bracelet, and the medication's bar code.
- Check the patient's history for hypersensitivity to the local anesthetic. If the patient isn't an infant, tell him which bone site will be infused. Inform him that he will receive a local anesthetic and will feel pressure from needle insertion.
- Wash your hands.
- Provide a sedative, if ordered, before the procedure.
- Position the patient based on the selected puncture site.
- Using sterile technique, the practitioner cleans the puncture site with an antiseptic pad and allows it to dry. He then covers the area with a sterile drape.
- Using sterile technique, hand the practitioner the 3- or 5-ml syringe with 1% lidocaine *so that he can anesthetize the infusion site.*
- The practitioner inserts the infusion needle through the skin and into the bone at an angle of 10 to 15 degrees from vertical. He advances it with a forward and backward rotary motion through the periosteum until it penetrates the marrow cavity. The needle should "give" suddenly as it enters the marrow and stand erect when released.
- Then the practitioner removes the obturator from the needle and attaches a 5-ml syringe. He aspirates some bone marrow *to confirm needle placement.*
- The practitioner replaces this syringe with a syringe containing 5 ml of heparin flush solution and flushes the cannula *to confirm needle placement and clear the cannula of clots and bone particles.*
- Next, the practitioner removes the syringe of flush solution and attaches I.V. tubing to the cannula *to allow infusion of medications and I.V. fluids.*
- Put on sterile gloves.
- Clean the infusion site with antiseptic pads, and then secure the site with tape and a sterile gauze dressing.
- Monitor vital signs, and check the infusion site for bleeding and extravasation.

Special considerations

- Facility policy may vary as to securing the site and dressing materials used. Some facilities may use transport dressings. Check your facility's policy and procedure manual.

- Intraosseous infusion should be discontinued as soon as conventional vascular access is established (within 2 to 4 hours, if possible). *Prolonged infusion significantly increases the risk of infection.*
- After the needle has been removed, place a sterile dressing over the injection site, and apply firm pressure to the site for 5 minutes.
- Intraosseous flow rates are determined by needle size and flow through the bone marrow. Fluids should flow freely if needle placement is correct. Normal saline solution has been given intraosseously at a rate of 600 ml/minute and up to 2,500 ml/hour when delivered under pressure of 300 mm Hg through a 13G needle.

Complications

Common complications include extravasation of fluid into subcutaneous tissue, resulting from incorrect needle placement; subperiosteal effusion, resulting from failure of fluid to enter the marrow space; and clotting in the needle, resulting from delayed infusion or failure to flush the needle after placement. Other complications include subcutaneous abscess, osteomyelitis, and epiphyseal injury.

Documentation

Record the time, date, location, and the patient's tolerance of the procedure. Document the amount of fluid infused on the intake and output record.

SELECTED REFERENCES

American Heart Association. "AHA Guidelines for Cardiopulmonary Resuscitation and Emergency Cardiovascular Care of Pediatric and Neonatal Patients: Pediatric Advanced Life Support." Available at *http://circ.ahajournals.org/content/vol112/24_suppl/.*

Buck, M. "Intraosseous Administration of Drugs in Infants and Children," *Pediatric Pharmacology* 12(12), December 2006.

DeBoer, S., et al. "Intraosseous Infusion: Not Just for Kids Anymore," *Emergency Medical Service* 34(3):54, 56-63, March 2005.

Fiorito, B.A., et al. "Intraosseous Access in the Setting of Pediatric Critical Care Transport," *Pediatric Critical Care Medicine* 6(1):505-503, January 2005.

Koschel, M.J. "Sternal Intraosseous Infusion: Emergency Vascular Access in Adults," *AJN* 105(1):66-68, January 2005.

Smith, R., et al. "The Utilisation of Intraosseous Infusion in the Resuscitation of Paediatric Major Trauma Patients," *Injury* 36(9):1034-1038, September 2005.

"Standard 63. Intraosseous Access Devices. Infusion Nursing Standards of Practice," *Journal of Infusion Nursing* 29(1S):S67-68, January-February 2006.

DRUG INFUSION THROUGH A SECONDARY I.V. LINE

A secondary I.V. line is a complete I.V. set—container, tubing, and microdrip or macrodrip system—connected to the lower Y-port (secondary port) of a primary line instead of to the I.V. catheter or needle. It can be used for continuous or intermittent drug infusion. When used continuously, a secondary I.V. line permits drug infusion and titration while the primary line maintains a constant total infusion rate.

When used intermittently, a secondary I.V. line is commonly called a *piggyback set.* In this case, the primary line maintains venous access between drug doses. Typically, a piggyback set includes a small I.V. container, short tubing, and a macrodrip system. This set connects to the primary line's upper Y-port, also called a piggyback port. Antibiotics are most commonly administered by intermittent (piggyback) infusion. To make this set work, the primary I.V. container must be positioned below the piggyback container. (The manufacturer provides an extension hook for this purpose.)

Most drugs can be piggybacked with a needle-free system, which consists of a blunt-tipped plastic insertion device and a rubber injection port. The port may be part of a special administration set or an adapter for existing administration sets. The rubber injection port has a preestablished slit that can open and reseal immediately. The needle-free system reduces the risk of accidental needle-stick injuries. I.V. pumps may be used to maintain constant infusion rates, especially with a drug such as lidocaine. A pump allows more accurate titration of drug dosage and helps maintain venous access.

Equipment

Patient's medication record and chart ▪ prescribed I.V. medication ▪ prescribed I.V. solution ▪ administration set with secondary injection port ▪ needleless adapter ▪ alcohol pads ▪ 1″ adhesive tape ▪ time tape ▪ labels ▪ infusion pump ▪ extension hook and appropriate solution for intermittent piggyback infusion ▪ optional: normal saline solution for infusion with incompatible solutions, sterile I.V. plug.

For intermittent infusion, the primary line typically has a piggyback port with a backcheck valve that stops the flow from the primary line during drug infusion and returns to the primary flow after infusion. A volume-control set can also be used with an intermittent infusion line. (For more information, see "Volume-control sets," page 348.)

Preparation of equipment

Verify the order on the patient's medication record by checking it against the practitioner's order. Wash your hands. Inspect the I.V. container for cracks, leaks, and contamination, and check drug compatibility with the primary solution. Verify the expiration date. Check to see whether the primary line has a secondary injection port. If it doesn't and the medication is to be given regularly, replace the I.V. set with one that has a secondary injection port.

If necessary, add the drug to the secondary I.V. solution. To do so, remove any seals from the secondary container, and wipe the main port with an alcohol pad. Inject the prescribed medication, and gently agitate the solution to mix the medication thoroughly. Properly label the I.V. mixture. Insert the administration set spike, and attach the needleless adapter. Open the flow clamp and prime the line. Then close the flow clamp.

Some medications are available in vials that are suitable for hanging directly on an I.V. pole. Instead of preparing medication and injecting it into a container, you can inject diluent directly into the medication vial. Then you can spike the vial, prime the tubing, and hang the set, as directed.

Implementation

- Confirm the patient's identity using two patient identifiers according to your facility's policy.
- If your facility uses a bar code scanning system, be sure to scan your ID badge, the patient's ID bracelet, and the medication's bar code.
- Assess the patient's I.V. site for pain, redness, swelling, and patency. If the I.V. shows signs of infiltration or phlebitis, remove it, and insert another I.V. catheter in a new site.
- If the drug is incompatible with the primary I.V. solution, replace the primary solution with a fluid that's compatible with both solutions, such as normal saline solution, and flush the line before starting the drug infusion. Many facility protocols require that the primary I.V. solution be removed and that a sterile I.V. plug be inserted into the container until it's ready to be rehung. *This maintains the sterility of the solution and prevents someone else from inadvertently restarting the incompatible solution before the line is flushed with normal saline solution.*
- Hang the secondary set's container, and wipe the injection port of the primary line with an alcohol pad.
- Insert the needleless adapter from the secondary line into the injection port, and secure it to the primary line.
- To run the secondary set's container by itself, lower the primary set's container with an extension hook. To run both containers simultaneously, place them at the same height. (See *Assembling a piggyback set.*)
- Open the clamp and adjust the drip rate. For continuous infusion, set the secondary solution to the desired drip rate; then adjust the primary solution *to achieve the desired total infusion rate.*

EQUIPMENT

Assembling a piggyback set

A piggyback set is useful for intermittent drug infusion. To work properly, the secondary set's container must be positioned higher than the primary set's container.

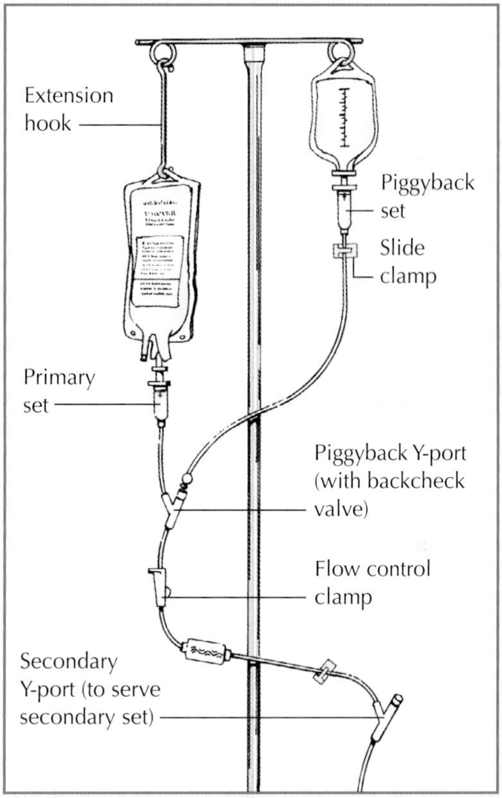

- For intermittent infusion, adjust the primary drip rate, as required, on completion of the secondary solution. If the secondary solution tubing is being reused, close the clamp on the tubing, and follow your facility's policy: Either remove the needleless adapter and replace it with a new one, or leave it securely taped in the injection port and label it with the time it was first used. In this case, also leave the empty container in place until you replace it with a new dose of medication at the prescribed time. If the tubing won't be reused, discard it appropriately with the I.V. container.

Special considerations

- If policy allows, use a pump for drug infusion. Put a time tape on the secondary container *to help prevent an inaccurate administration rate.*
- When reusing secondary tubing, change it according to your facility's policy, usually every 96 hours. Similarly, inspect the injection port for leakage with each use, and change it more often if needed.
- Unless you're piggybacking lipids, don't piggyback a secondary I.V. line to a total parenteral nutrition line *because of the risk of contamination.* Check your facility's policy for possible exceptions.

Complications

The patient may experience an adverse reaction to the infused drug. In addition, repeated punctures of the secondary injection port can damage the seal, possibly allowing leakage or contamination.

Documentation

Record the amount and type of drug and the amount of I.V. solution on the intake and output and medication records. Note the date, duration and rate of infusion, and patient's response, where applicable.

Selected references

Centers for Disease Control and Prevention. "Guidelines for the Prevention of Intravascular Device-Related Infections," *MMWR* 51(RR10):1-26, August 2002.

Fields, M., and Peterman, J. "Intravenous Medication Safety System Averts High Risk Medication Errors and Provides Actionable Data," *Nursing Administration Quarterly* 29(1):78-87, January-March 2005.

The Joint Commission. *Comprehensive Accreditation Manual for Hospitals: The Official Handbook.* Standard MM.1.10. 2007.

The Joint Commission. *Comprehensive Accreditation Manual for Hospitals: The Official Handbook.* Standard MM.3.10. 2007.

The Joint Commission. *Comprehensive Accreditation Manual for Hospitals: The Official Handbook.* Standard MM.4.10. 2007.

The Joint Commission. *Comprehensive Accreditation Manual for Hospitals: The Official Handbook.* Standard MM.4.20. 2007.

The Joint Commission. *Comprehensive Accreditation Manual for Hospitals: The Official Handbook.* Standard MM.4.30. 2007.

The Joint Commission. *Comprehensive Accreditation Manual for Hospitals: The Official Handbook.* Standard MM.5.10. 2007.

"Standard 29. Add-on Devices and Junction Securement. Infusion Nursing Standards of Practice," *Journal of Infusion Nursing* 29(1S):S32, January-February 2006.

"Standard 48. Administration Set Change-Primary and Secondary Continuous. Infusion Nursing Standards of Practice," *Journal of Infusion Nursing* 29(1S):S48, January-February 2006.

Drug administration through an intermittent infusion device

An intermittent infusion injection device, or saline lock, eliminates the need for multiple venipunctures or for maintaining venous access with a continuous I.V. infusion. This device allows intermittent administration by infusion or by the I.V. bolus injection method.

Dilute heparin or saline solutions are typically injected as the final step in this procedure to prevent clotting in the device. When heparin is used, the device must be flushed with normal saline solution before and after the prescribed medication is administered in case the heparin and the medication are incompatible. The device may then be reflushed with the heparin flush solution.

Equipment

Patient's medication record and chart ▪ gloves ▪ alcohol pads ▪ three 3-ml syringes with needleless adapter ▪ normal saline solution ▪ extra intermittent infusion device ▪ prescribed medication in an I.V. container with administration set and needle (for infusion) or in a syringe with needle (for I.V. bolus or push) ▪ tourniquet ▪ tape ▪ optional: dilute heparin solution, sterile bacteriostatic water.

The concentration of dilute heparin solution ranges from 10 to 100 units/ml. The solution is available in a cartridge-injection system in doses of 10 to 100 units/ml. If this system is used, substitute its syringe for the 3-ml syringe and the heparin cartridge for the heparin solution. Normal saline solution is available in a similar cartridge system.

Preparation of equipment

Verify the order on the patient's medication record by checking it against the practitioner's order. Wash your hands, and then wipe the tops of the normal saline solution, heparin flush solution, and medication containers with alcohol pads. Fill two of the 3-ml syringes (bearing 22G needles) with normal saline solution; if required by facility policy, draw 1 ml of heparin flush solution into the third syringe. If you'll be infusing medication, insert the administration set spike into the I.V. container, attach the needleless adapter, and prime the line. If you'll be giving an I.V. injection, fill a syringe with the prescribed medication.

Implementation

■ Confirm the patient's identity using two patient identifiers according to your facility's policy. Explain the procedure.
■ If your facility uses a bar code scanning system, be sure to scan your ID badge, the patient's ID bracelet, and the medication's bar code.
■ Put on gloves.
■ Assess the patient's I.V. site for redness, swelling, or pain. If necessary, remove the intermittent infusion device, and insert a new device in a new location.
■ Wipe the injection port of the intermittent infusion device with an alcohol pad, and insert the needleless adapter of a saline-filled syringe.
■ Aspirate the syringe and observe for blood *to verify the patency of the device.* If none appears, apply a tourniquet slightly above the site, keep it in place for about 1 minute, and then aspirate again. If blood still doesn't appear, remove the tourniquet and inject the normal saline solution slowly.
NURSING ALERT *Stop the injection immediately if you feel any resistance* because resistance indicates that the device is occluded. *If this occurs, insert a new saline lock.*
■ If you feel no resistance, watch for signs of infiltration (puffiness or pain at the site) as you slowly inject the saline solution. If these signs occur, insert a new intermittent infusion device.
■ If blood is aspirated, slowly inject the saline solution and observe for signs of infiltration. *The saline solution flushes out any residual heparin solution that might be incompatible with the medication.*
■ Withdraw the saline syringe and needleless adapter.

EQUIPMENT

Using a needleless system for intermittent infusions

You can use a needleless I.V. system, such as the CLAVE Needleless Connector (shown below), to administer intermittent infusion medication when you need to convert an I.V. line to a saline lock. To make the conversion:
■ clamp the I.V. tubing and remove the administration set from the catheter or needle hub
■ connect the adapter
■ inject the remaining dilute heparin or saline solution to fill the line and prevent clot formation.

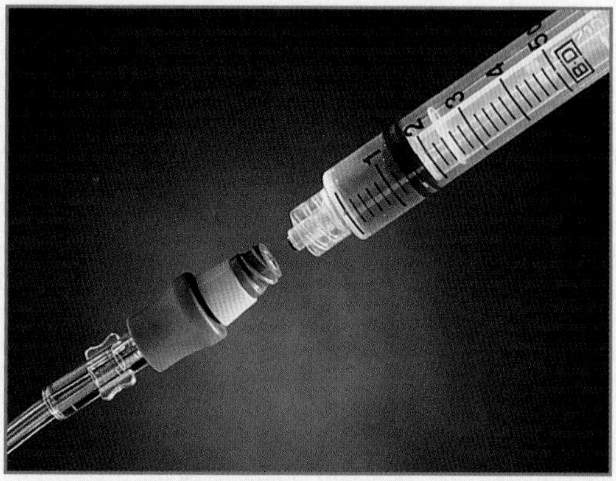

Administering I.V. bolus injections

■ Insert the needleless adapter and syringe with the medication for the I.V. bolus injection into the injection port of the device.
■ Inject the medication at the required rate. Then remove the needleless adapter and syringe from the injection port.
■ Insert the needleless adapter of the remaining saline-filled syringe into the injection port, and slowly inject the saline solution *to flush all medication through the device.*
■ Remove the needleless adapter and syringe, and insert and inject the heparin (or saline) flush solution *to prevent clotting in the device.*

Administering an infusion

■ Insert and secure the needleless adapter attached to the administration set.
■ Open the infusion line, and adjust the flow rate as necessary.
■ Infuse medication for the prescribed length of time; then flush the device with normal saline solution and heparin flush solution, as you would after a bolus or push injection, according to your facility's policy.
■ To administer fluids and drugs simultaneously or to administer a medication incompatible with the primary I.V. solution, you may want to use a needleless adapter. (See *Using a needleless system for intermittent infusions.*)

Special considerations

■ If you're giving a bolus injection of a drug that's *incompatible* with saline solution, such as diazepam, flush the device with bacteriostatic water.
■ Some facilities use diluted heparin solution (10 to 100 units/ml) *to prevent clotting in the cannula.* Others use 2 to 3 ml of normal saline solution or some other solution or dilution. Check your facility's policy.
■ Intermittent infusion devices should be changed regularly (usually every 72 hours), according to standard precautions guidelines and your facility's policy.

■ If you can't rotate injection sites because the patient has fragile veins, document this fact.

Complications

Infiltration and a specific reaction to the infused medication are the most common complications.

Documentation

Record the type and amount of drug administered and times of administration. Include all I.V. solutions used to dilute the medication and flush the line on the intake record. Also document the use of dilute heparin solution.

SELECTED REFERENCES

Centers for Disease Control and Prevention. "Guidelines for Prevention of Intravascular Catheter-Related Infections," *MMWR* 55(RR-1):1-26, August 2002.

Fields, M., and Peterman, J. "Intravenous Medication Safety System Averts High Risk Medication Errors and Provides Actionable Data," *Nursing Administration Quarterly* 29(1):78-87, January-March 2005.

The Joint Commission. *Comprehensive Accreditation Manual for Hospitals: The Official Handbook.* Standard MM.1.10. 2007.

The Joint Commission. *Comprehensive Accreditation Manual for Hospitals: The Official Handbook.* Standard MM.2.10. 2007.

The Joint Commission. *Comprehensive Accreditation Manual for Hospitals: The Official Handbook.* Standard MM.3.10. 2007.

The Joint Commission. *Comprehensive Accreditation Manual for Hospitals: The Official Handbook.* Standard MM.4.10. 2007.

The Joint Commission. *Comprehensive Accreditation Manual for Hospitals: The Official Handbook.* Standard MM.4.20. 2007.

The Joint Commission. *Comprehensive Accreditation Manual for Hospitals: The Official Handbook.* Standard MM.5.10. 2007.

The Joint Commission. *Comprehensive Accreditation Manual for Hospitals: The Official Handbook.* Standard MM.6.10. 2007.

The Joint Commission. *Comprehensive Accreditation Manual for Hospitals: The Official Handbook.* Standard MM.6.20. 2007.

The Joint Commission. *Comprehensive Accreditation Manual for Hospitals: The Official Handbook.* Standard MM.7.10. 2007.

Paparella, S. "Avoiding Disastrous Outcomes with Rapid Intravenous Push Medications," *Journal of Emergency Nursing* 30(5):478-80, October 2004.

"Standard 49. Catheter Removal. Infusion Nursing Standards of Practice," *Journal of Infusion Nursing* 29(1S):S51-S55, January-February 2006.

I.V. BOLUS INJECTION

The I.V. bolus injection method allows rapid drug administration. It can be used in an emergency to provide an immediate drug effect. It can also be used to administer drugs that can't be given I.M., to achieve peak drug levels in the bloodstream, and to deliver drugs that can't be diluted, such as diazepam, digoxin, and phenytoin. The term bolus usually refers to the concentration or amount of a drug. I.V. push is a technique for rapid I.V. injection.

Bolus doses of medication may be injected directly through an existing I.V. line, or through an implanted vascular access port (VAP). The medication administered by these methods usually takes effect rapidly, so the patient must be monitored for an adverse reaction, such as cardiac arrhythmia and anaphylaxis. I.V. bolus injections are contraindicated when rapid drug administration could cause life-threatening complications. For certain drugs, the safe rate of injection is specified by the manufacturer.

Equipment

Patient's medication record and chart ■ gloves ■ prescribed medication ■ syringe and needleless adaptor ■ diluent, if needed ■ tourniquet ■ antiseptic swab ■ tape ■ optional: second syringe (and needleless adapter) filled with normal saline solution.

A useful dosage form is the ready injectable. (See *Using a ready injectable.*)

Preparation of equipment

Verify the order on the patient's medication record by checking it against the practitioner's order. Know the actions, adverse effects, and administration rate of the medication to be injected. Draw up the prescribed medication in the syringe, and dilute it if necessary.

Implementation

■ Confirm the patient's identity using two patient identifiers according to your facility's policy, wash your hands, put on gloves, and explain the procedure.

■ If your facility uses a bar code scanning system, be sure to scan your ID badge, the patient's ID bracelet, and the medication's bar code.

Giving injections through an existing I.V. line

■ Check the compatibility of the medication with the I.V. solution.

■ Close the flow clamp, wipe the injection port with an antiseptic swab, and inject the medication. (Some I.V. lines have a secondary injection port or a T-connector; others have a needleless adapter or latex cap at the end of the I.V. tubing where the blunt-tipped administration device is attached.)

- Open the flow clamp and readjust the flow rate.
- If the drug isn't compatible with the I.V. solution, flush the line with normal saline solution before and after the injection. (For additional information, see "Intermittent infusion device insertion," page 360.)

Giving a bolus injection through a VAP

- Wash your hands, put on gloves, and clean the injection site with an alcohol or an antiseptic pad, starting at the center of the port and working outward in a circular motion over a 4″ to 5″ (10- to 12.7-cm) diameter. Do this three times.
- Palpate the area over the port *to locate the port septum.*
- Anchor the port between the thumb and first two fingers of your nondominant hand. Then, using your dominant hand, insert the needle into the appropriate area of the device and deliver the injection. (See "Vascular access device use," page 380.)

Special considerations

- *Because drugs administered by I.V. bolus or push injections are delivered directly into the circulatory system and can produce an immediate effect,* an acute allergic reaction or anaphylaxis can develop rapidly. If signs of anaphylaxis (dyspnea, cyanosis, seizures, and increasing respiratory distress) occur, notify the practitioner immediately, and begin emergency procedures, as necessary. Also watch for signs of extravasation (redness, swelling). If extravasation occurs, stop the injection, estimate the amount of infiltration, and notify the practitioner.
- If you're giving diazepam or chlordiazepoxide, flush the line with normal saline solution *to prevent drug precipitation resulting from incompatibility.*

Complications

Excessively rapid administration may cause adverse effects, depending on the medication administered.

Documentation

Record the amount and type of drug administered, time of injection, appearance of the site, duration of administration, and patient's tolerance of the procedure. Also note the drug's effect and any adverse reactions.

EQUIPMENT

Using a ready injectable

A commercially premeasured medication package with a syringe and needle, the ready injectable allows for rapid drug administration in an emergency. Preparing a ready injectable usually takes only 15 to 20 seconds. Other advantages include the reduced risk of breaking sterile technique during administration and the easy identification of medication and dose.

When giving commercially prefilled syringe, be sure to give the precise dose prescribed. For example, if a 50-mg/ml cartridge is supplied but the patient's prescribed dose is 25 mg, you must administer only 0.5 ml — half of the volume contained in the cartridge. Be alert for potential medication errors whenever dispensing medications in premeasured dosage forms.

Selected references

Hatcher, I., et al. "An Intravenous Medication Safety System: Preventing High-Risk Medication Errors at the Point of Care," *Journal of Nursing Administration* 34(10):437-39, October 2004.

The Joint Commission. *Comprehensive Accreditation Manual for Hospitals: The Official Handbook.* Standard MM.1.10. 2007.

The Joint Commission. *Comprehensive Accreditation Manual for Hospitals: The Official Handbook.* Standard MM.2.10. 2007.

The Joint Commission. *Comprehensive Accreditation Manual for Hospitals: The Official Handbook.* Standard MM.3.10. 2007.

The Joint Commission. *Comprehensive Accreditation Manual for Hospitals: The Official Handbook.* Standard MM.4.10. 2007.

The Joint Commission. *Comprehensive Accreditation Manual for Hospitals: The Official Handbook.* Standard MM.4.20. 2007.

The Joint Commission. *Comprehensive Accreditation Manual for Hospitals: The Official Handbook.* Standard MM.5.10. 2007.

The Joint Commission. *Comprehensive Accreditation Manual for Hospitals: The Official Handbook.* Standard MM.6.10. 2007.

The Joint Commission. *Comprehensive Accreditation Manual for Hospitals: The Official Handbook.* Standard MM.6.20. 2007.

The Joint Commission. *Comprehensive Accreditation Manual for Hospitals: The Official Handbook.* Standard MM.7.10. 2007.

Paparella, S. "Avoiding Disastrous Outcomes with Rapid Intravenous Push Medications," *Journal of Emergency Nursing* 30(5):478-80, October 2004.

"Standard 68. Parenteral Medication and Solution Administration. Infusion Nursing Standards of Practice," *Journal of Infusion Nursing* 29(1S):S74-S75, January-February 2006.

PATIENT-CONTROLLED ANALGESIA

Patient-controlled analgesia (PCA) is a drug delivery system providing I.V. analgesia, usually morphine, when the patient presses a call button at the end of a cord. Analgesia is provided at the level and time needed by the patient. The device prevents the patient from accidentally overdosing by imposing a lockout time between dose — usually 6 to 10 minutes. During this interval, the patient won't receive any analgesic, even if he pushes the button.

PCA is advantageous because it eliminates the need for I.M. analgesics. The pain relief is tailored to each patient's size and pain tolerance. PCA also provides the patient with a sense of control over pain and allows the patient to sleep at night with minimal daytime drowsiness. Additionally, postoperative deep breathing, coughing, and ambulation are improved, and opioid use is reduced when compared with those patients who don't receive PCA.

PCA is typically given to trauma patients postoperatively and to terminal cancer patients and others with chronic diseases. To receive PCA therapy, patients must be mentally alert and able to understand and comply with instructions and procedures. Additionally, patients should have no history of allergy to the analgesic. PCA therapy is contraindicated in patients with limited respiratory reserve, a history of drug abuse or chronic sedative or tranquilizer use, or a psychiatric disorder.

Equipment

PCA system and system specific tubing ▪ syringe with prescribed medication ▪ alcohol pads ▪ compatible I.V. solution if necessary ▪ clean gloves ▪ tape.

Preparation of equipment

Follow the manufacturer's instructions for setting up the device. Numerous types of devices are available. Obtain the medication, and verify the medication order with the practitioner's order. Gather the equipment, and bring it to the patient's bedside. Plug the PCA device into an electrical outlet. If the device is battery-operated, check to make sure that the battery is fully charged and working.

Wash your hands thoroughly. Connect device tubing to the medication syringe, and insert the syringe into the device. Make sure that the markings and labels on the syringe are readily visible. Prime the tubing to remove air from the system *to reduce the risk of an air embolism.*

Implementation

- Confirm the patient's identity using two patient identifiers according to your facility's policy.
- Provide privacy, and explain the procedure to the patient.
- Obtain baseline blood pressure, heart rate, and respiratory rate.
- Put on gloves.
- Assess the patient's I.V. access site. If the patient doesn't have I.V. access, start an I.V. line according to facility policy. Ensure the patency of the I.V. line.
- Wipe the connection port on the patient's I.V. line with an alcohol pad and then connect the PCA tubing to the patient's I.V. line or I.V. access device. Secure the connection with tape, if necessary.
- Program the device to deliver the prescribed parameters, such as loading dose, basal rate, bolus amount, and time lockout for boluses. Have a second nurse confirm these settings *to prevent possible errors.*
- Adjust the prescribed I.V. solution flow rate, if appropriate.
- Label the PCA pump, PCA tubing, and I.V. infusion tubing.
- Instruct the patient to push the button each time he has pain and needs relief.
- Monitor vital signs frequently during the initial loading dose and every 1 to 2 hours throughout therapy. Be aware of the amount the patient will receive when he activates the device and the maximum amount the patient can receive within a specified time (if an adjustable device is used). Have naloxone readily available *in case the patient develops respiratory depression from the drug.*
- Inspect the infusion site for changes; check the device function — including rate — periodically.
- Replace the medication syringe when empty.
- Remove gloves and discard used equipment appropriately.

Special considerations

- Encourage the patient to cough and deep breathe to promote ventilation.
- Monitor the I.V. insertion site for infiltration into the subcutaneous tissues and for catheter occlusion, *which may cause the drug to back up in the primary I.V. tubing.*
- If the analgesic nauseates the patient, administer an antiemetic as ordered.
- Assess the patient's pain using a pain rating scale before therapy and then periodically during therapy. Notify the practitioner if the patient's pain isn't being relieved.
- Before initiating PCA therapy, be sure to teach the patient how the device works. Allow the patient to practice with a sample device. Reinforce to the patient that he should

take enough analgesic to relieve acute pain but not enough to make him feel drowsy.

Complications

Respiratory depression may occur secondary to drug being administered. As with any I.V. infusion, I.V. infiltration is a risk.

Documentation

Record the date and time of PCA therapy initiation, the I.V. access device used and its location, baseline vital signs and pain assessment, medication doses (loading dose, individual doses, and time interval), and ongoing assessments of vital signs, pain, and I.V. site. Also document the patient's understanding and tolerance of the procedure and any patient teaching performed.

SELECTED REFERENCES

The Joint Commission. *Comprehensive Accreditation Manual for Hospitals: The Official Handbook.* Standard MM.1.10. 2007.

The Joint Commission. *Comprehensive Accreditation Manual for Hospitals: The Official Handbook.* Standard MM.2.10. 2007.

The Joint Commission. *Comprehensive Accreditation Manual for Hospitals: The Official Handbook.* Standard MM.3.10. 2007.

The Joint Commission. *Comprehensive Accreditation Manual for Hospitals: The Official Handbook.* Standard MM.4.10. 2007.

The Joint Commission. *Comprehensive Accreditation Manual for Hospitals: The Official Handbook.* Standard MM.4.20. 2007.

The Joint Commission. *Comprehensive Accreditation Manual for Hospitals: The Official Handbook.* Standard MM.5.10. 2007.

The Joint Commission. *Comprehensive Accreditation Manual for Hospitals: The Official Handbook.* Standard MM.6.10. 2007.

The Joint Commission. *Comprehensive Accreditation Manual for Hospitals: The Official Handbook.* Standard MM.6.20. 2007.

The Joint Commission. *Comprehensive Accreditation Manual for Hospitals: The Official Handbook.* Standard MM.7.10. 2007.

Pasero, C., and McCaffery, M. "Pain Control: Authorized and Unauthorized Use of PCA Pumps: Clarifying the Use of Patient-Controlled Analgesia, in Light of Recent Alerts," *AJN* 105(7):30-32, July 2005.

"Standard 67. Patient-Controlled Analgesia. Infusion Nursing Standards of Practice," *Journal of Infusion Nursing* 29(1S):S73, January-February 2006.

Weir, V.L. "Best-Practice Protocols: Preventing Adverse Drug Events," *Nursing Mangement* 36(9):24-30, September 2005.

Wuhrman, E., et al. "Authorized and Unauthorized ("PCA by Proxy") Dosing of Analgesic Infusion Pumps: Position Statement with Clinical Practice Recommendations," *Pain Management Nursing* 8(1):4-11, March 2007.

CHEMOTHERAPEUTIC DRUG PREPARATION AND HANDLING

When preparing chemotherapeutic drugs, take extra care, both for the patient's safety and for your own. Patients who receive chemotherapeutic drugs risk teratogenic, mutagenic, and carcinogenic effects, but the people who prepare and handle the drugs are at risk as well. Although the danger from handling these drugs hasn't been fully determined, chemotherapeutic drugs can increase the handler's risk of reproductive abnormalities. These drugs also pose environmental threats, and the best method for handling them hasn't been determined.

The Occupational Safety and Health Administration (OSHA) has set down guidelines for handling chemotherapeutic drugs. Although these guidelines are simply recommendations, adhering to them will help ensure both your safety and that of your environment.

The OSHA guidelines outline two basic requirements. The first is that all health care workers who handle chemotherapeutic drugs must be educated and trained. A key element of such training involves learning how to reduce your exposure when handling the drugs. The second requirement states that the drugs should be prepared in a class II biological safety cabinet. If one isn't available, OSHA recommends that a respirator be worn while mixing the drugs.

OSHA guidelines recommend that chemotherapeutic drugs be mixed in a properly enclosed and ventilated work area and that respiratory and skin protection be worn. Smoking, drinking, applying cosmetics, and eating where these drugs are prepared, stored, or used should be strictly prohibited, and sterile technique should be used while mixing the drugs.

Gloves, gowns, syringes or vials, and other materials that have been used in chemotherapy preparation and administration present a possible source of exposure or injury to the facility's staff, patients, and visitors. Therefore, use of properly labeled, sealed, and covered containers, handled only by trained and protected personnel, should be routine practice. Spills also represent a hazard, and all employees should be familiar with appropriate spill procedures for their own protection.

Equipment

Prescribed drug or drugs ▪ patient's medication record and chart ▪ long-sleeved gown ▪ latex surgical gloves ▪ face shield or goggles ■ plastic absorbent pad ■ alcohol pads ■ sterile gauze pads ■ shoe covers ■ impervious container with the label CAUTION: BIOHAZARD for the disposal of any unused drug or equipment ■ I.V. solution ■ diluent (if necessary) ■ medication labels ■ class II biological safety cabinet ■ disposable towel ■ 70% alcohol ■ hydrophobic filter ■ 18G needle ■ syringes and needles of various sizes ■ I.V. tubing with luer-lock fittings ■ chemotherapy HAZARD labels ■ soap ■ I.V. pump.

Have a chemotherapeutic spill kit available that includes water-resistant, nonpermeable, long-sleeved gown with cuffs and back closure ■ shoe covers ■ two pairs of latex gloves (for double gloving) ■ goggles ■ mask ■ disposable dustpan ■ plastic scraper (for collecting broken glass) ■ plastic-backed or absorbable towels ■ container of desiccant powder or granules (to absorb wet contents) ■ two disposable pads ■ punctureproof, leakproof container labeled BIOHAZARD WASTE ■ container of 70% alcohol for cleaning the spill area.

Implementation

■ Remember to wash your hands before and after drug preparation and administration.

■ Prepare the drugs in a class II biological safety cabinet.

■ Wear protective garments (such as a long-sleeved gown, gloves, and a face shield or goggles), as indicated by your facility's policy. Don't wear the garments outside the preparation area.

■ Before you prepare the drug (and after you finish), clean the internal surfaces of the cabinet with 70% alcohol and a disposable towel. Discard the towel in a leakproof chemical waste container.

■ Cover the work surface with a clean plastic absorbent pad *to minimize contamination by droplets or spills.* Change the pad at the end of the shift or whenever a spill occurs.

■ Consider all the equipment used in drug preparation as well as any unused drug as hazardous waste. Dispose of them according to your facility's policy.

■ Place all chemotherapeutic waste products in labeled, leakproof, sealable plastic bags or other appropriate impervious containers.

■ Prepare the drugs in accordance with current product instructions, paying attention to compatibility, stability, and reconstitution technique.

■ If a hood isn't available, prepare drugs in a well-ventilated work space, away from heating or cooling vents and other personnel. Vent vials with a hydrophobic filter, or use negative-pressure techniques. Also, use a needle with a hydrophobic filter to remove solution from a vial. To break an ampule, wrap a sterile gauze pad or alcohol pad around the neck of the ampule *to reduce the contamination risk.*

Special considerations

■ Take precautions to reduce your exposure to chemotherapeutic drugs. Systemic absorption can occur through ingestion of contaminated materials, skin contact, and inhalation. You can inhale a drug without realizing it, such as while opening a vial, clipping a needle, expelling air from a syringe, or discarding excess drug. You can also absorb a drug from handling contaminated stools or body fluids.

■ *For maximum protection,* mix all chemotherapeutic drugs in an approved class II biological safety cabinet. Also, prime all I.V. bags that contain chemotherapeutic drugs under the hood. Leave the hood blower on 24 hours per day, 7 days per week.

■ Make sure the biological safety cabinet is examined every 6 months, or any time the cabinet is moved, by a company specifically qualified to perform this work. If the cabinet passes certification, the certifying company will affix a sticker to the cabinet attesting to its approval.

■ Use only syringes and I.V. sets that have luer-lock fittings. Label all chemotherapeutic drugs with a CHEMOTHERAPY HAZARD label.

■ Don't clip needles, break syringes, or remove the needles from syringes. Use a gauze pad when removing syringes and needles from I.V. bags of chemotherapeutic drugs.

■ Place used syringes and needles in a punctureproof container, along with other sharp or breakable items.

■ When mixing chemotherapeutic drugs, wear latex surgical gloves and a gown of low-permeability fabric with a closed front and cuffed long sleeves. When working steadily with chemotherapeutic drugs, change gloves every 60 minutes. If you spill a drug solution or puncture or tear a glove, remove the gloves at once. Wash your hands before putting on new gloves and any time you remove your gloves.

■ If some of the drug comes in contact with your skin, wash the involved area thoroughly with soap (not a germicidal agent) and water. If eye contact occurs, flood the eye with water or an isotonic eyewash for at least 5 minutes while holding the eyelid open. Obtain a medical evaluation as soon as possible after accidental exposure.

■ If a major spill occurs, use a chemotherapeutic spill kit to clean the area.

■ Discard disposable gowns and gloves in an appropriately marked, waterproof receptacle when contaminated or when you leave the work area.

■ Don't place any food or drinks in the same refrigerator as chemotherapeutic drugs.

■ Become familiar with drug excretion patterns, and take appropriate precautions when handling a chemotherapy patient's body fluids.

■ Give male patients a urinal with a tight-fitting lid. Wear disposable latex surgical gloves when handling body fluids.

Before flushing the toilet, place a waterproof pad over the toilet bowl *to avoid splashing.* Wear gloves and a gown when handling linens soiled with body fluids. Place soiled linens in isolation linen bags designated for separate laundering.

- When providing home care, empty waste products into the toilet close to the water *to minimize splashing.* Close the lid and flush two or three times. Place soiled linens in a washable pillowcase; then launder them twice, separately from other household linens. Wear gloves when handling contaminated linens, bedclothes, or other materials.
- Women who are pregnant, trying to conceive, or breast-feeding should exercise caution when handling chemotherapeutic drugs.
- Don't eat, drink, smoke, or apply cosmetics in the drug preparation area.

Home care

When teaching your patient about handling chemotherapeutic drugs, discuss appropriate safety measures. If the patient will be receiving chemotherapy at home, teach him how to dispose of contaminated equipment. Tell the patient and his family to wear gloves whenever handling chemotherapy equipment and contaminated linens or bedclothes. Instruct them to place soiled linens in a separate washable pillowcase and to launder the pillowcase twice, with the soiled linens inside, separately from other linens.

All materials used for the treatment should be placed in a leakproof container and taken to a designated disposal area. The patient or his family should make arrangements with either a hospital or a private company for pickup and proper disposal of contaminated waste.

Complications

Chemotherapeutic drugs may be mutagenic. Chronic exposure to chemotherapeutic drugs may damage the liver or chromosomes. Direct exposure to these drugs may burn and damage the skin.

Documentation

Document each incident of exposure according to your facility's policy.

SELECTED REFERENCES

Brown, K., et al. *Chemotherapy and Biotherapy Guidelines and Recommendations for Practice.* Pittsburgh: Oncology Nursing Society, 2001.

Martin, S., and Larson, E. "Chemotherapeutic Handling Practices of Outpatient and Office-based Oncology Nursing," *Oncology Nursing Forum* 30(4):575-81, July-August 2003.

Saria, M.G., and Rome, S.I. "The ACE Project: Avoiding Chemotherapy Errors in a Blended Medical/Surgical/Oncology Unit," *Clinical Nurse Specialist* 19(2):80, March-April 2005.

"Standard 25. Disposal of Sharps, Hazardous Materials, and Hazardous Waste. Infusion Nursing Standards of Practice," *Journal of Infusion Nursing* 29(1S):S30, January-February 2006.

"Standard 26. Laminar Flow Hood. Infusion Nursing Standards of Practice," *Journal of Infusion Nursing* 29(1S):S28, January-February 2006.

"Standard 65. Antineoplastic and Biologic Therapy. Infusion Nursing Standards of Practice," *Journal of Infusion Nursing* 29(1S):S69-71, January-February 2006.

U.S. Department of Labor. Occupational Safety & Health Administration. "Controlling Occupational Exposure to Harmful Drugs," In: TED 1-0.15A, Section VI, chapter 2. OSHA Technical Manual. Washington, D.C.: OSHA, January 1999. Available at *www.osha.gov/dts/osta_vi/otm_vi_2.htm.*

Wilson, L. "Oncology Safety: Safe Environment/Safe Practice for Patients and Providers," *ONS News* 21(8 Suppl):29-30, 2006.

CHEMOTHERAPEUTIC DRUG ADMINISTRATION

Administration of chemotherapeutic drugs requires skills in addition to those used when giving other drugs. For example, some drugs require special equipment or must be given through an unusual route. Others become unstable after a while, and still others must be protected from light. Finally, the drug dosage must be exact to avoid possibly fatal complications. For these reasons, only specially trained nurses and physicians should give chemotherapeutic drugs.

Chemotherapeutic drugs may be administered through a number of routes. Although the I.V. route (using peripheral or central veins) is used most commonly, these drugs may also be given orally, subcutaneously, I.M., intra-arterially, into a body cavity, through a central venous catheter, through an Ommaya reservoir into the spinal canal. They may also be administered into an artery, the peritoneal cavity, or the pleural space. (See *Intraperitoneal chemotherapy: An alternative approach,* page 326.)

The administration route depends on the drug's pharmacodynamics and the tumor's characteristics. For example, if a malignant tumor is confined to one area, the drug may be administered through a localized, or regional, method. Regional administration allows delivery of a high drug dose directly to the tumor. This is particularly advantageous because many solid tumors don't respond to drug levels that are safe for systemic administration.

Chemotherapy may be administered to a patient whose cancer is believed to have been eradicated through surgery or radiation therapy. This treatment, known as *adjuvant chemotherapy,* helps to ensure that no undetectable metas-

Intraperitoneal chemotherapy: An alternative approach

Administering chemotherapeutic drugs into the peritoneal cavity has several benefits for patients with malignant ascites or ovarian cancer that has spread to the peritoneum. This technique passes drugs directly to the tumor area in the peritoneal cavity, exposing malignant cells to high concentrations of chemotherapy — up to 1,000 times the amount that can be safely given systemically. What's more, the semipermeable peritoneal membrane permits prolonged exposure of malignant cells to the drug.

Typically, intraperitoneal chemotherapy is performed using a peritoneal dialysis kit, but drugs can also be administered directly to the peritoneal cavity by using a Tenckhoff catheter (as shown at right). This method can be performed on an outpatient basis, if necessary; it uses equipment that's readily available on most units with oncology patients.

In this technique, the chemotherapy bag is connected directly to the Tenckhoff catheter with a length of I.V. tubing, the solution is infused, and the catheter and I.V. tubing are clamped. Then the patient is asked to change positions every 10 to 15 minutes for 1 hour *to move the solution around in the peritoneal cavity.*

After the prescribed dwell time, the chemotherapeutic drugs are drained into an I.V. bag. The patient is encouraged to change positions *to facilitate drainage.* Then the I.V. tubing and catheter are clamped, the I.V. tubing is removed, and a new intermittent infusion cap is fitted to the catheter. Finally, the catheter is flushed with a syringe of heparin flush solution.

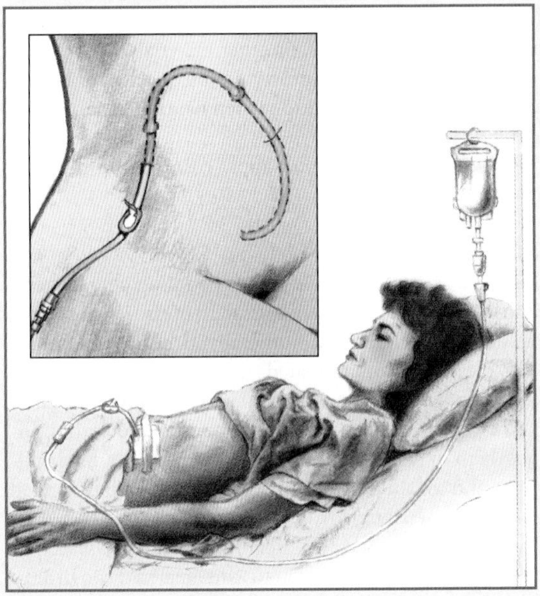

tasis exists. A patient may also receive chemotherapy before surgery or radiation therapy. This is called *induction chemotherapy* (or *neoadjuvant* or *synchronous chemotherapy*). Induction chemotherapy helps improve survival rates by shrinking a tumor before surgical excision or radiation therapy.

In general, chemotherapeutic drugs prove more effective when given in higher doses, but their adverse effects often limit the dosage. An exception to this rule is methotrexate. This drug is particularly effective against rapidly growing tumors, but it's also toxic to normal tissues that are growing and dividing rapidly. However, physicians have discovered that they can give a large dose of methotrexate to destroy cancer cells and then, before the drug has had a chance to permanently damage vital organs, give a dose of folinic acid as an antidote. The antidote stops the effects of methotrexate, thus preserving normal tissue.

Equipment
Prescribed drug ▪ gloves ▪ aluminum foil or a brown paper bag (if the drug is photosensitive) ▪ normal saline solution ▪ syringes and needleless adapters ▪ infusion pump ▪ impervious containers labeled CAUTION: BIOHAZARD.

Preparation of equipment
Verify the drug, dosage, and administration route by checking the medication record against the practitioner's order. Make sure you know the immediate and delayed adverse effects of the ordered drug. Follow administration guidelines for appropriate procedures in this chapter.

Implementation
- Confirm the patient's identity using two patient identifiers according to your facility's policy.
- Assess the patient's physical condition, and review his medical history.
- Make sure you understand what chemotherapeutic agent needs to be given and by what route, and provide the necessary teaching and support to the patient and his family.
- If your facility uses a bar code scanning system, be sure to scan your ID badge, the patient's ID bracelet, and the medication's bar code.

- Determine the best site to administer the drug. When selecting the site, consider drug compatibilities, frequency of administration, and vesicant potential of the drug. (See *Classifying chemotherapeutic drugs.*) For example, if the practitioner has ordered the intermittent administration of a vesicant drug, you can give it either by instilling the drug into the side port of an infusing I.V. line or by direct I.V. push through an intermittent infusion device. If the vesicant drug is to be infused continuously, you should administer it only through a central venous line or a vascular access device. On the other hand, nonvesicant agents (including irritants) may be given by direct I.V. push through an intermittent infusion device, through the side port of an infusing I.V. line, or as a continuous infusion.

  Check your facility's policy before administering a vesicant. *Because vein integrity decreases with time,* some facilities require that vesicants be administered *before* other drugs. Conversely, *because vesicants increase vein fragility,* some facilities require that vesicants be given *after* other drugs.
- Evaluate your patient's condition, paying particular attention to the results of recent laboratory studies, specifically the complete blood count, blood urea nitrogen level, platelet count, urine creatinine level, and liver function studies.
- Determine whether the patient has received chemotherapy before, and note the severity of any adverse effects.
- Check his drug history for medications that might interact with chemotherapy. As a rule, you shouldn't mix chemotherapeutic drugs with other medications. If you have questions or concerns about giving the chemotherapeutic drug, talk with the practitioner or pharmacist before you give it.
- Next, double-check the patient's chart for the complete chemotherapy protocol order, including the patient's name, drug's name and dosage, and route, rate, and frequency of administration. See if the drug's dosage depends on certain laboratory values. Be aware that some facilities require two nurses to verify the dosage order of high-alert medications and to check the drug and amount being administered.
- Check to see whether the practitioner has ordered an antiemetic, fluids, a diuretic, or electrolyte supplements to be given before, during, or after chemotherapy administration.
- Evaluate the patient's and his family's understanding of chemotherapy, and make sure the patient or a responsible family member has signed the consent form.
- Next, put on gloves. Keep them on through all stages of handling the drug, including preparation, priming the I.V. tubing, and administration.
- Before administering the drug, perform a new venipuncture proximal to the old site. Avoid giving chemotherapeutic drugs through an existing I.V. line. To identify an administration site, examine the patient's veins, starting with his hand and proceeding to his forearm.
- When an appropriate line is in place, infuse 10 to 20 ml of normal saline solution to test vein patency. Never test vein patency with a chemotherapeutic drug. Next, administer the drug as appropriate: nonvesicants by I.V. push or admixed in a bag of I.V. fluid; vesicants by I.V. push through a piggyback set connected to a rapidly infusing I.V. line.
- During I.V. administration, closely monitor the patient for signs of a hypersensitivity reaction or extravasation. Check

Classifying chemotherapeutic drugs

Chemotherapeutic drugs may be classified as irritants, vesicants, or nonvesicants.

Irritants

Irritants can cause a local venous response with or without a skin reaction. Chemotherapeutic irritants include:
- carboplatin (Paraplatin)
- carmustine (BiCNU)
- dacarbazine (DTIC-Dome)
- etoposide (VePesid)
- ifosfamide (Ifex)
- irinotecan (Camptosar)
- streptozocin (Zanosar)
- topotecan (Hycamtin).

Vesicants

Vesicants cause a reaction so severe that blisters form and tissue is damaged or destroyed. Chemotherapeutic vesicants include:
- dactinomycin (Cosmegen)
- daunorubicin (Cerubidine)
- doxorubicin (Adriamycin)
- idarubicin (Idamycin)
- mechlorethamine (Mustargen)
- mitomycin (Mutamycin)
- mitoxantrone (Novantrone)
- vinblastine (Velban)
- vincristine (Oncovin)
- vinorelbine (Navelbine).

Nonvesicants

Nonvesicants don't cause irritation or damage. Chemotherapeutic nonvesicants include:
- asparaginase (Elspar)
- bleomycin (Blenoxane)
- cyclophosphamide (Cytoxan)
- cytarabine (Cytosar-u)
- floxuridine (FUDR)
- fluorouracil (Efudex).

Managing extravasation

Extravasation — the infiltration of a vesicant drug into the surrounding tissue — can result from a punctured vein or leakage around a venipuncture site. If vesicant drugs or fluids extravasate, severe local tissue damage may result. This may cause prolonged healing, infection, cosmetic disgurement, and loss of function and may necessitate multiple debridements and, possibly, amputation.

Extravasation of vesicant drugs requires emergency treatment. Follow your facility's protocol. Essential steps include:

- Stop the I.V. flow, aspirate the remaining drug in the catheter, and remove the I.V. line, unless you need the needle to infiltrate the antidote.
- Estimate the amount of extravasated solution and notify the practitioner.
- Instill the appropriate antidote according to your facility's protocol.
- Elevate the extremity.
- Record the extravasation site, patient's symptoms, estimated amount of infiltrated solution, and treatment. Include the time you notified the practitioner and the practitioner's name. Continue documenting the appearance of the site and associated symptoms.
- Depending on your facility policy, apply either ice packs or warm compresses to the affected area. Ice is applied to all extravasated areas for 15 to 20 minutes every 4 to 6 hours for about 3 days. For etoposide and vinca alkaloids, apply dressings as ordered.
- If skin breakdown occurs, apply dressings, as ordered.
- If severe tissue damage occurs, plastic surgery and physical therapy may be needed.

for adequate blood return after 5 ml of the drug has been infused or according to your facility's guidelines.

- After infusion of the medication, infuse 20 ml of normal saline solution. Do this between administrations of different chemotherapeutic drugs and before discontinuing the I.V. line.
- Dispose of used needles and syringes carefully. *To prevent aerosol dispersion of chemotherapeutic drugs,* don't clip needles. Place them *intact* in an impervious container for incineration. Dispose of I.V. bags, bottles, gloves, and tubing in a properly labeled and covered trash container.
- Wash your hands thoroughly with soap and warm water after giving any chemotherapeutic drug, even though you have worn gloves.

Special considerations

- Observe the I.V. site frequently for signs of extravasation and an allergic reaction (swelling, redness, urticaria). If you suspect extravasation, stop the infusion immediately. Leave the I.V. catheter in place, and notify the practitioner. A conservative method for treating extravasation involves aspirating any residual drug from the tubing and I.V. catheter, instilling an I.V. antidote, and then removing the I.V. catheter. Afterward, you may apply heat or cold to the site and elevate the affected limb. (See *Managing extravasation.*)
- During infusion, some drugs need protection from direct sunlight *to avoid possible drug breakdown.* If this is the case, cover the vial with a brown paper bag or aluminum foil.
- When giving vesicants, avoid sites where damage to underlying tendons or nerves may occur (veins in the antecubital fossa, near the wrist, or in the dorsal surface of the hand).
- Use an infusion pump *to ensure drug delivery within the prescribed time and rate.*
- Observe the patient at regular intervals and after treatment for adverse reactions. Monitor his vital signs throughout the infusion *to assess any changes during chemotherapy administration.*
- Maintain a list of the types and amounts of drugs the patient has received. This is especially important if he has received drugs that have a cumulative effect and that can be toxic to such organs as the heart and kidneys.

Complications

Common adverse effects of chemotherapy are nausea and vomiting, ranging from mild to debilitating. Another major complication is bone marrow suppression, leading to neutropenia and thrombocytopenia. Other adverse effects include intestinal irritation, stomatitis, pulmonary fibrosis, cardiotoxicity, nephrotoxicity, neurotoxicity, hearing loss, anemia, alopecia, urticaria, radiation recall (if drugs are given with or soon after radiation therapy), anorexia, esophagitis, diarrhea, and constipation.

I.V. administration of chemotherapeutic drugs may also lead to extravasation, causing inflammation, ulceration, necrosis, and loss of vein patency.

Documentation

Record the location and description of the I.V. site before treatment or the presence of blood return during bolus administration. Also record the drugs and dosages administered, sequence of drug administration, needle type and size used, amount and type of flushing solution, and site's condition after treatment. Document any adverse reactions, the patient's tolerance of the treatment, and topics discussed with the patient and his family.

SELECTED REFERENCES

Brown, K., et al. *Chemotherapy and Biotherapy Guidelines and Recommendations for Practice.* Pittsburgh: Oncology Nursing Society, 2001.

"Standard 25. Disposal of Sharps, Hazardous Materials, and Hazardous Waste. Infusion Nursing Standards of Practice," *Journal of Infusion Nursing* 29(1S):S30, January-February 2006.

"Standard 26. Laminar Flow Hood. Infusion Nursing Standards of Practice," *Journal of Infusion Nursing* 29(1S):S28, January-February 2006.

"Standard 65. Antineoplastic and Biologic Therapy. Infusion Nursing Standards of Practice," *Journal of Infusion Nursing* 29(1S):S69-71, January-February 2006.

Tipton, J.M., et al. "Putting Evidence into Practice: Evidence-Based Interventions to Prevent, Manage, and Treat Chemotherapy-Induced Nausea and Vomiting," *Clinical Journal of Oncology Nursing* 11(1):69-78, February 2007.

U.S. Department of Labor. Occupational Safety & Health Administration. "Controlling Occupational Exposure to Harmful Drugs," In: TED 1-0.15A, Section VI, chapter 2. OSHA Technical Manual. Washington, D.C.: OSHA, January 1999. Available at *www.osha.gov/dts/osta_vi/otm_vi_2.htm.*

Wickham, R., et al. "Vesicant Extravasation Part II: Evidence-Based Management and Continuing Controversies," *Oncology Nursing Forum* 33(6):1143-150, November 2006.

Wilson, L. "Oncology Safety: Safe Environment/Safe Practice for Patients and Providers," *ONS News* 21(8 Suppl):29-30, 2006.

SPECIAL ADMINISTRATION TECHNIQUES

EPIDURAL ANALGESICS

In this procedure, the practitioner injects or infuses medication into the epidural space, which lies just outside the subarachnoid space where cerebrospinal fluid (CSF) flows. The drug diffuses slowly into the subarachnoid space of the spinal canal and then into the CSF, which carries it directly into the spinal area, bypassing the blood-brain barrier. In some cases, the medication is injected directly into the subarachnoid space. (See *Understanding intrathecal injections.*)

Understanding intrathecal injections

An intrathecal injection allows the physician to inject medication into the subarachnoid space of the spinal canal. Certain drugs — such as anti-infectives, or antineoplastics used to treat meningeal leukemia — are administered by this route because they can't readily penetrate the blood-brain barrier through the bloodstream. Intrathecal injection may also be used to deliver anesthetics, such as lidocaine, to achieve regional anesthesia (as in spinal anesthesia) and for pain management with medications such as preservative-free morphine.

An invasive procedure performed under sterile conditions by a physician with the nurse assisting, intrathecal injection requires informed patient consent. The injection site is usually between the third and fourth (or fourth and fifth) lumbar vertebrae, well below the spinal cord to avoid the risk of paralysis. This procedure may be preceded by aspiration of spinal fluid for laboratory analysis.

Contraindications to intrathecal injection include inflammation or infection at the puncture site, septicemia, and spinal deformities (especially when considered as an anesthesia route).

Epidural analgesia helps manage acute and chronic pain, including moderate to severe postoperative pain. It's especially useful in patients with cancer or degenerative joint disease. This procedure works well because opioid receptors are located along the entire spinal cord. Opioid drugs act directly on the receptors of the dorsal horn to produce localized analgesia without motor blockade. Opioids, such as preservative-free morphine, fentanyl, and hydromorphone, are administered as a bolus dose or by continuous infusion, either alone or in combination with a local anesthetic. Infusion through an epidural catheter is preferable because it allows a smaller drug dose to be given continuously.

The epidural catheter, inserted into the epidural space, eliminates the risks of multiple I.M. injections, minimizes adverse cerebral and systemic effects, and eliminates the analgesic peaks and valleys that usually occur with intermittent I.M. injections. (See *Placement of a permanent epidural catheter,* page 330.)

Typically, epidural catheter insertion is performed by an anesthesiologist using sterile technique. When the catheter

EQUIPMENT

Placement of a permanent epidural catheter

An epidural catheter is implanted beneath the patient's skin and inserted near the spinal cord at the first lumbar (L1) interspace. For temporary analgesic therapy (less than 1 week), the catheter may exit directly over the spine and be taped up the patient's back to the shoulder. For prolonged therapy, the catheter may be tunneled subcutaneously to an exit site on the patient's side or abdomen or over his shoulder.

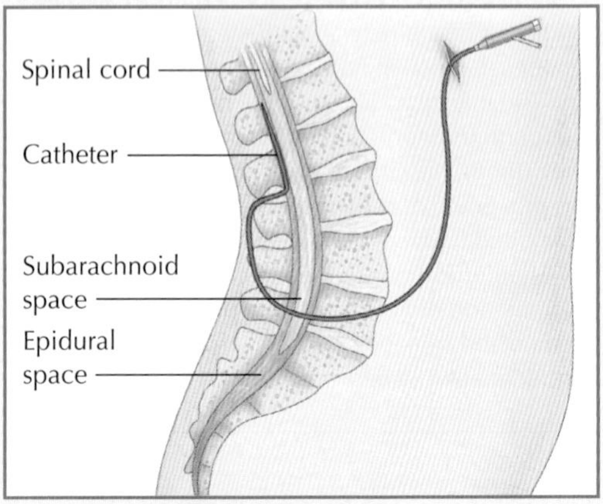

has been inserted, the nurse is responsible for monitoring the infusion and assessing the patient.

Epidural analgesia is contraindicated in patients who have local or systemic infection, neurologic disease, coagulopathy, spinal arthritis or a spinal deformity, hypotension, marked hypertension, or an allergy to the prescribed medication and in those who are undergoing anticoagulant therapy.

Equipment

Volume infusion device and epidural infusion tubing (depending on your facility's policy) ▪ patient's medication record and chart ▪ prescribed epidural solutions ▪ transparent dressing ▪ epidural tray ▪ labels for epidural infusion line ▪ silk tape ▪ optional: monitoring equipment for blood pressure and pulse, apnea monitor, pulse oximeter.

Have on hand the following drugs and equipment for emergency use: naloxone, 0.4 mg I.V.; ephedrine, 50 mg I.V. ▪ oxygen ▪ intubation set ▪ handheld resuscitation bag.

Preparation of equipment

Prepare the infusion device according to the manufacturer's instructions and your facility's policy. Obtain an epidural tray. Make sure that the pharmacy has been notified ahead of time regarding the medication order *because epidural solutions require special preparation.* Check the medication concentration and infusion rate against the practitioner's order. Label all medications and solutions on and off the sterile field.

Implementation

- Confirm the patient's identity using two patient identifiers according to your facility's policy.
- Explain the procedure and its potential complications to the patient. Tell him that he'll feel some pain as the catheter is inserted. Answer any questions he has. Make sure that a consent form has been properly signed and witnessed.
- Position the patient on his side in the knee-chest position, or have him sit on the edge of the bed and lean over a bedside table.
- After the catheter is in place, prime the infusion device, confirm the appropriate medication and infusion rate, and then adjust the device for the correct rate.
- Help the anesthesiologist connect the infusion tubing to the epidural catheter. Then connect the tubing to the infusion pump.
- Bridge-tape all connection sites, and apply an EPIDURAL INFUSION label to the catheter, infusion tubing, and infusion pump *to prevent accidental infusion of other drugs.* Then start the infusion.
- Tell the patient to immediately report any pain. Instruct him to use a pain scale from 0 to 10, with 0 denoting no pain and 10 denoting the worst pain imaginable. A response of 3 or less typically indicates tolerable pain. If the patient reports a higher pain score, the infusion rate may need to be increased. Call the practitioner or change the rate within prescribed limits.
- If ordered, place the patient on an apnea monitor for the first 24 hours after beginning the infusion.
- Change the dressing over the catheter's exit site every 24 to 48 hours, as needed, or as specified by your facility's policy. The dressing is usually transparent *to allow inspection of drainage* and commonly appears moist or slightly blood-tinged.
- The epidural generally isn't sutured in place, and it's important that you don't manipulate the catheter during a dressing change.
- Change the infusion tubing every 48 hours or as specified by your facility's policy.
- Change the epidural solution every 24 hours.

Special considerations

- Assess the patient's respiratory rate, blood pressure, and oxygen saturation every 2 hours for 8 hours and then every 4 hours for 8 hours during the first 24 hours after starting the infusion. Then assess the patient once per shift, depending on his condition or unless ordered otherwise. Your facility may require more frequent assessments. Notify the practitioner if the patient's respiratory rate is less than 10 breaths/minute or if his systolic blood pressure is less than 90 mm Hg.
- Assess the patient's sedation level, mental status, and pain-relief status every hour initially and then every 2 to 4 hours until adequate pain control is achieved. Notify the practitioner if the patient appears drowsy; experiences nausea and vomiting, refractory itching, or inability to void, *which are adverse effects of certain opioid analgesics;* or complains of unrelieved pain. A change in sedation level (the patient becoming somnolent) is an early indicator of the respiratory depressant effects of the opioid. Respiratory depression usually occurs during the first 24 hours and is treated with I.V. naloxone. Nausea, vomiting, and pruritus may also be treated with low-dose I.V. naloxone.
- Assess the patient's lower-extremity motor strength every 2 to 4 hours. If sensorimotor loss (numbness and leg weakness) occurs, large motor nerve fibers have been affected and the dose may need to be decreased. Notify the practitioner *because he may need to titrate the dosage in order to identify the dose that provides adequate pain control without causing excessive numbness and weakness.*
- Keep in mind that drugs given epidurally diffuse slowly and may cause adverse effects, including excessive sedation, up to 12 hours after the infusion has been discontinued.
- The patient should always have a peripheral I.V. line (either continuous infusion or heparin lock) open *to allow immediate administration of emergency drugs.*
- If CSF leaks into the dura mater at the initial puncture site, the patient usually experiences a headache. This postanalgesia headache worsens with postural changes, such as standing and sitting. The headache can be treated with a "blood patch," in which the patient's own blood (about 10 ml) is withdrawn from a peripheral vein and then injected into the epidural space. When the epidural needle is withdrawn, the patient is instructed to sit up. *Because the blood clots seal off the leaking area,* the blood patch should relieve the patient's headache immediately. The patient need not restrict his activity after this procedure.
- Typically, the anesthesiologist orders analgesics and removes the catheter. However, your facility's policy may allow a specially trained nurse to remove the catheter.
- If you feel resistance when removing the catheter, stop and call the practitioner for further orders.
- Be sure to save the catheter. *The practitioner will want to examine the catheter tip to rule out any damage during removal.*

Home care

Home use of epidural analgesia is possible only if the patient or a family member is willing and able to learn the care needed. The patient also must be willing and able to abstain from alcohol and street drugs *because these substances potentiate opioid action.*

Complications

Potential complications of epidural analgesic administration include adverse effects from opioids or local anesthetics, and catheter-related problems, such as infection, epidural hematoma, or catheter migration. Infection is treated with antibiotics. Epidural hematomas should be observed, and any increase in size should be reported to the practitioner.

Catheter migration occurs when the epidural catheter migrates out of the epidural space toward the skin. If this occurs, the patient will have decreased pain relief and leaking at the catheter site. Notify the practitioner because the infusion needs to be stopped and the catheter removed. Contact the practitioner for further pain management orders. The catheter can also migrate through the dura into the subarachnoid space if the epidural dose is too high for the smaller subarachnoid space, and the dose may eventually be toxic in high concentrations (the patient may show signs of increasing somnolence and eventually a decrease in respirations). Assess the patient and notify the practitioner immediately. The infusion needs to be stopped, the catheter removed, and the patient may need to be treated with I.V. naloxone and oxygen therapy.

Documentation

Record the patient's response to treatment, catheter patency, condition of the dressing and insertion site, vital signs, and assessment results. Also document the labeling of the epidural catheter, changing of the infusion bags, ordered analgesics, if any, and patient's response.

SELECTED REFERENCES

American Society of Anesthesiologists Task Force on Acute Pain Management. "Practice Guidelines for Acute Pain Management in the Perioperative Setting: An Updated Report by the American Society of Anesthesiologists Task Force on Acute Pain Management," *Anesthesiology* 100(6):1573-581, June 2004.

Anim-Somuah, M., et al. "Epidural Versus Non-Epidural or No Analgesia in Labour," *Cochrane Database of Systematic Review* Issue 4. Art.No.: CD000331, October 2005.

Coyne, P.J., et al. "Effectively Starting and Titrating Intrathecal Analgesic Therapy in Patients with Refractory Cancer Pain," *Clinical Journal of Oncology Nursing* 9(5):581-83, October 2005.

DePetri, L., et al. "The Use of Intrathecal Morphine for Postoperative Pain Relief after Liver Resection: A Comparison with Epidural Analgesia," *Anesthesia and Analgesia* 102(4):1157-163, April 2006.

Mordechai, M.M., and Brull, S.J. "Spinal Anesthesia," *Current Opinion in Anaesthesiology* 18(5):527-33, October 2005.

Ng, K., et al. "Spinal versus Epidural Anesthesia for Caesarean Section," *Cochrane Database of Systematic Review* Issue 2, Art No.: CD0037, 2004.

Rathmell, J.P., et al. "The Role of Intrathecal Drugs in the Treatment of Acute Pain," *Anesthesia and Analgesia* 101(Suppl 5):S30-43, November 2005.

Viscusi, E.R. "Emerging Techniques in the Management of Acute Pain: Epidural Analgesia," *Anesthesia and Analgesia* 101(Suppl 5):S23-29, November 2005.

OMMAYA RESERVOIR

Also known as a subcutaneous cerebrospinal fluid (CSF) reservoir, an Ommaya reservoir allows delivery of long-term drug therapy to the CSF by way of the brain's ventricles. The reservoir spares the patient repeated lumbar punctures to administer chemotherapeutic drugs, analgesics, antibiotics, and antifungals. It's most commonly used for chemotherapy and pain management, specifically for treating central nervous system (CNS) leukemia, malignant CNS disease, and meningeal carcinomatosis.

The reservoir is a mushroom-shaped silicone apparatus with an attached catheter. It's surgically implanted beneath the patient's scalp in the nondominant lobe, and the catheter is threaded into the ventricle through a burr hole in the skull. (See *How the Ommaya reservoir works.*) Besides providing convenient, comparatively painless access to CSF, the Ommaya reservoir permits consistent and predictable drug distribution throughout the subarachnoid space and CNS. It also allows for measurement of intracranial pressure (ICP).

Before reservoir insertion, the patient may receive a local or general anesthetic, depending on his condition and the physician's preference. After an X-ray confirms placement of the reservoir, a pressure dressing is applied for 24 hours, followed by a gauze dressing for another day or two. The sutures may be removed in about 10 days. However, the reservoir can be used within 48 hours to deliver drugs, obtain CSF pressure measurements, drain CSF, and withdraw CSF specimens.

The physician usually injects drugs into the Ommaya reservoir, but a specially trained nurse may perform this procedure if allowed by your facility's policy and the state's nurse practice act. This sterile procedure usually takes 15 to 30 minutes.

Equipment

Equipment varies but may include the following: preservative-free prescribed drug (at room temperature) ▪ sterile or chemotherapy gloves ▪ antiseptic solution ▪ sterile towel ▪ two 5- or 10-ml syringes ▪ 25G needle or 22G Huber needle ▪ sterile gauze pad ▪ collection tubes for CSF (if ordered) ▪ vial of bacteriostatic normal saline solution.

Preparation of equipment

Check the physician's order on the patient's chart. Wash your hands. Using the sterile towel, establish a sterile field near the patient. Prepare a syringe with the preservative-free drug to be instilled, and place it, the CSF collection tubes, and the normal saline solution on the sterile field. Label all medications, medication containers, and other solutions on and off the sterile field.

Implementation

- Confirm the patient's identity using two patient identifiers according to your facility's policy. Obtain baseline vital signs.
- If your patient is scheduled to receive an Ommaya reservoir, explain the procedure before reservoir insertion. Make sure the patient and his family understand the potential complications, and answer any questions they may have. Reassure the patient that any hair shaved for the implant will grow back and that only a coin-sized patch must remain shaved for injections. (Hair regrowth will be slower if the patient is receiving chemotherapy.)
- If your facility uses a bar code system, scan your ID badge, the patient's ID bracelet, and the medication's bar code.
- Position the patient so that he's either sitting or reclining. The head of the bed may be elevated or flat.
- Put on gloves, and prepare the patient's scalp with the antiseptic solution. Use a gauze pad to move the patient's hair and expose the reservoir.
- Placing the 25G needle at a 45-degree angle, insert it into the reservoir and aspirate 3 ml of clear CSF into a syringe. (If the aspirate isn't clear, check with the physician before continuing.)
- Continue to aspirate as many milliliters of CSF as you will instill of the drug. Then detach the syringe from the needle hub, attach the drug syringe, and instill the medication slowly, monitoring for headache, nausea, and dizziness. (Some facilities use the CSF instead of a preservative-free diluent to deliver the drug.)
- Cover the site with a sterile dressing, and apply gentle pressure for a moment or two until superficial bleeding stops.

- Instruct the patient to lie quietly for 15 to 30 minutes after the procedure. *This may prevent meningeal irritation leading to nausea and vomiting.*
- Monitor the patient for adverse drug reactions and signs of increased ICP, such as nausea, vomiting, pain, and dizziness. Assess for adverse reactions every 30 minutes for 2 hours, then every hour for 2 hours and, finally, every 4 hours.

Special considerations

- The physician may prescribe an antiemetic to be administered 30 minutes before the procedure *to control nausea and vomiting.*
- After the reservoir is implanted, the patient may resume normal activities. Instruct him to protect the site from bumps and traumatic injury while the incision heals. Tell him that unless complications develop, the reservoir may function for years.
- Instruct the patient and his family to notify the physician if signs of infection develop at the insertion site (for example, redness, swelling, tenderness, and drainage) or if the patient develops headache, neck stiffness, or fever, which may indicate a systemic infection.

Complications

Infection may develop but can usually be treated successfully by injection of antibiotics directly into the reservoir. Persistent infection may require removal of the reservoir. Catheter migration or blockage may cause symptoms of increased ICP, such as headache and nausea. If the physician suspects this problem, he may gently push and release the reservoir several times (a technique called *pumping*). With his finger on the patient's scalp, the physician can feel the reservoir refill. Slow filling suggests catheter migration or blockage, which must be confirmed by a computed tomography scan. Surgical correction is required.

Documentation

Record the appearance of the reservoir insertion site before and after access, the patient's tolerance of the procedure, the amount of CSF withdrawn and its appearance, and the name and dose of the drug instilled.

EQUIPMENT

How the Ommaya reservoir works

To insert an Ommaya reservoir, the physician drills a burr hole and inserts the device's catheter through the patient's nondominant frontal lobe into the lateral ventricle. The reservoir, which has a self-sealing silicone injection dome, rests over the burr hole under a scalp flap. This creates a slight, soft bulge on the scalp about the size of a quarter. Usually, drugs are injected into the dome with a syringe.

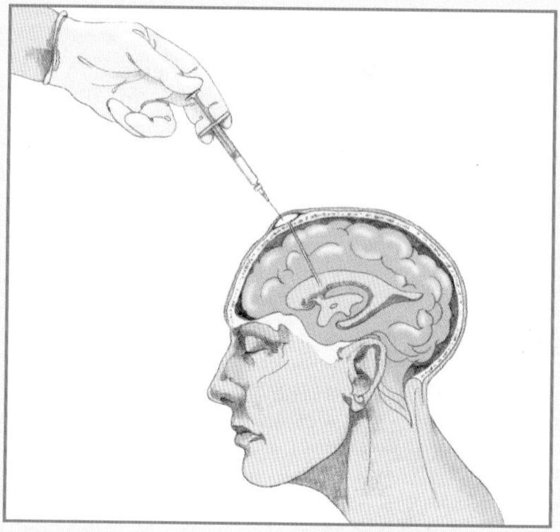

SELECTED REFERENCES

American Association of Neuroscience Nurses. *Core Curriculum for Neuroscience Nursing,* 4th ed. Philadelphia: W.B. Saunders, Co., 2004.

Dickerman, R.D., and Eisenberg, M.B. "Preassembled Method for Insertion of Ommaya Reservoir," *Journal of Surgical Oncology* 89(1):36-38, January 2005.

Ishii, K., et al. "Intracranial Ectopic Recurrence of Craniopharyngioma after Ommaya Reservoir Implantation," *Pediatric Neurosurgery* 40(5):230-33, September-October 2004.

ENDOTRACHEAL DRUGS

When an I.V. line isn't readily available, drugs can be administered into the respiratory system through an endotracheal (ET) tube. This route allows uninterrupted resuscitation efforts and avoids such complications as coronary artery laceration, cardiac tamponade, and pneumothorax, which can occur when emergency drugs are administered intracardially.

Drugs given endotracheally usually have a longer duration of action than drugs given I.V. because they're absorbed in the alveoli. For this reason, repeat doses and continuous

Administering endotracheal drugs

In an emergency, some drugs may be given through an endotracheal (ET) tube if I.V. access isn't available. They may be given using the syringe method or the adapter method.

Before injecting any drug, check for proper placement of the ET tube, using an end-tidal CO_2 detector or an esophageal detection device. Make sure that the patient is supine and that her head is level with or slightly higher than her trunk.

Syringe method

Remove the needle before injecting medication into the ET tube. Insert the tip of the syringe into the ET tube, and inject the drug deep into the tube (as shown below).

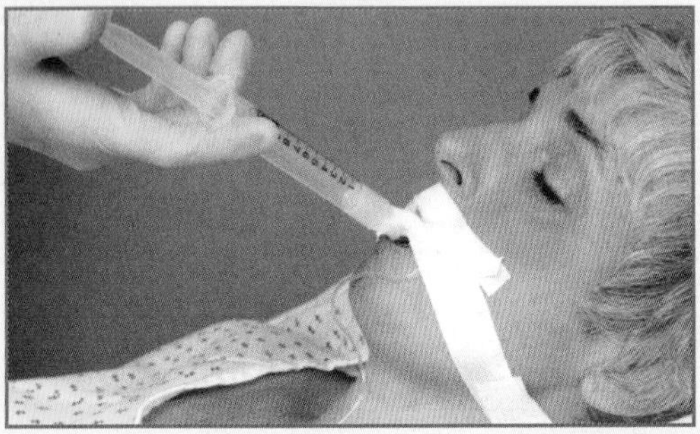

Adapter method

An adapter for ET drug administration provides a more closed system of drug delivery than the syringe method. A special adapter placed on the end of the ET tube (as shown below) allows needle insertion and drug delivery through the closed stopcock.

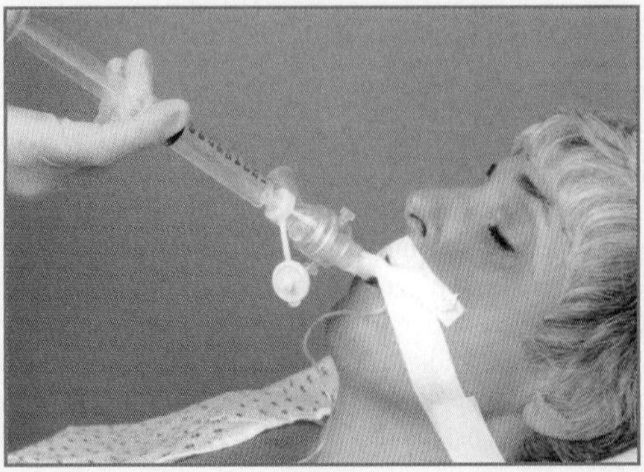

infusions must be adjusted to prevent adverse effects. Drugs most commonly given by this route include atropine, epinephrine, lidocaine, naloxone, and vasopressin.

Endotracheal drugs are usually administered in an emergency situation by a physician, an emergency medical technician, or a critical care nurse. Although guidelines may vary, depending on state, county, or city regulations, the basic administration method is the same. (See *Administering endotracheal drugs.*)

Endotracheal drugs may be given using the syringe method or the adapter method. Usually used for bronchoscopy suctioning, the swivel adapter can be placed on the end of the tube and, while ventilation continues through a bag-valve device, the drug can be delivered with a needle through the closed stopcock.

Equipment

ET tube ■ gloves ■ end-tidal carbon dioxide (CO_2) detection device or esophageal detection device ■ handheld resuscitation bag ■ prescribed drug ■ syringe or adapter ■ sterile water or normal saline solution.

Preparation of equipment

Verify the order on the patient's medication record by checking it against the practitioner's order. In an emergency situation, verify the practitioner's verbal order. Wash your hands. Check ET tube placement by using an end-tidal CO_2 or esophageal detection device.

Calculate the drug dose. Adult advanced cardiac life support guidelines recommend that drugs be administered at 2 to 2½ times the recommended I.V. dose. Next, draw the drug up into a syringe. Dilute it in 10 ml of sterile water or normal saline solution. *Dilution increases drug volume and contact with lung tissue.*

Implementation

- Put on gloves.
- Move the patient into the supine position, and make sure his head is level with or slightly higher than his trunk.
- Ventilate the patient three to five times with the resuscitation bag. Then remove the bag.
- Remove the needle from the syringe, and insert the tip of the syringe into the ET tube. Inject the drug deep into the tube.
- After injecting the drug, reattach the resuscitation bag, and ventilate the patient briskly. *This propels the drug into the lungs, oxygenates the patient, and clears the tube.*
- Discard the syringe in an appropriate sharps container.
- Remove and discard your gloves.

Special considerations

Be aware that the drug's onset of action may be quicker than it would be by I.V. administration. If the patient doesn't respond quickly, the practitioner may order a repeat dose.

Complications

Potential complications of endotracheal drug administration result from the prescribed drug, not the administration route.

Documentation

Record the date and time of drug administration, drug administered, and patient's response.

SELECTED REFERENCES

American Heart Association. "2005 Guidelines for Cardiopulmonary Resuscitation and Emergency Cardiovascular Care: Advanced Cardiac Life Support," *Circulation* 112(suppl IV):IV-58, December 2005.

Kockare, M., et al. "Comparison Between Direct Humdification and Nebulization of the Respiratory Tract at Mechanical Ventilation: Distribution of Saline Solution Studied by Gamma Camera," *Journal of Clinical Nursing* 15(3):301-307, March 2006.

INTRAPLEURAL DRUGS

An intrapleural drug is injected through the chest wall into the pleural space or instilled through a chest tube placed intrapleurally for drainage. Physicians use intrapleural administration to promote analgesia, treat spontaneous pneumothorax, resolve pleural effusions, and administer chemotherapy.

Intrapleurally administered drugs diffuse across the parietal pleura and innermost intercostal muscles to affect the intercostal nerves. During intrapleural injection of a drug, the needle passes through the intercostal muscles and parietal pleura on its way to the pleural space.

The internal intercostal muscle is a key landmark for needle placement. It resists the advancing needle, becoming the posterior intercostal membrane in the posterior chest region.

Drugs commonly given by intrapleural injection include tetracycline, streptokinase, anesthetics, and chemotherapeutic agents (to treat malignant pleural effusion or lung adenocarcinoma).

Contraindications for this route include pleural fibrosis or adhesions, which interfere with diffusion of the drug to the intended site; pleural inflammation; sepsis; and infection at the puncture site. Patients with bullous emphysema and those receiving respiratory therapy using positive end-expiratory pressure also shouldn't have intrapleural injections because the injections may exacerbate an already compromised pulmonary condition.

Equipment

An intrapleural drug is given through a #16 to #20 or #28 to #40 chest tube if the patient has empyema, pleural effusion, or pneumothorax. Otherwise, it's given through a 16G to 18G blunt-tipped intrapleural (epidural) needle and catheter. Accessory equipment depends on the type of access device the physician uses. All equipment must be sterile.

For intrapleural catheter insertion: Gloves ■ gauze ■ antiseptic solution ■ drape ■ local anesthetic, such as 1% lidocaine ■ 3- or 5-ml syringe with 22G 1" and 25G ⅝" needles ■ 18G needle or scalpel ■ 16G to 18G blunt-tipped intrapleural needle and catheter ■ saline-lubricated glass syringe ■ dressings ■ sutures ■ tape ■ blunt-tipped intrapleural needle ■ intrapleural catheter.

For chest tube insertion: Towels ■ gloves ■ gauze ■ antiseptic solution ■ 3- or 5-ml syringe ■ local anesthetic such as 1% lidocaine ■ 18G needle or scalpel ■ chest tube with or without trocar (#16 to #20 catheter for air or serous fluid, #28 to #40 catheter for blood, pus, or thick fluid) ■ two rubber-tipped clamps, if necessary ■ sutures ■ drain dressings ■ tape ■ thoracic drainage system and tubing.

For drug administration: Sterile gloves ■ sterile gauze pads ■ antiseptic solution ■ prescribed medication ■ appropriate-sized needles and syringes ■ 1% lidocaine, if necessary ■ dressings ■ tape ■ infusion pump ■ two rubber-tipped clamps, if necessary.

Implementation

- Confirm the patient's identity using two patient identifiers according to your facility's policy.
- Explain the procedure to the patient *to allay his fears.* Encourage him to follow instructions.

Inserting an intrapleural catheter

- The physician inserts the intrapleural catheter at the patient's bedside with the nurse assisting.
- Position the patient on his side with the affected side up. The physician inserts the catheter into the fourth to eighth intercostal space, 3" to 4" (7.5 to 10 cm) from the posterior midline. (See *Inserting an intrapleural catheter*, page 336.)
- The physician puts on sterile gloves, cleans around the puncture site with antiseptic-soaked gauze, and then covers the area with a sterile drape. Next, he fills the 3- or 5-ml syringe with local anesthetic and injects it into the skin and deep tissues.
- The physician punctures the skin with the 18G needle or scalpel, which helps the blunt-tipped intrapleural needle

Inserting an intrapleural catheter

In intrapleural administration, the physician injects a drug into the pleural space using a catheter.

Help the patient lie on one side with the affected side up. The physician inserts a needle into the fourth to eighth intercostal space, 3" to 4" (7.5 to 10 cm) from the posterior midline. He then advances the needle medially over the superior edge of the patient's rib through the intercostal muscles until it tangentially penetrates the parietal pleura, as shown. The catheter is advanced into the pleural space through the needle, which is then removed.

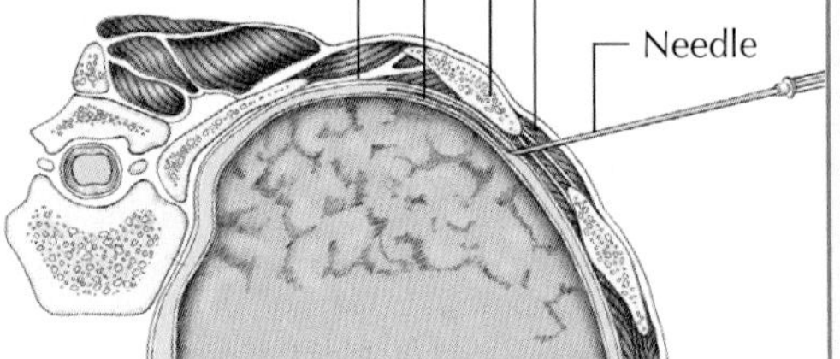

penetrate the skin over the superior edge of the lower rib in the chosen interspace. Keeping the bevel tilted upward, he directs the needle medially at a 30- to 40-degree angle to the skin. When the needle tip punctures the posterior intercostal membrane, he removes the stylet and attaches a saline-lubricated glass syringe containing 2 to 4 cc of air to the needle hub.

- During puncture, tell the patient to hold his breath (or momentarily disconnect him from mechanical ventilation) until the needle is removed *to help prevent the needle from injuring lung tissue.*
- The physician advances the needle slowly. When the needle punctures the parietal pleura, negative intrapleural pressure moves the plunger outward. He then removes the syringe from the needle and threads the intrapleural catheter through the needle until he has advanced it about 2" (5 cm) into the pleural space. Without removing the catheter, he carefully withdraws the needle.
- Tell the patient that he can breathe again (or reconnect mechanical ventilation).
- After inserting the catheter, the physician coils it *to prevent kinking* and then sutures it securely to the patient's skin. He confirms placement by aspirating the catheter. Resistance indicates correct placement in the pleural space; aspirated blood means that the catheter probably is misplaced in a blood vessel, and aspirated air means that it's probably in a lung. He will then order a chest X-ray *to detect pneumothorax.*
- Apply a sterile dressing over the insertion site *to prevent catheter dislodgment.* Take the patient's vital signs every 15 minutes for the first hour after the procedure and then as needed.

Inserting a chest tube

- The physician inserts the chest tube with the nurse assisting. (For more information on chest tube insertion, see chapter 8, Respiratory care.)
- First, position the patient with the affected side up, and drape him with sterile towels.
- The physician puts on gloves and cleans the appropriate site with antiseptic-soaked gauze. If the patient has a pneumothorax, the physician uses the second intercostal space as the access site *because air rises to the top of the pleural space.* If the patient has a hemothorax or pleural effusion, the physician uses the sixth to eighth intercostal space *because fluid settles to the bottom of the pleural space.*
- The physician fills the syringe with a local anesthetic and injects it into the site. He makes a small incision with the 18G needle or scalpel, inserts the appropriate-sized chest tube, and immediately connects it to the thoracic drainage system or clamps it close to the patient's chest. He then sutures the tube to the patient's skin.
- Tape the chest tube to the patient's chest distal to the insertion site *to help prevent accidental dislodgment.* Also tape the junction of the chest tube and drainage tube *to prevent their separation.* Apply sterile drain dressings, and tape them to the site.
- After insertion, the physician checks tube placement with an X-ray. Check the patient's vital signs every 15 minutes for 1 hour and then as needed. Auscultate his lungs at least every 4 hours *to assess air exchange in the affected lung.* Diminished or absent breath sounds mean that the lung hasn't reexpanded.

Administering the medication

- The physician injects medication through the intrapleural catheter or chest tube with the nurse assisting.
- If the patient will receive chemotherapy, expect to give an antiemetic at least 30 minutes before.
- Position the patient with the affected side up. Help the physician move the dressing away from the intrapleural

catheter or chest tube and clamp the drainage tube, if present.

- The physician disinfects the access port of the catheter or chest tube with antiseptic-soaked gauze. Draw up the appropriate medication dose, and hand it to the physician with the vial for verification.
- The physician injects the medication. If it's an anesthetic, he gives a bolus or loading dose initially and then a continuous infusion. For tetracycline, he mixes it with an anesthetic such as lidocaine *to alleviate pain during injection.*
- Reapply the dressings around the catheter. Monitor the patient closely during and after drug administration *to gauge the effectiveness of drug therapy and to check for complications and adverse effects.*

Special considerations

- Make sure the patient has signed a consent form.
- Before catheter insertion, ask the patient to urinate *to promote comfort.*
- If the patient is receiving a continuous infusion, label the solution bag clearly. Cover all injection ports so that other drugs aren't injected into the pleural space accidentally.
- If the chest tube dislodges, cover the site at once with a sterile gauze pad, and tape it in place. Stay with the patient, monitor his vital signs, and observe carefully for signs and symptoms of tension pneumothorax: hypotension, distended jugular veins, absent breath sounds, tracheal shift, hypoxemia, dyspnea, tachypnea, diaphoresis, chest pain, and weak, rapid pulse. Have another nurse call the physician and gather the equipment for reinsertion.
- Keep rubber-tipped clamps at the bedside. If a commercial chest tube system cracks or a tube disconnects, use the clamps to clamp the chest tube close to the insertion site temporarily. Be sure to observe the patient closely for signs of tension pneumothorax *because no air can escape from the pleural space while the tube is clamped.*
- You can wrap a piece of petroleum gauze around the chest tube at the insertion site to make an airtight seal; then apply the sterile dressing.

Complications

Pneumothorax or tension pneumothorax may occur if the physician accidentally injects air into the pleural cavity. These complications are more likely to occur in a patient who is on mechanical ventilation.

Accidental catheter placement in the lung can lead to respiratory distress; catheter placement within a vessel can increase the medication's effects. With catheter fracture, lung puncture may occur. Laceration of intercostal vessels can cause bleeding.

Local anesthetic toxicity can lead to tinnitus, metallic taste, light-headedness, somnolence, visual and auditory disturbances, restlessness, delirium, slurred speech, nystagmus, muscle tremor, seizures, arrhythmias, and cardiovascular collapse. A local anesthetic containing epinephrine can cause tachycardia and hypertension.

Intrapleural chemotherapeutic drugs can irritate the pleura chemically and cause such systemic effects as neutropenia and thrombocytopenia. Administering intrapleural tetracycline without an anesthetic can cause pain.

The insertion site can become infected. However, meticulous skin preparation, strict sterile technique, and sterile dressings usually prevent infection.

Documentation

Document the date, time, and site of catheter insertion, the physician's name, and the patient's tolerance of the procedure. Document the drug administered, drug dosage, patient's response to the treatment, and condition of the catheter insertion site.

SELECTED REFERENCES

Maskell, N., et al. "Intrapleural Streptokinase for Pleural Infection," *British Medical Journal* 332(7540):552, March 2006.

Ren, S., et al. "Intrapleural Staphylococcal Superantigen Induces Resolution of Malignant Pleural Effusions and a Survival Benefit in Non-Small Cell Lung Cancer," *Chest* 126(5):1529-539, November 2004.

Tokuda, Y., et al. "Intrapleural Fibrinolytic Agents for Empyema and Complicated Parapneumonic Effusions: A Meta-Analysis," *Chest* 129(3):783-90, March 2006.

DRUG IMPLANTS

A method of drug delivery involves implanting drugs beneath the skin — subdermally or subcutaneously — as well as targeting specific tissues with radiation implants.

With subdermal implants, flexible capsules are placed under the skin. Most often, various hormones are administered subdermally. Small Silastic capsules filled with the hormone are placed under the skin of the patient's upper arm, and the drug then diffuses through the capsule walls continuously.

With subcutaneous implants, drug pellets are injected into the skin's subcutaneous layer. The drug is then stored in one area of the body, called a depot. A treatment for prostate cancer cells calls for implants of goserelin acetate, a synthetic form of luteinizing hormone. By inhibiting pituitary gland secretion, goserelin implants reduce testosterone levels to those previously achieved only through castration. This reduction causes tumor regression and suppression of symptoms.

Equipment

For subdermal implants: Sterile surgical drapes ▪ sterile gloves ▪ antiseptic solution ▪ local anesthetic ▪ set of implants ▪ needles ▪ 5-ml syringe ▪ #11 scalpel ▪ #10 trocar ▪ forceps ▪ sutures ▪ sterile gauze ▪ tape.

For subcutaneous implants: Alcohol pad ▪ drug implant in a preloaded syringe ▪ local anesthetic (for some patients).

Implementation

- Explain the procedure and its benefits and risks to the patient, and show him a set of implants.

Inserting subdermal implants

- Assist the patient into a supine position on the examination table. During the procedure, stay and provide support as necessary.
- After anesthetizing the upper portion of the nondominant arm, the practitioner will use a trocar to insert each capsule through a 2-mm incision. After insertion, he'll remove the trocar and palpate the area. He'll then close the incision and cover it with a dry compress and sterile gauze.

Inserting subcutaneous implants

- Help the patient into the supine position, and drape him so that his abdomen is accessible. Remove the syringe from the package, and make sure you can see the drug in the chamber. Clean a small area on the patient's upper abdominal wall with the alcohol pad.
- As you stretch the skin at the injection site with one hand, grip the needle with the fingers of your other hand around the barrel of the syringe. Insert the needle into subcutaneous fat at a 45-degree angle. Don't attempt to aspirate. If blood appears in the syringe, withdraw the needle and inject a new preloaded syringe and needle at another site.
- Next, change the direction of the needle so that it's parallel to the abdominal wall. With the barrel hub touching the patient's skin, push the needle in. Then withdraw it about ½" (1.3 cm) *to create a space for the drug.* Depress the plunger. Withdraw the needle and bandage the site.
- Inspect the tip of the needle. If you can see the metal tip of the plunger, the drug has been discharged.

Special considerations

Special care may be necessary, depending on the type of implant used.

Subdermal implants

- Tell the patient to resume normal activities but to protect the site during the first few days after implantation. Advise him not to bump the insertion site and to keep the area dry and covered with a gauze bandage for 3 days.
- Tell the patient to report signs of bleeding or infection at the insertion site.
- Tell the patient to notify the practitioner immediately if one of the implanted capsules falls out before the skin heals over the implants. If it's a contraceptive implant, it may no longer be effective. Advise the patient to use alternative means of contraception until she sees the practitioner. If pregnancy is suspected, the implants must be removed immediately.

Subcutaneous implants

- Be aware that if an implant must be removed, the practitioner will order an X-ray to locate it.
- Tell the patient to check the administration site for signs of infection or bleeding.
- Goserelin implants must be changed every 28 days. Female patients should be advised to use a nonhormonal form of contraception.

Complications

Complications vary, depending on the type of implant used.

Subdermal implants

Possible reactions to hormones include hyperpigmentation at the insertion site, menstrual irregularities, headache, nervousness, nausea, dizziness, adnexal enlargement, dermatitis, acne, appetite and weight changes, mastalgia, hirsutism, and alopecia. More serious reactions include breast abnormalities, mammographic changes, diabetes, elevated cholesterol or triglyceride levels, hypertension, seizures, depression, and gallbladder, heart, or kidney disease.

Subcutaneous implants

Goserelin implants may cause anemia, lethargy, pain, dizziness, insomnia, anxiety, depression, headache, chills, fever, edema, heart failure, arrhythmias, stroke, hypertension, peripheral vascular disease, nausea, vomiting, diarrhea, impotence, renal insufficiency, urinary obstruction, rash, sweating, hot flashes, gout, hyperglycemia, weight increase, and breast swelling and tenderness.

Documentation

For subdermal and subcutaneous implants, document the name of the drug, insertion or administration site, date and time of insertion, and patient's response to the procedure. Note the date that implants should be removed and a new set inserted or the date of the next administration, as appropriate.

SELECTED REFERENCES

The Joint Commission. *Comprehensive Accreditation Manual for Hospitals: The Official Handbook.* Standard MM.4.30. 2007.

The Joint Commission. *Comprehensive Accreditation Manual for Hospitals: The Official Handbook.* Standard MM.5.10. 2007.

The Joint Commission. *Comprehensive Accreditation Manual for Hospitals: The Official Handbook.* Standard MM.5.20. 2007.

The Joint Commission. *Comprehensive Accreditation Manual for Hospitals: The Official Handbook.* Standard MM.6.20. 2007.

Taylor, C., et al. *Fundamentals of Nursing: The Art and Science of Nursing Care,* 6th ed. Philadelphia: Lippincott Williams & Wilkins, 2008.

IONTOPHORESIS

Iontophoresis is a technique for delivering dermal analgesia quickly (in 10 to 20 minutes) with minimal discomfort and without distorting the tissue. The Numby 900 iontophoretic drug-delivery system is a handheld device with two electrodes that uses a mild electric current to deliver charged ions of lidocaine 2% with epinephrine 1:100,000 solution into the skin. The device is powered by a 9-volt battery.

Because iontophoresis acts quickly, it's an excellent choice for numbing an I.V. injection site, especially in children.

Equipment

Dose-control device with battery ▪ drug-delivery electrode kit ▪ lidocaine 2% with epinephrine 1: 100,000 solution ▪ alcohol pads ▪ syringe with needle ▪ gloves ▪ tongue blade.

Implementation

- Confirm the patient's identity using two patient identifiers according to your facility's policy
- Ask the patient — or if the patient is a child, ask the parents — if he has any allergies or sensitivity to medications. Avoid using iontophoresis in patients with implanted devices such as a pacemaker.
- Explain the procedure to the patient, and tell him that he may feel tingling or warmth under the electrode pads while they're on the skin.
- Assess the patient for appropriate electrode placement. You'll place a medication-delivery electrode over the intended I.V. insertion site. The second electrode, which drives drug ions into the skin, must be applied over a muscle 4″ to 6″ (10 to 15 cm) away.
- Put on gloves. Examine the patients' skin, and select intact electrode placement sites, avoiding areas with pimples, unhealed wounds, or ingrown hairs. With alcohol pads, briskly rub an area slightly larger than the electrode at each site.
- Remove the paper flap from the back of the drug-delivery electrode.
- Draw up the lidocaine with epinephrine in a syringe. Remove the needle from the syringe and saturate the medication pad with the amount of lidocaine and epinephrine solution indicated on the electrode pad (as shown below).

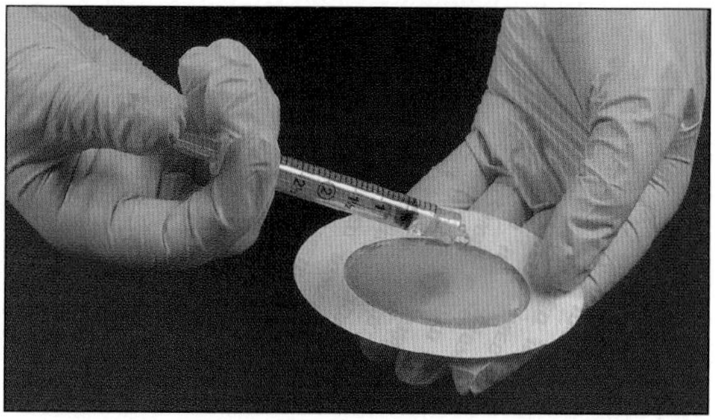

The amount of lidocaine and epinephrine solution required to saturate the pad varies with pad size: For a standard-sized pad, use about 1 ml; for a large pad, use about 2.5 ml.

- Remove the remaining backing from the drug-delivery pad, and apply the pad to the selected site. Remove the backing from the grounding electrode, and apply it to the second prepared site.
- Connect the lead clips: red (positive charge) to the drug-delivery electrode and black (negative charge) to the grounding electrode.
- Turn on the device (as shown below).

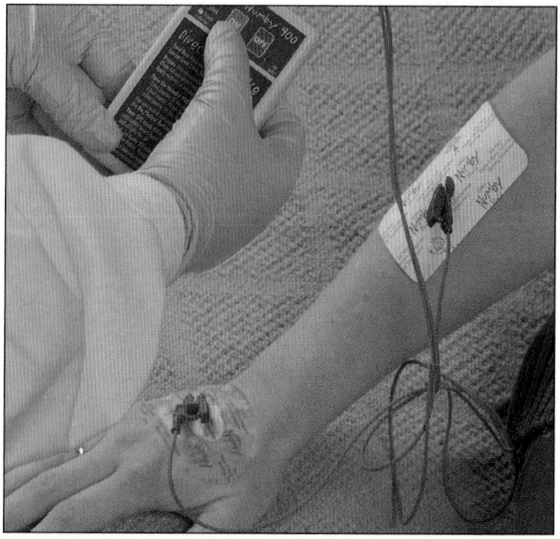

As indicated by the green light, the device will automatically operate at the lowest current, 2 milliamperes (mA), unless you increase the level to 3 or 4 mA by pressing the ON button. If your patient has discomfort at a higher setting, reduce the current by pushing the ON button until the appropriate light indicates the desired level. The device is calibrated to deliver a dose of 40mA, after which it will automatically stop. If the setting remains at 4 mA, treatment is completed in 10 minutes. However, if you decrease the setting because the patient has discomfort, the device will automatically adjust to a longer treatment time to deliver the entire dose.

- After the dose has been delivered, remove the electrodes. Assess the skin at the drug-delivery site for numbness by touching it with a blunt object such as a tongue blade.
- Promptly prepare the site and perform the venipuncture *because the numbness may only last a few minutes,*
- Discard your supplies and gloves, and wash your hands.

Special considerations

- *To avoid interfering with energy emissions,* don't tape or compress the electrodes.
- If you need to stop the treatment for any reason, press the OFF button and hold it. The lights will indicate decreasing current levels, then the device will beep and turn off. Don't disconnect the lead clips or the electrodes until all signals have stopped *because the device is still transmitting energy until it turns off.*

Complications

Allergic reaction may occur in patients sensitive to lidocaine or epinephrine.

Documentation

Document the treatment, the sites used, and whether analgesia was achieved. Also document an allergic response, if any.

SELECTED REFERENCES

Becker, B., et al. "Ultrasound with Topical Anesthetic Rapidly Decreases Pain of Intravenous Cannulation," *Academy of Emergency Medicine* 12(4):289-95, April 2005.

Gokoglu, F., et al. "Evaluation of Iontophoresis and Local Corticosteroid Injection in the Treatment of Carpal Tunnel Syndrome," *American Journal of Physician Medicine and Rehabilitation* 84(2):92-96, February 2005.

Pasero, C. "Lidocaine Iontophoresis for Dermal Procedure Analgesia," *Journal of Perianesthesia Nursing* 21(1):48-52, February 2006.

"Standard 40. Local Anesthesia. Infusion Nursing Standards of Practice," *Journal of Infusion Nursing* 29(1S):S41, January-February 2006.

Viscusi, E.R., et al. "An Clontophoretic Fentanyl Patient-Activated Analgesic Delivery System for Postoperative Pain: A Double-blind, Placebo-controlled Trial," *Anesthesia and Analgesia* 102(1):188-84, January 2006.

6 ■ Intravascular therapy

INTRODUCTION

More than 80% of hospitalized patients receive some form of I.V. therapy. Although you may not be called on to insert all types of I.V. lines, you'll be responsible for maintaining the lines and preventing complications throughout therapy. You'll also be responsible for helping the practitioner perform minor surgical procedures, such as insertion of central venous (CV) and arterial lines.

This chapter explains the administration methods and primary uses of I.V. therapy. You'll review how to prepare for I.V. therapy; how to insert, maintain, and remove specific I.V. lines and devices; how to control infection and maintain flow rates; and how to monitor the patient's response to therapy. You'll also learn about patient-teaching responsibilities and home care issues.

I.V. DELIVERY METHODS

The factors involved in choosing an I.V. delivery method include the therapy's purpose and duration; the patient's diagnosis, age, and health history; and the condition of his veins. For example, in peripheral I.V. therapy, you'll administer I.V. solutions through a vein in the arm, hand, leg, or foot — typically, for short-term or intermittent therapy.

In CV therapy, you'll give I.V. solutions through a central vein such as the superior vena cava. These lines are often inserted through the subclavian and the internal or external jugular veins. This method is typically used for patients who need a large volume of fluid or a hypertonic solution, caustic drug, or high-calorie parenteral nutrition solution. Midline and peripherally inserted central catheters are used both in home care and in health care facilities. Implanted vascular access devices provide a variation on CV infusion. The infused solution enters a central vein through an access device surgically implanted in a subcutaneous pocket. This method is used for patients who require long-term (6 months or longer) I.V. therapy.

Uses of I.V. therapy

The most common uses of I.V. therapy are maintaining and restoring fluid and electrolyte balance, administering drugs, transfusing blood, and delivering parenteral nutrition.

The I.V. route allows rapid, effective drug administration. Commonly infused drugs include antibiotics, thrombolytics, antineoplastic agents, cardiovascular drugs, anticonvulsants, and patient-controlled analgesics. Drugs can be infused rapidly (I.V. push) or over time.

With blood transfusion, your nursing responsibilities include administering blood and blood components as well as monitoring patients receiving therapy. Transfusion aims to maintain adequate blood volume, increase the blood's oxygen-carrying capacity, and maintain hemostasis.

Parenteral nutrition is the administration of nutrients by the I.V. route. Low-concentration parenteral nutrition solutions are administered through a peripheral vein; more highly concentrated ones are administered through a central vein. If you're caring for a patient who is receiving parenteral nutrition, you'll need to know how to recognize changes in fluid and electrolyte status, glucose tolerance, amino acid, mineral, and vitamin levels. You'll also need to judge your patient's response to the nutrient solution and to detect early signs of complications.

Patient teaching

Many patients are apprehensive about I.V. therapy. To allay their fears, you can provide information that explains and clarifies this therapy. Use pamphlets and videotapes if available. If possible, show the patient the actual equipment, and explain how it will be used during therapy.

Allow the patient to express fears and concerns, and convey reassurance by answering his questions fully. You may want to involve a family member or caregiver in these discussions to further reassure the patient.

Home I.V. therapy

More and more patients are receiving I.V. therapy at home. Home therapy benefits patients by making them feel more comfortable and allowing them to perform many of their normal activities. Its lower cost benefits both patients and health care facilities.

Home care patients may receive fluids or medications such as antibiotics, antifungals, chemotherapeutic agents, insulin, and analgesics. Some blood products have been given at home after an initial transfusion in a health care facility.

Candidates for home I.V. therapy should be selected carefully. Such patients must be willing and able to administer therapy safely, learn the potential complications and interventions, understand the basics of asepsis, and obtain the necessary supplies. Patients who need help must enlist a home caregiver, such as a family member or friend, to assist them in administering I.V. therapy.

When teaching the home care patient, demonstrate procedures and answer any questions. Have the patient or family members give return demonstrations whenever possible. Teaching should begin in the facility and be completed before the patient is discharged. You may want to include a family member or caregiver in your patient teaching.

Documentation

You need to document I.V. therapy for many reasons. First, an accurate description of your care provides legal protection for you and the facility. Furthermore, thorough documentation furnishes health care insurers with the records they need of the equipment and supplies used. You may document I.V. therapy on progress notes, a special I.V. therapy sheet or flowchart, or a nursing plan of care on the patient's chart. You also must document it on the intake and output sheet.

PERIPHERAL I.V. THERAPY

MEDICATION ERROR REDUCTION

The National Coordinating Council for Medication Error Reporting and Prevention defines a medication error as "any preventable event that may cause or lead to inappropriate medication use or patient harm while the medication is in the control of the health care professional, patient, or consumer. Such events may be related to professional practice, health care products, procedures, and systems, including prescribing; order communication; product labeling, packaging, and nomenclature; compounding; dispensing; distribution; administration; education; monitoring; and use."

A 1999 report by the Institute of Medicine (IOM) found that medication errors are the most common cause of medical errors in the hospital and affect 3.7% of patients. Medical errors accounted for 44,000 to 98,000 deaths each year, with the total cost of medical errors estimated at $17 to $29 billion annually.

To reduce medication errors, the Institute for Safe Medication Practices recommends that health care facilities set up a multidisciplinary team. At a minimum, the team should be comprised of front-line practitioners — physicians, pharmacists, and nurses who have intimate knowledge of the medication use processes; a strong facilitator, such as a risk management or quality improvement professional, to handle the day-to-day team issues; a representative from high-level administration for support and quick decision-making; and another practitioner who's willing to help promote medication safety initiatives. The team's goals should include:

- promoting a nonpunitive approach to reducing medication errors and increasing detection and reporting of medication errors
- educating practitioners about the system-based causes of errors and their prevention and exploring the cause of medication errors
- responding to potentially hazardous situations (such as medication labeling) before errors occur
- recommending and facilitating hospital-wide, system-based changes to prevent medication errors.

Key nursing steps in reducing errors

Taking the following steps can help reduce the risk of medication errors.

Know your patient

Studies have shown that preventable adverse drug events occur because the practitioner doesn't know enough about the patient — for example, awareness of a patient's drug allergies — before prescribing, dispensing, and administering medications. Having information about the patient helps the primary care provider determine appropriate medications, dosages, and administration routes. Information such as height, weight, allergies, medical history, and pregnancy status as well as vital signs and laboratory values are key to monitoring the effects of medications and the underlying disease process. This information should be communicated to the pharmacist *so that he can properly screen all medication orders before dispensing them.*

Properly identify your patient

Knowing your patient isn't enough to prevent a medication error. Each time you administer a medication, you must confirm the patient's identity using two patient identifiers, aside from the patient's room number, according to your facility's policy.

Know the medications

Keeping abreast of new drug therapies is important. Not knowing about current therapies can be as risky as not knowing your patient. Most serious medication errors occur because the patient receives the wrong medication or the wrong dose. Errors in medication dosing usually occur due to miscommunication or miscalculation. To get up-to-date information about medications, use various sources, such as textbooks, a controlled drug formulary, drug protocols, dosing scales and order sets, medication administration records, and communication with your in-house pharmacy.

Communicate

Miscommunication is one of the major causes of medication errors. It could result from:

- absence of a standardized prescribing vocabulary. At least 1 in 10 medication errors is directly related to the use of incorrect drug names, confusing use of dosage forms, or misunderstood abbreviations. The Joint Commission's National Patient Safety Goals require the use of standardized abbreviations, acronyms, and symbols. *Using a standardized prescribing vocabulary eliminates the use of acronyms, "coined names," and confusing abbreviations, which aids in preventing medication errors.*

- incorrect decimal point placement. This could cause serious harm to the patient. When the dose is less than 1, a zero should always precede the decimal, and a zero should never appear after a whole number — for example, 2 mg shouldn't appear as 2.0 mg *because if the decimal point is missed, the patient could receive 10 times the prescribed dose.*
- verbal orders. Although convenient for the prescriber, verbal orders can easily be misheard and should only be used in an emergency. The protocol for verbal orders should include safety checks, such as having another nurse on the phone when taking a verbal order by telephone, restating the patient's name, spelling out the drug name, and repeating the dosage to the prescriber. After receiving the verbal order, you should immediately write it in the patient's chart. In instances when the prescriber attempts to give a verbal order while visiting a patient, request that he write the order in the patient's chart instead.
- intimidation. This can commonly hinder effective communication between health care professionals. The problem may be compounded further if the facility doesn't have a policy on how to settle disagreements about the safety of orders. It's important to speak up and get answers about any order that doesn't seem to be right.

Watch for drugs that sound alike

Confusion over drug names that sound alike is one of the most common reasons pharmacies dispense and nurses administer the wrong drug. Adding to the problem are label packaging and confusing labels. One way to reduce the risk of dispensing and administering the wrong drug is to store drugs with similar packaging separate from one another.

Improper labeling coupled with the lack of a unit-dose system also contribute to faulty drug identification. To avoid this factor, ask the pharmacist to send up prefilled, prelabeled syringes of medications, such as heparin, sodium chloride solution flushes, and opioids. In addition, use blank labels that can be easily added to the needles, even if you intend to administer the medication right away. Otherwise, prepare the patient's medication at the bedside and administer it right away.

The IOM has developed strategies to improve medication safety. Some key strategies are:

- implementing a standard process for medication doses, dose timing, and dose scales in a given patient care unit
- standardizing prescription writing and prescribing rules (for example, including the purpose of the prescribed medication)
- using pharmaceutical software
- having a central pharmacy supply dispense high-risk I.V. medications such as chemotherapeutic drugs
- limiting the type of medications stored on patient care units
- including the pharmacist on patient rounds in the units.

In general, implementing simple strategies and working with a team to improve medication prescription, administration, and dispensing of drugs helps reduce medication errors. When medication orders don't seem quite right, pharmacists, nurses, and practitioners must take the extra step to verify an order before a medication is prescribed, dispensed, or administered to a patient.

SELECTED REFERENCES

Bond, C.A., et al. "Medication Errors in United States Hospitals," *Pharmacotherapy* 21(9):1023-36, July 2001.

Bullock, J., et al. "Standardizing IV Infusion Medication Concentrations to Reduce Variability in Medication Errors," *Critical Care Nursing Clinics of North America* 18(4):515-21, December 2006.

Eisehauer, L.A., et al. "Nurses' Reported Thinking during Medication Administration," *Journal of Nursing Scholarship* 39(1):82-87, 2007.

Hairon, N. "Preventing Medication Errors and Improving Patient Safety," *Nursing Times* 103(15):21-22, April 2007.

The Joint Commission. 2005 National Patient Safety Goals. *Comprehensive Accreditation Manual for Hospitals: The Official Handbook,* November 2005.

Mahlmeister, L.R. "Best Practices in Medication Administration: Preventing Adverse Drug Events in Perinatal Settings," *Journal of Perinatal and Neonatal Nursing* 21(1):6-8, January-March 2007.

PERIPHERAL I.V. THERAPY PREPARATION

Selection and preparation of appropriate equipment are essential for accurate delivery of an I.V. solution. Selection of an I.V. administration set depends on the rate and type of infusion desired and the type of I.V. solution container used. Two types of drip sets are available: the macrodrip and the microdrip. The macrodrip set can deliver a solution in large quantities at rapid rates because it delivers a larger amount with each drop than the microdrip set. The microdrip set, used for pediatric patients and certain adult patients who require small or closely regulated amounts of I.V. solution, delivers a smaller quantity with each drop.

Administration tubing with a secondary injection port permits separate or simultaneous infusion of two solutions; tubing with a piggyback port and a backcheck valve permits intermittent infusion of a secondary solution and, on its completion, a return to infusion of the primary solution. Vented I.V. tubing is selected for solutions in nonvented bottles; nonvented tubing is selected for solutions in bags or vented bottles. Assembly of I.V. equipment requires sterile technique to prevent contamination, which can cause local or systemic infection.

According to Infusion Nurses Society Standards, primary and secondary set should be changed every 72 hours, using sterile technique and immediately upon suspected contamination or when the integrity of the system has been compromised.

Equipment

I.V. solution ▪ alcohol pad ▪ I.V. administration set ▪ in-line filter, if needed ▪ I.V. pole ▪ medication and label, if necessary.

Preparation of equipment

Verify the type, volume, and expiration date of the I.V. solution. Discard outdated solution. If the solution is contained in a glass bottle, inspect the bottle for chips and cracks; if it's in a plastic bag, squeeze the bag to detect leaks. Examine the I.V. solution for particles, abnormal discoloration, and cloudiness. If present, discard the solution, and notify the pharmacy or dispensing department. If ordered, add medication to the solution, and place a completed medication-added label on the container. Remove the administration set from its box, and check for cracks, holes, and missing clamps.

Implementation

- Wash your hands thoroughly *to prevent introducing contaminants during preparation.*
- Slide the flow clamp of the administration set tubing down to the drip chamber or injection port, and close the clamp.

Preparing a bag

- Place the bag on a flat, stable surface, or hang it on an I.V. pole.
- Remove the protective cap, or tear the tab from the tubing insertion port.
- Remove the protective cap from the administration set spike, as shown top of next column.

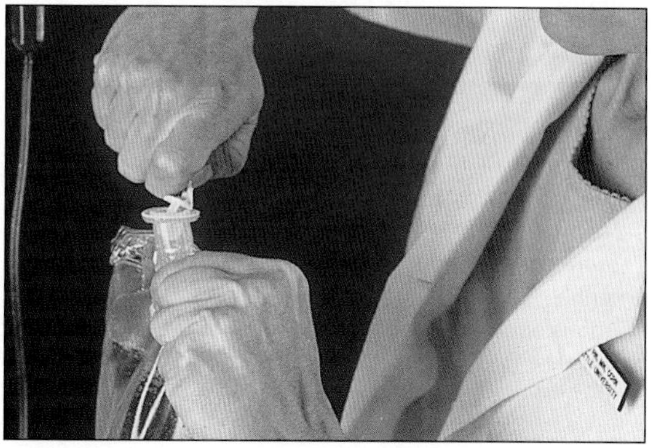

- Holding the port firmly with one hand, insert the spike with your other hand, as shown below.

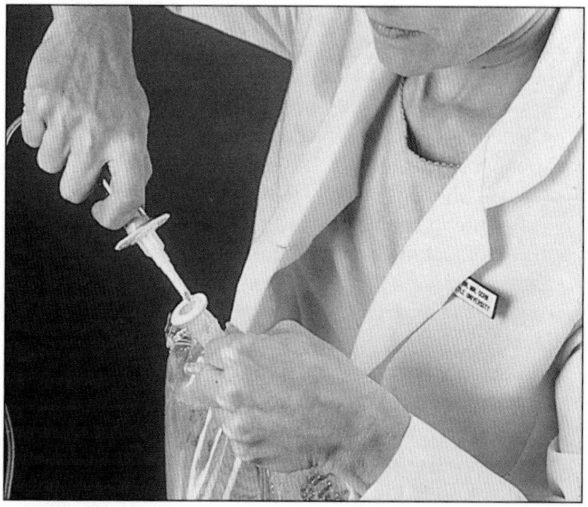

- Hang the bag on the I.V. pole, if you haven't already, and squeeze the drip chamber until it is half full, as shown below.

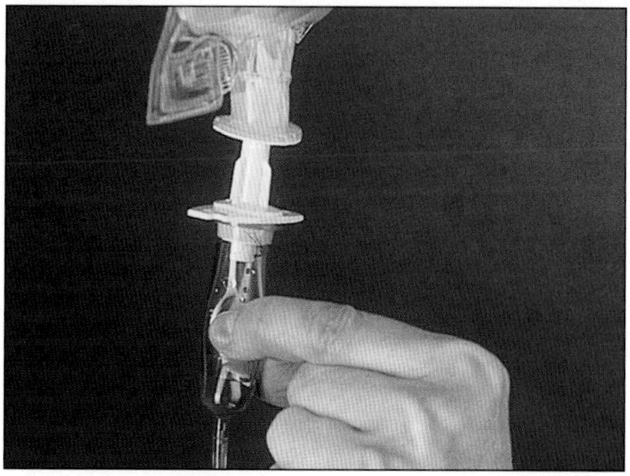

When to use an in-line filter

An in-line filter removes pathogens and particles from I.V. solutions, *helping to reduce the risk of infusion phlebitis*. However, *because in-line filters are expensive and their installation is cumbersome and time-consuming*, they aren't used routinely. Many facilities allow use of an in-line filter only when administering an admixture. If you're unsure of whether to use a filter, check your facility's policy or follow this list of do's and don'ts.

Do's

Use an in-line filter:

- when administering solutions to an immunodeficient patient.
- when administering total parenteral nutrition.
- when using additives comprising many separate particles, such as antibiotics requiring reconstitution, or when administering several additives.
- when using rubber injection ports or plastic diaphragms repeatedly.
- when phlebitis is likely to occur.

Be sure to change the in-line filter according to the manufacturer's recommendations. *If you don't, bacteria trapped in the filter releases endotoxin, a pyrogen small enough to pass through the filter into the bloodstream.*

Use an add-on filter of larger pore size (1.2 microns) when infusing lipid emulsions and albumin mixed with nutritional solutions.

If a positive-pressure electronic infusion device is used, consider the pound per square inch (psi) rating of the filter. If the psi from the infusion device exceeds that of the filter, the filter will crack or break under the pressure.

Don'ts

Don't use an in-line filter:

- when administering solutions with large particles *that will clog a filter and stop I.V. flow,* such as suspensions, lipid emulsions, and high-molecular-volume plasma expanders. These require specialized filters.
- when administering a drug dose of 5 mg or less *because the filter may absorb it.*

Preparing a nonvented bottle

- Remove the bottle's metal cap and inner disk, if present.
- Place the bottle on a stable surface, and wipe the rubber stopper with an alcohol pad.
- Remove the protective cap from the administration set spike, and push the spike through the center of the bottle's rubber stopper. Avoid twisting or angling the spike *to prevent pieces of the stopper from breaking off and falling into the solution.*
- Invert the bottle. If its vacuum is intact, you'll hear a hissing sound and see air bubbles rise (this may not occur if you've already added medication). If the vacuum isn't intact, discard the bottle and begin again.
- Hang the bottle on the I.V. pole, and squeeze the drip chamber until it's half full.

Preparing a vented bottle

- Remove the bottle's metal cap and latex diaphragm *to release the vacuum.* If the vacuum isn't intact (except after medication has been added), discard the bottle and begin again.
- Place the bottle on a stable surface, and wipe the rubber stopper with an alcohol pad.
- Remove the protective cap from the administration set spike, and push the spike through the insertion port next to the air vent tube opening.
- Hang the bottle on the I.V. pole, and squeeze the drip chamber until it's half full.

Priming the I.V. tubing

- If necessary, attach a filter to the opposite end of the I.V. tubing, and follow the manufacturer's instructions for filling and priming it. Purge the tubing before attaching the filter *to avoid forcing air into the filter and, possibly, clogging some filter channels.* Most filters are positioned with the distal end of the tubing facing upward *so that the solution will completely wet the filter membrane and all air bubbles will be eliminated from the line.* (See *When to use an in-line filter.*)
- If you aren't using a filter, aim the distal end of the tubing over a wastebasket or sink and slowly open the flow clamp. (Most distal tube coverings allow the solution to flow without having to remove the protective cover.)
- Leave the clamp open until the I.V. solution flows through the entire length of tubing *to release trapped air bubbles and force out all the air.*
- Invert all Y-ports and backcheck valves and tap them, if necessary, *to fill them with solution.*
- After priming the tubing, close the clamp. Then loop the tubing over the I.V. pole.
- Label the container with the patient's name and room number, date and time, container number, ordered rate and duration of infusion, and your initials.

Special considerations

- Before initiation of I.V. therapy, the patient should be told what to expect. (See *Teaching about I.V. therapy.*)

Teaching about I.V. therapy

Many patients are apprehensive about peripheral I.V. therapy. So before you begin therapy, tell your patient what to expect before, during, and after the procedure *to reduce anxiety and make therapy easier.*

Before insertion

- Describe the procedure. Tell him that "intravenous" means inside the vein and that a plastic catheter will be placed in his vein. Explain that fluids containing nutrients or medications will flow from a bag or bottle through a length of tubing and then through the plastic catheter into his vein.
- Tell him about how long the catheter will stay in place. Explain that the practitioner will decide how much and what type of fluid the patient needs.
- If the patient will receive a local anesthetic at the insertion site, ask him if he's allergic to lidocaine. If in doubt, use another anesthetic. Tell him that this injection will numb the site *to reduce the pain of I.V. device insertion.*
- If no anesthetic will be used, tell the patient that he may feel transient pain at the insertion site but that the discomfort will stop when the catheter is in place.
- Tell him that I.V. fluid may feel cold at first but that this sensation should last only a few minutes.

During therapy

- Tell the patient to report any discomfort after the catheter has been inserted and the fluid has begun flowing.
- Explain any restrictions as ordered. As appropriate, tell the patient that he may be able to walk and, depending on the insertion site and the device, to shower or take a tub bath during therapy.
- Teach him how to care for the I.V. line. Tell him not to pull at the insertion site or tubing, not to remove the container from the I.V. pole, and not to kink the tubing or lie on it. Instruct him to call a nurse if the flow rate suddenly slows or speeds up.

At removal

- Explain that removing a peripheral I.V. line is a simple procedure. Tell the patient that pressure will be applied to the site until the bleeding stops. Reassure him that when the device is out and the bleeding stops, he'll be able to use the affected arm or leg as before therapy.

- Always use sterile technique when preparing I.V. solutions. If you contaminate the administration set or container, replace it with a new one *to prevent introducing contaminants into the system.*
- If necessary, you can use vented tubing with a vented bottle. To do this, don't remove the latex diaphragm. Instead, insert the spike into the larger indentation in the diaphragm.
- Change I.V. tubing every 72 hours or according to your facility's policy or more frequently if you suspect contamination. Change the filter according to the manufacturer's recommendations or sooner if it becomes clogged.

Documentation

Document the type of solution used and any additives added to the solution.

SELECTED REFERENCES

Hadaway, L.C. "Reopen the Pipeline for I.V. Therapy," *Nursing* 35(8):54-61, August 2005.

Higgins, D. "Priming an I.V. Infusion Set," *Nursing Times* 100(47):32-33, November 2004.

"Standard 11. Patient Education. Infusion Nursing Standards of Practice," *Journal of Infusion Nursing* 29(1S):S19-20, January-February 2006.

"Standard 14. Documentation. Infusion Nursing Standards of Practice," *Journal of Infusion Nursing* 29(1S):S22-S23, January-February 2006.

"Standard 15. Product Evaluation, Integrity, and Defect Reporting. Infusion Nursing Standards of Practice," *Journal of Infusion Nursing* 29(1S):S22-S23, January-February 2006.

"Standard 16. Product Labeling. Infusion Nursing Standards of Practice," *Journal of Infusion Nursing* 29(1S):S23-S24, January-February 2006.

"Standard 19. Infection Control. Infusion Nursing Standards of Practice," *Journal of Infusion Nursing* 29(1S):S25-S26, January-February 2006.

"Standard 20. Hand Hygiene. Infusion Nursing Standards of Practice," *Journal of Infusion Nursing* 29(1S):S27-S28, January-February 2006.

"Standard 32. Filters. Infusion Nursing Standards of Practice," *Journal of Infusion Nursing* 29(1S):S33-34, January-February 2006.

"Standard 48. Administration Set Change. Infusion Nursing Standards of Practice," *Journal of Infusion Nursing* 29(1S):S48-S51, January-February 2006.

Taylor, C., et al. *Fundamentals of Nursing: The Art and Science of Nursing Care,* 6th ed. Philadelphia: Lippincott Williams & Wilkins, 2008.

Zahourek, R. "Nursing the I.V. Tubing," *AJN* 105(10):15, October 2005.

Volume-control sets

A volume-control set — an I.V. line with a graduated chamber — delivers precise amounts of fluid and shuts off when the fluid is exhausted, preventing air from entering the I.V. line. It may be used as a secondary line in adults for intermittent infusion of medication.

PEDIATRIC ALERT *A volume-control set is used as a primary line in children for continuous infusion of fluids or medication.*

Equipment

Volume-control set ▪ I.V. pole (for setting up a primary I.V. line) ▪ I.V. solution ▪ 19G to 21G 1″ needle or needle-free adapter ▪ antimicrobial swab ▪ medication in labeled syringe ▪ tape ▪ label.

Although various models of volume-control sets are available, each one consists of a graduated fluid chamber (120 to 250 ml) with a spike and a filtered air line on top and administration tubing underneath. Floating-valve sets have a valve at the bottom that closes when the chamber empties; membrane-filter sets have a rigid filter at the bottom that, when wet, prevents the passage of air.

Preparation of equipment

Ensure the sterility of all equipment, and inspect it carefully *to ensure the absence of flaws.* Take the equipment to the patient's bedside.

Implementation

- Confirm the patient's identity using two patient identifiers according to your facility's policy.
- Wash your hands, and explain the procedure to the patient.
- If an I.V. line is already in place, observe its insertion site for signs of infiltration and infection.
- Remove the volume-control set from its box, and close all the clamps.
- Remove the protective cap from the volume-control set spike, insert the spike into the I.V. solution container, and hang the container on the I.V. pole.
- Open the air vent clamp and close the upper slide clamp. Then open the lower clamp on the I.V. tubing, slide it upward until it's slightly below the drip chamber, and close the clamp.
- Open the upper clamp, until the fluid chamber fills with about 30 ml of solution. Then close the clamp, and carefully squeeze the drip chamber until it is half full.
- Keeping the drip chamber flat, close the lower clamp. Now release the drip chamber so that it fills halfway.
- Open the lower clamp, prime the tubing, and close the clamp. To use the set as a primary line, insert the distal end of the tubing into the catheter or needle hub.
- To use the set as a secondary line, wipe the Y-port of the primary tubing with an antimicrobial swab, and attach the distal end of the tubing to the Y-port of the primary tubing, following the manufacturer's instructions.
- To add medication, wipe the injection port on the volume-control set with an antimicrobial swab, and inject the medication, as shown below.

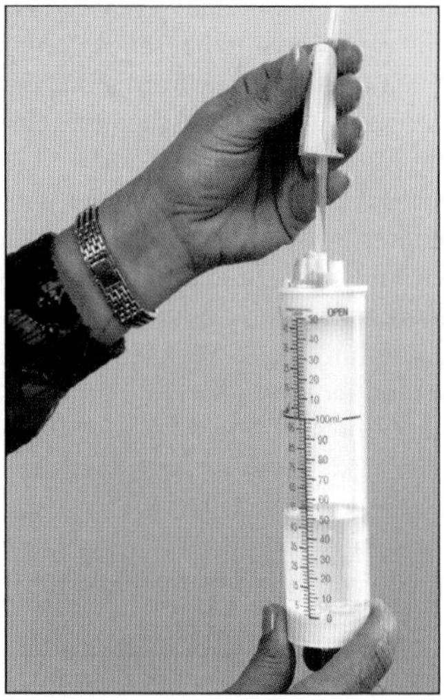

- Place a label on the chamber, indicating the drug, dose, and date. Don't write directly on the chamber because the plastic absorbs ink.
- Open the upper clamp, fill the fluid chamber with the prescribed amount of solution (as shown below), and close the clamp. Gently rotate the chamber *to mix the medication.*

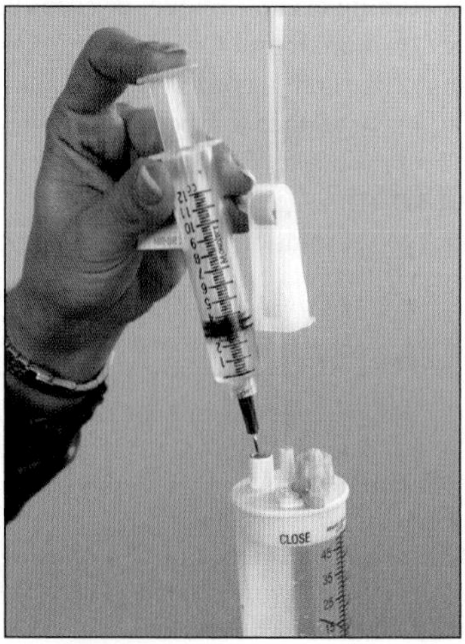

- Turn off the primary solution (if present) or lower the drip rate *to maintain an open line.*
- Open the lower clamp on the volume-control set, and adjust the drip rate as ordered. After completion of the infusion, open the upper clamp and let 10 ml of I.V. solution flow into the chamber and through the tubing *to flush them.*
- If you're using the volume-control set as a secondary I.V. line, close the lower clamp, and reset the flow rate of the primary line. If you're using the set as a primary I.V. line, close the lower clamp, refill the chamber to the prescribed amount, and begin the infusion again.

Special considerations

- Always check compatibility of the medication and the I.V. solution. If you're using a membrane-filter set, avoid administering suspensions, lipid emulsions, blood, or blood components through it.
- The diaphragm may stick after repeated use. If it does, close the air vent and upper clamp, invert the drip chamber, and squeeze it. If the diaphragm opens, reopen the clamp and continue to use the set.
- If the drip chamber overfills, immediately close the upper clamp and air vent, invert the chamber, and squeeze the excess fluid from the drip chamber back into the graduated fluid chamber.

Documentation

If you add a drug to the volume-control set, record the amount and type of medication, amount of fluid used to dilute it, and date and time of infusion.

SELECTED REFERENCES

"Standard 15. Product Evaluation, Integrity, and Defect Report. Infusion Nursing Standards of Practice," *Journal of Infusion Nursing* 29(1S):S23, January-February 2006.

"Standard 48. Administration Set Change. Infusion Nursing Standards of Practice," *Journal of Infusion Nursing* 29(1S):S48-51, January-February 2006.

"Standard 68. Parenteral Medication and Solution Administration. Infusion Nursing Standards of Practice," *Journal of Infusion Nursing* 29(1S):S74-75, January-February 2006.

Weinstein, S.M. *Plumer's Principles and Practices of Intravenous Therapy,* 8th ed. Philadelphia: Lippincott Williams & Wilkins, 2007.

PERIPHERAL I.V. CATHETER INSERTION

Peripheral I.V. catheter insertion involves selection of a venipuncture device and an insertion site, application of a tourniquet, preparation of the site, and venipuncture. Selection of a venipuncture device and site depends on the type of solution to be used; frequency and duration of infusion; patency and location of accessible veins; the patient's age, size, and condition; and, when possible, the patient's preference.

If possible, choose a vein in the nondominant arm or hand. Preferred venipuncture sites are the cephalic and basilic veins in the lower arm and the veins in the dorsum of the hand; least favorable are the leg and foot veins because of the increased risk of thrombophlebitis. Antecubital veins can be used if no other venous access is available. Subsequent venipunctures should be performed proximal to a previously used or injured vein.

A peripheral catheter allows administration of fluids, medication, blood, and blood components and maintains I.V. access to the patient. Insertion is contraindicated in a sclerotic vein, an edematous or impaired arm or hand, or a postmastectomy arm and in patients with a mastectomy, burns, or an arteriovenous fistula. If the catheter has to be inserted in the mastectomy arm or one with impaired circulation, the practitioner should be contacted and an order written before starting therapy.

Equipment

Antimicrobial solution ▪ gloves ▪ tourniquet (rubber tubing or a blood pressure cuff) ▪ I.V. access devices ▪ I.V. solution with attached and primed administration set ▪ I.V. pole ▪ sharps container ▪ sterile 2″ × 2″ gauze pads, a transparent semipermeable dressing, or a catheter securement device ▪ 1″ hypoallergenic ▪ optional: arm board, roller gauze, tube gauze, warm packs, scissors.

Commercial venipuncture kits come with or without an I.V. access device. (See *Comparing venous access devices,* page 350.) In many facilities, venipuncture equipment is kept on a tray or cart, *which allows choice of correct access devices and easy replacement of contaminated items.*

Preparation of equipment

Check the information on the label of the I.V. solution container, including the patient's name and room number, type of solution, time and date of its preparation, preparer's name, and ordered infusion rate. Compare the practitioner's orders with the solution label *to verify that the solution is the correct one.* Then select the smallest-gauge device that's appropriate for the infusion (unless subsequent therapy will require a larger one). *Smaller gauges cause less trauma to veins, allow greater blood flow around their tips, and reduce the risk of phlebitis.*

If you're using a winged infusion set, connect the adapter to the administration set, and unclamp the line until fluid flows from the open end of the needle cover. Then close the

- Aggressively push the needle directly through the skin and into the vein in one motion. Check the flashback chamber behind the hub for blood return, *signifying that the vein has been properly accessed.* (You may not see a blood return in a small vein.)
- Then level the insertion device slightly by lifting the tip of the device up *to prevent puncturing the back wall of the vein with the access device.*
- If you're using a winged infusion set, advance the needle fully, if possible, and hold it in place. Release the tourniquet, open the administration set clamp slightly, and check for free flow or infiltration.
- If you're using an over-the-needle cannula, advance the device to at least half its length *to ensure that the cannula itself—not just the introducer needle—has entered the vein.* Then remove the tourniquet.
- Grasp the cannula hub to hold it in the vein, and withdraw the needle. As you withdraw it, press lightly on the catheter tip *to prevent bleeding* (as shown below).

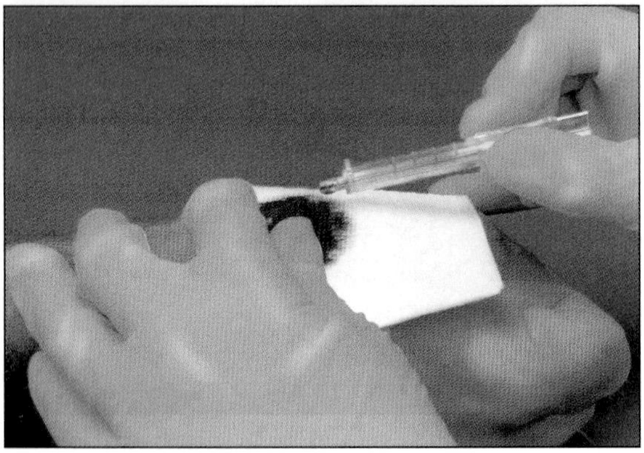

- Advance the cannula up to the hub or until you meet resistance.
- To advance the cannula while infusing I.V. solution, release the tourniquet and remove the inner needle. Using sterile technique, attach the I.V. tubing and begin the infusion. While stabilizing the vein with one hand, use the other to advance the catheter into the vein. When the catheter is advanced, decrease the I.V. flow rate. *This method reduces the risk of puncturing the vein's opposite wall because the catheter is advanced without the steel needle and because the rapid flow dilates the vein.*
- To advance the cannula before starting the infusion, first release the tourniquet. While stabilizing the vein and needle with one hand, use the other to advance the catheter off the needle and further into the vein up to the hub (as shown top of next column). Next, remove the inner needle and, using sterile technique, quickly attach the I.V. tubing. *This method often results in less blood being spilled.*

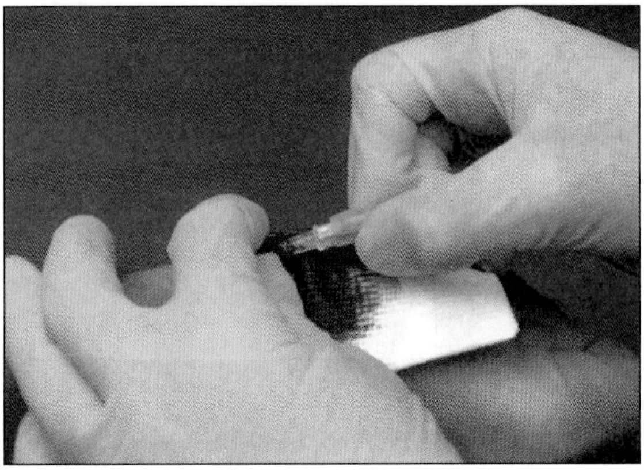

Dressing the site

- After the venous access device has been inserted, clean the skin completely. If necessary, dispose of the stylet in a sharps container. Then regulate the flow rate.
- You may use a transparent semipermeable dressing *to secure the device.* If possible, use a commercial catheter securement device to secure the catheter. (See *How to apply a transparent semipermeable dressing.*)
- If you don't use a transparent dressing, cover the site with a sterile gauze pad or small adhesive bandage.
- Loop the I.V. tubing on the patient's limb, and secure the tubing with tape. *The loop allows some slack to prevent dislodgment of the cannula from tension on the line.* (See *Methods of taping a venous access site,* page 354.)
- Label the last piece of tape with the type, gauge of needle, and length of cannula; date and time of insertion; and your initials. Adjust the flow rate as ordered.
- If the puncture site is near a movable joint, place an arm board under the joint, and secure it with roller gauze or tape *to provide stability because excessive movement can dislodge the venous access device and increase the risk of thrombophlebitis and infection.*
- When an arm board is used, check frequently for impaired circulation distal to the infusion site.

Removing a peripheral I.V. line

- A peripheral I.V. line is removed on completion of therapy, for cannula site changes, and for suspected infection or infiltration; the procedure usually requires gloves, a sterile gauze pad, and an adhesive bandage.
- To remove the I.V. line, first clamp the I.V. tubing *to stop the flow of solution.* Then gently remove the transparent dressing and all tape from the skin.
- Using sterile technique, open the gauze pad and adhesive bandage, and place them within reach. Put on gloves. Hold the sterile gauze pad over the puncture site with one hand,

and use your other hand to withdraw the cannula slowly and smoothly, keeping it parallel to the skin.

- Inspect the cannula tip; if it isn't smooth, assess the patient immediately, and notify the practitioner.
- Using the gauze pad, apply firm pressure over the puncture site for 1 to 2 minutes after removal or until bleeding has stopped.
- Clean the site and apply the adhesive bandage or, if blood oozes, apply a pressure bandage.
- If drainage appears at the puncture site, swab the tip of the device across an agar plate, or cut the tip into a sterile container using sterile scissors, and send it to the laboratory to be cultured according to your facility's policy. (*A draining site may or may not be infected.*) Then clean the area, apply a sterile dressing, and notify the practitioner.
- Instruct the patient to restrict activity for about 10 minutes and to leave the dressing in place for at least 1 hour. If the patient experiences lingering tenderness at the site, apply warm packs and notify the practitioner.

Special considerations

ELDER ALERT ***Apply the tourniquet carefully to avoid pinching the skin. If necessary, apply it over the patient's gown. Make sure skin preparation materials are at room temperature to avoid vasoconstriction resulting from lower temperatures.***

- If the patient is allergic to iodine-containing compounds, clean the skin with alcohol.
- If you fail to see blood flashback after the needle enters the vein, pull back slightly and rotate the device. If you still fail to see flashback, remove the cannula and try again, or proceed according to your facility's policy.
- Change a gauze or transparent dressing whenever you change the administration set (every 48 hours or according to your facility's policy).
- Be sure to rotate the I.V. site, every 72 hours or according to your facility's policy.

How to apply a transparent semipermeable dressing

To secure the I.V. insertion site, you can apply a transparent semipermeable dressing as follows:

- Make sure the insertion site is clean and dry.
- Remove the dressing from the package and, using sterile technique, remove the protective seal. Avoid touching the sterile surface.
- Place the dressing directly over the insertion site and the hub, as shown below. Don't cover the tubing. Also, don't stretch the dressing *because doing so may cause itching.*

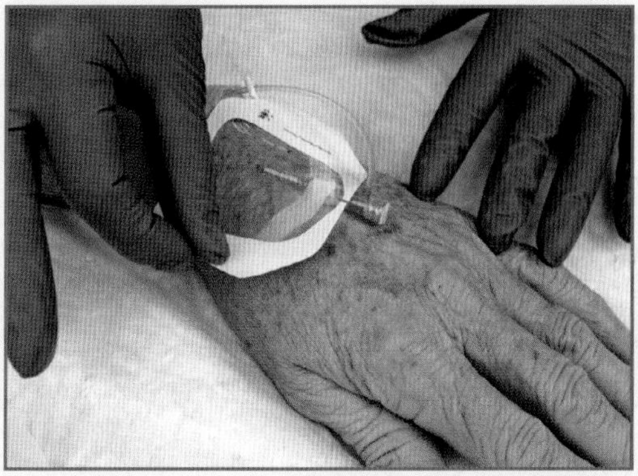

- Tuck the dressing around and under the cannula hub *to make the site impervious to microorganisms.*
- To remove the dressing, grasp one corner, and then lift and stretch it. If removal is difficult, try loosening the edges with alcohol or water.

Home care

Most patients who receive I.V. therapy at home have a central venous line. But if you're caring for a patient going home with a peripheral line, you should teach him how to care for the I.V. site and identify certain complications. If the patient must observe movement restrictions, make sure he understands them.

Teach the patient how to examine the site, and instruct him to notify the practitioner or home care nurse if redness, swelling, or discomfort develops or if the dressing becomes moist.

Also tell the patient to report any problems with the I.V. line, for instance, if the solution stops infusing or if an alarm goes off on an infusion pump. Explain that the I.V. site will be changed at established intervals by a home care nurse.

If the patient is using an intermittent infusion device, teach him how and when to flush it. Finally, teach the patient to document daily whether the I.V. site is free from pain, swelling, and redness.

Complications

Peripheral line complications can result from the needle or catheter (infection, phlebitis, and embolism) or from the solution (circulatory overload, infiltration, sepsis, and allergic reaction). (See *Risks of peripheral I.V. therapy,* pages 355 to 359.)

Methods of taping a venous access site

If you'll be using tape to secure the access device to the insertion site, use one of the basic methods described below. Use sterile tape if you'll be placing a transparent dressing over the tape.

Chevron method

- Cut a long strip of ½″ tape, and place it sticky side up under the cannula and parallel to the short strip of tape.
- Cross the ends of the tape over the cannula so that the tape sticks to the patient's skin (as shown below).
- Apply a piece of 1″ (2.5-cm) tape across the two wings of the chevron.
- Loop the tubing, and secure it with another piece of 1″ tape. When the dressing is secured, apply a label. On the label, write the date and time of insertion, type and gauge of the needle, and your initials.

U method

- Cut a 2″ (5-cm) strip of ½″ tape. With the sticky side up, place it under the hub of the cannula.
- Bring each side of the tape up, folding it over the wings of the cannula in a U shape (as shown below). Press it down parallel to the hub.
- Apply tape to stabilize the catheter.
- When a dressing is secured, apply a label. On the label, write the date and time of insertion, type and gauge of the needle or cannula, and your initials.

H method

- Cut three strips of 1″ tape.
- Place one strip of tape over each wing, keeping the tape parallel to the cannula (as shown below).
- Now place the other strip of tape perpendicular to the first two. Put it either directly on top of the wings or just below the wings, directly on top of the tubing.
- Make sure the cannula is secure; then apply a dressing and a label. On the label, write the date and time of insertion, type and gauge of needle or cannula, and your initials.

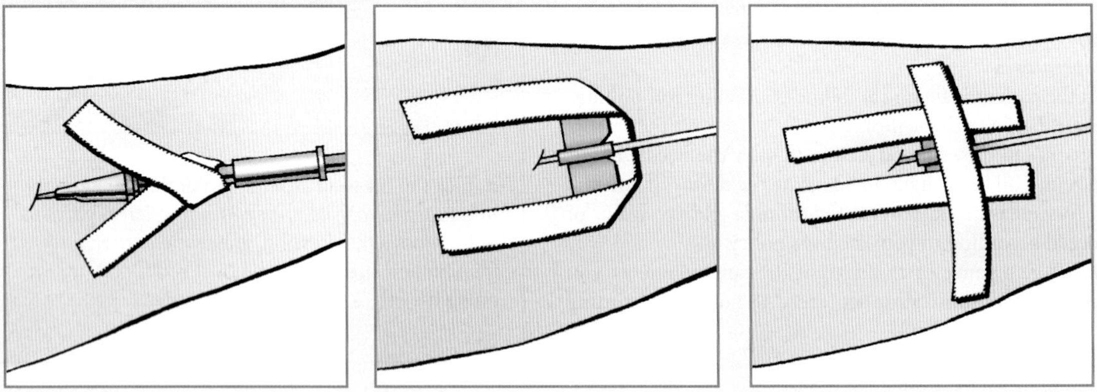

Documentation

In your notes or on the appropriate I.V. sheets, record the date and time of the venipuncture; type, gauge, and length of the cannula; anatomic location of the insertion site; and reason the site was changed.

Also document the number of attempts at venipuncture (if you made more than one), type and flow rate of the I.V. solution, name and amount of medication in the solution (if any), any adverse reactions and actions taken to correct them, patient teaching and evidence of patient understanding, and your initials.

SELECTED REFERENCES

Centers for Disease Control and Prevention. "Guidelines for the Prevention of Intravascular Device-Related Infections," *MMWR* 51(RR-10):1-26, August 2002.

Rosenthal, K. "Tailor Your I.V. Insertion Techniques Special Populations," *Nursing* 35(5):36-41, May 2005.

Rosenthal, K. "Get a Hold on Costs and Safety with Securement Devices," *Nursing Management* 36(5):52-54, May 2005.

"Standard 36. Tourniquet. Infusion Nursing Standards of Practice," *Journal of Infusion Nursing* 29(1S):S36, January-February 2006.

(Text continues on page 360.)

Risks of peripheral I.V. therapy

COMPLICATION	SIGNS AND SYMPTOMS	POSSIBLE CAUSES	NURSING INTERVENTIONS
LOCAL COMPLICATIONS			
Phlebitis	■ Tenderness at tip of and proximal to venous access device ■ Redness at tip of cannula and along vein ■ Puffy area over vein ■ Vein hard on palpation ■ Elevated temperature	■ Poor blood flow around venous access device ■ Friction from cannula movement in vein ■ Venous access device left in vein too long ■ Drug or solution with high or low pH or high osmolarity ■ Clotting at cannula tip	■ Remove venous access device. ■ Apply warm soaks. ■ Notify practitioner. ■ Document patient's condition and your interventions. ***Prevention*** ■ Restart infusion using larger vein for irrigating solution, or restart with smaller-gauge device *to ensure adequate blood flow.* ■ Tape device securely *to prevent motion.*
Infiltration	■ Swelling at and above I.V. site (may extend along entire limb) ■ Discomfort, burning, or pain at site (may be painless) ■ Tight feeling at site ■ Decreased skin temperature around site ■ Blanching at site ■ Continuing fluid infusion even when vein is occluded (although rate may decrease) ■ Absent blood black flow ■ Slower infusion rate	■ Venous access device dislodged from vein, or perforated vein	■ Stop infusion. Infiltrate site with an antidote, if appropriate. ■ Apply ice (early) or warm soaks (later) *to aid absorption.* Elevate limb. ■ Check for pulse and capillary refill periodically *to assess circulation.* ■ Restart infusion above infiltration site or in another limb. ■ Document patient's condition and your interventions. ***Prevention*** ■ Check I.V. site frequently. ■ Don't obscure area above site with tape. ■ Teach patient to observe I.V. site and report pain or swelling.

(continued)

Risks of peripheral I.V. therapy *(continued)*

Complication	Signs and symptoms	Possible causes	Nursing interventions
Local complications *(continued)*			
Cannula dislodgment	■ Cannula partly backed out of vein ■ Solution infiltrating	■ Loosened tape, or tubing snagged in bed linens, resulting in partial retraction of cannula; pulled out by confused patient	■ If no infiltration occurs, retape without pushing cannula back into vein. If pulled out, apply pressure to I.V. site with sterile dressing. ***Prevention*** ■ Tape venipuncture device securely on insertion.
Occlusion	■ Infusion doesn't flow ■ Infusion pump alarms indicating occlusion ■ Discomfort at infusion site	■ I.V. flow interrupted ■ Saline lock not flushed ■ Blood backflow in line when patient walks ■ Line clamped too long ■ Hypercoaguble patient	■ Use mild flush injection. Don't force it. If unsuccessful, remove I.V. line and reinsert a new one. ***Prevention*** ■ Maintain I.V. flow rate. ■ Flush promptly after intermittent piggyback administration. ■ Have patient walk with his arm bent at the elbow *to reduce risk of blood backflow.*
Vein irritation or pain at I.V. site	■ Pain during infusion ■ Possible blanching if vasospasm occurs ■ Red skin over vein during infusion ■ Rapidly developing signs of phlebitis	■ Solution with high or low pH or high osmolarity, such phenytoin, and some antibiotics (vancomycin and nafcillin)	■ Decrease the flow rate. ■ Try using an electronic flow device *to achieve a steady flow.* ***Prevention*** ■ Dilute solutions before administration. For example, give antibiotics in 250-ml solution rather than 100-ml solution. If drug has low pH, ask pharmacist if drug can be buffered with sodium bicarbonate. (Refer to your facility's policy.) ■ If long-term therapy of irritating drug is planned, ask practitioner to use central I.V. line.
Hematoma	■ Tenderness at venipuncture site ■ Bruised area around site ■ Inability to advance or flush I.V. line	■ Vein punctured through opposite wall at time of insertion ■ Leakage of blood from needle displacement	■ Remove venous access device. ■ Apply pressure and warm soaks to affected area. ■ Recheck for bleeding. ■ Document patient's condition and your interventions. ***Prevention*** ■ Choose a vein that can accommodate the size of venous access device. ■ Release tourniquet as soon as insertion is successful.

Risks of peripheral I.V. therapy *(continued)*

COMPLICATION	SIGNS AND SYMPTOMS	POSSIBLE CAUSES	NURSING INTERVENTIONS
LOCAL COMPLICATIONS *(continued)*			
Severed cannula	■ Leakage from cannula shaft	■ Cannula inadvertently cut by scissors ■ Reinsertion of needle into cannula	■ If broken part is visible, attempt to retrieve it. If unsuccessful, notify the practitioner. ■ If portion of cannula enters bloodstream, place tourniquet above I.V. site *to prevent progression of broken part.* ■ Notify practitioner and radiology department. ■ Document patient's condition and your interventions. ***Prevention*** ■ Don't use scissors around I.V. site. ■ Never reinsert needle into cannula. ■ Remove unsuccessfully inserted cannula and needle together.
Venous spasm	■ Pain along vein ■ Flow rate sluggish when clamp completely open ■ Blanched skin over vein	■ Severe vein irritation from irritating drugs or fluids ■ Administration of cold fluids or blood ■ Very rapid flow rate (with fluids at room temperature)	■ Apply warm soaks over vein and surrounding area. ■ Decrease flow rate. ***Prevention*** ■ Use a blood warmer for blood or packed red blood cells.
Vasovagal reaction	■ Sudden collapse of vein during venipuncture ■ Sudden pallor, sweating, faintness, dizziness, and nausea ■ Decreased blood pressure	■ Vasospasm from anxiety or pain	■ Lower head of bed. ■ Have patient take deep breaths. ■ Check vital signs. ***Prevention*** ■ Prepare patient for therapy *to relieve his anxiety.* ■ Use local anesthetic *to prevent pain.*
Thrombosis	■ Painful, reddened, and swollen vein ■ Sluggish or stopped I.V. flow	■ Injury to endothelial cells of vein wall, allowing platelets to adhere and thrombi to form	■ Remove venous access device; restart infusion in opposite limb if possible. ■ Apply warm soaks. ■ Watch for I.V. therapy–related infection; *thrombi provide an excellent environment for bacterial growth.* ***Prevention*** ■ Use proper venipuncture techniques *to reduce injury to vein.*

(continued)

Risks of peripheral I.V. therapy *(continued)*

Complication	Signs and symptoms	Possible causes	Nursing interventions
Local complications *(continued)*			
Thrombophlebitis	■ Severe discomfort ■ Reddened, swollen, and hardened vein	■ Thrombosis and inflammation	■ Same as for thrombosis. ***Prevention*** ■ Check site frequently. Remove venous access device at first sign of redness and tenderness.
Nerve, tendon, or ligament damage	■ Extreme pain (similar to electrical shock when nerve is punctured) ■ Numbness and muscle contraction ■ Delayed effects, including paralysis, numbness, and deformity	■ Improper venipuncture technique, resulting in injury to surrounding nerves, tendons, or ligaments ■ Tight taping or improper splinting with arm board	■ Stop procedure and remove device. ***Prevention*** ■ Don't repeatedly penetrate tissues with venous access device. ■ Don't apply excessive pressure when taping; don't encircle limb with tape. ■ Pad arm boards and tape, securing arm boards if possible.
Systemic complications			
Systemic infection (septicemia or bacteremia)	■ Fever, chills, and malaise for no apparent reason ■ Contaminated I.V. site, usually with no visible signs of infection at site	■ Failure to maintain sterile technique during insertion or site care ■ Severe phlebitis, which can set up ideal conditions for organism growth ■ Poor taping that permits venous access device to move, which can introduce organisms into bloodstream ■ Prolonged indwelling time of device ■ Weak immune system	■ Notify the practitioner. ■ Administer medications as prescribed. ■ Culture the site and device. ■ Monitor vital signs. ***Prevention*** ■ Use scrupulous sterile technique when handling solutions and tubing, inserting venous access device, and discontinuing infusion. ■ Secure all connections. ■ Change I.V. solutions, tubing, and venous access device at recommended times. ■ Use I.V. filters.

Risks of peripheral I.V. therapy *(continued)*

COMPLICATION	SIGNS AND SYMPTOMS	POSSIBLE CAUSES	NURSING INTERVENTIONS
SYSTEMIC COMPLICATIONS *(continued)*			
Allergic reaction	▪ Itching ▪ Watery eyes and nose ▪ Bronchospasm ▪ Wheezing ▪ Urticarial rash ▪ Edema at I.V. site ▪ Anaphylactic reaction (flushing, chills, anxiety, itching, palpitations, paresthesia, wheezing, seizures, cardiac arrest) after exposure	▪ Allergens such as medications	▪ If reaction occurs, stop infusion immediately, and infuse normal saline solution. ▪ Maintain a patent airway. ▪ Notify the practitioner. ▪ Administer antihistaminic steroid, anti-inflammatory, and antipyretic drugs, as prescribed. ▪ Give epinephrine as prescribed. Repeat as needed and prescribed. ▪ Administer cortisone if prescribed. ***Prevention*** ▪ Obtain patient's allergy history. Be aware of crossallergies. ▪ Assist with test dosing. ▪ Monitor patient carefully during first 15 minutes of administration of a new drug.
Circulatory overload	▪ Discomfort ▪ Jugular vein engorgement ▪ Respiratory distress ▪ Increased blood pressure ▪ Crackles ▪ Increased difference between fluid intake and output	▪ Roller clamp loosened to allow run-on infusion ▪ Flow rate too rapid ▪ Miscalculation of fluid requirements	▪ Raise the head of the bed. ▪ Administer oxygen as needed. ▪ Slow infusion rate; don't remove I.V. line. ▪ Notify the practitioner. ▪ Administer medications (probably furosemide) as prescribed. ***Prevention*** ▪ Use pump or rate minder for elderly or compromised patients. ▪ Recheck calculations of fluid requirements. ▪ Monitor infusion frequently.
Air embolism	▪ Respiratory distress ▪ Unequal breath sounds ▪ Weak pulse ▪ Increased central venous pressure ▪ Decreased blood pressure ▪ Loss of consciousness	▪ Solution container empty ▪ Solution container empties, and added container pushes air down the line (if line wasn't purged first) ▪ Tubing disconnected from venous access device or I.V. bag	▪ Discontinue infusion. ▪ Place patient on his left side in Trendelenburg's position *to allow air to enter right atrium.* ▪ Administer oxygen. ▪ Notify the practitioner. ▪ Document patient's condition and your interventions. ***Prevention*** ▪ Purge tubing of air completely before starting infusion. ▪ Use air-detection device on pump or air-eliminating filter proximal to I.V. site. ▪ Secure connections

"Standard 37. Site Selection. Infusion Nursing Standards of Practice," *Journal of Infusion Nursing* 29(1S):S37-39, January-February 2006.

"Standard 38. Catheter Selection. Infusion Nursing Standards of Practice," *Journal of Infusion Nursing* 29(1S):S38-40, January-February 2006.

"Standard 39. Hair Removal. Infusion Nursing Standards of Practice," *Journal of Infusion Nursing* 29(1S):S40-41, January-February 2006.

"Standard 40. Local Anesthesia. Infusion Nursing Standards of Practice," *Journal of Infusion Nursing* 29(1S):S41, January-February 2006.

"Standard 41. Access Site Preparation. Infusion Nursing Standards of Practice," *Journal of Infusion Nursing* 29(1S):S41-42, January-February 2006.

"Standard 42. Catheter Placement. Infusion Nursing Standards of Practice," *Journal of Infusion Nursing* 29(1S):S42-44, January-February 2006.

"Standard 43. Catheter Stabilization. Infusion Nursing Standards of Practice," *Journal of Infusion Nursing* 29(1S):S44, January-February 2006.

"Standard 44. Dressings. Infusion Nursing Standards of Practice," *Journal of Infusion Nursing* 29(1S):S44-45, January-February 2006.

"Standard 49. Catheter Removal. Infusion Nursing Standards of Practice," *Journal of Infusion Nursing* 29(1S):S51-54, January-February 2006.

"Standard 52. Discontinuation of Therapy. Infusion Nursing Standards of Practice," *Journal of Infusion Nursing* 29(1S):S58, January-February 2006.

"Standard 53. Phlebitis. Infusion Nursing Standards of Practice," *Journal of Infusion Nursing* 29(1S):S58-59, January-February 2006.

"Standard 54. Infiltration. Infusion Nursing Standards of Practice," *Journal of Infusion Nursing* 29(1S):S59, January-February 2006.

"Standard 58. Culturing for Suspected Infusion-Related Infections. Infusion Nursing Standards of Practice," *Journal of Infusion Nursing* 29(1S):S63-64, January-February 2006.

INTERMITTENT INFUSION DEVICE INSERTION

Also called a *saline* or *heparin lock,* an intermittent infusion device consists of a cannula with an injection cap attached. Filled with dilute heparin or saline solution to prevent blood clot formation, the device maintains venous access in patients who are receiving I.V. medication regularly or intermittently but who don't require continuous infusion. An intermittent infusion device is superior to an I.V. line that is maintained at a moderately slow infusion rate because it minimizes the risk of fluid overload and electrolyte imbalance. It also cuts costs, reduces the risk of contamination by eliminating I.V. solution containers and administration sets, increases patient comfort and mobility, reduces patient anxiety and, if inserted in a large vein, allows collection of multiple blood samples without repeated venipuncture.

Equipment

Intermittent infusion device ▪ needleless system device ▪ normal saline solution ▪ tourniquet ▪ antimicrobial solution ▪ venipuncture equipment ▪ transparent semipermeable dressing ▪ tape.

Prefilled saline cartridges are available for use in a syringe cartridge holder.

Implementation

- Wash your hands thoroughly *to prevent contamination of the venipuncture site.*
- Confirm the patient's identity using two patient identifiers according to your facility's policy.
- Explain the procedure to the patient, and describe the purpose of the intermittent infusion device.
- Remove the set from its packaging, wipe the port with an antimicrobial swab, and inject normal saline solution to fill the tubing and needleless system. *This removes air from the system, preventing formation of an air embolus.*
- Select a venipuncture site, and clean it with antimicrobial solution, wiping outward from the site in a circular motion.
- Perform the venipuncture, and ensure correct needle placement in the vein. Then release the tourniquet. (See "Peripheral I.V. catheter insertion," page 349, for complete instructions.)
- Tape the set in place. Loop the tubing, if applicable, *so that the injection port is free and easily accessible.*
- Apply a transparent semipermeable dressing. On a dressing label, write the time, date, and your initials, and place the label on the dressing.
- Remove and discard your gloves.
- Inject normal saline solution every 8 to 24 hours or according to your facility's policy *to maintain the patency of the intermittent infusion device.* Inject the heparin slowly *to prevent stinging.*

Special considerations

- When accessing an intermittent infusion device, be sure to stabilize the device *to prevent dislodging it from the vein.*
- If the patient feels a burning sensation during the injection of saline, stop the injection and check cannula placement. If the cannula is in the vein, inject the saline at a slower rate *to minimize irritation.* If the needle isn't in the vein, remove and discard it. Then select a new venipuncture site and, using fresh equipment, restart the procedure.
- Change the intermittent infusion device every 48 to 72 hours, according to your facility's policy, using a new venipuncture site. Some facilities use a transparent semi-

permeable dressing. *This allows more patient freedom and better observation of the injection site.*

■ If the practitioner orders an I.V. infusion discontinued and an intermittent infusion device inserted in its place, convert the existing line by disconnecting the I.V. tubing and inserting a male adapter cap into the device. (See *Converting an I.V. line to an intermittent infusion device.*)

Home care

If you're caring for a patient who will be going home with a peripheral line, teach him how to care for the I.V. site and identify complications. If he must observe movement restrictions, make sure he understands which movements to avoid.

Because the patient may have special drug delivery equipment that differs from the type used in the facility, be sure to demonstrate the equipment and have the patient give a return demonstration.

Teach the patient to examine the site and to notify the nurse if the dressing becomes moist, if blood appears in the tubing, or if redness, swelling, or discomfort develops.

Also tell the patient to report any problems with the I.V. line, for instance, if the solution stops infusing or if an alarm goes off on the infusion pump. Explain that the I.V. site will be changed at established intervals by a home care nurse.

Teach the patient or caregiver how and when to flush the device. Finally, teach the patient to document daily whether the I.V. site is free from pain, swelling, and redness.

Complications

Use of an intermittent infusion device has the same potential complications as the use of a peripheral I.V. line. (See "Peripheral I.V. catheter insertion," page 349.)

Documentation

Record the date and time of insertion; type and gauge of the needle and length of the cannula; anatomic location of the insertion site; patient's tolerance of the procedure; and date and time of each saline or heparin flush.

Converting an I.V. line to an intermittent infusion device

Many types of adapter caps (shown below) allow you to convert an existing I.V. line to an intermittent infusion device. To make the conversion, follow these steps:

■ Prime the male adapter plug with normal saline solution.

■ Clamp the I.V. tubing, and remove the administration set from the cannula hub.

■ Insert the male adapter cap.

■ Flush the access with the remaining solution to prevent clot formation.

Short male adapter

This short luer-lock adapter cap twists into place.

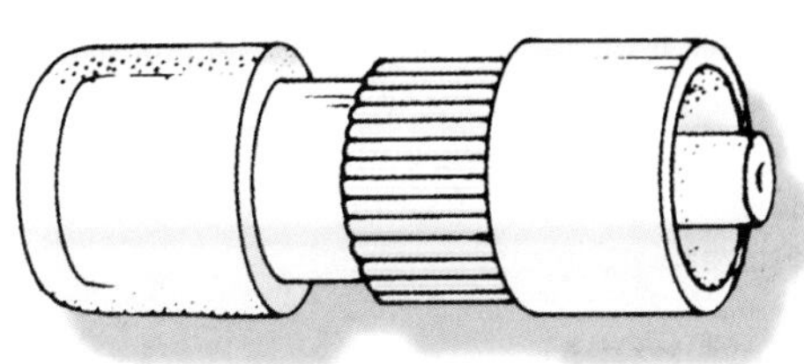

SELECTED REFERENCES

Campbell, S.G., et al. "How Often Should Peripheral Intravenous Catheters in Ambulatory Patients Be Flushed?" *Journal of Infusion Nursing* 28(6):399-404, November-December 2005.

Fujita. T., et al. "Normal Saline Flushing for Maintenance of Peripheral Intravenous Sites," *Journal of Clinical Nursing* 15(1):103-104, January 2006.

Mok. E., et al. "A Randomized Controlled Trial for Maintaining Peripheral Intravenous Lock in Children," *International Journal of Nursing Practice* 13(1):33-45, February 2007.

"Standard 29. Add-on Devices and Junction Securement. Infusion Nursing Standards of Practice," *Journal of Infusion Nursing* 29(1S):S32, January-February 2006.

"Standard 50. Flushing. Infusion Nursing Standards of Practice," *Journal of Infusion Nursing* 29(1S):S52, January-February 2006.

PERIPHERAL I.V. CATHETER MAINTENANCE

Routine maintenance of I.V. sites and systems includes regular assessment and rotation of the site and periodic changes of the dressing, tubing, and solution. These measures help prevent complications, such as thrombophlebitis and infection. They should be performed according to your facility's policy.

Typically, gauze I.V. dressing are changed every 48 hours or whenever the dressing becomes wet, soiled, or nonocclusive. Transparet semipermeable dressings are changed whenever I.V. tubing is changed. I.V. tubing is changed every 72 hours or according to policy, and I.V. solution is changed every 24 hours or as needed. The site should be assessed every 2 hours if a transparent semipermeable dressing is used or with every dressing change otherwise and should be rotated every 72 hours. Sometimes limited venous access prevents frequent site changes; if so, be sure to assess the site frequently.

Equipment

For dressing changes: Sterile gloves ▪ antimicrobial solution ▪ adhesive bandage, sterile 2″ × 2″ gauze pad, or transparent semipermeable dressing ▪ 1″ adhesive tape.

For solution changes: Solution container ▪ alcohol pad.

For tubing changes: I.V. administration set ▪ sterile gloves ▪ sterile 2″ × 2″ gauze pad ▪ adhesive tape for labeling ▪ optional: hemostats.

For I.V. site change: Commercial kits containing the equipment for dressing changes are available.

Preparation of equipment

If your facility keeps I.V. equipment and dressings in a tray or cart, have it nearby, if possible, *because you may have to select a new venipuncture site, depending on the current site's condition.* If you're changing both the solution and the tubing, attach and prime the I.V. administration set before entering the patient's room.

Implementation

- Confirm the patient's identity using two patient identifiers according to your facility's policy.
- Wash your hands thoroughly *to prevent the spread of microorganisms.* Remember to wear sterile gloves whenever working near the venipuncture site.
- Explain the procedure to the patient *to allay his fears and ensure cooperation.*

Changing the dressing

- Remove the old dressing (as shown below), open all supply packages, and put on gloves.

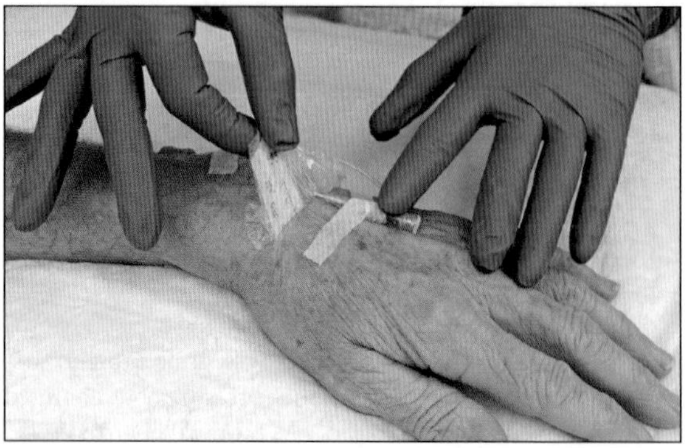

- Hold the cannula in place with your nondominant hand (as shown below) *to prevent accidental movement or dislodgment, which could puncture the vein and cause infiltration.*

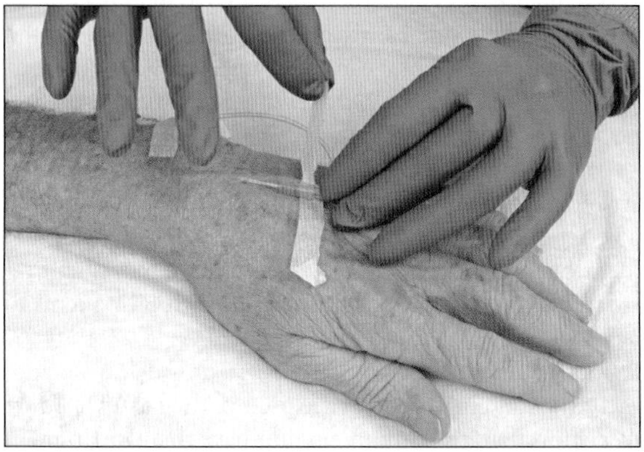

- Assess the venipuncture site for signs of infection (redness and pain at the puncture site), infiltration (coolness, blanching, and edema at the site), and thrombophlebitis (redness, firmness, pain along the path of the vein, and edema). If any such signs are present, cover the area with a sterile 2″ × 2″ gauze pad and remove the catheter. Apply pressure to the area until the bleeding stops, and apply an adhesive bandage. Then using fresh equipment and solution, start the I.V. in another appropriate site, preferably on the opposite extremity.
- If the venipuncture site is intact, stabilize the cannula and carefully clean around the puncture site with antimicrobial solution (as shown below). Work in a circular motion outward from the site *to avoid introducing bacteria into the clean area.* Allow the area to dry completely.

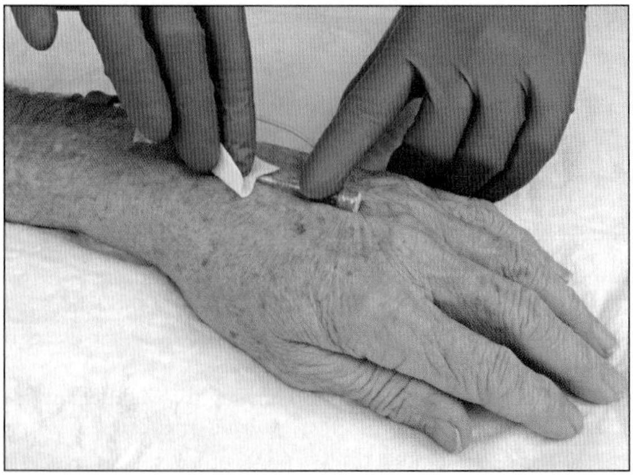

- Cover the site with transparent semipermeable dressing (as shown top of next page). *The transparent dressing allows*

visualization of the insertion site and maintains sterility. It's placed over the insertion site to halfway up the cannula.

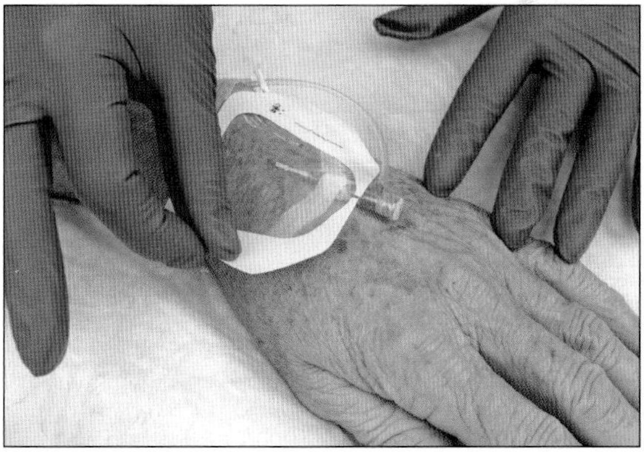

■ Label the dressing with the date and time of the procedure (as shown below).

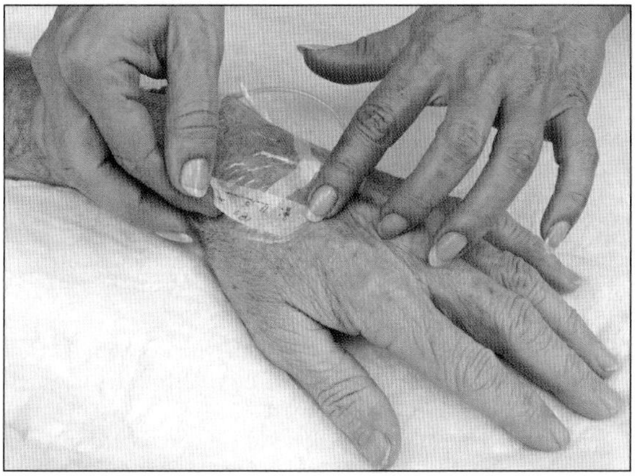

Changing the solution

■ Wash your hands.
■ Inspect the new solution container for cracks, leaks, and other damage. Check the solution for discoloration, turbidity, and particulates. Note the date and time the solution was mixed and its expiration date.
■ Clamp the tubing when inverting it *to prevent air from entering the tubing.* Keep the drip chamber half full.
■ If you're replacing a bag, remove the seal or tab from the new bag, and remove the old bag from the pole. Remove the spike, insert it into the new bag, and adjust the flow rate.
■ If you're replacing a bottle, remove the cap and seal from the new bottle, and wipe the rubber port with an alcohol pad. Clamp the line, remove the spike from the old bottle, and insert the spike into the new bottle. Then hang the new bottle and adjust the flow rate.

Changing the tubing

■ Reduce the I.V. flow rate, remove the old spike from the container, and hang it on the I.V. pole. Place the cover of the new spike loosely over the old one.
■ Keeping the old spike in an upright position above the patient's heart level, insert the new spike into the I.V. container (as shown below).

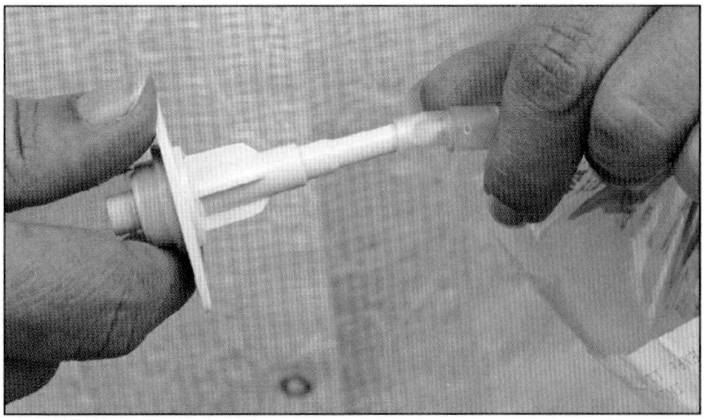

■ Prime the system. Hang the new I.V. container and primed set on the pole, and grasp the new adapter in one hand. Then stop the flow rate in the old tubing.
■ Put on sterile gloves.
■ Place a sterile gauze pad under the needle or cannula hub *to create a sterile field.* Press one of your fingers over the cannula to prevent bleeding.
■ Gently disconnect the old tubing (as shown below), being careful not to dislodge or move the I.V. device. (If you have trouble disconnecting the old tubing, use a hemostat to hold the hub securely while twisting the tubing *to remove it.* Or use one hemostat on the venipuncture device and another on the hard plastic end of the tubing. Then pull the hemostats in opposite directions. Don't clamp the hemostats shut; *this could crack the tubing adapter or the venipuncture device.*)

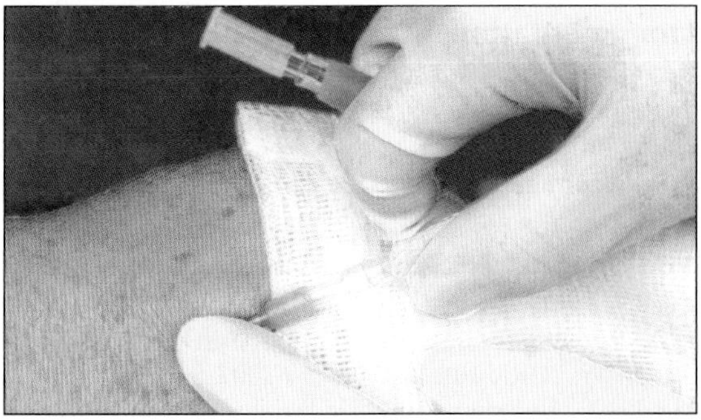

- Remove the protective cap from the new tubing, and connect the new adapter to the cannula. Hold the hub securely *to prevent dislodging the needle or cannula tip.*
- Observe for blood backflow into the new tubing *to verify that the needle or cannula is still in place.* (You may not be able to do this with small-gauge cannulas.)
- Adjust the clamp to maintain the appropriate flow rate (as shown below).

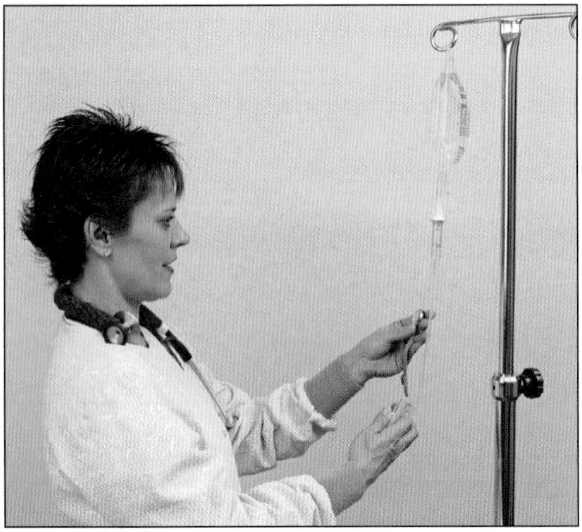

- Retape the cannula hub and I.V. tubing, and recheck the I.V. flow rate *because taping may alter it.*
- Label the new tubing and container with the date and time. Label the solution container with a time strip.

Special considerations

- Check the prescribed I.V. flow rate before each solution change *to prevent errors.*
- If you crack the adapter or hub (or if you accidentally dislodge the cannula from the vein), remove the cannula. Apply pressure and an adhesive bandage to stop any bleeding. Perform a venipuncture at another site and restart the I.V.

Documentation

Record the time, date, and rate and type of solution (and any additives) on the I.V. flowchart. Also record this information, dressing or tubing changes, and appearance of the site in your notes.

SELECTED REFERENCES

Centers for Disease Control and Prevention. "Guidelines for the Prevention of Intravascular Catheter-Related infections," *MMWR* 51(RR-10): 1-26, August 2002.

Hindley, G. "Infection Control in Peripheral Cannulae," *Nursing Standards* 18(27):37-40, March 2004.

The Joint Commission. *Comprehensive Accreditation Manual for Hospitals: The Official Handbook.* Standard MM.4.20. 2007.

The Joint Commission. *Comprehensive Accreditation Manual for Hospitals: The Official Handbook.* Standard MM.4.30. 2007

The Joint Commission. *Comprehensive Accreditation Manual for Hospitals: The Official Handbook.* Standard MM.5.10. 2007.

"Standard 14. Documentation. Infusion Nursing Standards of Practice," *Journal of Infusion Nursing* 29(1S):S22-23, January-February 2006.

"Standard 16. Product Labeling. Infusion Nursing Standards of Practice," *Journal of Infusion Nursing* 29(1S):S23-24, January-February 2006.

"Standard 23. Expiration and Beyond-Use Dates. Infusion Nursing Standards of Practice," *Journal of Infusion Nursing* 29(1S):S29, January-February 2006.

"Standard 44. Dressings. Infusion Nursing Standards of Practice," *Journal of Infusion Nursing* 29(1S):S44-S45, January-February 2006.

"Standard 48. Administration Set Change. Infusion Nursing Standards of Practice," *Journal of Infusion Nursing* 29(1S):S48-49, January-February 2006.

"Standard 51. Catheter Site Care. Infusion Nursing Standards of Practice," *Journal of Infusion Nursing* 29(1S): S57-56, January-February 2006.

"Standard 53. Phlebitis. Infusion Nursing Standards of Practice," *Journal of Infusion Nursing* 29(1S):S58-59, January-February 2006.

"Standard 54. Infiltration. Infusion Nursing Standards of Practice," *Journal of Infusion Nursing* 29(1S):S59-60, January-February 2006.

"Standard 55. Extravasation. Infusion Nursing Standards of Practice," *Journal of Infusion Nursing* 29(1S):S61-62, January-February 2006.

"Standard 56. Infection. Infusion Nursing Standards of Practice," *Journal of Infusion Nursing* 29(1S):S62-63, January-February 2006.

CENTRAL VENOUS THERAPY

CENTRAL VENOUS CATHETER USE

A central venous catheter (CVC) is a sterile catheter that's inserted through a large vein such as the subclavian vein or the jugular vein and the tip of the catheter is placed in the superior vena cava. (See *Central venous catheter pathways.*)

CVCs allow long-term administration in situations requiring safe, repeated access to the venous system for administration of drugs, fluids and nutrition, and blood products.

Central venous catheter pathways

The illustrations below show several common pathways for central venous catheter (CVC) insertion. Typically, a CVC is inserted in the subclavian vein or the internal jugular vein. The catheter may terminate in the superior vena cava or, rarely, the right atrium.

Insertion: Subclavian vein
Termination: Superior vena cava

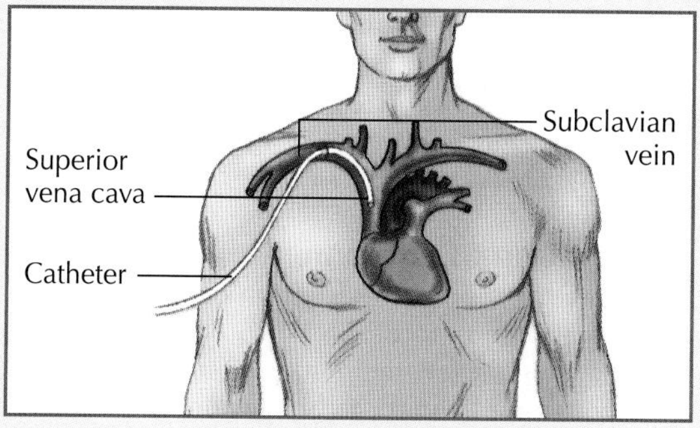

Insertion: Subclavian vein
Termination: Right atrium

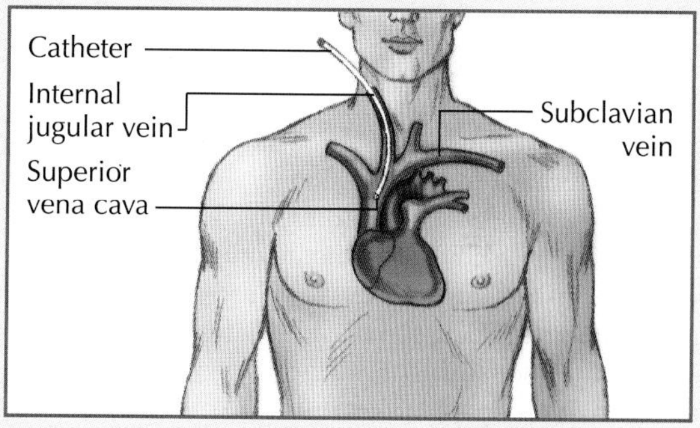

Insertion: Internal jugular vein
Termination: Superior vena cava

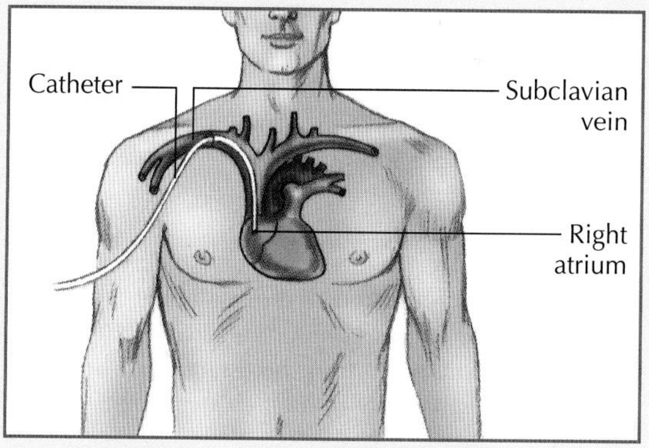

Insertion: Through a subcutaneous tunnel to the subclavian vein (Dacron cuff helps hold catheter in place)
Termination: Superior vena cava

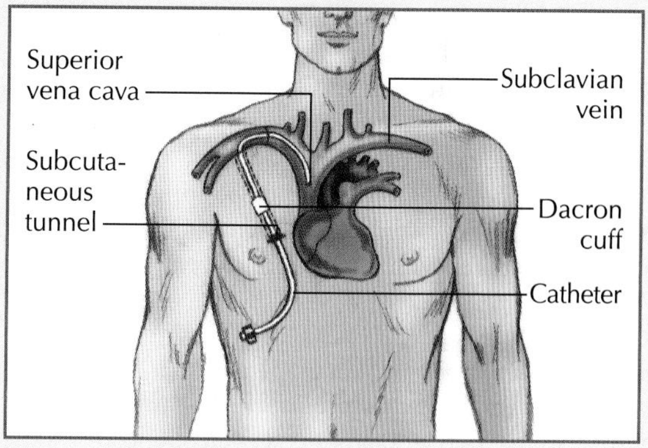

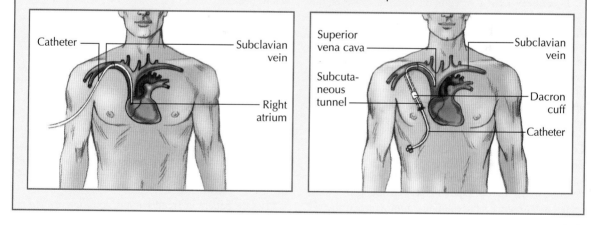

Other benefits of CV therapy include ease in monitoring CV pressure, drawing blood samples, administering large fluid volumes and irritating substances (such as total parenteral nutrition), and providing long-term venous access. Because multiple blood samples can be drawn through it without repeated venipuncture, the use of a CVC decreases the patient's anxiety and preserves or restores peripheral veins. However, CV therapy also increases the risk of complications, such as pneumothorax, sepsis, thrombus formation, and vessel and adjacent organ perforation (all life-threatening conditions). Also, the CV catheter may decrease patient mobility, is difficult to insert, and costs more than a peripheral I.V. catheter.

Site selection for a CV catheter should be considered a medical act. A catheter should be chosen with the minimum number of lumens needed for patient care. There also seems to be a lower incidence of infection when the subclavian route is chosen over the internal jugular or femoral sites. The femoral vein should be used with caution, with the distal tip terminating in the inferior vena cava. Nursing assessment should include the patient's condition, infusion history, and duration and type of therapy.

The type of catheter (tunneled, implanted, or percutaneously inserted) to be used is determined by the patient's condition, length of therapy, and type of medication to be infused. A single lumen catheter should be used unless additional therapies are required. An X-ray should be taken before initiation of therapy to confirm proper catheter placement and intermittently to verify that the catheter tip is in the superior vena cava.

A sterile dressing, either gauze or transparent semipermeable membrane, should be applied and maintained on the CVC. Topical antibiotic ointment or cream isn't recommended for use on the insertion site due to the potential of promoting a fungal infection or antimicrobial resistance. The edges of the gauze dressing should be covered with an occlusive material and should routinely be changed every 48 hours and immediately if the integrity of the dressing is compromised. The optimal interval for changing transparent semipermeable dressings depends on the dressing material's age and the patient's condition. Gauze used in conjunction with a transparent membrane should be changed every 48 hours. Good hand hygiene and aseptic technique during insertion and care decreases the risk of catheter-related infection.

If a catheter-related infection is suspected, however, the catheter should be cultured. If a complication is suspected, the catheter should be removed immediately. A practitioner or nurse usually performs CVC removal, either at the end of therapy or at the onset of complications. Caution should be used in the removal of a CVC, including precautions to prevent air embolism. Pressure should be applied to the site until bleeding stops, antiseptic ointment should be applied, and the site covered with a sterile occlusive dressing.

Equipment

For insertion of a CVC: Skin preparation kit, if necessary ▪ sterile gloves and gowns ▪ blanket ▪ linen-saver pad ▪ sterile towel ▪ large sterile drape ▪ masks ▪ alcohol pads ▪ antiseptic swab ▪ normal saline solution ▪ 3-ml syringe with 25G 1″ needle ▪ 1% or 2% injectable lidocaine ▪ dextrose 5% in water ▪ syringes for blood sample collection ▪ suture material ▪ two 14G or 16G CVCs ▪ I.V. solution with administration set prepared for use ▪ infusion pump as needed ▪ sterile 4″ × 4″ gauze ▪ 1″ adhesive tape ▪ sterile scissors ▪ heparin or normal saline flushes as needed ▪ transparent semipermeable dressing ▪ sterile marker ▪ sterile labels.

For flushing a catheter: Heparin flush solution ▪ antimicrobial swab.

For changing an injection cap: Alcohol pad ▪ injection cap ▪ padded clamp.

For obtaining a blood sample: Gloves ▪ alcohol pad ▪ 10-ml vial of normal saline solution ▪ heparin flush solution, as needed ▪ 2 10-ml syringes with needless hub (or other size syringe as appropriate) ▪ blood collection tubes ▪ laboratory slip ▪ labels ▪ BIOHAZARD transport bag.

For removal of a CVC: Clean gloves ▪ sterile suture removal set ▪ alcohol padsvsterile gloves ▪ antimicrobial swab ▪ sterile 4″ × 4″gauze ▪ forceps ▪ tape ▪ sterile, plastic adhesive-backed dressing or transparent semipermeable dressing ▪ agar plate, if necessary for culture ▪ antiseptic ointment.

Some facilities have prepared trays containing most of the equipment for catheter insertion. The type of catheter selected depends on the type of therapy to be used. (See *Guide to central venous catheters.*)

Preparation of equipment

Before insertion of a CVC, confirm catheter type and size with the practitioner; usually, a 14G or 16G catheter is selected. Set up the I.V. solution, and prime the administration set using strict sterile technique. Attach the line to the infusion pump, if ordered. Recheck all connections *to make sure they're tight.* Label all medications, medication containers, and other solutions on and off the sterile filed. As ordered, notify the radiology department that a chest X-ray will be needed.

Implementation

- Confirm the patient's identity using two patient identifiers according to your facility's policy.
- Wash your hands thoroughly *to prevent the spread of microorganisms.*

Inserting a CVC

- Reinforce the practitioner's explanation of the procedure, and answer the patient's questions. Ensure that the patient has signed a consent form, if necessary, and check his history for hypersensitivity to iodine, latex, or the local anesthetic.
- Place the patient in Trendelenburg's position *to dilate the veins and reduce the risk of air embolism.*
- For subclavian insertion, place a rolled blanket lengthwise between the shoulders *to increase venous distention.* For jugular insertion, place a rolled blanket under the opposite shoulder *to extend the neck, making anatomic landmarks more visible.* Place a linen-saver pad under the patient *to prevent soiling the bed.*
- Turn the patient's head away from the site *to prevent possible contamination from airborne pathogens and to make the site more accessible.* Or, if dictated by your facility's policy,

EQUIPMENT

Guide to central venous catheters

The various types of central venous catheters differ in their design, composition, and indications for use. This chart outlines the advantages, disadvantages, and nursing considerations for several commonly used catheters.

TYPE	DESCRIPTION	INDICATIONS	ADVANTAGES AND DISADVANTAGES	NURSING CONSIDERTATIONS
Groshong catheter	■ Silicone rubber ■ About 35″ (88.9 cm) long ■ Closed end with pressure-sensitive three-way valve ■ Dacron cuff ■ Single or double lumen ■ Tunneled 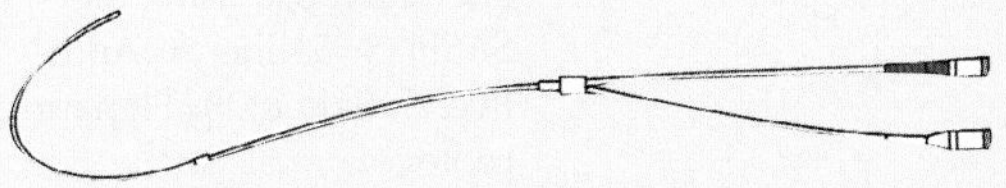	■ Long-term central venous (CV) access ■ Patient with heparin allergy	***Advantages*** ■ Less thrombogenic ■ Pressure-sensitive three-way valve eliminates heparin flushes ■ Dacron cuff anchors catheter and prevents bacterial migration ***Disadvantages*** ■ Requires surgical insertion ■ Tears and kinks easily ■ Blunt end makes it difficult to clear substances from its tip	■ Two surgical sites require dressing after insertion. ■ Handle catheter gently. ■ Check the external portion frequently for kinks and leaks. ■ Repair kit is available. ■ Remember to flush with enough saline solution to clear the catheter, especially after drawing or administering blood. ■ Change end caps weekly.
Short-term single-lumen catheter	■ Silastic rubber or polyurethane ■ About 8″ (20.3 cm) long ■ Lumen gauge varies 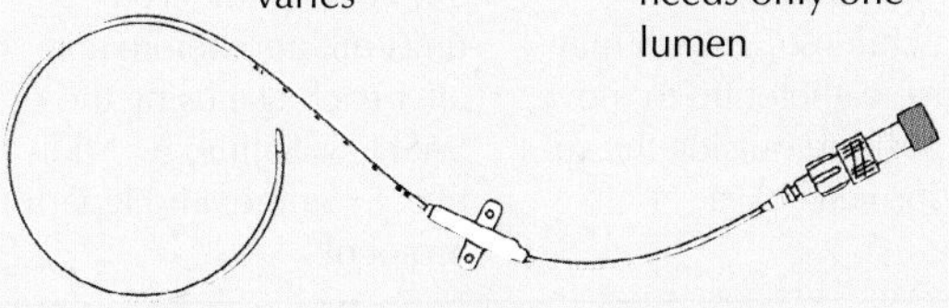	■ Short-term CV access ■ Emergency access ■ Patient who needs only one lumen	***Advantages*** ■ Easily inserted at bedside ■ Easily removed ■ Stiffness aids central venous pressure (CVP) monitoring ***Disadvantages*** ■ Limited functions ■ Should be changed every 3 to 7 days (frequency may depend on facility's policy)	■ Assess frequently for signs of infection and clot formation.
Short-term multilumen catheter	■ Silastic rubber or polyurethane ■ Two, three, or four lumens exiting at ¾″ (2-cm) intervals ■ Lumen gauges vary 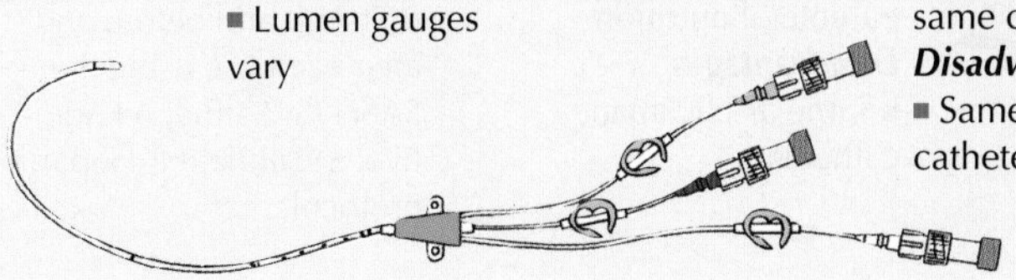	■ Short-term CV access ■ Patient with limited insertion sites who requires multiple infusions	***Advantages*** ■ Same as single-lumen catheter ■ Allows infusion of multiple (even incompatible) solutions through the same catheter ***Disadvantages*** ■ Same as single-lumen catheter	■ Know gauge and purpose of each lumen. ■ Use the same lumen for the same task.

(continued)

Guide to central venous catheters *(continued)*

Type	Description	Indications	Advantages and disadvantages	Nursing considerations
Hickman catheter 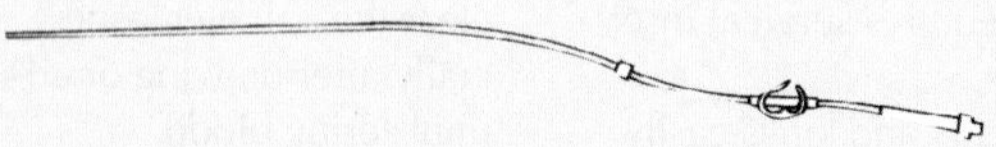	▪ Silicone rubber ▪ About 35″ (89 cm) long ▪ Open end with clamp ▪ Dacron cuff 11¾″ (29.8 cm) from hub ▪ Tunneled	▪ Long-term CV access ▪ Home therapy	***Advantages*** ▪ Dacron cuff prevents excess motion and migration of bacteria ▪ Clamps eliminate need for Valsalva's maneuver ***Disadvantages*** ▪ Requires surgical insertion ▪ Open end ▪ Requires physician for removal ▪ Tears and kinks easily	▪ Two surgical sites require dressing after insertion. ▪ Handle catheter gently. ▪ Observe frequently for kinks and tears. ▪ Repair kit is available. ▪ Clamp catheter with a nonserrated clamp any time it becomes disconnected or opens. ▪ When not in use, flush the catheter daily with 3 to 5 ml of heparin (10 units/ml) and before and after each use using the SASH (S=Saline; A=Additive; S=Saline; H=Heparin) protocol.
Broviac catheter 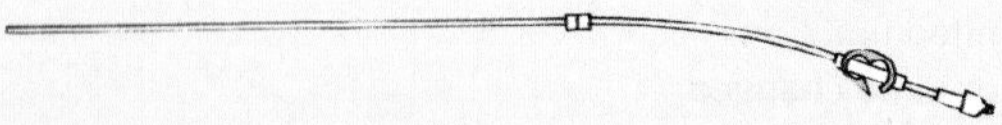	▪ Identical to Hickman except smaller inner lumen	▪ Long-term CV access ▪ Patient with small central vessels (pediatric or geriatric)	***Advantages*** ▪ Smaller lumen for better comfort ***Disadvantages*** ▪ Small lumen may limit uses ▪ Single lumen ▪ In children, growth may cause catheter tip to move its position outside the superior vena cava	▪ Check your facility's policy before drawing blood or administering blood or blood products. ▪ When not in use, flush the catheter daily with 3 to 5 ml of heparin (10 units/ml) and before and after each use using the SASH (S=Saline; A=Additive; S=Saline; H=Heparin) protocol.
Hickman/ Broviac catheter 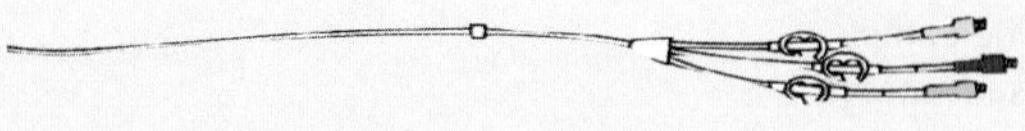	▪ Hickman and Broviac catheters combined	▪ Long-term CV access ▪ Patient who requires multiple infusions	***Advantages*** ▪ Double-lumen Hickman catheter allows sampling and administration of blood ▪ Broviac lumen delivers I.V. fluids, including total parenteral nutrition ***Disadvantages*** ▪ Same as Hickman catheter	▪ Know the purpose and function of each lumen. ▪ Label lumens to prevent confusion. ▪ When not in use, flush the catheter daily with 3 to 5 ml of heparin (10 units/ml) and before and after each use using the SASH (S=Saline; A=Additive; S=Saline; H=Heparin) protocol.

place a mask on the patient unless this increases his anxiety or is contraindicated because of his respiratory status.

- Prepare the insertion site. You may need to wash the skin with soap and water first. Make sure the skin is free of hair *because hair can harbor microorganisms.* Clip the hair close to the skin rather than shaving. *Shaving may cause skin irritation and create multiple small open wounds, increasing the risk of infection.*
- Establish a sterile field on a table, using a sterile towel or the wrapping from the instrument tray.
- Put on a mask and sterile gloves and gown, and clean the area around the insertion site with an antiseptic swab.
- After the practitioner puts on a sterile mask, gown, and gloves and drapes the area with a large sterile drape to create a sterile field, open the packaging of the 3-ml syringe and 25G needle, and give the syringe to him, using sterile technique.
- Wipe the top of the lidocaine vial with an alcohol pad and invert it. The practitioner then fills the 3-ml syringe and injects the anesthetic into the site (as shown below).

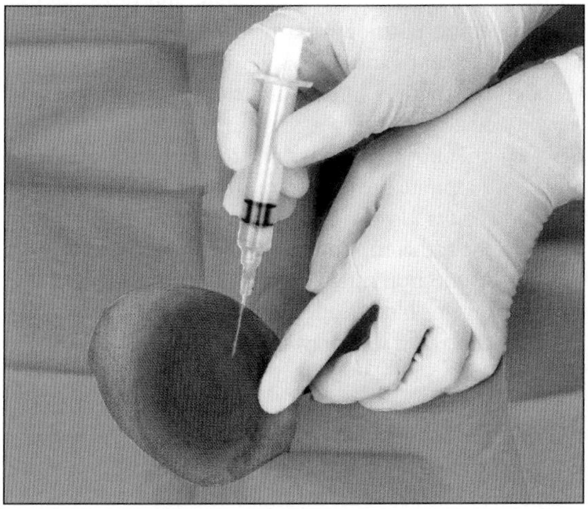

- Open the catheter package and give the catheter to the practitioner, using sterile technique. The practitioner then inserts the catheter.
- During this time, prepare the I.V. administration set for immediate attachment to the catheter hub. Ask the patient to perform Valsalva's maneuver while the practitioner attaches the I.V. line to the catheter hub. *This increases intrathoracic pressure, reducing the possibility of an air embolus.* (See *Valsalva's maneuver.*)
- After the practitioner attaches the I.V. line to the catheter hub, set the flow rate at a keep-vein-open rate to maintain venous access. (Alternatively, the catheter may be capped and flushed with heparin.) The practitioner then sutures the catheter in place.

Valsalva's maneuver

Increased intrathoracic pressure reduces the risk of air embolus during insertion and removal of a central venous catheter. A simple way to achieve this is to ask the patient to perform Valsalva's maneuver: forced exhalation against a closed airway. Instruct the patient to take a deep breath and hold it, and then to bear down for 10 seconds. Then tell the patient to exhale and breathe quietly.

Valsalva's maneuver raises intrathoracic pressure from its normal level of 3 to 4 mm Hg to levels of 60 mm Hg or higher. It also slows the pulse rate, decreases the return of blood to the heart, and increases venous pressure.

This maneuver is contraindicated in patients with increased intracranial pressure. It also shouldn't be taught to patients who aren't alert or cooperative.

- After an X-ray confirms correct catheter placement in the superior vena cava, set the flow rate as ordered.
- Use antimicrobial solution *to remove dried blood that could harbor microorganism.* Secure the catheter with adhesive tape, and apply a sterile 4″ × 4″ gauze. You may also apply a transparent semipermeable dressing (as shown below) either alone or over the gauze. Expect some serosanguineous drainage during the first 24 hours.

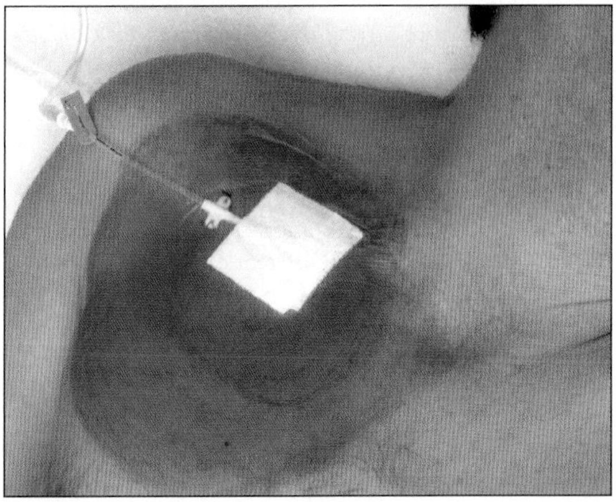

- Label the dressing with the time and date of catheter insertion and catheter length (as shown top of next page), if not imprinted on the catheter.

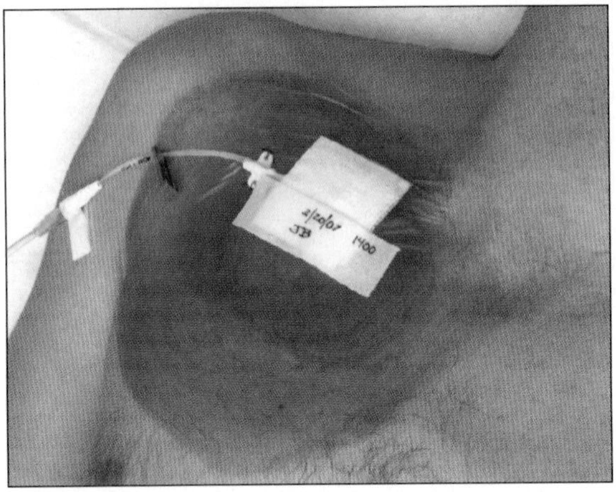

- Place the patient in a comfortable position and reassess his status.

Flushing the catheter

- *To maintain patency,* flush the catheter routinely according to your facility's policy. If the system is being maintained as a saline lock and the infusions are intermittent, the flushing procedure will vary according to policy, the medication administration schedule, and the type of catheter.
- All lumens of a multilumen catheter must be flushed regularly. Most facilities use a heparin flush solution available in premixed 10-ml multidose vials. Recommended concentrations vary from 10 to 100 units of heparin per milliliter. Use normal saline solution instead of heparin to maintain patency in three-way valved devices, such as the Groshong type, *because research suggests that heparin isn't always needed to keep the line open.*
- The recommended frequency for flushing CVCs varies from once every 8 hours to once weekly.
- The recommended amount of flushing solution also varies. Most facilities recommend using 3 to 5 ml of solution to flush the catheter, although some facility policies call for as much as 10 ml of solution. Different catheters require different amounts of solution.
- To perform the flushing procedure, start by cleaning the cap or needleless access port with an antimicrobial swab. Allow the cap to dry.
- Access the cap, and aspirate 3 to 5 ml of blood *to confirm the proper function and patency of the CVC.*
- Inject the recommended type and amount of flush solution.
- After flushing the catheter, maintain positive pressure by keeping your thumb on the plunger of the syringe while withdrawing the syringe. *This prevents blood backflow and clotting in the line.* If flushing a valved catheter, close the clamp before the last of the flush solution leaves the syringe.

Changing the injection cap

- CVCs used for intermittent infusions have needle-free injection caps (short luer-lock devices similar to the heparin lock adapters used for peripheral I.V. infusion therapy). These caps must be luer-lock types *to prevent inadvertent disconnection and an air embolism.* These caps contain a small amount of empty space, so you don't have to preflush the cap before connecting it.
- The frequency of cap changes varies according to your facility's policy and how often the cap is used; however, if the integrity of the product is compromised, it should be changed immediately. Use strict sterile technique when changing the cap.
- Clean the connection site with an alcohol pad.
- Instruct the patient to perform Valsalva's maneuver while you quickly disconnect the old cap and connect the new cap using sterile technique. If he can't perform this maneuver, use a padded clamp *to prevent air from entering the catheter.*

Obtaining a blood sample from a CVC

- Explain the procedure to the patient, and place the patient in a supine position with the head slightly elevated.
- Wash your hands and put on gloves.
- Clamp the catheter lumen, and clean the injection surface with an alcohol pad.
- Attach an empty 10 ml-syringe to the hub, release the clamp, and aspirate the discard volume *to clear the catheter of dead space and blood diluted by flush solution.*
- Clamp the catheter, and remove the syringe for discard.
- Wipe the injection surface with alcohol, and connect the empty syringe or blood collection tube to the catheter, release the clamp, and withdraw the blood sample. If using a blood collection tube with a rubber diaphragm, swab the area with alcohol before using.
- Clamp the catheter and remove the syringe.
- Wipe the injection surface with alcohol, and connect the syringe with normal saline solution.
- Open the clamp and flush with solution. Close the clamp.
- Repeat the flushing procedure with a heparin flush solution as per your facility's policy if the patient does not have a continuous infusion prescribed.
- If you used a syringe instead of a blood collection tube, attach a needle to the syringe with the blood sample, and inject the blood into the appropriate blood collection tube after wiping it with an alcohol swab.
- Label the specimens with the name, room number, and date and time of collection.

Removing a CVC

- If you'll be removing the CVC, first check the patient's record for the most recent placement (confirmed by an X-ray) *to trace the catheter's path as it exits the body.* Make sure assistance is available if a complication (such as uncontrolled bleeding) occurs during catheter removal. *(Some vessels, such as the subclavian vein, can be difficult to compress.)* Before you remove the catheter, explain the procedure to the patient.

- Place the patient in a supine position *to prevent an air embolism.*
- Wash your hands, and put on clean gloves and a mask.
- Turn off all infusions, and prepare a sterile field using a sterile drape.
- Remove and discard the old dressing, and change to sterile gloves.
- Inspect the site for signs of drainage and inflammation. Clean the site with antimicrobial solution.
- Clip the sutures and, using forceps, remove the catheter in a slow, even motion. Have the patient perform Valsalva's maneuver as the catheter is withdrawn *to prevent an air embolism.*
- Apply pressure with a sterile gauze pad immediately after removing the catheter.
- Apply antiseptic ointment to the insertion site *to seal it.* Cover the site with a gauze pad, and tape a transparent semipermeable dressing over the gauze. Label the dressing with the date and time of the removal and your initials. Keep the site covered until epithelization has occurred.
- Inspect the catheter tip and measure the length of the catheter *to ensure that the catheter has been completely removed.* If you suspect that the catheter hasn't been completely removed, notify the practitoner immediately, and monitor the patient closely for signs of distress. If you suspect an infection, swab the catheter on a fresh agar plate, and send it to the laboratory for culture.
- Dispose of the I.V. tubing and equipment properly.

Special considerations

NURSING ALERT *Be alert for such signs of air embolism as sudden onset of pallor, cyanosis, dyspnea, coughing, and tachycardia, progressing to syncope and shock. If any of these signs occur, place the patient on his left side in Trendelenburg's position, and notify the practitioner.*

- After insertion, also watch for signs of pneumothorax, such as shortness of breath, uneven chest movement, tachycardia, and chest pain. Notify the practitioner immediately if such signs appear.
- Change the dressing every 48 hours if a gauze dressing is used and a transparent dressing every 7 days, according to your facility's policy, or whenever it becomes moist or soiled. Change the tubing every 72 hours and solution every 24 hours or according to your facility's policy while the CVC is in place. Dressing, tubing, and solution changes for a CVC should be performed using sterile technique. (See *Key steps in changing a central venous dressing.*) Assess the site for signs

Key steps in changing a central venous dressing

Expect to change your patient's central venous (CV) dressing every 48 hours if it's a gauze dressing and at least every 7 days if it's transparent. Many facilities specify dressing changes whenever the dressing becomes soiled, moist, or loose. The following illustrations show the key steps you'll perform.

First, put on clean gloves, and remove the old dressing by pulling it toward the exit site of a long-term catheter or toward the insertion site of a short-term catheter. *This technique helps you avoid pulling out the line.* Remove and discard your gloves.

Next, put on sterile gloves, and clean the skin around the site three times using an alcohol pad. Start at the center and move outward, using a circular motion.

Allow the skin to dry, and clean the site with antimicrobial swabs.

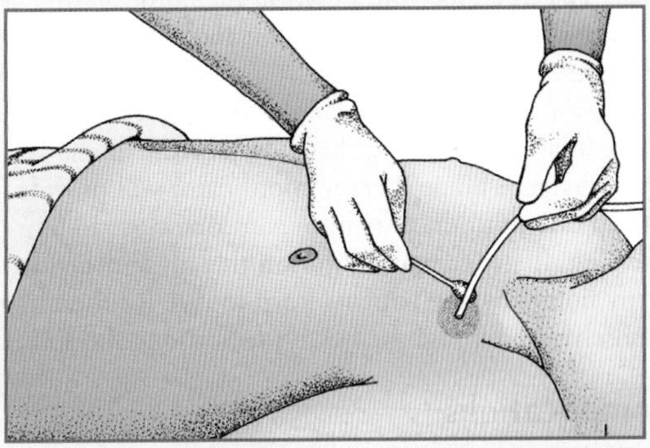

After the solution has dried, cover the site with a dressing, such as a transparent semipermeable dressing shown below. Write the time and date on the dressing.

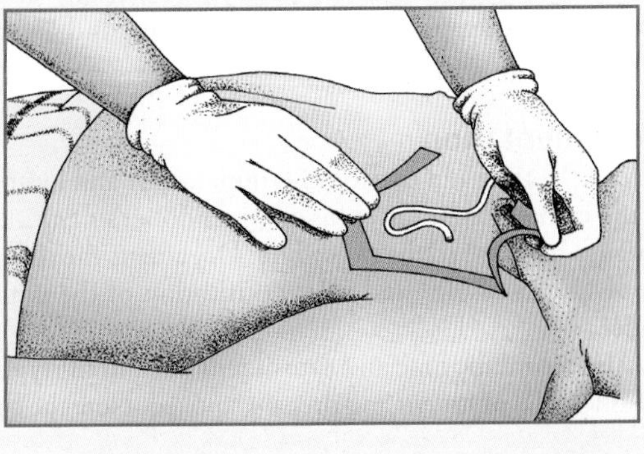

of infection, such as discharge, inflammation, and tenderness.

■ *To prevent an air embolism,* close the catheter clamp or have the patient perform Valsalva's maneuver each time the catheter hub is open to air. (A Groshong catheter doesn't require clamping *because it has an internal valve.)*

■ If you have trouble aspirating blood, the catheter tip may be poorly positioned. Ask the patient to cough, reposition him on his side, raise his arms above his head, or put him in a sitting position.

Home care

Long-term use of a CVC allows patients to receive all types of infusion therapies at home. These catheters have a much longer life because they are less thrombogenic and less prone to infection than short-term devices.

A candidate for home therapy must have a family member or friend who can safely and competently administer the I.V. fluids, a backup helper, a suitable home environment, a telephone, transportation, adequate reading skills, and the ability to prepare, handle, store, and dispose of the equipment. The care procedures used in the home are the same as those used in the facility, except the patient uses clean technique instead of sterile.

Because the overall goal of home therapy is patient safety, your patient teaching must begin well before discharge. After discharge, a home therapy coordinator will provide follow-up care until the patient or someone close to him can provide catheter care and infusion therapy independently. Many home therapy patients learn to care for the catheter themselves and infuse their own medications and solution.

Complications

Complications can occur at any time during infusion therapy. Traumatic complications such as pneumothorax typically occur on catheter insertion but may not be noticed until after the procedure is completed. Systemic complications such as sepsis typically occur later during infusion therapy. Other complications include phlebitis (especially in peripheral CV therapy), thrombus formation, and air embolism. (See *Risks of central venous therapy.*)

Documentation

Record the time and date of insertion, length and location of the catheter, solution infused, practitioner's name, and patient's response to the procedure. Document the time of the X-ray, its results, and your notification of the practitioner.

Also record the time and date of removal and the type of antimicrobial ointment and dressing applied. Note the condition of the catheter insertion site and collection of a culture specimen.

Selected references

Brungs, S.M., and Render M.L. "Using Evidence-Based Practice to Reduce Central Line Infections," *Clinical Journal of Oncology Nursing* 10(6):723-25, December 2006.

Centers for Disease Control and Prevention. "Guidelines for the Prevention of Intravascular Catheter-Related Infections," *MMWR* 51(RR-10):1-26, August 2002.

Crawford, A.G., et al. "Cost-Benefit Analysis of Chlorhexidine Gluconate Dressing in the Prevention of Catheter-Related Bloodstream Infections," *Infection Control and Hospital Epidemiology* 25(8):668-74, August 2004.

Hadaway, L. "Keeping Central Line Infection at Bay," *Nursing* 36(4):58-63, April 2006.

Ingram, P., et al. "The Safe Removal of Central Venous Catheters," *Nursing Standards* 20(49):42-46, August 2006.

Lynn-McHale Wiegand, D.J., and Carlson, K.K. *AACN Procedure Manual for Critical Care,* 5th ed. Philadelphia: W.B. Saunders Co., 2005.

Posa, P.J., et al. "Elimination of Central Line-Associated Bloodstream Infections: Application of the Evidence," *AACN Advanced Critical Care* 17(4):446-54, October-December 2006.

"Standard 35. Injection and Access Caps. Infusion Nursing Standards of Practice," *Journal of Infusion Nursing* 29(1S):S35-S36, January-February 2006.

"Standard 37. Site Selection. Infusion Nursing Standards of Practice," *Journal of Infusion Nursing* 29(1S):S37-S39, January-February 2006.

"Standard 38. Catheter Selection. Infusion Nursing Standards of Practice," *Journal of Infusion Nursing* 29(1S):S39-S40, January-February 2006.

"Standard 39. Hair Removal. Infusion Nursing Standards of Practice," *Journal of Infusion Nursing* 29(1S):S40-S41, January-February 2006.

"Standard 40. Local Anesthesia. Infusion Nursing Standards of Practice," *Journal of Infusion Nursing* 29(1S):S41, January-February 2006.

"Standard 41. Access Site Preparation. Infusion Nursing Standards of Practice," *Journal of Infusion Nursing* 29(1S):S41-S42, January-February 2006.

"Standard 44. Dressings. Infusion Nursing Standards of Practice," *Journal of Infusion Nursing* 29(1S):S44-S45, January-February 2006.

"Standard 50. Flushing. Infusion Nursing Standards of Practice," *Journal of Infusion Nursing* 29(1S):S55-S57, January-February 2006.

"Standard 51. Catheter Site Care. Infusion Nursing Standards of Practice," *Journal of Infusion Nursing* 29(1S):S57-S58, January-February 2006.

"Standard 66. Phlebotomy. Infusion Nursing Standards of Practice," *Journal of Infusion Nursing* 29(1S):S71-S73, January-February 2006.

Risks of central venous therapy

Problem	Signs and symptoms	Possible causes	Nursing interventions
Infection	■ Redness, warmth, tenderness, swelling at insertion or exit site ■ Possible exudate of purulent material ■ Local rash or pustules ■ Fever, chills, malaise ■ Leukocytosis ■ Nausea and vomiting ■ Elevated urine glucose level	■ Failure to maintain sterile technique during catheter insertion or care ■ Failure to comply with dressing change protocol ■ Wet or soiled dressing remaining on site ■ Immunosuppression ■ Irritated suture line ■ Contaminated catheter or solution ■ Frequent accessing of catheter or long-term use of single I.V. access site	■ Monitor temperature frequently. ■ Monitor vital signs closely. ■ Culture the site. ■ Redress aseptically. ■ Treat systemically with antibiotics or antifungals, depending on culture results and practitioner's order. ■ Catheter may be removed. ■ Draw central and peripheral blood cultures; if the same organism appears in both, then catheter is primary source and should be removed. ■ If cultures don't match but are positive, the catheter may be removed or the infection may be treated through the catheter. ■ If the catheter is removed, culture its tip. ■ Document interventions. ***Prevention*** ■ Maintain sterile technique. Use sterile gloves, masks, and gowns when appropriate. ■ Observe dressing-change protocols. ■ Teach about restrictions on swimming, bathing, and so on. (With adequate white blood cell count, the practitioner may allow these activities.) ■ Change wet or soiled dressing immediately. ■ Change dressing more frequently if catheter is located in femoral area or near tracheostomy. Perform tracheostomy care after catheter care. ■ Examine solution for cloudiness and turbidity before infusing; check fluid container for leaks. ■ Monitor urine glucose level in patients receiving total parenteral nutrition (TPN); if greater than 2+, suspect early sepsis. ■ Use a 0.22-micron filter (or a 1.2-micron filter for 3-in-1 TPN solutions). ■ Catheter may be changed frequently. ■ Keep the system closed as much as possible.

(continued)

Risks of central venous therapy *(continued)*

PROBLEM	SIGNS AND SYMPTOMS	POSSIBLE CAUSES	NURSING INTERVENTIONS
Pneumothorax, hemothorax, chylothorax, hydrothorax	■ Decreased breath sounds on affected side ■ With hemothorax, decreased hemoglobin level because of blood pooling ■ Abnormal chest X-ray	■ Repeated or long-term use of same vein ■ Preexisting cardiovascular disease ■ Lung puncture by catheter during insertion or exchange over a guidewire ■ Large blood vessel puncture with bleeding inside or outside the lung ■ Lymph node puncture with leakage of lymph fluid ■ Infusion of solution into chest area through infiltrated catheter	■ Notify practitioner. ■ Remove catheter or assist with removal. ■ Administer oxygen as ordered. ■ Set up and assist with chest tube insertion. ■ Document interventions. ***Prevention*** ■ Position patient head down with a rolled towel between his scapulae to dilate and expose the internal jugular or subclavian vein as much as possible during catheter insertion. ■ Assess for early signs of fluid infiltration (swelling in the shoulder, neck, chest, and arm). ■ Ensure that the patient is immobilized and prepared for insertion. Active patients may need to be sedated or taken to the operating room. ■ Minimize patient activity after insertion, especially with a peripheral catheter.
Air embolism	■ Respiratory distress ■ Unequal breath sounds ■ Weak pulse ■ Increased central venous (CV) pressure ■ Decreased blood pressure ■ Alteration or loss of consciousness	■ Intake of air into the CV system during catheter insertion or tubing changes, or inadvertent opening, cutting, or breaking of catheter	■ Clamp catheter immediately. ■ Turn patient on his left side, head down, so that air can enter the right atrium. Maintain this position for 20 to 30 minutes. ■ Don't recommend Valsalva's maneuver because a large air intake worsens the condition. ■ Administer oxygen. ■ Notify the practitioner. ■ Document interventions. ***Prevention*** ■ Purge all air from tubing before hookup. ■ Teach patient to perform Valsalva's maneuver during catheter insertion and tubing changes. ■ Use air-eliminating filters. ■ Use an infusion device with air detection capability. ■ Use luer-lock tubing, tape the connections, or use locking devices for all connections.

Risks of central venous therapy *(continued)*

PROBLEM	SIGNS AND SYMPTOMS	POSSIBLE CAUSES	NURSING INTERVENTIONS
Thrombosis	■ Edema at puncture site ■ Erythema ■ Ipsilateral swelling of arm, neck, and face ■ Pain along vein ■ Fever, malaise ■ Chest pain ■ Dyspnea ■ Cyanosis	■ Sluggish flow rate ■ Composition of catheter material (polyvinyl chloride catheters are more thrombogenic) ■ Hematopoietic status of patient ■ Preexisting limb edema ■ Infusion of irritating solutions	■ Notify practitioner. ■ Possibly remove catheter. ■ Possibly infuse anticoagulant doses of heparin. ■ Verify thrombosis with diagnostic studies. ■ Apply warm, wet compresses locally. ■ Don't use limb on affected side for subsequent venipuncture. ■ Document interventions. ***Prevention*** ■ Maintain steady flow rate with infusion pump, or flush catheter at regular intervals. ■ Use catheters made of less thrombogenic materials or catheters coated to prevent thrombosis. ■ Dilute irritating solutions. ■ Use a 0.22-micron filter for infusions.

PERIPHERALLY INSERTED CENTRAL CATHETER USE

Peripheral central venous (CV) therapy involves the insertion of a catheter into a peripheral vein instead of a central vein, but the catheter tip still lies in the CV circulation. A peripherally inserted central catheter (PICC) usually enters at the basilic vein and terminates in the subclavian vein or superior vena cava. A specially trained nurse may insert PICCs. New catheters have longer needles and smaller lumens, facilitating this procedure. For a patient who needs CV therapy for 1 to 6 months or who requires repeated venous access, a PICC may be the best option.

PICCs are commonly used in home I.V. therapy but may also be used with chest injury; chest, neck, or shoulder burns; compromised respiratory function; proximity of a surgical site to the CV line placement site; and if a practitioner isn't available to insert a CV line. With any of these conditions, a PICC helps avoid complications that may occur with a CV line.

Infusions commonly given by a PICC include total parenteral nutrition, chemotherapy, antibiotics, opioids, and analgesics. PICC therapy works best when introduced early in treatment; it shouldn't be considered as a last resort for patients with sclerotic or repeatedly punctured veins.

Before PICC insertion, anatomical measurements should be taken to determine the length of the catheter required to ensure full advancement of the catheter with tip placement in the superior vena cava. PICCs may range from 16G to 23G in diameter and from 16″ to 24″ (40.5 to 61 cm) in length. (See *Understanding PICC lines,* page 376.)

The patient receiving PICC therapy must have a peripheral vein large enough to accept a 14G or 16G introducer needle and a 3.8G to 4.8G catheter.

Site selection should be routinely initiated in the region of the antecubital fossa; veins that should be considered for PICC insertion are the cephalic, basilic, and median cubital veins.

If your state nurse practice act permits, you may insert a PICC if you show sufficient knowledge of vascular access devices. To prove your competence in PICC insertion, it's recommended that you complete an 8-hour workshop and demonstrate three successful catheter insertions. You may have to demonstrate competence every year.

Equipment

Catheter insertion kit ■ antiseptic solution ■ antiseptic ointment ■ 3-ml vial of heparin (100 units/ml) ■ injection port with short extension tubing ■ sterile and clean measuring tape ■ vial of normal saline solution ■ sterile gauze pads ■ tape ■ linen-saver pad ■ sterile drapes ■ tourniquet ■ sterile transparent semipermeable dressing ■ sterile marker ■ ster-

Understanding PICC lines

Description
- Silicone rubber
- 20" to 24" (51 to 61 cm) long; available in 14G, 16G, 18G, 20G, 22G, and 24G

Indications
- Long term central venous (CV) access
- Patient with poor central access
- Patient at high risk for complications from insertion at CV access sites
- Patient who needs CV access but faces or has had head and neck surgery

Advantages
- Peripherally inserted
- Can be inserted at the bedside with minimal complications
- May be inserted by a trained, skilled, competent registered nurse in most states

Disadvantages
- May occlude smaller peripheral vessels
- May be difficult to keep immobile

Nursing considerations
- Check frequently for signs of phlebitis and thrombus formation.
- Insert the catheter above the antecubital fossa.
- Use an arm board, if necessary.
- The catheter may alter CV pressure measurements.

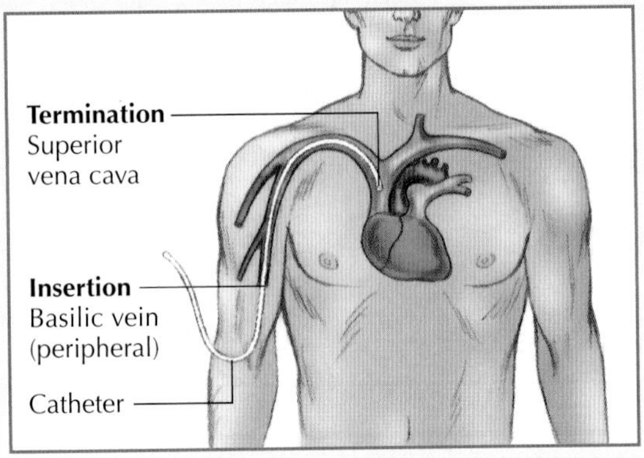

ile labels ▪ two pairs of sterile gloves ▪ sterile gown ▪ mask ▪ goggles ▪ clean gloves.

Preparation of equipment
Gather the necessary supplies. If you're administering PICC therapy in the patient's home, bring everything with you.

Implementation
- Confirm the patient's identity using two patient identifiers according to your facility's policy.
- Describe the procedure to the patient, and answer his questions.
- Wash your hands.
- Prepare the sterile field. Label all medications, medication containers, and other solutions on and off the sterile field.

Inserting a PICC
- Select the insertion site, and place the tourniquet on the patient's arm. Assess the antecubital fossa.
- Remove the tourniquet.
- Determine catheter tip placement or the spot at which the catheter tip will rest after insertion.
- For placement in the superior vena cava, measure the distance from the insertion site to the shoulder and from the shoulder to the sternal notch. Then add 3" (7.6 cm) to the measurement (as shown below).

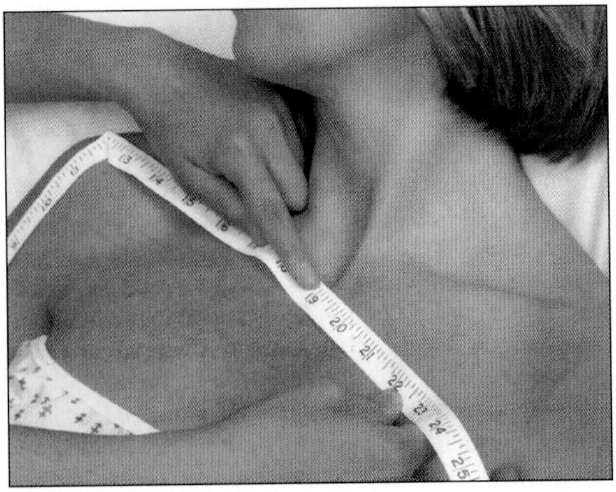

- Have the patient lie in a supine position with her arm at a 90-degree angle to her body. Place a linen-saver pad under her arm.

- Open the PICC tray and drop the rest of the sterile items onto the sterile field. Put on the sterile gown, mask, goggles, and sterile gloves.
- Using the sterile measuring tape, cut the distal end of the catheter according to specific manufacturer's recommendations and guidelines, using the equipment provided by the manufacturer (as shown below).

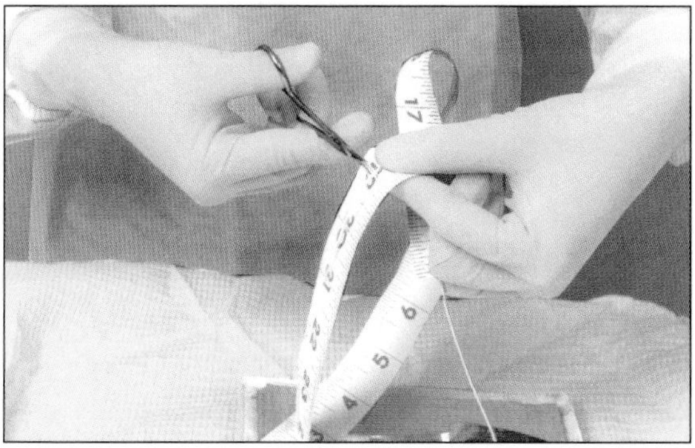

- Using sterile technique, withdraw 5 ml of the normal saline solution and flush the extension tubing and the cap (as shown below).

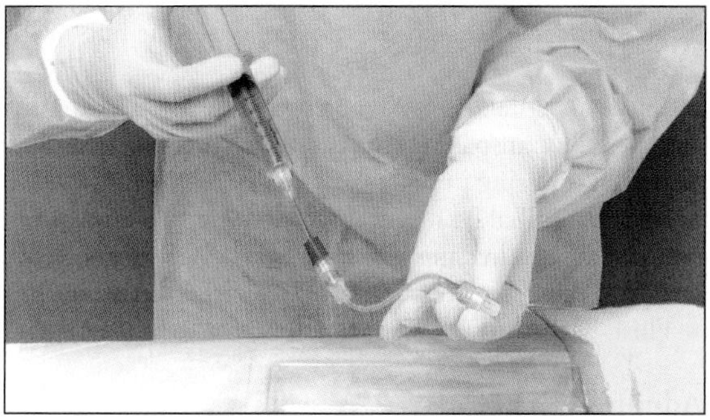

- Remove the needle from the syringe. Attach the syringe to the hub of the catheter and flush (as shown below).

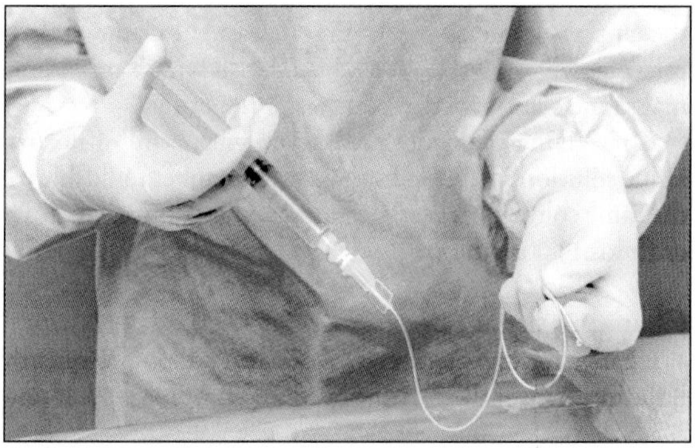

- Prepare the insertion site using an antiseptic solution. Allow the area to dry. Be sure not to touch the intended insertion site.
- Take your gloves off. Then apply the tourniquet about 4" (10 cm) above the antecubital fossa.
- Put on a new pair of sterile gloves. Then place a sterile drape under the patient's arm and another on top of her arm. Drop a sterile 4″ × 4″ gauze pad over the tourniquet.
- Stabilize the patient's vein. Insert the catheter introducer at a 10-degree angle, directly into the vein (as shown below).

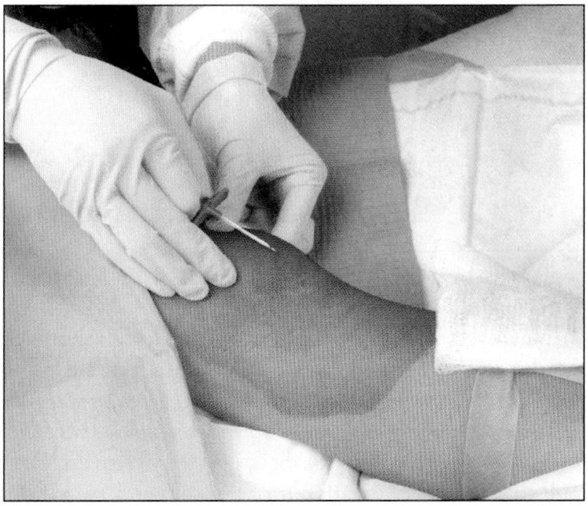

- After successful vein entry, you should see a blood return in the flashback chamber. Without changing the needle's position, gently advance the plastic introducer sheath until you're sure the tip is well within the vein.
- Carefully withdraw the needle while holding the introducer still. *To minimize blood loss,* try applying finger pressure on the vein just beyond the distal end of the introducer sheath (as shown below).

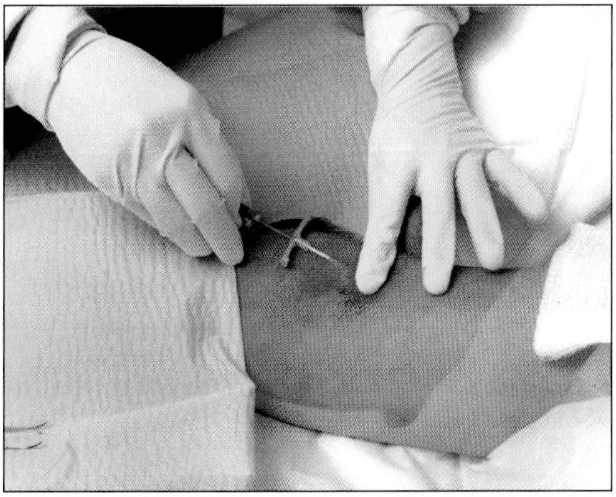

■ Using sterile forceps, insert the catheter into the introducer sheath, and advance it into the vein 2″ to 4″ (as shown below).

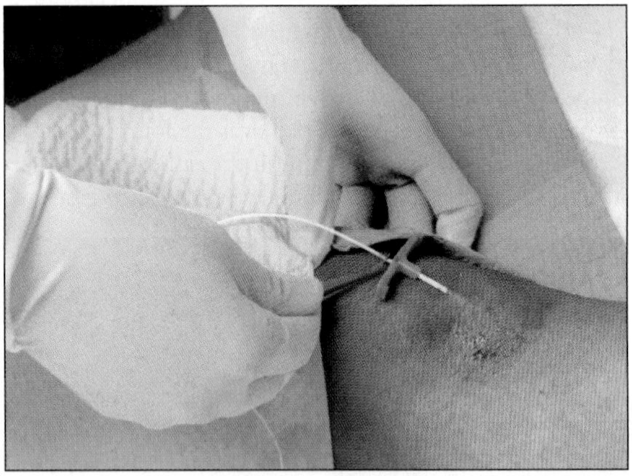

■ Remove the tourniquet, using a sterile 4″ × 4″ gauze pad *to maintain sterile technique.*

■ When you have advanced the catheter to the shoulder, ask the patient to turn her head toward the affected arm and place her chin on her chest. *This will occlude the jugular vein and ease the catheter's advancement into the subclavian vein.*

■ Advance the catheter until about 4″ (10 cm) remain. Then pull the introducer sheath out of the vein and away from the venipuncture site (as shown below).

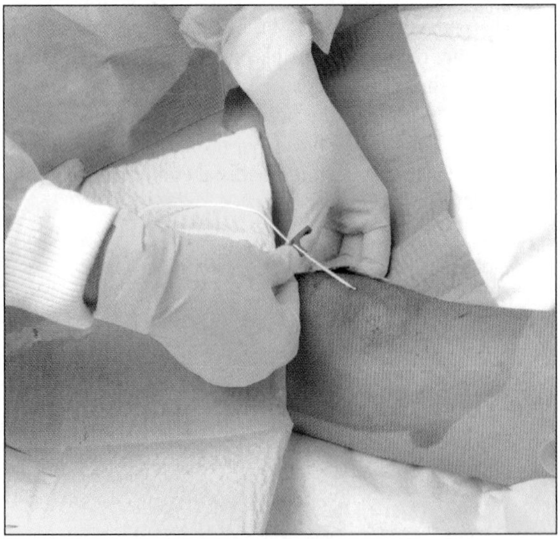

■ Grasp the tabs of the introducer sheath, and flex them toward its distal end *to split the sheath.*

■ Pull the tabs apart and away from the catheter until the sheath is completely split (as shown below). Discard the sheath.

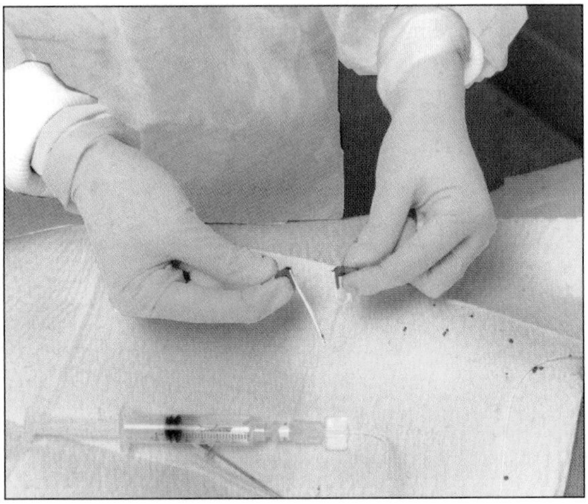

■ Continue to advance the catheter until it's completely inserted. Flush with normal saline solution followed by heparin, according to your facility's policy.

■ With the patient's arm below heart level, remove the syringe. Connect the capped extension set to the hub of the catheter.

■ Apply a sterile 2″ × 2″ gauze pad directly over the site and a sterile transparent semipermeable dressing over that. Leave this dressing in place for 24 hours.

■ After the initial 24 hours, apply a new sterile transparent semipermeable dressing. The gauze pad is no longer necessary. You can place Steri-Strips over the catheter wings.

■ Flush with heparin, according to your facility's policy.

Administering drugs

■ As with any CV line, be sure to check for blood return and flush with normal saline solution before administering a drug through a PICC line.

■ Clamp the 7″ (17.8-cm) extension tubing, and connect the empty syringe to the tubing. Release the clamp and aspirate slowly *to verify blood return.* Flush with 3 ml of normal saline solution; then administer the drug.

■ After giving the drug, flush again with 3 ml of normal saline solution in a 10-ml syringe. (Remember to flush with the same solution between infusions of incompatible drugs or fluids.) Close the clamp.

Changing the dressing

■ Change the dressing every 2 to 7 days and more frequently if the integrity of the dressing becomes compromised. If possible, choose a transparent semipermeable dressing, *which has a high moisture-vapor transmission rate.* Use sterile technique.

- Wash your hands and assemble the necessary supplies. Position the patient with her arm extended away from her body at a 45- to 90-degree angle so that the insertion site is below heart level *to reduce the risk of air embolism.* Put on a sterile mask.
- Open a package of sterile gloves, and use the inside of the package as a sterile field. Then open the transparent semipermeable dressing and drop it onto the field. Put on clean gloves, and remove the old dressing by holding your left thumb on the catheter and stretching the dressing parallel to the skin. Repeat the last step with your right thumb holding the catheter. Free the remaining section of the dressing from the catheter by peeling toward the insertion site from the distal end to the proximal end *to prevent catheter dislodgment.* Remove the clean gloves.
- Put on sterile gloves. Clean the area thoroughly with antimicrobial solution, starting at the insertion site and working outward. Allow to dry.
- Apply the dressing carefully. Secure the tubing to the edge of the dressing over the tape with ¼″ adhesive tape.

Removing a PICC

- You'll remove a PICC when therapy is complete, if the catheter becomes damaged or broken and can't be repaired or, possibly, if the line becomes occluded. Measure the catheter after you remove it *to ensure that the line has been removed intact.*
- Assemble the necessary equipment at the patient's bedside.
- Explain the procedure to the patient. Wash your hands. Place a linen-saver pad under the patient's arm.
- Remove the tape holding the extension tubing. Open two sterile gauze pads on a clean, flat surface. Put on clean gloves. Stabilize the catheter at the hub with one hand. Without dislodging the catheter, use your other hand to gently remove the dressing by pulling it toward the insertion site.
- Next, withdraw the catheter with smooth, gentle pressure in small increments. It should come out easily. If you feel resistance, stop. Apply slight tension to the line by taping it down. Apply a warm moist pack, then try to remove it again in a few minutes. If you still feel resistance after the second attempt, notify the practitioner for further instructions.
- When you successfully remove the catheter, apply manual pressure to the site with a sterile gauze pad for 1 minute.
- Measure and inspect the catheter. If any part has broken off during removal, notify the practitioner immediately, and monitor the patient for signs of distress.
- Cover the site with antiseptic ointment, and tape a new folded gauze pad in place. Dispose of used items properly, and wash your hands.

Special considerations

- For a patient receiving intermittent PICC therapy, flush the catheter with 6 ml of normal saline solution and 3 ml of heparin (100 units/ml) after each use. For catheters that aren't being used routinely, flushing every 12 hours with 3 ml (100 units/ml) heparin will maintain patency.
- You can use a declotting agent, such as urokinase, to clear a clotted PICC, but make sure you read the manufacturer's recommendations first.
- Remember to add an extension set to all PICCs *so you can start and stop an infusion away from the insertion site.* An extension set will also make using a PICC easier for the patient who will be administering infusions herself.
- If a patient will be receiving blood or blood products through the PICC, use at least an 18G cannula.
- Assess the catheter insertion site through the transparent semipermeable dressing every 24 hours. Look at the catheter and cannula pathway, and check for bleeding, redness, drainage, and swelling. Ask your patient if she's having pain associated with therapy. Although oozing is common for the first 24 hours after insertion, excessive bleeding after that should be evaluated.

NURSING ALERT ***If a portion of the catheter breaks during removal, immediately apply a tourniquet to the upper arm, close to the axilla,*** **to prevent advancement of the catheter piece into the right atrium.** ***Then check the patient's radial pulse. If you don't detect the radial pulse, the tourniquet is too tight. Keep the tourniquet in place until an X-ray can be obtained, the practitioner is notified, and surgical retrieval is attempted.***

Complications

PICC therapy causes fewer and less severe complications than conventional CV therapy. Catheter breakage on removal is probably the most common complication. Catheter occlusion is also relatively common. Air embolism, always a potential risk of venipuncture, poses less danger in PICC therapy than in traditional CV therapy *because the line is inserted below heart level.*

Catheter tip migration may occur with vigorous flushing. Patients receiving chemotherapy are most vulnerable to this complication *because of frequent nausea and vomiting and subsequent changes in intrathoracic pressure.*

Documentation

Document the entire procedure, including any problems with catheter placement. Also document the size, length, and type of catheter as well as the insertion location.

Selected references

Brungs, S.M., and Render M.L. "Using Evidence-Based Practice to Reduce Central Line Infections," *Clinical Journal of Oncology Nursing* 10(6):723-25, December 2006.

Centers for Disease Control and Prevention. "Guidelines for the Prevention of Intravascular Catheter-Related Infections," *MMWR* 51(RR-10):1-26, August 2002.

Hadaway, L. "Keeping Central Line Infection at Bay," *Nursing* 36(4):58-63, April 2006.

Oncology Nursing Society. *Access Device Guidelines: Recommendations for Nursing Practice and Education,* 2nd ed. Pittsburgh: Oncology Nursing Society, 2004.

Saldar, N., and Maki, D. "Risk of Catheter-Related Bloodstream Infection with Peripherally Inserted Central Venous Catheters Used in Hospitalized Patients," *Chest* 128(2):489-95, August 2005.

"Standard 37. Site Selection. Infusion Nursing Standards of Practice," *Journal of Infusion Nursing* 29(1S):S37-S39, January-February 2006.

"Standard 38. Catheter Selection. Infusion Nursing Standards of Practice," *Journal of Infusion Nursing* 29(1S):S39-S40, January-February 2006.

"Standard 39. Hair Removal. Infusion Nursing Standards of Practice," *Journal of Infusion Nursing* 29(1S):S40-S41, January-February 2006.

"Standard 40. Local Anesthesia. Infusion Nursing Standards of Practice," *Journal of Infusion Nursing* 29(1S):S41, January-February 2006.

"Standard 41. Access Site Preparation. Infusion Nursing Standards of Practice," *Journal of Infusion Nursing* 29(1S):S41-S42, January-February 2006.

"Standard 44. Dressings. Infusion Nursing Standards of Practice," *Journal of Infusion Nursing* 29(1S):S44-S45, January-February 2006.

"Standard 51. Catheter Site Care. Infusion Nursing Standards of Practice," *Journal of Infusion Nursing* 29(1S):S57-S58, January-February 2006.

Vascular access device use

Surgically implanted under local anesthesia by a physician, a vascular access device consists of a silicone catheter attached to a reservoir, which is covered with a self-sealing silicone rubber septum. It is used most commonly when an external central venous catheter (CVC) isn't desirable for long-term I.V. therapy. The most common type of vascular access device is a vascular access port (VAP). One- and two-piece units with single or double lumens are available. (See *Understanding vascular access ports.*)

VAPs come in two basic types: top entry, the most commonly used, and side entry. The VAP reservoir can be made of titanium, stainless steel, or molded plastic. The type and lumen size selected depend on the patient's needs.

Implanted in a pocket under the skin, a VAP functions much like a long-term CVC, except that it has no external parts. The attached indwelling catheter tunnels through the subcutaneous tissue so that the catheter tip lies in a central vein, for example, the subclavian vein. A VAP can also be used for arterial access or be implanted into the epidural space, peritoneum, or pericardial or pleural cavity.

Typically, VAPs deliver intermittent infusions. They're used to deliver chemotherapy and other drugs, I.V. fluids, and blood. They can also be used to obtain blood samples.

VAPs offer several advantages, including minimal activity restrictions, few steps for the patient to perform, and few dressing changes (except when used to maintain continuous infusions or intermittent infusion devices). Implanted devices are easier to maintain than external devices. For instance, they require heparinization only once after each use (or periodically if not in use). They also pose less risk of infection because they have no exit site to serve as an entry for microorganisms.

VAPs create only a slight protrusion under the skin, so many patients find them easier to accept than external infusion devices. Because they're implanted, however, they may be harder for the patient to manage, particularly if he'll be administering drugs or fluids frequently. And because accessing the device requires inserting a needle through subcutaneous tissue, patients who fear or dislike needle punctures may be uncomfortable using a VAP and may require a local anesthetic. In addition, implantation and removal of the device require surgery and hospitalization. The cost of VAPs makes them worthwhile only for patients who require infusion therapy for at least 6 months.

Implanted VAPs are contraindicated in patients who have been unable to tolerate other implanted devices and in those who may develop an allergic reaction.

Equipment

To implant a VAP: Noncoring needles (a noncoring needle has a deflected point, which slices the port's septum) of appropriate type and gauge with attached extension set tubing ▪ VAP ▪ sterile gloves ▪ mask ▪ alcohol pads ▪ antiseptic cleaning swabs ▪ local anesthetic (lidocaine without epinephrine) ▪ ice pack ▪ 10- and 20-ml syringes ▪ normal saline and heparin flush solutions ▪ I.V. solution ▪ sterile dressings ▪ luer-lock injection cap ▪ clamp ▪ adhesive skin closures ▪ suture removal set.

To access the VAP: Noncoring needles of appropriate type and gauge with attached extension set tubing ▪ sterile gloves ▪ antiseptic cleaning swab ▪ local anesthetic (lidocaine without epinephrine), as needed ▪ ice pack ▪ two 10-ml syringes ▪ normal saline solution ▪ transparent semipermeable dressing ▪ luer-lock injection cap.

To administer a bolus injection: Noncoring needle of appropriate type and gauge ▪ attached extension set ▪ clamp ▪ 10-ml syringe filled with normal saline solution ▪ syringe containing the prescribed medication ▪ optional: sterile syringe filled with heparin flush solution.

To administer a continuous infusion: Prescribed I.V. solution or drug ▪ .V. administration set ▪ filter, if ordered ▪ noncoring needle of appropriate type and gauge ▪ attached extension set ▪ clamp ▪ 10-ml syringe filled with normal saline solution ▪ adhesive tape ▪ sterile 2″ × 2″ gauze pad ▪ sterile tape ▪ transparent semipermeable dressing.

Some facilities use an implantable port access kit.

Preparation of equipment

Confirm the size and type of the device and the insertion site with the physician. Attach the tubing to the solution container, prime the tubing with fluid, fill the syringes with saline or heparin flush solution, and prime the noncoring needle with extension set. All priming must be done using strict sterile technique, and all tubing must be free of air. After you've primed the tubing, recheck all connections for tightness. Make sure all open ends are covered with sealed caps.

Implementation

- Wash your hands *to prevent spreading microorganisms.*

Assisting with implantation of a VAP

- Reinforce to the patient the physician's explanation of the procedure, its benefit to the patient, and what's expected of him during and after implantation.
- Although the physician is responsible for obtaining consent for the procedure, make sure the written document is signed, witnessed, and on the chart.
- Allay the patient's fears and answer questions about movement restrictions, cosmetic concerns, and management regimens.
- Check the patient's history for hypersensitivity to local anesthetics or iodine.
- The physician will surgically implant the VAP, probably using a local anesthetic (similar to insertion of a CVC). Occasionally, a patient may receive a general anesthetic for VAP implantation.
- During the implantation procedure, you may be responsible for handing equipment and supplies to the physician. First, the physician makes a small incision and introduces the catheter, typically into the superior vena cava through the subclavian, jugular, or cephalic vein. After fluoroscopy verifies correct placement of the catheter tip, the physician creates a subcutaneous pocket over a bony prominence in the chest wall. Then he tunnels the catheter to the pocket.

EQUIPMENT

Understanding vascular access ports

A vascular access port (VAP) is typically used to deliver intermittent infusions of medication, chemotherapy, and blood products. VAPs offer several advantages over external central venous therapy. Because the device is completely covered by the patient's skin, the risk of extrinsic contamination is reduced. In addition, patients may prefer this type of central line because it doesn't alter the body image and requires less routine catheter care.

The VAP consists of a catheter connected to a small reservoir. A septum designed to withstand multiple punctures seals the reservoir. To access the port, a special noncoring needle is inserted perpendicular to the reservoir.

Accessing VAP

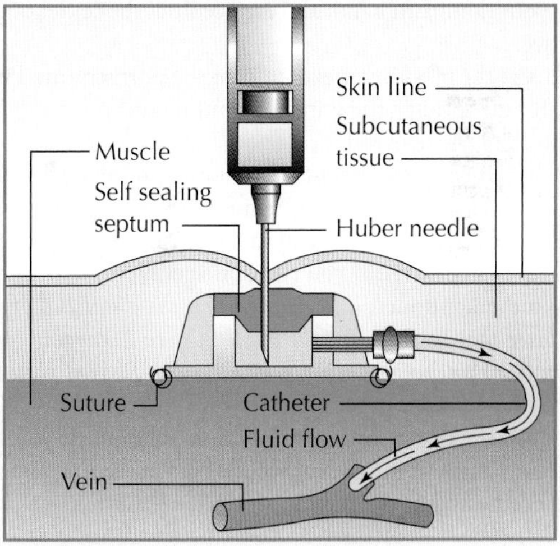

Next, he connects the catheter to the reservoir, places the reservoir in the pocket, and flushes it with heparin solution. Finally, he sutures the reservoir to the underlying fascia and closes the incision.

Preparing to access the port

- The VAP can be used immediately after placement, although some edema and tenderness may persist for about 72 hours. *This makes the device initially difficult to palpate and slightly uncomfortable for the patient.*

■ Prepare to access the port, following the specific steps for top-entry or side-entry ports.
■ Using sterile technique, inspect the area around the port for signs of infection and skin breakdown.
■ Place an ice pack over the area for several minutes *to alleviate possible discomfort from the needle puncture.* Alternatively, administer a local anesthetic after cleaning the area.
■ Wash your hands thoroughly. Put on sterile gloves, and wear them throughout the procedure.
■ Clean the area with an antiseptic swab, starting at the center of the port and working outward with a firm, circular motion over a 4″ × 4″ (10- to 12.5-cm) diameter. Repeat this procedure twice.
■ If facility policy calls for a local anesthetic, check the patient's record for possible allergies. As indicated, anesthetize the insertion site by injecting 0.1 ml of lidocaine (without epinephrine).

Accessing a top-entry port

■ Palpate the area over the port to find the port septum.
■ Anchor the port with your nondominant hand. Then, using your dominant hand, aim the needle at the center of the device.
■ Insert the needle perpendicular to the port septum. Push the needle through the skin and septum until you reach the bottom of the reservoir.
■ Check needle placement by aspirating for blood return.
■ If you can't obtain blood, remove the needle and repeat the procedure. Ask the patient to raise his arms and perform Valsalva's maneuver. If you still don't get blood return, notify the practitioner; *a fibrin sleeve on the distal end of the catheter may be occluding the opening.* (See *Managing common vascular access port problems.* See also *Risks of vascular access port therapy,* page 384.)
■ Flush the device with normal saline solution. If you detect swelling or if the patient reports pain at the site, remove the needle and notify the practitioner.

Accessing a side-entry port

■ To gain access to a side-entry port, follow the same procedure as with a top-entry port, but insert the needle parallel to the reservoir instead of perpendicular to it.

Administering a bolus injection

■ Attach the 10-ml syringe filled with saline solution to the end of the extension set of the noncoring needle, and remove all the air. Check for blood return. Then flush the port with normal saline solution according to your facility's policy.
■ Clamp the extension set and remove the saline syringe.
■ Connect the medication syringe to the extension set. Open the clamp and inject the drug as ordered.
■ Examine the skin surrounding the needle for signs of infiltration, such as swelling and tenderness. If you note these signs, stop the injection and intervene appropriately.
■ When the injection is complete, clamp the extension set and remove the medication syringe.
■ Open the clamp and flush with 5 ml of normal saline solution after each drug injection *to minimize drug incompatibility reactions.*
■ Flush with heparin solution according to your facility's policy.

Administering a continuous infusion

■ Remove all air from the extension set of the noncoring needle by priming it with an attached syringe of normal saline solution.
■ Flush the port system with normal saline solution. Clamp the extension set and remove the syringe.
■ Connect the administration set, and secure the connections with sterile tape if necessary.
■ Unclamp the extension set and begin the infusion.
■ Affix the needle to the skin. Then apply a transparent semipermeable dressing. (See *Continuous infusion: Securing the needle,* page 385.)
■ Examine the site carefully for infiltration. If the patient complains of stinging, burning, or pain at the site, discontinue the infusion and intervene appropriately.
■ When the solution container is empty, obtain a new I.V. solution container as ordered.
■ Flush with normal saline solution followed by heparin solution according to your facility's policy.

Special considerations

■ After implantation, monitor the site for signs of hematoma and bleeding. Edema and tenderness may persist for about 72 hours. The incision site requires routine postoperative care for 7 to 10 days. You'll also need to assess the implantation site for signs of infection, device rotation, and skin erosion. You don't need to apply a dressing to the wound site except during infusions or to maintain an intermittent infusion device.
■ While the patient is hospitalized, a luer-lock injection cap may be attached to the end of the extension set to provide ready access for intermittent infusions. *Besides saving nursing time, a luer-lock cap reduces the discomfort of accessing the port and prolongs the life of the port septum by decreasing the number of needle punctures.*
■ If your patient is receiving a continuous or prolonged infusion, change the transparent dressing and needle every 7 days. However, any dressing should be changed immediately

TROUBLESHOOTING

Managing common vascular access port problems

PROBLEMS AND POSSIBLE CAUSES	NURSING INTERVENTIONS
INABILITY TO FLUSH THE DEVICE OR DRAW BLOOD	
Kinked tubing or closed clamp	■ Check tubing or clamp.
Catheter lodged against vessel wall	■ Reposition the patient. ■ Teach the patient to change his position *to free the catheter from the vessel wall.* ■ Raise the arm that's on the same side as the catheter. ■ Roll the patient to his opposite side. ■ Have the patient cough, sit up, or take a deep breath. ■ Infuse 10 ml of normal saline solution into the catheter. ■ Regain access to the catheter or vascular access port (VAP) using a new needle.
Incorrect needle placement or needle not advanced through septum	■ Regain access to the device. ■ Teach the home care patient to push down firmly on the noncoring needle device in the septum and to verify needle placement by aspirating for blood return.
Clot formation	■ Assess patency by trying to flush the VAP while the patient changes position. ■ Notify the practitioner; obtain an order for instillation of a fibrinolytic agent. ■ Teach the patient to recognize clot formation, to notify the practitioner if it occurs, and to avoid forcibly flushing the VAP.
Kinked catheter, catheter migration, or port rotation	■ Notify the practitioner immediately. ■ Tell the patient to notify the practitioner if he has trouble using the VAP.
INABILITY TO PALPATE THE DEVICE	
Deeply implanted port	■ Note portal chamber scar. ■ Use deep palpation technique. ■ Ask another nurse to try locating the VAP. ■ Use a 1½" or 2" (3.8- or 5-cm) noncoring needle to gain access to the VAP.

if its integrity is compromised. You'll also need to change the tubing and solution, as you would for a long-term CV infusion. If your patient is receiving an intermittent infusion, flush the port periodically with heparin solution. When the VAP isn't being used, flush it every 4 weeks. During the course of therapy, you may have to clear a clotted VAP as ordered.

■ If clotting threatens to occlude the VAP, the practitioner may order a fibrinolytic agent to clear the catheter. *Because such agents increase the risk of bleeding,* this may be contraindicated in patients who have had surgery within the

Risks of vascular access port therapy

Complication	Signs and symptoms	Possible causes	Nursing interventions
Site infection or skin breakdown	■ Erythema and warmth at vascular access port (VAP) site ■ Oozing or purulent drainage at VAP site or pocket ■ Fever	■ Infected incision or VAP pocket ■ Poor postoperative healing	■ Assess the site daily for redness; note any drainage. ■ Notify the practitioner. ■ Administer antibiotics as prescribed. ■ Apply warm soaks for 20 minutes four times per day. ***Prevention*** ■ Teach the patient to inspect for and report redness, swelling, drainage, or skin breakdown at VAP site.
Extravasation	■ Burning sensation or swelling in subcutaneous tissue	■ Needle dislodged into subcutaneous tissue ■ Needle incorrectly placed in VAP ■ Needle position not confirmed; needle pulled out of septum ■ Use of vesicant drugs ■ Rupture of catheter along tunnel route	■ Stop the infusion, but don't remove the needle. ■ Notify the practitioner; prepare to administer an antidote, if ordered. ***Prevention*** ■ Teach the patient how to gain access to the device, verify its placement, and secure the needle before initiating an infusion.
Thrombosis	■ Inability to flush VAP or administer infusion	■ Frequent blood sampling ■ Infusion of packed red blood cells (RBCs)	■ Notify the practitioner; obtain an order to administer a fibrinolytic agent. ***Prevention*** ■ Flush the VAP thoroughly right after obtaining a blood sample. ■ Administer packed RBCs as a piggyback with normal saline solution and use an infusion pump; flush with saline solution between units.
Fibrin sheath formation	■ Blocked VAP and catheter lumen ■ Inability to flush VAP or administer infusion ■ Possibly swelling, tenderness, and erythema in neck, chest, and shoulder	■ Adherence of platelets to catheter	■ Notify the practitioner; prepare to administer a thrombolytic agent. ***Prevention*** ■ Use the port only to infuse fluids and medications; don't use it to obtain blood samples. ■ Administer only compatible substances through the port.

past 10 days, those who have active internal bleeding such as GI bleeding, and those who have experienced central nervous system damage, such as infarction, hemorrhage, traumatic injury, surgery, or primary or metastatic disease, within the past 2 months.

- Besides performing routine care measures, you must be prepared to handle several common problems that may arise during an infusion with a VAP. These common problems include an inability to flush the VAP, withdraw blood from it, or palpate it.

Home care

If your patient is going home, he'll need thorough teaching about procedures as well as follow-up visits from a home care nurse *to ensure safety and successful treatment.* If he'll be accessing the port himself, explain that the most uncomfortable part of the procedure is the actual insertion of the needle into the skin.

When the needle has penetrated the skin, the patient will feel mostly pressure. Eventually, the skin over the port will become desensitized from frequent needle punctures. Until then, the patient may want to use a topical anesthetic.

Stress the importance of pushing the needle into the port until the patient feels the needle bevel touch the back of the port. Many patients tend to stop short of the back of the port, leaving the needle bevel in the rubber septum.

Also stress the importance of monthly flushes when no more infusions are scheduled. If possible, instruct a family member in all aspects of care.

Complications

A patient who has a VAP faces risks similar to those associated with CVCs. They include infection, thrombus formation, and occlusion.

Documentation

Record your assessment findings and interventions, according to your facility's policy. Include the following information: type, amount, rate, and duration of the infusion; appearance of the site; and any adverse reactions and nursing interventions.

Also keep a record of all needle and dressing changes for continuous infusions; blood samples obtained, including the type and amount; and patient-teaching topics covered. Finally, document the removal of the infusion needle, status of the site, use of heparin flush, and any problems you found and resolved.

SELECTED REFERENCES

Centers for Disease Control and Prevention. "Guidelines for the Prevention of Intravascular Device-Related Infections," *MMWR* 51(RR10):1-26, August 2002.

Continuous infusion: Securing the needle

When starting a continuous infusion, you must secure the right-angle, noncoring needle to the skin. If the needle hub is flush with the skin, apply a transparent, semipermeable dressing over the entire site. If the needle hub isn't flush with the skin, place a folded sterile dressing under the hub, as shown below. Then apply adhesive skin closures across it.

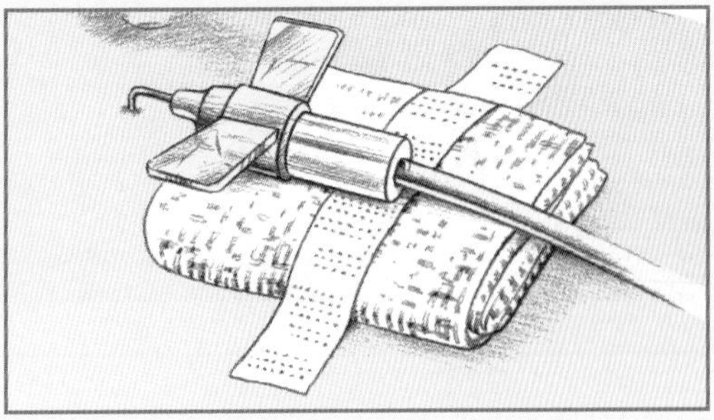

Secure the needle and tubing, using the chevron taping technique using sterile tape.

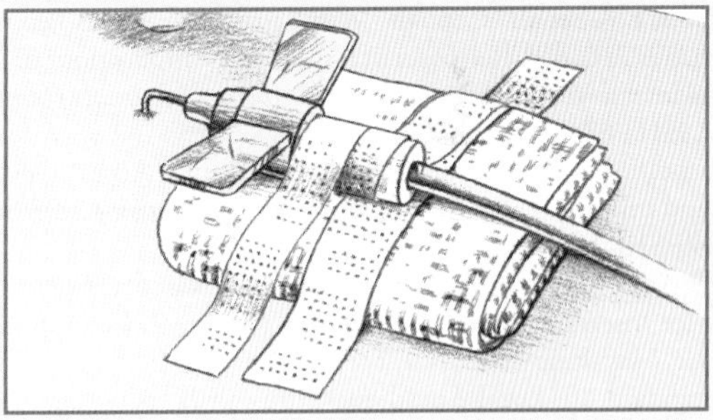

Apply a transparent semipermeable dressing over the entire site.

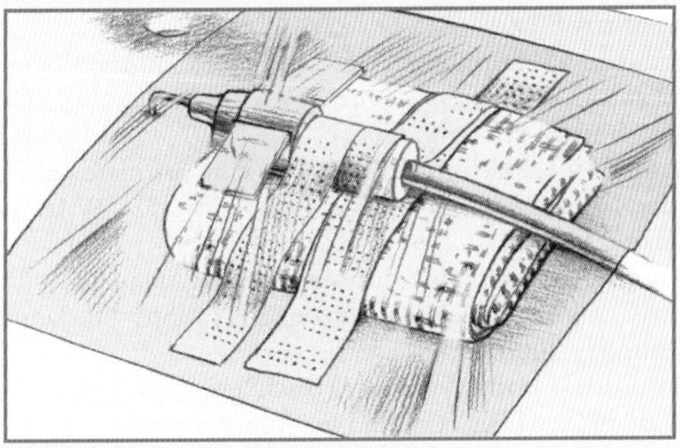

EQUIPMENT

Using I.V. clamps

With a roller clamp, you can increase or decrease the flow through the I.V. line by turning a wheel.

Roller clamp

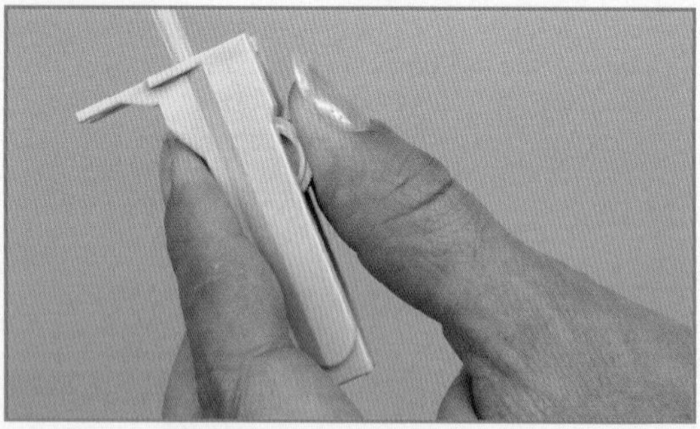

With a slide clamp, you can open or close the line by moving the clamp horizontally. However, you can't make fine adjustments to the flow rate.

Slide clamp

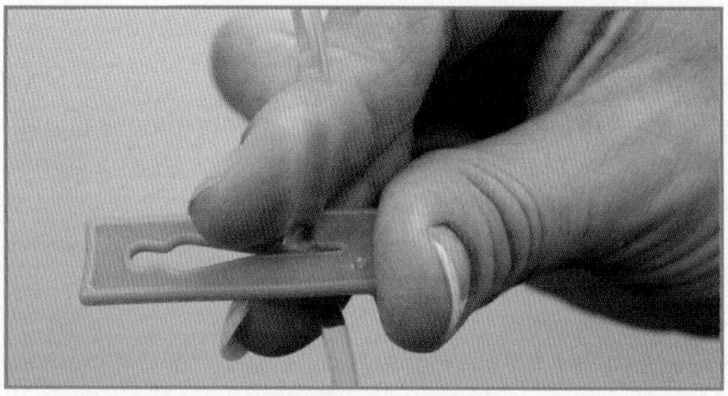

Earhart, A. "Diagnostic Tools and Therapeutic Interventions That May Influence the Integrity of Vascular and Nonvascular Access Devices," *Journal of Infusion Nursing* 28(3 Suppl):S13-17, May-June 2005.

Jablon, L.K., et al. "Cephalic Vein Cut-Down Versus Percutaneous Access: A Retrospective Study of Complications of Implantable Venous Access Devices," *American Journal of Surgery* 192(1):63-67, July 2006.

Masoorli, S. "Legal Issues Related to Vascular Access Devices and Infusion Therapy," *Journal of Infusion Nursing* 28(3 Suppl):S18-21, May-June 2006.

Pieger-Mooney, S. "Innovations in Central Vascular Access Device Insertion," *Journal of Infusion Nursing* 28(3 Suppl):S7-12, May-June 2005.

"Standard 40. Local Anesthesia. Infusion Nursing Standards of Practice," *Journal of Infusion Nursing* 29(1S):S41, January-February 2006.

"Standard 44. Dressings. Infusion Nursing Standards of Practice," *Journal of Infusion Nursing* 29(1S):S44-45, January-February 2006.

"Standard 45. Implanted Ports and Pumps. Infusion Nursing Standards of Practice," *Journal of Infusion Nursing* 29(1S):S44-45, January-February 2006.

"Standard 53. Phlebitis. Infusion Nursing Standards of Practice," *Journal of Infusion Nursing* 29(1S):S58-59, January-February 2006.

"Standard 54. Infiltration. Infusion Nursing Standards of Practice," *Journal of Infusion Nursing* 29(1S):S59-60, January-February 2006.

Tilton, D. "Central Venous Access Device Infections in the Critical Care Unit," *Critical Care Nursing Quarterly* 29(2):117-22, April-June 2006.

Warren, D.K., et al. "A Multicenter Intervention to Prevent Catheter-Associated Bloodstream Infections," *Infection Control and Hospital Epidemiology* 27(7):662-69, July 2006.

INFUSION RATE MANAGEMENT

I.V. INFUSION RATES AND MANUAL CONTROL

Calculated from a practitioner's orders, infusion rate is usually expressed as the total volume of I.V. solution infused over a prescribed interval or as the total volume given in milliliters per hour. Many devices can regulate the infusion of I.V. solution, including clamps, the flow regulator (or rate minder), and the volumetric pump. (See *Using I.V. clamps.*)

When regulated by a clamp, the infusion rate is usually measured in drops per minute; by a volumetric pump, in milliliters per hour. The infusion regulator can be set to deliver the desired amount of solution, also in milliliters per hour. Less accurate than infusion pumps, infusion regulators are most reliable when used with inactive adult patients. With any device, flow rate can be easily monitored by using a time tape, which indicates the prescribed solution level at hourly intervals.

Calculating flow rates

When calculating the flow rate of I.V. solutions, remember that the number of drops required to deliver 1 ml varies with the type and manufacturer of the administration set used. The illustration on the left shows a standard (macrodrip) set, which delivers from 10 to 20 drops/ml. The illustration in the center shows a pediatric (microdrip) set, which delivers about 60 drops/ml. The illustration on the right shows a blood transfusion set, which delivers about 10 drops/ml.

To calculate the flow rate, you must know the calibration of the drip rate for each manufacturer's product. Use this formula to calculate specific drip rates:

$$\frac{\text{Volume of infusion (in ml)}}{\text{time of infusion (in minutes)}} \times \text{drip factor (in drops/ml)} = \text{drops/minute}$$

Macrodrip set

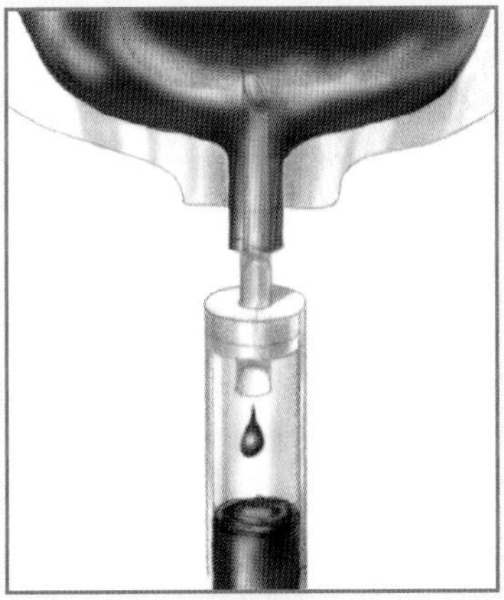

Microdrip set

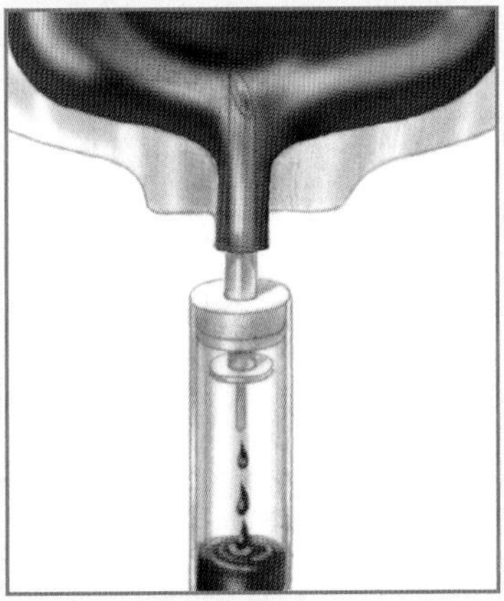

Blood transfusion set

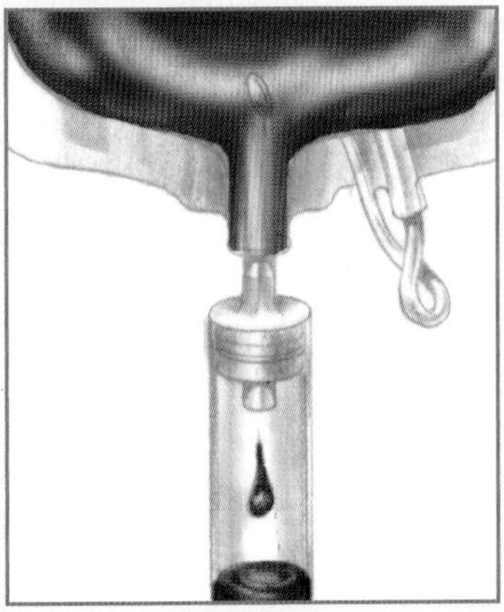

Equipment

I.V. administration set with clamp ▪ 1″ paper or adhesive tape (or premarked time tape) ▪ infusion pump (if infusing medication) ▪ watch with second hand ▪ drip rate chart, as necessary ▪ pen.

Standard macrodrip sets deliver from 10 to 20 drops/ml, depending on the manufacturer; microdrip sets, 60 drops/ml; and blood transfusion sets, 10 drops/ml. A commercially available adapter can convert a macrodrip set to a microdrip system.

Implementation

- The infusion rate requires close monitoring and correction *because such factors as venous spasm, venous pressure changes, patient movement or manipulation of the clamp, and bent or kinked tubing can cause the rate to vary markedly.*

Calculating and setting the drip rate

- Follow the steps in *Calculating flow rates*, to determine the proper drip rate, or use your unit's drip rate chart.
- After calculating the desired drip rate, remove your watch, and hold it next to the drip chamber *so that you can observe the watch and drops simultaneously.*
- Release the clamp to the approximate drip rate. Then count drops for 1 minute *to account for flow irregularities.*
- Adjust the clamp, as necessary, and count drops for 1 minute. Continue to adjust the clamp and count drops until the correct rate is achieved.

Making a time tape

- Calculate the number of milliliters to be infused per hour. Place a piece of tape vertically on the container alongside the volume-increment markers.
- Starting at the current solution level, move down the number of milliliters to be infused in 1 hour, and mark the appropriate time and a horizontal line on the tape at this level. Then continue to mark 1-hour intervals until you reach the bottom of the container.
- Check the flow rate every 15 minutes until stable, then every hour or according to your facility policy's; adjust as needed.

TROUBLESHOOTING

Managing I.V. flow rate deviations

PROBLEM	POSSIBLE CAUSES	NURSING INTERVENTIONS
Flow rate too slow	■ Venous spasm after insertion	■ Apply warm soaks over site.
	■ Venous obstruction from bending arm	■ Secure with an arm board if necessary.
	■ Pressure change (decreasing fluid in bottle causes solution to run slower because of decreasing pressure)	■ Readjust flow rate.
	■ Elevated blood pressure	■ Readjust flow rate. Use infusion pump *to ensure correct flow rate.*
	■ Cold solution	■ Allow solution to warm to room temperature before hanging.
	■ Change in solution viscosity from medication added	■ Readjust flow rate.
	■ I.V. container too low or patient's arm or leg too high	■ Hang container higher or remind patient to keep his arm below heart level.
	■ Bevel against vein wall (positional cannulation)	■ Withdraw needle slightly, or place a folded 2″ × 2″ gauze pad over or under catheter hub *to change angle.*
	■ Excess tubing dangling below insertion site	■ Replace tubing with shorter piece, or tape excess tubing to I.V. pole, below flow clamp. (Make sure tubing isn't kinked.)
	■ Cannula too small	■ Remove cannula in use, and insert a larger-bore cannula, or use an infusion pump.
	■ Infiltration or clotted cannula	■ Remove cannula in use and insert a new cannula.
	■ Kinked tubing	■ Check tubing over its entire length, and unkink it.
	■ Clogged filter	■ Remove filter, and replace it with a new one.
	■ Tubing memory (tubing compressed at clamped area)	■ Massage or milk tubing by pinching and wrapping it around a pencil four or five times. Quickly pull pencil out of coiled tubing.

■ With each check, inspect the I.V. site for complications, and assess the patient's response to therapy.

Special considerations

■ If the infusion rate slows significantly, a slight rate increase may be necessary. If the rate must be increased by more than 30%, consult the practitioner. When infusing drugs, use an

Managing I.V. flow rate deviations *(continued)*

Problem	Possible causes	Nursing interventions
Flow rate too fast	■ Patient or visitor manipulated clamp	■ Instruct patient not to touch clamp. Place tape over it. Restrain patient, or administer I.V. solution with infusion pump, if necessary.
	■ Tubing disconnected from catheter	■ Wipe distal end of tubing with alcohol, reinsert firmly into catheter hub, and tape at connection site. Use tubing with luer-lock connections.
	■ Change in patient position	■ Administer I.V. solution with infusion pump *to ensure correct flow rate.*
	■ Bevel against vein wall (positional cannulation)	■ Manipulate cannula, and place a 2″ × 2″ gauze pad under or over catheter hub *to change the angle.* Reset flow clamp at desired rate. If necessary, remove cannula and reinsert.
	■ Flow clamp drifted because of patient movement	■ Place tape below clamp.

I.V. pump, if possible, *to avoid flow rate inaccuracies.* Always use a pump or controller when infusing solutions by way of a central line.

■ Large-volume solution containers have about 10% more fluid than the amount indicated on the bag *to allow for tubing purges.* Thus, a 1,000-ml bag or bottle contains an additional 100 ml; similarly, a 500-ml container holds an extra 50 ml; and a 250-ml container, 25 ml.

Complications

An excessively slow flow rate may cause insufficient intake of fluids, drugs, and nutrients; an excessively rapid rate of fluid or drug infusion may cause circulatory overload — possibly leading to heart failure and pulmonary edema — as well as adverse drug effects. (See *Managing I.V. flow rate deviations.*)

Documentation

Record the original flow rate when setting up a peripheral line. If you adjust the rate, record the change, date and time, and your initials.

Selected references

"Standard 14. Documentation. Infusion Nursing Standards of Practice," *Journal of Infusion Nursing* 29(1S):S22-23, January-February 2006.

"Standard 33. Flow-Control Devices. Infusion Nursing Standards of Practice," *Journal of Infusion Nursing* 29(1S):S34-35, January-February 2006.

Weinstein, S.M. *Plumer's Principles and Practices of Intravenous Therapy,* 8th ed. Philadelphia: Lippincott Williams & Wilkins, 2007.

I.V. pumps

Various types of I.V. pumps electronically regulate the flow of I.V. solutions or drugs with great accuracy.

Volumetric pumps, used for high-pressure infusion of drugs or for highly accurate delivery of fluids or drugs, have mechanisms to propel the solution at the desired rate under pressure. (Pressure is brought to bear only when gravity flow rates are insufficient to maintain preset infusion rates.) The peristaltic pump applies pressure to the I.V. tubing to force the solution through it. (Not all peristaltic pumps are volumetric; some count drops.) The piston-cylinder pump pushes the solution through special disposable cassettes. Most of these pumps operate at high pressures (up to 45 psi), delivering from 1 to 999 ml/hour with about 98% accuracy. (Some pumps operate at 10 to 25 psi.) The portable syringe pump, another type of volumetric pump, delivers very small amounts of fluid over a long period. It's used for administering fluids to infants and for delivering intra-arterial drugs.

EQUIPMENT

Infusion pumps

Infusion pumps electronically regulate the flow of I.V. solutions and drugs. You'll use them when a precise flow rate is needed; for example, when administering total parenteral nutrition solutions and chemotherapeutic or cardiovascular agents.

Infusion pump

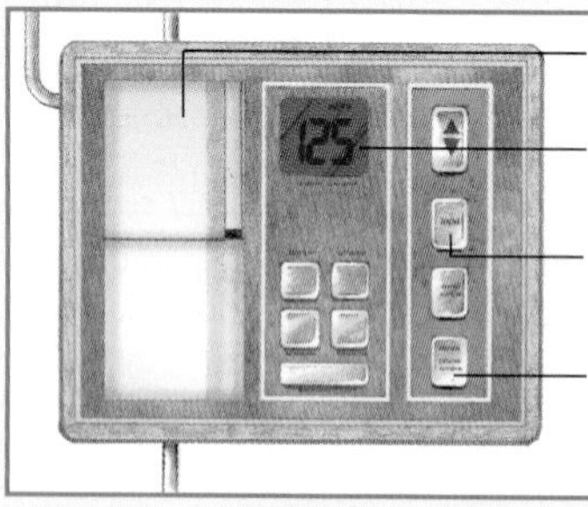

Other specialized devices include bar code automated programming devices, the controlled-release infusion system, secondary syringe converter, and patient-controlled analgesia.

Pumps have various detectors and alarms that automatically signal or respond to the completion of an infusion, air in the line, low battery power, and occlusion or inability to deliver at the set rate. Depending on the problem, these devices may sound or flash an alarm, shut off, or switch to a keep-vein-open rate.

Equipment

Peristaltic pump ▪ I.V. pole ▪ I.V. solution ▪ sterile administration set ▪ sterile peristaltic tubing or cassette, if needed ▪ alcohol pads ▪ adhesive tape. Tubing and cassettes vary among manufacturers. (See *Infusion pumps*.)

Preparation of equipment

Attach the pump to the I.V. pole. Then swab the port on the I.V. container with alcohol, insert the administration set spike, and fill the drip chamber completely *to prevent air bubbles from entering the tubing.* Next, prime the tubing and close the clamp. Follow the manufacturer's instructions for placement of tubing.

Implementation

- Position the pump on the same side of the bed as the I.V. or anticipated venipuncture site *to avoid crisscrossing I.V. lines over the patient.* If necessary, perform the venipuncture.
- Plug in the machine, and attach its tubing to the needle or catheter hub.
- Depending on the machine, turn it on and press the START button. Set the appropriate dials on the front panel to the desired infusion rate and volume. Always set the volume dial at 50 ml less than the prescribed volume or 50 ml less than the volume in the container *so that you can hang a new container before the old one empties.*
- If your facility uses a bar code automated pump, scan your ID badge, the patient's ID bracelet, and the patient ID on the medication bag *to ensure that the right patient is receiving the infusion.*
- Confirm that the right information is displayed on the pump, then push the RUN button.
- Check the patency of the I.V. line, and watch for infiltration.
- Tape all connections.
- Turn on the alarm switches. Then explain the alarm system to the patient *to prevent anxiety when a change in the infusion activates the alarm.*

Special considerations

- Monitor the pump and the patient frequently *to ensure the device's correct operation and flow rate and to detect infiltration and such complications as infection and air embolism.*
- If electrical power fails, the pumps automatically switch to battery power.
- Check the manufacturer's recommendations before administering opaque fluids, such as blood, *because some pumps fail to detect opaque fluids and others may cause hemolysis of infused blood.*
- Remove I.V. solutions from the refrigerator 1 hour before infusing them to help release small gas bubbles from the solutions. *Small bubbles in the solution can join to form larger bubbles, which can activate the pump's air-in-line alarm.*

Home care

Make sure the patient and his family understand the purpose of using the pump. If necessary, demonstrate how the device works. Also demonstrate how to maintain the system (tubing, solution, and site assessment and care) until you're confident that the patient and family can proceed safely. As time permits, have the patient repeat the demonstration. Discuss which complications to watch for, such as infiltration, and review measures to take if complications occur. Schedule a teaching session with the patient or family *so you can answer questions they may have about the procedure before the patient's discharge.*

Complications

Complications associated with I.V. pumps are the same as those associated with peripheral lines. (See "Peripheral I.V. catheter insertion," page 349.) Keep in mind that infiltration can develop rapidly with infusion by a volumetric pump because the increased subcutaneous pressure won't slow the infusion rate until significant edema occurs.

Documentation

In addition to routine documentation of the I.V. infusion, record the use of a pump on the I.V. record and in your notes.

SELECTED REFERENCES

The Joint Commission. *Comprehensive Accreditation Manual for Hospitals: The Official Handbook.* Standard MM.6.10. 2007.

"Standard 14. Documentation. Infusion Nursing Standards of Practice," *Journal of Infusion Nursing* 29(1S):S22-23, January-February 2006.

"Standard 33. Flow-Control Devices. Infusion Nursing Standards of Practice," *Journal of Infusion Nursing* 29(1S):S34-35, January-February 2006.

Weinstein, S.M. *Plumer's Principles and Practices of Intravenous Therapy,* 8th ed. Philadelphia: Lippincott Williams & Wilkins, 2007.

PARENTERAL NUTRITION

PARENTERAL NUTRITION

When a patient can't meet his nutritional needs by oral or enteral feedings, he may require I.V. nutritional support, or parenteral nutrition. The patient's diagnosis, history, and prognosis determine the need for parenteral nutrition. Generally, this treatment is prescribed for any patient who can't absorb nutrients through the GI tract for more than 10 days. More specific indications include:

- debilitating illness lasting longer than 2 weeks
- loss of 10% or more of pre-illness weight
- serum albumin level below 3.5 g/dl
- excessive nitrogen loss from wound infection, fistulas, or abscesses
- renal or hepatic failure
- a nonfunctioning GI tract for 5 to 7 days in a severely catabolic patient.

Common illnesses that can trigger the need for parenteral nutrition include inflammatory bowel disease, radiation enteritis, severe diarrhea, intractable vomiting, and moderate to severe pancreatitis. A massive small-bowel resection, bone marrow transplantation, high-dose chemotherapy or radiation therapy, and major surgery can also hinder a patient's ability to absorb nutrients and require parenteral nutrition.

Infants with congenital or acquired disorders may need parenteral nutrition to promote growth and development. Specific disorders that may require parenteral nutrition include tracheoesophageal fistula, gastroschisis, duodenal atresia, cystic fibrosis, meconium ileus, diaphragmatic hernia, volvulus, malrotation of the gut, and annular pancreas.

Parenteral nutrition shouldn't be given to patients with a normally functioning GI tract, and it has limited value for well-nourished patients whose GI tract will resume normal function within 10 days. It may also be inappropriate for patients with a poor prognosis or if the risks of parenteral nutrition outweigh the benefits.

Parenteral nutrition may be given through a peripheral or central venous (CV) line. Depending on the solution, it may be used to boost the patient's caloric intake, to supply full caloric needs, or to surpass the patient's caloric requirements.

The type of parenteral solution prescribed depends on the patient's condition and metabolic needs and on the administration route. The solution usually contains protein, carbohydrates, electrolytes, vitamins, and trace minerals. A lipid emulsion provides the necessary fat. (See *Types of parenteral nutrition,* pages 392 and 393.)

Total parenteral nutrition (TPN) refers to any nutrient solution, including lipids, given through a CV line. Peripheral parenteral nutrition (PPN), which is given through a peripheral line, supplies full caloric needs while avoiding the risks that accompany a CV line. To keep from sclerosing the vein through which it's administered, the dextrose in PPN solution must be limited to 10% or less. Therefore, the success of PPN depends on the patient's tolerance for the large volume of fluid necessary to supply his nutritional needs.

Often, you'll need to increase the glucose content beyond the level a peripheral vein can handle. For example, most TPN solutions are six times more concentrated than blood. As a result, they must be delivered into a vein with a high rate of blood flow to dilute the solution.

The most common delivery route for TPN is through a central venous catheter (CVC) into the superior vena cava. The catheter may also be placed through the infraclavicular approach or, less commonly, through the supraclavicular, internal jugular, or antecubital fossa approach.

(Text continues on page 394.)

Types of parenteral nutrition

Type	Solution components per liter	Uses	Special considerations
Standard I.V. therapy	■ Dextrose, water, electrolytes in varying amounts; for example: – Dextrose 5% in water (D_5W) = 170 calories/L – $D_{10}W$ = 340 calories/L – Normal saline = 0 calories ■ Vitamins as ordered	■ Less than 1 week as nutrition source ■ Maintains hydration (main function) ■ Facilitates and maintains normal metabolic function	■ Nutritionally incomplete; doesn't provide sufficient calories to maintain adequate nutritional status
Total parenteral nutrition (TPN) by way of central venous (CV) line	■ $D_{15}W$ to $D_{25}W$ (1 L dextrose 25% = 850 nonprotein calories) ■ Crystalline amino acids 2.5% to 8.5% ■ Electrolytes, vitamins, trace elements, and insulin, as ordered ■ Lipid emulsion 10% to 20% (usually infused as a separate solution)	■ 2 weeks or more ■ For patients with large caloric and nutrient needs ■ Provides calories, restores nitrogen balance, and replaces essential vitamins, electrolytes, minerals, and trace elements ■ Promotes tissue synthesis, wound healing, and normal metabolic function ■ Allows bowel rest and healing; reduces activity in the gallbladder, pancreas, and small intestine ■ Improves tolerance of surgery	***Basic solution*** ■ Nutritionally complete ■ Requires minor surgical procedure for CV line insertion (can be done at bedside by the practitioner) ■ Highly hypertonic solution ■ May cause metabolic complications (glucose intolerance, electrolyte imbalance, essential fatty acid deficiency) ***I.V. lipid emulsion*** ■ May not be used effectively in severely stressed patients (especially burn patients) ■ May interfere with immune mechanisms; in patients suffering respiratory compromise, reduces carbon dioxide buildup ■ Given by way of CV line; irritates peripheral vein in long-term use
Protein-sparing therapy	■ Crystalline amino acids in same amounts as TPN ■ Electrolytes, vitamins, minerals, and trace elements, as ordered	■ 2 weeks or less ■ May preserve body protein in a stable patient ■ Augments oral and tube feedings	■ Nutritionally complete ■ Requires little mixing ■ May be started or stopped any time during the hospital stay ■ Other I.V. fluids, medications, and blood by-products may be administered through the same I.V. line ■ Not as likely to cause phlebitis as peripheral parenteral nutrition ■ Adds a major expense; has limited benefits ■ Special formulations for neonates and patients with renal or hepatic failure

Types of parenteral nutrition *(continued)*

Type	Solution components per liter	Uses	Special considerations
Total nutrient admixture	■ One day's nutrients are contained in a single, 3-L bag (also called 3:1 solution) ■ Combines lipid emulsion with other parenteral solution components	■ 2 weeks or more ■ For relatively stable patients because solution components can be adjusted just once daily ■ For other uses, see TPN (previous page)	■ See TPN (previous page) ■ Reduces need to handle bag, cutting risk of contamination ■ Decreases nursing time and reduces need for infusion sets and electronic devices, lowering facility costs, increasing patient mobility, and allowing easier adjustment to home care ■ Has limited use because not all types and amounts of components are compatible ■ Precludes use of certain infusion pumps because they can't accurately deliver large volumes of solution; precludes use of standard I.V. tubing filters because a 0.22-micron filter blocks lipid and albumin molecules
Peripheral parenteral nutrition (PPN)	■ D_5W to $D_{10}W$ ■ Crystalline amino acids 2.5% to 5% ■ Electrolytes, minerals, vitamins, and trace elements, as ordered ■ Lipid emulsion 10% or 20% (1 L of dextrose 10% and amino acids 3.5% infused at the same time as 1 L of lipid emulsion = 1,440 nonprotein calories) ■ Heparin or hydrocortisone as ordered	■ 2 weeks or less ■ Provides up to 2,000 calories/day ■ Maintains adequate nutritional status in patients who can tolerate relatively high fluid volume, in those who usually resume bowel function and oral feedings after a few days, and in those who are susceptible to infections associated with the CV catheter	***Basic solution*** ■ Nutritionally complete for a short time ■ Can't be used long term in nutritionally depleted patients ■ Can't be used in volume-restricted patients because PPN requires large fluid volume ■ For weight maintenance, not weight gain ■ Avoids insertion and care of CV line but requires adequate venous access; site must be changed every 72 hours ■ Delivers less hypertonic solutions than CV line TPN ■ May cause phlebitis and increases risk of metabolic complications ■ Less chance of metabolic complications than with CV line TPN ***I.V. lipid emulsion*** ■ As effective as dextrose for caloric source ■ Diminishes phlebitis if infused at the same time as basic nutrient solution ■ Irritates vein in long-term use ■ Reduces carbon dioxide buildup in pulmonary compromise

Equipment

Bag or bottle of prescribed parenteral nutrition solution ▪ sterile I.V. tubing with attached extension tubing ▪ 0.22-micron filter (or 1.2-micron filter if solution contains lipids or albumin) ▪ reflux valve ▪ time tape ▪ alcohol pads ▪ electronic infusion pump ▪ portable glucose monitor ▪ scale ▪ intake and output record ▪ sterile gloves ▪ optional: mask

Preparation of equipment

Make sure the solution, the patient, and the equipment are ready. Remove the solution from the refrigerator at least 1 hour before use *to avoid pain, hypothermia, venous spasm, and venous constriction, which can result from delivery of a chilled solution.* Check the solution against the practitioner's order for correct patient name, expiration date, and formula components. Observe the container for cracks and the solution for cloudiness, turbidity, and particles. If any of these is present, return the solution to the pharmacy. If you'll be administering a total nutrient admixture solution, look for a brown layer on the solution, *which indicates that the lipid emulsion has "cracked," or separated from the solution.* If you see a brown layer, return the solution to the pharmacy.

When you're ready to administer the solution, explain the procedure to the patient. Check the name on the solution container against the name on the patient's wristband. Confirm the patient's identity using two patient identifiers according to your facility's policy. Then put on gloves and, if specified by facility policy, a mask. Throughout the procedure, use strict sterile technique.

In sequence, connect the pump tubing, the micron filter with attached extension tubing (if the tubing doesn't contain an in-line filter), and the reflux valve. Insert the filter as close to the catheter site as possible. Next, squeeze the I.V. drip chamber and, holding it upright, insert the tubing spike into the I.V. bag or bottle. Then release the drip chamber. Squeezing the drip chamber before spiking an I.V. bottle *prevents accidental dripping of the parenteral nutrition solution.* An I.V. bag, however, shouldn't drip.

Next, prime the tubing. Invert the filter at the distal end of the tubing, and open the roller clamp. Let the solution fill the tubing and the filter. Gently tap it *to dislodge air bubbles trapped in the Y-ports.* If indicated, attach a time tape to the parenteral nutrition container *for accurate measurement of fluid intake.* Record the date and time you hung the fluid, and initial the parenteral nutrition solution container. Next, attach the setup to the infusion pump, and prepare it according to the manufacturer's instructions. Remove and discard your gloves.

With the patient in the supine position, flush the catheter with heparin or normal saline solution, according to your facility's policy. Then put on gloves, and clean the catheter injection cap with an alcohol pad.

Implementation

- If you'll be attaching the container of parenteral nutrition solution to a CV line, clamp the CV line before disconnecting it *to prevent air from entering the catheter.* If a clamp isn't available, ask the patient to perform Valsalva's maneuver just as you change the tubing, if possible. Or, if the patient is being mechanically ventilated, change the I.V. tubing immediately after the machine delivers a breath at peak inspiration. *Both of these measures increase intrathoracic pressure and prevent air embolism.*
- Using sterile technique, attach the tubing to the designated luer-locking port. After connecting the tubing, remove the clamp, if applicable.
- Set the infusion pump at the ordered flow rate, and start the infusion. Make sure the catheter junction is secure.
- Tag the tubing with the date and time of change.

Starting the infusion

- *Because parenteral nutrition solution often contains a large amount of glucose,* you may need to start the infusion slowly to allow the patient's pancreatic beta cells time to increase their output of insulin. Depending on the patient's tolerance, parenteral nutrition is usually initiated at a rate of 40 to 50 ml/hour and then advanced by 25 ml/hour every 6 hours (as tolerated) until the desired infusion rate is achieved. However, when the glucose concentration is low, as occurs in most PPN formulas, you can initiate the rate necessary to infuse the complete 24-hour volume and discontinue the solution without tapering.
- You may allow a container of parenteral nutrition solution to hang for 24 hours.

Changing solutions

- Prepare the new solution and I.V. tubing as described earlier. Put on sterile gloves. Remove the protective caps from the solution containers, and wipe the tops of the containers with alcohol pads.
- Turn off the infusion pump, and close the flow clamps. Using strict sterile technique, remove the spike from the solution container that's hanging, and insert it into the new container.
- Hang the new container and tubing alongside the old. Turn on the infusion pump, set the flow rate, and open the flow clamp completely.
- If you'll be attaching the solution to a peripheral line, examine the skin above the insertion site for redness and warmth, and assess for pain. If you suspect phlebitis, remove the existing I.V. line, and start a line in a different vein. Also insert a new line if the I.V. catheter has been in place for 72 hours or more *to reduce the risk of phlebitis and infiltration.*
- Next, turn off the infusion pump, and close the flow clamp on the old tubing. Disconnect the tubing from the catheter

hub and connect the new tubing. Open the flow clamp on the new container to a moderately slow rate.

- Remove the old tubing from the infusion pump, and insert the new tubing according to the manufacturer's instructions. Then turn on the infusion pump, set it to the desired flow rate, and open the flow clamp completely. Remove the old equipment and dispose of it properly.

Special considerations

- Always infuse a parenteral nutrition solution at a constant rate without interruption *to avoid blood glucose fluctuations.* If the infusion slows, consult the practitioner before changing the infusion rate.
- Monitor the patient's vital signs every 4 hours or more often if necessary. Watch for an increased temperature, *an early sign of catheter-related sepsis.* (See *Correcting common parenteral nutrition problems,* pages 396 to 398.)
- Check the patient's blood glucose every 6 hours. Some patients may require supplementary insulin, which the pharmacist may add directly to the solution. The patient may require additional subcutaneous doses.
- *Because most patients receiving parenteral nutrition are in a protein-wasted state,* the therapy causes marked changes in fluid and electrolyte status and in levels of glucose, amino acids, minerals, and vitamins. Therefore, record daily intake and output accurately. Specify the volume and type of each fluid, and calculate the daily caloric intake.
- Monitor the results of routine laboratory tests, and report abnormal findings to the practitioner *to allow for appropriate changes in the parenteral nutrition solution.* Such tests typically include measurement of serum electrolyte, calcium, blood urea nitrogen, creatinine, and blood glucose levels at least three times weekly; serum magnesium and phosphorus levels twice weekly; liver function studies, complete blood count and differential, and serum albumin and transferrin levels weekly; and urine nitrogen balance and creatinine-height index studies weekly. A serum zinc level is obtained at the start of parenteral nutrition therapy. The practitioner may also order serum prealbumin levels, total lymphocyte count, amino acid levels, fatty acid-phospholipid fraction, skin testing, and expired gas analysis. (Also see "Patient monitoring during parenteral nutrition," page 400.)
- Physically assess the patient daily. If ordered, measure arm circumference and skin-fold thickness over the triceps. Weigh him at the same time each morning after he voids; he should be weighed in similar clothing and on the same scale. Suspect fluid imbalance if he gains more than 1 lb (0.5 kg) daily.
- Change the dressing over the catheter according to your facility's policy or whenever the dressing becomes wet, soiled, or nonocclusive. Always use strict sterile technique. When performing dressing changes, watch for signs of phlebitis and catheter retraction from the vein. Measure the catheter length from the insertion site to the hub for verification.
- Change the tubing and filters every 24 hours or according to your facility's policy.
- Closely monitor the catheter site for swelling, *which may indicate infiltration.* Extravasation of parenteral nutrition solution can lead to tissue necrosis.
- Use caution when using the parenteral nutrition line for other functions. Don't use a single-lumen CVC to infuse blood or blood products, to give a bolus injection, to administer simultaneous I.V. solutions, to measure CV pressure, or to draw blood for laboratory tests.
- Provide regular mouth care. Also provide emotional support. Keep in mind that patients commonly associate eating with positive feelings and become disturbed when they can't eat.
- Teach the patient the potential adverse effects and complications of parenteral nutrition. Encourage the patient to inspect his mouth regularly for signs of parotitis, glossitis, and oral lesions. Tell him that he may have fewer bowel movements while receiving parenteral nutrition therapy. Encourage him to remain physically active *to help his body use the nutrients more fully.*

Home care

Patients who require prolonged or indefinite parenteral nutrition may be able to receive the therapy at home. Home parenteral nutrition reduces the need for long hospitalizations and allows the patient to resume many of his normal activities. Meet with a home care patient before discharge *to make sure he knows how to perform the administration procedure and how to handle complications.*

Complications

Catheter-related sepsis is the most serious complication of parenteral nutrition. Although rare, a malpositioned subclavian or jugular vein catheter may lead to thrombosis or sepsis.

An air embolism, a potentially fatal complication, can occur during I.V. tubing changes if the tubing is inadvertently disconnected. It may also result from undetected hairline cracks in the tubing. Extravasation of parenteral nutrition solution can cause necrosis and then sloughing of the epidermis and dermis.

Documentation

Document the times of the dressing, filter, and solution changes; the condition of the catheter insertion site; your

(Text continues on page 398.)

Correcting common parenteral nutrition problems

Complication	Signs and symptoms	Interventions
Metabolic problems		
Hepatic dysfunction	Elevated serum aspartate aminotransferase, alkaline phosphatase, and bilirubin levels	■ Reduce total caloric intake and dextrose intake, making up lost calories by administering lipid emulsion. ■ Change to cyclical infusion. ■ Use specific hepatic formulations only if the patient has encephalopathy.
Hypercapnia	Heightened oxygen consumption, increased carbon dioxide production, measured respiratory quotient of 1 or greater	■ Reduce total caloric and dextrose intake and balance dextrose and fat calories.
Hyperglycemia	Fatigue, restlessness, confusion, anxiety, weakness, polyuria, dehydration, elevated serum glucose levels and, in severe hyperglycemia, delirium or coma	■ Restrict dextrose intake by decreasing either the rate of infusion or the dextrose concentration. ■ Compensate for calorie loss by administering lipid emulsion. ■ Begin insulin therapy.
Hyperosmolarity	Confusion, lethargy, seizures, hyperosmolar hyperglycemic nonketotic syndrome, hyperglycemia, dehydration, and glycosuria	■ Discontinue dextrose infusion. ■ Administer insulin and half-normal saline solution with 10 to 20 mEq/L of potassium to rehydrate the patient.
Hypocalcemia	Polyuria, dehydration, and elevated blood and urine glucose levels	■ Increase calcium supplements.
Hypoglycemia	Sweating, shaking, and irritability after infusion has stopped	■ Increase dextrose intake or decrease exogenous insulin intake.
Hypokalemia	Muscle weakness, paralysis, paresthesia, and arrhythmias	■ Increase potassium supplements.
Hypomagnesemia	Tingling around mouth, paresthesia in fingers, mental changes, and hyperreflexia	■ Increase magnesium supplements.
Hypophosphatemia	Irritability, weakness, paresthesia, coma, and respiratory arrest	■ Increase phosphate supplements.
Zinc deficiency	Dermatitis, alopecia, apathy, depression, taste changes, confusion, poor wound healing, and diarrhea	■ Increase zinc supplements.

Correcting common parenteral nutrition problems *(continued)*

COMPLICATION	SIGNS AND SYMPTOMS	INTERVENTIONS
METABOLIC PROBLEMS *(continued)*		
Metabolic acidosis	Elevated serum chloride level, reduced serum bicarbonate level	■ Increase acetate and decrease chloride in parenteral nutrition solution.
Metabolic alkalosis	Reduced serum chloride level, elevated serum bicarbonate level	■ Decrease acetate and increase chloride in parenteral nutrition solution.
MECHANICAL PROBLEMS		
Clotted I.V. catheter	Interrupted flow rate, resistance to flushing and blood withdrawal	■ Attempt to aspirate clot. If unsuccessful, instill a fibrinolytic agent to clear catheter lumen as ordered.
Cracked or broken tubing	Fluid leaking from tubing	■ Apply a padded hemostat above break *to prevent air from entering line.*
Dislodged catheter	Catheter out of vein	■ Apply pressure to site with sterile gauze pad.
Too-rapid infusion	Nausea, headache, and lethargy	■ Adjust infusion rate and, if applicable, check infusion pump.
OTHER PROBLEMS		
Air embolism	Apprehension, chest pain, tachycardia, hypotension, cyanosis, seizures, loss of consciousness, and cardiac arrest	■ Clamp catheter. Place patient in a steep, left lateral Trendelenburg position. Administer oxygen as ordered. If cardiac arrest occurs, begin cardiopulmonary resuscitation. ■ When catheter is removed, cover insertion site with dressing for 24 to 48 hours.
Extravasation	Swelling and pain around insertion site	■ Stop infusion, and assess patient for cardiopulmonary abnormalities; chest X-ray may be required.
Phlebitis	Pain, tenderness, redness, and warmth	■ Apply gentle heat to area and, if possible, elevate insertion site.
Pneumothorax and hydrothorax	Dyspnea, chest pain, cyanosis, and decreased breath sounds	■ Assist with chest tube insertion, and apply suction as ordered.
Septicemia	Red and swollen catheter site, chills, fever, and leukocytosis	■ Remove catheter and culture the tip. Obtain a blood culture if patient has a fever. Give appropriate antibiotics.

(continued)

Correcting common parenteral nutrition problems *(continued)*

Complication	Signs and symptoms	Interventions
Other problems *(continued)*		
Thrombosis	Erythema and edema at insertion site; ipsilateral swelling of arm, neck, face, and upper chest; pain at insertion site and along vein; malaise; fever; and tachycardia	▪ Remove catheter promptly. ▪ If not contraindicated, systemic thrombolytic therapy may be used. ▪ Apply warm compresses to insertion site, and elevate affected extremity. ▪ Venous flow studies may be done.

observations of the patient's condition; and any complications and interventions.

Selected references

American Society for Parenteral and Enteral Nutrition. *Nutritional Support Nursing Core Curriculum,* 3rd ed. Columbus, Ohio: ASPEN, 1996.

"Standard 14. Documentation. Infusion Nursing Standards of Practice," *Journal of Infusion Nursing* 29(1S):S22-S23, January-February 2006.

"Standard 15. Product Evaluation, Integrity, and Defect Reporting. Infusion Nursing Standards of Practice," *Journal of Infusion Nursing* 29(1S):S22-S23, January-February 2006.

"Standard 16. Product Labeling. Infusion Nursing Standards of Practice," *Journal of Infusion Nursing* 29(1S):S23-S24, January-February 2006.

"Standard 19. Infection Control. Infusion Nursing Standards of Practice," *Journal of Infusion Nursing* 29(1S):S25-S26, January-February 2006.

"Standard 20. Hand Hygiene. Infusion Nursing Standards of Practice," *Journal of Infusion Nursing* 29(1S):S27-S28, January-February 2006.

"Standard 22. Stability and Compatibility of Parenteral Products. Infusion Nursing Standards of Practice," *Journal of Infusion Nursing* 29(1S):S28-29, January-February 2006.

"Standard 32. Filters Infusion Nursing Standards of Practice," *Journal of Infusion Nursing* 29(15):S33-S34, January-February 2006.

"Standard 48. Administration Set Change. Infusion Nursing Standards of Practice," *Journal of Infusion Nursing* 29(1S):S48-51, January-February 2006.

"Standard 68. Parenteral Nutrition. Infusion Nursing Standards of Practice," *Journal of Infusion Nursing* 29(1S):S74-75, January-February 2006.

"Standard 69. Parenteral Nutrition. Infusion Nursing Standards of Practice," *Journal of Infusion Nursing* 29(1S):S75-76, January-February 2006.

Sudakin, T. "Supporting Nutrition with T.E.N. or T.P.N.," *Nursing* 36(12Pt1):52-55, December 2006.

Weinstein, S.M. *Plumer's Principles and Practice of Intravenous Therapy,* 8th ed. Philadelphia: Lippincott Williams & Wilkins, 2007.

Lipid emulsions

Given as separate solution in conjunction with parenteral nutrition, lipid emulsions are a source of calories and essential fatty acids. A deficiency in essential fatty acids can hinder wound healing, adversely affect the production of red blood cells, and impair prostaglandin synthesis.

Lipid emulsions may also be given alone. They can be administered through either a peripheral or a central venous line, although central venous access is preferred if the infusion is ordered for more than 48 hours.

Lipid emulsions are contraindicated in patients who have a condition that disrupts normal fat metabolism, such as pathologic hyperlipidemia, lipid nephrosis, or acute pancreatitis. They must be used cautiously in patients who have liver disease, pulmonary disease, anemia, or coagulation disorders and in those who are at risk for developing a fat embolism. They can't be given to patients with severe egg allergies.

Equipment

Lipid emulsion ▪ I.V. administration set with vented spike (a separate adapter may be used if an administration set with vented spike isn't available) ▪ access pin with reflux valve ▪ tape ▪ time tape ▪ alcohol pads.

If administering the lipid emulsion as part of a 3-in-1 solution, also obtain a filter that's 1.2 microns or greater because lipids will clog a smaller filter.

Preparation of equipment

Inspect the lipid emulsion for opacity and consistency of color and texture. If the emulsion looks frothy or oily or contains particles or if you think its stability or sterility is questionable, return the bottle to the pharmacy. *To prevent aggregation of fat globules,* don't shake the lipid container excessively. Protect the emulsion from freezing, and never add anything to it. Make sure you have the correct lipid emulsion, and verify the practitioner's order and the patient's identity.

Implementation

- Explain the procedure to the patient *to promote his cooperation.*

Connecting the tubing

- First, connect the I.V. tubing to the access pin. Access pins with reflux valves take the place of needles when connecting piggyback tubing to primary tubing.
- Close the flow clamp on the I.V. tubing. Check that all connections are secure.
- Using sterile technique, remove the protective cap from the lipid emulsion bottle, and wipe the rubber stopper with an alcohol pad.
- Hold the bottle upright and, using strict sterile technique, insert the vented spike through the inner circle of the rubber stopper.
- Invert the bottle, and squeeze the drip chamber until it fills to the level indicated in the tubing package instructions.
- Open the flow clamp and prime the tubing. Gently tap the tubing *to dislodge air bubbles trapped in the Y-ports.* If necessary, attach a time tape to the lipid emulsion container *to monitor fluid intake.*
- Label the tubing, noting the date and time the tubing was hung.
- Wipe the access port on the primary tubing with an alcohol swab. Connect the tubing to the primary tubing below the inline filter.

Starting the infusion

- If this is the patient's first lipid infusion, administer a test dose at the rate of 1 ml/minute for 30 minutes.
- Monitor the patient's vital signs, and watch for signs and symptoms of an adverse reaction, such as fever; flushing, sweating, or chills; a pressure sensation over the eyes; nausea; vomiting; headache; chest and back pain; tachycardia; dyspnea; and cyanosis. An allergic reaction is usually due either to the source of lipids or to eggs, which occur in the emulsion as egg phospholipids, an emulsifying agent.
- If the patient has no adverse reactions to the test dose, begin the infusion at the prescribed rate. Use an infusion pump whenever infusing lipids.

Special considerations

- Always maintain strict sterile technique while preparing and handling equipment.
- Observe the patient's reaction to the lipid emulsion. Most patients report a feeling of satiety; some complain of an unpleasant metallic taste.
- Change the I.V. tubing and the lipid emulsion container every 24 hours.
- Monitor the patient for hair and skin changes. Also, closely monitor his lipid tolerance rate. Cloudy plasma in a centrifuged sample of citrated blood indicates that the lipids haven't been cleared from the patient's bloodstream.
- A lipid emulsion may clear from the blood at an accelerated rate in patients with full-thickness burns, multiple traumatic injuries, or a metabolic imbalance. *This is because catecholamines, adrenocortical hormones, thyroxine, and growth hormone enhance lipolysis and embolization of fatty acids.*
- Obtain weekly laboratory tests, as ordered. The usual tests include liver function studies, prothrombin time, platelet count, and serum triglyceride levels. Whenever possible, draw blood for triglyceride levels at least 6 hours after the completion of the lipid emulsion infusion *to avoid falsely elevated results.*
- *A lipid emulsion is an excellent medium for bacterial growth.* Therefore, never rehang a partially empty bottle of emulsion.

Complications

Immediate or early adverse reactions to lipid emulsion therapy, which occur in fewer than 1% of patients, include fever, dyspnea, cyanosis, nausea, vomiting, headache, flushing, diaphoresis, lethargy, syncope, chest and back pain, slight pressure over the eyes, irritation at the infusion site, hyperlipidemia, hypercoagulability, and thrombocytopenia.

PEDIATRIC ALERT *Thrombocytopenia has been reported in infants receiving a 20% I.V. lipid emulsion.*

Delayed but uncommon complications associated with prolonged administration of lipid emulsion include hepatomegaly, splenomegaly, jaundice secondary to central lobular cholestasis, and blood dyscrasias (such as thrombocytopenia, leukopenia, and transient increases in liver function studies). Dry or scaly skin, thinning hair, abnormal liver function studies, and thrombocytopenia may indicate a deficiency of essential fatty acids. For unknown reasons, some patients develop brown pigmentation in the reticuloendothelial system.

PEDIATRIC ALERT *In premature or low-birth-weight neonates, peripheral parenteral nutrition with a lipid emulsion may cause lipids to accumulate in the infants' lungs.*

Report any adverse reactions to the patient's practitioner so that he can change the parenteral nutrition regimen as needed.

Documentation

Record the times of all dressing changes and solution changes, the condition of the catheter insertion site, your observations of the patient's condition, and any complications and resulting treatments.

SELECTED REFERENCES

American Society for Parenteral and Enteral Nutrition. *Nutritional Support Nursing Core Curriculum,* 3rd ed. Columbus, Ohio: ASPEN, 1996.

"Standard 14. Documentation. Infusion Nursing Standards of Practice," *Journal of Infusion Nursing* 29(1S):S22-S23, January-February 2006.

"Standard 15. Product Evaluation, Integrity, and Defect Reporting. Infusion Nursing Standards of Practice," *Journal of Infusion Nursing* 29(1S):S22-S23, January-February 2006.

"Standard 22. Stability and Compatibility of Parenteral Products. Infusion Nursing Standards of Practice," *Journal of Infusion Nursing* 29(1S):S28-29, January-February 2006.

"Standard 48. Administration Set Change. Infusion Nursing Standards of Practice," *Journal of Infusion Nursing* 29(1S):S48-51, January-February 2006.

"Standard 68. Parenteral Nutrition. Infusion Nursing Standards of Practice," *Journal of Infusion Nursing* 29(1S):S74-75, January-February 2006.

"Standard 69. Parenteral Nutrition. Infusion Nursing Standards of Practice," *Journal of Infusion Nursing* 29(1S):S75-76, January-February 2006.

Sudakin, T. "Supporting Nutrition with T.E.N. or T.P.N.," *Nursing* 36(12Pt1):52-55, December 2006.

Weinstein, S.M. *Plumer's Principles and Practice of Intravenous Therapy,* 8th ed. Philadelphia: Lippincott Williams & Wilkins, 2007.

PATIENT MONITORING DURING PARENTERAL NUTRITION

Parenteral nutrition (PN) requires careful monitoring. Because the typical patient is in a protein-wasting state, PN therapy causes marked changes in fluid and electrolyte status and in glucose, amino acid, mineral, and vitamin levels. If the patient displays an adverse reaction or signs of complications, the regimen can be changed as needed.

Assessment of the patient's nutritional status includes a physical examination, anthropometric measurements, biochemical determinations, and tests of cell-mediated immunity. Assessment of the patient's condition to detect complications requires recognition of the signs and symptoms of possible complications, understanding of laboratory test results, and careful record keeping.

Because the PN solution is high in glucose content, the infusion must start slowly to allow the patient's pancreatic beta cells to adapt to it by increasing insulin output. Within the first 3 to 5 days of PN, the typical adult patient can tolerate 3 L of solution daily without adverse reactions. Lipid emulsions also require monitoring.

During PN administration, the nurse should be especially observant of signs of metabolic and electrolyte disturbances and should also assess the catheter site daily for signs and symptoms of infection or other catheter-related problems.

Equipment

PN solution and administration equipment ▪ blood glucose meter ▪ stethoscope ▪ sphygmomanometer ▪ watch with second hand ▪ scale ▪ input and output chart ▪ time tape ▪ additional equipment for nutritional assessment as ordered.

Preparation of equipment

For information on preparing the infusion pump and PN solution, see appropriate sections of this chapter. Attach a time tape to the PN container *to allow approximate measurement of fluid intake.* Make sure each bag or bottle has a label listing the expiration date, glucose concentration, and total volume of solution. (If the bag or bottle is damaged and you don't have an immediate replacement, hang a bag of dextrose 10% in water until the new container is ready.)

Implementation

- Explain the procedure to the patient *to diminish his anxiety and encourage cooperation.* Instruct him to inform you if he experiences any unusual sensations during the infusion.
- Record vital signs every 4 hours or more often if necessary *because increased temperature is one of the earliest signs of catheter-related sepsis.*
- Perform I.V. site care and dressing changes at least three times a week (once per week for transparent semipermeable dressings) or whenever the dressing becomes wet, soiled, or nonocclusive. Use strict sterile technique.
- Physically assess the patient daily. If ordered, measure arm circumference and skin-fold thickness over the triceps.
- Weigh the patient at the same time each morning (after voiding), in similar clothing, and on the same scale. Compare this data with his fluid intake and output record. *Weight gain, especially early in treatment, may indicate fluid overload rather than increasing fat and protein stores.* A patient should not gain more than 3 lb (1.4 kg) per week; a gain of 1 lb (0.5 kg) a week is a reasonable goal for most patients. Suspect fluid imbalance if the patient gains more than 1 lb daily. Assess for peripheral and pulmonary edema.
- Monitor the patient for signs and symptoms of glucose metabolism disturbance, fluid and electrolyte imbalances,

and nutritional aberrations. Remember that some patients may require supplemental insulin for the duration of PN; the pharmacy usually adds insulin directly to the PN solution, but additional subcutaneous insulin by sliding scale may be required.

- Monitor levels of electrolytes and protein frequently—daily at first for electrolytes and twice weekly for serum albumin. Later, as the patient's condition stabilizes, you won't need to monitor these values quite as closely. (Be aware that in a severely dehydrated patient, albumin levels may drop initially as treatment restores hydration.)
- Pay close attention to magnesium and calcium levels. If these electrolytes have been added to the PN solution, the dose may need adjusting to maintain normal serum levels. Assess the patient for signs and symptoms of magnesium and calcium imbalances.
- Monitor serum glucose levels every 6 hours initially and then once a day, and stay alert for signs and symptoms of hyperglycemia, such as thirst and polyuria. Periodically confirm blood glucose meter readings with laboratory tests.
- Check kidney function by monitoring blood urea nitrogen and creatinine levels; *increases can indicate excess amino acid intake.* Also assess nitrogen balance with 24-hour urine collection.
- Assess liver function by periodically monitoring liver enzyme, bilirubin, triglyceride, and cholesterol levels. *Abnormal values may indicate an intolerance or excess of lipid emulsions or a problem with metabolizing the protein or glucose in the PN formula.*
- Change the I.V. administration set every 24 hours. Use aseptic technique, and coordinate the change with a solution change. Keep in mind that the tubing, injection caps, stopcocks, catheter, and even the patient's skin are potential sources of microbial contamination. The catheter hub, where most manipulations take place, is especially vulnerable. (The PN formula itself, which is prepared aseptically in the pharmacy, is seldom the source of infection.)
- Monitor for signs of inflammation, infection, and sepsis, the most common complications of PN. Microbial contamination of the venous access device is the usual cause. Watch for redness and drainage at the venous access site, and monitor the patient for fever and other signs and symptoms of sepsis.
- While weaning the patient from PN, document his dietary intake and work with the nutritionist to determine the total calorie and protein intake. Also teach other health care staff caring for the patient the importance of recording food intake. Use percentages of food consumed ("ate 50% of a baked potato") instead of subjective descriptions ("had a good appetite") *to provide a more accurate account of patient intake.*
- Provide emotional support. Keep in mind that patients often associate eating with positive feelings and become disturbed when eating is prohibited.
- Provide frequent mouth care.
- Keep the patient active *to enable him to use nutrients more fully.*
- When discontinuing PN, decrease the infusion rate slowly, depending on the patient's current glucose intake, *to minimize the risk of hyperinsulinemia and resulting hypoglycemia.* Weaning usually takes place over 24 to 48 hours but can be completed in 4 to 6 hours if the patient receives sufficient oral or I.V. carbohydrates.

Special considerations

- Always maintain strict sterile technique when handling the equipment used to administer therapy. *Because the PN solution serves as a medium for bacterial and fungal growth and the central venous (CV) line provides systemic access,* the patient risks infection and sepsis.
- When using a filter, position it as close to the access site as possible. Check the filter's porosity and pounds per square inch (psi) capacity *to make sure it exceeds the number of psi exerted by the infusion pump.*
- Don't let PN solutions hang for more than 24 hours.
- Be careful when using the PN line for other functions. If using a single-lumen CV catheter, don't use the line to infuse blood or blood products, to give a bolus injection, to administer simultaneous I.V. solutions, to measure CV pressure, or to draw blood for laboratory tests. Never add medication to a PN solution container. Also, don't use a three-way stopcock, if possible, *because add-on devices increase the risk of infection.*
- When a patient is severely malnourished, starting PN may spark "refeeding syndrome," which includes a rapid drop in potassium, magnesium, and phosphorus levels. *To avoid compromising cardiac function,* initiate feeding slowly and monitor the patient's blood values especially closely until they stabilize.

Complications

Catheter-related, metabolic, and mechanical complications can occur during PN administration.

Documentation

Record serial monitoring indexes on the appropriate flowchart to determine the patient's progress and response. Note any abnormal, adverse, or altered responses.

SELECTED REFERENCES

"Standard 23. Expiration and Beyond-Use Dates. Infusion Nursing Standards of Practice," *Journal of Infusion Nursing* 29(1S):S29, January-February 2006.

"Standard 29. Add-On Devices and Junction Securement. Infusion Nursing Standards of Practice," *Journal of Infusion Nursing* 29(1S):S32, January-February 2006.
"Standard 48. Administration Set Change. Infusion Nursing Standards of Practice," *Journal of Infusion Nursing* 29(1S):S48-51, January-February 2006.
"Standard 69. Parenteral Nutrition. Infusion Nursing Standards of Practice," *Journal of Infusion Nursing* 29(1S):S75-76, January-February 2006.
Sudakin, T. "Supporting Nutrition with T.E.N. or T.P.N.," *Nursing* 36(12Pt1):52-55, December 2006.
Weinstein, S.M. *Plumer's Principles and Practice of Intravenous Therapy*, 8th ed. Philadelphia: Lippincott Williams & Wilkins, 2007.

Preparation for home parenteral nutrition

Home parenteral nutrition (HPN) makes possible prolonged or indefinite I.V. total parenteral nutrition (TPN). This technique has dramatically improved the health of patients with such chronic conditions as Crohn's disease and malabsorption syndrome, those with such acute conditions as incomplete bowel obstruction, and those receiving chemotherapy. It has also decreased the duration of hospitalization. Although peripheral parenteral nutrition may be administered at home, long-term TPN is the primary home care therapy. Preparation for HPN usually necessitates extensive patient teaching and, when possible, instructions for the patient's family. Follow up by home health nurses to continue education and the care plan is preferred, and appropriate referrals should be made as soon as possible.

Some patients receiving HPN can ingest part of their caloric requirements during the day and require 8 to 10 hours of infusion nightly to supply the remaining nutrients. If all the patient's nutrition must be received I.V., a continuous infusion may be necessary. For intermittent and continuous infusion, patient teaching must include techniques for proper care.

Equipment

Teaching aids (including audiovisual teaching aids and mannequins), as available ▪ I.V. infusion apparatus ▪ dressings ▪ TPN solution ▪ volumetric infusion pump ▪ portable I.V. pole.

Implementation

- Assess the patient's ability to perform the care routines necessary for HPN, and determine whether family members or friends can assist with or perform them. Consider the patient's motivation, mental aptitude, job or other daily activities, and home environment as well as the accessibility of hospitals, home nursing services, and other health care support systems.
- Formulate a patient-teaching plan based on your assessment and the patient's expectations. Make sure the plan incorporates goals, specifies criteria for meeting them, and proceeds from simple to complex tasks *to allow the patient to develop confidence.* Avoid placing time limits on goals *because learning ability and mastery of tasks requiring manual dexterity vary from patient to patient.*
- If desired, develop a written contract between you and the patient that specifies the goals of HPN and the means to achieve them. Revise the contract, as necessary, to reflect changes in the patient's needs and performance. *A contractual relationship enhances the patient's independence, minimizes conflict and frustration between patient and nurse, encourages open communication, and promotes a cooperative patient-nurse relationship.*
- Conduct patient-teaching sessions in a quiet area and, if possible, arrange to have a family member present. *Family members who understand the patient's pathophysiology, medical management, and progress tend to be less anxious, more satisfied with the quality of health care, and better able to acknowledge the limitations and constraints of HPN.*
- Use various teaching aids *to accommodate differences in patients' abilities.* When teaching the mature patient, use an extensively illustrated manual (if available) that includes goals, equipment, procedures with rationales, suggested learning activities, and evaluations of HPN equipment. Give demonstrations with mannequins (if available) and real equipment *to involve the patient actively and reduce anxiety about performing HPN tasks.* Stimulate his interest with audiovisual teaching aids.
- Offer positive feedback during all teaching phases.
- Before discharge, critically evaluate the patient's ability to perform HPN tasks and ensure that all essential learning goals have been met.
- Remind the patient to change the catheter site dressing as ordered or whenever it becomes soiled and to change administration tubing as scheduled. Tell him to wash gently around the site and to take only sponge baths. Tell him he may be allowed to remove his dressing to bathe or shower after the implanted catheter has been in place for 10 days.
- Also remind the patient to prevent contact between the catheter and granular or lint-producing surfaces *to avoid local tissue reaction from airborne particles and surface contaminants.*
- Discuss a suitable TPN schedule with the patient, considering his nutritional needs as well as his lifestyle. Emphasize his adherence to the prescribed schedule and volume *to prevent glucose imbalance.*

■ Arrange for a home care agency to help the patient adjust to HPN and resolve any difficulties (including how to obtain supplies), or notify the facility's discharge planner *so that the appropriate referrals can be made.*

Special considerations

■ Suggest that the patient wear a medical identification bracelet or subscribe to a medical alert service. Tell the patient that a nurse from the home health care team will always be available in case of emergency.

■ Refer the patient to social services; *the financial burden of long-term or permanent HPN can be devastating, even for a patient with health insurance.*

ELDER ALERT *Inform the elderly patient that Medicare may assume the cost of supplies and pharmaceuticals if he meets eligibility requirements.*

Documentation

Record your patient-teaching measures and the patient's learning progress in your notes. Document discharge plans and any referrals made.

SELECTED REFERENCES

De Burgoa, L.J., et al. "Examination of Factors that Lead to Complications for New Home Parenteral Nutrition Patients," *Journal of Infusion Nursing* 29(2):74-80, March-April 2006.

"Standard 11. Patient Education. Infusion Nursing Standards of Practice," *Journal of Infusion Nursing* 29(1S):S19-20, January-February 2006.

"Standard 22. Stability and Compatibility of Parenteral Products. Infusion Nursing Standards of Practice," *Journal of Infusion Nursing* 29(1S):S28-S29, January-February 2006.

"Standard 23. Expiration and Beyond-Use Dates. Infusion Nursing Standards of Practice," *Journal of Infusion Nursing* 29(1S):S29, January-February 2006.

"Standard 29. Add-On Devices and Junction Securement. Infusion Nursing Standards of Practice," *Journal of Infusion Nursing* 29(1S):S32, January-February 2006.

"Standard 48. Administration Set Change. Infusion Nursing Standards of Practice," *Journal of Infusion Nursing* 29(1S):S48-51, January-February 2006.

"Standard 68. Parenteral Medication and Solution Administration. Infusion Nursing Standards of Practice," *Journal of Infusion Nursing* 29(15):S74-745, January-February 2006.

"Standard 69. Parenteral Nutrition. Infusion Nursing Standards of Practice," *Journal of Infusion Nursing* 29(1S):S75-76, January-February 2006.

Sudakin, T. "Supporting Nutrition with T.E.N. or T.P.N.," *Nursing* 36(12Pt1):52-55, December 2006.

Weinstein, S.M. *Plumer's Principles and Practice of Intravenous Therapy*, 8th ed. Philadelphia: Lippincott Williams & Wilkins, 2007.

BLOOD AND BLOOD COMPONENTS

TRANSFUSION OF WHOLE BLOOD AND PACKED CELLS

Whole blood transfusion replenishes the volume and the oxygen-carrying capacity of the circulatory system by increasing the mass of circulating red cells. Transfusion of packed red blood cells (RBCs), from which 80% of the plasma has been removed, restores only the oxygen-carrying capacity. After plasma is removed, the resulting component has a hematocrit of 65% to 80% and a usual volume of 250 to 300 ml.

Each unit of whole blood or RBCs contains enough hemoglobin to raise the hemoglobin concentration in an average-sized adult 1 g/dl. Both types of transfusion treat decreased hemoglobin level and hematocrit. Whole blood is usually used only when decreased levels result from hemorrhage; packed RBCs are used when such depressed levels accompany normal blood volume to avoid possible fluid and circulatory overload. (See *Transfusing blood and selected components,* pages 404 to 406.) Whole blood and packed RBCs contain cellular debris, requiring in-line filtration during administration.

Before starting the transfusion, positive patient identification, the therapy's appropriateness, blood compatibility, practitioner's order, and signed consent form should be verified by the nurse. In addition to confirming patient identity with the appropriate blood or blood component identification numbers, the patient's identity must also also be verified using two patient identifiers, aside from the patient's room number, according to your facility's policy.

Blood and blood components should be filtered and transfused through an appropriate blood administration set. Straight-line and Y-type blood administration sets are commonly used. Although filters come in mesh and microaggregate types, the latter type is preferred, especially when transfusing multiple units of blood. Highly effective leukocyte removal filters are available for use when transfusing blood and packed RBCs. The use of these filters can postpone sensitization to transfusion therapy.

Administer packed RBCs with a Y-type set. Using a straight-line set forces you to piggyback the tubing so you can stop the transfusion if necessary but still keep the vein open. Piggybacking increases the chance of harmful microorganisms entering the tubing as you're connecting the blood line to the established line.

(Text continues on page 406.)

Transfusing blood and selected components

Blood component	Indications	Compatibility	Nursing considerations
Whole blood			
Complete (pure) blood	■ To restore blood volume lost from hemorrhaging, trauma, or burns ■ Exchange transfusion in sickle cell disease	■ ABO identical: Group A receives A; group B receives B; group AB receives AB; group O receives O ■ Rh type must match	■ Remember that whole blood is seldom administered. ■ Use blood administration tubing to infuse within 4 hours. ■ Closely monitor patient volume status for volume overload. ■ Warm blood if giving a large quantity. ■ Use only with normal saline solution.
Packed red blood cells (RBCs)			
Same RBC mass as whole blood but with 80% of the plasma removed	■ To restore or maintain oxygen-carrying capacity ■ To correct anemia and surgical blood loss ■ To increase RBC mass ■ Red cell exchange	■ Group A receives A or O ■ Group B receives B or O ■ Group AB receives AB, A, B, or O ■ Group O receives O ■ Rh type must match ■ Same as packed RBCs ■ Rh type must match	■ Use blood administration tubing to infuse over more than 4 hours. ■ Use only with normal saline solution. ■ Avoid administering packed RBCs for anemic conditions correctable by nutritional or drug therapy.
Leukocyte-poor RBCs			
Same as packed RBCs with about 70% of the leukocytes removed	■ Same as packed RBCs ■ To prevent febrile reactions from leukocyte antibodies ■ To treat immunocompromised patients ■ To restore RBCs to patients who have had two or more nonhemolytic febrile reactions	■ Same as packed RBCs ■ Rh type must match	■ Use blood administration tubing. ■ May require a 40-micron filter suitable for hard-spun, leukocyte-poor RBCs. ■ Other considerations are same as those for packed RBCs. Cells expire 24 hours after washing.

Transfusing blood and selected components *(continued)*

BLOOD COMPONENT	INDICATIONS	COMPATIBILITY	NURSING CONSIDERATIONS
White blood cells (leukocytes)			
Whole blood with all the RBCs and about 80% of the plasma removed	■ To treat sepsis that's unresponsive to antibiotics (especially if patient has positive blood cultures or a persistent fever exceeding 101° F [38.3° C]) and life-threatening granulocytopenia (granulocyte count less than 500/µl)	■ Same as packed RBCs ■ Compatibility with human leukocyte antigen (HLA) preferable but not necessary unless patient is sensitized to HLA from previous transfusion ■ Rh type must match	■ Use a blood administration set. Give 1 unit daily for 4 to 6 days or until infection resolves. ■ As prescribed, premedicate with antihistamines, acetominophen (Tylenol), or steroids. ■ If fever occurs, administer an antipyretic, don't discontinue transfusion; instead, reduce flow rate, as ordered, for patient comfort. ■ Because reactions are common, administer slowly over 2 to 4 hours. Check patient's vital signs and assess him every 15 minutes throughout transfusion. ■ Give transfusion with antibiotics to treat infection.
Platelets			
Platelet sediment from RBCs or plasma platelets	■ To treat bleeding caused by decreased circulating platelets or functionally abnormal platelets ■ To improve platelet count preoperatively in a patient whose count is 50,000/µl or less	■ ABO compatibility identical; Rh-negative recipients should receive Rh-negative platelets	■ Use a blood filter or leukocyte-reduction filter. ■ As prescribed, premedicate with antipyretics and antihistamines if patient's history includes a platelet transfusion reaction or to reduce chills, fever, and allergic reactions. ■ Use single donor platelets if patient has a need for repeated transfusions. ■ Platelets aren't used to treat autoimmune thrombocytopenia or thrombocytopenic purpura unless patient has a life-threatening hemorrhage.
Fresh frozen plasma (FFP)			
Uncoagulated plasma separated from RBCs and rich in coagulation factors V, VIII, and IX	■ To treat postoperative hemorrhage ■ To correct an undetermined coagulation factor deficiency ■ To replace a specific factor when that factor isn't available ■ Warfarin reversal	■ ABO compatibility required ■ Rh match not required	■ Use a blood administration set, and administer infusion rapidly. ■ Keep in mind that large-volume transfusions of FFP may require correction for hypocalcemia because citric acid in FFP binds calcium. ■ Must be infused within 24 hours of being thawed.

(continued)

Transfusing blood and selected components *(continued)*

Blood component	Indications	Compatibility	Nursing considerations
Albumin 5% (buffered saline); albumin 25% (salt-poor)			
A small plasma protein prepared by fractionating pooled plasma	■ To replace volume lost because of shock from burns, trauma, surgery, or infections ■ To treat hypoproteinemia (with or without edema)	■ Not required	■ Use administration set supplied by manufacturer and set rate based on patient's condition and response. ■ Keep in mind that albumin is contraindicated in severe anemia. ■ Administer cautiously in cardiac and pulmonary disease because heart failure may result from circulatory overload.
Factor VIII concentrate (antihemophilic factor)			
Cold insoluble portion of plasma recovered from FFP	■ To treat a patient with hemophilia A ■ To treat a patient with von Willebrand's disease	■ ABO compatibility not required	■ Administer by I.V. injection using a filter needle, or use administration set supplied by manufacturer.
Cryoprecipitate			
Insoluble plasma portion of FFP containing fibrinogen, factor VIIIc, factor VIIvWF, factor XIII and fibronectin	■ To treat factor VIII deficiency and fibrinogen disorders ■ To treat significant factor XIII deficiency	■ ABO compatibility required ■ Rh match not required	■ Administer with a blood administration set. ■ Add normal saline solution to each bag of cryoprecipitate, as necessary, to facilitate infusion. ■ Keep in mind that cryoprecipitate must be administered within 6 hours of thawing. ■ Before administration, check laboratory studies to confirm a deficiency of one of specific clotting factors present in cryoprecipitate. ■ Be aware that patients with hemophilia A or von Willebrand's disease should only be treated with cryoprecipitate when appropriate factor VIII concentrates aren't available.

Single units of whole blood or blood components should be transfused within a 4-hour period. The start of the transfusion should begin within 30 minutes from the time the blood is released from the blood bank. No medications should be added to the blood other than normal saline solution. Patients should also be monitored 15 minutes after the start of therapy and at 15- to 30-minute intervals throughout the transfusion.

Multiple-lead tubing minimizes the risk of contamination, especially when transfusing multiple units of blood (a straight-line set would require multiple piggybacking). A Y-type set gives you the option of adding normal saline solution to packed cells—decreasing their viscosity— if the patient can tolerate the added fluid volume.

Hemoglobin replacement products (or blood substitutes) may be an alternative to blood transfusions. The replacement product is derived from human RBCs. It carries the benefits of decreased viral and bacterial transmission, reduced risk of allergic or immune reactions, universal compatibility with all blood types, efficient oxygen delivery to vital organs and tissues, and an extended shelf life of at least 1 year (compared with 42 days for donor blood). Successful transfusions have been performed in clinical trials with cardiac bypass patients. However, these products don't provide blood cells with clotting factors or the ability to fight infection.

Equipment

Blood administration set (170 to 260-micron filter and tubing with drip chamber for blood, or combined set) ■ I.V. pole ■ gloves ■ gown ■ face shield ■ multiple-lead tubing ■ whole blood or packed RBCs ■ 250 ml of normal saline solution ■ venipuncture equipment, if necessary (should include 20G or larger catheter) ■ optional: ice bag, warm compresses.

Straight-line and Y-type blood administration sets are commonly used. Although filters come in mesh and microaggregate types, the latter type is preferred, especially when transfusing multiple units of blood. Highly effective leukocyte removal filters are available for use when transfusing blood and packed RBCs. *The use of these filters can postpone sensitization to transfusion therapy.*

Administer packed RBCs with a Y-type set. Using a straight-line set forces you to piggyback the tubing so you can stop the transfusion if necessary but still keep the vein open. Piggybacking increases the chance of harmful microorganisms entering the tubing as you're connecting the blood line to the established line.

Multiple-lead tubing minimizes the risk of contamination, especially when transfusing multiple units of blood (a straight-line set would require multiple piggybacking). A Y-type set gives you the option of adding normal saline solution to packed cells—decreasing their viscosity—if the patient can tolerate the added fluid volume.

Preparation of equipment

Avoid obtaining either whole blood or packed RBCs until you're ready to begin the transfusion. Prepare the equipment when you're ready to start the infusion.

Implementation

- Confirm the patient's identity using two patient identifiers according to your facility's policy.
- Explain the procedure to the patient. Explain possible signs and symptoms of a transfusion reaction (chills, rash, fever, flank or back pain, dizziness, or blood in urine) and to report these possible signs and symptoms to the nurse. Make sure he has signed an informed consent form before transfusion therapy is initiated.
- Record the patient's baseline vital signs.
- Obtain whole blood or packed RBCs from the blood bank within 30 minutes of the transfusion start time. Check the expiration date on the blood bag, and observe for abnormal color, RBC clumping, gas bubbles, and extraneous material. Return outdated or abnormal blood to the blood bank.
- Compare the patient's confirmed identity with those on the blood bag label. Check the blood bag identification number, ABO blood group, and Rh compatibility. Also, compare the patient's blood bank identification number, if present, with the number on the blood bag. Identification of blood and blood products is performed at the patient's bedside by two licensed professionals, according to the facility's policy.
- Put on gloves, a gown, and a face shield.
- Using a blood administration set, close all the clamps on the set. Then insert the spike of the line you're using for the normal saline solution into the bag of saline solution. Next, open the port on the blood bag, and insert the spike of the line you're using to administer the blood or cellular component into the port. Hang the bag of normal saline solution and blood or cellular component on the I.V. pole, open the clamp on the line of saline solution, and squeeze the drip chamber until it's half full. Then remove the adapter cover at the tip of the blood administration set, open the main flow clamp, and prime the tubing with saline solution.
- If you're administering packed RBCs with a blood administration set, you can add saline solution to the bag *to dilute the cells* by closing the clamp between the patient and the drip chamber and opening the clamp from the blood. Then lower the blood bag below the saline container and let 30 to 50 ml of saline solution flow into the packed cells. Finally, close the clamp to the blood bag, rehang the bag, rotate it gently *to mix the cells and saline solution,* and close the clamp to the saline container.
- If the patient doesn't have an I.V. line in place, perform a venipuncture, using a 20G or larger-diameter catheter. Avoid using an existing line if the needle or catheter lumen is smaller than 20G. Central venous access devices may also be used for transfusion therapy.
- If you're administering whole blood, gently invert the bag several times *to mix the cells.*
- Attach the prepared blood administration set to the venipuncture device, and flush it with normal saline solution. Then close the clamp to the saline solution, and open

the clamp between the blood bag and the patient. Adjust the flow rate to no greater than 5 ml/minute for the first 15 minutes of the transfusion *to observe for a possible transfusion reaction.*

- Remain with the patient, and watch for signs of a transfusion reaction. If such signs develop, record vital signs and stop the transfusion. Infuse saline solution at a moderately slow infusion rate, and notify the practitioner at once. If no signs of a reaction appear within 15 minutes, you'll need to adjust the flow rate to no graeter than 5 ml/minute for the first 15 minutes of the transfusion *to observe for a possible transfusion reaction.*
- It's undesirable for RBC preparations to remain at room temperature for more than 4 hours. If the infusion rate must be so slow that the entire unit can't be infused within 4 hours, it may be appropriate to have the blood bank divide the unit and keep one portion refrigerated until it can be administered.
- After completing the transfusion, you'll need to put on gloves and remove and discard the used infusion equipment. Then remember to reconnect the original I.V. fluid, if necessary, or discontinue the I.V. infusion.
- Return the empty blood bag to the blood bank, if facility policy dictates, and discard the tubing and filter.
- Record the patient's vital signs.

Special considerations

- Although some microaggregate filters can be used for up to 10 units of blood, always replace the filter and tubing if more than 1 hour elapses between transfusions. When administering multiple units of blood under pressure, use a blood warmer *to avoid hypothermia.* Blood components may be warmed to no more than 107.6° F (42° C).
- For rapid blood replacement, you may need to use a pressure bag. Be aware that excessive pressure may develop, leading to broken blood vessels and extravasation, with hematoma and hemolysis of the infusing RBCs.
- If the transfusion stops, take these steps as needed:

–Check that the I.V. container is at least 3′ (1 m) above the level of the I.V. site.

–Make sure the flow clamp is open and that the blood completely covers the filter. If it doesn't, squeeze the drip chamber until it does.

–Gently rock the bag back and forth, agitating blood cells that may have settled.

–Untape the dressing over the I.V. site to check cannula placement. Reposition the cannula if necessary.

–Flush the line with saline solution, and restart the transfusion. Using a Y-type set, close the flow clamp to the patient, and lower the blood bag. Next, open the saline clamp, and allow some saline solution to flow into the blood bag. Rehang the blood bag, open the flow clamp to the patient, and reset the flow rate.

–If a hematoma develops at the I.V. site, immediately stop the infusion. Remove the I.V. cannula. Notify the practitioner, and expect to place ice on the site intermittently for 8 hours; then apply warm compresses. Follow your facility's policy.

–If the blood bag empties before the next one arrives, administer normal saline solution slowly. If you're using a Y-type set, close the blood-line clamp, open the saline clamp, and let the saline run slowly until the new blood arrives. Decrease the flow rate or clamp the line before attaching the new unit of blood.

Complications

Despite improvements in crossmatching precautions, transfusion reactions can still occur. Unlike a transfusion reaction, an infectious disease transmitted during a transfusion may go undetected until days, weeks, or even months later, when it produces signs and symptoms. Measures to prevent disease transmission include laboratory testing of blood products and careful screening of potential donors, neither of which is guaranteed.

Hepatitis C accounts for most posttransfusion hepatitis cases. The tests that detect hepatitis B and hepatitis C can produce false-negative results and may allow some hepatitis cases to go undetected.

When testing for antibodies to human immunodeficiency virus (HIV), keep in mind that antibodies don't appear until 6 to 12 weeks after exposure. The American Association of Blood Banks estimates the risk of acquiring HIV from a single blood transfusion is between 1 in 40,000 to 1 in 153,000.

Many blood banks screen blood for cytomegalovirus (CMV). Blood with CMV is especially dangerous for an immunosuppressed, seronegative patient. Blood banks also test blood for syphilis, but refrigerating blood virtually eliminates the risk of transfusion-related syphilis.

Circulatory overload and hemolytic, allergic, febrile, and pyogenic reactions can result from any transfusion. Coagulation disturbances, citrate intoxication, hyperkalemia, acid-base imbalance, loss of 2,3-diphosphoglycerate, ammonia intoxication, and hypothermia can result from massive transfusion.

Documentation

Record the date and time of the transfusion, the type and amount of transfusion product, the patient's vital signs, your check of all identification data, and the patient's response. Document any transfusion reaction and treatment. (See *Documenting blood transfusions.*)

Documenting blood transfusions

Whether you administer blood or blood components, you must use proper identification and crossmatching procedures.

After matching the patient's name, medical record number, blood group (or type) and Rh factor (the patient's and the donor's), the cross match data, and the blood bank identification number with the label on the blood bag, you'll need to clearly record that you did so. The blood or blood component must be identified and documented properly by two health care professionals as well.

On the transfusion record, document:

- date and time the transfusion was started and completed
- name of the health care professional who verified the information
- catheter type and gauge
- total amount of the transfusion
- patient's vital signs before and after the transfusion
- any infusion device used
- flow rate and if blood warming unit was used.

If the patient receives his own blood, document in the intake and output records:

- amount of autologous blood retrieved
- amount of autologous blood infused
- laboratory data during and after the autotransfusion
- patient's pretransfusion and posttransfusion vital signs.

Pay particular attention to:

- patient's coagulation profile
- hemoglobin level, hematocrit, and arterial blood gas and calcium levels.

SELECTED REFERENCES

American Association of Blood Banks. *Technical Manual,* 13th ed. Bethesda, Md.: AABB, 1999.

Hainsworth, T. "Guidance for Preventing Errors in Administering Blood Transfusions," *Nursing Times* 100(27):30-31, July 2004.

Rana, R. "Evidence-Based Red Cell Transfusion in the Critically Ill: Quality Improvement Using Computerized Physician Order Entry," *Critical Care Medicine* 34(7):1892-897, July 2006.

"Standard 32. Filters. Infusion Nursing Standards of Practice," *Journal of Infusion Nursing* 29(1S):S33-34, January-February 2006.

"Standard 34. Blood and Fluid Warmers. Infusion Nursing Standards of Practice," *Journal of Infusion Nursing* 29(1S):S35, January-February 2006.

"Standard 48. Administration Set Change. Infusion Nursing Standards of Practice," *Journal of Infusion Nursing* 29(1S):S48-51, January-February 2006.

"Standard 70. Transfusion Therapy. Infusion Nursing Standards of Practice," *Journal of Infusion Nursing* 29(1S):S76-77, January-February 2006.

TRANSFUSION REACTION MANAGEMENT

A transfusion reaction typically stems from a major antigen-antibody reaction and can result from a single or massive transfusion of blood or blood products. Although many reactions occur during transfusion or within 96 hours afterward, infectious diseases transmitted during a transfusion may go undetected until days, weeks, or months later, when signs and symptoms appear.

A transfusion reaction requires immediate recognition and prompt nursing action to prevent further complications and, possibly, death — particularly if the patient is unconscious or so heavily sedated that he can't report the common symptoms. (See *Guide to transfusion reactions,* pages 410 to 412.)

Equipment

Normal saline solution ■ I.V. administration set ■ sterile urine specimen container ■ needle, syringe, and tubes for blood samples ■ transfusion reaction report form ■ optional: oxygen, epinephrine, hypothermia blanket, leukocyte removal filter.

Implementation

- As soon as you suspect an adverse reaction, stop the transfusion, and start the saline infusion at a keep-vein-open rate *to maintain venous access.* Don't discard the blood bag or administration set.
- Notify the practitioner.
- Monitor vital signs every 15 minutes or as indicated by the severity and type of reaction.
- Compare the labels on all blood containers with corresponding patient identification forms *to verify that the transfusion was the correct blood or blood product.*

(Text continues on page 413.)

Guide to transfusion reactions

Any patient receiving a transfusion of processed blood products risks certain complications; for example, hemosiderosis and hypothermia. The chart below describes *endogenous reactions*—those caused by an antigen-antibody reaction in the recipient, and *exogenous reactions*—those caused by external factors in administered blood.

REACTION AND CAUSES	SIGNS AND SYMPTOMS	NURSING INTERVENTIONS
ENDOGENOUS		
Allergic		
■ Allergen in donor blood ■ Donor blood hypersensitive to certain drugs	■ Anaphylaxis (chills, facial swelling, laryngeal edema, pruritus, urticaria, wheezing), fever, nausea, and vomiting	■ Administer antihistamines as prescribed. ■ Monitor patient for anaphylactic reaction, and administer epinephrine and corticosteroids if indicated. ■ As prescribed, premedicate patient with diphenhydramine before subsequent transfusion. ■ Observe patient closely for first 30 minutes of transfusion.
Bacterial contamination		
■ Organisms that can survive cold, such as *Pseudomonas* and *Staphylococcus*	■ Chills, fever, vomiting, abdominal cramping, diarrhea, shock, signs of renal failure	■ Provide broad-spectrum antibiotics, corticosteroids, or epinephrine as prescribed. ■ Maintain strict blood storage control. ■ Change blood administration set and filter every 4 hours or after every 2 units. ■ Infuse each unit of blood over 2 to 4 hours; stop the infusion if the time span exceeds 4 hours. ■ Maintain sterile technique during administration. ■ Inspect blood before transfusion for air, clots, and dark purple color.
Febrile		
■ Bacterial lipopolysaccharides ■ Antileukocyte recipient antibodies directed against donor white blood cells	■ Temperature up to 104° F (40° C), chills, headache, facial flushing, palpitations, cough, chest tightness, increased pulse rate, flank pain	■ Relieve symptoms with an antipyretic, an antihistamine, or meperidine, as prescribed. ■ If the patient requires further transfusions, use frozen RBCs, add a special leukocyte removal filter to the blood line, or premedicate him with acetaminophen, as prescribed, before starting another transfusion. ■ Premedicate patient with an antipyretic, an antihistamine and, possibly, a steroid.
Hemolytic		
■ ABO or Rh incompatibility ■ Intradonor incompatibility ■ Improper crossmatching ■ Improperly stored blood	■ Chest pain, dyspnea, facial flushing, fever, chills, shaking, hypotension, flank pain, hemoglobinuria, oliguria, bloody oozing at the infusion site or surgical incision site, burning sensation along vein receiving blood, shock, renal failure	■ Monitor blood pressure. ■ Manage shock with I.V. fluids, oxygen, epinephrine, a diuretic, and a vasopressor, as prescribed. ■ Obtain posttransfusion-reaction blood samples and urine specimens for analysis. ■ Observe for signs of hemorrhage resulting from disseminated intravascular coagulation. ■ Before the transfusion, check donor and recipient blood types to ensure blood compatibility.

Guide to transfusion reactions *(continued)*

Reaction and causes	Signs and symptoms	Nursing interventions
Endogenous *(continued)*		
Plasma protein incompatibility		
■ Immunoglobulin-A incompatibility	■ Abdominal pain, diarrhea, dyspnea, chills, fever, flushing, hypotension	■ Administer oxygen, fluids, epinephrine, or a corticosteroid, as prescribed.
Exogenous		
Bleeding tendencies		
■ Low platelet count in stored blood, causing thrombocytopenia	■ Abnormal bleeding and oozing from a cut, a break in the skin surface, or the gums; abnormal bruising and petechiae	■ Administer platelets, fresh frozen plasma, or cryoprecipitate, as prescribed. ■ Monitor platelet count. ■ Use only fresh blood (less than 7 days old) when possible.
Circulatory overload		
■ May result from infusing blood too rapidly or in large volumes	■ Increased plasma volume, back pain, chest tightness, chills, fever, dyspnea, flushed feeling, headache, hypertension, increased central venous pressure and jugular vein pressure	■ Monitor blood pressure. ■ Use packed red blood cells (RBCs) instead of whole blood. ■ Administer diuretics as prescribed. ■ Transfuse blood slowly.
Elevated blood ammonia level		
■ Increased ammonia level in stored donor blood	■ Confusion, forgetfulness, lethargy	■ Monitor ammonia level in blood. ■ Decrease the amount of protein in the patient's diet. ■ If indicated, give neomycin.
Hemosiderosis		
■ Increased level of hemosiderin (iron-containing pigment) from RBC destruction, especially after many transfusions	■ Iron plasma level exceeding 200 mg/dl	■ Perform a phlebotomy to remove excess iron. ■ Administer blood only when absolutely necessary.

(continued)

Guide to transfusion reactions *(continued)*

Reaction and causes	Signs and symptoms	Nursing interventions
Exogenous *(continued)*		
Hypocalcemia		
■ Citrate toxicity occurs when citrate-treated blood is infused rapidly. Citrate binds with calcium, causing a calcium deficiency, or normal citrate metabolism becomes impeded by hepatic disease.	■ Arrhythmias, hypotension, muscle cramps, nausea, vomiting, seizures, tingling in fingers	■ Slow or stop the transfusion, depending on the patient's reaction. Expect a more severe reaction in hypothermic patients or patients with elevated potassium levels. ■ Slowly administer calcium gluconate I.V., if prescribed.
Hypothermia		
■ Rapid infusion of large amounts of cold blood, which decreases body temperature	■ Chills; shaking; hypotension; arrhythmias, especially bradycardia; cardiac arrest, if core temperature falls below 86° F (30° C)	■ Stop the transfusion. ■ Warm the patient with blankets. ■ Obtain an electrocardiogram (ECG). ■ Warm blood to 95° to 98° F(35° to 36.7 ° C)— especially before massive transfusions.
Increased oxygen affinity for hemoglobin		
■ Decreased level of 2,3-diphosphoglycerate in stored blood, causing an increase in the oxygen's hemoglobin affinity. When this occurs, oxygen stays in the bloodstream and isn't released into body tissues.	■ Depressed respiratory rate, especially in patients with chronic lung disease	■ Monitor arterial blood gas values, and provide respiratory support as needed.
Potassium intoxication		
■ An abnormally high level of potassium in stored plasma caused by hemolysis of RBCs	■ Diarrhea, intestinal colic, flaccidity, muscle twitching, oliguria, renal failure, bradycardia progressing to cardiac arrest, ECG changes with tall, peaked T waves	■ Obtain an ECG. ■ Administer sodium polystyrene sulfonate (Kayexalate) orally or by enema. ■ Administer dextrose 50% and insulin, bicarbonate, or calcium, as prescribed, to force potassium into cells. ■ Use fresh blood when administering massive transfusions.

■ Notify the blood bank of a possible transfusion reaction and collect blood samples, as ordered. Immediately send the samples, all transfusion containers (even if empty), and the administration set to the blood bank. *The blood bank will test these materials to further evaluate the reaction.*
■ Collect the first posttransfusion urine specimen, mark the collection slip "Possible transfusion reaction," and send it to the laboratory immediately. *The laboratory tests this urine specimen for the presence of hemoglobin (Hb), which indicates a hemolytic reaction.*
■ Closely monitor intake and output. Note evidence of oliguria or anuria *because Hb deposition in the renal tubules can cause renal damage.*
■ If prescribed, administer oxygen, epinephrine, or other drugs and apply a hypothermia blanket *to reduce fever.*
■ Make the patient as comfortable as possible, and provide reassurance as necessary.

Special considerations

■ Treat all transfusion reactions as serious until proven otherwise. If the practitioner anticipates a transfusion reaction, such as one that may occur in a leukemia patient, he may order prophylactic treatment with antihistamines or antipyretics to precede blood administration.
■ *To avoid a possible febrile reaction,* the practitioner may order the blood washed to remove as many leukocytes as possible, or a leukocyte removal filter may be used during the transfusion.

Documentation

Record the time and date of the transfusion reaction, type and amount of infused blood or blood products, clinical signs of the transfusion reaction in order of occurrence, patient's vital signs, specimens sent to the laboratory for analysis, treatment given, and patient's response to treatment. If required by your facility's policy, complete the transfusion reaction form.

SELECTED REFERENCES

American Association of Blood Banks. *Technical Manual,* 13th ed. Bethesda, Md.: AABB, 1999.
"Documenting a Transfusion Reaction," *Nursing* 35(3):25, March 2005.
The Joint Commission. *Comprehensive Accreditation Manual for Hospitals: The Official Handbook.* Standard PI.2.20. 2007.
Knippen, M. "Transfusion-related Acute Lung Injury," *AJN* 106(6):61-64, June 2006.
Nowlin, A. "Your Guide to Safe Transfusions," *RN* 69(3):24ac1-24ac5, March 2006.
"Standard 48. Administration Set Change. Infusion Nursing Standards of Practice," *Journal of Infusion Nursing* 29(1S):S48-51, January-February 2006.
"Standard 70. Transfusion Therapy. Infusion Nursing Standards of Practice," *Journal of Infusion Nursing* 29(1S):S76-77, January-February 2006.

AUTOLOGOUS BLOOD TRANSFUSION

Also called *autotransfusion,* autologous transfusion is the collection, filtration, and reinfusion of the patient's own blood. Today, with the concern over acquired immunodeficiency syndrome and other blood-borne diseases, the use of autologous transfusion is on the rise.

Indications for autologous transfusion include:
■ elective surgery (blood donated over time)
■ nonelective surgery (blood withdrawn immediately before surgery)
■ perioperative and emergency blood salvage during and after thoracic or cardiovascular surgery and hip, knee, or liver resection and during surgery for ruptured ectopic pregnancy and hemothorax
■ perioperative and emergency blood salvage for traumatic injury of the lungs, liver, chest wall, heart, pulmonary vessels, spleen, kidneys, inferior vena cava, and iliac, portal, or subclavian veins.

Autologous transfusion has several advantages over transfusion of bank blood. Transfusion reactions don't occur, diseases aren't transmitted, anticoagulants aren't added (except in postoperative autotransfusion, when acid citrate dextrose or citrate phosphate dextrose is added), and the blood supply isn't depleted. Also, unlike bank blood, autologous blood contains normal levels of 2,3-diphosphoglycerate, which is helpful in tissue oxygenation.

Autologous transfusion is performed before, during, or after surgery and after traumatic injury. The three techniques used are preoperative blood donation, perioperative blood donation, and acute normovolemic hemodilution.

Preoperative blood donation is commonly recommended for patients scheduled for orthopedic surgery, which causes large blood loss. The donation period begins 4 to 6 weeks before surgery. Donated autologous blood can be stored frozen up to 3 years.

Perioperative blood donation (sometimes called intraoperative or postoperative) is used in vascular and orthopedic surgery and in treatment of traumatic injury. Blood may be collected during surgery or up to 12 hours afterward. (Considerable bleeding may follow vascular and orthopedic surgery.) The blood is transfused immediately after collection or processed (washed) before infusion. Blood obtained postoperatively may be collected from chest tubes, mediastinal drains, or wound drains (placed in the surgical wound during surgery). Commonly inserted during orthopedic surgery, wound drains can be used when enough uncontaminated blood is recovered from a closed wound to be reinfused.

Acute normovolemic hemodilution is used mainly in open-heart surgery. One or 2 units of blood are drawn immediately before or after anesthesia induction. The blood is replaced with a crystalloid or colloid solution, such as lactated Ringer's solution or dextran 40, to produce normovolemic anemia. The blood is reinfused right after surgery. The combination of reduced hemoglobin and the replacement solution causes the patient to lose fewer red blood cells during surgery.

The equipment and procedures presented here are for preoperative and perioperative blood donation only. Acute normovolemic hemodilution is performed the same way as preoperative blood donation, and blood collected this way is reinfused the same way as any other transfusion.

Contraindications to autotransfusion include active infection, malignant neoplasms, coagulopathies, anemia, and patients whose blood has been contaminated by bowel content.

Equipment

For preoperative blood donation: Gloves ▪ gown ▪ mask ▪ antiseptic cleaning swabs ▪ tourniquet ▪ rubber ball ▪ large-bore needle for venipuncture ▪ collection bags ▪ I.V. line ▪ in-line filter for reinfusion ▪ I.V. fluids, if needed.

For perioperative blood donation: Autologous transfusion system ▪ gloves ▪ gown ▪ mask ▪ 250 ml normal saline solution ▪ blood administration tubing ▪ wall suction with pressure gauge.

Implementation

The steps to take depend on the circumstances of the autologous transfusion.

- Confirm patient's identity using two patient identifiers according to your facility's policy.

For preoperative blood donation

- Explain autologous transfusion to the patient, including what it is, how it's performed, how often he can donate blood (every 7 days), and how much he can donate (1 unit every week until 3 to 7 days before surgery).
- To prevent hypovolemia, tell the patient to drink plenty of fluids before donating blood.
- Warn him that he may feel light-headed during the donation but that the problem can be treated without further compromise.
- Check the patient's hemoglobin level, which must be 11 g/dl or higher to donate blood.
- Check and record vital signs before blood donation.
- Help the patient into a supine position.
- Prepare the collection bags according to the manufacturer's instructions.
- Prepare the I.V. fluids, if ordered.
- Perform a venipuncture with a large-bore catheter, and connect the collecting system per the manufacturer's instructions.
- Monitor the patient for adverse reactions to the venipuncture, and administer replacement fluids, if ordered.
- When collection is complete, discontinue the I.V. catheter, and perform site care according to your facility's protocol.
- Recheck the patient's vital signs after the donation is complete.
- Send a blood sample to the laboratory to be checked for the patient's coagulation profile and hemoglobin, hematocrit, and calcium levels.
- Clearly label the collecting bag with the patient's name, identifying numbers, and AUTOLOGOUS USE ONLY notation. *(This way, the blood will not be subjected to rigorous blood bank testing or be accidentally given to another patient.)*

For perioperative blood donation

- Call the transfusionist to set up the autotransfusion device and connect the tubing to the setup according to your facility's protocol and the autotransfusion manufacturer's instructions.
- Put on gown, gloves, and face shield. Follow standard precautions.
- Make sure the collection chamber and the blood transfer bag are clearly marked with the patient's name, identifying numbers, and an AUTOLOGOUS BLOOD label.
- Take and record the patient's vital signs.
- Check that the patient has a patent, acceptable venous access site available for blood administration according to your facility's policy. The access may be either peripheral or central and must be 20G or larger. (See "Transfusion of whole blood and packed cells," page 403.)
- Insert one spike of the standard Y-type blood administration set into the 250 ml bag of normal saline solution. Close all clamps. Hang the setup on an I.V. pole.
- The transfusionist will begin the shed blood collection according to your facility's protocol and the autotransfusion manufacturer's instructions. (Some devices process and centrifuge the blood automatically.)
- Monitor the patient and the blood collection.
- When enough blood has been collected to reinfuse, spike the blood transfer bag with the open port of the standard blood administration I.V. set. Remove all air from the blood transfer bag, and hang the bag on the I.V. pole.

Managing problems of autologous transfusion

PROBLEM	POSSIBLE CAUSES	NURSING INTERVENTIONS
Citrate toxicity (rare, unpredictable)	■ Chelating effect on calcium of citrate in phosphate dextrose (CPD) ■ Predisposing factors, including hyperkalemia, hypocalcemia, acidosis, hypothermia, myocardial dysfunction, and liver or kidney problems	■ Watch for hypotension, arrhythmias, and myocardial contractility. ■ Prophylactic calcium chloride may be administered if more than 2,000 ml of CPD-anticoagulated blood is given over 20 minutes. ■ Stop infusing CPD and correct acidosis. Measure arterial blood gas values and serum calcium levels frequently to assess for toxicity.
Coagulation	■ Not enough anticoagulant ■ Blood not defibrinated in mediastinum	■ Add CPD or another regional anticoagulant at a ratio of 7 parts blood to 1 part anticoagulant. Keep blood and CPD mixed by shaking collection bottle regularly. ■ Check for anticoagulant reversal. Strip chest tubes as needed.
Coagulopathies	■ Reduced platelet and fibrinogen levels ■ Platelets caught in filters ■ Enhanced levels of fibrin split products	■ Patients receiving autologous transfusions of more than 4,000 ml of blood may also need transfusion of fresh frozen plasma or platelet concentrate.
Emboli	■ Microaggregate debris ■ Air	■ Don't use equipment with roller pumps or pressure infusion systems. Before reinfusion, remove air from blood bags. ■ Reinfuse with a 20- to 40-unit microaggregate filter.
Hemolysis	■ Trauma to blood caused by turbulence or roller pumps	■ Don't skim operative field or use equipment with roller pumps. When collecting blood from chest tubes, keep vacuum below 30 mm Hg; when aspirating from a surgical site, keep vacuum below 60 mm Hg.
Sepsis	■ Lack of sterile technique ■ Contaminated blood	■ Give broad-spectrum antibiotics. Use strict sterile technique. Reinfuse patient within 4 hours. ■ Don't infuse blood from infected areas or blood that contains feces, urine, or other contaminants.

- Open the clamp from the normal saline solution, and prime the filter and tubing. Close the clamp from the normal saline solution. Remove all air from the tubing.
- Open the clamp from the blood transfer bag to the drip chamber of the blood administration set, and prime the filter and tubing with blood.
- Attach the blood tubing to the venous access site.
- Begin the reinfusion according to your facility's policy.
- Make sure the reinfusion is completed within your facility's recommended time frame.
- After the reinfusion is complete, record the patient's vital signs.
- When the necessary reinfusion is complete, either you or the transfusionist may disconnect the blood collection setup from the patient's drains according to your facility's policy.

■ Recheck the laboratory data for coagulation profile and hemoglobin, hematocrit, and calcium levels after the reinfusion is complete or as ordered by the practitioner.

Special considerations

Preoperative blood donation

■ In the 4 to 6 weeks prior to surgery, the patient may be prescribed iron supplements *to prevent depletion of his iron stores.*

■ Monitor the patient closely during and after the donation. *Although vasovagal reactions are usually mild and easy to treat, they can quickly progress to severe reactions such as loss of consciousness and seizures.*

■ Have the patient remain supine for 10 minutes after the donation. If he feels lightheaded or dizzy when he gets up, advise him to sit down immediately and to lower his head between his knees, or to lie down with his head lower than his body, until his symptoms resolve.

■ Instruct the patient to drink more fluids than usual for a few hours after the donation and to eat heartily at his next meal.

■ Instruct the patient to monitor his I.V. site for a few hours after the donation. If some bleeding occurs, he should apply firm pressure for 5 to 10 minutes. If the bleeding continues, tell him to notify his practitioner.

Perioperative blood donation

■ If multiple units are to be reinfused, change the blood administration setup and filter as needed according to your facility's policy.

■ The closed, continuous circuit of the perioperative autotransfusion may make the procedures acceptable for use by some Jehovah's Witnesses.

■ Clotting factors may need to be replaced if large volumes of blood are reinfused.

Complications

Autologous transfusion may cause hemolysis, air and particulate emboli, coagulation, thrombocytopenia, vasovagal reactions (from transient hypotension and bradycardia), and hypovolemia (especially in elderly patients). (See *Managing problems of autologous transfusion*, page 415.)

Documentation

Document the amount of blood the patient donated and had reinfused and how he tolerated each procedure.

Selected references

Dzik, W.H., et al. "Patient Safety and Blood Transfusion: New Solutions," *Transfusion Medicine Reviews* 17(3):169-180, July 2003.

Kirschman, R.A. "Finding Alternatives to Blood Transfusion," *Nursing* 34(6):58-62, June 2004.

Maglish Ehrman, B.L. "Blood Conservation Strategies in Cardiovascular Surgery," *Dimensions in Critical Care Nursing* 23(6):244-52, June 2004.

Murphy, G.J., et al. "Safety Efficacy and Cost of Intraoperative Cell Salvage and Autotransfusion After Off Pump Coronary Bypass Surgery," *Journal of Thoracic and Cardiovascular Surgery* 130(1):20-28, July 2005.

Rock, G., et al. "The Development of an Optimized Autologous Blood Donation Program," *Transfusion and Apheresis Science* 33(3):325-31, November 2005.

7 ■ Cardiovascular care

Introduction

Cardiovascular disorders, the leading cause of death in the United States, affect millions of Americans each year. The responsibility of caring for patients with these disorders pervades nearly every area of nursing practice. As a result, cardiovascular care ranks as one of the most rapidly growing areas of nursing. In addition, it's one of the most rapidly changing fields, with the continuing proliferation of new diagnostic tests, new drugs and other treatments, and sophisticated monitoring equipment. Consequently, nurses face a constant challenge to keep up with the latest developments.

Patient teaching

Today, nurses assume much of the responsibility for preparing patients physically and psychologically for their hospitalization and ongoing care. Specifically, they play a pivotal role in teaching patients and their families about test and procedure preparation and follow-up care, drugs and other treatments, disease prevention, and lifestyle modification. Through patient teaching, nurses can help patients reduce stress and comply with prescribed therapy.

Monitoring

Cardiac and hemodynamic monitoring represent critical cardiovascular care responsibilities. Cardiac monitoring involves either hardwire or telemetric systems that continuously record the patient's cardiac activity. This makes monitoring useful not only for assessing cardiac rhythm, but also for gauging a patient's response to drug therapy and for preventing complications associated with diagnostic and therapeutic procedures. Once used only in critical care areas, cardiac monitoring is now performed in high-risk obstetric, general medical, pediatric, and transplantation departments.

Similarly, hemodynamic monitoring has become more widely used since its inception in the 1970s. It uses invasive techniques to measure pressure, flow, and resistance within the cardiovascular system. Made with a pulmonary artery (PA) catheter, these measurements are used to guide therapy. Hemodynamic monitoring includes pulmonary artery pressure monitoring, cardiac output measurement, right ventricular ejection fraction and volume measurement, temporary pacing through the PA catheter, and continuous evaluation of mixed venous oxygen saturation.

Treatment

In cardiovascular emergencies, nurses may perform or assist with cardiopulmonary resuscitation, defibrillation, cardioversion, and temporary pacing. Carrying out these lifesaving procedures calls for in-depth knowledge of cardiovascular anatomy, physiology, and equipment as well as sound assessment and intervention techniques. Only nurses with up-to-date information and sharpened skills can provide safe, effective patient care.

MONITORING

ELECTROCARDIOGRAPHY

One of the most valuable and frequently used diagnostic tools, electrocardiography displays the heart's electrical activity as waveforms. Impulses moving through the heart's conduction system create electric currents that can be monitored on the body's surface. Electrodes attached to the skin can detect these electric currents and transmit them to an instrument that produces a record (the electrocardiogram [ECG]) of cardiac activity.

Electrocardiography can be used to identify myocardial ischemia and infarction, rhythm and conduction disturbances, chamber enlargement, electrolyte imbalances, and the effects of drugs on the heart. To determine which patient would benefit from an ECG, the American Heart Association (AHA) and the American College of Cardiology (ACC) have set guidelines for ECG use. These guidelines classify patients into three groups: patients with known cardiovascular disease or dysfunction; patients who are suspected of having, or who are at increased risk for developing, cardiovascular disease or dysfunction; and patients with no apparent or suspected heart disease or dysfunction.

The standard 12-lead ECG uses a series of electrodes placed on the extremities and the chest wall to assess the heart from 12 different views (leads). The 12 leads consist of three standard bipolar limb leads (designated I, II, III), three unipolar augmented leads (aV_R, aV_L, aV_F), and six unipolar precordial leads (V_1 to V_6). The limb leads and augmented leads show the heart from the frontal plane. The precordial leads show the heart from the horizontal plane. (See *Understanding ECG leads.*)

The ECG device measures and averages the differences between the electrical potential of the electrode sites for each lead and graphs them over time. This creates the standard ECG complex, called PQRST. The P wave represents atrial depolarization; the QRS complex, ventricular depolarization; and the T wave, ventricular repolarization. (See *Reviewing ECG waveforms and components,* page 420.)

Variations of standard ECG include exercise ECG (stress ECG) and ambulatory ECG (Holter monitoring). Exercise ECG monitors heart rate, blood pressure, and ECG waveforms as the patient walks on a treadmill or pedals a stationary bicycle. For patients unable to perform exercises,

Understanding ECG leads

Each of the leads on a 12-lead electrocardiogram (ECG) views the heart from a different angle. These illustrations show the direction of electrical activity (depolarization) monitored by each lead and the 12 views of the heart.

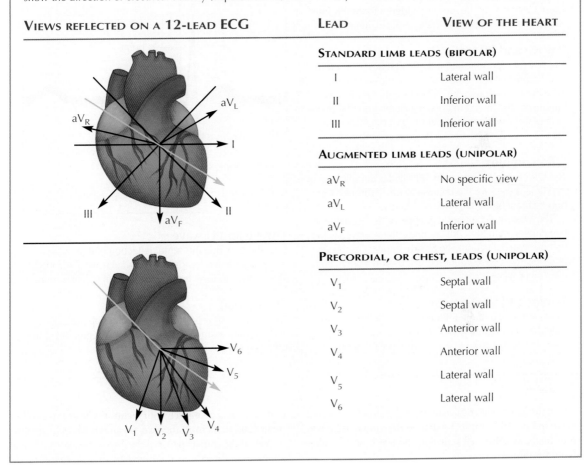

VIEWS REFLECTED ON A 12-LEAD ECG

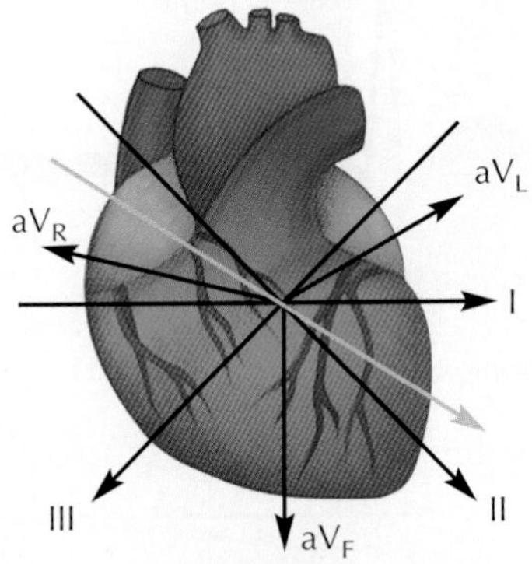

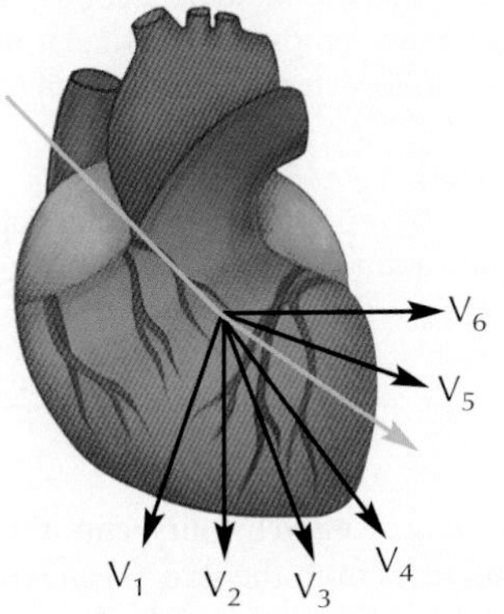

LEAD	VIEW OF THE HEART
STANDARD LIMB LEADS (BIPOLAR)	
I	Lateral wall
II	Inferior wall
III	Inferior wall
AUGMENTED LIMB LEADS (UNIPOLAR)	
aV_R	No specific view
aV_L	Lateral wall
aV_F	Inferior wall
PRECORDIAL, OR CHEST, LEADS (UNIPOLAR)	
V_1	Septal wall
V_2	Septal wall
V_3	Anterior wall
V_4	Anterior wall
V_5	Lateral wall
V_6	Lateral wall

pharmacologic agents—such as adenosine or dobutamine—can be used to produce the same cardiovascular stress brought on by exercise to allow for testing. For ambulatory ECG, the patient wears a portable Holter monitor to record heart activity continually over 24 hours.

Today, ECG is typically accomplished using a multichannel method. All electrodes are attached to the patient at once, and the machine prints a simultaneous view of all leads.

Equipment

ECG machine ▪ recording paper ▪ disposable pregelled electrodes ▪ 4″ × 4″ gauze pads ▪ optional: clippers, marking pen.

Preparation of equipment

Place the ECG machine close to the patient's bed, and plug the power cord into the wall outlet. If the patient is already connected to a cardiac monitor, remove the electrodes *to accommodate the precordial leads and minimize electrical interference on the ECG tracing.* Keep the patient away from objects that might cause electrical interference, such as equipment, fixtures, and power cords.

Implementation

- Confirm the patient's identity using two patient identifiers according to your facility's policy.
- As you set up the machine to record a 12-lead ECG, explain the procedure to the patient. Tell him that the test

Reviewing ECG waveforms and components

An electrocardiogram (ECG) waveform has three basic components: the P wave, QRS complex, and T wave. These elements can be further divided into the PR interval, J point, ST segment, U wave, and QT interval.

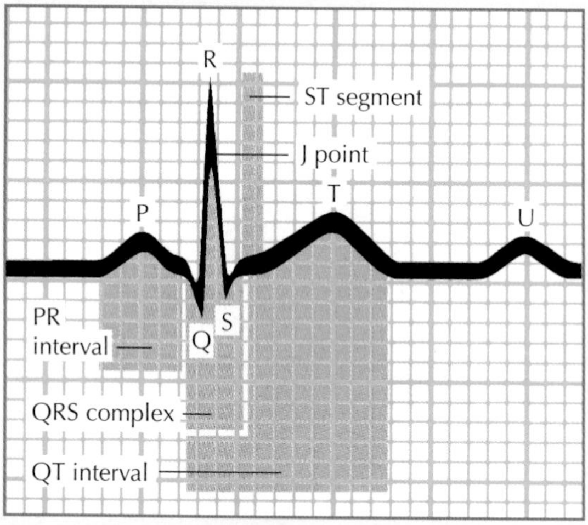

P wave and PR interval

The P wave represents atrial depolarization. The PR interval represents the time it takes an impulse to travel from the atria through the atrioventricular nodes and bundle of His. The PR interval measures from the beginning of the P wave to the beginning of the QRS complex.

QRS complex

The QRS complex represents ventricular depolarization (the time it takes for the impulse to travel through the bundle branches to the Purkinje fibers).

The Q wave, when present, appears as the first negative deflection in the QRS complex; the R wave, as the first positive deflection. The S wave appears as the second negative deflection or the first negative deflection after the R wave.

J point and ST segment

Marking the end of the QRS complex, the J point also indicates the beginning of the ST segment. The ST segment represents part of ventricular repolarization.

T wave and U wave

Usually following the same deflection pattern as the P wave, the T wave represents ventricular repolarization. The U wave follows the T wave, but isn't always seen.

QT interval

The QT interval represents ventricular depolarization and repolarization. It extends from the beginning of the QRS complex to the end of the T wave.

records the heart's electrical activity, and it may be repeated at certain intervals. Emphasize that no electrical current will enter his body. Also, tell him that the test typically takes about 5 minutes.

- Have the patient lie in a supine position in the center of the bed with his arms at his sides. You may raise the head of the bed *to promote his comfort.* Expose his arms and legs, and drape him appropriately. His arms and legs should be relaxed *to minimize muscle trembling, which can cause electrical interference.*
- If the bed is too narrow, place the patient's hands under his buttocks *to prevent muscle tension.* Also use this technique if the patient is shivering or trembling. Make sure his feet aren't touching the bed board.
- Select flat, fleshy areas to place the electrodes. Avoid muscular and bony areas. If the patient has an amputated limb, choose a site on the stump.
- If an area is excessively hairy, clip it. Clean excess oil or other substances from the skin *to enhance electrode contact.*
- Peel off the contact paper of the disposable electrodes, and apply them directly to the prepared site. *To guarantee the best connection to the leadwire,* position disposable electrodes on the legs with the lead connection pointing superiorly.
- Connect the limb leadwires to the electrodes. Make sure the metal parts of the electrodes are clean and bright. *Dirty or corroded electrodes prevent a good electrical connection.*
- You'll see that the tip of each leadwire is lettered and color-coded for easy identification. The white or RA leadwire goes to the right arm; the green or RL leadwire, to the right leg; the red or LL leadwire, to the left leg; the black or LA leadwire, to the left arm; and the brown or V_1 to V_6 leadwires, to the chest.
- Now, expose the patient's chest. Put a disposable electrode at each electrode position. (See *Positioning chest electrodes.*)

If your patient is a woman, be sure to place the chest electrodes below the breast tissue. In a large-breasted woman, you may need to displace the breast tissue laterally.

- Check to see that the paper speed selector is set to the standard 25 mm/second and that the machine is set to full voltage. The machine will record a normal standardization mark — a square that's the height of two large squares or 10 small squares on the recording paper. Then, if necessary, enter the appropriate patient identification data.
- If any part of the waveform extends beyond the paper when you record the ECG, adjust the normal standardization to half-standardization. Note this adjustment on the ECG strip *because this will need to be considered in interpreting the results.*
- Now you're ready to begin the recording. Ask the patient to relax and breathe normally. Tell him to lie still and not to talk when you record his ECG. Then press the AUTO button. Observe the tracing quality. The machine will record all 12 leads automatically, recording three consecutive leads simultaneously. Some machines have a display screen *so you can preview waveforms before the machine records them on paper.*
- When the machine finishes recording the 12-lead ECG, remove the electrodes and clean the patient's skin. After disconnecting the leadwires from the electrodes, dispose of or clean the electrodes, as indicated.
- If serial ECGs are expected, consider marking the electrode positions on the patient's skin. *Consistent lead placement enhances the comparison of serial ECGs and eliminates inaccuracy due to lead placement.*

Positioning chest electrodes

To ensure accurate test results, position chest electrodes as follows:

V_1: Fourth intercostal space at right sternal border
V_2: Fourth intercostal space at left sternal border
V_3: Halfway between V_2 and V_4
V_4: Fifth intercostal space at midclavicular line
V_5: Fifth intercostal space at anterior axillary line (halfway between V_4 and V_6)
V_6: Fifth intercostal space at midaxillary line, level with V_4

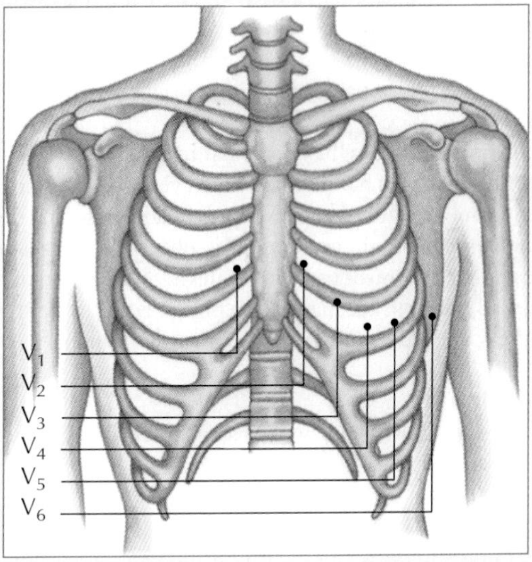

Special considerations

- Small areas of hair on the patient's chest or extremities may be clipped, but this usually isn't necessary.
- If the patient's skin is exceptionally oily, scaly, or diaphoretic, rub the electrode site with a dry 4" × 4" gauze or alcohol pad before applying the electrode *to help reduce interference in the tracing.* During the procedure, ask the patient to breathe normally. If his respirations distort the recording, ask him to hold his breath briefly *to reduce baseline wander in the tracing.*
- If the patient has a pacemaker, you can perform an ECG with or without a magnet, according to the practitioner's orders. Be sure to note the presence of a pacemaker and the use of the magnet on the strip.

Documentation

Label the ECG recording with the patient's name, room number, and facility identification number. Document in your notes the test's date and time as well as significant responses by the patient. Record the date, time, and patient's name and room number on the ECG itself. Note any appropriate clinical information on the ECG.

SELECTED REFERENCES

American College of Cardiology and American Heart Association. "ACC/AHA Clinical Competence Statement on Electrocardiography and Ambulatory Electrocardiography," *Circulation* 104:3169-178, December 2001.

Lynn-McHale Wiegand, D.J., and Carlson, K.K., eds. *AACN Procedure Manual for Critical Care,* 5th ed. Philadelphia: W.B. Saunders Co., 2005.

Noordzij, P.G., et al. "Prognostic Value of Routine Preoperative Electrocardiography in Patients Undergoing Noncardiac Surgery," *American Journal of Cardiology* 97(7):1103-106, April 2006.

RIGHT CHEST LEAD ELECTROCARDIOGRAPHY

Unlike a standard 12-lead electrocardiogram (ECG), used primarily to evaluate left ventricular function, a right chest lead ECG reflects right ventricular function and provides clues to damage or dysfunction in this chamber. You might need to perform a right chest lead ECG for a patient with an inferior wall myocardial infarction (MI) and suspected right ventricular involvement. Between 25% and 50% of patients with this type of MI have right ventricular involvement.

Early identification of a right ventricular MI is essential because this type of MI is associated with significant morbidity and mortality. ST-segment elevation of 1 mm or more in the right precordial lead (V_{4R}) indicates a right ventricular MI.

Treatment for a right ventricular infarction differs from that for other MIs. For instance, in left ventricular MI, treatment involves withholding I.V. fluids or administering them judiciously to prevent heart failure. Conversely, in right ventricular MI, treatment usually requires administration of I.V. fluids to maintain adequate filling pressures on the right side of the heart and to support left ventricular filling.

Equipment

Multichannel ECG machine ▪ paper ▪ pregelled disposable electrodes ▪ several 4″ × 4″ gauze pads.

Implementation

- Confirm the patient's identity using two patient identifiers according to your facility's policy.
- Take the equipment to the patient's bedside, and explain the procedure to him. Inform him that the practitioner has ordered a right chest lead ECG, a procedure that involves placing electrodes on his wrists, ankles, and chest. Reassure him that the test is painless and takes only a few minutes, during which he'll need to lie quietly on his back.
- Make sure the paper speed is set at 25 mm/second and the amplitude at 1 mV/10 mm.
- Place the patient in a supine position or, if he has difficulty lying flat, in semi-Fowler's position. Provide privacy and expose his arms, chest, and legs. (Cover a female patient's chest with a drape until you apply the chest leads.)
- Examine the patient's wrists and ankles for the best areas to place the electrodes. Choose flat and fleshy (not bony or muscular), hairless areas such as the inner aspects of the wrists and ankles. Clean the sites with the gauze pads *to promote good skin contact.*
- Connect the leadwires to the electrodes. The leadwires are color-coded and lettered. Place the white or right arm (RA) wire on the right arm; the black or left arm (LA) wire on the left arm; the green or right leg (RL) wire on the right leg; and the red or left leg (LL) wire on the left leg.
- Then examine the patient's chest *to locate the correct sites for chest lead placement* (as shown below). If the patient is a woman, place the electrodes under the breast tissue.

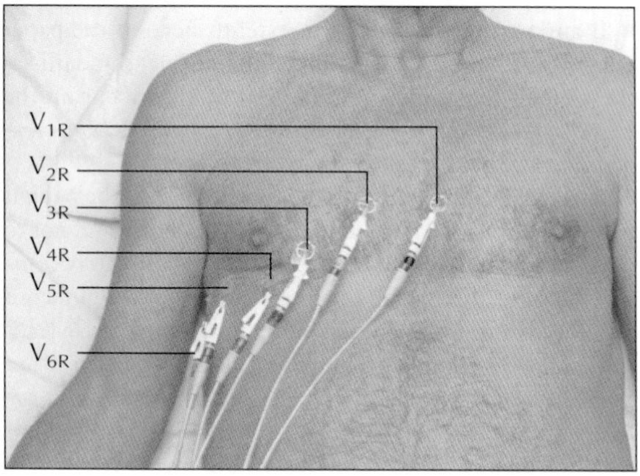

- Use your fingers to feel between the patient's ribs (the intercostal spaces). Start at the second intercostal space on the left (the notch felt at the top of the sternum, where the manubrium joins the body of the sternum). Count down two spaces to the fourth intercostal space. Then apply a disposable electrode to the site and attach leadwire V_{1R} to that electrode.
- Move your fingers across the sternum to the fourth intercostal space on the right side of the sternum. Apply a disposable electrode to that site and attach lead V_{2R}.
- Move your finger down to the fifth intercostal space and over to the midclavicular line. Place a disposable electrode here and attach lead V_{4R}.
- Visually draw a line between V_{2R} and V_{4R}. Apply a disposable electrode midway on this line and attach lead V_{3R}.
- Move your finger horizontally from V_{4R} to the right midaxillary line. Apply a disposable electrode to this site and attach lead V_{6R}.
- Move your fingers along the same horizontal line to the midpoint between V_{4R} and V_{6R}. This is the right anterior midaxillary line. Apply a disposable electrode to this site and attach lead V_{5R}.
- Turn on the ECG machine. Ask the patient to breathe normally but to refrain from talking during the recording *so that muscle movement won't distort the tracing.* Enter any appropriate patient information required by the machine you're using. If necessary, standardize the machine. This will

cause a square tracing of 10 mm (two large squares) to appear on the ECG paper when the machine is set for 1 mV (1 mV = 10 mm).

- Press the AUTO key. The ECG machine will record all 12 leads automatically. Check your facility's policy for the number of readings to obtain. (Some facilities require at least two ECGs *so that one copy can be sent out for interpretation while the other remains at the bedside.*)
- When you're finished recording the ECG, turn off the machine. Clearly label the ECG with the patient's name, the date, and the time. Also label the tracing "Right chest ECG" *to distinguish it from a standard 12-lead ECG.* Make sure the leads are correctly labeled: V_{1R} through V_{6R}. Remove the electrodes and help the patient get comfortable.
- If serial right chest lead ECGs are anticipated, consider marking the electrode sites on the patient's skin *to facilitate consistent placement.*

Special considerations

For best results, place the electrodes symmetrically on the limbs. If the patient's wrist or ankle is covered by a dressing, or if the patient is an amputee, choose an area that's available on both sides.

Documentation

Document the procedure in your nurse's notes, and document the patient's tolerance of the procedure. Place a copy of the tracing on the patient's chart.

SELECTED REFERENCES

Carter, T., and Ellis, K. "Right Ventricular Infarction," *Critical Care Nurse* 25(2):52-62, April 2005.

Lynn-McHale Wiegand, D.J., and Carlson, K.K., eds. *AACN Procedure Manual for Critical Care*, 5th ed. Philadelphia: W.B. Saunders Co., 2005.

POSTERIOR CHEST LEAD ELECTROCARDIOGRAPHY

Because of the location of the heart's posterior surface, changes associated with myocardial damage aren't apparent on a standard 12-lead electrocardiogram (ECG). Studies have shown that the addition of posterior leads V_7, V_8, and V_9 to the 12-lead ECG increases the sensitivity and specificity of identifying a posterior wall myocardial infarction (MI) and may provide clues to posterior wall infarction so that appropriate treatment can begin.

Usually, the posterior lead ECG is performed with a standard ECG and only involves recording the additional posterior leads. ST-segment elevation of 1 mm or more in at least two posterior leads indicates a posterior wall MI.

Equipment

Multichannel ECG machine with recording paper ▪ disposable pregelled electrodes ▪ 4″ × 4″ gauze pads ▪ optional: electric clippers, moist cloth.

Implementation

- Confirm the patient's identity using two patient identifiers according to your facility's policy.
- Prepare the electrode sites according to the manufacturer's instructions. *To ensure good skin contact,* clip the site if the patient has considerable back hair.
- These leads are placed opposite the anterior leads V_4, V_5, and V_6, on the left side of the patient's back, following the same horizontal line. Begin by attaching a disposable electrode to the V_7 position on the left posterior axillary line, at the same horizontal level as V_6, at the fifth intercostal space. Then attach the V_4 leadwire to the V_7 electrode.
- Next, attach a disposable electrode to the patient's back at the V_8 position on the left midscapular line at the same horizontal level as lead V_6, at the fifth intercostal space, and attach at the V_5 leadwire to this electrode.
- Finally, attach a disposable electrode to the patient's back at the V_9 position, just left of the spinal column at the fifth intercostal space. Then attach the V_6 leadwire to the V_9 electrode. (See *Placing electrodes for posterior ECG,* page 424.)
- All leads will print out as a straight line except those labeled V_4, V_5, and V_6. Relabel those leads V_7, V_8, and V_9 respectively.
- When the ECG is complete, remove the electrodes and clean the patient's skin with a gauze pad or a moist cloth. If you think you may need more than one posterior lead ECG, use a marking pen to mark the electrode sites on his skin *to permit accurate comparison for future tracings.*

Special considerations

- The number of leads may vary according to the cardiologist's preference. (If right posterior leads are requested, position the patient on his left side. These leads, known as V_{7R}, V_{8R}, and V_{9R}, are located at the same landmarks on the right side of the patient's back.)
- Some ECG machines won't operate unless you connect all leadwires. In that case, you may need to connect the limb leadwires and the leadwires for V_1, V_2, and V_3.

Documentation

Document the procedure in your nurse's notes. Make sure the patient's name, age, room number, time, date, and practitioner's name are clearly written on the ECG along with the relabeled lead tracings. Document any patient teaching you may have performed as well as the patient's tolerance of the procedure.

Placing electrodes for posterior ECG

To ensure an accurate electrocardiogram (ECG) reading, make sure that the posterior leads V_7, V_8, and V_9 are placed at the same level horizontally as the V_6 lead at the fifth intercostal space. Place lead V_7 at the posterior axillary line, lead V_9 at the paraspinal line, and lead V_8 halfway between leads V_7 and V_9.

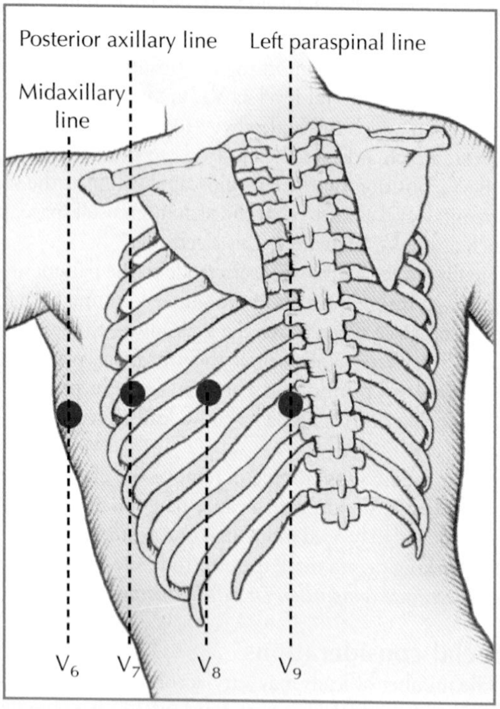

SELECTED REFERENCES

Alinier, G., et al. "12-lead ECG Training: The Way Forward," *Nurse Education Today* 26(1):87-92, January 2006.

Goldich, G. "Understanding the 12-lead ECG, Part I," *Nursing* 36(11):36-41, November 2006.

Goldich, G. "Understanding the 12-lead ECG, Part II: Learn to Recognize Bundle Branch Block, Myocardial Infarction, and Common Dysrhythmias," *Nursing* 36(12):36-41, December 2006.

Jevon, P. "Cardiac Monitoring, Part 2: Recording a 12-lead ECG," *Nursing Times* 103(2):26-27, January 2007.

Lynn-McHale Wiegand, D.J., and Carlson, K.K., eds. *AACN Procedure Manual for Critical Care,* 5th ed. Philadelphia: W.B. Saunders Co., 2005.

SIGNAL-AVERAGED ELECTROCARDIOGRAPHY

Signal-averaged electrocardiography helps to identify patients at risk for sustained ventricular tachycardia. Because this cardiac arrhythmia can be a precursor of sudden death after a myocardial infarction (MI), the results of a signal-averaged electrocardiogram (ECG) can allow appropriate preventive measures.

Through a computer-based ECG, signal averaging detects low-amplitude signals or late electrical potentials, which reflect slow conduction or disorganized ventricular activity through abnormal or infarcted regions of the ventricles. The signal-averaged ECG is developed by recording the noise-free surface ECG in three specialized leads for several hundred beats.

Signal averaging enhances signals that would otherwise be missed because of increased amplitude and sensitivity to ventricular activity. For instance, on the standard 12-lead ECG, "noise" created by muscle tissue, electronic artifacts, and electrodes masks late potentials, which have a low amplitude.

This procedure identifies the risk of sustained ventricular tachycardia in patients with malignant ventricular tachycardia, a history of MI, unexplained syncope, nonischemic congestive cardiomyopathy, or nonsustained ventricular tachycardia.

Equipment

Signal-averaged ECG machine ▪ signal-averaged computer ▪ record of patient's surface ECG for 200 to 300 QRS complexes ▪ three bipolar electrodes or leads ▪ alcohol pads ▪ clippers.

Implementation

- Confirm the patient's identity using two patient identifiers according to your facility's policy.
- Inform the patient that this procedure will take 10 to 30 minutes and will help the practitioner determine his risk for a certain type of arrhythmia. If appropriate, mention that it may be done along with other tests, such as echocardiography, Holter monitoring, and a stress test.
- Ensure a quiet environment with no interruption during the test.
- Place the patient in the supine position, and tell him to lie as still as possible. Tell him he shouldn't speak and should breathe normally during the procedure.
- If the patient has hair on his chest, clip the hair, then rub the patient's chest with alcohol and dry it before placing the electrodes on it.

- Place the leads in the X, Y, and Z orthogonal positions. (See *Placing electrodes for signal-averaged ECG.*)
- The ECG machine gathers input from these leads and amplifies, filters, and samples the signals. The computer collects and stores data for analysis. The crucial values are those showing QRS complex duration, duration of the portion of the QRS complex with an amplitude under 40 mV, and the root mean square voltage of the last 40 msec.

Special considerations

- *Because muscle movements may cause a false-positive result,* patients who are restless or in respiratory distress are poor candidates for signal-averaged ECG. Proper electrode placement and skin preparation are essential to this procedure.
- Results indicating low-amplitude signals include a QRS complex duration greater than 110 msec, a duration of more than 40 msec for the amplitude portion under 40 mV, and a root mean square voltage of less than 25 mV during the last 40 msec of the QRS complex. However, all three factors need not be present to consider the result positive or negative. The final interpretation hinges on individualized patient factors.
- Results of signal-averaged ECG help the practitioner determine whether the patient is a candidate for invasive procedures, such as electrophysiologic testing or angiography.
- Keep in mind that the significance of signal-averaged ECG results in patients with bundle-branch heart block is unknown *because myocardial activation doesn't follow the usual sequence in these patients.*

Documentation

Document the time of the procedure, why the procedure was done, and how the patient tolerated it.

Placing electrodes for signal-averaged ECG

To prepare your patient for a signal-averaged electrocardiography (ECG), place the electrodes in the X, Y, and Z orthogonal positions. These positions bisect one another to provide a three-dimensional, composite view of ventricular activation.

Anterior chest

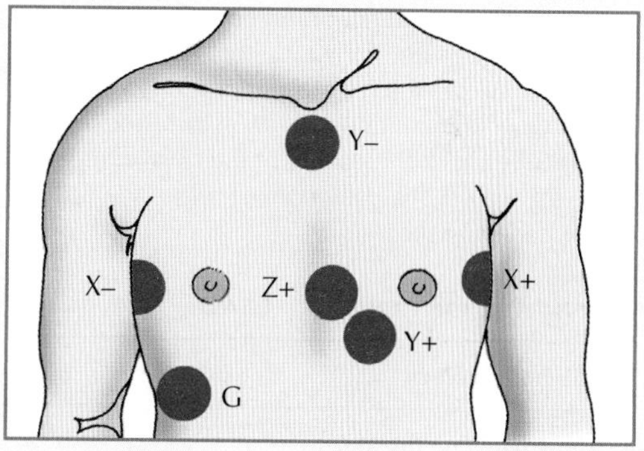

Posterior chest

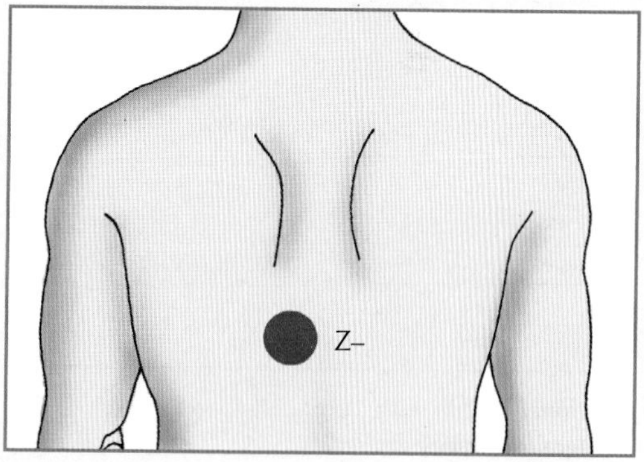

Key

X+ Fourth intercostal space, midaxillary line, left side
X– Fourth intercostal space, midaxillary line, right side
Y+ Standard V_3 position (or proximal left leg)
Y– Superior aspect of manubrium
Z+ Standard V_2 position
Z– V_2 position, posterior
G Ground, eighth rib on right side

SELECTED REFERENCES

Archbold, R.A. "The Signal Averaged P-wave to Predict Atrial Fibrillation after Cardiac Surgery," *Annals of Thoracic Surgery* 81(1):406-407, January 2006.

Chiu, C., et al. "Diagnosis and Treatment of Idiopathic Ventricular Tachycardia," *AACN Clinical Issues* 15(3):449-61, July 2005.

Hohnloser, S.H. "Usefulness of Microvolt T-wave Alternans for Prediction of Ventricular Tachyarrhythmic Events in Patients with Dilated Cardiomyopathy: Results from a Prospective Observational Study," *Journal of the American College of Cardiology* 41(12):2220-224, June 2003.

Matsyshuta, S., et al. "High Frequent QRS Potentials as a Marker of Cardiac Dysfunction after Cardiac Surgery," *Annals of Thoracic Surgery* 77(4):1293-297, April 2004.

Yamada, T., et al. "Usefulness of Spatial Dispersion of QRS Duration in Predicting Mortality in Patients with Mild to Moderated Chronic Heart Failure," *American Journal of Cardiology* 94(7):960-63, October 2004.

CARDIAC MONITORING

Because it allows continuous observation of the heart's electrical activity, cardiac monitoring is used in patients with conduction disturbances and in those at risk for life-threatening arrhythmias. Like other forms of electrocardiography, cardiac monitoring uses electrodes placed on the patient's chest to transmit electrical signals that are converted into a tracing of cardiac rhythm on an oscilloscope.

Two types of monitoring may be performed: hardwire or telemetry. In *hardwire monitoring*, the patient is connected to a monitor at the bedside. The rhythm display appears at the bedside, but it may also be transmitted to a console at a remote location. *Telemetry* uses a small transmitter connected to the ambulatory patient to send electrical signals to another location, where they're displayed on a monitor. Battery powered and portable, telemetry frees the patient from cumbersome wires and cables and lets him be comfortably mobile and safely isolated from the electrical leakage and accidental shock occasionally associated with hardwire monitoring. Telemetry is especially useful for monitoring arrhythmias that occur during sleep, rest, exercise, or stressful situations. However, unlike hardwire monitoring, telemetry can monitor only cardiac rate and rhythm.

Regardless of the type, cardiac monitors can display the patient's heart rate and rhythm, produce a printed record of cardiac rhythm, and sound an alarm if the heart rate exceeds or falls below specified limits. Monitors also recognize and count abnormal heartbeats as well as changes. For example, a relatively new technique, ST-segment monitoring, helps detect myocardial ischemia, electrolyte imbalance, coronary artery spasm, and hypoxic events. The ST segment represents early ventricular repolarization, and changes in this waveform component reflect alterations in myocardial oxygenation. Any monitoring lead that views an ischemic heart region will reveal ST-segment changes. The monitor's software establishes a template of the patient's normal QRST pattern from the selected leads; then the monitor displays ST-segment changes. Some monitors display such changes continuously, others only on command. (See *Lead selection.*)

Lead selection

Your patient's clinical condition determines the leads you'll monitor. *Note:* If the monitor can detect arrhythmias, know which leads perform this function. Even if you don't continuously monitor these leads, periodically check the quality of their waveforms *because the arrhythmia detection algorithm will fail without adequate waveforms.*

CLINICAL CONCERN	LEAD
Bundle-branch block	V_1 or V_6
Ischemia based on the area of infarction or site of percutaneous coronary intervention	
Anterior	V_3, V_4
Septal	V_1, V_2
Lateral	I, aV_L, V_5, V_6
Inferior	II, III, aV_F
Right ventricle	V_{4R}
Junctional rhythm with retrograde P waves	II
Optimal view of atrial activity	I, II, or Lewis lead
Ventricular ectopy, wide complex tachycardia	V_1 (may use V_6 along with V_1)
Ventricular pacing	V_1 or II

Equipment

Cardiac monitor ▪ leadwires ▪ patient cable ▪ disposable pregelled electrodes (number of electrodes varies from three to five, depending on patient's needs) ▪ alcohol pads ▪ 4″ × 4″ gauze pads ▪ optional: clippers, washcloth.

For telemetry: Transmitter ▪ transmitter pouch ▪ telemetry battery pack, leads, and electrodes.

Preparation of equipment

Plug the cardiac monitor into an electrical outlet and turn it on *to warm up the unit while you prepare the equipment and the patient.* Insert the cable into the appropriate socket in the monitor. Connect the leadwires to the cable. In some systems, the leadwires are permanently secured to the cable. Each leadwire should indicate the location for attachment to the patient: right arm (RA), left arm (LA), right leg (RL), left leg (LL), and ground (C or V). This should appear on the leadwire — if it's permanently connected — or at the connection of the leadwires and cable to the patient. Then connect an electrode to each of the leadwires, carefully checking that each leadwire is in its correct outlet.

For telemetry monitoring, insert a new battery into the transmitter. Be sure to match the poles on the battery with the polar markings on the transmitter case. By pressing the button at the top of the unit, test the battery's charge and test the unit to ensure that the battery is operational. If the leadwires aren't permanently affixed to the telemetry unit, attach them securely. If they must be attached individually, be sure to connect each one to the correct outlet.

Implementation

- Confirm the patient's identity using two patient identifiers according to your facility's policy.
- Explain the procedure to the patient, provide privacy, and ask the patient to expose his chest. Wash your hands.
- Determine electrode positions on the patient's chest, based on which system and lead you're using. (See *Positioning monitoring leads,* pages 428 and 429.)
- If the leadwires and patient cable aren't permanently attached, verify that the electrode placement corresponds to the label on the patient cable.
- If necessary, clip the hair from an area about 4" (10 cm) in diameter around each electrode site. Clean the area with an alcohol pad and dry it completely *to remove skin secretions that may interfere with electrode function.* Gently abrade the dried area by rubbing it briskly until it reddens *to remove dead skin cells and to promote better electrical contact with living cells.* (Some electrodes have a small, rough patch for abrading the skin; otherwise, use a dry washcloth or a dry gauze pad.)
- Remove the backing from the pregelled electrode. Check the gel for moistness. If the gel is dry, discard it and replace it with a fresh electrode.
- Apply the electrode to the site and press firmly *to ensure a tight seal.* Repeat with the remaining electrodes.
- When all the electrodes are in place, check for a tracing on the cardiac monitor. Assess the quality of the electrocardiogram (ECG). (See *Identifying cardiac monitor problems,* page 430.)
- *To verify that each beat is being detected by the monitor,* compare the digital heart rate display with your count of the patient's heart rate.
- If necessary, use the gain control *to adjust the size of the rhythm tracing,* and use the position control *to adjust the waveform position on the recording paper.*
- Set the upper and lower limits of the heart rate alarm, based on unit policy. Turn the alarm on.

For telemetry monitoring

- Wash your hands. Explain the procedure to the patient and provide privacy.
- Expose the patient's chest, and select the lead arrangement. Remove the backing from one of the gelled electrodes. Check the gel for moistness. If it's dry, discard the electrode and obtain a new one.
- Apply the electrode to the appropriate site by pressing one side of the electrode against the patient's skin, pulling gently, and then pressing the other side against the skin. Press your fingers in a circular motion around the electrode *to fix the gel and stabilize the electrode.* Repeat for each electrode.
- Attach an electrode to the end of each leadwire.
- Place the transmitter in the pouch. Tie the pouch strings around the patient's neck and waist, making sure that the pouch fits snugly without causing him discomfort. If no pouch is available, place the transmitter in the patient's bathrobe pocket.
- Check the patient's waveform for clarity, position, and size. Adjust the gain and baseline as needed. (If necessary, ask the patient to remain resting or sitting in his room while you locate his telemetry monitor at the central station.)
- To obtain a rhythm strip, press the RECORD key at the central station. Label the strip with the patient's name and room number, date, and time. Also identify the rhythm. Place the rhythm strip in the appropriate location in the patient's chart.

Special considerations

- Make sure all electrical equipment and outlets are grounded *to avoid electric shock and interference (artifacts).* Also ensure that the patient is clean and dry *to prevent electric shock.*
- Avoid opening the electrode packages until just before using *to prevent the gel from drying out.*
- Avoid placing the electrodes on bony prominences, hairy locations, areas where defibrillator pads will be placed, or areas for chest compression.
- If the patient's skin is very oily, scaly, or diaphoretic, rub the electrode site with a dry 4" × 4" gauze pad before applying the electrode *to help reduce interference in the tracing.* Have the patient breathe normally during the procedure. If his respirations distort the recording, ask him to hold his breath briefly *to reduce baseline wander in the tracing.*
- Assess skin integrity, and reposition the electrodes every 24 hours or as necessary.
- If the patient is being monitored by telemetry, show him how the transmitter works. If applicable, show him the button that will produce an ECG recording at the central station. Teach him how to push the button whenever he has symptoms. *This causes the central console to print a rhythm*

(Text continues on page 431.)

Positioning monitoring leads

This chart shows the correct electrode positions for some of the monitoring leads you'll use most often. For each lead, you'll see electrode placement for a five-leadwire system, a three-leadwire system, and a telemetry system.

In the two hardwire systems, the electrode positions for one lead may be identical to the electrode positions for another lead. In this case, you simply change the lead selector switch to the setting that corresponds to the lead you want. In some cases, you'll need to reposition the electrodes.

In the telemetry system, you can create the same lead with two electrodes that you do with three, simply by eliminating the ground electrode.

The illustrations below use these abbreviations: RA, right arm; LA, left arm; RL, right leg; LL, left leg; C, chest; and G, ground.

FIVE-LEADWIRE SYSTEM | **THREE-LEADWIRE SYSTEM** | **TELEMETRY SYSTEM**

LEAD I

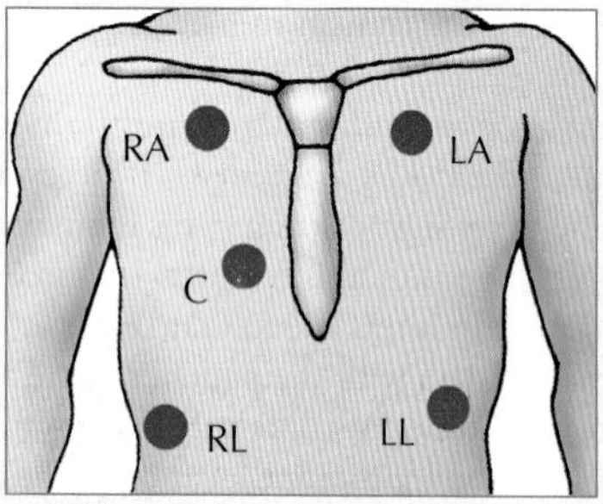

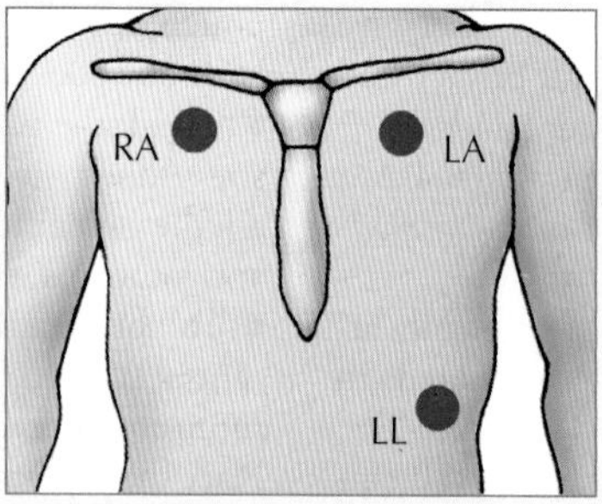

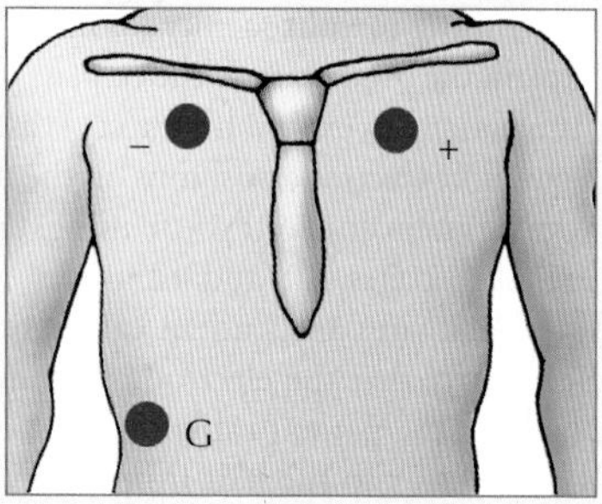

LEAD II

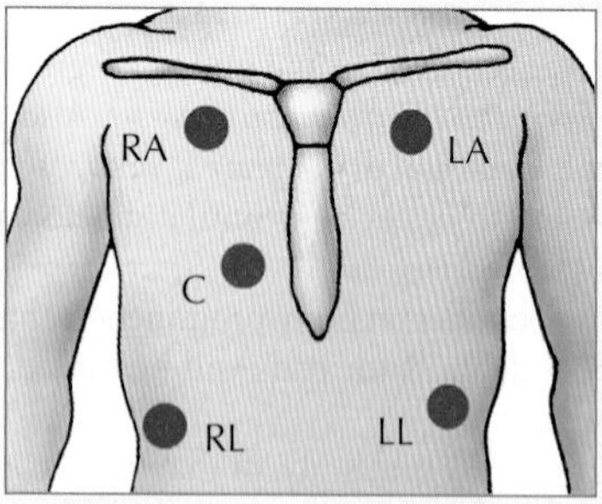

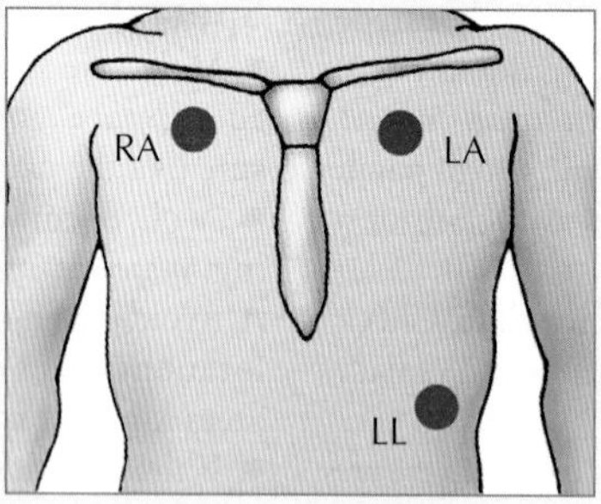

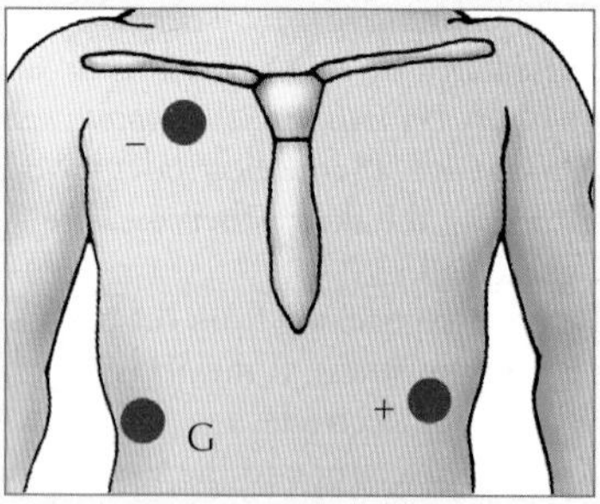

LEAD III

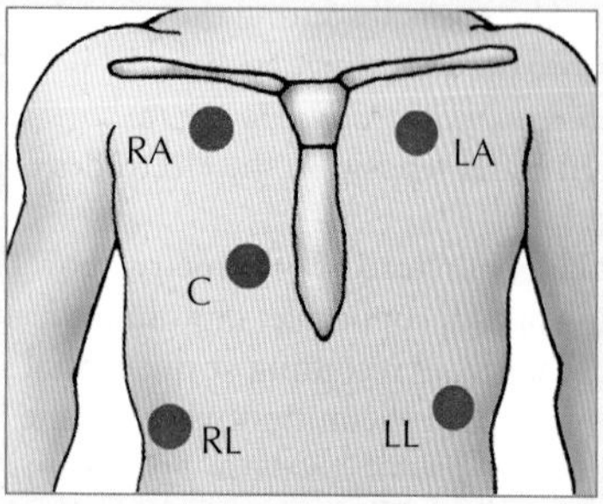

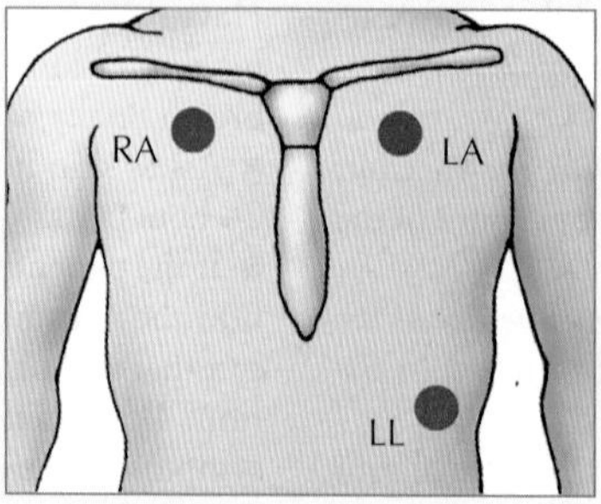

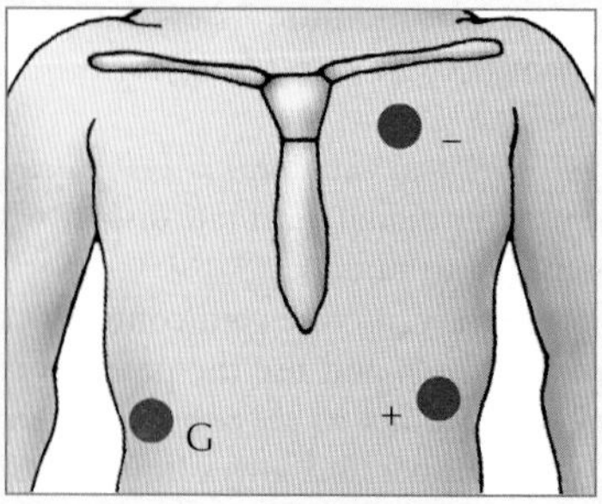

Positioning monitoring leads *(continued)*

FIVE-LEADWIRE SYSTEM | **THREE-LEADWIRE SYSTEM** | **TELEMETRY SYSTEM**

LEAD MCL_1

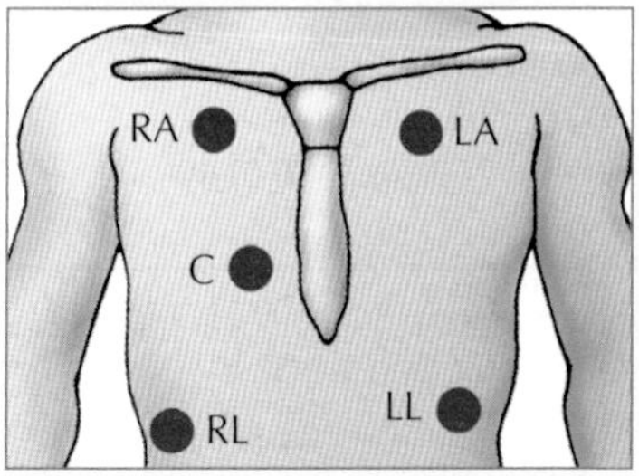

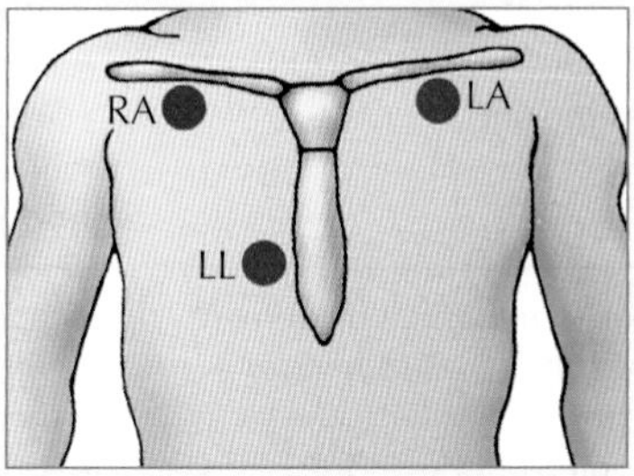

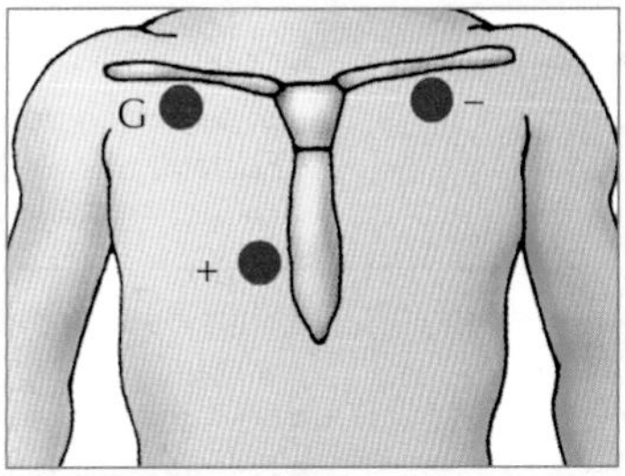

LEAD MCL_6

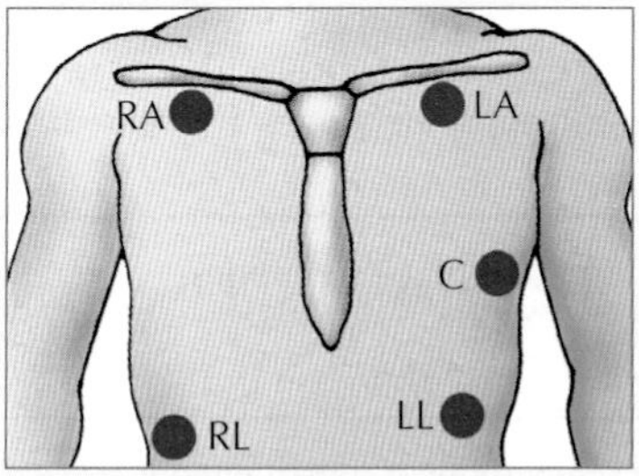

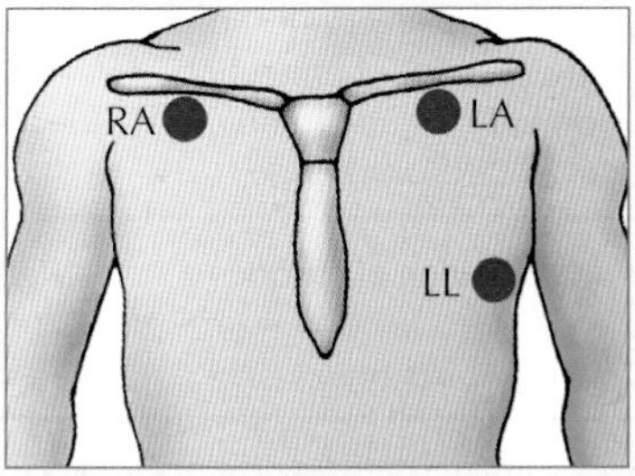

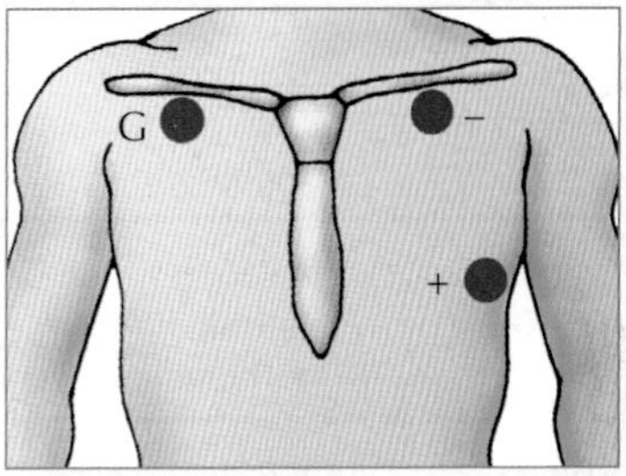

STERNAL LEAD

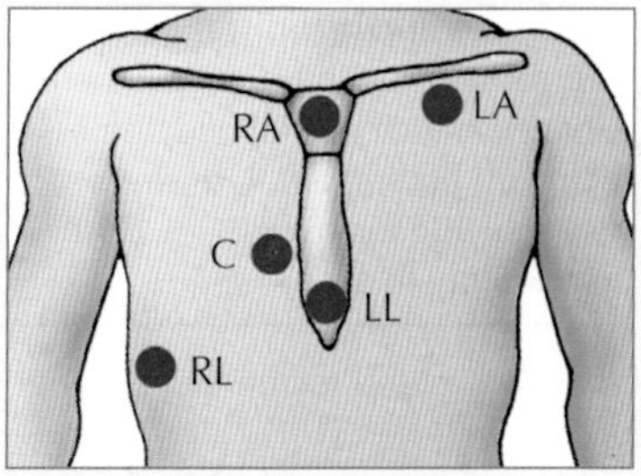

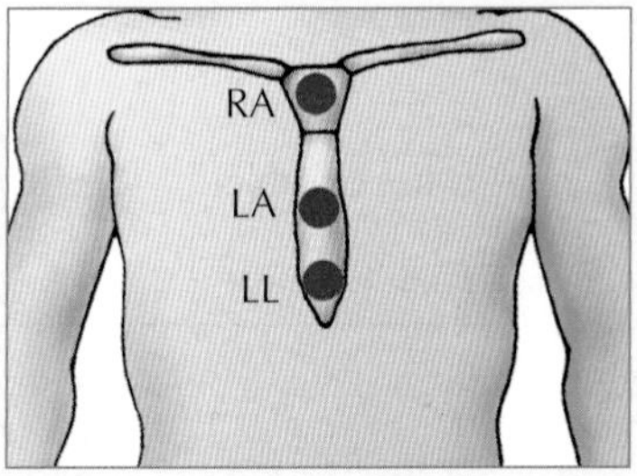

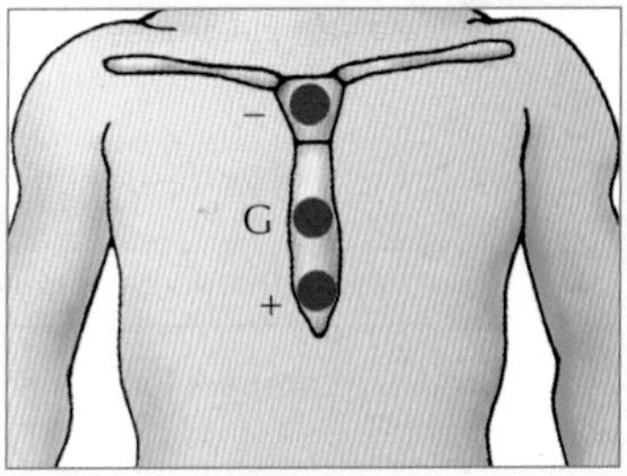

LEWIS LEAD

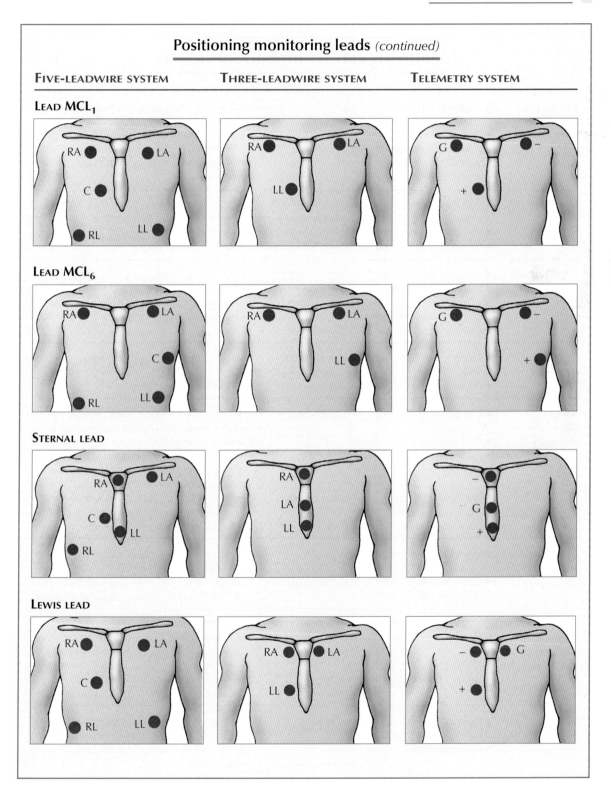

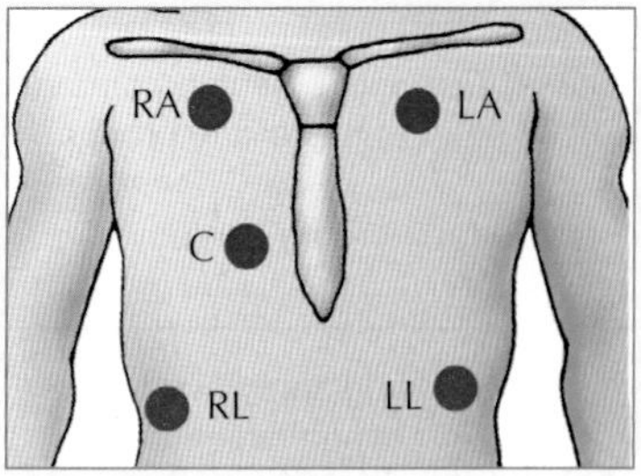

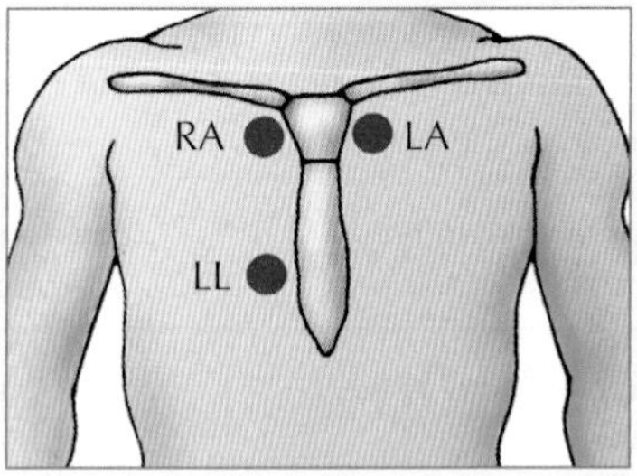

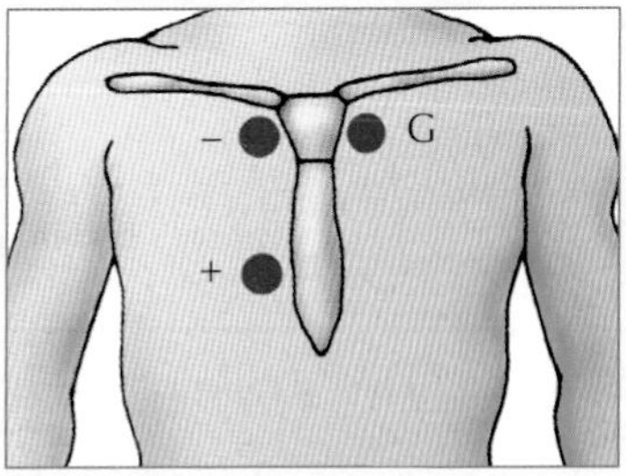

TROUBLESHOOTING

Identifying cardiac monitor problems

PROBLEM	POSSIBLE CAUSES	NURSING INTERVENTIONS
False–high-rate alarm	■ Monitor interpreting large T waves as QRS complexes, *which doubles the rate* ■ Skeletal muscle activity	■ Reposition electrodes to lead where QRS complexes are taller than T waves. ■ Place electrodes away from major muscle masses.
False–low-rate alarm	■ Shift in electrical axis from patient movement, *making QRS complexes too small to register* ■ Low amplitude of QRS ■ Poor contact between electrode and skin	■ Reapply electrodes. Set gain so height of complex is greater than 1 mV. ■ Increase gain. ■ Reapply electrodes.
Low amplitude	■ Gain dial set too low ■ Poor contact between skin and electrodes; dried gel; broken or loose leadwires; poor connection between patient and monitor; malfunctioning monitor; physiologic loss of QRS amplitude	■ Increase gain. ■ Check connections on all leadwires and monitoring cable. Replace electrodes, as necessary. Reapply electrodes, if required.
Wandering baseline	■ Poor position or contact between electrodes and skin ■ Thoracic movement with respirations	■ Reposition or replace electrodes. ■ Reposition electrodes.
Artifact (waveform interference)	■ Patient having seizures, chills, or anxiety ■ Patient movement ■ Electrodes applied improperly ■ Static electricity ■ Electrical short circuit in leadwires or cable ■ Interference from decreased room humidity	■ Notify practitioner and treat patient, as ordered. Keep patient warm and reassure him. ■ Help patient relax. ■ Check electrodes and reapply, if necessary. ■ Make sure cables don't have exposed connectors. Change static-causing bedclothes. ■ Replace broken equipment. Use stress loops when applying leadwires. ■ Regulate humidity to 40%.
Broken leadwires or cable	■ Stress loops not used on leadwires ■ Cables and leadwires cleaned with alcohol or acetone, *causing brittleness*	■ Replace leadwires and retape them, using stress loops. ■ Clean cable and leadwires with soapy water. *Do not allow cable ends to become wet.* Replace cable, as needed.
60-cycle interference (fuzzy baseline)	■ Electrical interference from other equipment in room ■ Patient's bed improperly grounded	■ Attach all electrical equipment to common ground. Check plugs to make sure prongs aren't loose. ■ Attach bed ground to room's common ground.
Skin excoriation under electrode	■ Patient allergic to electrode adhesive ■ Electrode on skin too long	■ Remove electrodes and apply hypoallergenic electrodes and hypoallergenic tape. ■ Remove electrode, clean site, and reapply electrode at new site.

strip. Tell the patient to remove the transmitter if he takes a shower or bath, but stress that he should let you know before he removes the unit.

Documentation

Record in your nurse's notes the date and time that monitoring begins and the monitoring lead used. Document a rhythm strip at least every 8 hours and with any changes in the patient's condition (or as stated by your facility's policy). Label the rhythm strip with the patient's name and room number, the date, the time, the lead recorded, and the rhythm interpreted.

SELECTED REFERENCES

American Heart Association. "Practice Standard for Electrocardiographic Monitoring in Hospital Settings," *Circulation* 110(17):2721-746, October 2004.

Jevon, P. "Cardiac Monitoring. Part 1—Electrocardiography (ECG)" *Nursing Times* 103(1):26-27, January 2007.

Lynn-McHale Wiegand, D.J., and Carlson, K.K., eds. *AACN Procedure Manual for Critical Care,* 5th ed. Philadelphia: W.B. Saunders Co., 2005.

ST-SEGMENT MONITORING

A sensitive indicator of myocardial damage, the ST segment is normally flat or isoelectric. A depressed ST segment may result from cardiac glycosides, myocardial ischemia, or a subendocardial infarction. An elevated ST segment suggests myocardial infarction.

Continuous ST-segment monitoring is helpful for patients with acute coronary syndromes and for those who have received thrombolytic therapy or have undergone coronary angioplasty or cardiac surgery. ST-segment monitoring allows early detection of reocclusion. It's also useful for patients who have had previous episodes of cardiac ischemia without chest pain, those who have difficulty distinguishing between cardiac pain and pain from other sources, and those who have difficulty communicating. ST-segment monitoring gives the practitioner the ability to identify and reverse ischemia by starting early interventions.

Because ischemia typically occurs in a single area of the heart muscle, some electrocardiogram (ECG) leads can't detect it. Select the most appropriate lead by examining ECG tracings obtained during an ischemic episode. Use the leads that show ischemia for ST-segment monitoring. ST-segment monitoring isn't useful for patients with left- or right-bundle branch block, ventricular paced rhythm, or who are restless.

Changes in the ST segment

Closely monitoring the ST segment on a patient's electrocardiogram can help you detect ischemia or injury before infarction develops.

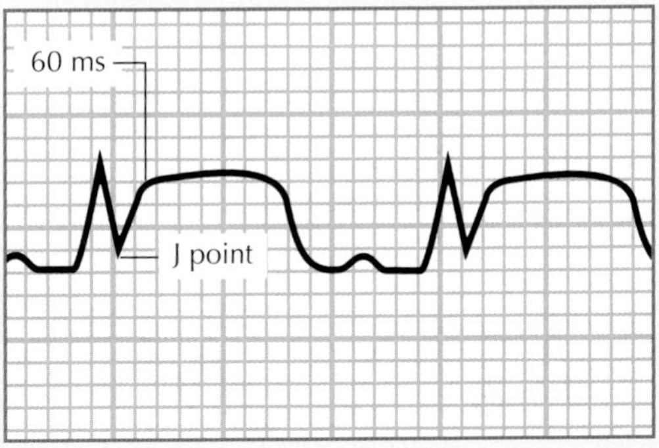

Equipment

ECG electrodes ▪ gauze pads ▪ ECG monitor cable ▪ leadwires ▪ alcohol pads ▪ cardiac monitor programmed for ST-segment monitoring.

Preparation of equipment

Plug the cardiac monitor into an electrical outlet and turn it on *to warm up while you prepare equipment and patient.*

Implementation

- Confirm the patient's identity using two patient identifiers according to your facility's policy.
- Bring the equipment to the patient's bedside and explain the procedure to him. Provide privacy.
- Wash your hands. If the patient isn't already on a monitor, turn on the device and attach the cable.
- Select the sites for electrode placement and prepare the patient's skin for attachment as you would for continuous cardiac monitoring or a 12-lead ECG. Attach the leadwires to the electrodes and position the electrodes on the patient's skin in the appropriate positions.
- Activate ST-segment monitoring by pressing the MONITORING PROCEDURES key and then the ST key. Activate individual ST parameters by pressing the ON/OFF parameter key.
- Select the appropriate ECG for each ST channel to be monitored by pressing the PARAMETERS key and then the key labeled ECG.
- Identify ECG complexes as prompted by the monitor.
- Adjust the ST point to 60 msec after the J point. (See *Changes in the ST segment.*)

Understanding changes in the ST segment

Closely monitoring the ST segment can help detect ischemia or injury before infarction develops.

ST-segment elevation

An ST segment is considered elevated when it's 1 mm or more above the baseline. An elevated ST segment may indicate myocardial injury.

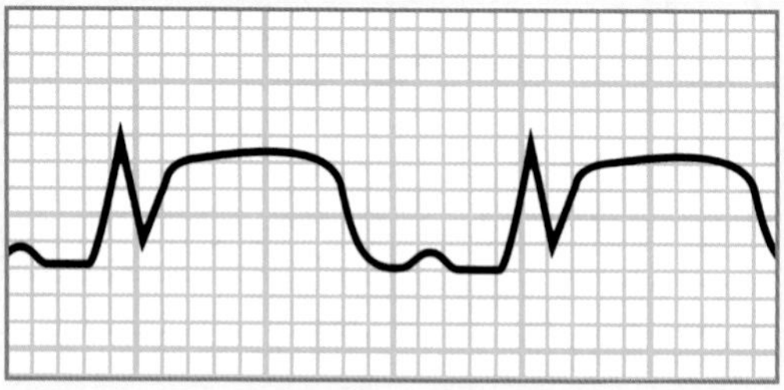

ST-segment depression

An ST segment is considered depressed when it's 0.5 mm or more below the baseline. A depressed ST segment may indicate myocardial ischemia or digoxin toxicity.

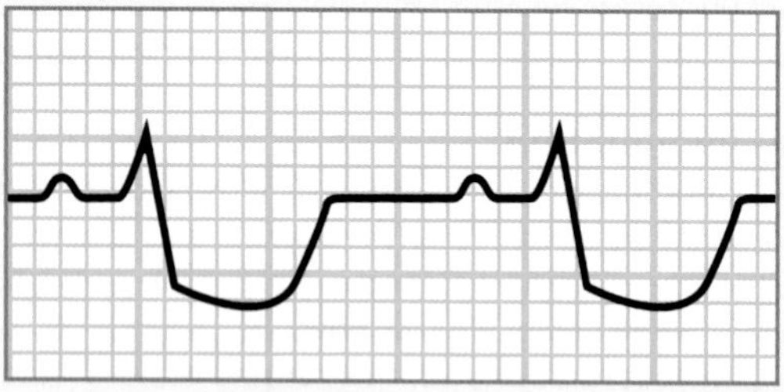

- Set the alarm limits for each ST-segment parameter by manipulating the high and low limit keys.
- Press the key labeled STANDARD DISPLAY to return to the display screen.
- Assess the waveform shown on the monitor.

Special considerations

- Be sure to abrade the patient's skin gently *to ensure electrode adhesion and promote electrical conductivity.*
- If monitoring only one lead, choose the lead most likely to show arrhythmias and ST-segment changes.

NURSING ALERT *Always give precedence to the lead that shows arrhythmias.*

- Verify limit parameters for the patient with the practitioner. Typically, when a limit is surpassed for more than 1 minute, visual and audible alarms are activated.
- Evaluate the monitor for ST-segment depression or elevation. (See *Understanding changes in the ST segment.*)
- If ischemia is noted, obtain a 12-lead ECG and assess the patient for signs and symptoms of acute ischemia, such as arrhythmias, angina, and hemodynamic changes.

Documentation

Document the leads being monitored and the ST measurement points in the patient's medical record.

SELECTED REFERENCES

Drew, B.J., et al. "AHA Scientific Statement: Practice Standards for Electrocardiographic Monitoring in Hospital Settings: An American Heart Association Scientific Statement from the Councils on Cardiovascular Nursing, Clinical Cardiology, and Cardiovascular Disease in the Young: Endorsed by the International Society of Computerized Electrocardiography and the American Association of Critical-Care Nurses," *Journal of Cardiovascular Nursing* 20(2):76-106, March-April 2005.

Flanders, S.A. "Continuous ST-segment Monitoring: Raising the Bar," *Critical Care Nursing Clinics of North America* 18(2):169-77, June 2006.

Krucoff, M.W., et al. "Clinical Utility of Serial and Continuous ST-segment Recovery Assessment in Patients with Acute ST-elevation Myocardial Infarction: Assessing the Dynamics of Epicardial and Myocardial Reperfusion," *Circulation* 110(25):e533-39, December 2004.

Landesberg, G., et al. "Myocardial Ischemia, Cardiac Troponin, and Long-term Survival of High-cardiac Risk Critically Ill Intensive Care Unit Patients," *Critical Care Medicine* 33(6):1281-287, June 2005.

Lynn-McHale Wiegand, D.J., and Carlson, K.K., eds. *AACN Procedure Manual for Critical Care,* 5th ed. Philadelphia: W.B. Saunders Co., 2005.

PULSE AMPLITUDE MONITORING

Determining the presence and strength of peripheral pulses, an essential part of cardiovascular assessment, helps you to evaluate the adequacy of peripheral perfusion. A pulse amplitude monitor simplifies this procedure. A sensor taped to the patient's skin over a pulse point sends signals to a monitor, which measures the amplitude of the pulse and displays it as a waveform on a screen. The system continuously monitors the patient's peripheral pulse so you can perform other patient care duties.

The pulse amplitude monitor can be used after peripheral vascular reconstruction on the upper or lower extremities or after percutaneous transluminal peripheral or coronary angioplasty (either with the sheaths in place or after they've been removed).

Because the sensor monitors only relatively flat pulse points, it can't be used for the posterior tibial pulse point. Also, movement distorts the waveform, so the patient must remain as still as possible during monitoring. The patient shouldn't have lesions on the skin where the pulse will be monitored because the sensor must be placed directly on this site. The sensor and tape could irritate the lesion, or the lesion could impair transmission of the pulse amplitude. If the patient has a strong peripheral pulse, you'll see an adequate waveform.

Equipment

Pulse amplitude display monitor with sensor.

Preparation of equipment

Plug the monitor into a grounded outlet. Although the monitor has battery power for up to 24 hours, it should be plugged in when the battery isn't needed.

Turn on the monitor and allow it to warm up, which may take up to 10 seconds. Plug the sensor cable into the monitor; then tap the sensor gently. *If tapping causes interference on the display screen, you can assume that the sensor-monitor connection is functioning properly.*

Implementation

- Confirm the patient's identity using two patient identifiers according to your facility's policy.
- Explain to the patient how the pulse amplitude monitor works.
- Locate the pulse you want to monitor. Mention that you'll tape the sensor to a selected site, usually the foot.
- Place the sensor over the strongest point of the pulse you're going to monitor. While observing the display screen, move the sensor until you see a strong upright waveform.
- Without moving the sensor from this site, peel off the adhesive strips and affix the sensor securely to the patient's foot. The sensor must maintain proper skin contact, so be sure to tape it firmly.
- Adjust the height of the pulse wave signal to half the height of the display screen. *This will give the waveform room to fluctuate as the pulse amplitude increases and decreases.*
- Set the low and high waveform amplitude alarms *so you'll be alerted to any waveform changes.*

Discontinuing monitor use

- Turn the machine off but keep it plugged in.
- Peel the sensor tapes from the patient's skin.
- Discard the sensor and, if necessary, wipe the monitor with a mild soap solution.

Special considerations

- Be aware that although the waveform displayed by a pulse amplitude monitor may resemble an electrocardiogram or blood pressure waveform, it isn't the same.
- Don't apply much pressure on the pulse sensor film or press on it with a sharp object *because such stress may warp or destroy the sensor.*
- Never place the sensor over an open wound or ulcerated skin.
- If waveform amplitude decreases, assess the patient's leg for capillary refill time, temperature, color, and sensation. The amplitude change may stem from a malfunction in the monitor itself (such as a low battery) or from a thrombus, a hematoma, or a significant change in the patient's hemodynamic status.
- If the display screen is blank when you turn on the machine, make sure the monitor is plugged in. If it's plugged in but the screen remains blank, the screen may need repair.
- If the screen is functioning but no waveform appears on it, first check the sensor-monitor connection. Then check the sensor by gently tapping it to see if interference appears on the screen. If the sensor is working properly, relocate the peripheral pulse on the patient's foot, and reapply the sensor. If your interventions don't work, the screen may need servicing.

Documentation

Print out a strip of the patient's waveform, and place the strip in the patient's medical record during every shift and whenever you note a change in the waveform or the patient's condition. Along the left side of the strip, you'll see a reference scale used to measure pulse amplitude height. Include this scale in your documentation. Also indicate the site where the sensor was placed.

SELECTED REFERENCES

Lee, H.S., et al. "Digital Blood Flow after Radial Artery Harvest for Coronary Artery Bypass Grafting," *Annals of Thoracic Surgery* 77(6):2071-2074, June 2004.

Sanderson, P.M., et al. "Advanced Patient Monitoring Displays: Tools for Continuous Informing," *Anesthesia and Analgesia* 101(1):161-68, July 2005.

THORACIC ELECTRICAL BIOIMPEDANCE MONITORING

A noninvasive alternative for tracking hemodynamic status, thoracic electrical bioimpedance monitoring, also known as *impedance cardiography,* provides information about a patient's cardiac index, preload, afterload, contractility, cardiac output, and blood flow.

In this procedure, electrodes are placed on the patient's thorax and serve two purposes: to send harmless low-level electricity through the patient's body and to detect return electrical signals. These signals, which are interruptions in the electrical flow, come from changes in the volume and velocity of blood as it flows through the aorta. The bioimpedance monitor interprets the signals as a waveform. Cardiac output is then computed from this waveform and the electrocardiogram (ECG).

Thoracic electrical bioimpedance monitoring eliminates the risk of infection, bleeding, pneumothorax, emboli, and arrhythmias associated with traditional invasive monitoring. The accuracy of results obtained through this method proves comparable to that obtained by thermodilution; further, the bioimpedance monitor automatically updates information every 2nd to 10th heartbeat.

Equipment

Thoracic electrical bioimpedance unit ▪ color-coded leadwires ▪ connecting cable ▪ four sets of thoracic electrical bioimpedance electrodes ▪ three ECG electrodes ▪ 4″ × 4″ gauze pads ▪ tape measure ▪ gloves.

Preparation of equipment

Explain the procedure to the patient. Wash your hands and put on gloves. Plug the thoracic electrical bioimpedance unit into a power supply; then press the POWER button. The initial display screen will appear, at which point you'll enter the patient's name, identification number, gender, central venous pressure, blood pressure, and height and weight.

Implementation

- Confirm the patient's identity using two patient identifiers according to your facility's policy.
- Help the patient onto his back with the head of the bed elevated no more than 30 degrees.
- Provide privacy and expose his chest. Then, wet some 4″ × 4″ gauze pads with warm water and clean the skin on each side of his neck from the base of the neck to 2″ (5 cm) above the base. Also clean the skin on both sides of the chest at the midaxillary line directly across the xiphoid process. *To ensure that you have cleaned a large enough area for electrode placement,* clean at least two fingerbreadths above and below the site.
- Place one electrode set vertically on the side of the neck in line with the ear. Make sure that the bottom of the electrode set isn't lower than the junction of the shoulder at the base of the neck.
- Place the second set of electrodes on the opposite side of the neck in line with the ear and about 180 degrees from the first set.
- Place the remaining two sets of electrodes on either side of the patient's chest. *To determine the correct locations,* draw a line with your finger from the xiphoid process to the midaxillary line on one side of the chest. This is the site for the first chest electrode. Make sure that the top portion of the electrode is at the level of the xiphoid process.
- Attach ECG electrodes and try different lead selections until you obtain a consistent QRS signal. Don't remove the patient from the primary monitor. *The regular system must be maintained to ensure monitoring at the central station and to keep the alarms intact.*
- Attach the leadwires to the thoracic electrical bioimpedance electrodes and the ECG electrodes.
- Next, measure the distance between the bottom of an electrode set on one side of the patient's neck and the top of an electrode set on the same side of his chest. This distance, the thorax length, is the numeric value required by the monitor's computer to calculate accurate stroke volume. Enter this value on the patient data screen. Return to the waveform screen.

Special considerations

- Baseline bioimpedance values may be reduced in patients who have conditions characterized by increased fluid in the chest, such as pulmonary edema and pleural effusion.
- Bioimpedance values may be lower than thermodilution values in patients with tachycardia and other arrhythmias.

Documentation

Note the waveforms and values on the monitor and document the values by pressing PRINT on the waveform screen. Place the strip in the patient's chart.

SELECTED REFERENCES

Albert, N.M. "Bioimpedance Cardiography Measurements of Cardiac Output and Other Cardiovascular Parameters," *Critical Care Clinics of North America* 18(2):195-202, June 2006.

Albert, N.M. "Equivalence of the Bioimpedance and Thermodilution Methods in Measuring Cardiac Output in Hospitalized Patients with Advanced, Decompensated Chronic Heart Failure," *American Journal of Critical Care* 13(6):469-76, November 2004.

Brown, C.V., et al. "The Effect of Obesity on Bioimpedance Cardiac Index," *American Journal of Surgery* 189(5):547-50, May 2005.

DeMarzo, A.P., et al. "Using Impedance Cardiography to Assess Left Ventricular Systolic Function via Postural Change in Patients with Heart Failure," *Progress in Cardiovascular Nursing* 20(4):163-67, Fall 2005.

Lynn-McHale Wiegand, D.J., and Carlson, K.K., eds. *AACN Procedure Manual for Critical Care,* 5th ed. Philadelphia: W.B. Saunders Co., 2005.

Packer, M., et al. "Utility of Impedance Cardiography for the Identification of Short-Term Risk of Clinical Decompensation in Stable Patients with Chronic Heart Failure," *Journal of American College of Cardiology* 47(11):2245-252, June 2006.

Parry, M.J., and McFetridge-Durdle, J. "Ambulatory Impedance Cardiography: A Systematic Review," *Nursing Research* 55(4):283-91, July-August 2006.

TRANSDUCER SYSTEM SETUP

The exact type of transducer system used depends on the patient's needs and the practitioner's preference. Some systems monitor pressure continuously, whereas others monitor pressure intermittently. Single-pressure transducers monitor only one type of pressure — for example, pulmonary artery pressure (PAP). Multiple-pressure transducers can monitor two or more types of pressure, such as PAP and central venous pressure.

Equipment

Bag of heparin flush solution (usually 500 ml normal saline solution with 500 or 1,000 units heparin) ▪ pressure infusion bag ▪ medication-added label ▪ preassembled disposable pressure tubing with flush device and disposable transducer ▪ monitor and monitor cable ▪ I.V. pole with transducer mount ▪ carpenter's level ▪ nonvented stopcock caps ▪ sterile gauze package.

Preparation of equipment

Turn the monitor on before gathering the equipment *to give it sufficient time to warm up.* Gather the equipment you'll need.

Implementation

- Confirm the patient's identity using two patient identifiers according to your facility's policy.
- Wash your hands.

To set up and zero a single-pressure transducer system, perform the following steps:

Setting up the system

- Follow your facility's policy on adding heparin to the flush solution. If your patient has a history of bleeding or clotting problems, use heparin with caution. Add the ordered amount of heparin to the solution — usually, 1 to 2 units of heparin/ml of solution — and then label the bag.
- Put the pressure module into the monitor, if necessary, and connect the transducer cable to the monitor.
- Remove the preassembled pressure tubing from the package. If necessary, connect the pressure tubing to the transducer. Tighten all tubing connections.
- Position all stopcocks so the flush solution flows through the entire system. Then roll the tubing's flow regulator to the OFF position.
- Spike the flush solution bag with the tubing, invert the bag, open the roller clamp, and squeeze all the air through the drip chamber. Then, compress the tubing's drip chamber, filling it no more than halfway with the flush solution.
- Place the flush solution bag into the pressure infuser bag. To do this, hang the pressure infuser bag on the I.V. pole, and then position the flush solution bag inside the pressure infuser bag. Don't inflate the pressure bag *because priming the tubing under pressure can cause air bubbles to enter the system.*
- Open the tubing's flow regulator, uncoil the tube if you haven't already done so, and remove the protective cap at the end of the pressure tubing. Squeeze the continuous flush device slowly to prime the entire system, including the stopcock ports, with the flush solution.
- As the solution nears the disposable transducer, hold the transducer at a 45-degree angle (as shown below). *This forces the solution to flow upward to the transducer. In doing so, the solution forces any air out of the system.*

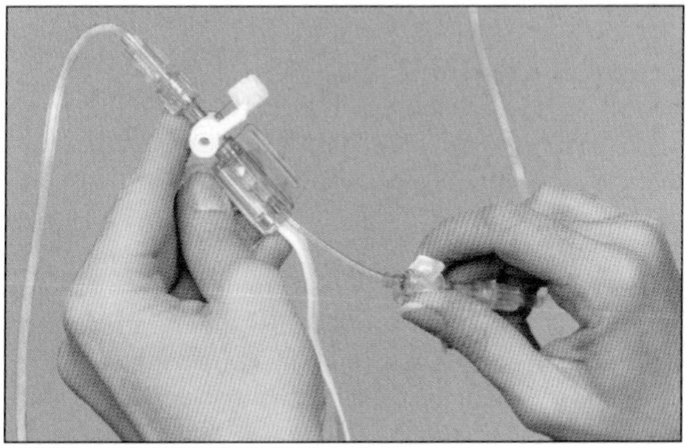

- When the solution nears a stopcock, open the stopcock to air, allowing the solution to flow into the stopcock (as shown top of next page). When the stopcock fills, close it to air and turn it open to the remainder of the tubing. Do this for each stopcock.

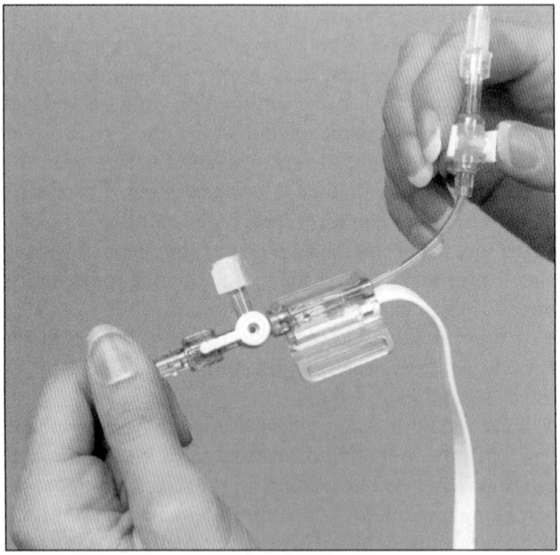

■ After removing the air from the stopcock, replace the vented cap with a nonvented cap *to prevent air from entering the system.*
■ After you've completely primed the system, replace the protective cap at the end of the tubing.
■ Inflate the pressure infusion bag to 300 mm Hg. *This bag keeps the pressure in the arterial line higher than the patient's systolic pressure, preventing blood backflow into the tubing and ensuring a continuous flow rate.* When you inflate the pressure bag, take care that the drip chamber doesn't completely fill with fluid. Afterward, flush the system again *to remove all air bubbles.*
■ If you're going to mount the transducer on an I.V. pole, insert the device into its holder.

Zeroing the system

■ Now you're ready for a preliminary zeroing of the transducer. *To ensure accuracy,* position the patient and the transducer on the same level each time you zero the transducer or record a pressure. Typically, the patient lies flat in bed, if he can tolerate that position.
■ Next, use the carpenter's level to position the air-reference stopcock or the air-fluid interface of the transducer level with the phlebostatic axis (midway between the posterior chest and the sternum at the fourth intercostal space, midaxillary line). Alternatively, you may level the air-reference stopcock or the air-fluid interface to the same position as the catheter tip.
■ After leveling the transducer, turn the stopcock next to the transducer off to the patient and open to air. Remove the cap to the stopcock port. Place the cap inside an opened sterile gauze package *to prevent contamination.*
■ Now zero the transducer. To do so, follow the manufacturer's directions for zeroing.
■ When you have finished zeroing, turn the stopcock on the transducer so that it's closed to air and open to the patient. This is the monitoring position. Replace the cap on the stopcock. You're then ready to attach the single-pressure transducer to the patient's catheter. Now you've assembled a single-pressure transducer system. The photograph below shows how the system will look.

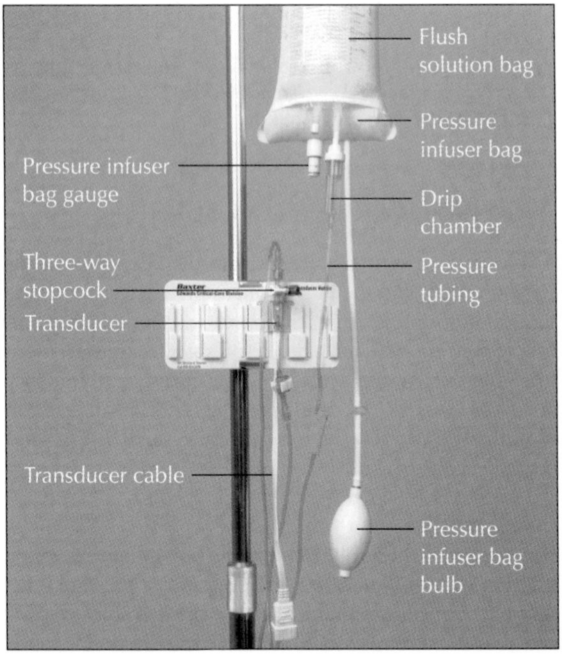

Special considerations

■ You may use any of several methods to set up a multiple-pressure transducer system. The easiest way is to add to the single-pressure system. You'll also need another bag of heparin flush solution in a second pressure infuser bag. Then you'll prime the tubing, mount the second transducer, and connect an additional cable to the monitor. Finally, you'll zero the second transducer.
■ Alternatively, your facility may use a Y-type tubing setup with two attached pressure transducers. This method requires only one bag of heparin flush solution. To set up the system, proceed as you would for a single transducer, with this exception: First, prime one branch of the Y-type tubing and then the other. Next, attach two cables to the monitor in the modules for each pressure that you'll be measuring. Finally, zero each transducer.

■ Change the heparin flush bag and the tubing every 96 hours or according to your facility's policy.

Documentation

Document the patient's position for zeroing *so that other health care team members can replicate the placement.* Document the flush solution used and the date and time of tubing changes.

SELECTED REFERENCES

"Evaluation of the Effects of Heparinized and Nonheparinized Flush Solution on the Patency of Arterial Pressure Monitoring Lines: The AACN Thunder Project. By the American Association of Critical Care Nurses," *American Journal of Critical Care* 2(1):3-15, January 1993.

Garland, J.S., et al. "The 2002 Hospital Infection Control Practices Advisory Committee Centers for Disease Control and Prevention Guideline for Prevention of Intravascular Device-related Infections," *Pediatrics* 110(5):1009-1013, November 2002.

Lynn-McHale Wiegand, D.J., and Carlson, K.K., eds. *AACN Procedure Manual for Critical Care,* 5th ed. Philadelphia: W.B. Saunders Co., 2005.

"Standard 48. Administration Set Change. Infusion Nursing Standards of Practice," *Journal of Infusion Nursing* 29(1S):S48-51, January-February 2006.

ARTERIAL PRESSURE MONITORING

Direct arterial pressure monitoring permits continuous measurement of systolic, diastolic, and mean pressures and allows arterial blood sampling. Because direct measurement reflects systemic vascular resistance as well as blood flow, it's generally more accurate than indirect methods (such as palpation and auscultation of Korotkoff's, or audible pulse, sounds), which are based on blood flow.

Direct monitoring is indicated when highly accurate or frequent blood pressure measurements are required—for example, in patients with low cardiac output and high systemic vascular resistance. It may also be used for hospitalized patients who are obese or have severe edema, if these conditions make indirect measurement hard to perform. In addition, it may be used for patients who are receiving titrated doses of vasoactive drugs or who need frequent blood sampling.

An arterial pressure monitoring system can be open or closed. An *open system* is one where you attach a syringe to the stopcock and withdraw 5 to 10 ml of blood for waste, which is then discarded and not returned to the patient. A *closed system* has an attached reservoir where you can withdraw the waste. When you're finished drawing the blood samples, you can return the blood in the reservoir to the patient.

Equipment

For catheter insertion: Gloves ■ gown ■ mask ■ protective eyewear ■ sterile gloves ■ 16G to 20G catheter (type and length depend on the insertion site, patient's size, and other anticipated uses of the line) ■ preassembled preparation kit (if available) ■ sterile drapes ■ sheet protector ■ sterile towels ■ prepared pressure transducer system ■ ordered local anesthetic ■ sutures ■ syringe and needle (21G to 25G, 1″) ■ I.V. pole ■ tubing and medication labels ■ site care kit (containing sterile dressing and hypoallergenic tape) ■ armboard ■ soft limb restraint, as needed ■ optional: electric clipper (for femoral artery insertion).

For blood sample collection: If an *open system* is in place: gloves ■ gown ■ mask ■ sterile 4″ × 4″ gauze pads ■ protective eyewear ■ sheet protector ■ Vacutainer ■ needleless Vacutainer luerlock adapter needle ■ appropriate blood specimen collection tubes ■ laboratory request forms and labels ■ sterile dead-end cap.

If a *closed system* is in place: gloves ■ gown ■ mask ■ protective eyewear ■ closed system cannula ■ syringes of appropriate size and number for ordered laboratory tests ■ laboratory request forms and labels ■ alcohol swab ■ blood transfer unit ■ appropriate blood specimen collection tubes.

For arterial line tubing changes: Gloves ■ gown ■ mask ■ protective eyewear ■ sheet protector ■ preassembled arterial pressure tubing with flush device and disposable pressure transducer ■ sterile gloves ■ 500-ml bag of I.V. flush solution (usually normal saline solution) ■ 500 or 1,000 units of heparin ■ syringe and needle (21G to 25G, 1″) ■ alcohol swabs ■ medication label ■ pressure bag ■ site care kit ■ tubing labels.

For arterial catheter removal: Gloves ■ mask ■ gown ■ protective eyewear ■ two sterile 4″ × 4″ gauze pads ■ sheet protector ■ sterile suture removal set ■ dressing ■ alcohol swabs ■ hypoallergenic tape ■ sterile container (if catheter-tip culture is ordered).

Preparation of equipment

Before setting up and priming the monitoring system, wash your hands thoroughly. Maintain asepsis by wearing personal protective equipment throughout preparation. (For instructions on setting up and priming the monitoring system, see "Transducer system setup," page 435.) Label all medications, medication containers, and other solutions on and off the sterile field.

When you have completed equipment preparation, set the alarms on the bedside monitor according to your facility's policy.

Implementation

- Confirm the patient's identity using two patient identifiers according to your facility's policy.
- Maintain asepsis by wearing personal protective equipment throughout all procedures described.
- Position the patient for easy access to the catheter insertion site. Place a sheet protector under the site.

Inserting an arterial catheter

- Explain the procedure to the patient and his family, including the purpose of arterial pressure monitoring and the anticipated duration of catheter placement. Make sure the patient signs a consent form. If he can't sign, ask a responsible family member to give written consent.
- Check the patient's history for an allergy or a hypersensitivity to iodine, heparin, or the ordered local anesthetic.
- If the catheter will be inserted into the radial artery, perform Allen's test *to assess collateral circulation in the hand.* (See "Arterial puncture for blood gas analysis," page 196.)
- Using a preassembled preparation kit, the practitioner prepares and anesthetizes the insertion site. He covers the surrounding area with either sterile drapes or towels. The catheter is then inserted into the artery and attached to the fluid-filled pressure tubing.
- While the practitioner holds the catheter in place, activate the fast-flush release *to flush blood from the catheter.* After each fast-flush operation, observe the drip chamber *to verify that the continuous flush rate is as desired.* A waveform should appear on the bedside monitor.
- The practitioner may suture the catheter in place, or you may secure it with hypoallergenic tape. Cover the insertion site with a dressing, as specified by your facility's policy.
- Immobilize the insertion site. With a radial or brachial site, use an arm board and soft wrist restraint (if the patient's condition so requires). With a femoral site, assess the need for an ankle restraint; maintain the patient on bed rest, with the head of the bed raised no more than 30 degrees, *to prevent the catheter from kinking.* Level the zeroing stopcock of the transducer with the phlebostatic axis. Then zero the system to atmospheric pressure.
- Activate monitor alarms, as appropriate.

Obtaining a blood sample from an open system

- Assemble the equipment, taking care not to contaminate the equipment.
- Attach the needleless luerlock adapter needle to the Vacutainer.
- Turn off or temporarily silence the monitor alarms, depending on your facility's policy. (Some facilities require that alarms be left on.)
- Locate the blood sampling port of the stopcock nearest the patient. Remove the dead-end cap from the stopcock.
- Connect the needleless adapter of the Vacutainer into the sampling port of the stopcock and turn the stopcock off to the flush solution. Attach a blood specimen collection tube for the discard sample into the stopcock. (*This sample is discarded because it's diluted with flush solution.*) Follow your facility's policy on how much discard blood to collect. In most cases, you'll withdraw 5 to 10 ml.
- Remove the discard-specimen blood collection tube from the Vacutainer.
- Attach each blood specimen collection tube into the Vacutainer, keeping the stopcock turned off to the flush solution. Because the Vacutainer is a nonvented system, there won't be any backflow of blood from the patient. If the practitioner has ordered coagulation tests, obtain blood for this sample from the final syringe *to prevent dilution from the flush device.*
- After you've obtained blood for the final sample, turn the stopcock off to the sampling port and activate the fast-flush release *to clear the tubing.*
- Turn the stopcock off to the patient and attach an empty blood specimen collection tube, or place a sterile 4″ × 4″ gauze pad beneath the sampling port of the stopcock and activate the fast-flush release *to clear stopcock port of any remaining blood.*
- Turn the stopcock off to the stopcock port, and remove the Vacutainer. Place a new sterile dead-end cap on the blood sampling port. Reactivate the monitor alarms.
- Label all blood specimen collection tubes with correct labels. Send all samples to the laboratory with appropriate documentation.
- Check the monitor for return of the arterial waveform and pressure reading. (See *Understanding the arterial waveform.*)

Obtaining a blood sample from a closed system

- Assemble the equipment, maintaining sterile technique. Locate the closed-system reservoir and blood sampling site.
- Deactivate or temporarily silence monitor alarms. (However, some facilities require that alarms be left on.)
- Holding the reservoir upright, grasp the flexures and slowly fill the reservoir with blood over a 3- to 5-second period. *(This blood serves as discard blood.)* If you feel resistance, reposition the affected extremity, and check the catheter site for obvious problems (such as kinking). Then resume blood withdrawal.
- Turn the one-way valve off to the reservoir by turning the handle perpendicular to the tubing. Clean the sampling site with an alcohol swab. Using a syringe with an attached cannula, insert the cannula into the sampling site. (Make sure

Understanding the arterial waveform

Normal arterial blood pressure produces a characteristic waveform, representing ventricular systole and diastole. The waveform has five distinct components: the anacrotic limb, systolic peak, dicrotic limb, dicrotic notch, and end diastole.

The *anacrotic limb* marks the waveform's initial upstroke, which results as blood is rapidly ejected from the ventricle through the open aortic valve into the aorta. The rapid ejection causes a sharp rise in arterial pressure, which appears as the waveform's highest point. This is called the *systolic peak.*

As blood continues into the peripheral vessels, arterial pressure falls, and the waveform begins a downward trend. This part is called the *dicrotic limb.* Arterial pressure usually will continue to fall until pressure in the ventricle is less than pressure in the aortic root. When this occurs, the aortic valve closes. This event appears as a small notch (the *dicrotic notch*) on the waveform's downside. When the aortic valve closes, diastole begins, progressing until the aortic root pressure gradually descends to its lowest point. On the waveform, this is known as *end diastole.*

Normal arterial waveform

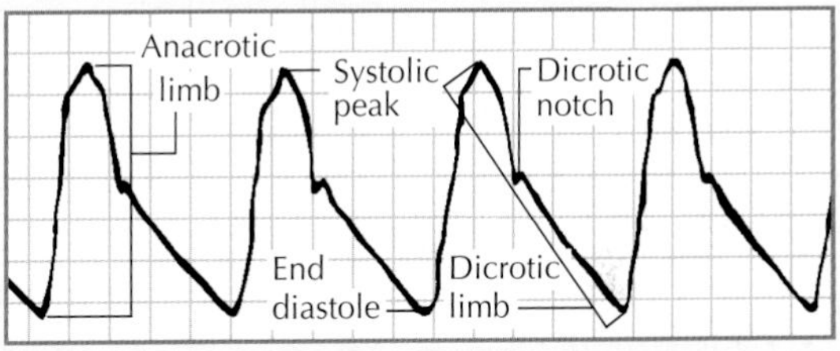

the plunger is depressed to the bottom of the syringe barrel.) Slowly fill the syringe. Repeat the procedure as needed to fill the required number of syringes. Then grasp the cannula near the sampling site, and remove the syringe and cannula as one unit. If the practitioner has ordered coagulation tests, obtain blood for those tests from the final syringe *to prevent dilution from the flush solution.*
- After filling the syringes, turn the one-way valve to its original position, parallel to the tubing. Smoothly and evenly push down on the plunger until the flexures lock in place in the fully closed position and all fluid has been reinfused. The fluid should be reinfused over a 3- to 5-second period. Then activate the fast-flush release *to clear blood from the tubing and reservoir.*
- Clean the sampling site with an alcohol swab. Reactivate the monitor alarms. Using the blood transfer unit, transfer blood samples to the appropriate blood specimen collection tubes, labeling them according to your facility's policy. Send all samples to the laboratory with appropriate documentation.

Changing arterial line tubing
- Wash your hands and follow standard precautions. Assemble the new pressure monitoring system.
- Consult your facility's policy and procedure manual *to determine how much tubing length to change.*
- Position the patient for easy access to the catheter site. Place a sheet protector under the site.
- Inflate the pressure bag to 300 mm Hg, and check it for air leaks. Then release the pressure.
- Prepare the I.V. flush solution, and prime the pressure tubing and transducer system. At this time, add both medication and tubing labels. Apply 300 mm Hg of pressure to the system. Then hang the I.V. bag on a pole.
- Remove the dressing from the catheter insertion site, taking care not to dislodge the catheter or cause vessel trauma. Turn off or temporarily silence the monitor alarms. (However, some facilities require that alarms be left on.)
- Turn off the flow clamp of the tubing segment that you'll change. Disconnect the tubing from the catheter hub, taking care not to dislodge the catheter. Immediately insert new tubing into the catheter hub. Secure the tubing and then activate the fast-flush release to clear it.
- Reactivate the monitor alarms. Apply an appropriate dressing.
- Level the zeroing stopcock of the transducer with the phlebostatic axis, and zero the system to atmospheric pressure.

Removing an arterial line
- Consult your facility's policy *to determine whether you're permitted to perform this procedure.*
- Check the patient's coagulation studies prior to removal of the catheter *to determine if pressure will need to be held for a longer time in order to achieve hemostasis.*
- Explain the procedure to the patient.
- Assemble all equipment. Wash your hands. Observe standard precautions, including wearing personal protective equipment, for this procedure.

Recognizing abnormal waveforms

Understanding a normal arterial waveform is relatively straightforward. An abnormal waveform, however, is more difficult to decipher. Abnormal patterns and markings may provide important diagnostic clues to the patient's cardiovascular status, or they may simply signal trouble in the monitor. Use this chart to help you recognize and resolve waveform abnormalities.

Abnormality	Possible causes	Nursing interventions
Alternating high and low waves in a regular pattern 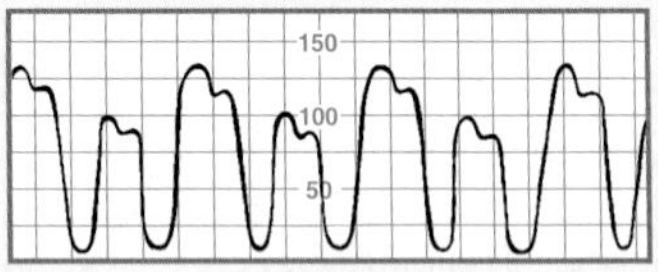 	Ventricular bigeminy Cardiac tamponade	■ Check the patient's electrocardiogram to confirm ventricular bigeminy. The tracing should reflect premature ventricular contractions every second beat. ■ Assess the patient for signs of tamponade.
Flattened waveform 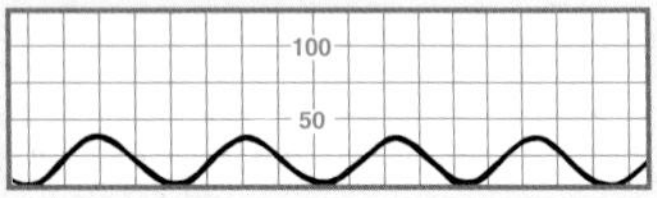 	Overdamped waveform or hypotensive patient	■ Check the dynamic response or square wave test. An overdampened waveform should be suspected if a slurred upstroke occurs at the beginning of the wave and after the initial downstroke if there's a loss of oscillations. Check for kinks or obstructions in the line or tubing. Clear the line of air or blood. Repeat the square wave test *to verify optimal waveform*. ■ If the square wave test indicates optimal waveform, assess and treat the patient for hypotension.
Slightly rounded waveform with consistent variations in systolic height 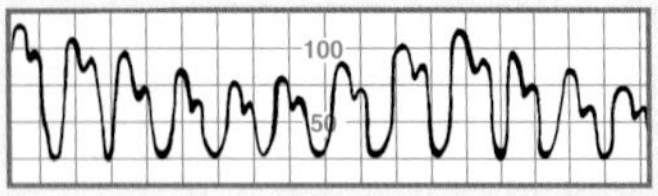 	Patient on ventilator with positive end-expiratory pressure	■ Check the patient's systolic blood pressure regularly. The difference between the highest and lowest systolic pressure reading should be less than 10 mm Hg. If the difference exceeds that amount, suspect pulsus paradoxus, possibly from cardiac tamponade.
Slow upstroke 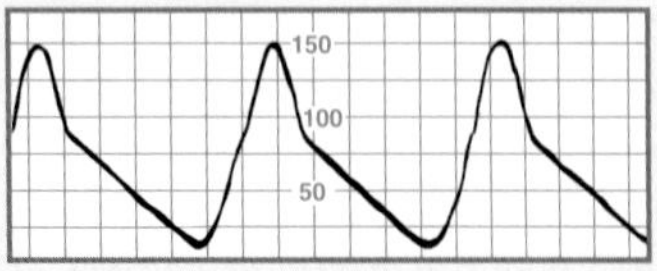 	Aortic stenosis	■ Check the patient's heart sounds for signs of aortic stenosis. Also notify the practitioner, who will document suspected aortic stenosis in his notes.
Diminished amplitude on inspiration 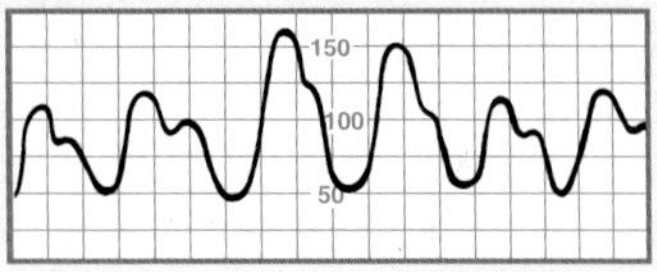 	Pulsus paradoxus, possibly from cardiac tamponade, constrictive pericarditis, or lung disease	■ Note systolic pressure during inspiration and expiration. If inspiratory pressure is at least 10 mm Hg less than expiratory pressure, call the practitioner. ■ If you're also monitoring pulmonary artery pressure, observe for a diastolic plateau. This occurs when the mean central venous pressure (right atrial pressure), mean pulmonary artery pressure, and mean pulmonary artery wedge pressure (pulmonary artery obstructive pressure) are within 5 mm Hg of one another.

- Record the patient's systolic, diastolic, and mean blood pressures. If a manual, indirect blood pressure hasn't been assessed recently, obtain one now *to establish a new baseline.*
- Turn off the monitor alarms. Then turn off the flow clamp to the flush solution.
- Carefully remove the dressing over the insertion site. Remove any sutures, using the suture removal kit, and then carefully check that all sutures have been removed.
- Withdraw the catheter using a gentle, steady motion. Keep the catheter parallel to the artery during withdrawal *to reduce the risk of traumatic injury.*
- Immediately after withdrawing the catheter, apply pressure to the site with a sterile 4" × 4" gauze pad. Maintain pressure for at least 5 minutes (longer if bleeding or oozing persists). Apply additional pressure to a femoral site or if the patient has coagulopathy or is receiving anticoagulants. In some facilities, a compression device may be used to apply pressure to the femoral site.
- Apply a pressure dressing to the site *to help prevent rebleeding.*
- If the practitioner has ordered a culture of the catheter tip (*to diagnose a suspected infection*), gently place the catheter tip on a 4" × 4" sterile gauze pad. When the bleeding is under control, hold the catheter over the sterile container. Using sterile scissors, cut the tip so it falls into the sterile container. Label the specimen and send it to the laboratory.
- Observe the site for bleeding. Assess circulation in the extremity distal to the site by evaluating color, pulses, and sensation. Repeat this assessment every 15 minutes for the first 4 hours, every 30 minutes for the next 2 hours, then hourly for the next 6 hours.

Special considerations

- Observing the pressure waveform on the monitor can enhance assessment of arterial pressure. An abnormal waveform may reflect an arrhythmia (such as atrial fibrillation) or other cardiovascular problems, such as aortic stenosis, aortic insufficiency, pulsus alternans, or pulsus paradoxus. (See *Recognizing abnormal waveforms.*)
- Assess the site for signs of infection, such as redness and swelling. Notify the practitioner if you see these signs.
- Change the pressure tubing every 96 hours, or according to your facility's policy. Change the dressing at the catheter site at intervals specified by your facility's policy.
- Be aware that erroneous pressure readings may result from a catheter that's clotted or positional, loose connections, addition of extra stopcocks or extension tubing, inadvertent entry of air into the system, or improper calibrating, leveling, or zeroing of the monitoring system. If the catheter lumen clots, the flush system may be improperly pressurized. Regularly assess the amount of flush solution in the I.V. bag, and maintain 300 mm Hg of pressure in the pressure bag.

Complications

Direct arterial pressure monitoring can cause such complications as arterial bleeding, infection, air embolism, arterial spasm, or thrombosis.

Documentation

Document the date of system setup *so that all caregivers will know when to change the components.* Document the dynamic response or square wave test every 8 to 12 hours *to verify the accuracy of the waveforms and readings.* (See *Square wave test,* page 442.)

Document systolic, diastolic, and mean pressure readings as well. Record circulation in the extremity distal to the site by assessing color, pulses, and sensation. Carefully document the amount of flush solution infused *to avoid hypervolemia and volume overload, and to ensure accurate assessment of the patient's fluid status.*

Make sure the position of the patient is documented when each blood pressure reading is obtained. *This is important for determining trends.*

Document the date and time the catheter was removed, how long pressure was held, and any complications encountered.

SELECTED REFERENCES

Centers for Disease Control and Prevention. "Guidelines for the Prevention of Intravascular Catheter-Related Infections." *MMWR* 51(RR-10):1-26, August 2002.

Giuliano, K.K., and Kleinpell, R. "The Use of Common Continuous Monitoring Parameters: A Quality Indicator for Critically Ill Patients with Sepsis," *AACN Clinical Issues* 16(2):140-48, April-June 2005.

Lynn-McHale Wiegand, D.J., and Carlson, K.K., eds. *AACN Procedure Manual for Critical Care,* 5th ed. Philadelphia: W.B. Saunders Co., 2005.

Murphy, G.S., et al. "Retrograde Air Embolization during Routine Radial Artery Catheter Flushing in Adult Cardiac Surgical Patients: An Ultrasound Study," *Anesthesiology* 101(3):614-19, September 2004.

"Standard 48. Administration Set Change. Infusion Nursing Standards of Practice," *Journal of Infusion Nursing* 29(1S):S48-51, January-February 2006.

Task Force of the American College of Critical Care Medicine, Society of Critical Medicine. "Practice Parameters for Hemodynamic Support of Sepsis in Adult Patients: 2004 Update," *Critical Care Medicine* 32(9):1928-948, September 2004.

Square wave test

When using a pressure monitoring system, you must ensure and document the system's accuracy. Along with leveling and zeroing the system to atmospheric pressure at the phlebostatic axis and interpreting waveforms, you can ensure accuracy by performing the square wave test (or dynamic response test). To perform the test:

- Activate the fast-flush device for 1 second, and then release. Obtain a graphic printout.
- Observe for the desired response: the pressure wave rises rapidly, squares off, and is followed by a series of oscillations. (See illustration below.)
- Know that these oscillations should have an initial downstroke, which extends below the baseline and just 1 to 2 oscillations after the initial downstroke. Usually, but not always, the first upstroke is about one-third the height of the initial downstroke.
- Be aware that the intervals between oscillations should be no more than 0.04 to 0.08 second (1 to 2 small boxes).

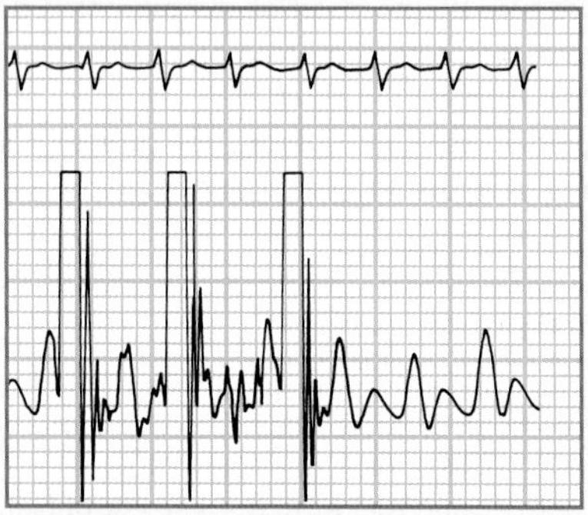

Underdamped square wave

If you observe extra oscillations after the initial downstroke or more than 0.08 second between oscillations, the waveform is underdamped. (See illustration at top of next column.) This can cause falsely high-pressure readings and artifact in the waveforms. It can be corrected by:

- removing excess tubing or extra stopcocks from the system
- inserting a damping device (available from pressure tubing companies)
- dampening the wave by inserting a small air bubble at the transducer stopcock.

Repeat the square wave test, read the pressure waveform, and then remove the small air bubble.

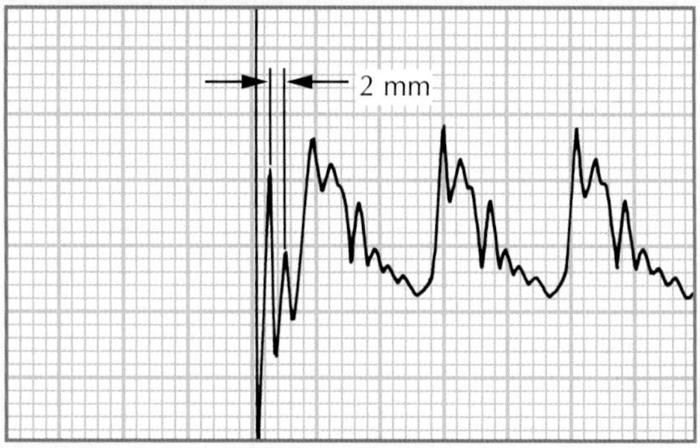

Overdamped square wave

If you observe a slurred upstroke at the beginning of the square wave and a loss of oscillations after the initial downstroke, the waveform is overdamped. (See illustration below.) This can cause falsely low pressure readings, and you can lose the sharpness of waveform peaks and the dicrotic notch. It can be corrected by:

- clearing the line of any blood or air
- checking to make sure there are no kinks or obstructions in the line
- ensuring that you're using short, low-compliance tubing.

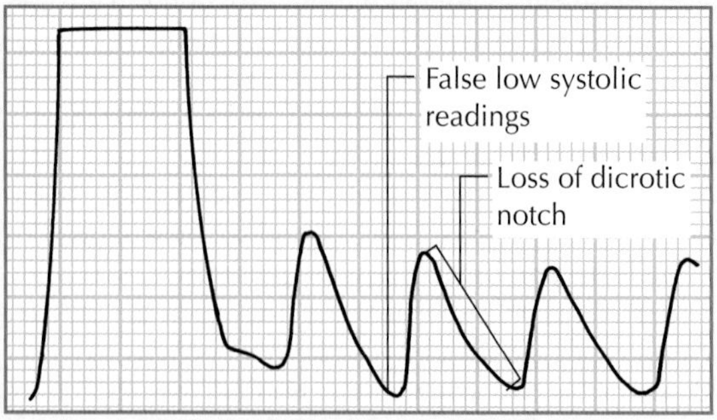

Adapted with permission from Quaal, S.J. "Improving the Accuracy of Pulmonary Artery Catheter Measurements," *Journal of Cardiovascular Nursing* 15(2):71-82, January 2001. © 2001 Aspen Publishers.

PAP AND PAWP MONITORING

Continuous pulmonary artery pressure (PAP) and intermittent pulmonary artery wedge pressure (PAWP) measurements provide important information about left ventricular function and preload. You can use this information not only for monitoring but also for aiding diagnosis, refining your assessment, guiding interventions, and projecting patient outcomes.

Nearly all acutely ill patients are candidates for PAP monitoring—especially those who are hemodynamically unstable, who need fluid management or continuous cardiopulmonary assessment, or who are receiving multiple or frequently administered cardioactive drugs. There are several clinical conditions for which the use of a pulmonary artery (PA) catheter is generally recommended. These include:

- assessment of intravascular volume, particularly in patients with severe pulmonary edema, heart failure, or oliguric renal failure
- guide for therapy in severe refractory shock or multiorgan failure
- guide for therapy to maximize oxygen delivery to tissues in selected patients.

The original PAP monitoring catheter, which had two lumens, was invented by two physicians, Swan and Ganz. The device still bears their name (Swan-Ganz catheter) but is commonly referred to as a PA catheter. Current versions have up to six lumens, allowing more hemodynamic information to be gathered. In addition to distal and proximal lumens used to measure pressures, a PA catheter has a balloon inflation lumen that inflates the balloon for PAWP measurement and a thermistor connector lumen that allows cardiac output measurement. Some catheters also have a pacemaker wire lumen that provides a port for pacemaker electrodes and measures continuous mixed venous oxygen saturation. (See *PA catheters: From basic to complex*, page 444.)

Fluoroscopy usually isn't required during catheter insertion because the catheter is flow directed, following venous blood flow from the right heart chambers into the pulmonary artery. Also, the pulmonary artery, right atrium, and right ventricle produce characteristic pressures and waveforms that can be observed on the monitor to help track catheter-tip location. Marks on the catheter shaft, with 10-cm graduations, assist tracking by showing how far the catheter is inserted.

The PA catheter is inserted into the heart's right side with the distal tip lying in the pulmonary artery. Left-sided pressures can be assessed indirectly.

No specific contraindications for PAP monitoring exist. However, some patients undergoing it require special precautions. These include elderly patients with pulmonary hypertension, those with left bundle-branch heart block, and those for whom a systemic infection would be life-threatening.

Equipment

Balloon-tipped, flow-directed PA catheter ▪ prepared pressure transducer system ▪ sterile gloves ▪ I.V. solutions ▪ alcohol pads ▪ medication-added label ▪ monitor and monitor cable ▪ I.V. pole with transducer mount ▪ emergency resuscitation equipment ▪ electrocardiogram (ECG) monitor ▪ ECG electrodes ▪ armboard (for antecubital insertion) ▪ lead aprons (if fluoroscope is necessary) ▪ sterile marker ▪ sterile labels ▪ sutures ▪ sterile 4″ × 4″ gauze pads or dry, occlusive dressing material ▪ prepackaged introducer kit ▪ optional: dextrose 5% in water, electric clippers (for femoral insertion site), small sterile basin, sterile water.

If a prepackaged introducer kit is unavailable, obtain the following: an introducer (one size larger than the catheter) ▪ sterile tray containing instruments for procedure ▪ masks ▪ sterile gowns ▪ sterile gloves ▪ sterile drape ▪ 2% chlorhexidine solution ▪ sutures ▪ two 10-ml syringes ▪ local anesthetic (1% to 2% lidocaine) ▪ one 5-ml syringe ▪ 25G ½″ needle ▪ 1″ and 3″ tape.

Preparation of equipment

To obtain reliable pressure values and clear waveforms, the pressure monitoring system and bedside monitor must be properly calibrated and zeroed. Make sure the monitor has the correct pressure modules; then calibrate it according to the manufacturer's instructions. (For instructions, see "Transducer system setup," page 435.)

Turn the monitor on before gathering the equipment *to give it time to warm up*. Be sure to check the operations manual for the monitor you're using; some older monitors may need 20 minutes to warm up.

Prepare the pressure monitoring system according to policy. Your facility's guidelines may also specify whether to mount the transducer on the I.V. pole or tape it to the patient and whether to add heparin to the flush. *To manage complications from catheter insertion,* be sure to have emergency resuscitation equipment on hand (defibrillator, oxygen, and supplies for intubation and emergency drug administration).

Prepare a sterile field for insertion of the introducer and catheter. Label all medications, medication containers, and solutions on and off the sterile field.

Implementation

- Confirm the patient's identity using two patient identifiers according to your facility's policy.
- Check the patient's chart for heparin sensitivity, which contraindicates adding heparin to the flush solution.

EQUIPMENT

PA catheters: From basic to complex

Depending on the intended uses, pulmonary artery (PA) catheters may be simple or complex. A basic PA catheter has a distal and a proximal lumen, a thermistor, and a balloon inflation gate valve. The *distal lumen,* which exits in the pulmonary artery, monitors PA pressure. Its hub usually is marked P DISTAL or is color-coded yellow. The *proximal lumen* exits in the right atrium or vena cava, depending on the size of the patient's heart. It monitors right atrial pressure and can be used as the injected solution lumen for cardiac output determination and infusing solutions. The proximal lumen hub usually is marked PROXIMAL or is color-coded blue.

The *thermistor,* located about 1½" (4 cm) from the distal tip, measures temperature (aiding core temperature evaluation) and allows cardiac output measurement. The thermistor connector attaches to a cardiac output connector cable, then to a cardiac output monitor. Typically, it's red.

The *balloon inflation gate valve* is used for inflating the balloon tip with air. A stopcock connection, typically color-coded red, may be used.

Additional lumens

Complex PA catheters have additional lumens used to obtain other hemodynamic data or permit certain interventions. For instance, *a proximal infusion port,* which exits in the right atrium or vena cava, allows additional fluid administration. A *right ventricular lumen,* exiting in the right ventricle, allows fluid administration, right ventricular pressure measurement, or use of a temporary ventricular pacing lead.

Other complex PA catheters have additional right atrial and right ventricular lumens for atrioventricular pacing. A *right ventricular ejection fraction test-response thermistor,* with PA and right ventricular sensing electrodes, allows volumetric and ejection fraction measurements. Fiber-optic filaments, such as those used in pulse oximetry, exit into the pulmonary artery and permit measurement of continuous mixed venous oxygen saturation.

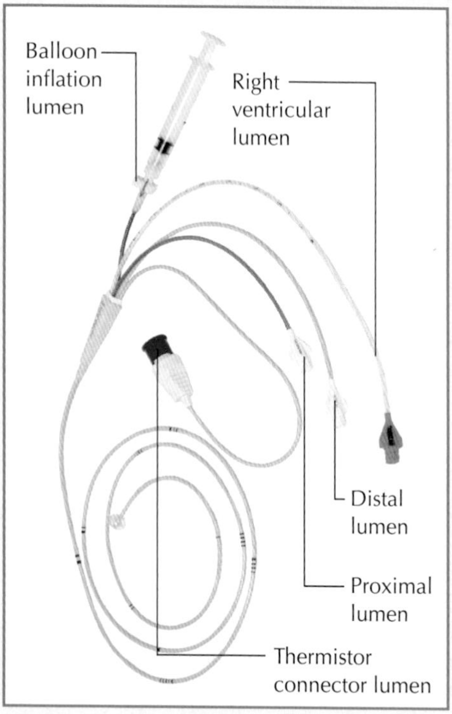

■ If the patient is alert, explain the procedure to him *to reduce his anxiety.* Reassure him that the catheter poses little danger and rarely causes pain. Tell him that if he feels pain at the introducer insertion site, the physician will order an analgesic or a sedative.

■ Be sure to tell the patient and his family not to be alarmed if they see the pressure waveform on the monitor "move around." Explain that the cause is usually artifact.

Positioning the patient for catheter placement

■ Position the patient at the proper height and angle. If the physician will use a superior approach for percutaneous insertion (most commonly using the internal jugular or subclavian vein), place the patient flat or in a slight Trendelenburg position. Remove the patient's pillow *to help engorge the vessel and prevent air embolism.* Turn his head to the side opposite the insertion site.

■ If the physician will use an inferior approach to access a femoral vein, position the patient flat. Be aware that with this approach, certain catheters are harder to insert and may require more manipulation.

Preparing the catheter

■ Maintain aseptic technique and use standard precautions throughout catheter preparation and insertion.

■ Wash your hands. Then clean the insertion site with a 2% chlorhexidine solution and drape it.
■ Put on a mask. Help the physician put on a sterile mask, gown, and gloves.
■ Open the outer packaging of the catheter, revealing the inner sterile wrapping. Using sterile technique, the physician opens the inner wrapping and picks up the catheter. Take the catheter lumen hubs as he hands them to you.
■ *To remove air from the catheter and verify its patency,* flush the catheter. In the more common flushing method, you connect the syringes aseptically to the appropriate pressure lines, and then flush them before insertion. *This method makes pressure waveforms easier to identify on the monitor during insertion.*
■ Alternatively, you may flush the lumens after catheter insertion with sterile I.V. solution from sterile syringes attached to the lumens. Leave the filled syringes on during insertion.
■ If the system has multiple pressure lines (such as a distal line to monitor PAP and a proximal line to monitor right atrial pressure), make sure the distal PA lumen hub is attached to the pressure line that will be observed on the monitor. *Inadvertently attaching the distal PA line to the proximal lumen hub will prevent the proper waveform from appearing during insertion.*
■ *To verify the integrity of the balloon,* the physician inflates it with air (usually 1.5 cc) before handing you the lumens to attach to the pressure monitoring system. He then observes the balloon for symmetrical shape. He may also submerge it in a small, sterile basin filled with sterile water and observe it for bubbles, *which indicate a leak.*

Inserting the catheter

■ Assist the physician as he inserts the introducer to access the vessel. He may perform a cutdown or (more commonly) insert the catheter percutaneously, as with a modified Seldinger technique.
■ After the introducer is placed and the catheter lumens are flushed, the physician inserts the catheter through the introducer. In the internal jugular or subclavian approach, he inserts the catheter into the end of the introducer sheath with the balloon deflated, directing the curl of the catheter toward the patient's midline.
■ As insertion begins, observe the bedside monitor for waveform variations. (See *Normal PA waveforms,* page 446.)
■ Observe the diastolic values carefully during insertion. Make sure the scale is appropriate for lower pressures. A scale of 0 to 20 mm Hg or 0 to 40 mm Hg (more common) is preferred. (With a higher scale, such as 0 to 100 or 0 to 250 mm Hg, waveforms appear too small and the location of the catheter tip will be hard to identify.)
■ When the catheter exits the end of the introducer sheath and reaches the junction of the superior vena cava and right atrium (at the 15- to 20-cm mark on the catheter shaft), the monitor shows oscillations that correspond to the patient's respirations. The balloon is then inflated with the recommended volume of air *to allow normal blood flow and aid catheter insertion.*
■ Using a gentle, smooth motion, the physician advances the catheter through the heart chambers, moving rapidly to the pulmonary artery *because prolonged manipulation may reduce catheter stiffness.*
■ When the mark on the catheter shaft reaches 15 to 20 cm, the catheter enters the right atrium. The waveform shows two small, upright waves; pressure is low (between 2 and 4 mm Hg). Read pressure values in the mean mode *because systolic and diastolic values are similar.*
■ The physician advances the catheter into the right ventricle, working quickly *to minimize irritation.* The waveform now shows sharp systolic upstrokes and lower diastolic dips. Depending on the size of the patient's heart, the catheter should reach the 30- to 35-cm mark. (The smaller the heart, the shorter the catheter length needed to reach the right ventricle.) Record both systolic and diastolic pressures. Systolic pressure normally ranges from 15 to 25 mm Hg; diastolic pressure, from 0 to 8 mm Hg.
■ As the catheter floats into the pulmonary artery, note that the upstroke from right ventricular systole is smoother, and systolic pressure is nearly the same as right ventricular systolic pressure. Record systolic, diastolic, and mean pressures (typically ranging from 8 to 15 mm Hg). A dicrotic notch on the diastolic portion of the waveform indicates pulmonic valve closure.

Wedging the catheter

■ To obtain a wedge tracing, the physician lets the inflated balloon float downstream with the blood flow to a smaller, more distal branch of the pulmonary artery. Here, the catheter lodges, or wedges, causing occlusion of right ventricular and PA diastolic pressures. The tracing resembles the right atrial tracing *because the catheter tip is recording left atrial pressure.* The waveform shows two small uprises. Record PAWP in the mean mode (usually between 6 and 12 mm Hg).
■ A PAWP waveform, or wedge tracing, appears when the catheter has been inserted 45 to 50 cm. (In a large heart, a longer catheter length—up to 55 cm—typically is required. However, a catheter should never be inserted more than 60 cm.) Usually, 30 to 45 seconds elapse from the time the physician inserts the introducer until the wedge tracing appears.
■ The physician deflates the balloon, and the catheter drifts out of the wedge position and into the pulmonary artery, its normal resting place.
■ If the appropriate waveforms don't appear at the expected times during catheter insertion, the catheter may be coiled

Normal PA waveforms

During pulmonary artery (PA) catheter insertion, the waveforms on the monitor change as the catheter advances through the heart.

Right atrium

When the catheter tip enters the right atrium, the first heart chamber on its route, a waveform like the one shown below appears on the monitor. Note the two small upright waves. The *a* waves represent the right ventricular end-diastolic pressure; the *v* waves, right atrial filling.

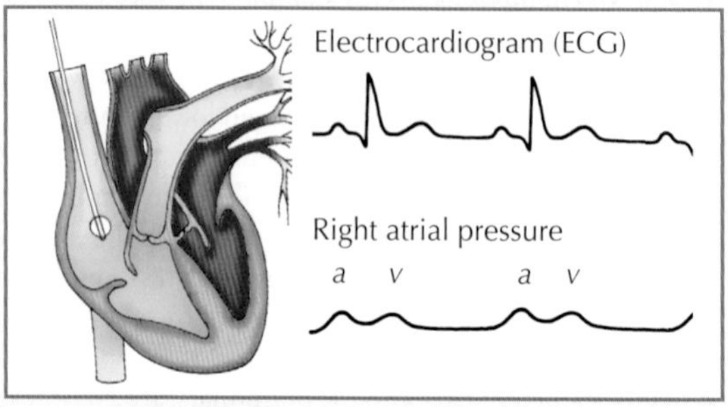

Right ventricle

As the catheter tip reaches the right ventricle, you'll see a waveform with sharp systolic upstrokes and lower diastolic dips, as shown below.

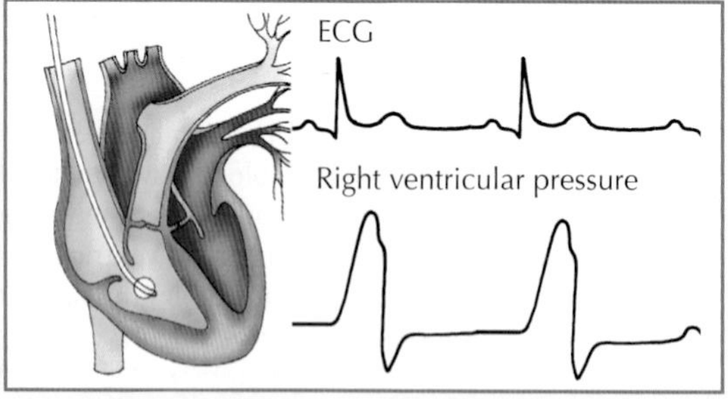

Pulmonary artery

The catheter then floats into the pulmonary artery, causing a pulmonary artery pressure (PAP) waveform such as the one shown below. Note that the upstroke is smoother than on the right ventricle waveform. The dicrotic notch indicates pulmonic valve closure.

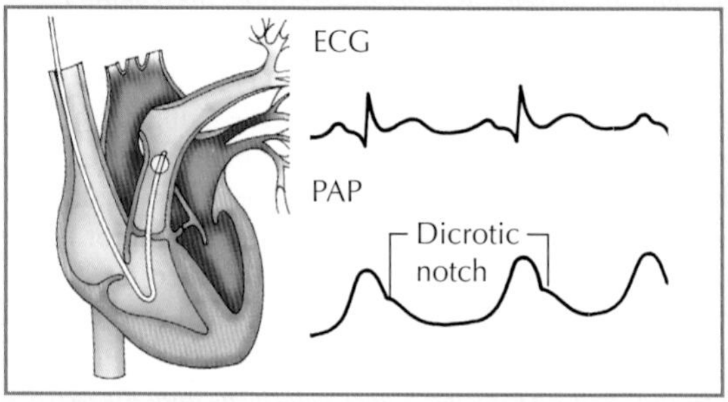

PAWP

Floating into a distal branch of the pulmonary artery, the balloon wedges where the vessel becomes too narrow for it to pass. The monitor now shows a pulmonary artery wedge pressure (PAWP) waveform, with two small upright waves, as shown below. The *a* wave represents left ventricular end-diastolic pressure; the *v* wave, left atrial filling. The balloon is then deflated, and the catheter is left in the pulmonary artery.

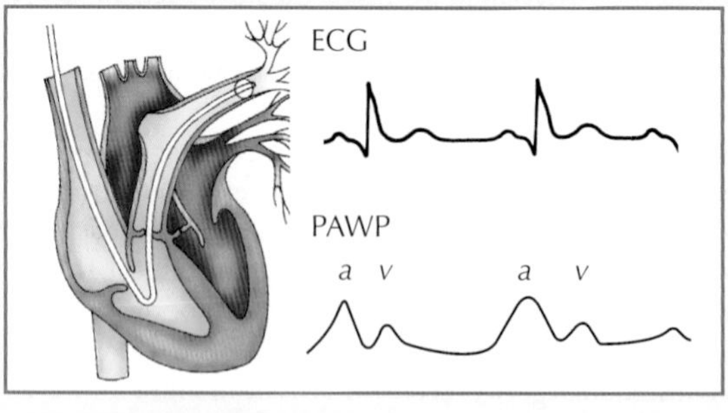

in the right atrium and ventricle. To correct this problem, deflate the balloon. To do this, unlock the gate valve or turn the stopcock to the ON position and then detach the syringe from the balloon inflation port. Back pressure in the pulmonary artery causes the balloon to deflate on its own. (Active air withdrawal may compromise balloon integrity.) *To verify balloon deflation,* observe the monitor for return of the PA tracing.

- Typically, the physician orders a portable chest X-ray *to confirm catheter position.*
- Apply a sterile occlusive dressing to the insertion site.

Obtaining intermittent PAP values

- After inserting the catheter and recording initial pressure readings, record subsequent PAP values and monitor waveforms. These values will be used to calculate other important hemodynamic indices. *To ensure accurate values,* make sure the transducer is properly leveled and zeroed at the phlebostatic axis.
- If possible, obtain PAP values at end expiration (when the patient completely exhales). *At this time, intrathoracic pressure approaches atmospheric pressure and has the least effect on PAP.* If you obtain a reading during other phases of the respiratory cycle, respiratory interference may occur. For instance, during inspiration, when intrathoracic pressure drops, PAP may be false-low *because the negative pressure is transmitted to the catheter.* During expiration, when intrathoracic pressure rises, PAP may be false-high.
- For patients with a rapid respiratory rate and subsequent variations, you may have trouble identifying end expiration. The monitor displays an average of the digital readings obtained over time as well as those readings obtained during a full respiratory cycle. If possible, obtain a printout. Use the averaged values obtained through the full respiratory cycle. *To analyze trends accurately,* be sure to record values at consistent times during the respiratory cycle.

Taking a PAWP reading

- PAWP is recorded by inflating the balloon and letting it float in a distal artery. Some facilities allow only physicians or specially trained nurses to take a PAWP reading *because of the risk of PA rupture—a rare but life-threatening complication.* If your facility permits you to perform this procedure, do so with extreme caution and make sure you're thoroughly familiar with intracardiac waveform interpretation.
- To begin, verify that the transducer is properly leveled and zeroed. Detach the syringe from the balloon inflation hub. Draw 1.5 cc of air into the syringe, and then reattach the syringe to the hub. Watching the monitor, inject the air through the hub slowly and smoothly. When you see a wedge tracing on the monitor, immediately stop inflating the balloon.

NURSING ALERT ***Never inflate the balloon beyond the volume needed to obtain a wedge tracing.***

- Take the pressure reading at end expiration. Note the amount of air needed to change the PA tracing to a wedge tracing (normally, 1.25 to 1.5 cc). If the wedge tracing appeared with the injection of less than 1.25 cc, suspect that the catheter has migrated into a more distal branch and requires repositioning. If the balloon is in a more distal branch, the tracings may move up the oscilloscope, indicating that the catheter tip is recording balloon pressure rather than PAWP. This may lead to PA rupture.
- Detach the syringe from the balloon inflation port and allow the balloon to deflate on its own. Observe the waveform tracing and make sure the tracing returns from the wedge tracing to the normal PA tracing.

Removing the catheter

- To assist the practitioner, inspect the chest X-ray for signs of catheter kinking or knotting. (In some states, you may be permitted to remove a PA catheter yourself under an advanced collaborative standard of practice.)
- Obtain the patient's baseline vital signs, and note the ECG pattern.
- Explain the procedure to the patient. Place the head of the bed flat, unless ordered otherwise. If the catheter was inserted using a superior approach, turn the patient's head to the side opposite the insertion site. Gently remove the dressing.
- Remove sutures securing the catheter unless the introducer is left in place.
- Turn all stopcocks off to the patient. (You may turn stopcocks on to the distal port if you wish to observe waveforms. However, use caution *because this may cause an air embolism.*)
- Put on sterile gloves. After verifying that the balloon is deflated, withdraw the catheter slowly and smoothly. If you feel resistance, stop immediately, stay with the patient, and notify the practitioner.
- Watch the ECG monitor for arrhythmias.
- If the introducer was removed, apply pressure to the site, and check it frequently for signs of bleeding. Dress the site again, as necessary. If the introducer is left in place, observe the diaphragm for any blood backflow, *which verifies the integrity of the hemostasis valve.*
- Return all equipment to the appropriate location. You may turn off the bedside pressure modules but leave the ECG module on.
- Reassure the patient and his family that he'll be observed closely. Make sure he understands that the catheter was removed because his condition has improved and he no longer needs it.

Special considerations

- Advise the patient to use caution when moving about in bed *to avoid dislodging the catheter.*
- Never leave the balloon inflated *because this may cause pulmonary infarction.* To determine if the balloon is inflated, check the monitor for a wedge tracing, which indicates inflation. (A PA tracing confirms balloon deflation.) (See *Troubleshooting the PAP monitoring system,* pages 448 and 449.)
- Never inflate the balloon with more than the recommended air volume (specified on the catheter shaft) *because this may cause loss of elasticity or balloon rupture.* With appropriate in-

TROUBLESHOOTING

Troubleshooting the PAP monitoring system

When your patient has a pulmonary artery (PA) catheter, many common problems can develop. Use this table to help you recognize and resolve such problems.

Abnormality	Causes	Nursing interventions
No waveform on monitor	■ Transducer not open to catheter ■ Transducer or monitor set up improperly ■ Defective or cracked transducer ■ Clotted catheter tip ■ Large leak in the system; loose connections	■ Check the stopcock, calibration, and scale mechanisms of the system. ■ Tighten all connections. ■ Rezero the setup. ■ Replace the transducer.
Overdamped waveform	■ Air bubble or blood clots within the catheter or tubing ■ Catheter tip lodged in the vessel wall ■ Kinked or knotted catheter or tubing ■ Small leak in the system due to a loose connection	■ Remove air bubbles observed in the catheter tubing and transducer. ■ Restore patency to a clotted catheter by gently aspirating the clot with a syringe. (*Note:* Never irrigate the line as a first step.) ■ Correct a lodged catheter by repositioning the patient or by having him cough and breathe deeply.
Changed waveform configuration (noisy or erratic tracings)	■ Incorrectly positioned catheter ■ Loose connections in the setup ■ Faulty electrical circuitry	■ Reposition the patient. ■ Assist with chest X-ray *to verify catheter location.* ■ Check and tighten connections in the catheter and transducer apparatus.
Ventricular irritability	■ Irritation of the ventricular endocardium or heart valves by the catheter	■ Notify the physician. (*Note:* The physician may prevent this problem during insertion by keeping the balloon inflated when advancing the catheter through the heart.) ■ Administer antiarrhythmics, as ordered.
Right ventricular waveform	■ Migration of the PA catheter into the right ventricle	■ Notify the physician immediately. The catheter may need to be repositioned.
Catheter fling	■ Excessive catheter movement that may result from an arrhythmia, excessive respiratory effort, hyperdynamic circulation, excessive catheter length in the right ventricle, or location of the catheter tip near the pulmonic valve	■ Notify the physician for catheter repositioning.
Falsely increased or decreased pulmonary artery pressure (PAP) readings	■ System not properly leveled or zeroed ■ Patient's body or bed repositioned without releveling or rezeroing the system	■ Reposition the transducer level with the phlebostatic axis. ■ Rezero the monitor.

Troubleshooting the PAP monitoring system *(continued)*

Abnormality	Causes	Nursing interventions
Continuous pulmonary artery wedge pressure (PAWP) waveform	■ Catheter migration ■ Balloon still inflated	■ Reposition the patient or have him cough and breathe deeply. ■ Keep the balloon inflated for no longer than two respiratory cycles or 15 seconds.
Missing PAWP waveform	■ Malpositioned catheter ■ Insufficient air in the balloon tip ■ Ruptured balloon	■ Reposition the patient. (Don't aspirate the balloon.) ■ Reinflate the balloon adequately. (Remove the syringe from the balloon lumen, wait for the balloon to deflate passively, and then instill the correct volume of air.) ■ Assess the balloon's competence. (Note resistance during inflation, feel how the syringe's plunger springs back after the balloon inflates, and check for blood leaking from the balloon lumen.) ■ If the balloon has ruptured, turn the patient onto his left side, tape the balloon-inflation port, and notify the physician.

flation volume, the balloon floats easily through the heart chambers and rests in the main branch of the pulmonary artery, producing accurate waveforms. Never inflate the balloon with fluids *because they may not be able to be retrieved from inside the balloon, preventing deflation.*

- Be aware that the catheter may slip back into the right ventricle. *Because the tip may irritate the ventricle,* check the monitor for a right ventricular waveform to detect this problem promptly.
- *To minimize valvular trauma,* make sure the balloon is deflated whenever the catheter is withdrawn from the pulmonary artery to the right ventricle or from the right ventricle to the right atrium.
- Change the dressing whenever it's moist, or every 48 hours for a gauze dressing, every 7 days for a transparent dressing, or according to your facility's policy. Change the pressure tubing every 48 hours and the flush solution every 24 hours.
- Perform and document the dynamic response or square wave test every 8 to 12 hours *to validate the optimal waveform.*

Complications

Complications of PA catheter insertion include PA perforation, pulmonary infarction, catheter knotting, local or systemic infection, cardiac arrhythmias, and heparin-induced thrombocytopenia.

Documentation

Document the date and time of catheter insertion, the physician who performed the procedure, the catheter insertion site, pressure waveforms and values for the various heart chambers, balloon inflation volume required to obtain a wedge tracing, any arrhythmias occurring during or after the procedure, type of flush solution used and its heparin concentration (if any), type of dressing applied, and the patient's tolerance of the procedure. Remember to initial and date the dressing.

After catheter removal, document the patient's tolerance of the removal procedure, and note any problems encountered during removal.

Selected references

American Society of Anesthesiologists. "Practice Guidelines for Pulmonary Artery Catheterization: An Updated Report by the American Society of Anesthesiologist Task Force," *Anesthesiology* 99(40):988-1014, October 2003.

Binanay, C. "Evaluation Study of Congestive Heart Failure and Pulmonary Artery Catheterization Effectiveness: The ESCAPE trial," *JAMA* 294(13):1625-633, October 2005.

Bridges, E.J. "Pulmonary Artery Pressure Monitoring: When, How, and What Else to Use," *AACN Advanced Critical Care* 17(3):286-303, July-September 2006.

Centers for Disease Control and Prevention. "Guidelines for the Prevention of Intravascular Catheter-related Infections," *MMWR* 51(RR-10):1-26, August 2002.

Friese, R.S., et al. "Pulmonary Artery Catheter Use is Associated with Reduced Mortality in Severely Injured Patients: A National Trauma Data Bank Analysis of 53,312 Patients," *Critical Care Medicine* 34(6):1597-601, June 2006.

Georghiou, G.P., et al. "Knotting of a Pulmonary Artery Catheter in the Superior Vena Cava: Surgical Removal and a Word of Caution," *Heart* 90(5):e28, May 2004.

Lynn-McHale Wiegand, D.J., and Carlson, K.K., eds. *AACN Procedure Manual for Critical Care,* 5th ed. Philadelphia: W.B. Saunders Co., 2005.

Shah, M.R., et al. "Impact of the Pulmonary Artery Catheter in Critically Ill Patients: Meta-analysis of Randomized Clinical Trials," *JAMA* 294(13):1664-670, October 2005.

Task Force of the American College of Critical Care Medicine, Society of Critical Medicine. "Practice Parameters for Hemodynamic Support of Sepsis in Adult Patients: 2004 Update," *Critical Care Medicine* 32(9):1928-948, September 2004.

CENTRAL VENOUS PRESSURE MONITORING

In central venous pressure (CVP) monitoring, the practitioner inserts a catheter through a vein and advances it until its tip lies in or near the right atrium. Because no major valves lie at the junction of the vena cava and right atrium, pressure at end diastole reflects back to the catheter. When connected to a manometer, the catheter measures CVP, an index of right ventricular function.

CVP monitoring helps to assess cardiac function, to evaluate venous return to the heart, and to indirectly gauge how well the heart is pumping. The central venous (CV) line also provides access to a large vessel for rapid, high-volume fluid administration and allows frequent blood withdrawal for laboratory samples.

CVP can be monitored intermittently or continuously. There are three accepted methods for measuring pressure in the right atrium: using a water manometer attached to a CV catheter, using the proximal lumen of a pulmonary artery (PA) catheter, or using a line placed directly into the right atrium and attached to a transducer system. CVP is recorded in millimeters of mercury (mm Hg). When measured by a water manometer, CVP is reported in centimeters of water (cm H_2O).

Normal CVP ranges from 2 to 6 mm Hg (5 to 10 cm H_2O). Any condition that alters venous return, circulating blood volume, or cardiac performance may affect CVP. If circulating volume increases (such as with enhanced venous return to the heart), CVP rises. If circulating volume decreases (such as with reduced venous return), CVP drops.

Equipment

For intermittent CVP monitoring: Disposable CVP manometer set ▪ leveling device (such as a rod from a reusable CVP pole holder or a carpenter's level or rule) ▪ additional stopcock (to attach the CVP manometer to the catheter) ▪ extension tubing (if needed) ▪ I.V. pole ▪ I.V. solution ▪ I.V. drip chamber and tubing ▪ dressing materials ▪ tape.

For continuous CVP monitoring: Pressure monitoring kit with disposable pressure transducer ▪ leveling device ▪ bedside pressure module ▪ continuous I.V. flush solution ▪ pressure bag.

For withdrawing blood samples through the CV line: Appropriate number of syringes for the ordered tests ▪ 5- or 10-ml syringe for the discard sample. (Syringe size depends on the tests ordered.)

For using an intermittent CV line: Syringe with normal saline solution ▪ syringe with heparin flush solution.

For removing a CV catheter: Sterile gloves ▪ suture removal set ▪ sterile gauze pads ▪ antimicrobial ointment ▪ dressing ▪ tape.

Implementation

▪ Confirm the patient's identity using two patient identifiers according to your facility's policy.

▪ Gather the necessary equipment. Explain the procedure to the patient *to reduce his anxiety.*

▪ Assist the practitioner as he inserts the CV catheter. (The procedure is similar to that used for pulmonary artery pressure monitoring, except that the catheter is advanced only as far as the superior vena cava.)

Obtaining intermittent CVP readings with a water manometer

▪ With the CV line in place, position the patient flat. Align the base of the manometer with the previously determined zero reference point by using a leveling device. *Because CVP reflects right atrial pressure,* you must align the right atrium (the zero reference point) with the zero mark on the manometer. To find the right atrium, locate the fourth intercostal space at the midaxillary line. This is the phlebostatic axis. Mark the appropriate place on the patient's chest *so that all subsequent recordings will be made using the same location.*

▪ If the patient can't tolerate a flat position, place him in semi-Fowler's position. Use the same degree of elevation for all subsequent measurements.

▪ Attach the water manometer to an I.V. pole or place it next to the patient's chest. Make sure the zero reference point

Measuring CVP with a water manometer

To ensure accurate central venous pressure (CVP) readings, make sure the manometer base is aligned with the patient's right atrium (the zero reference point). The manometer set usually contains a leveling rod to allow you to determine this quickly.

After adjusting the manometer's position, examine the typical three-way stopcock. By turning it to any position shown, you can control the direction of fluid flow. Four-way stopcocks are also available.

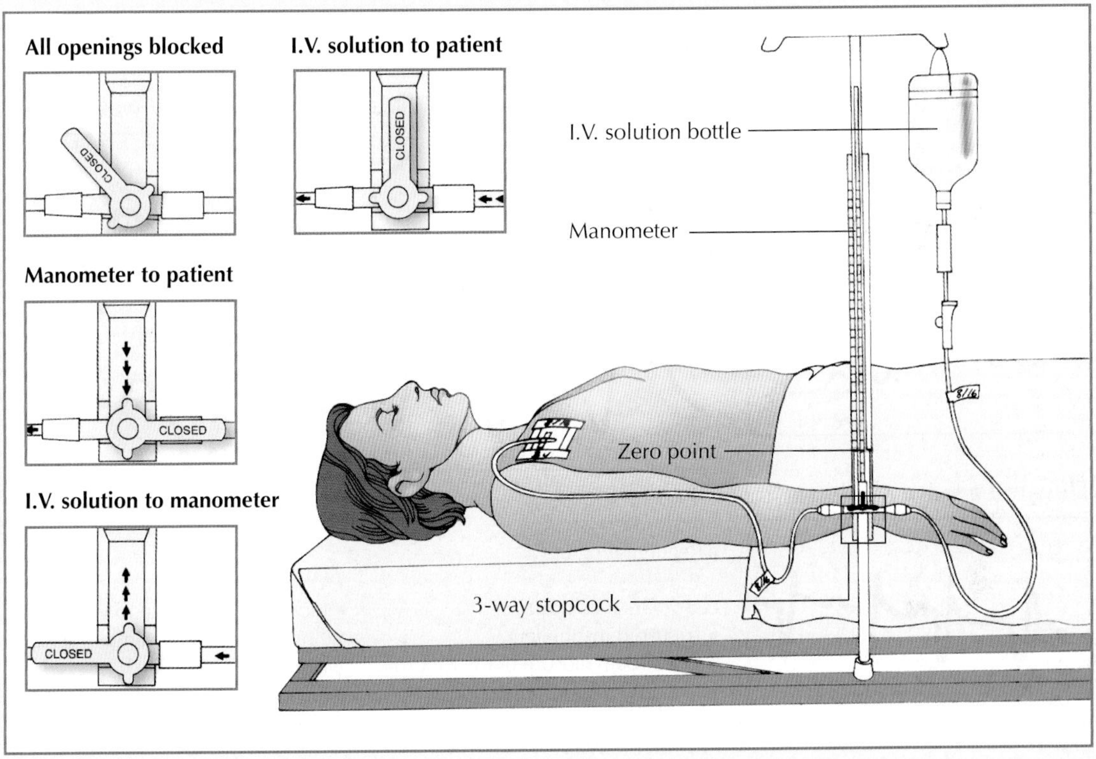

is level with the right atrium. (See *Measuring CVP with a water manometer.*)

- Verify that the water manometer is connected to the I.V. tubing. Typically, markings on the manometer range from –2 to 38 cm H_2O. *However, manufacturer's markings may differ,* so be sure to read the directions before setting up the manometer and obtaining readings.
- Turn the stopcock off to the patient, and slowly fill the manometer with I.V. solution until the fluid level is 10 to 20 cm H_2O higher than the patient's expected CVP value. Don't overfill the tube *because fluid that spills over the top can become a source of contamination.*
- Turn the stopcock off to the I.V. solution and open to the patient. The fluid level in the manometer will drop. When the fluid level comes to rest, it will fluctuate slightly with respirations. Expect it to drop during inspiration and to rise during expiration.
- Record CVP at the end of expiration, *when intrathoracic pressure has a negligible effect.* Depending on the type of water manometer used, note the value either at the bottom of the meniscus or at the midline of the small floating ball.
- After you've obtained the CVP value, turn the stopcock to resume the I.V. infusion. Adjust the I.V. drip rate as required.
- Place the patient in a comfortable position.

Differentiating normal from abnormal CVP waveforms

These illustrations show a normal central venous pressure (CVP) waveform and abnormal CVP waveforms, along with possible causes of abnormal waveforms.

Normal waveforms

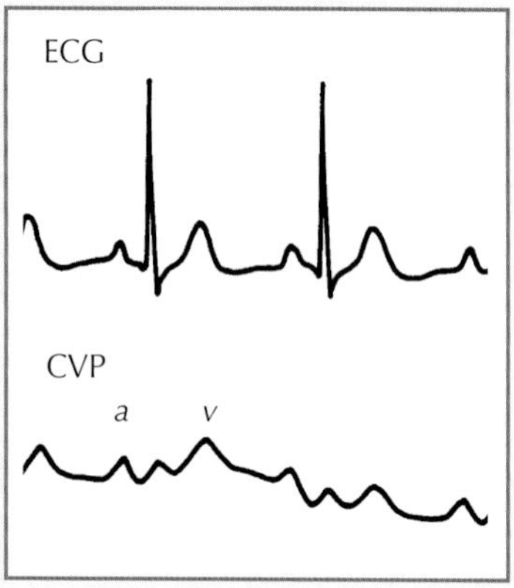

Elevated *a* wave

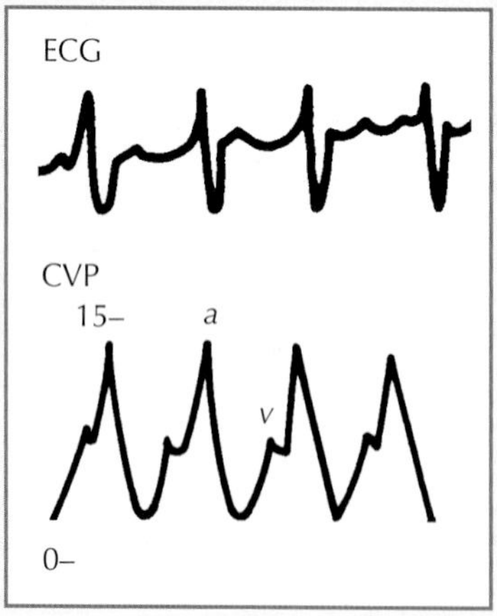

Physiologic causes
- Increased resistance to ventricular filling
- Increased atrial contraction

Associated conditions
- Heart failure
- Tricuspid stenosis
- Pulmonary hypertension

Elevated *v* wave

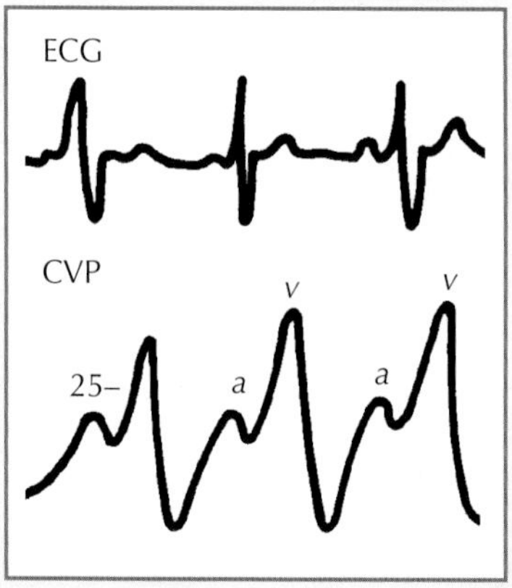

Physiologic causes
- Regurgitating flow

Associated conditions
- Tricuspid insufficiency
- Inadequate closure of the tricuspid valve due to heart failure

Absent *a* wave

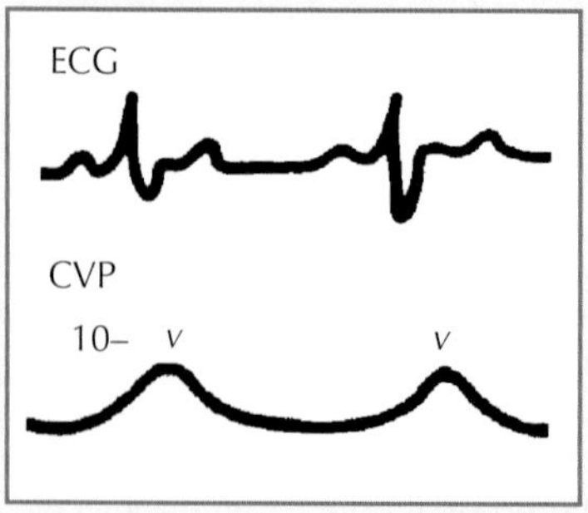

Physiologic causes
- Decreased or absent atrial contraction

Associated conditions
- Atrial fibrillation
- Junctional arrhythmias
- Ventricular pacing

Elevated *a* and *v* waves

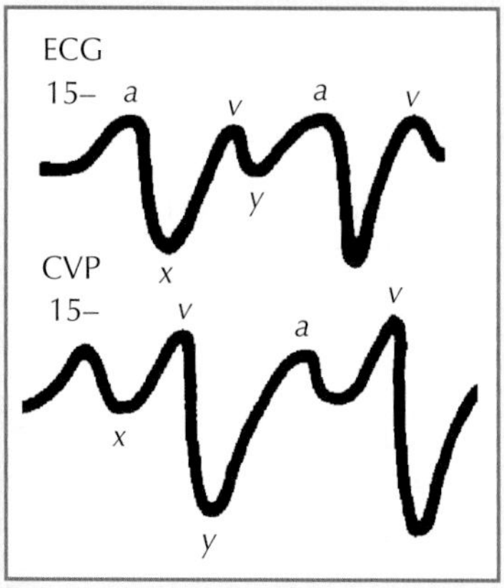

Physiologic causes
- Increased resistance to ventricular filling, which causes an elevated *a* wave
- Functional regurgitation, which causes an elevated *v* wave

Associated conditions
- Cardiac tamponade (smaller *y* descent than *x* descent)
- Constrictive pericardial disease (*y* descent exceeds *x* descent)
- Heart failure
- Hypervolemia
- Atrial hypertrophy

Obtaining continuous CVP readings with a water manometer
- Make sure the stopcock is turned so that the I.V. solution port, CVP column port, and patient port are open. Be aware that with this stopcock position, infusion of the I.V. solution increases CVP. Therefore, expect higher readings than those taken with the stopcock turned off to the I.V. solution. If the I.V. solution infuses at a constant rate, CVP will

change as the patient's condition changes, although the initial reading will be higher. Assess the patient closely for changes.

Obtaining continuous CVP readings with a pressure monitoring system

- Make sure the CV line or the proximal lumen of a PA catheter is attached to the system. (If the patient has a CV line with multiple lumens, one lumen may be dedicated to continuous CVP monitoring and the other lumens used for fluid administration.)
- Set up a pressure transducer system. (See "Transducer system setup," page 435.) Connect noncompliant pressure tubing from the CVP catheter hub to the transducer. Then connect the flush solution container to a flush device.
- To obtain values, position the patient flat. If he can't tolerate this position, use semi-Fowler's position. Locate the level of the right atrium by identifying the phlebostatic axis. Zero the transducer, leveling the transducer air-fluid interface stopcock with the right atrium. Read the CVP value from the digital display on the monitor, and note the waveform. Make sure the patient is still when the reading is taken *to prevent artifact.* Be sure to use this position for all subsequent readings.

Removing a CV line

- You may assist the practitioner in removing a CV line. (In some states, a nurse is permitted to remove the catheter with a practitioner's order or when acting under advanced collaborative standards of practice.)
- If the head of the bed is elevated, *to minimize the risk of air embolism during catheter removal,* place the patient in Trendelenburg's position if the line was inserted using a superior approach. If he can't tolerate this, position him flat.
- Turn the patient's head to the side opposite the catheter insertion site. Remove the dressing and expose the insertion site. If sutures are in place, remove them carefully.
- Turn the I.V. solution off.
- Put on sterile gloves.
- Pull the catheter out in a slow, smooth motion and then apply pressure to the insertion site.
- Clean the insertion site, apply antimicrobial ointment, and cover it with a dressing as ordered. Remove your gloves and wash your hands.
- Assess the patient for signs of respiratory distress, *which may indicate an air embolism.*

Special considerations

- As ordered, arrange for daily chest X-rays *to check catheter placement.*
- Care for the insertion site according to your facility's policy. Change a gauze dressing every 48 hours, a transparent dressing every 7 days, whenever the dressing becomes moist, or according to your facility's policy.
- Be sure to wash your hands before performing dressing changes and to use sterile technique and sterile gloves when re-dressing the site. When removing the old dressing, observe for signs of infection, such as redness, and note any patient complaints of tenderness. Cover the site with a sterile gauze dressing or a clear occlusive dressing.
- After the initial CVP reading, reevaluate readings frequently *to establish a baseline for the patient.* Authorities recommend obtaining readings at 15-, 30-, and 60-minute intervals to establish a baseline. If the patient's CVP fluctuates by more than 2 cm H_2O, suspect a change in his clinical status and report this finding to the practitioner. (See *Differentiating normal from abnormal CVP waveforms.*)
- Change the I.V. solution every 24 hours and the I.V. tubing every 96 hours, according to your facility's policy. Label the I.V. solution, tubing, and dressing with the date, time, and your initials.

Complications

Complications of CVP monitoring include pneumothorax (which typically occurs upon catheter insertion), sepsis, thrombus, vessel or adjacent organ puncture, and air embolism.

Documentation

Document all dressing, tubing, and solution changes. Document the patient's tolerance of the procedure, the date and time of catheter removal, and the type of dressing applied. Note the condition of the catheter insertion site and whether a culture specimen was collected. Note any complications and actions taken.

SELECTED REFERENCES

Brungs, S.M., and Render, M.L. " Using Evidence-based Practice to Reduce Central Line Infections," *Clinical Journal of Oncology Nursing* 10(6):723-25, December 2006.

Danks, L.A. "Central Venous Catheters: A Review of Skin Cleansing and Dressings," *British Journal of Nursing* 15(12):650-54, June-July 2006.

Day, M.W. "Tension Pneumothorax from Central Line Placement," *Nursing* 36(11):80, November 2006.

Hadaway, L.C. "Keeping Central Line Infection at Bay," *Nursing* 36(4):58-63, April 2006.

Ho, A.M., et al. "Accuracy of Central Venous Pressure Monitoring during Simultaneous Continuous Infusion through the Same Catheter," *Anaesthesia* 60(10):1027-1030, October 2005.

Lynn-McHale Wiegand, D.J., and Carlson, K.K., eds. *AACN Procedure Manual for Critical Care,* 5th ed. Philadelphia: W.B. Saunders Co., 2005.

Posa, P., et al. "Elimination of Central Line-associated Bloodstream Infections: Application of the Evidence," *AACN Advanced Critical Care* 17(4):446-54, October-December 2006.
Weinstein, S. *Plumer's Principles & Practice of Intravenous Therapy,* 8th ed. Philadelphia: Lippincott Williams & Wilkins, 2007.

CARDIAC OUTPUT MEASUREMENT

Cardiac output (CO) — the amount of blood ejected by the heart — helps evaluate cardiac function. Each ventricle has a CO of 4 to 6 L/minute. The most widely used method of calculating this measurement is the bolus thermodilution technique. Performed at the patient's bedside, the thermodilution technique is the most practical method of evaluating the cardiac status of critically ill patients and those suspected of having cardiac disease. (See *A closer look at the thermodilution method.*)

To measure CO, a quantity of solution colder than the patient's blood is injected into the right atrium via a port on a pulmonary artery (PA) catheter. This indicator solution mixes with the blood as it travels through the right ventricle into the pulmonary artery, and a thermistor on the catheter registers the change in temperature of the flowing blood. A computer then plots the temperature change over time as a curve, and calculates flow based on the area under the curve. (See *Analyzing thermodilution curves.*)

Iced or room-temperature injectant may be used. The choice should be based on your facility's policy as well as the patient's status. The accuracy of the bolus thermodilution technique depends on the computer being able to differentiate the temperature change caused by the injectant in the pulmonary artery and the temperature changes in the pulmonary artery. Because iced injectant is colder than room-temperature injectant, it provides a stronger signal to be detected.

Typically, however, room-temperature injectant is more convenient and provides equally accurate measurements. Iced injectant may be more accurate in patients with high or low CO, hypothermic patients, or when smaller volumes of injectant must be used (3 to 5 ml), as in patients with volume restrictions or in children.

Equipment

Thermodilution PA catheter in position ▪ output computer and cables (or a module for the bedside cardiac monitor)

A closer look at the thermodilution method

This illustration shows the path of the injectant solution through the heart during thermodilution cardiac output monitoring.

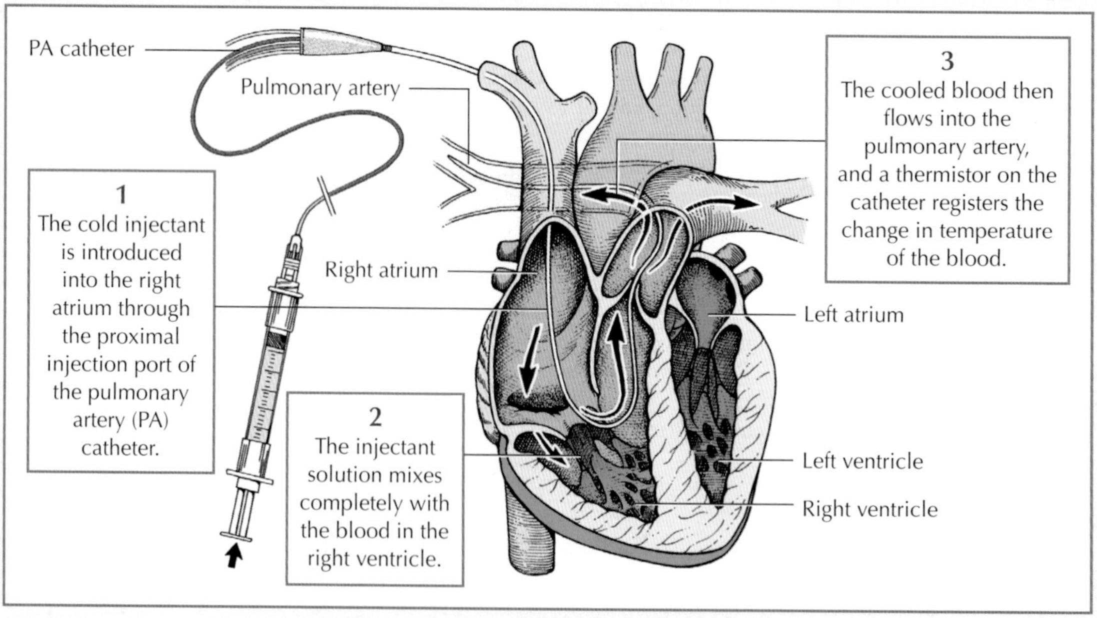

■ closed or open injectant delivery system ■ 10-ml syringe ■ 500-ml bag of dextrose 5% in water or normal saline solution ■ crushed ice and water (if iced injectant is used).

Some bedside cardiac monitors measure CO continuously, using either an invasive or a noninvasive method. If your bedside monitor doesn't have this capability, you'll need a freestanding CO computer.

Analyzing thermodilution curves

The thermodilution curve provides valuable information about cardiac output (CO), injection technique, and equipment problems. When studying the curve, keep in mind that the area under the curve is inversely proportionate to CO: The smaller the area under the curve, the higher the CO; the larger the area under the curve, the lower the CO.

Besides providing a record of CO, the curve may indicate problems related to technique, such as erratic or slow injectant instillations, or other problems, such as respiratory variations or electrical interference. The curves below correspond to those typically seen in clinical practice.

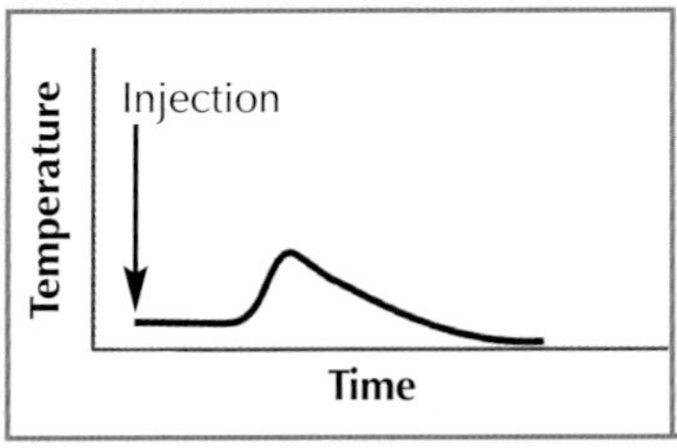

Normal thermodilution curve

With an accurate monitoring system and a patient who has adequate CO, the thermodilution curve begins with a smooth, rapid upstroke and is followed by a smooth, gradual downslope. The curve shown at left indicates that the injectant instillation time was within the recommended 4 seconds and that the temperature curve returned to baseline blood temperature.

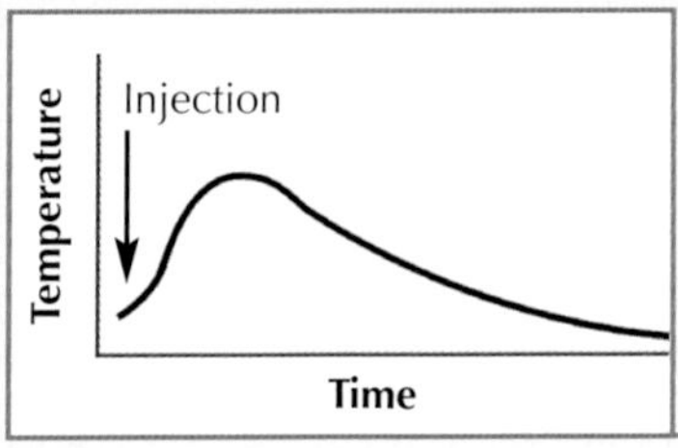

Low CO curve

A thermodilution curve representing low CO shows a rapid, smooth upstroke (from proper injection technique). However, because the heart is ejecting blood less efficiently from the ventricles, the injectant warms slowly and takes longer to be ejected from the ventricle. Consequently, the curve takes longer to return to baseline. This slow return produces a larger area under the curve, corresponding to low CO.

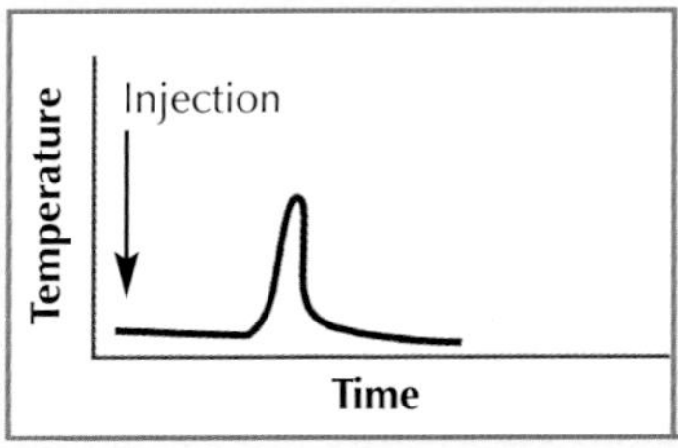

High CO curve

Again, the curve has a rapid, smooth upstroke from proper injection technique. But because the ventricles are ejecting blood too forcefully, the injectant moves through the heart quickly and the curve returns to baseline more rapidly. The smaller area under the curve suggests higher CO.

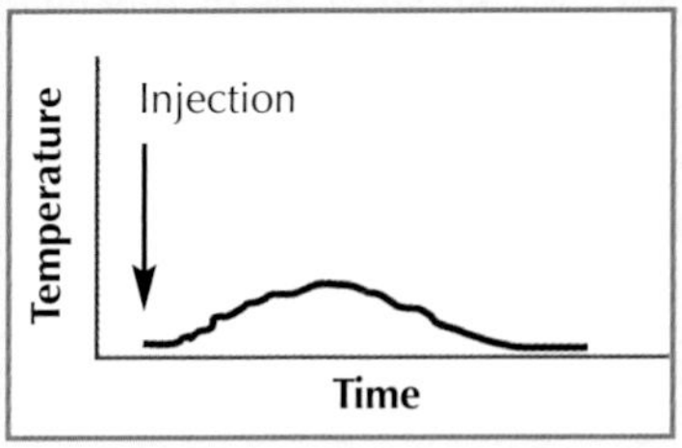

Curve reflecting poor technique

This curve results from an uneven and too slow (taking more than 4 seconds) administration of injectant. The uneven and slower than normal upstroke and the larger area under the curve erroneously indicate low CO. A kinked catheter, unsteady hands during the injection, or improper placement of the injectant lumen in the introducer sheath may also cause this type of curve.

Preparation of equipment

Wash your hands thoroughly, and assemble the equipment at the patient's bedside. Insert the closed injectant system tubing into the 500-ml bag of I.V. solution. Connect the 10-ml syringe to the system tubing, and prime the tubing with I.V. solution until it's free of air. Then clamp the tubing. Confirm the patient's identity using two patient identifiers according to your facility's policy. The steps that follow differ, depending on the temperature of the injectant.

Iced injectant: After clamping the tubing, place the coiled segment into the Styrofoam container and add crushed ice and water to cover the entire coil. Let the solution cool for 15 to 20 minutes. The rest of the steps are the same as those for the room-temperature injectant closed delivery system.

Room-temperature injectant: After clamping the tubing, connect the primed system to the stopcock of the proximal injectant lumen of the PA catheter. Next, connect the temperature probe from the CO computer to the closed injectant system's flow-through housing device. Connect the CO computer cable to the thermistor connector on the PA catheter and verify the blood temperature reading. Finally, turn on the CO computer and enter the correct computation constant, as provided by the catheter's manufacturer. The constant is determined by the volume and temperature of the injectant as well as the size and type of catheter.

PEDIATRIC ALERT *For children, you'll need to adjust the computation constant to reflect a smaller volume and a smaller catheter size.*

Implementation

- Make sure your patient is in a comfortable position. Tell him not to move during the procedure *because movement can cause an error in measurement.*
- Explain to the patient that the procedure will help determine how well his heart is pumping and that he'll feel no discomfort.

For iced injectant

- Unclamp the I.V. tubing and withdraw 5 ml of solution into the syringe.

PEDIATRIC ALERT *With children, use 3 ml or less.*

- Inject the solution to flow past the temperature sensor while observing the injectant temperature that registers on the computer. Verify that the injectant temperature is between 43° and 54° F (6.1° and 12.2° C).
- Verify the presence of a PA waveform on the cardiac monitor.
- Withdraw exactly 10 ml of cooled solution before reclamping the tubing.
- Turn the stopcock at the catheter injectant hub to open a fluid path between the injectant lumen of the PA catheter and the syringe.
- Press the START button on the CO computer, or wait for the INJECT message to flash.
- Inject the solution smoothly within 4 seconds, making sure it doesn't leak at the connectors.
- If available, analyze the contour of the thermodilution washout curve on a strip chart recorder for a rapid upstroke and a gradual, smooth return to baseline.
- Wait 1 minute between injections, and repeat the procedure until three values are within 10% to 15% of the median value. Compute the average, and record the patient's CO.
- Return the stopcock to its original position, and make sure the injectant delivery system tubing is clamped.
- Verify the presence of a PA waveform on the cardiac monitor.
- Discontinue CO measurements when the patient is hemodynamically stable and weaned from his vasoactive and inotropic medications. You can leave the PA catheter inserted for pressure measurements.
- Disconnect and discard the injectant delivery system and the I.V. bag. Cover exposed stopcocks with air-occlusive caps.
- Monitor the patient for signs and symptoms of inadequate perfusion, including restlessness, fatigue, changes in level of consciousness (LOC), decreased capillary refill time, diminished peripheral pulses, oliguria, and pale, cool skin.

For room-temperature injectant

- Verify the presence of a PA waveform on the cardiac monitor.
- Unclamp the I.V. tubing and withdraw exactly 10 ml of solution. Reclamp the tubing.
- Turn the stopcock at the catheter injectant hub to open a fluid path between the injectant lumen of the PA catheter and the syringe.
- Press the START button on the CO computer, or wait for an INJECT message to flash.
- Inject the solution smoothly within 4 seconds, making sure it doesn't leak at the connectors.
- If available, analyze the contour of the thermodilution washout curve on a strip chart recorder for a rapid upstroke and a gradual, smooth return to the baseline.
- Repeat these steps until three values are within 10% to 15% of the median value. Compute the average, and record the patient's CO.
- Return the stopcock to its original position, and make sure the injectant delivery system tubing is clamped.

■ Verify the presence of a PA waveform on the cardiac monitor.
■ Discontinue CO measurements when the patient is hemodynamically stable and weaned from his vasoactive and inotropic medications. You can leave the PA catheter inserted for pressure measurements.
■ Disconnect and discard the injectant delivery system and the I.V. bag. Cover exposed stopcocks with air-occlusive caps.
■ Monitor the patient for signs and symptoms of inadequate perfusion, including restlessness, fatigue, changes in LOC, decreased capillary refill time, diminished peripheral pulses, oliguria, and pale, cool skin.

Special considerations

■ The normal range for CO is 4 to 8 L/minute. The adequacy of a patient's CO is better assessed by calculating his cardiac index (CI), adjusted for his body size.
■ To calculate the patient's CI, divide his CO by his body surface area (BSA), a function of height and weight. For example, a CO of 4 L/minute might be adequate for a 65″, 120-lb (165-cm, 54-kg) patient (normally a BSA of 1.59 and a CI of 2.5) but would be inadequate for a 74″, 230-lb (188-cm, 104-kg) patient (normally a BSA of 2.26 and a CI of 1.8). The normal CI for adults ranges from 2.5 to 4.2 L/minute/m^2; for pregnant women, 3.5 to 6.5 L/minute/m^2.
PEDIATRIC ALERT *Normal CI for infants and children is 3.5 to 4 L/minute/m^2.*

ELDER ALERT *Normal CI for elderly adults is 2 to 2.5 L/minute/m^2.*
■ Add the fluid volume injected for CO determinations to the patient's total intake. Injectant delivery of 30 ml/hour will contribute 720 ml to the patient's 24-hour intake.
■ After CO measurement, make sure the clamp on the injectant bag is secured *to prevent inadvertent delivery of the injectant to the patient.*

Documentation

Document your patient's CO, CI, and other hemodynamic values and vital signs at the time of measurement. Note the patient's position during measurement and other unusual occurrences, such as bradycardia or neurologic changes.

SELECTED REFERENCES

Bridges, E.J. "Pulmonary Artery Pressure Monitoring: When, How and What Else to Use," *AACN Advanced Critical Care* 17(3):286-303, July-September 2006.

Engoren, M., and Barbee, D. "Comparison of Cardiac Output Determination by Bioimpedance, Thermodilution, and the Fick Method," *American Journal of Critical Care* 14(1):40-45, January 2005.

Johnson, K.L. "Diagnostic Measures to Evaluate Oxygenation in Critically Ill Adults: Implications and Limitations," *AACN Clinical Issues* 15(4):506-24, October- December 2004.

Payen, D., and Gayat, E. "Which General Intensive Care Unit Patients can Benefit from Placement of the Pulmonary Artery Catheter?" *Critical Care* 10(Suppl 3):S7, 2006.

TREATMENTS

PERMANENT PACEMAKER CARE

Designed to operate for 3 to 20 years, a permanent pacemaker is a self-contained device. The cardiologist implants the pacemaker in a pocket beneath the patient's skin. This is usually done in the operating room or cardiac catheterization laboratory. Nursing responsibilities involve monitoring the electrocardiogram (ECG) and maintaining sterile technique.

Permanent pacemakers function in the demand mode, allowing the patient's heart to beat on its own but preventing it from falling below a preset rate. Pacing electrodes can be placed in the atria, ventricles, or both chambers (atrioventricular sequential, dual chamber). (See *Understanding pacemaker codes,* page 458.) The most common pacing codes are VVI for single-chamber pacing and DDD for dual-chamber pacing. To keep the patient healthy and active, newer generation pacemakers have been specially designed to increase the heart rate with exercise.

Candidates for permanent pacemakers include patients with myocardial infarction and persistent bradyarrhythmia and patients with complete heart block or slow ventricular rates stemming from congenital or degenerative heart disease or cardiac surgery. Patients who suffer Stokes-Adams syndrome as well as those with Wolff-Parkinson-White syndrome or sick sinus syndrome may also benefit from permanent pacemaker implantation. Permanent pacemakers are also being used in patients other than those with symptomatic bradycardia. These include patients with hypertrophic cardiomyopathy, dilated cardiomyopathy, atrial fibrillation, neurocardiogenic syndrome, and long QT syndrome.

A biventricular pacemaker is also available for patients with heart failure. This device differs from a standard pacemaker in that it has three leads instead of one or two. One lead is placed in the right atrium, one in the right ventricle, and one in the left ventricle. The leads simultaneously stimulate the right and left ventricles, allowing the ventricles to coordinate their pumping action and making the heart more efficient.

Understanding pacemaker codes

A permanent pacemaker's three-letter (or sometimes five-letter) code simply refers to how it's programmed. The first letter represents the chamber that's paced; the second letter, the chamber that's sensed; and the third letter, how the pulse generator responds. In five-letter codes, the fourth letter denotes the pacemaker's programmability, and the fifth letter denotes the pacemaker's response to tachycardia. Typically, only the first three letters are used.

First letter	Second letter	Third letter	Fourth letter	Fifth letter
A = atrium V = ventricle D = dual (both chambers) O = not applicable	A = atrium V = ventricle D = dual (both chambers) O = not applicable	I = inhibited T = triggered D = dual (inhibited and triggered) O = not applicable	P = basic functions programmable M = multiple programmable parameters C = communicating functions such as telemetry R = rate responsiveness	P = pacing ability S = shock D = dual ability to shock and pace 0 = none

Examples of two common programming codes

DDD
Pace: atrium and ventricle
Sense: atrium and ventricle
Response: inhibited and triggered
This is a fully automatic, or universal, pacemaker.

VVI
Pace: ventricle
Sense: ventricle
Response: inhibited
This is a demand pacemaker, inhibited.

Equipment

Sphygmomanometer ▪ stethoscope ▪ ECG monitor and strip-chart recorder ▪ sterile dressing tray ▪ antimicrobial ointment ▪ clippers ▪ sterile gauze dressing ▪ hypoallergenic tape ▪ sedatives ▪ alcohol pads ▪ emergency resuscitation equipment ▪ I.V. catheter, tubing, and I.V. solution.

Implementation

- Confirm the patient's identity using two patient identifiers according to your facility's policy.
- Explain the procedure to the patient. Provide and review literature from the manufacturer or the American Heart Association *so he can learn about the pacemaker and how it works.* Emphasize that the pacemaker merely augments his natural heart rate.
- Make sure the patient or a responsible family member signs a consent form, and ask the patient if he's allergic to anesthetics or iodine.

Preoperative care

- For pacemaker insertion, clip hair from the patient's chest from the axilla to the midline and from the clavicle to the nipple line on the side selected by the physician, as ordered.
- Establish an I.V. line at a keep-vein-open rate.
- Obtain baseline vital signs and a baseline ECG.
- Provide sedation as ordered.

Postoperative care

- Monitor the patient's ECG *to check for arrhythmias and ensure correct pacemaker functioning.*
- Monitor the I.V. flow rate; the I.V. line is usually kept in place for 24 to 48 hours postoperatively *to allow for possible emergency treatment of arrhythmias.*
- Check the dressing for signs of bleeding and infection (swelling, redness, or exudate). The practitioner may order prophylactic antibiotics for up to 7 days after the implantation.
- Change the dressing and apply antimicrobial ointment at least once every 24 to 48 hours, or according to the practitioner's orders and your facility's policy. If the dressing be-

Teaching the patient who has a permanent pacemaker

If your patient is going home with a permanent pacemaker, teach him about daily care, safety and activity guidelines, and other precautions as detailed below.

Daily care

- Clean your pacemaker site gently with soap and water when you take a shower or a bath. Leave the incision exposed to the air.
- Inspect your skin around the incision. A slight bulge is normal, but call your practitioner if you feel discomfort or notice swelling, redness, a discharge, or other problems.
- Check your pulse for 1 minute as your practitioner showed you—on the side of your neck, inside your elbow, or on the thumb side of your wrist. Your pulse rate should be the same as your pacemaker rate or faster. Contact your practitioner if you think your heart is beating too fast or too slow.
- Take your medications, including those for pain, as prescribed. Even with a pacemaker, you still need the medication your practitioner ordered.

Safety and activity

- Keep your pacemaker instruction booklet handy, and carry your pacemaker identification card at all times. This card has your pacemaker model number and other information needed by health care personnel who treat you.
- You can resume most of your usual activities when you feel comfortable doing so, but don't drive until the cardiologist gives you permission. Also avoid heavy lifting and stretching exercises for at least 6 to 8 weeks or as directed by the cardiologist.
- Try to use both arms equally to prevent stiffness. Check with the cardiologist before you golf, swim, play tennis, or perform other strenuous activities.

Electromagnetic interference

- Today's pacemakers are designed and insulated to eliminate most electrical interference. You can safely operate common household electrical devices, including microwave ovens, razors, and sewing machines. You can ride in or operate a motor vehicle without it affecting your pacemaker.
- Take care to avoid direct contact with large running motors, high-powered CB radios and other similar equipment, welding machinery, and radar devices.
- If your pacemaker activates the metal detector in an airport, show your pacemaker identification card to the security official. Patients with an implantable cardioverter-defibrillator/pacemaker continuation device should identify themselves to the security official and bypass the metal detector.
- *Because the metal in your pacemaker makes you ineligible for certain diagnostic studies, such as magnetic resonance imaging,* be sure to inform your practitioners, dentist, and other health care personnel that you have a pacemaker.

Special precautions

- If you feel light-headed or dizzy when you're near electrical equipment, moving away from the device should restore normal pacemaker function. Ask your practitioner about particular electrical devices.
- Notify your practitioner if you experience signs of pacemaker failure, such as palpitations, a fast heart rate, a slow heart rate (5 to 10 beats less than the pacemaker's setting), dizziness, fainting, shortness of breath, swollen ankles or feet, anxiety, forgetfulness, or confusion.

Checkups

- Be sure to schedule and keep regular checkup appointments with your practitioner.
- If your practitioner checks your pacemaker status by telephone, keep your transmission schedule and instructions in a handy place.

comes soiled or the site is exposed to air, change the dressing immediately, regardless of when you last changed it.

- Check vital signs and level of consciousness (LOC) every 15 minutes for the first hour, every hour for the next 4 hours, every 4 hours for the next 48 hours, and then once every shift.

ELDER ALERT *Confused, elderly patients with second-degree heart block won't show immediate improvement in LOC.*

Special considerations

- Provide the patient with an identification card that lists the pacemaker type and manufacturer, serial number, pacemaker rate setting, date implanted, and cardiologist's name. (See *Teaching the patient who has a permanent pacemaker.*) The markings, along with the shape of the generator, may assist in determining the manufacturer of the generator and pacemaker battery. This may be helpful if the patient has lost the permanent pacemaker identification card.

- Watch for signs of pacemaker malfunction.

Complications

Insertion of a permanent pacemaker places the patient at risk for certain complications, such as infection, lead displacement, a perforated ventricle, cardiac tamponade, or lead fracture and disconnection.

NURSING ALERT *Watch for signs and symptoms of a perforated ventricle, with resultant cardiac tamponade: persistent hiccups, distant heart sounds, pulsus paradoxus, hypotension with narrow pulse pressure, increased venous pressure, cyanosis, distended jugular veins, decreased urine output, restlessness, or complaints of fullness in the chest. If the patient develops any of these, notify the practitioner immediately.*

Documentation

Document the type of pacemaker used, the serial number and the manufacturer's name, the pacing rate, the date of implantation, and the cardiologist's name. Note whether the pacemaker successfully treated the patient's arrhythmias and the condition of the incision site.

SELECTED REFERENCES

American College of Cardiology and the American Heart Association. "2002 Guideline Update for Implantation of Cardiac Pacemakers and Antiarrhythmia Devices." Available at *www.americanheart.org.*

American College of Cardiology and the American Heart Association. "ACC/AHA/NASPE 2002 Guideline Update for Implantation of Cardiac Pacemakers and Antiarrhythmia Devices: Summary Article," *Circulation* 106:2145-161, October 2002.

Borer, A., et al. "Prevention of Infections Associated with Permanent Cardiac Antiarrhythmic Devices by Implementation of a Comprehensive Infection Control Program," *Infection Control and Hospital Epidemiology* 25(6):492-96, June 2004.

Cotter, J., et al. "Helping Patients Who Need a Permanent Pacemaker," *Nursing* 36(8):50-54, August 2004.

TEMPORARY PACEMAKER INSERTION AND CARE

Usually inserted in an emergency, a temporary pacemaker consists of an external, battery-powered pulse generator and a lead or electrode system. Four types of temporary pacemakers exist: transcutaneous, transvenous, transthoracic, and epicardial.

In a life-threatening situation when time is critical, a *transcutaneous pacemaker* is the best choice. (See *Indications for transcutaneous pacing.*) This device works by sending an electrical impulse from the pulse generator to the patient's heart by way of two electrodes, which are placed on the front and back of the patient's chest. Transcutaneous pacing is quick and effective, but it's used only until the physician can institute transvenous pacing.

Transcutaneous pacing is recommended by the 2005 AHA guidelines for cardiopulmonary resuscitation (CPR) and emergency cardiovascular care for symptomatic bradycardia when a pulse is present. If transcutaneous pacing doesn't correct the problem, transvenous pacing is indicated. Transvenous pacing involves threading an electrode catheter through a vein into the patient's right atrium or right ventricle. The electrode then attaches to an external pulse generator. As a result, the pulse generator can provide an electrical stimulus directly to the endocardium. This is the most common type of pacemaker.

However, a physician may choose to insert a *transthoracic pacemaker* as an elective surgical procedure or as an emergency measure during CPR. To insert this type of pacemaker, the physician performs a procedure similar to pericardiocentesis, in which he uses a cardiac needle to pass an electrode through the chest wall and into the right ventricle. This procedure carries a significant risk of coronary artery laceration and cardiac tamponade.

During cardiac surgery, the surgeon may insert electrodes through the epicardium of the right ventricle and, if he wants to institute atrioventricular sequential pacing, the right atrium. From there, the electrodes pass through the chest wall, where they remain available if temporary pacing becomes necessary. This is called *epicardial pacing.*

In addition to helping to correct conduction disturbances, a temporary pacemaker may help diagnose conduction abnormalities. For example, during a cardiac catheterization or electrophysiology study, a physician may use a temporary pacemaker to localize conduction defects. In the process, he may also learn whether the patient risks developing an arrhythmia.

Among the contraindications to pacemaker therapy are electromechanical dissociation and ventricular fibrillation.

Equipment

For transcutaneous pacing: Transcutaneous pacing generator ▪ transcutaneous pacing electrodes ▪ cardiac monitor with electrocardiogram (ECG) electrodes ▪ clippers.

For all other types of temporary pacing: Temporary pacemaker generator with new battery ▪ guide wire or introducer ▪ electrode catheter ▪ sterile gloves ▪ sterile dressings ▪ sterile marker ▪ sterile labels ▪ adhesive tape ▪ antiseptic solution ▪ emergency cardiac drugs ▪ intubation equipment ▪ defibrillator ▪ cardiac monitor with strip-chart recorder

▪ equipment to start a peripheral I.V. line, if appropriate ▪ I.V. fluids ▪ sedative ▪ electric clippers, if needed.

For transvenous pacing: All equipment listed for temporary pacing ▪ bridging cable ▪ percutaneous introducer tray or venous cutdown tray ▪ sterile gowns ▪ linen-saver pad ▪ antimicrobial soap ▪ alcohol pads ▪ vial of 1% lidocaine ▪ 5-ml syringe ▪ fluoroscopy equipment, if necessary, including protective apron ▪ fenestrated drape ▪ prepackaged cutdown tray (for antecubital vein placement only) ▪ sutures.

For transthoracic pacing: All equipment listed for temporary pacing ▪ transthoracic or cardiac needle.

For epicardial pacing: All equipment listed for temporary pacing ▪ atrial epicardial wires ▪ ventricular epicardial wires ▪ sterile rubber finger cot ▪ sterile dressing materials (if the wires won't be connected to a pulse generator).

Implementation

▪ If applicable, explain the procedure to the patient.
▪ Obtain emergency cardiac drugs and intubation equipment and have them readily available.

For transcutaneous pacing

▪ If necessary, clip the hair over the areas of electrode placement. However, don't shave the area. *If you nick the skin, the current from the pulse generator could cause discomfort and the nicks could become irritated or infected after the electrodes are applied.*
▪ Attach monitoring electrodes to the patient in lead I, II, or III position. Do this even if the patient is already on telemetry monitoring *because you'll need to connect the electrodes to the pacemaker.* If you select the lead II position, adjust the LL electrode placement to accommodate the anterior pacing electrode and the patient's anatomy.
▪ Plug the patient cable into the ECG input connection on the front of the pacing generator. Set the selector switch to the MONITOR ON position.
▪ You should see the ECG waveform on the monitor. Adjust the R-wave beeper volume to a suitable level, and activate the alarm by pressing the ALARM ON button. Set the alarm for 10 to 20 beats lower and 20 to 30 beats higher than the intrinsic rate.
▪ Press the START/STOP button for a printout of the waveform.
▪ Now you're ready to apply the two pacing electrodes. First, make sure the patient's skin is clean and dry *to ensure good skin contact.*
▪ Pull off the protective strip from one electrode, and apply the electrode on the left side of the back, just below the scapula and to the left of the spine.
▪ Pull off the protective strip from the second electrode, and apply it to the skin in the anterior position — to the left side of the precordium in the usual V_2 to V_5 position. (See *Proper electrode placement,* page 462.)
▪ Now you're ready to pace the heart. After making sure the energy output in milliamperes (mA) is on 0, connect the electrode cable to the monitor output cable.
▪ Check the waveform, looking for a tall QRS complex in lead II.
▪ Next, turn the selector switch to PACER ON. Tell the patient that he may feel a thumping or twitching sensation. Reassure him that you'll give him medication if he can't tolerate the discomfort.
▪ Now set the rate dial to 10 to 20 beats higher than the patient's intrinsic rhythm. Look for pacer artifact or spikes, which will appear as you increase the rate. If the patient doesn't have an intrinsic rhythm, set the rate at 60.
▪ Slowly increase the amount of energy delivered to the heart by adjusting the OUTPUT mA dial. Do this until capture is achieved — you'll see a pacer spike followed by a widened QRS complex that resembles a premature ventricular contraction (PVC). This is the pacing threshold. *To ensure consistent capture,* increase output by 10%. Don't go any higher *because you could cause the patient needless discomfort.*

Indications for transcutaneous pacing

The American Heart Association recommends transcutaneous pacing for these indications:

Class I

▪ Symptomatic bradycardia with hemodynamic instability unresponsive to atropine
▪ High degree block (Mobitz type II second-degree block or third-degree atrioventricular block)

Class IIa

▪ Bradycardia with an escape rhythm unresponsive to drug therapy
▪ Cardiac arrest with profound bradycardia, or pulseless electrical activity due to drug overdose, acidosis, or electrolyte abnormalities

Class IIb

Supraventricular or ventricular tachycardia refractory to drug therapy or cardioversion

Note: Overdrive pacing should be used for these patients.

Proper electrode placement

Place the two pacing electrodes for a noninvasive temporary pacemaker at heart level on the patient's chest and back (as shown below). This placement ensures that the electrical stimulus must travel only a short distance to the heart.

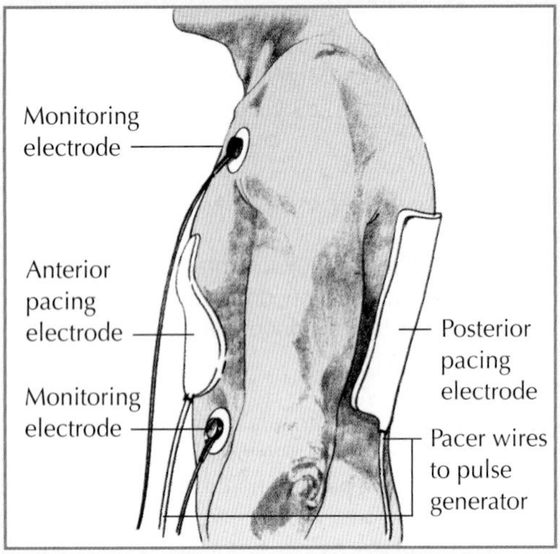

■ With full capture, the patient's heart rate should be approximately the same as the pacemaker rate set on the machine. The usual pacing threshold is between 40 and 80 mA.

For transvenous pacing

■ Check the patient's history for hypersensitivity to local anesthetics. Then attach the cardiac monitor to the patient and obtain a baseline assessment, including the patient's vital signs, skin color, level of consciousness (LOC), heart rate and rhythm, and emotional state.

■ Insert a peripheral I.V. line if the patient doesn't already have one. Begin an I.V. infusion of dextrose 5% in water at a keep-vein-open rate.

■ Insert a new battery into the external pacemaker generator, and test it to make sure it has a strong charge. Connect the bridging cable to the generator, and align the positive and negative poles. *This cable allows slack between the electrode catheter and the generator, reducing the risk of accidental catheter displacement.*

■ Place the patient in the supine position. If necessary, clip the hair around the insertion site.

■ Open the supply tray while maintaining a sterile field. Label all medications, medication containers, and other solutions on and off the sterile field.

■ Using sterile technique, clean the insertion site with antimicrobial soap and then wipe the area with antiseptic solution. Cover the insertion site with a fenestrated drape. *Because fluoroscopy may be used during the placement of leadwires,* put on a protective apron.

■ After anesthetizing the insertion site with 1% lidocaine, the physician will puncture the brachial, femoral, subclavian, or jugular vein. Then he'll insert a guide wire or an introducer and advance the electrode catheter.

■ As the catheter advances, watch the cardiac monitor. When the electrode catheter reaches the right atrium, you'll notice large P waves and small QRS complexes. Then, as the catheter reaches the right ventricle, the P waves will become smaller while the QRS complexes enlarge. When the catheter touches the right ventricular endocardium, expect to see elevated ST segments, PVCs, or both.

■ When the electrode catheter is in the right ventricle, it will send an impulse to the myocardium, causing depolarization. If the patient needs atrial pacing, either alone or with ventricular pacing, the physician may place an electrode in the right atrium.

■ Meanwhile, continuously monitor the patient's cardiac status and treat any arrhythmias, as appropriate. Also assess the patient for jaw pain and earache; *these symptoms indicate that the electrode catheter has missed the superior vena cava and has moved into the neck instead.*

■ When the electrode catheter is in place, attach the catheter leads to the bridging cable, lining up the positive and negative poles.

■ Check the battery's charge by pressing the BATTERY TEST button.

■ Set the pacemaker as ordered.

■ The physician will then suture the catheter to the insertion site. Afterward, put on sterile gloves and apply a sterile dressing to the site. Label the dressing with the date and time of application.

For transthoracic pacing

■ Clean the skin to the left of the xiphoid process with antiseptic solution. Work quickly *because CPR must be interrupted for the procedure.*

■ After interrupting CPR, the physician will insert a transthoracic needle through the patient's chest wall to the left of the xiphoid process into the right ventricle. He'll then follow the needle with the electrode catheter.

■ Connect the electrode catheter to the generator, lining up the positive and negative poles. Watch the cardiac monitor for signs of ventricular pacing and capture.

■ After the physician sutures the electrode catheter into place, use sterile technique to apply a sterile 4″ × 4″ gauze dressing to the site. Tape the dressing securely, and label it with the date and time of application.
■ Check the patient's peripheral pulses and vital signs *to assess cardiac output.* If you can't palpate a pulse, continue performing CPR.
■ If the patient has a palpable pulse, assess the patient's vital signs, ECG, and LOC.

For epicardial pacing
■ During your preoperative teaching, inform the patient that epicardial pacemaker wires may be placed during cardiac surgery.
■ During cardiac surgery, the physician will hook epicardial wires into the epicardium just before the end of the surgery. Depending on the patient's condition, the physician may insert either atrial or ventricular wires or both.
■ If indicated, connect the electrode catheter to the generator, lining up the positive and negative poles. Set the pacemaker as ordered.
■ If the wires won't be connected to an external pulse generator, place them in a sterile rubber finger cot. Then cover both the wires and the insertion site with a sterile, occlusive dressing. *This will help protect the patient from microshock as well as infection.*

Special considerations
■ Take care to prevent microshock. This includes warning the patient not to use electrical equipment that isn't grounded, such as telephones, electric shavers, televisions, or lamps.
■ Other safety measures you'll want to take include placing a plastic cover supplied by the manufacturer over the pacemaker controls *to avoid an accidental setting change.* Also, insulate the pacemaker by placing the pacing unit in a dry, rubber surgical glove. If the patient needs emergency defibrillation, make sure the pacemaker can withstand the procedure. If you're unsure, disconnect the pulse generator *to avoid damage.*
■ When using a transcutaneous pacemaker, don't place the electrodes over a bony area *because bone conducts current poorly.* With female patients, place the anterior electrode under the patient's breast but not over her diaphragm. If the physician inserts the electrode through the brachial or femoral vein, immobilize the patient's arm or leg *to avoid putting stress on the pacing wires.*
■ After insertion of any temporary pacemaker, assess the patient's vital signs, skin color, LOC, and peripheral pulses *to determine the effectiveness of the paced rhythm.* Perform a 12-lead ECG to serve as a baseline, and then perform additional ECGs daily or with clinical changes. Also, if possible, obtain a rhythm strip before, during, and after pacemaker placement; any time that pacemaker settings are changed; and whenever the patient receives treatment because of a complication due to the pacemaker.
■ Continuously monitor the ECG reading, noting capture, sensing, rate, intrinsic beats, and competition of paced and intrinsic rhythms. If the pacemaker is sensing correctly, the sense indicator on the pulse generator should flash with each beat. (See *When a temporary pacemaker malfunctions,* pages 464 and 465.)
■ If the patient has epicardial pacing wires in place, clean the insertion site with antiseptic solution and change the dressing daily. At the same time, monitor the site for signs of infection. Always keep the pulse generator nearby *in case pacing becomes necessary.*

Complications
Complications associated with pacemaker therapy include microshock, equipment failure, and competitive or fatal arrhythmias. Transcutaneous pacemakers may also cause skin breakdown and muscle pain and twitching when the pacemaker fires. Transvenous pacemakers may cause such complications as pneumothorax or hemothorax, cardiac perforation and tamponade, diaphragmatic stimulation, pulmonary embolism, thrombophlebitis, and infection. Also, if the physician threads the electrode through the antecubital or femoral vein, venous spasm, thrombophlebitis, or lead displacement may result.

Complications associated with transthoracic pacemakers include pneumothorax, cardiac tamponade, emboli, sepsis, lacerations of the myocardium or coronary artery, and perforations of a cardiac chamber. Epicardial pacemakers carry a risk of infection, cardiac arrest, and diaphragmatic stimulation.

Documentation
Record the reason for pacing, the time it started, and the locations of the electrodes. For a transvenous or transthoracic pacemaker, note the date, the time, and reason for the temporary pacemaker.

For any temporary pacemaker, record the pacemaker settings. Note the patient's response to the procedure, along with any complications and the interventions taken. If possible, obtain rhythm strips before, during, and after pacemaker placement, and whenever pacemaker settings are changed or when the patient receives treatment for a complication caused by the pacemaker. As you monitor the patient, record his response to temporary pacing and note any changes in his condition.

TROUBLESHOOTING

When a temporary pacemaker malfunctions

Occasionally, a temporary pacemaker may fail to function appropriately. When this occurs, you'll need to take immediate action to correct the problem. Take the steps described below when your patient's pacemaker fails to pace, capture, or sense intrinsic beats.

Failure to pace

This happens when the pacemaker either doesn't fire or fires too often. The pulse generator may not be working properly, or it may not be conducting the impulse to the patient.

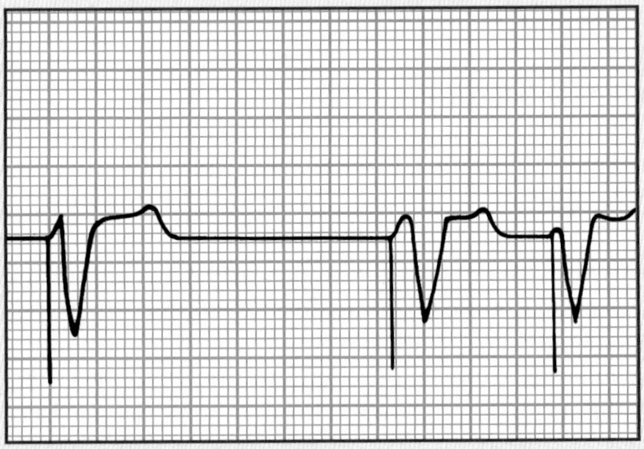

Nursing interventions

- If the pacing or sensing indicator flashes, check the connections to the cable and the position of the pacing electrode in the patient (by X-ray). The cable may have come loose, or the electrode may have been dislodged, pulled out, or broken.
- If the pulse generator is turned on but the indicators still aren't flashing, change the battery. If that doesn't help, use a different pulse generator.
- Check the settings if the pacemaker is firing too rapidly. If they're correct, or if altering them (according to your facility's policy or the physician's order) doesn't help, change the pulse generator.

Failure to capture

Here, you see pacemaker spikes but the heart isn't responding. This may be caused by changes in the pacing threshold from ischemia, an electrolyte imbalance (high or low potassium or magnesium levels), acidosis, an adverse reaction to a medication, a perforated ventricle, fibrosis, or the position of the electrode.

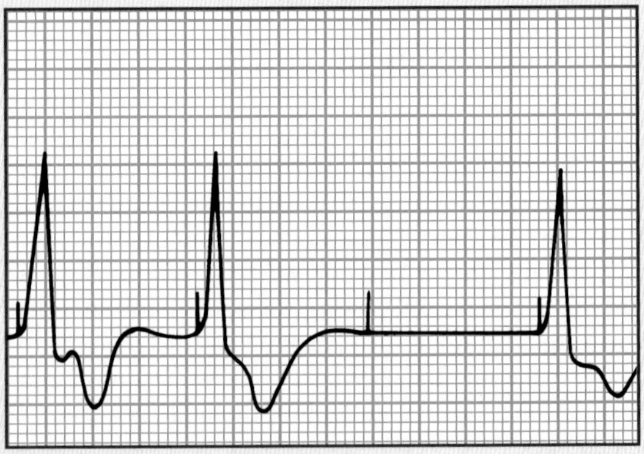

Nursing interventions

- If the patient's condition has changed, notify the physician and ask him for new settings.
- If pacemaker settings have been altered by the patient (or his family members), return them to their correct positions. Then make sure the face of the pacemaker is covered with a plastic shield. Tell the patient and his family members not to touch the dials.
- If the heart isn't responding, try any or all of these suggestions: Carefully check all connections, making sure they're placed properly and securely; increase the milliamperes slowly (acording to your facility's policy or the physician's order); turn the patient on his left side, then on his right (if turning him to the left didn't help); and schedule an anteroposterior or lateral chest X-ray to determine the position of the electrode.

When a temporary pacemaker malfunctions *(continued)*

Failure to sense intrinsic beats

This could cause ventricular tachycardia or ventricular fibrillation if the pacemaker fires on the vulnerable T wave. This could be caused by the pacemaker sensing an external stimulus as a QRS complex, which could lead to asystole, or by the pacemaker not being sensitive enough, which means it could fire anywhere within the cardiac cycle.

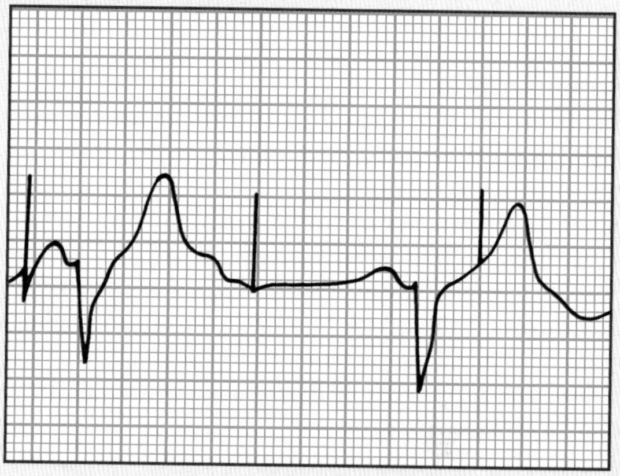

Nursing interventions

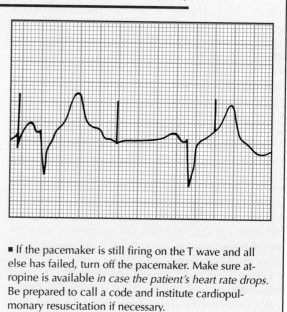

- If the pacing is undersensing, turn the sensitivity control completely to the right. If it's oversensing, turn it slightly to the left.
- If the pacemaker isn't functioning correctly, change the battery or the pulse generator.
- Remove items in the room causng electromechanical interference (razors, radios, cautery devices). Check the ground wires on the bed and other equipment for obvious damage. Unplug each piece and see if the inteference stops. When you locate the cause, notify the staff engineer and ask him to check it.
- If the pacemaker is still firing on the T wave and all else has failed, turn off the pacemaker. Make sure atropine is available *in case the patient's heart rate drops.* Be prepared to call a code and institute cardiopulmonary resuscitation if necessary.

SELECTED REFERENCES

American Association for Respiratory Care. "Clinical Practice Guideline. Resuscitation and Defibrillation in the Health Care Setting—2004 Revision and Update," *Respiratory Care* 89(9):1085-99, September 2004.

American Heart Association. "2005 AHA Guidelines for Cardiopulmonary Resuscitation and Emergency Cardiovascular Care: International Consensus on Science," *Circulation* 112(22 Suppl): IV-1-IV-221, November 2005.

Craig, K. "How to Provide Transcutaneous Pacing," *Nursing* 35(10):52-53, October 2005.

Lynn-McHale Wiegand, D.J., and Carlson, K.K., eds. *AACN Procedure Manual for Critical Care,* 5th ed. Philadelphia: W.B. Saunders Co., 2005.

Overbay, D., and Criddle, L. "Mastering Temporary Invasive Cardiac Pacing," *Critical Care Nurse* 24(3):25-32, June 2004.

EPICARDIAL PACEMAKER WIRE REMOVAL

Epicardial pacing wires are commonly positioned on the epicardial (outer) surface of the heart after cardiac surgery to diagnose and treat arrhythmias, which may be caused by electrolyte imbalances, inflammation, injury, edema, and hypothermia. Depending on the needs of the patient, the surgeon usually places positive and negative electrodes on both the right atrium and the right ventricle. These electrodes are loosely sutured to the epicardial surface and brought out through the chest wall through small incisions.

In the event that pacing is required, epicardial pacing wires are connected to the pulse generator of a temporary pacemaker. When the patient becomes hemodynamically stable, the wires can be removed. Complications following epicardial pacing wire removal occur more frequently in patients with a history of heart failure and repeat heart surgery. Historically, only physicians or physician assistants were allowed to remove epicardial pacing wires; however, specially trained critical care nurses can now safely remove them.

Equipment

Nonsterile gloves ▪ gown ▪ goggles or face shield with mask ▪ sterile gauze ▪ tape ▪ suture removal kit ▪ cardiac monitor ▪ emergency cart, including temporary transcutaneous or transvenous pacing equipment, should be immediately available.

Preparation of equipment

Wash your hands and bring the equipment to the patient's bedside. Using sterile technique, open the suture removal kit and gauze packages and place them within reach.

Implementation

- Verify the order in the patient's chart for epicardial wire removal *to assure the right procedure is being performed on the right patient at the right time.*
- Confirm the patient's identity using two patient identifiers according to your facility's policy.
- Explain the procedure to the patient *to reduce anxiety and enhance cooperation,* and tell him that a burning or pulling sensation is normal but he shouldn't feel pain.
- Administer an analgesic 20 to 30 minutes before the procedure *to promote patient comfort.*
- Check laboratory data for coagulation and electrolyte results to be sure they are within normal limits *to reduce the risk of bleeding and cardiac arrhythmias.* Notify the physician of any abnormal values.
- Obtain vital signs and an electrocardiogram (ECG) rhythm strip, and assess cardiovascular status *to ensure the patient is stable prior to removal of pacing wires and to provide a baseline for comparison.*
- Check the medication record to ensure the patient isn't receiving anticoagulants *to reduce the risk of hemorrhage following the procedure.*
- Check that the emergency cart, with temporary transcutaneous or transvenous pacing equipment, is readily available.
- Confirm that the patient has patent I.V. access in case emergency fluids or medications are required.
- Put on goggles, mask, gloves, and gown.
- Place the patient in a supine position so that the wires are readily accessible and the patient is properly positioned *if emergency measures become necessary.*
- Carefully remove any tape and dressing covering the wires.
- Cut the sutures at the appropriate place and remove them.
- Grasp a wire and slowly and gently pull to uncoil it from the epicardium. If you feel resistance, stop and notify the physician.
- While pulling each wire, observe the cardiac monitor for arrhythmias.
- Inspect the pacing wire for a small piece of tissue at the tip *indicating that the entire wire was removed intact.*
- If bleeding is noted at the exit site, apply pressure.
- Observe the site, noting any drainage, redness, or skin breakdown.
- Place sterile gauze pads over the exit sites and secure with tape.
- Dispose of soiled supplies according to your facility's policy *to reduce the risk of transmission of microorganisms.*
- Check vital signs and for arrhythmias and clinical findings of cardiac tamponade every 15 minutes for the first hour, every 30 minutes for the next 2 hours, and then hourly for the following 2 hours *to assess hemodynamic stability.*

Special considerations

- Pacing wires should be removed at least 24 hours prior to discharge *so the patient can be monitored for complications.*
- *Because these pacing wires provide a direct electrical route to the heart,* prevent microshocks by wearing gloves when handling the wires.

Complications

Monitor for signs and symptoms of life-threatening cardiac tamponade, such as Beck's triad (hypotension, muffled heart tones, and jugular vein distention), tachycardia, decreased peripheral pulses, and dyspnea. Cardiac tamponade may not be immediately evident if the bleeding is slow; therefore, close monitoring for up to 2 hours may be needed. Other complications include infection, hemorrhage, hematoma, arrhythmias, hemodynamic instability, myocardial ischemia, and graft site trauma.

Documentation

Record the date, time, and name of the person removing the wires. If an analgesic was administered, record the name, dose, route, and time it was given and the patient's rating of his level of pain (on a 0-to-10 scale). Describe the condition of the insertion sites, the ease with which the wires were removed, and whether any tissue was noted at the end of the wires. Include vital signs, ECG strip, and patient assessment before, during, and after the procedure. Record how the site was dressed. Note the patient's tolerance of the procedure. If any adverse effects occurred, note the time and name of the physician notified, orders given, nursing interventions, and the patient's response. Document frequent assessments on a frequent vital sign assessment sheet, according to your facility's policy. Include any patient and family teaching provided.

SELECTED REFERENCES

Lynn-McHale Wiegand, D.J., and Carlson, K.K., eds. *AACN Procedure Manual for Critical Care,* 5th ed. Philadelphia: W.B. Saunders Co., 2005.

Overbay, D., and Criddle, L. "Mastering Temporary Invasive Cardiac Pacing," *Critical Care Nurse* 24(3):25-32, June 2004.

Reade, M.C. "Temporary Epicardial Pacing after Cardiac Surgery: A Practical Review. Part 1: General Considerations in the

Management of Epicardial Pacing," *Anaesthesia* 62(3): 264–71, March 2007.

Roschkov, S., and Jensen, L. "Coronary Artery Bypass Graft Patients' Pain Perception during Epicardial Pacing Wire Removal," *Canadian Journal of Cardiovascular Nursing* 14(3):32-38, 2004.

Timothy, P.R., and Rodeman, B.J. "Temporary Pacemakers in Critically Ill Patients: Assessment and Management Strategies," *AACN Clinical Issues* 15(3):305-25, July-September 2004.

CODE MANAGEMENT

The goals of any code are to restore the patient's spontaneous heartbeat and respirations and to prevent hypoxic damage to the brain and other vital organs. Fulfilling these goals requires a team approach. Ideally, the team should consist of health care workers trained in advanced cardiac life support (ACLS), although nurses trained in basic life support (BLS) may also be a part of the team. Sponsored by the American Heart Association (AHA), the ACLS course incorporates BLS skills with advanced resuscitation techniques. BLS and ACLS procedures and protocols should be performed according to the 2005 AHA guidelines.

In most health care facilities, ACLS-trained nurses provide the first resuscitative efforts to cardiac arrest patients, commonly administering cardiac medications and performing defibrillation before the practitioner's arrival. Because ventricular fibrillation commonly precedes sudden cardiac arrest, initial resuscitative efforts focus on rapid recognition of arrhythmias and, when indicated, defibrillation. If monitoring equipment isn't available, you should simply perform BLS measures. Of course, the scope of your responsibilities in any situation depends on your facility's policies and procedures and your state's nurse practice act.

A code may be called for patients with absent pulse, apnea, VF, ventricular tachycardia, or asystole. Some facilities allow family members to be present during a code; check your facility's policy regarding this issue.

The 2005 AHA guidelines for cardiopulmonary resuscitation (CPR) and emergency cardiovascular care stress the importance of good BLS care as the foundation of ACLS. Basic CPR and early defibrillation are of primary importance because they can significantly increase the patient's chances of survival. Drug therapy is the second priority. Recommended priorities include:

- starting CPR
- attempting defibrillation
- establishing I.V. access
- considering drug therapy
- inserting an advanced airway.

The 2005 AHA guidelines also stress that compressions shouldn't be interrupted unless a shock is being delivered or a rhythm check is being performed.

Health care providers shouldn't attempt to check for a pulse after a shock is delivered, but the pulse check should occur after five cycles of CPR, if a rhythm is detected.

Equipment

Oral, nasal, and endotracheal (ET) airways ▪ one-way valve masks ▪ oxygen source ▪ oxygen flowmeter ▪ intubation supplies, including end-tidal carbon dioxide detector or esophageal detector ▪ handheld resuscitation bag ▪ suction supplies ▪ nasogastric (NG) tube ▪ goggles, masks, and gloves ▪ cardiac arrest board ▪ peripheral I.V. supplies, including 14G and 18G peripheral I.V. catheters ▪ central I.V. supplies, including an 18G thin-wall catheter, a 6-cm needle catheter, and a 16G 15- to 20-cm catheter ▪ I.V. administration sets (including macrodrip and microdrip) ▪ I.V. fluids, including dextrose 5% in water (D_5W), normal saline solution, and lactated Ringer's solution ▪ electrocardiogram (ECG) monitor and leads ▪ cardioverter-defibrillator ▪ conductive medium ▪ cardiac drugs, including adenosine, epinephrine, lidocaine, procainamide, vasopressin, amiodarone, atropine, isoproterenol, dopamine, calcium chloride, and dobutamine.

Preparation of equipment

Because effective emergency care depends on reliable and accessible equipment, the equipment as well as the personnel must be ready for a code at any time. (See *Organizing your crash cart,* page 468.) You should also be familiar with the cardiac drugs you may have to administer. (See *Common emergency cardiac drugs,* pages 469 to 471.)

Always be aware of your patient's code status as defined by the practitioner's orders, the patient's advance directives, and family wishes. If the practitioner has ordered a "no code," make sure he has written and signed the order. If possible, have the patient or a responsible family member cosign the order.

In some cases, you may need to consider whether the family wishes to be present during a code. If they want to be present and if a nurse or clergyman can remain with them, consider allowing them to remain during the code.

Implementation

- If you're the first to arrive at the site of a code, call for help, and instruct another person to retrieve the emergency equipment. Then, assess the patient's level of consciousness (LOC); assess airway, breathing, and circulation; and then begin CPR. Use a pocket mask, if available, to ventilate the patient.

EQUIPMENT

Organizing your crash cart

When responding to a code, you can't waste time searching the drawers of your crash cart for the equipment you need. One way to make sure you know the precise location of everything is to follow the ABCD plan to maintain an organized crash cart. Label the crash cart drawers with the letters A, B, C, and D, and fill them as described below.

A: Airway control drawer

The airway control drawer should contain all the equipment necessary for maintaining a patient's airway, including:

- oral, nasal, and endotracheal (ET) airways
- an intubation tray containing a laryngoscope and blades
- an extra laryngoscope
- lidocaine ointment
- tape or ET tube securement device
- a 10-ml syringe to inflate the ET balloon
- extra batteries and light bulbs
- suction devices.

B: Breathing drawer

The breathing drawer should contain all of the equipment needed to support the patient's ventilation and oxygenation. Maintain gastric compression with nasogastric tubes. Support oxygenation with:

- nasal cannulas
- face masks
- Venturi masks.

C: Circulation drawer

In the circulation drawer, place anything needed to start a central or peripheral I.V. line, such as:

- catheters
- tubing
- start kits
- pump tubing
- 250-ml or 500-ml bags of I.V. solutions (dextrose 5% in water and normal saline solution).

D: Drug drawer

The drug drawer should contain all medications needed for advanced cardiac life support.

- When the emergency equipment arrives, have the second BLS provider place the cardiac arrest board under the patient and assist with two-rescuer CPR. Meanwhile, have the nurse assigned to the patient relate the patient's medical history and describe the events leading to cardiac arrest.
- A third person, either a nurse certified in BLS or a respiratory therapist, will then attach the handheld resuscitation bag to the oxygen source and begin to ventilate the patient with 100% oxygen.
- When the ACLS-trained nurse arrives, she'll expose the patient's chest and apply defibrillator pads. She'll then apply the paddles to the patient's chest to obtain a "quick look" at the patient's cardiac rhythm. If the patient is in VF, ACLS protocol calls for defibrillation as soon as possible with 360 joules. Then, resume CPR immediately. A rhythm check isn't done at this time. After five cycles of CPR and if a rhythm is detected, perform a pulse check. (See *ACLS pulseless arrest algorithm,* pages 472 and 473.) The ACLS-trained nurse will act as code leader until the practitioner arrives.
- If not already in place, apply ECG electrodes and attach the patient to the defibrillator's cardiac monitor. Avoid placing electrodes on bony prominences or hairy areas. Also avoid the areas where the defibrillator pads will be placed and where chest compressions will be given.
- After five cycles of CPR, the patient's rhythm will be checked and, if necessary, another shock will be given at the same dose; you'll then continue CPR while the defibrillator is charging. After another five cycles of CPR, the patient's rhythm will be checked, and another shock will be given at the same dose, if necessary.
- As CPR continues, you or an ACLS-trained nurse will then start two peripheral I.V. lines with large-bore I.V. catheters. Be sure to use only a large vein, such as the antecubital vein, *to allow for rapid fluid administration and to prevent drug extravasation.*
- As soon as the I.V. catheter is in place, begin an infusion of normal saline solution *to help prevent circulatory collapse.* D_5W continues to be acceptable but the latest ACLS guidelines encourage the use of normal saline solution *because D_5W can produce hyperglycemic effects during a cardiac arrest.*
- While one nurse starts the I.V. lines, the other nurse will set up portable or wall suction equipment and suction the patient's oral secretions, as necessary, *to maintain an open airway.*
- The ACLS-trained nurse will then prepare and administer emergency cardiac drugs as needed. Keep in mind that drugs administered through a central line reach the myocardium more quickly than those administered through a peripheral line.

Common emergency cardiac drugs

You may be called on to administer a variety of cardiac drugs during a code. This table lists the most commonly used emergency cardiac drugs, along with their actions, indications, and dosage.

Drug	Actions	Indications	Typical adult dosage
Adenosine	■ Slows conduction through atrioventricular (AV) node; may interrupt reentry through AV node ■ Shortens duration of atrial action potential during supraventricular tachycardia	■ Supraventricular tachycardia, including those associated with accessory bypass tracts (Wolff-Parkinson-White syndrome)	■ 6 mg I.V. push over 1 to 3 seconds initially; may be increased to 12 mg if conversion hasn't occurred within 2 minutes; may repeat 12 mg in 1 to 2 minutes, if needed. Each dose should quickly be followed by a 20-ml saline flush. ■ *Caution*: Slower-than-recommended administration decreases drug's effectiveness.
Amiodarone	■ Thought to prolong the refractory period and action potential, duration	■ Supraventricular tachycardia ■ Persistent ventricular tachycardia (VT) or venricular fibrillation (VF)	■ For wide complex tachycardia, 150 mg over 10 minutes, followed by 1 mg/minute infusion for 6 hours, then 0.5 mg/minute. ■ For cardiac arrest, 300 mg I.V. push or I.O.; repeat 150 mg I.V. push in 3 to 5 minutes. Dilute in 20 to 30 ml dextrose 5% in water (D_5W). Maximum dose: 2.2. g I.V./24 hours.
Atropine	■ Accelerates AV conduction and heart rate by blocking vagal nerve	■ Symptomatic bradycardia ■ Asystole ■ AV block ■ Pulseless electrical activity (PEA) (slow rate)	■ 0.5 to 1 mg I.V. push (for asystole or PEA, 1 mg); repeated every 3 to 5 minutes until heart rate exceeds 60 beats/minute (up to 3 mg total). ■ *Caution*: Excessive increases in heart rate may worsen ischemia in patients with acute myocardial infarction.
Dobutamine	■ Increases myocardial contractility without raising oxygen demand	■ Heart failure ■ Cardiogenic shock	■ 2 to 20 mcg/kg/minute by continuous I.V. infusion. Titrate so heart rate isn't greater than 10% of baseline. ■ *Caution:* Don't administer in same I.V. line with alkaline solution.
Dopamine	■ Produces inotropic effect, increasing cardiac output, blood pressure, and renal perfusion	■ Hypotension (except when caused by hypovolemia)	■ Continuous I.V. infusion at 2 to 4 mcg/kg/minute initially; can be increased to 20 mcg/kg/minute, as needed. *Note:* Always dilute and give I.V. drip, never I.V. push. Titrate to patient response. ■ *Caution*: Don't administer in same I.V. line with alkaline solution.

(continued)

Common emergency cardiac drugs *(continued)*

DRUG	ACTIONS	INDICATIONS	TYPICAL ADULT DOSAGE
Epinephrine	■ Increases heart rate, peripheral resistance, and blood flow to heart (enhancing myocardial and cerebral oxygenation) ■ Strengthens myocardial contractility ■ Increases coronary perfusion pressure during cardiopulmonary resuscitation	■ VF ■ Pulseless VT ■ Asystole ■ Hypotension (secondary agent) ■ PEA ■ Symptomatic bradycardia	■ 10 ml of 1:10,000 solution (1 mg) I.V. push or I.O. initially; may be repeated every 3 to 5 minutes, as needed. After each dose, flush with 20 ml of I.V. fluid if administered peripherally. ■ 2 to 2½ times the I.V. dose endotracheally if no I.V. line is available. *Note:* 1:1,000 solution contains 1 mg/ml, so it must be diluted in 9 ml of normal saline solution to provide 1 mg/10 ml. ■ For hypotension, 1 mg/500 ml of D_5W by continuous infusion, starting at 1 mcg/minute and titrated to desired effect (2 to 10 mcg/minute). ■ *Caution*: Don't administer in same I.V. line with alkaline solution.
Isoproterenol	■ Enhances automaticity and accelerates conduction ■ Increases heart rate and cardiac contractility, but exacerbates ischemia and arrhythmias in patients with ischemic heart disease	■ Indicated only for temporary control of severe bradycardia unresponsive to atropine (while awaiting pacemaker insertion) ■ Torsades de Pointes	■ Continuous I.V. infusion at 2 to 10 mcg/minute titrated p.r.n. to obtain an adequate heart rate. Monitor heart rate and blood pressure carefully. ■ *Caution:* Doses that increase heart rate to greater than 130 beats/minute may induce ventricular arrhythmias.
Lidocaine	■ Depresses automaticity and conduction of ectopic impulses in ventricles, especially in ischemic tissue ■ Raises fibrillation threshold, especially in an ischemic heart	■ Frequent premature ventricular contractions (PVCs) ■ VT ■ VF	■ 1 to 1.5 mg/kg (usually 50 to 75 mg) I.V. push or I.O. initially; may be followed by 0.5 to 0.75 mg/kg bolus dose every 5 to 10 minutes up to total of 3 mg/kg. ■ Continuous I.V. infusion of 2 g/500 ml of D_5W (1 to 4 mg/minute) to prevent recurrence of lethal arrhythmias; may be reduced by 50% after 24 hours.
Magnesium sulfate	■ Mechanism of action is unclear but drug may help in cardiac arrest associated with refractory VT or VF	■ Cardiac arrest associated with refractory VT or VF ■ Torsades de Pointes ■ Ventricular arrhythmias due to digoxin toxicity	■ For cardiac arrest associated with Torsades de Pointes, 1 to 2 g I.V. in 10 ml of D_5W over 5 to 20 minutes. ■ For Torsades de Pointes without cardiac arrest, 1 to 2 g in 50 to 100 ml of D_5W over 5 to 60 minutes; follow with 0.5 to 1 g/hour I.V. ■ *Caution:* If hypotension develops, slow or stop infusion.

Common emergency cardiac drugs *(continued)*

DRUG	ACTIONS	INDICATIONS	TYPICAL ADULT DOSAGE
Procainamide	■ Depresses automaticity and conduction ■ Prolongs refraction in the atria and ventricles	■ PVCs ■ VT ■ Supraventricular arrhythmias	■ 20 mg/minute up to a total of 17 mg/kg, followed by maintenance dose of 1 to 4 mg/minute by I.V. infusion.
Vasopressin	■ Causes peripheral vasoconstriction	■ Refractory VF ■ Pulseless VT ■ VF	■ 40 units I.V. or I.O. as a single dose, one time only.
Verapamil	■ Slows conduction through AV node ■ Causes vasodilation ■ Produces negative inotropic effect on heart, depressing myocardial contractility	■ Paroxysmal supraventricular tachycardia with narrow QRS complex and rate control in atrial fibrillation	■ 2.5 to 5 mg I.V. push over 2 minutes initially (over 3 minutes in older adult); repeat dose of 5 to 10 mg every 15 to 30 minutes, if needed, for a total dose of 20 mg. ■ *Caution:* Monitor ECG and blood pressure.

- The ACLS pulseless arrest algorithm shows the timing of drug administration and shock administration. Drug doses should be given immediately after a rhythm check.
- If the patient doesn't have an accessible I.V. line, you may administer such medications as epinephrine, lidocaine, vasopressin, and atropine through an ET tube. To do so, dilute the drugs in 10 ml of normal saline solution or sterile water and then instill them into the patient's ET tube. Afterward, ventilate the patient manually *to improve absorption by distributing the drug throughout the bronchial tree.*
- The ACLS-trained nurse will also prepare for, and assist with, ET intubation or other advanced airway. Compression interruption should be minimized during advanced airway placement.
- Suction the patient as needed. After the patient has been intubated, the practitioner should use clinical assessment and confirmation devices to check ET tube placement. Assessment includes visualizing chest expansion, auscultation of equal breath sounds, and auscultation of breath sounds over the epigastrium. Devices used to check tube placement include exhaled carbon dioxide detectors and esophageal detectors. When the tube is correctly positioned, tape it securely. *To serve as a reference,* mark the point on the tube level with the patient's lips.
- Meanwhile, other members of the code team should keep a written record of the events. Other duties include prompting participants about when to perform certain activities (such as when to check a pulse or take vital signs), overseeing the effectiveness of CPR, and keeping track of the time between therapies. Each team member should know what each participant's role is *to prevent duplicating effort.* Finally, someone from the team should make sure the primary nurse's other patients are reassigned to another nurse.
- If the family is present during the code, have someone, such as a clergy member or social worker, remain with them. Be sure to keep the family regularly informed of the patient's status.
- If the family isn't at the facility, contact them as soon as possible. Encourage them not to drive to the facility, but offer to call someone who can give them a ride.

Special considerations

- When the patient's condition has stabilized, assess his LOC, breath sounds, heart sounds, peripheral perfusion, bowel sounds, and urine output. Measure his vital signs every 15 minutes, and monitor his cardiac rhythm continuously.
- Make sure the patient receives an adequate supply of oxygen, whether through a mask or a ventilator.
- Check the infusion rates of all I.V. fluids, and use infusion pumps to deliver vasoactive drugs. *To evaluate the effectiveness of fluid therapy,* insert an indwelling catheter if the patient doesn't already have one. Also insert an NG tube *to relieve or prevent gastric distention.*

(Text continues on page 474.)

ACLS pulseless arrest algorithm

This American Heart Association algorithm outlines the steps an advanced cardiac life support (ACLS)-certified nurse should take to treat rhythms that produce cardiac arrest, such as ventricular fibrillation (VF), rapid ventricular tachycardia (VT), pulseless electrical activity, and asystole. If you aren't ACLS-certified, the algorithm will help you know what to expect in such an emergency.

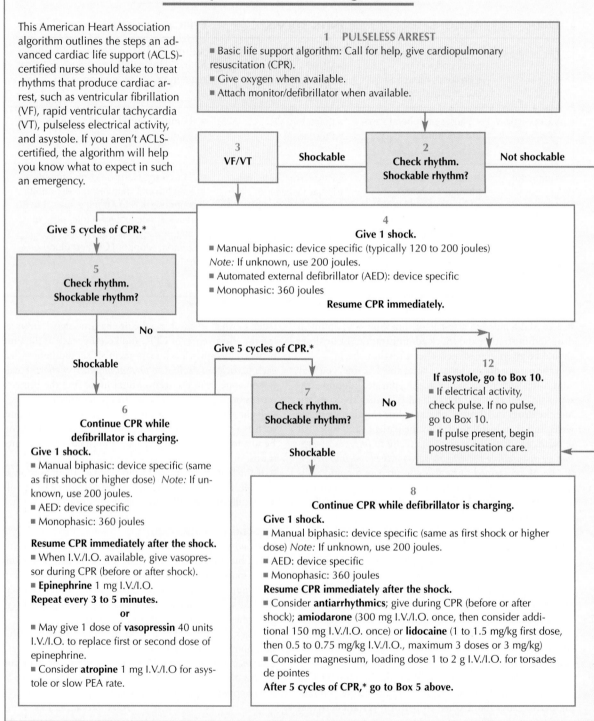

1 PULSELESS ARREST
- Basic life support algorithm: Call for help, give cardiopulmonary resuscitation (CPR).
- Give oxygen when available.
- Attach monitor/defibrillator when available.

2 Check rhythm. Shockable rhythm?

Shockable → 3; Not shockable → 12

3 VF/VT

4 Give 1 shock.
- Manual biphasic: device specific (typically 120 to 200 joules) *Note:* If unknown, use 200 joules.
- Automated external defibrillator (AED): device specific
- Monophasic: 360 joules

Resume CPR immediately.

Give 5 cycles of CPR.*

5 Check rhythm. Shockable rhythm?

No → 12; Shockable → 6

6 Continue CPR while defibrillator is charging.

Give 1 shock.
- Manual biphasic: device specific (same as first shock or higher dose) *Note:* If unknown, use 200 joules.
- AED: device specific
- Monophasic: 360 joules

Resume CPR immediately after the shock.
- When I.V./I.O. available, give vasopressor during CPR (before or after shock).
- **Epinephrine** 1 mg I.V./I.O.

Repeat every 3 to 5 minutes.

or
- May give 1 dose of **vasopressin** 40 units I.V./I.O. to replace first or second dose of epinephrine.
- Consider **atropine** 1 mg I.V./I.O for asystole or slow PEA rate.

Give 5 cycles of CPR.*

7 Check rhythm. Shockable rhythm?

No → 12; Shockable → 8

8 Continue CPR while defibrillator is charging.

Give 1 shock.
- Manual biphasic: device specific (same as first shock or higher dose) *Note:* If unknown, use 200 joules.
- AED: device specific
- Monophasic: 360 joules

Resume CPR immediately after the shock.
- Consider **antiarrhythmics**; give during CPR (before or after shock); **amiodarone** (300 mg I.V./I.O. once, then consider additional 150 mg I.V./I.O. once) or **lidocaine** (1 to 1.5 mg/kg first dose, then 0.5 to 0.75 mg/kg I.V./I.O., maximum 3 doses or 3 mg/kg)
- Consider magnesium, loading dose 1 to 2 g I.V./I.O. for torsades de pointes

After 5 cycles of CPR,* go to Box 5 above.

12 If asystole, go to Box 10.
- If electrical activity, check pulse. If no pulse, go to Box 10.
- If pulse present, begin postresuscitation care.

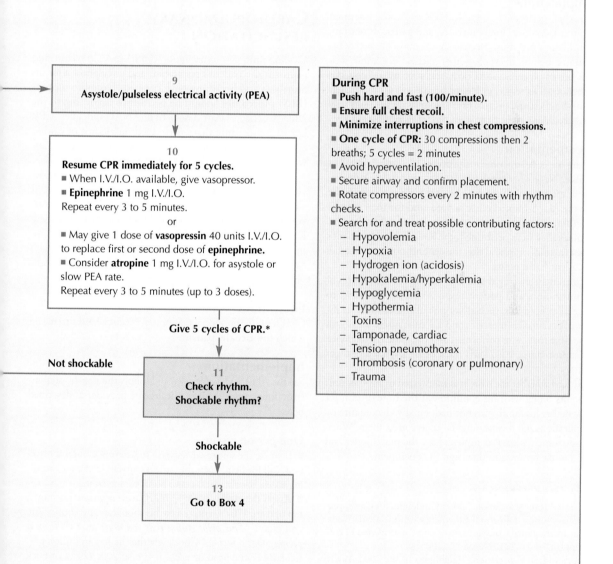

9
Asystole/pulseless electrical activity (PEA)

10
Resume CPR immediately for 5 cycles.
- When I.V./I.O. available, give vasopressor.
- **Epinephrine** 1 mg I.V./I.O.
Repeat every 3 to 5 minutes.
or
- May give 1 dose of **vasopressin** 40 units I.V./I.O. to replace first or second dose of **epinephrine.**
- Consider **atropine** 1 mg I.V./I.O. for asystole or slow PEA rate.
Repeat every 3 to 5 minutes (up to 3 doses).

Give 5 cycles of CPR.*

11
Check rhythm.
Shockable rhythm?

Not shockable

Shockable

13
Go to Box 4

During CPR
- **Push hard and fast (100/minute).**
- **Ensure full chest recoil.**
- **Minimize interruptions in chest compressions.**
- **One cycle of CPR:** 30 compressions then 2 breaths; 5 cycles = 2 minutes
- Avoid hyperventilation.
- Secure airway and confirm placement.
- Rotate compressors every 2 minutes with rhythm checks.
- Search for and treat possible contributing factors:
  - Hypovolemia
  - Hypoxia
  - Hydrogen ion (acidosis)
  - Hypokalemia/hyperkalemia
  - Hypoglycemia
  - Hypothermia
  - Toxins
  - Tamponade, cardiac
  - Tension pneumothorax
  - Thrombosis (coronary or pulmonary)
  - Trauma

*After an advanced airway is placed, rescuers no longer deliver "cycles" of CPR. Give continuous chest compressions without pauses for breaths. Give 8 to 10 breaths/minute. Check rhythm every 2 minutes.

- If appropriate, reassure the patient and explain what's happening. Allow the patient's family to visit as soon as possible. If the patient dies, notify the family and allow them to see the patient as soon as possible.
- To make sure your code team performs optimally, schedule a time to review the code.

Complications

Even when performed correctly, CPR can cause fractured ribs, liver laceration, lung puncture, and gastric distention. Defibrillation can cause electric shock, and emergency intubation can result in esophageal or tracheal laceration, subcutaneous emphysema, or accidental right mainstem bronchus intubation. (Decreased or absent breath sounds on the left side of the chest and normal breath sounds on the right may signal accidental right mainstem bronchus intubation.)

Documentation

During the code, document the events in as much detail as possible. Note whether the arrest was witnessed or unwitnessed, the time of the arrest, the time CPR was begun, the time the ACLS-trained nurse arrived, and the total resuscitation time. Also document the number of defibrillations, the times they were performed, the joule level, the patient's cardiac rhythm before and after the defibrillation, and whether the patient had a pulse.

Document all drug therapy, including dosages, routes of administration, and patient response. You'll also want to record all procedures, such as peripheral and central line insertion, pacemaker insertion, and ET tube insertion as well as the time they were performed and the patient's tolerance of the procedures. Also keep track of all arterial blood gas results.

Record whether the patient is transferred to another unit or facility along with his condition at the time of transfer and whether his family was notified. Finally, document any complications and the measures taken to correct them. When your documentation is complete, have the practitioner and ACLS nurse review and then sign the document.

SELECTED REFERENCES

American Heart Association. "2005 Guidelines for Cardiopulmonary Resuscitation and Emergency Cardiovascular Care: The International Consensus on Science," *Circulation* 112(22 Suppl):IV-1-IV-221, November 2005.

American Heart Association. "Highlights of the 2005 American Heart Association Guidelines for Cardiopulmonary Resuscitation and Emergency Cardiovascular Care," *Currents* 16(4):1-27, Winter 2005-2006.

Emergency Nurses Association. "Family Presence at the Bedside during Invasive Procedures or Resuscitation. Position Statement." Available at *www.ena.org/about/position/PDFs/4E6C256B26994E319F66C65748BFBDBF.pdf.*

Halm, M.A. "Family Presence during Resuscitation: A Critical Review of the Literature," *American Journal of Critical Care* 14(6):494-511, November 2005.

CARDIOPULMONARY RESUSCITATION

Cardiopulmonary resuscitation (CPR) seeks to restore and maintain the patient's respiration and circulation after his heartbeat and breathing have stopped. Basic life support (BLS) procedures should be performed according to the 2005 American Heart Association (AHA) guidelines. CPR is a BLS procedure that's performed on victims of cardiac arrest. Another BLS procedure is clearing the obstructed airway. (See "Obstructed airway management," page 526.)

Most adults who experience sudden cardiac arrest develop ventricular fibrillation and require defibrillation; CPR alone doesn't improve their chances of survival. Therefore, you must assess the victim and then contact emergency medical services (EMS) or call a code *before* starting CPR. Timing is critical because early access to EMS, early CPR, and early defibrillation greatly improve a patient's chances of survival.

Equipment

CPR requires no special equipment except a hard surface on which to place the patient.

Implementation

See the AHA's *BLS algorithm* and follow the step-by-step instructions for CPR for the healthcare provider as described here.

One-person rescue

- If you're the sole rescuer, expect to determine unresponsiveness, call for help, open the patient's airway, check for breathing, assess for circulation, and begin compressions.
- Assess the victim *to determine if he's unconscious* (as shown top of page 476). Gently shake his shoulders and shout, "Are you okay?" *This helps ensure that you don't start CPR on a person who's conscious.* Check whether he has an injury, particularly to the head or neck. If you suspect a head or neck injury, move him as little as possible *to reduce the risk of paralysis.*

BLS algorithm

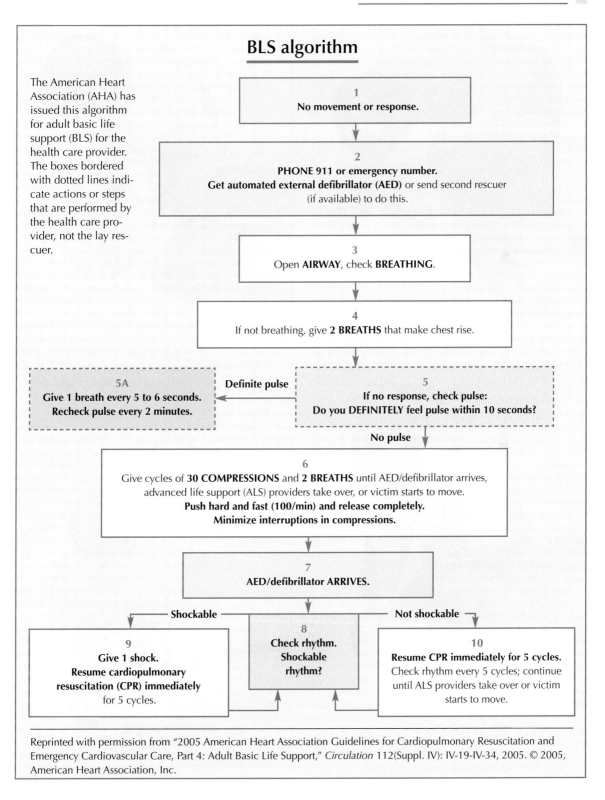

The American Heart Association (AHA) has issued this algorithm for adult basic life support (BLS) for the health care provider. The boxes bordered with dotted lines indicate actions or steps that are performed by the health care provider, not the lay rescuer.

1
No movement or response.

2
PHONE 911 or emergency number.
Get automated external defibrillator (AED) or send second rescuer (if available) to do this.

3
Open **AIRWAY**, check **BREATHING**.

4
If not breathing, give **2 BREATHS** that make chest rise.

5
If no response, check pulse:
Do you DEFINITELY feel pulse within 10 seconds?

Definite pulse →

5A
Give 1 breath every 5 to 6 seconds.
Recheck pulse every 2 minutes.

No pulse →

6
Give cycles of **30 COMPRESSIONS** and **2 BREATHS** until AED/defibrillator arrives, advanced life support (ALS) providers take over, or victim starts to move.
Push hard and fast (100/min) and release completely.
Minimize interruptions in compressions.

7
AED/defibrillator ARRIVES.

8
Check rhythm.
Shockable rhythm?

Shockable →

9
Give 1 shock.
Resume cardiopulmonary resuscitation (CPR) immediately for 5 cycles.

Not shockable →

10
Resume CPR immediately for 5 cycles.
Check rhythm every 5 cycles; continue until ALS providers take over or victim starts to move.

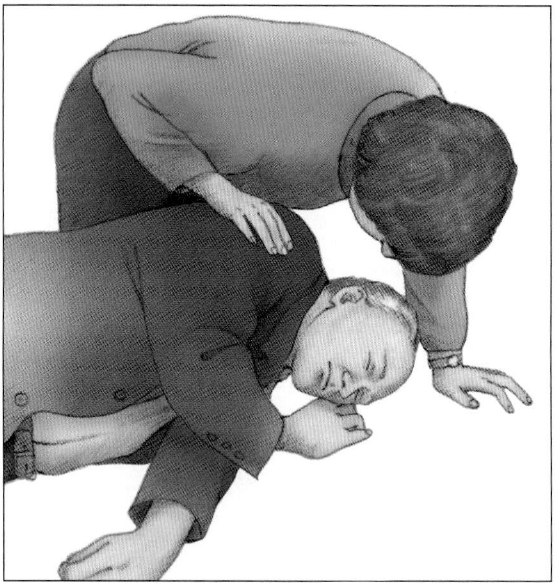

■ Call out for help. Send someone to contact the EMS or call a code, and get the automated external defibrillator (AED). Place the victim in a supine position on a hard, flat surface. When moving him, roll his head and torso as a unit (as shown below). Avoid twisting or pulling his neck, shoulders, or hips.

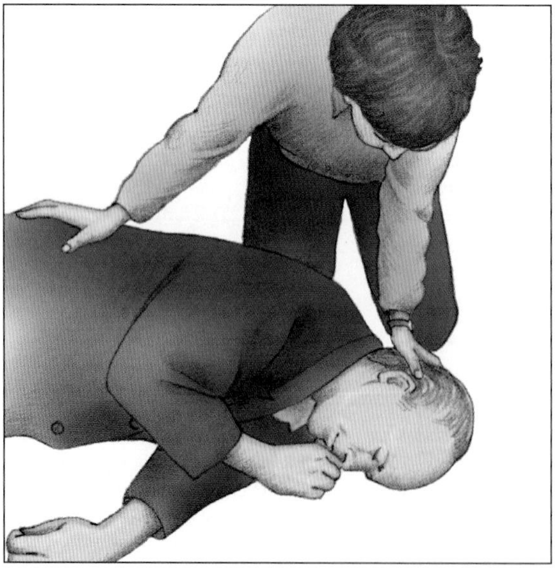

■ Kneel near his shoulders (as shown top of next column). This position will give you easy access to his head and chest.

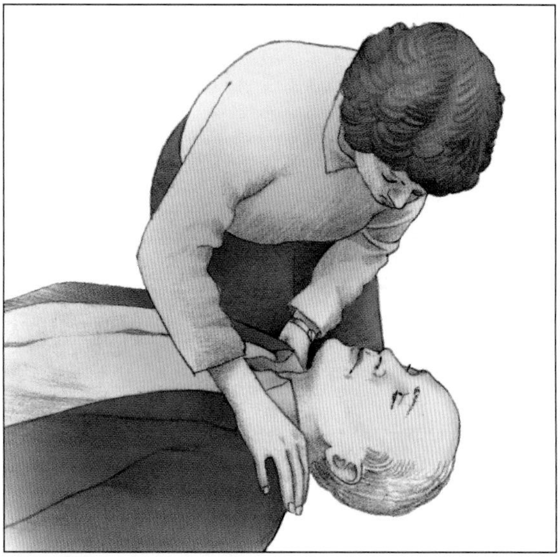

■ In many cases, the muscles controlling the victim's tongue will be relaxed, causing the tongue to obstruct the airway. If the victim doesn't appear to have a neck injury, use the *head-tilt, chin-lift maneuver* to open his airway. To accomplish this, first place your hand that's closer to the victim's head on his forehead. Then apply firm pressure. The pressure should be firm enough to tilt the victim's head back. Next, place the fingertips of your other hand under the bony part of his lower jaw near the chin. Now lift the victim's chin (as shown below). At the same time, keep his mouth partially open.

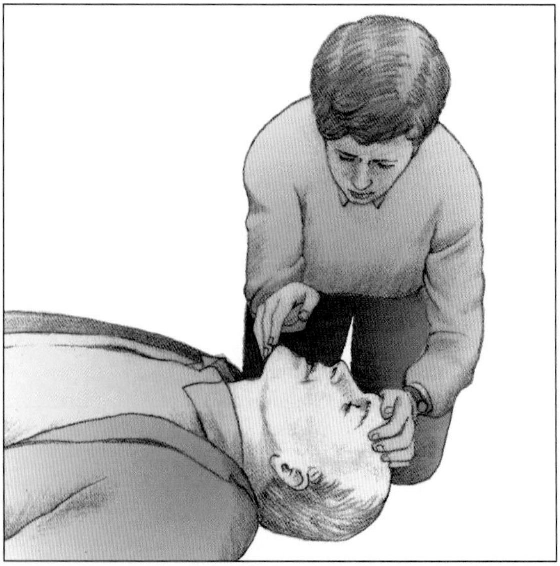

NURSING ALERT *Avoid placing your fingertips on the soft tissue under the victim's chin* because this maneuver may inadvertently obstruct the airway you're trying to open.

■ If you suspect a neck injury, use the *jaw-thrust maneuver* instead of the *head-tilt, chin-lift maneuver* without head extension. Kneel at the victim's head with your elbows on the ground. Rest your thumbs on his lower jaw near the corners of the mouth, pointing your thumbs toward his feet. Then place your fingertips around the lower jaw. To open the airway, lift the lower jaw with your fingertips (as shown below).

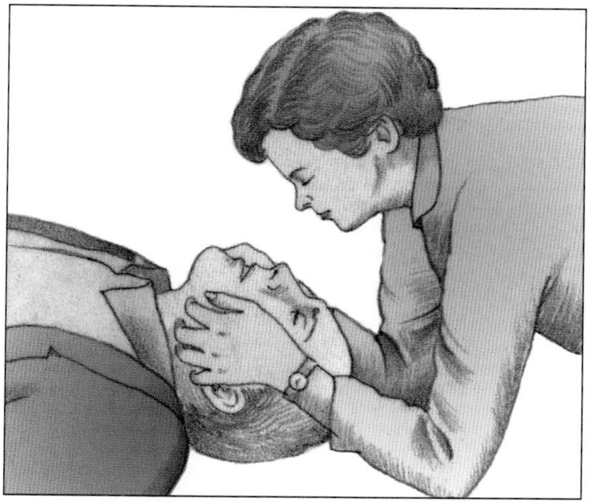

■ While maintaining the open airway, look, listen, and feel for breathing. Place your ear over the victim's mouth and nose (as shown below). Now, listen for the sound of air moving, and note whether his chest rises and falls. You may also feel airflow on your cheek. If he starts to breathe, keep the airway open and continue checking his breathing until help arrives.

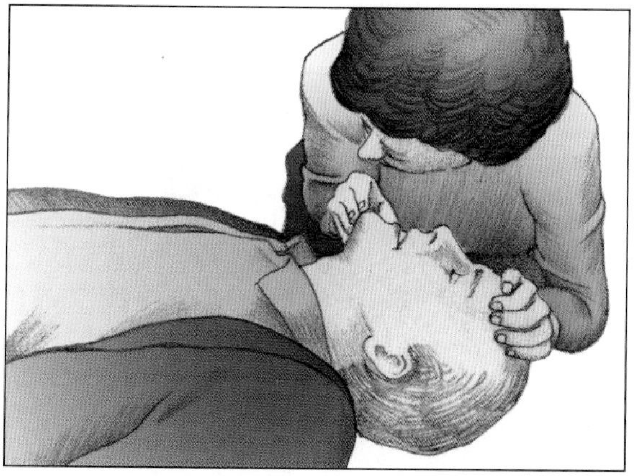

■ If you don't detect adequate breathing within 10 seconds after you open his airway, begin rescue breathing. Pinch his nostrils shut with the thumb and index finger of the hand you've had on his forehead (as shown below).

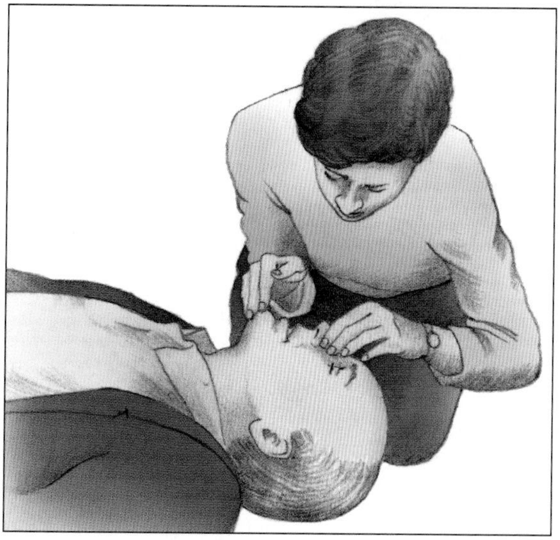

■ Take a regular (not deep) breath and place your mouth over the victim's mouth, creating a tight seal (as shown below). Give two breaths, each over 1 second. Each ventilation should have enough volume to produce a visible chest rise.

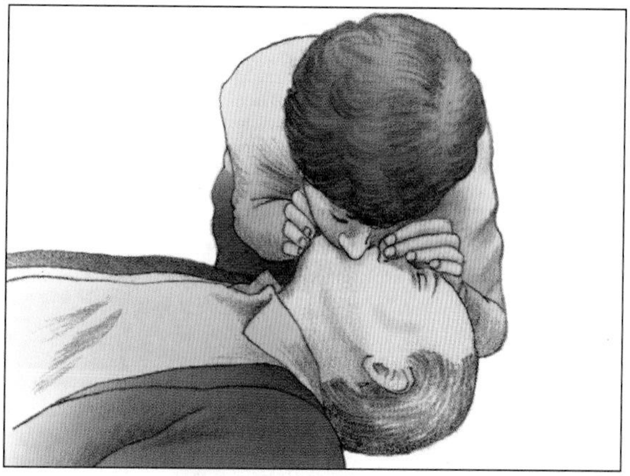

■ If the first ventilation isn't successful, reposition the victim's head and try again. If you still aren't successful, he may have a foreign-body airway obstruction. Check for loose dentures. If dentures or any other objects are blocking the airway, follow the procedure for clearing an airway obstruction.

■ Keep one hand on the victim's forehead so his airway remains open. With your other hand, palpate the carotid artery that's closer to you (as shown below). To do this, place your index and middle fingers in the groove between the trachea and the sternocleidomastoid muscle. Palpate for 10 seconds.

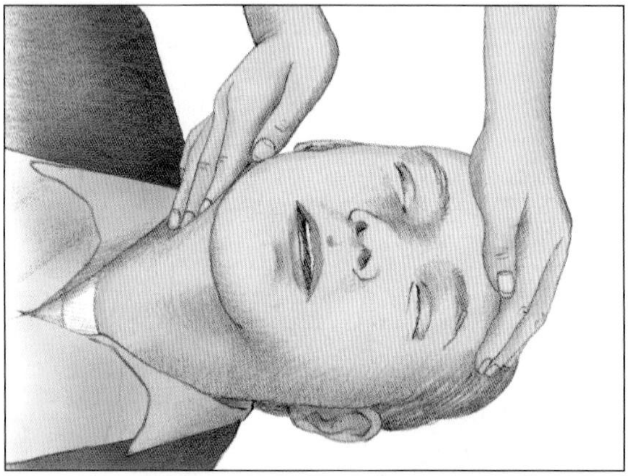

■ If you detect a pulse, don't begin chest compressions. Instead, perform rescue breathing by giving the victim 10 to 12 ventilations per minute (or one every 5 to 6 seconds). Each breath should be given over 1 second and cause a visible chest rise. After 2 minutes, recheck his pulse but spend only 10 seconds doing so.

■ If there's no pulse, start giving chest compressions. Make sure the patient is lying on a hard surface. Make sure your knees are apart *for a wide base of support.* Using the hand closer to his feet, locate the lower margin of the rib cage (as shown below). Then move your fingertips along the margin to the notch where the ribs meet the sternum.

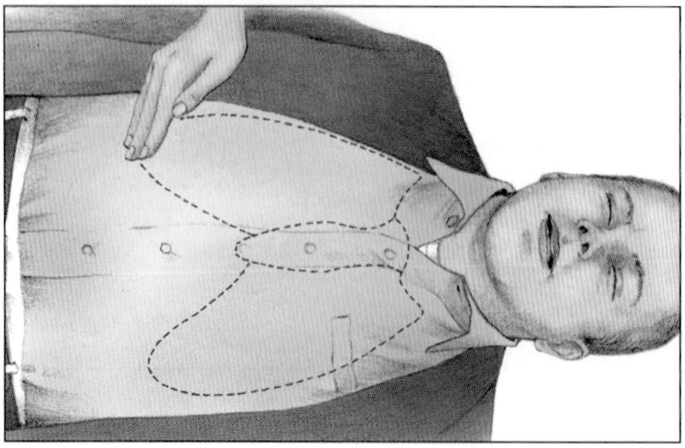

■ Place your middle finger on the notch and your index finger next to your middle finger (as shown top of next column). The long axis of the heel of your hand will be aligned with the long axis of the sternum (as shown) in the center of the chest between the nipples.

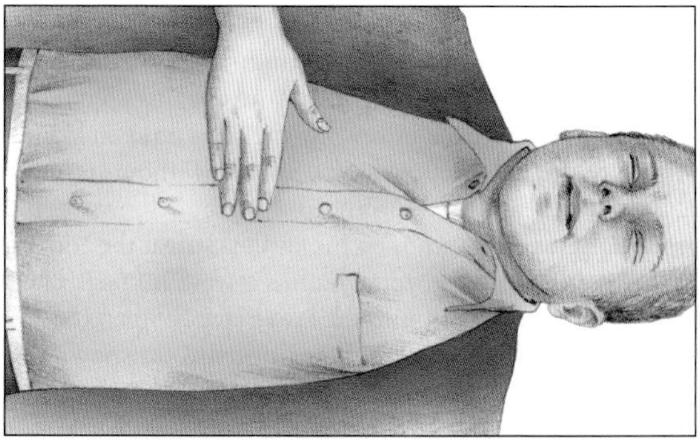

■ Put the heel of your other hand on the sternum, next to the index finger. The long axis of the heel of your hand will be aligned with the long axis of the sternum (as shown below).

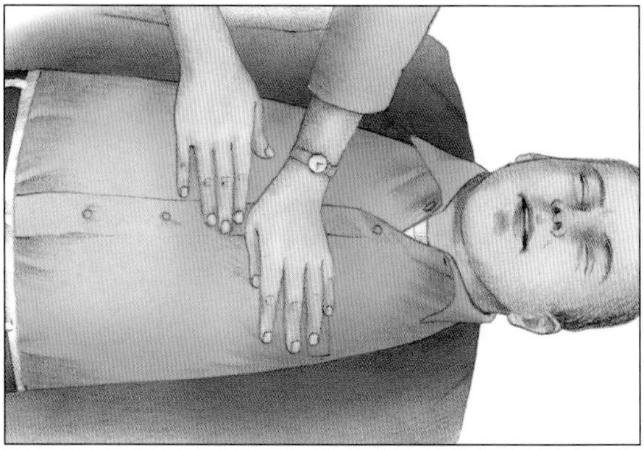

■ Take the first hand off the notch and put it on top of the hand on the sternum. Make sure you have one hand directly on top of the other and your fingers aren't on his chest (as shown below). This position will keep the force of the compression on the sternum and reduce the risk of a rib fracture, lung puncture, or liver laceration.

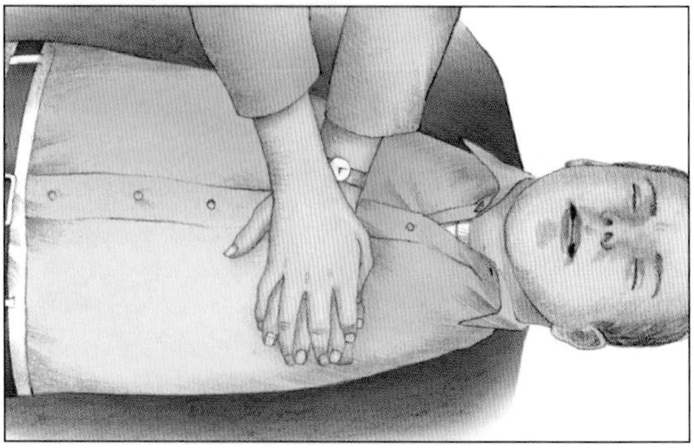

■ With your elbows locked, arms straight, and your shoulders directly over your hands (as shown below), you're ready to give chest compressions. Using the weight of your upper body, compress the victim's sternum 1½″ to 2″ (3.8 to 5 cm), delivering the pressure through the heels of your hands. After each compression, release the pressure and allow the chest to return to its normal position so that the heart can fill with blood. Don't change your hand position during compressions—you might injure the victim.

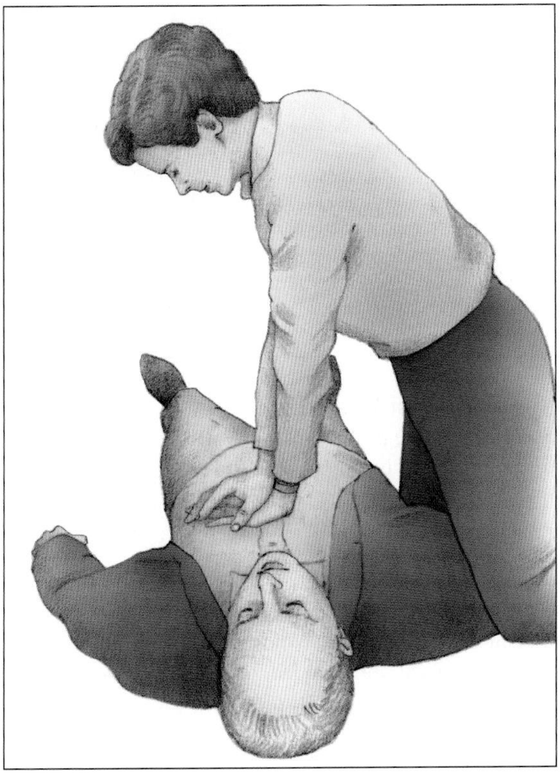

■ Give 30 chest compressions at a rate of approximately 100 per minute. Push hard and fast. Open the airway and give two ventilations. Then find the proper hand position again and deliver 30 more compressions.

■ Continue chest compressions until the EMS arrives or another rescuer arrives with the AED. Health care providers should interrupt chest compressions as infrequently as possible. Interruptions should last for no more than 10 seconds except for special interventions, such as use of the AED or insertion of an airway.

Two-person rescue

If another rescuer arrives while you're giving CPR, follow these steps:

■ If the EMS team hasn't arrived, tell the second rescuer to repeat the call for help. If he isn't a health care professional, ask him to stand by. Then, after about 2 minutes or five cycles of compressions and ventilations, you should switch. The switch should occur in less than 5 seconds (as shown below).

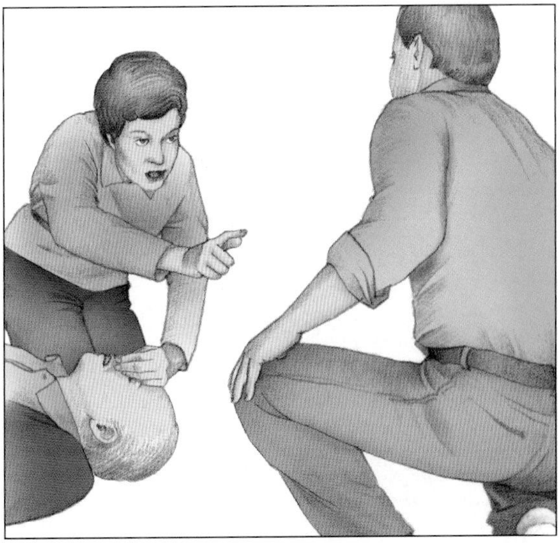

■ If the rescuer is another health care professional, the two of you can perform two-person CPR. He should start assisting after you've finished five cycles of 30 compressions, two ventilations, and a pulse check.

■ The second rescuer should get into place opposite you. While you're checking for a pulse, he should be finding the proper hand placement for delivering chest compressions (as shown below).

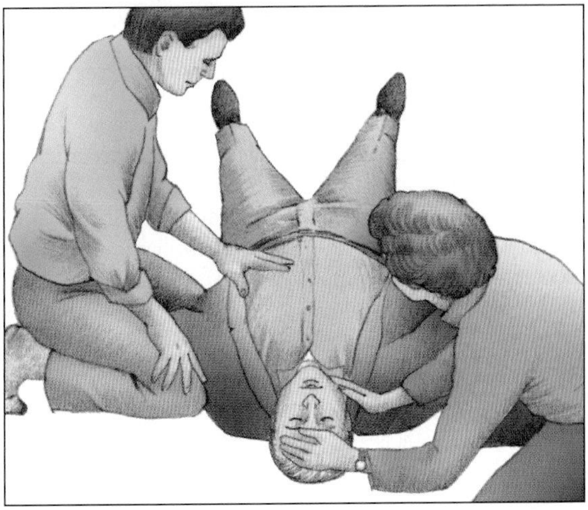

■ If you don't detect a pulse, say, "No pulse, continue CPR" and give two ventilations. Then the second rescuer should begin delivering compressions at a rate of 100 per minute. Compressions and ventilations should be administered at a ratio of 30 compressions to two ventilations. The compressor (at this point, the second rescuer) should count out loud *so the ventilator can anticipate when to give ventilations. To ensure that the ventilations are effective,* watch for a visible chest rise (as shown below).

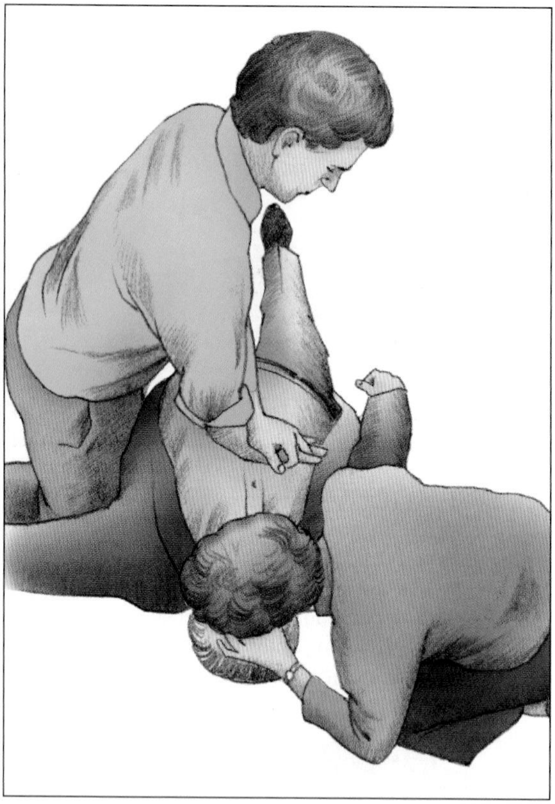

■ The compressor role should switch after five cycles of compressions and ventilations. The switch should occur in less than 5 seconds.

■ As shown top of next column, both of you should continue giving CPR until an AED or defibrillator arrives, the advanced cardiac life support (ACLS) provider takes over, or the victim starts to move.

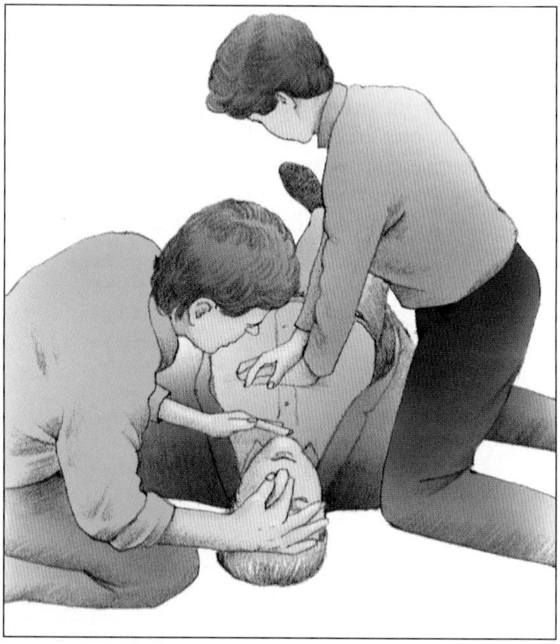

Special considerations

Some health care professionals may hesitate to give mouth-to-mouth rescue breaths. For this reason, the AHA recommends that all health care professionals learn how to use disposable airway equipment.

Complications

CPR can cause certain complications—especially if the compressor doesn't place her hands properly on the sternum. These complications include fractured ribs, a lacerated liver, and punctured lungs. Gastric distention, a common complication, results from giving too much air during ventilation. (See *Potential hazards of CPR.*)

Documentation

Whenever you perform CPR, document why you initiated it, whether the victim suffered from cardiac or respiratory arrest, when you found the victim and started CPR, and how long the victim received CPR. Note his response and any complications. Also include any interventions taken to correct complications.

If the victim also received ACLS, document which interventions were performed, who performed them, when they were performed, and what equipment was used.

SELECTED REFERENCES

American Association for Respiratory Care. "Clinical Practice Guideline. Resuscitation and Defibrillation in the Health-

Potential hazards of CPR

Cardiopulmonary resuscitation (CPR) can cause various complications, including injury to bones and vital organs. This chart describes the causes of CPR hazards and lists preventive steps.

HAZARD	CAUSES	ASSESSMENT FINDINGS	PREVENTIVE MEASURES
Sternum and rib fractures	▪ Osteoporosis ▪ Malnutrition ▪ Improper hand placement	▪ Paradoxical chest movement ▪ Chest pain or tenderness that increases with inspiration ▪ Crepitus ▪ Palpation of movable bony fragments over the sternum ▪ On palpation, sternum feels unattached to surrounding ribs	***While performing CPR*** ▪ Don't rest your hands or fingers on the patient's ribs. ▪ Interlock your fingers. ▪ Keep your bottom hand in contact with the chest, but release pressure after each compression. ▪ Compress the sternum at the recommended depth for the patient's age.
Pneumothorax, hemothorax, or both	▪ Lung puncture from fractured rib	▪ Chest pain and dyspnea ▪ Decreased or absent breath sounds over the affected lung ▪ Tracheal deviation from midline ▪ Hypotension ▪ Hyperresonance to percussion over the affected area along with shoulder pain	▪ Follow the measures listed for sternum and rib fractures.
Injury to the heart and great vessels (pericardial tamponade, atrial or ventricular rupture, vessel laceration, cardiac contusion, punctures of the heart chambers)	▪ Improperly performed chest compressions ▪ Transvenous or transthoracic pacing attempts ▪ Central line placement during resuscitation ▪ Intracardiac drug administration	▪ Jugular vein distention ▪ Muffled heart sounds ▪ Pulsus paradoxus ▪ Narrowed pulse pressure ▪ Electrical alternans (decreased electrical amplitude of every other QRS complex) ▪ Adventitious heart sounds ▪ Hypotension ▪ Electrocardiogram changes (arrhythmias, ST-segment elevation, T-wave inversion, and marked decrease in QRS voltage)	▪ Perform chest compressions properly.
Organ laceration (primarily liver and spleen)	▪ Forceful compression ▪ Sharp edge of a fractured rib or xiphoid process	▪ Persistent right upper quadrant tenderness (liver injury) ▪ Persistent left upper quadrant tenderness (splenic injury) ▪ Increasing abdominal girth	▪ Follow the measures listed for sternum and rib fractures.

(continued)

Potential hazards of CPR *(continued)*

HAZARD	CAUSES	ASSESSMENT FINDINGS	PREVENTIVE MEASURES
Aspiration of stomach contents	■ Gastric distention and an elevated diaphragm from high ventilatory pressures	■ Fever, hypoxia, and dyspnea ■ Auscultation of wheezes and crackles ■ Increased white blood cell count ■ Changes in color and odor of lung secretions	■ Intubate early. ■ Insert a nasogastric tube and apply suction, if gastric distention is marked.

Care Setting—2004 Revision and Update," *Respiratory Care* 89(9):1085-1099, September 2004.

American Heart Association. "2005 Guidelines for Cardiopulmonary Resuscitation and Emergency Cardiovascular Care: The International Consensus on Science," *Circulation* 112(22 Suppl):IV-1-IV-221, November 2005.

American Heart Association. "Highlights of the 2005 American Heart Association Guidelines for Cardiopulmonary Resuscitation and Emergency Cardiovascular Care," *Currents* 16(4):1-27, Winter 2005-2006.

Craig, K.J., and Hopkins-Pepe, L. "Understanding the New AHA Guidelines, Part I," *Nursing* 36(4):53, April 2006.

Yannopoulos, D., et al. "Clinical and Hemodynamic Comparison of 15:2 and 30:2 Compression-to-ventilation Ratios for Cardiopulmonary Resuscitation," *Critical Care Medicine* 34(5):1444-449, May 2006.

DEFIBRILLATION

The 2005 American Heart Association guidelines identity defibrillation as the standard treatment for ventricular fibrillation (VF), after cardiopulmonary resuscitation (CPR). CPR prolongs VF and prolongs the time that defibrillation can occur. CPR alone isn't likely to correct VF; therefore, early defibrillation is critical. Defibrillation involves using electrode paddles to direct an electric current through the patient's heart. The current causes the myocardium to depolarize, which, in turn, encourages the sinoatrial node to resume control of the heart's electrical activity. Successful defibrillation depends on the appropriate selection of energy to generate sufficient flow through the heart to achieve defibrillation while minimizing injury to the heart.

Modern defibrillators deliver current in waveforms and are available in monophasic and biphasic models. Defibrillators with monophasic waveforms deliver current in one direction. Few monophasic waveform defibrillators are being manufactured, but some are still in use. Biphasic waveforms deliver current that flows in a positive direction for a specific duration and then reverses and flows in a negative direction for the remaining time of electrical discharge. Lower energy shocks are required and have been shown to be as effective as the higher energy shocks used with monophasic waveform defibrillators in terminating VF.

Because VF leads to death if not corrected, the success of defibrillation depends on early recognition and quick treatment of this arrhythmia. In addition to treating VF, defibrillation may also be used to treat ventricular tachycardia (VT) that doesn't produce a pulse.

Patients with a history of VF may be candidates for an implantable cardioverter-defibrillator, a sophisticated device that automatically discharges an electric current when it senses a ventricular tachyarrhythmia. (See *Understanding the ICD.*)

Equipment

Defibrillator with electrocardiogram (ECG) monitor and recorder ■ oxygen therapy equipment ■ handheld resuscitation bag ■ airway equipment ■ emergency pacing equipment ■ emergency cardiac medications ■ blood pressure monitoring equipment.

Preparation of equipment

Make sure that the defibrillation pads are attached to the defibrillator. If the pads aren't pregelled, be sure to have conductive gel or paste on hand to place on the patient before placing the pads or paddles.

Implementation

- Assess the patient *to determine if he lacks a pulse.* Call for help and perform CPR until the defibrillator and other emergency equipment arrive.
- If the defibrillator has "quick-look" capability, place the paddles on the patient's chest *to quickly view his cardiac rhythm.* Otherwise, connect the monitoring leads of the defibrillator to the patient, and assess his cardiac rhythm.

- Expose the patient's chest, and apply the defibrillator pads at the paddle placement positions. For anterolateral placement, place one paddle to the right of the upper sternum, just below the right clavicle, and the other over the fifth or sixth intercostal space at the left anterior axillary line. For anteroposterior placement, place the anterior pad directly over the heart at the precordium, to the left of the lower sternal border. Place the posterior pad under the patient's body beneath the heart and immediately below the scapulae (but not under the vertebral column).

NURSING ALERT *Never place the defibrillator pads directly over an implanted pacemaker.* This may damage the pacemaker.

- Turn on the defibrillator and, if performing external defibrillation, set the energy level for 360 joules for an adult patient when using a monophasic defibrillator. Use clinically appropriate energy levels for biphasic defibrillators (usually 120 to 200 joules).
- Charge the pads by pressing the charge buttons, which are located either on the machine or on the pads themselves.
- Press the paddles firmly against the patient's chest, using 25 lb (11 kg) of pressure.
- Reassess the patient's cardiac rhythm.
- If the patient remains in VF or pulseless VT, instruct all personnel to stand clear of the patient and the bed. Visually verify that all personnel are clear of the patient and the bed before discharging the current.
- Discharge the current by pressing both paddle charge buttons simultaneously.
- Resume CPR immediately and give five cycles.
- Reassess the patient's cardiac rhythm.
- If necessary, prepare to defibrillate a second time. Instruct someone to reset the energy level on the defibrillator to 360 joules or the biphasic energy equivalent and continue CPR while the defibrillator is charging. Announce that you're preparing to defibrillate, and follow the procedure described above.
- Resume CPR immediately for five cycles. Begin administering appropriate medications, such as epinephrine or vasopressin.
- Reassess the patient. If defibrillation is again necessary, instruct someone to reset the energy level to 360 joules or the biphasic energy equivalent. Then follow the same procedure as before.
- Resume CPR immediately for five cycles. Continue to administer medications, adding antiarrhythmics or magnesium, as appropriate.
- If defibrillation restores a normal rhythm, check the patient's central and peripheral pulses and obtain a blood pressure reading, heart rate, and respiratory rate. Assess the patient's level of consciousness, cardiac rhythm, breath sounds, skin color, and urine output. Obtain baseline arterial blood gas levels and a 12-lead ECG. Provide supplemental oxygen, ventilation, and medications, as needed. Check the patient's chest for electrical burns and treat them, as ordered, with corticosteroid or lanolin-based creams. Also prepare the defibrillator for immediate reuse.

Understanding the ICD

The implantable cardioverter-defibrillator (ICD) has a programmable pulse generator and lead system that monitors the heart's activity, detects ventricular bradyarrhythmias and tachyarrhythmias, and responds with appropriate therapies. The range of therapies includes antitachycardia and bradycardia pacing, cardioversion, and defibrillation. Newer defibrillators also have the ability to pace both the atrium and the ventricle.

Implantation of the ICD is similar to that of a permanent pacemaker. The cardiologist positions the lead (or leads) transvenously in the endocardium of the right ventricle (and the right atrium, if both chambers require pacing). The lead connects to a generator box, which is implanted in the right or left upper chest near the clavicle.

ICD implantation has the same complications that may occur with permanent pacemaker insertion. In addition, inappropriate cardioversion, ineffective cardioversion/defibrillation, and device deactivation may occur. Causes may include T-wave oversensing, lead fracture, lead insulation breakage, electrocautery, magnetic resonance imaging, and electromagnetic interference. Use of a magnet over the ICD will inhibit further shocks until the underlying cause is diagnosed and treated. The bradycardiac pacing function will still activate should the patient require it.

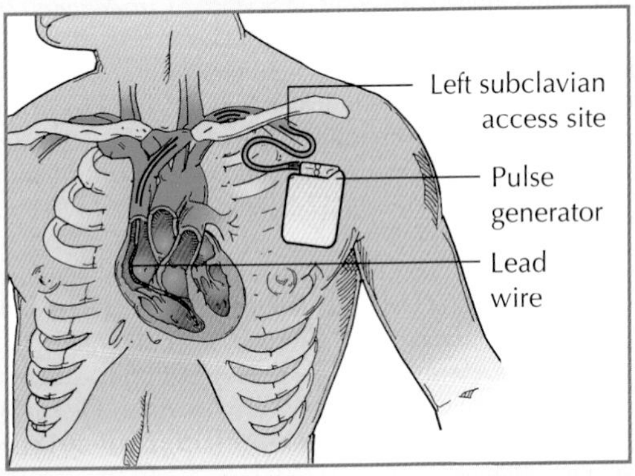

Special considerations

- Defibrillators vary from one manufacturer to the next, so familiarize yourself with your facility's equipment. Defibrillator operation should be checked at least once per shift and after each use.
- Defibrillation can be affected by several factors, including paddle size and placement, condition of the patient's myocardium, duration of the arrhythmia, chest resistance, and the number of countershocks.
- Remove any transdermal medications from the chest (and back if using anterior-posterior placement) *because the medication may interfere with the conduction of the current or produce a chest burn.*

Complications

Defibrillation can cause accidental electric shock to those providing care. Use of an insufficient amount of conductive medium can lead to skin burns.

Documentation

Document the procedure, including the patient's ECG rhythms both before and after defibrillation; the number of times defibrillation was performed; the voltage used during each attempt; whether a pulse returned; the dosage, route, and time of drug administration; whether CPR was used; how the airway was maintained; and the patient's outcome.

Selected references

American Heart Association. "2005 Guidelines for Cardiopulmonary Resuscitation and Emergency Cardiovascular Care: The International Consensus on Science," *Circulation* 112(22 Suppl):IV-1-IV-221, November 2005.

American Heart Association. "Highlights of the 2005 American Heart Association Guidelines for CPR and ECG," *Currents* 16(4):1-27, Winter 2005-2006.

Koster, R.W., et al. "Definition of Successful Defibrillation," *Critical Care Medicine* 34(12 Suppl):5423-426, December 2006.

Kudenchuk, P.J., et al. "Transthoracic Incremental Monophasic versus Biphasic Defibrillation by Emergency Responders (TIMBER): A Randomized Comparison of Monophasic with Biphasic Waveform Ascending Energy Defibrillation for the Resuscitation of Out-of-Hospital Cardiac Arrest Due to Ventricular Fibrillation," *Circulation* 114(19):2010-2018, November 2006.

Lynn-McHale Wiegand, D.J., and Carlson, K.K., eds. *AACN Procedure Manual for Critical Care,* 5th ed. Philadelphia: W.B. Saunders Co., 2005.

AUTOMATED EXTERNAL DEFIBRILLATION

Automated external defibrillators (AEDs) are commonly used today to meet the need for early defibrillation, which is currently considered the most effective treatment for ventricular fibrillation (VF). Some facilities now require an AED in every noncritical care unit. Their use is also common in such public places as shopping malls, sports stadiums, and airplanes. Instruction in using the AED is required as part of basic life support (BLS) and advanced cardiac life support (ACLS) training.

Studies have shown that established public access to defibrillation programs (laypersons who are trained to use an AED) have a survival rate of 41% to 74% from sudden cardiac arrest with VF when cardiopulmonary resuscitation (CPR) is initiated immediately and defibrillation occurs within 3 to 5 minutes.

The 2005 American Heart Association guidelines for CPR and emergency cardiovascular care recommend the integration of CPR with the use of an AED. The guidelines recommend that:

- early defibrillation is appropriate. Compression before defibrillation may be considered when emergency medical services arrival is greater than 4 to 5 minutes.
- one shock followed by immediate CPR—beginning with chest compressions—should be used. The rhythm should be checked after five cycles of CPR, or after 2 minutes.
- if more than one rescuer is present, one rescuer should start CPR while the other prepares the AED.
- AEDs can be used in children ages 1 to 8. For this age-group, an AED with a pediatric dose attenuator system should be used, if available.
- health care providers should be trained, equipped, and retrained to perform defibrillation.

AEDs provide early defibrillation—even when no health care provider is present. The AED interprets the victim's cardiac rhythm and gives the operator step-by-step directions on how to proceed if defibrillation is indicated. Most AEDs have a "quick-look" feature that allows visualization of the rhythm with the paddles before electrodes are connected.

The AED is equipped with a microcomputer that senses and analyzes a patient's heart rhythm at the push of a button. Then it audibly or visually prompts you to deliver a shock. AED models all have the same basic function but offer different operating options. For example, all AEDs communicate directions via messages on a display screen, give voice commands, or both. Some AEDs simultaneously display a patient's heart rhythm.

All devices record your interactions with the patient during defibrillation, either on a cassette tape or in a solid-state memory module. Some AEDs have an integral printer for immediate event documentation. Your facility's policy determines who's responsible for reviewing all AED interactions; the patient's practitioner always has that option. Local and state regulations govern who's responsible for collecting AED case data for reporting purposes.

There are two types of defibrillators: one with monophasic waveforms and the other with biphasic waveforms. Monophasic waveform defibrillators were introduced first and many are still in use today. When using this type of defibrillator, the initial shock should be set at 360 joules, with second and subsequent shocks also set at 360 joules.

Biphasic waveforms are used in most AEDs and manual defibrillators. When using this type of defibrillator, an energy setting of 120 to 200 joules should be used for the first shock and the same, or higher setting, for second and subsequent shocks. The optimal energy level for a biphasic waveform defibrillator hasn't been determined. The optimal dose for each device that has proven most effective in eliminating VF should be noted on the defibrillator.

Equipment

AED ▪ two prepackaged electrodes.

Implementation

- After discovering that your patient is unresponsive to your questions, pulseless, and apneic, follow BLS and ACLS protocols. Then ask a colleague to bring the AED into the patient's room and set it up before the code team arrives.
- Open the foil packets containing the two electrode pads. Attach the white electrode cable connector to one pad and the red electrode cable connector to the other. The electrode pads aren't site-specific.
- Expose the patient's chest. Remove the plastic backing film from the electrode pads, and place the electrode pad attached to the white cable connector on the right upper portion of the patient's chest, just beneath his clavicle.
- Place the pad attached to the red cable connector to the left of the heart's apex. To help remember where to place the pads, think "white—right, red—ribs." (Placement for both electrode pads is the same as for manual defibrillation or cardioversion.)
- Firmly press the device's ON button, and wait while the machine performs a brief self-test. Most AEDs signal their readiness by a computerized voice that says "Stand clear" or by emitting a series of loud beeps. (If the AED isn't functioning properly, it will convey the message "Don't use the AED. Remove and continue CPR.") Remember to report any AED malfunctions in accordance with your facility's procedure.
- Now the machine is ready to analyze the patient's heart rhythm. Ask everyone to stand clear, and press the ANALYZE button when the machine prompts you to. Be careful not to touch or move the patient while the AED is in analysis mode. (If you get the message "Check electrodes," make sure the electrodes are correctly placed and the patient cable is securely attached; then press the ANALYZE button again.)
- In 15 to 30 seconds, the AED will analyze the patient's rhythm. When the patient needs a shock, the AED will display a "Stand clear" message and emit a beep that changes into a steady tone as it's charging.
- When an AED is fully charged and ready to deliver a shock, it will prompt you to press the SHOCK button. (Some fully automatic AED models automatically deliver a shock within 15 seconds after analyzing the patient's rhythm. If a shock isn't needed, the AED will display "No shock indicated" and prompt you to "Check patient.")
- Make sure no one is touching the patient or his bed, and call out "Stand clear." Then press the SHOCK button on the AED. Most AEDs are ready to deliver a shock within 15 seconds.
- After the first shock, continue CPR, beginning with five cycles of chest compressions for about 2 minutes. Don't delay compressions to recheck rhythm or pulse. After five cycles of CPR, the AED should analyze the rhythm and deliver another shock, if indicated.
- If a nonshockable rhythm is detected, the AED should instruct you to resume CPR. Then continue the algorithm sequence until the code team leader arrives.
- After the code, remove and transcribe the AED's computer memory module or tape, or prompt the AED to print a rhythm strip with code data. Follow your facility's policy for analyzing and storing code data.

Special considerations

- Defibrillators vary from one manufacturer to the next, so be sure to familiarize yourself with your facility's equipment.
- Defibrillator operation should be checked at least every 8 hours and after each use.

Complications

Defibrillation can cause accidental electric shock to those providing care. Using an insufficient amount of conduction medium can lead to skin burns.

Documentation

After using an AED, give a synopsis to the code team leader. Remember to report the following:

- the patient's name, age, medical history, and chief complaint
- the time you found the patient in cardiac arrest
- when you started CPR
- when you applied the AED
- how many shocks the patient received
- when the patient regained a pulse at any point
- what postarrest care was given, if any
- physical assessment findings.

Later, be sure to document the code on the appropriate form.

SELECTED REFERENCES

American Heart Association. "2005 American Heart Association Guidelines for Cardiopulmonary Resuscitation and Emergency Cardiovascular Care: International Consensus on Science," *Circulation* 112(22 Suppl):IV-1-IV-221, November 2005.

American Heart Association. "Highlights of the 2005 American Heart Association Guidelines for Cardiopulmonary Resuscitation and Emergency Cardiovascular Care," *Currents* 16(4):1-27, Winter 2005-2006.

Hazinski, M.F., et al. "Lay Rescuer Automated External Defibrillator ("Public Access Defibrillation") Programs: Lessons Learned from an International Multicenter Trial," *Circulation* 111(24):3336-340, June 2005.

Sanna, T., et al. "Home Defibrillation: A Feasibility Study in Myocardial Infarction Survivors at Intermediate Risk of Sudden Death," *American Heart Journal* 152(4):685; e1-7, October 2006.

Valenzuela, T.D., et al. "Interruptions of Chest Compressions during Emergency Medical Systems Resuscitation," *Circulation* 112(9):1259-265, August 2005.

SYNCHRONIZED CARDIOVERSION

Used to treat tachyarrhythmias, cardioversion delivers an electric charge to the myocardium at the peak of the R wave. This causes immediate depolarization, interrupting reentry circuits and allowing the sinoatrial node to resume control. Synchronizing the electric charge with the R wave ensures that the current won't be delivered on the vulnerable T wave and thus disrupt repolarization.

Synchronized cardioversion is the treatment of choice for arrhythmias that don't respond to vagal massage or drug therapy, such as atrial tachycardia, atrial flutter, atrial fibrillation, and symptomatic ventricular tachycardia.

Cardioversion should be performed according to the 2005 American Heart Association (AHA) guidelines and should be preceded by assessing the patient's cardiac and metabolic status. This assessment should include electrolyte values, particularly potassium values, which should be in the normal range, and knowledge of renal function (creatinine level), which guides the dosage of adjunctive medications. The serum digoxin level should be in the nontoxic range. When possible, the patient should be in optimal functional status at the time of the procedure. Arterial blood gas (ABG) analysis may be relevant in the patient with chronic lung disease. Written informed consent should be obtained from the patient after appropriate discussion of the procedure. The procedure should be carried out in an area where a general anesthetic or sedative agent can be administered and, if necessary, CPR measures can be conducted.

Cardioversion may be an elective or urgent procedure, depending on how well the patient tolerates the arrhythmia. For example, if the patient is hemodynamically unstable, he would require urgent cardioversion. Remember that, when preparing for cardioversion, the patient's condition can deteriorate quickly, necessitating immediate defibrillation.

The AHA recommends immediate synchronized cardioversion for treatment of symptomatic (unstable) tachycardias. If the patient is stable, a 12-lead electrocardiogram (ECG) is done to further classify the tachycardia. Unstable signs include altered mental status, shock or hypotension, and ongoing chest pain.

Equipment

Cardioverter-defibrillator ▪ conductive medium pads ▪ anterior, posterior, or transverse paddles ▪ ECG monitor with recorder ▪ sedative ▪ oxygen therapy equipment ▪ airway ▪ handheld resuscitation bag ▪ emergency pacing equipment ▪ emergency cardiac medications ▪ automatic blood pressure cuff (if available) ▪ pulse oximeter (if available).

Implementation

- Test the cardioverter-defibrillator and make sure that it works. Attach the oxygen tubing and oxygen delivery device to the oxygen source. Make sure that you have an airway and a handheld resuscitation bag readily available for use. Also make sure that you have emergency pacing equipment available *in case the patient develops asystole or bradycardia during the cardioversion.*
- Confirm the patient's identity using two patient identifiers according to your facility's policy.
- Explain the procedure to the patient, and make sure he has signed a consent form.
- Check the patient's recent serum potassium and magnesium levels and ABG results. Also check recent digoxin levels. *Although digitalized patients may undergo cardioversion, they tend to require lower energy levels to convert.* If the patient takes digoxin, withhold the dose on the day of the procedure.

■ If possible, withhold all food and fluids for 6 to 12 hours before the procedure.
■ Obtain a 12-lead ECG *to serve as a baseline.*
■ Check to see if the practitioner has ordered administration of any cardiac drugs before the procedure. Also verify that the patient has a patent I.V. site to administer the sedative.
■ Connect the patient to a pulse oximeter and automatic blood pressure cuff, if available.
■ Consider administering oxygen for 5 to 10 minutes before the cardioversion *to promote myocardial oxygenation.* If the patient wears dentures, evaluate whether they support his airway or might cause an airway obstruction. If they might cause an obstruction, remove them.
■ Place the patient in the supine position, and assess his vital signs, level of consciousness (LOC), cardiac rhythm, and peripheral pulses.
■ Remove any oxygen delivery device just before cardioversion *to avoid possible combustion.*
■ Have epinephrine, lidocaine, and atropine at the patient's bedside.
■ Administer a sedative, as ordered. The patient should be heavily sedated but still able to breathe adequately.
■ Carefully monitor the patient's blood pressure and respiratory rate until he recovers.
■ Press the POWER button to turn on the defibrillator. Next, push the SYNC button *to synchronize the machine with the patient's QRS complexes.* Make sure the SYNC button flashes with each of the patient's QRS complexes. You should also see a bright green flag flash on the monitor.
■ Turn the ENERGY SELECT dial to the ordered amount of energy. Advanced cardiac life support protocols call for an initial shock of 50 to 100 joules for a patient with unstable supraventricular tachycardia, 100 to 200 joules for a patient with atrial fibrillation, 50 to 100 joules for a patient with atrial flutter, and 100 joules for a patient who has monomorphic ventricular tachycardia with a pulse. If there's no response with the first shock, the health care provider should increase the joules in a step-wise manner.
■ Remove the paddles from the machine, and prepare them as you would if you were defibrillating the patient. Place the conductive gel pads or paddles in the same positions as you would to defibrillate.
■ Make sure everyone stands away from the bed; then push the discharge buttons. Hold the paddles in place and wait for the energy to be discharged—*the machine has to synchronize the discharge with the QRS complex.*
■ Check the waveform on the monitor. If the arrhythmia fails to convert, repeat the procedure two or three more times at 3-minute intervals. Gradually increase the energy level with each additional countershock.
■ After the cardioversion, frequently assess the patient's LOC and respiratory status, including airway patency, respiratory rate and depth, and the need for supplemental oxygen. *Because the patient will be heavily sedated, he may require airway support.*
■ Record a postcardioversion 12-lead ECG, and monitor the patient's ECG rhythm for 2 hours. Check the patient's chest for electrical burns.

Special considerations

■ If the patient is attached to a bedside or telemetry monitor, disconnect the unit before cardioversion. *The electric current it generates could damage the equipment.*
■ Be aware that improper synchronization may result if the patient's ECG tracing contains artifact-like spikes, such as peaked T waves or bundle-branch heart blocks when the R′ wave may be taller than the R wave.
■ Although the electric shock of cardioversion won't usually damage an implanted pacemaker, avoid placing the paddles directly over the pacemaker.
■ Remove any patches with metallic backings such as nitroglycerin patches. *This backing may cause a ring during cardioversion.*
■ Reset the synchronization mode after each cardioversion because many defibrillators automatically default back to the unsynchronized mode.

Complications

Common complications following cardioversion include transient, harmless arrhythmias such as atrial, ventricular, and junctional premature beats. Serious ventricular arrhythmias such as ventricular fibrillation may also occur. However, this type of arrhythmia is more likely to result from high amounts of electrical energy, digoxin toxicity, severe heart disease, electrolyte imbalance, or improper synchronization with the R wave.

Documentation

Document the procedure, including the voltage delivered with each attempt, rhythm strips before and after the procedure, and how the patient tolerated the procedure.

SELECTED REFERENCES

American Heart Association. "2005 AHA Guidelines for Cardiopulmonary Resuscitation and Emergency Cardiovascular Care: International Consensus on Science, " *Circulation* 112 (22 Suppl): IV-1-IV-221, November 2005.
American Heart Association. "ACC/AHA/ECS 2006 Guidelines for the Management of Patients with Atrial Fibrillation," *Circulation* 114:257-354, August 2006.
Hagens, V.E., et al. "Determinants of Sudden Cardiac Death in Patients with Persistent Atrial Fibrillation in the Rate Con-

trol Versus Electrical Cardioversion (RACE) Study," *American Journal of Cardiology* 98(7):929-32, October 2006.
"Managing Atrial Fibrillation," *Harvard Women's Health Watch* 13(12):4-6, August 2006.
Tracy, C.M., et al. "American College of Cardiology/American Heart Association 2006 Update of the Clinical Competence Statement on Invasive Electrophysiology Studies, Catheter Ablation, and Cardioversion: A Report of the American College of Cardiology/American Heart Association/American College of Physicians Task Force on Clinical Competence and Training Developed in Collaboration with the Heart Rhythm Society," *American College of Cardiology* 48(7):1503-517, October 2006.

VAGAL MANEUVERS

When a patient suffers sinus, atrial, or junctional tachyarrhythmias, vagal maneuvers—Valsalva's maneuver and carotid sinus massage—can slow his heart rate. These maneuvers work by stimulating nerve endings, which respond as they would to an increase in blood pressure. They send this message to the brain stem, which in turn stimulates the autonomic nervous system to increase vagal tone and decrease the heart rate.

In *Valsalva's maneuver,* the patient holds his breath and bears down, raising his intrathoracic pressure. When this pressure increase is transmitted to the heart and great vessels, venous return, stroke volume, and systolic blood pressure decrease. Within seconds, the baroreceptors respond to these changes by increasing the heart rate and causing peripheral vasoconstriction.

When the patient exhales at the end of the maneuver, his blood pressure rises to its previous level. This increase, combined with the peripheral vasoconstriction caused by bearing down, stimulates the vagus nerve, decreasing the heart rate.

In *carotid sinus massage,* manual pressure applied to the left or right carotid sinus slows the heart rate. This method is used both to diagnose and treat tachyarrhythmias. The patient's response to carotid sinus massage depends on the type of arrhythmia. If he has sinus tachycardia, his heart rate will slow gradually during the procedure and speed up again after it. If he has atrial tachycardia, the arrhythmia may stop and the heart rate may remain slow because the procedure increases atrioventricular (AV) block. With atrial fibrillation or flutter, the ventricular rate may not change; AV block may even worsen. With paroxysmal atrial tachycardia, reversion to sinus rhythm occurs only 20% of the time. Nonparoxysmal tachycardia and ventricular tachycardia (VT) won't respond.

Vagal maneuvers are contraindicated for patients with severe coronary artery disease, acute myocardial infarction, or hypovolemia. Carotid sinus massage is contraindicated for patients with cardiac glycoside toxicity or cerebrovascular disease and for patients who have had carotid surgery.

Although usually performed by a physician, vagal maneuvers may also be done by a specially prepared nurse under a physician's supervision.

ELDER ALERT **Because older patients commonly have undiagnosed atherosclerosis and carotid bruits aren't always present even with significant atherosclerosis,** ***most experts avoid carotid sinus massage in elderly and late middle-age patients. In these patients, experts agree that Valsalva's maneuver should be used.***

Equipment

Crash cart with emergency medications and airway equipment ▪ electrocardiogram (ECG) monitor and electrodes ▪ I.V. catheter ▪ insertion supplies ▪ dextrose 5% in water (D_5W) ▪ optional: clippers if needed, cardiotonic drugs.

Implementation

- Confirm the patient's identity using two patient identifiers according to your facility's policy.
- Explain the procedure to the patient *to ease his fears and promote cooperation.* Ask him to let you know if he feels light-headed.
- Place the patient in a supine position. Insert an I.V. line, if necessary. Then administer D_5W at a keep-vein-open rate, as ordered. *This line will be used if emergency drugs become necessary.*
- Prepare the patient's skin, including clipping the hair if necessary, and attach ECG electrodes. Adjust the size of the ECG complexes on the monitor *so that you can see the arrhythmia clearly.*

Valsalva's maneuver

- Ask the patient to take a deep breath and bear down, as if he were trying to defecate. If he doesn't feel light-headed or dizzy and if no new arrhythmias occur, have him hold his breath and bear down for 10 seconds.
- If he does feel dizzy or light-headed or if you see a new arrhythmia on the monitor—asystole for more than 6 seconds, frequent premature ventricular contractions (PVCs), or VT or ventricular fibrillation—allow him to exhale and stop bearing down.
- After 10 seconds, ask him to exhale and breathe quietly. If the maneuver was successful, the monitor will show his heart rate slowing before he exhales.

Carotid sinus massage

- Begin by obtaining a rhythm strip, using the lead that shows the strongest P waves.

Location and technique for carotid sinus massage

Before applying manual pressure to the patient's right carotid sinus, locate the bifurcation of the carotid artery on the right side of the neck. Turn the patient's head slightly to the left and hyperextend the neck. This brings the carotid artery closer to the skin and moves the sternocleidomastoid muscle away from the carotid artery.

Then using a circular motion, gently massage the right carotid sinus between your fingers and the transverse processes of the spine for 3 to 5 seconds. Don't massage for more than 5 seconds *to avoid risking life-threatening complications.*

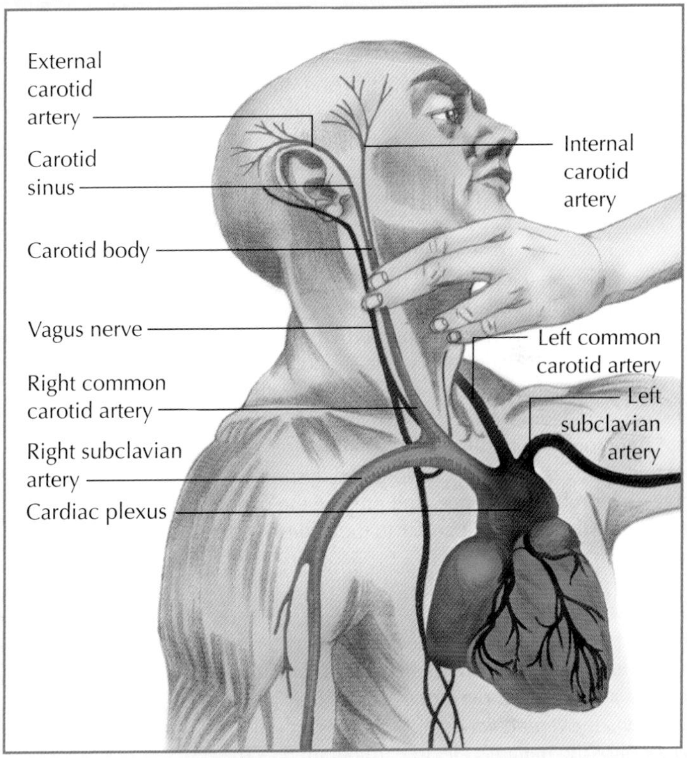

- Auscultate both carotid sinuses. If you detect bruits, inform the practitioner and don't perform carotid sinus massage. If you don't detect bruits, proceed as ordered. (See *Location and technique for carotid sinus massage.*)
- Monitor the ECG throughout the procedure. Stop massaging when the ventricular rate slows sufficiently to permit diagnosis of the rhythm. Or, stop as soon as any evidence of a rhythm change appears. Have the crash cart handy to give emergency treatment if a dangerous arrhythmia occurs.
- If the procedure has no effect within 5 seconds, stop massaging the right carotid sinus and begin to massage the left. If this also fails, administer cardiotonic drugs, as ordered.

Special considerations

- Remember that a brief period of asystole—from 3 to 6 seconds—and several PVCs may precede conversion to normal sinus rhythm.
- If the vagal maneuver succeeded in slowing the patient's heart rate and converting the arrhythmia, continue monitoring him for several hours.

Complications

Use caution when performing carotid sinus massage on elderly patients, patients receiving cardiac glycosides, and patients with heart block, hypertension, coronary artery disease, diabetes mellitus, or hyperkalemia. *The procedure may cause arterial pressure to plummet in these patients,* although it usually rises quickly afterward.

ELDER ALERT *Elderly patients with heart disease are especially susceptible to the adverse effects of vagal maneuvers.*

Vagal maneuvers can occasionally cause bradycardia or complete heart block, so monitor the patient's cardiac rhythm closely. (See *Adverse effects of vagal maneuvers,* page 490.)

Documentation

Record the date and time of the procedure, who performed it, and why it was necessary. Note the patient's response, any complications, and the interventions taken. If possible, obtain a rhythm strip before, during, and after the procedure.

Adverse effects of vagal maneuvers

Both Valsalva's maneuver and carotid sinus massage are useful for slowing heart rate. However, they can cause complications, some of which are life-threatening.

Valsalva's maneuver

This maneuver can cause bradycardia, accompanied by a decrease in cardiac output, possibly leading to syncope. The bradycardia will usually pass quickly; if it doesn't or if it advances to complete heart block or asystole, begin basic life support (BLS) followed, if necessary, by advanced cardiac life support (ACLS).

Valsalva's maneuver can mobilize venous thrombi and cause bleeding. Monitor the patient for signs and symptoms of vascular occlusion, including neurologic changes, chest discomfort, and dyspnea. Report such problems at once, and prepare the patient for diagnostic testing or transfer to the intensive care unit (ICU), as ordered.

Carotid sinus massage

Because carotid sinus massage can cause ventricular fibrillation, ventricular tachycardia, and standstill as well as worsening atrioventricular block that leads to junctional or ventricular escape rhythms, you'll need to monitor the patient's electrocardiogram (ECG) closely. If his ECG indicates complete heart block or asystole, start BLS at once, followed by ACLS. If emergency medications don't convert the complete heart block, the patient may need a temporary pacemaker.

Carotid sinus massage can cause cerebral damage from inadequate tissue perfusion, especially in elderly patients. It can also cause a stroke, either from decreased perfusion caused by total carotid artery blockage or from migrating endothelial plaque loosened by carotid sinus compression. Watch the patient carefully during and after the procedure for changes in neurologic status. If you note any, tell the practitioner at once and prepare the patient for further diagnostic tests or transfer to the ICU, as ordered.

SELECTED REFERENCES

American Association of Critical-Care Nurses Standards. Available at *ww.aacn.org/AACN/practice.nsf/Files/acstds/$file/130300StdsAcute.pdf.*

American Heart Association. "2005 AHA Guidelines for Cardiopulmonary Resuscitation and Emergency Cardiovascular Care: International Consensus on Science," *Circulation* 112 (22 Suppl):IV-1-IV-221, November 2005.

Deepak, S.M., et al. "Ventricular Fibrillation Induced by Carotid Sinus Massage without Preceding Bradycardia," *Europace* 7(6):638-40, November 2005.

Farwell, D.J., and Sulke, A.N. "A Randomized Prospective Comparison of Three Protocols for Head-up Tilt Testing and Carotid Sinus Massage," *International Journal of Cardiology* 105(3):241-49, February 2006.

Felker, G.M., et al. "The Valsalva Maneuver: A Bedside 'Biomarker' for Heart Failure," *American Journal of Medicine* 119(2):117-22, February 2006.

PERICARDIOCENTESIS

In pericardiocentesis, a needle is used to aspirate pericardial fluid for analysis. The procedure is both therapeutic and diagnostic, and is most useful as an emergency measure to relieve cardiac tamponade. It can also provide a fluid sample to confirm and identify the cause of pericardial effusion (excess pericardial fluid) and help determine appropriate therapy.

Normally, small amounts of plasma-derived fluid within the pericardium lubricate the heart and reduce friction. Excess pericardial fluid may accumulate after inflammation, cardiac surgery, rupture, or penetrating trauma (gunshot or stab wounds) of the pericardium. Rapidly forming effusions, such as those that develop after cardiac surgery or penetrating trauma, may induce cardiac tamponade, a potentially lethal syndrome marked by increased intrapericardial pressure. Cardiac tamponade prevents complete ventricular filling, thus reducing cardiac output. Slowly forming effusions, such as those in pericarditis, typically pose less immediate danger.

The pericardium normally contains 10 to 50 ml of sterile fluid. Pericardial fluid is clear and straw-colored without evidence of pathogens, blood, or malignant cells. The white blood cell count in the fluid is usually less than 1,000/µl. Its glucose concentration should approximate the glucose levels in the blood. Pericardial effusions are typically classified as transudates or exudates. (See *Pericardial effusions: Transudates and exudates.*)

Equipment

Prepackaged pericardiocentesis tray ▪ antiseptic solution ▪ 7-ml sterile test tubes ▪ sterile specimen container for culture ▪ sterile 4″ × 4″ gauze pads ▪ sterile bandage ▪ electrocardiogram (ECG) or bedside monitor ▪ pulse oximeter ▪ defibrillator and emergency drugs ▪ gloves ▪ protective eyewear ▪ sterile gloves ▪ sterile marker ▪ sterile label.

If a prepackaged tray isn't available, obtain the following: 1% procaine or 1% lidocaine for local anesthetic ▪ sterile needles (25G for anesthetic and 14G, 16G, and 18G 4" or 5" cardiac needles) ▪ 50-ml syringe with luer-lock tip ▪ Kelly clamp ▪ alligator clip ▪ three-way stopcock ▪ sterile syringe for anesthetic.

Preparation of equipment

Needle insertion is generally guided by ECG or echocardiogram. Connect the patient to the bedside monitor, which is set to read lead V_1 and the pulse oximeter. Make sure the defibrillator and emergency drugs are nearby.

Implementation

- Confirm the patient's identity using two patient identifiers according to your facility's policy.
- Explain the procedure to the patient *to ease his anxiety and ensure his cooperation.* Answer any questions he may have. Make sure an informed consent form has been signed.
- Inform the patient that he will feel some pressure when the needle is inserted into the pericardial sac.
- Wash your hands.
- Open the equipment tray on an overbed table, being careful not to contaminate the sterile field when you open the wrapper.
- Label all medications, medication containers, and other solutions on and off the sterile field.
- Provide adequate lighting at the puncture site and adjust the height of the patient's bed *to allow the physician to perform the procedure comfortably.*
- Position the patient in the supine position with the thorax elevated 60 degrees.
- Wash your hands again and put on gloves and protective eyewear.
- The physician cleans the skin with sterile gauze pads soaked in antiseptic solution from the left costal margin to the xiphoid process.
- If no ampule of anesthetic is included on the equipment tray, clean the injection port of a multidose vial of anesthetic with an alcohol pad. Then invert the vial 45 degrees so that the physician can insert a 25G needle attached to a syringe and withdraw the anesthetic for injection.
- Before the physician injects the anesthetic, tell the patient he'll experience a transient burning sensation and local pain.
- The physician attaches a 50-ml syringe to one end of a three-way stopcock and the cardiac needle to the other. The V_1 lead (precordial lead wire) of the ECG may be attached to the hub of the aspirating needle using the alligator clips *to help determine whether the needle has come in contact with the epicardium during the procedure.*

Pericardial effusions: Transudates and exudates

Transudates are protein-poor effusions that usually arise from mechanical factors altering fluid formation or resorption, such as increased hydrostatic pressure, decreased plasma oncotic pressure, or obstruction of the pericardial lymphatic drainage system by a tumor.

Most exudates result from inflammation and contain large amounts of protein. Inflammation damages the capillary membrane, allowing protein molecules to leak into the pericardial fluid.

Both effusion types occur in pericarditis, neoplasms, acute myocardial infarction, tuberculosis, rheumatoid disease, and systemic lupus erythematosus.

- The physician inserts the needle through the chest wall into the pericardial sac, maintaining gentle aspiration until fluid appears in the syringe. The needle is angled 35 to 45 degrees toward the tip of the right scapula between the left costal margin and the xiphoid process. *This subxiphoid approach minimizes the risk of lacerating the coronary vessels or the pleura.*
- When the needle is positioned properly, the physician attaches a Kelly clamp to the skin surface *so that the needle won't advance any farther.*
- Assist the physician during the aspiration of the pericardial fluid and label and number the specimen tubes. (See *Aspirating pericardial fluid,* page 492.)
- Clean the top of the culture and sensitivity tube with antiseptic solution *to reduce the risk of extrinsic contamination.* If bacterial culture and sensitivity tests are scheduled, record on the laboratory request any antimicrobial drugs the patient is receiving. If anaerobic organisms are suspected, consult the laboratory about proper collection technique *to avoid exposing the aspirate to air.* Send all specimens to the laboratory immediately.
- When the needle is withdrawn, apply pressure to the site immediately with sterile gauze pads for 3 to 5 minutes. Then apply a sterile bandage.
- Obtain a portable chest X-ray immediately after the procedure.
- Assess for complications and check blood pressure, pulse, respirations, oxygen saturation, and heart sounds every 15 minutes until stable, then every 30 minutes for 2 hours, every hour for 4 hours, and every 4 hours thereafter. Your

Aspirating pericardial fluid

In pericardiocentesis, a needle and syringe are inserted through the chest wall into the pericardial sac (as shown below). Electrocardiogram (ECG) monitoring, with a leadwire attached to the needle and electrodes placed on the limbs (right arm [RA], left arm [LA], and left leg [LL]), helps ensure proper needle placement and avoids damage to the heart.

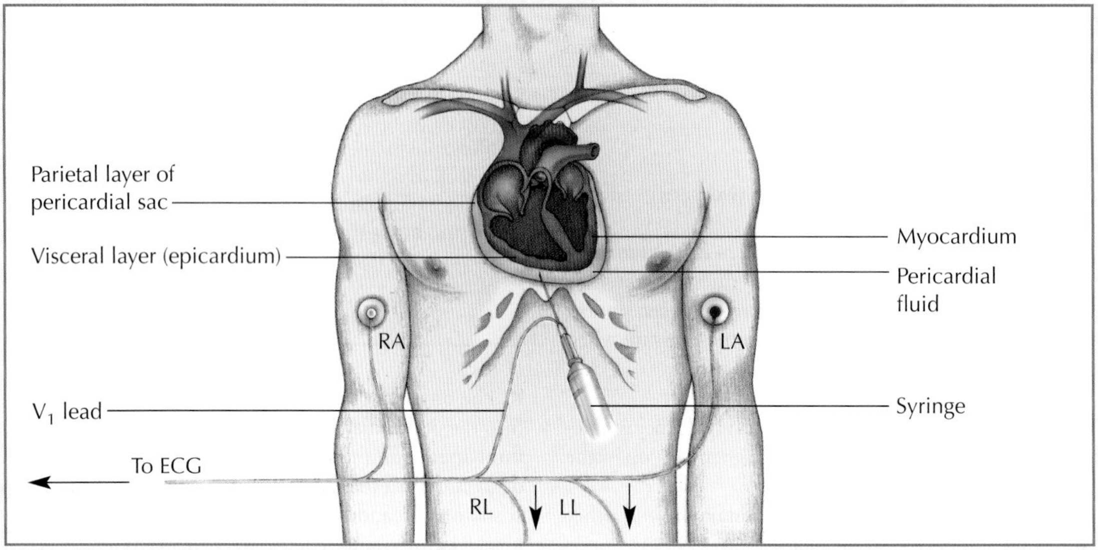

facility may require more frequent monitoring. Reassure the patient that such monitoring is routine.

- Monitor continually for cardiac arrhythmias, and document rhythm strips according to your facility's policy and procedure.
- Return all equipment to the proper location, and dispose of equipment according to your facility's policy.

Special considerations

- Carefully observe the ECG tracing when the cardiac needle is being inserted *because ST-segment elevation indicates that the needle has reached the epicardial surface and should be retracted slightly.* Likewise, an abnormally shaped QRS complex may indicate perforation of the myocardium. Premature ventricular contractions usually indicate that the needle has touched the ventricular wall.
- Watch for grossly bloody fluid aspirate, which may indicate inadvertent puncture of a cardiac chamber.
- After the procedure, be alert for respiratory and cardiac distress. Watch especially for signs of cardiac tamponade, including muffled and distant heart, distended neck veins, paradoxical pulse, and shock. Cardiac tamponade may result from rapid accumulation of pericardial fluid or puncture of a coronary vessel, causing bleeding into the pericardial sac.

Complications

Pericardiocentesis should be performed cautiously *because of the risk of potentially fatal complications, such as laceration of a coronary artery or the myocardium;* other possible complications include ventricular fibrillation or vasovagal arrest, pleural infection, and accidental puncture of the lung, liver, or stomach. *To minimize the risk of complications,* echocardiography should precede pericardiocentesis to determine the effusion site. Generally, surgical drainage and biopsy are safer than pericardiocentesis.

Documentation

Record the initiation and completion time of the procedure, the patient's response, vital signs, cardiac rhythm, and any medications administered. Document the amount, color and consistency of the fluid, the number of specimen tubes collected, and the time of transport to the laboratory. Document patient and family education and any complications and interventions.

SELECTED REFERENCES

Ben-Horin, S., et al. "The Composition of Normal Pericardial Fluid and its Implications for Diagnosing Pericardial Effusions," *American Journal of Medicine* 118(6):636-40, June 2005.

Cubero, G.I., et al. "Pericardial Effusion: Clinical and Analytical Parameters Clues," *International Journal of Cardiology* 108(3):404-405, April 2006.

Humphreys, M. "Pericardial Conditions: Signs, Symptoms, and Electrocardiogram Changes," *Emergency Nursing* 14(1):30-36, April 2006.

Little, W.C., and Freeman, G.L. "Pericardial Disease," *Circulation* 113(12):1622-632, March 2006.

Lynn-McHale Wiegand, D.J., and Carlson, K.K., eds. *AACN Procedure Manual for Critical Care,* 5th ed. Philadelphia: W.B. Saunders Co., 2005.

VENTRICULAR ASSIST DEVICE CARE

A temporary life-sustaining treatment for a failing heart, the ventricular assist device (VAD) diverts systemic blood flow from a diseased ventricle into a centrifugal pump. It maintains cardiac output, reduces ventricular work, and allows the myocardium to rest and contractility to improve. Although used most commonly to assist the left ventricle, this device may also assist the right ventricle or both ventricles. (See *VAD: Help for the failing heart,* page 494.)

Candidates for VAD include patients with massive myocardial infarction, irreversible cardiomyopathy, ventricular arrhythmias, acute myocarditis, an inability to be weaned from cardiopulmonary bypass, valvular disease, or bacterial endocarditis and those who have experienced a heart transplant rejection. The device may also be used in those awaiting a heart transplant.

Indications for VAD therapy include bridge to transplant, bridge to recovery, and destination therapy.

Destination therapy supports patients with VAD therapy until the end of their life — as an alternate to heart transplant for end-stage heart failure. Potential future indications for VAD therapy may include permanent support for a failing heart.

Equipment

The VAD is inserted in the operating room.

Implementation

- Before surgery, explain to the patient that food and fluid intake must be restricted and that you will continuously monitor his cardiac function (using an electrocardiogram, a pulmonary artery catheter, and an arterial line). Offer the patient reassurance. Before sending him to the operating room, make sure he has signed a consent form.
- If time permits, clip the hair on the patient's chest and scrub it with an antiseptic solution.
- When the patient returns from surgery, administer analgesics as ordered.
- Frequently monitor vital signs, intake, and output.
- Keep VAD exit sites immobile. The patient should be encouraged to rehabilitate as soon as clinically able.
- Monitor pulmonary artery pressures. If you have been trained to adjust the pump, maintain cardiac output at 5 to 8 L/minute, central venous pressure at 8 to 16 mm Hg, pulmonary artery wedge pressure at 10 to 20 mm Hg, mean arterial pressure at more than 60 mm Hg, and left atrial pressure between 4 and 12 mm Hg.
- Assess the patient who has a left VAD for signs and symptoms of right-sided heart failure.
- Monitor the patient for signs and symptoms of poor perfusion and ineffective pumping, including arrhythmias, hypotension, slow capillary refill, cool skin, oliguria or anuria, confusion, anxiety, and restlessness.
- Administer heparin, as ordered and depending on the recommendation of the VAD system being used, *to prevent clotting in the pump head and thrombus formation.* Check for bleeding, especially at the operative sites. Monitor laboratory studies, as ordered, especially complete blood count and coagulation studies. Follow your facility's anticoagulation protocol *because thromboembolism is a risk for the duration of VAD use.*
- Assess the patient's incisions and the cannula insertion sites for signs of infection. Monitor the white blood cell count and differential daily, and take rectal or core temperature every 4 hours. Maintain stability of all device exit sites *to promote tissue healing and decrease the risk of infection.*
- Change the dressing over the cannula sites daily or according to your facility's policy.
- Provide supportive care, including range-of-motion exercises and mouth and skin care.
- If VAD support is to be continued for a prolonged period, follow your facility's protocol for assessments, dressings, and patient mobility as the patient's condition progresses.
- If the patient is going home with the device, give explicit discharge instructions based on the VAD system used.

Special considerations

- If the patient with an acute indication for a VAD fails to show improved ventricular function in a few days, the patient may need a transplant. If so, provide psychological support for the patient and his family. You may also be asked to initiate the transplant process by contacting the appropriate agency.
- The psychological effects of the VAD can produce stress in the patient, his family, and his close friends. If appropriate, refer them to other support personnel.

VAD: Help for the failing heart

The ventricular assist device (VAD) functions somewhat like an artificial heart. The major difference is that the VAD assists the heart, whereas the artificial heart replaces it. The VAD is designed to aid one or both ventricles. The pumping chambers themselves aren't usually implanted in the patient.

The permanent VAD is implanted in the patient's chest cavity, although it still provides only temporary support. The device receives power through the skin by a belt of electrical transformer coils (worn externally as a portable battery pack). It can also operate off an implanted, rechargeable battery for up to 1 hour at a time.

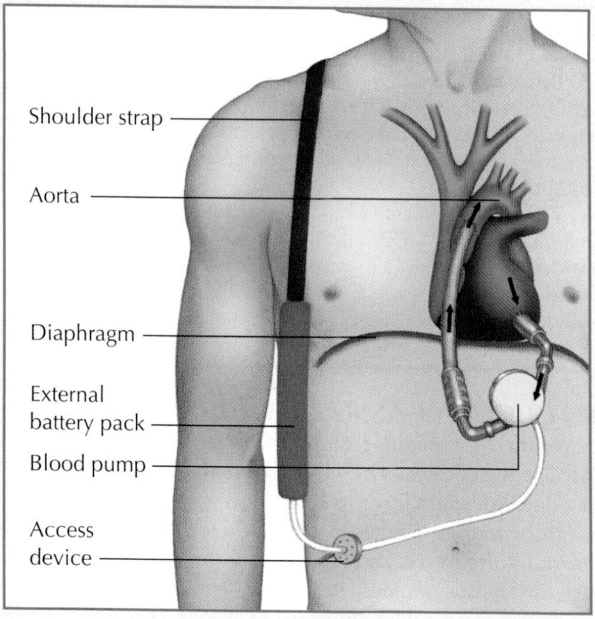

- Understand that the patient with a VAD as a bridge to transplant may have a prolonged wait for heart transplant. Maintaining or improving the patient's physical condition during this wait will improve post-transplant recovery and outcomes.

Complications

The VAD carries a high risk of complications, including damaged blood cells, which can increase the likelihood of thrombus formation and subsequent pulmonary embolism or stroke. Other risks include infection and device failure.

Documentation

Note the patient's condition following insertion of the VAD. Document any pump adjustments as well as any complications and interventions.

SELECTED REFERENCES

Birks, E.J., et al. "Left Ventricular Assist Device and Drug Therapy for the Reversal of Heart Failure," *New England Journal of Medicine* 355(18):1873-884, November 2006.

Fitzsimmons, C.L. "Sensitivity, Ventricular Assist Devices, and the Waiting Game in Heart Transplantation: What's New?" *Critical Care Nursing Quarterly* 27(1):65-77, January-March 2004.

Helton, T.J., et al. "Haemodynamic Monitoring with a Left Ventricular Assist Device," *Heart* 91(10):1261, October 2005.

Hipkins, M. et al. "Care of Patients with Heart Failure and the Use of Ventricular Assist Devices," *Professional Nurse* 19(12):34-36, August 2004.

Lietz, K., and Miller, L.W. "Will Left Ventricular Assist Device Therapy Replace Heart Transplantation in the Foreseeable Future?" *Current Opinion in Internal Medicine* 4(3): 291-96, June 2005.

Simon, M.A., et al. "Myocardial Recovery Using Ventricular Assist Devices," *Circulation* 112(9 Suppl):I32-36, August 2005.

INTRA-AORTIC BALLOON COUNTERPULSATION

Providing temporary support for the heart's left ventricle, intra-aortic balloon counterpulsation (IABC) mechanically displaces blood within the aorta by means of an intra-aortic balloon attached to an external pump console. The balloon is usually inserted through the common femoral artery and

How the intra-aortic balloon pump works

Made of polyurethane, the intra-aortic balloon is attached to an external pump console by means of a large-lumen catheter. The illustrations here show the direction of blood flow when the pump inflates and deflates the balloon.

Balloon inflation

The balloon inflates as the aortic valve closes and diastole begins. Diastole increases perfusion to the coronary arteries.

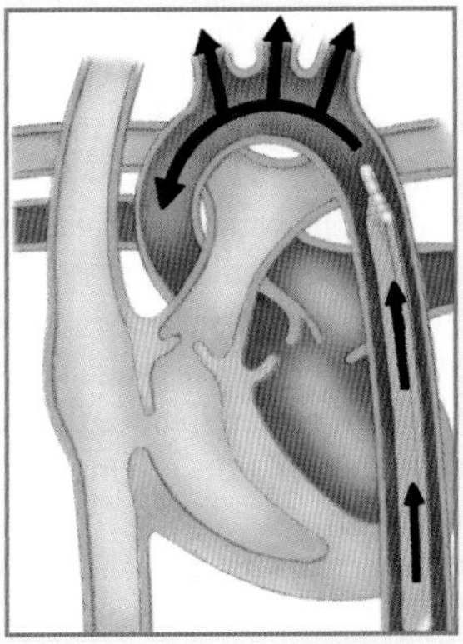

Balloon deflation

The balloon deflates before ventricular ejection, when the aortic valve opens. This permits ejection of blood from the left ventricle against a lowered resistance. As a result, aortic end-diastolic pressure and afterload decrease and cardiac output rises.

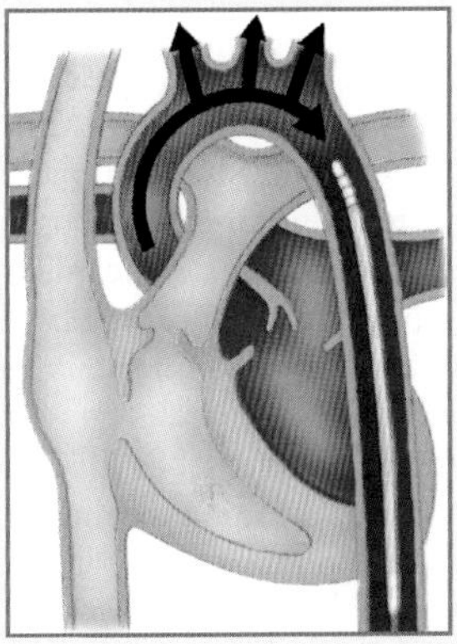

positioned with its tip just distal to the left subclavian artery. It monitors myocardial perfusion and the effects of drugs on myocardial function and perfusion. When used correctly, IABC improves two key aspects of myocardial physiology: It increases the supply of oxygen-rich blood to the myocardium, and it decreases myocardial oxygen demand. (See *How the intra-aortic balloon pump works.*)

IABC is recommended for patients with a wide range of low-cardiac-output disorders or cardiac instability, including refractory angina, ventricular arrhythmias associated with ischemia, and pump failure caused by cardiogenic shock, intraoperative myocardial infarction (MI), or low cardiac output after bypass surgery. IABC is also indicated for patients with low cardiac output secondary to acute mechanical defects after an MI (such as ventricular septal defect, papillary muscle rupture, or left ventricular aneurysm).

Perioperatively, the technique is used to support and stabilize patients with a suspected high-grade lesion who are undergoing such procedures as angioplasty, thrombolytic therapy, cardiac surgery, and cardiac catheterization.

IABC is contraindicated in patients with severe aortic regurgitation, aortic aneurysm, or severe peripheral vascular disease.

Equipment

IABC console and balloon catheters ▪ insertion kit ▪ gas supply (usually helium) ▪ electrocardiogram (ECG) monitor ▪ two sets of ECG electrodes ▪ sedative ▪ pain medication ▪ heparin flush solution, transducer, and flush setup ▪ temporary pacemaker setup ▪ sterile drape ▪ sterile gloves ▪ gown ▪ mask ▪ sutures ▪ suction setup ▪ oxygen setup and equipment, as appropriate ▪ defibrillator and emergency medications ▪ fluoroscope ▪ indwelling urinary catheter ▪ urinometer ▪ arterial blood gas (ABG) kits and tubes for laboratory studies ▪ antiseptic swabs ▪ dressing materials ▪ 4″ × 4″ gauze pads ▪ clippers ▪ optional: defibrillator, atropine, I.V. heparin, low-molecular-weight dextran.

If the balloon will be surgically inserted, you will also need a Dacron graft.

Preparation of equipment

Obtain the IABC console and gas supply. Make sure that the gas supply is full, and attach it to the console, following the manufacturer's recommendations. Prepare the transducer with heparin flush solution, as appropriate. Complete any other preparation for the IABC console, as indicated by your facility's policy and the instruction manual.

Implementation

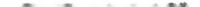

- Confirm the patient's identity using two patient identifiers according to your facility's policy.
- Explain to the patient that the physician will place a special balloon catheter in his aorta *to help his heart pump more easily.* Briefly explain the insertion procedure, and mention that the catheter will be connected to a large console next to his bed. Tell him that the balloon will temporarily reduce his heart's work load *to promote rapid healing of the ventric-*

ular muscle. Let him know that it will be removed after his heart can resume an adequate workload.

Preparing for intra-aortic balloon insertion

- Make sure the patient or a family member understands and signs a consent form. Verify that the form is attached to his chart.
- Obtain the patient's baseline vital signs, including pulmonary artery pressure (PAP). (A pulmonary artery [PA] line should already be in place.) Attach the patient to an ECG machine for continuous monitoring. Be sure to apply chest electrodes in a standard lead II position — or in whatever position produces the largest R wave — *because the R wave triggers balloon inflation and deflation.* Obtain a baseline ECG.
- Attach another set of ECG electrodes to the patient unless the ECG pattern is being transmitted from the patient's bedside monitor to the balloon pump monitor through a phone cable. Administer oxygen as ordered and as necessary.
- Make sure the patient has an arterial line, a PA line, and a peripheral I.V. line in place. The arterial line is used for withdrawing blood samples, monitoring blood pressure, and assessing the timing and effectiveness of therapy. The PA line allows measurement of PAP, aspiration of blood samples, and cardiac output studies. Increased PAP indicates increased myocardial workload and ineffective balloon pumping. Cardiac output studies are usually performed with and without the balloon to check the patient's progress. The central lumen of the intra-aortic balloon, used to monitor central aortic pressure, produces an augmented pressure waveform that allows you to check for proper timing of the inflation-deflation cycle and demonstrates the effects of counterpulsation, elevated diastolic pressure, and reduced end-diastolic and systolic pressures. (See *Interpreting intra-aortic balloon waveforms.*)
- Insert an indwelling catheter with a urinometer *so you can measure the patient's urine output and assess his fluid balance and renal function. To reduce the risk of infection,* clip hair bilaterally from the lower abdomen to the lower thigh, including the pubic area.
- Observe and record the patient's peripheral leg pulse, and document sensation, movement, color, and temperature of the legs.
- Administer a sedative, as ordered.
- Have the defibrillator, suction setup, temporary pacemaker setup, and emergency medications readily available *in case the patient develops complications during insertion such as an arrhythmia.*
- Open the insertion tray using sterile technique and place on a bedside table within easy reach for the physician.
- Before the physician inserts the balloon, he puts on sterile gloves, gown, and mask. He cleans the site with antiseptic solution and drapes the area with a sterile drape.

Inserting the intra-aortic balloon percutaneously

- The physician may insert the balloon percutaneously through the femoral artery into the descending thoracic aorta, using a modified Seldinger technique. First, he accesses the vessel with an 18G angiography needle and removes the inner stylet.
- Then he passes the guide wire through the needle and removes the needle.
- Next, the physician passes an introducer (dilator and sheath assembly) over the guide wire into the vessel until about 1″ (2.5 cm) remains above the insertion site. He then removes the inner dilator, leaving the introducer sheath and guide wire in place.
- After passing the balloon over the guide wire into the introducer sheath, the physician advances the catheter into position, ⅜″ to ¾″ (1 to 2 cm) distal to the left subclavian artery under fluoroscopic guidance.
- The physician attaches the balloon to the control system to initiate counterpulsation. The balloon catheter then unfurls.
- The physician will clean the insertion site and apply a sterile dressing.
- Obtain a chest X-ray to verify correct balloon placement.

Inserting the intra-aortic balloon surgically

- If the physician chooses not to insert the catheter percutaneously, he usually inserts it by femoral arteriotomy. (See *Surgical insertion sites for the intra-aortic balloon,* page 499.)
- After making an incision and isolating the femoral artery, the physician attaches a Dacron graft to a small opening in the arterial wall.
- He then passes the catheter through this graft. Using fluoroscopic guidance as necessary, he advances the catheter up the descending thoracic aorta and places the catheter tip between the left subclavian artery and the renal arteries.
- The physician sews the Dacron graft around the catheter at the insertion point and connects the other end of the catheter to the pump console.
- If the balloon can't be inserted through the femoral artery, the physician inserts it in an antegrade direction through the anterior wall of the ascending aorta. He positions it ⅜″ to ¾″ beyond the left subclavian artery and brings the catheter out through the chest wall.

Monitoring the patient with an intra-aortic balloon

NURSING ALERT *If the control system malfunctions or becomes inoperable, don't let the balloon catheter remain*

Interpreting intra-aortic balloon waveforms

During intra-aortic balloon counterpulsation, you can use electrocardiogram and arterial pressure waveforms to determine whether the balloon pump is functioning properly.

Normal inflation-deflation timing

Balloon inflation occurs after aortic valve closure; deflation, during isovolumetric contraction, just before the aortic valve opens. In a properly timed waveform, like the one shown at right, the inflation point lies at or slightly above the dicrotic notch. Both inflation and deflation cause a sharp V. Peak diastolic pressure exceeds peak systolic pressure; peak systolic pressure exceeds assisted peak systolic pressure.

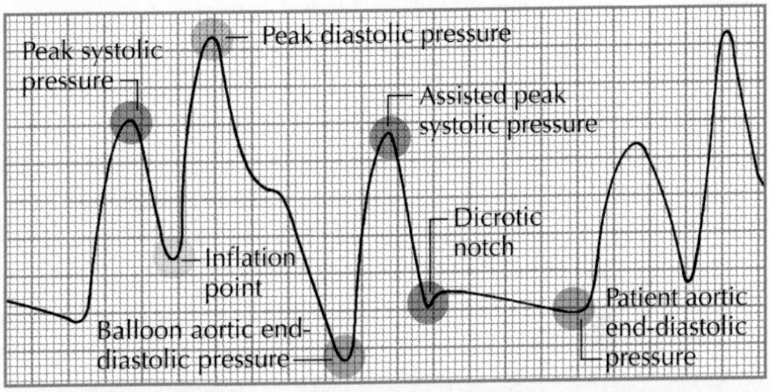

Early inflation

With *early inflation,* the inflation point lies before the dicrotic notch. Early inflation dangerously increases myocardial stress and decreases cardiac output.

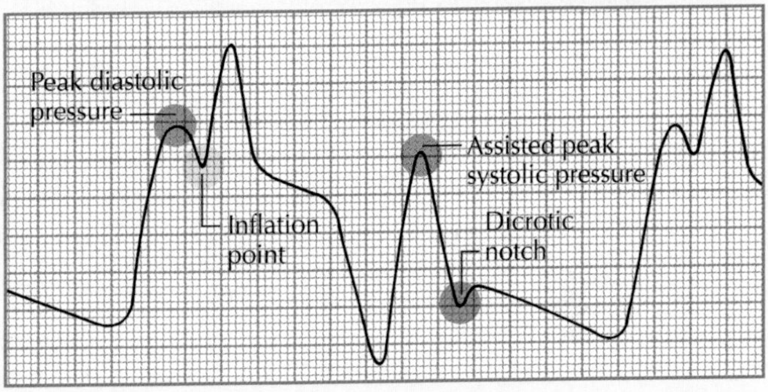

Early deflation

With *early deflation,* a U shape appears and peak systolic pressure is less than or equal to assisted peak systolic pressure. This won't decrease afterload or myocardial oxygen consumption.

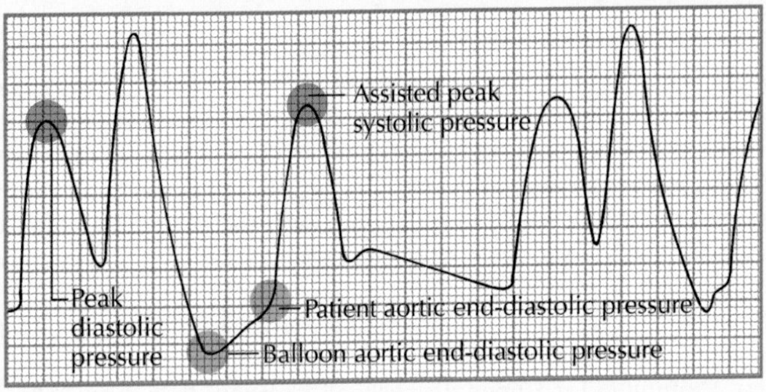

(continued)

Interpreting intra-aortic balloon waveforms *(continued)*

Late inflation

With *late inflation*, the dicrotic notch precedes the inflation point, and the notch and the inflation point create a W shape. This can lead to a reduction in peak diastolic pressure, coronary and systemic perfusion augmentation time, and augmented coronary perfusion pressure.

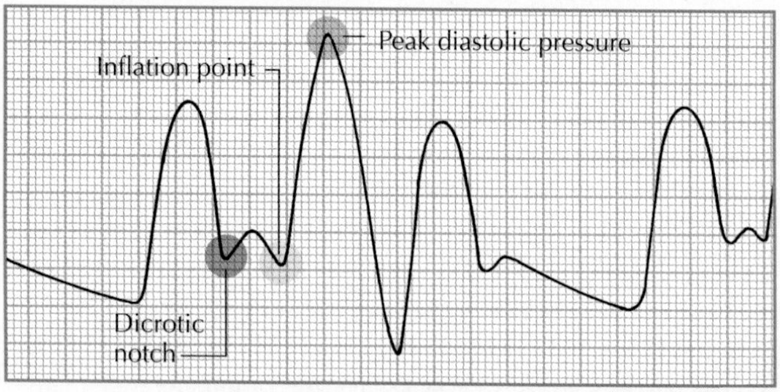

Late deflation

With *late deflation*, peak systolic pressure exceeds assisted peak systolic pressure. This threatens the patient by increasing afterload, myocardial oxygen consumption, cardiac workload, and preload. It occurs when the balloon has been inflated for too long.

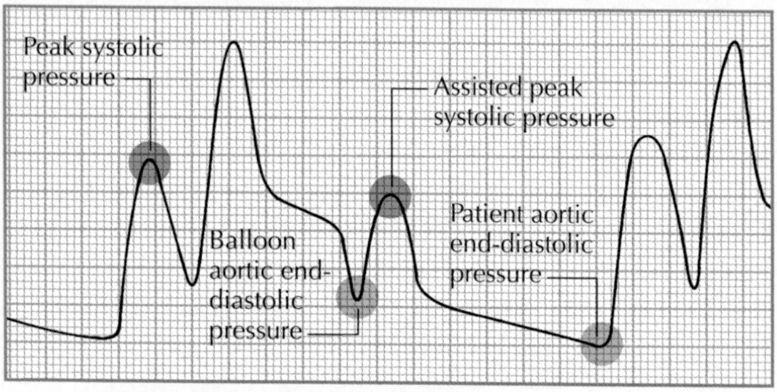

dormant for more than 30 minutes. Get another control system and attach it to the balloon; then resume pumping. In the meantime, inflate the balloon manually, using a 60-ml syringe and room air a minimum of once every 5 minutes, to prevent thrombus formation in the catheter.

- Assess and record pedal and posterior tibial pulses as well as color, sensation, and temperature in the affected limb every 15 minutes for 1 hour, then hourly. Notify the physician immediately if you detect circulatory changes; *the balloon may need to be removed.*
- Observe and record the patient's baseline arm pulses, arm sensation and movement, and arm color and temperature every 15 minutes for 1 hour after balloon insertion, then every 2 hours while the balloon is in place. *Loss of left arm pulses may indicate upward balloon displacement.* Notify the physician of any changes.
- Monitor the patient's urine output every hour. Note baseline blood urea nitrogen (BUN) and serum creatinine levels, and monitor these levels daily. *Changes in urine output, BUN, and serum creatinine levels may signal reduced renal perfusion from downward balloon displacement.*
- Auscultate and record bowel sounds every 4 hours. Check for abdominal distention and tenderness as well as changes in the patient's elimination patterns.
- Measure the patient's temperature every 1 to 4 hours. If it's elevated, obtain blood samples for a culture, send them to the laboratory immediately, and notify the physician. Culture any drainage at the insertion site.
- Monitor the patient's hematologic status. Observe for bleeding gums, blood in the urine or stools, petechiae, and bleeding at the insertion site. Monitor his platelet count, hemoglobin levels, and hematocrit daily. Expect to administer blood products *to maintain hematocrit at 30%.* If the platelet count drops, expect to administer platelets.
- Monitor partial thromboplastin time (PTT) every 6 hours while the heparin dose is adjusted *to maintain PTT at 1½ to 2 times the normal value,* then every 12 to 24 hours while the balloon remains in place.
- Measure PAP and pulmonary artery wedge pressure (PAWP) every 1 to 2 hours, as ordered. A rising PAWP reflects preload, signaling increased ventricular pressure and workload; notify the physician if this occurs. Some patients

require I.V. nitroprusside during IABC *to reduce preload and afterload.*

- Obtain samples for ABG analysis, as ordered.
- Monitor serum electrolyte levels — especially sodium and potassium — to assess the patient's fluid and electrolyte balance and help prevent arrhythmias.

NURSING ALERT *Watch for signs and symptoms of a dissecting aortic aneurysm: a blood pressure differential between the left and right arms, elevated blood pressure, syncope, pallor, diaphoresis, dyspnea, a throbbing abdominal mass, a reduced red blood cell count with an elevated white blood cell count, and pain in the chest, abdomen, or back. Notify the physician immediately if you detect these complications.*

Weaning the patient from IABC

- Assess the cardiac index, systemic blood pressure, and PAWP *to help the physician evaluate the patient's readiness for weaning*— usually about 24 hours after balloon insertion. The patient's hemodynamic status should be stable on minimal doses of inotropic agents, such as dopamine or dobutamine.
- To begin weaning, gradually decrease the frequency of balloon augmentation to 1:2 and 1:4, as ordered. Although your facility has its own weaning protocol, be aware that assist frequency is usually maintained for 1 hour or longer. If the patient's hemodynamic indices remain stable during this time, weaning may continue.
- Avoid leaving the patient on a low augmentation setting for more than 2 hours *to prevent embolus formation.*
- Assess the patient's tolerance of weaning. Signs and symptoms of poor tolerance include confusion and disorientation, urine output below 30 ml/hour, cold and clammy skin, chest pain, arrhythmias, ischemic ECG changes, and elevated PAP. If the patient develops any of these problems, notify the physician at once.

Removing the intra-aortic balloon

- The balloon is removed when the patient's hemodynamic status remains stable after the frequency of balloon augmentation is decreased. The control system is turned off and the connective tubing is disconnected from the catheter *to ensure balloon deflation.*
- The physician withdraws the balloon until the proximal end of the catheter contacts the distal end of the introducer sheath.
- The physician then applies pressure below the puncture site and removes the balloon and introducer sheath as a unit, allowing a few seconds of free bleeding *to prevent thrombus formation.*

Surgical insertion sites for the intra-aortic balloon

If an intra-aortic balloon can't be inserted percutaneously, the physician will insert it surgically, using a femoral or transthoracic approach.

Femoral approach

Insertion through the femoral artery requires a cutdown and an arteriotomy. The physician passes the balloon through a Dacron graft that has been sewn to the artery.

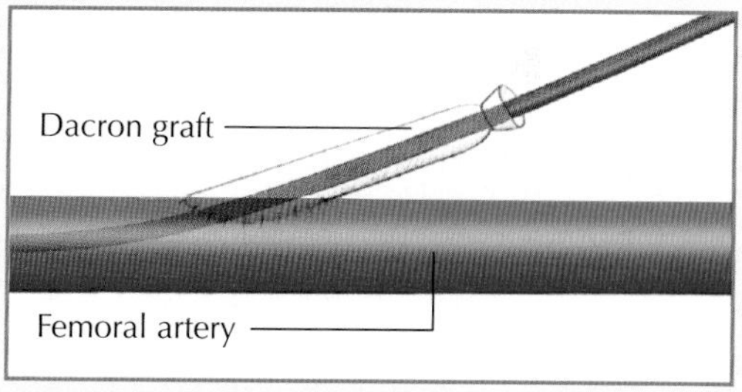

Transthoracic approach

If femoral insertion is unsuccessful, the physician may use a transthoracic approach. He inserts the balloon in an antegrade direction through the subclavian artery and then positions it in the descending thoracic aorta.

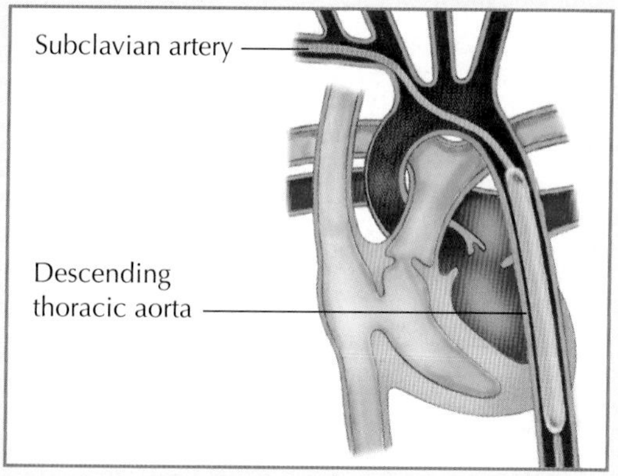

- *To promote distal bleedback,* the physician applies pressure above the puncture site.
- Apply direct pressure to the site for 30 minutes or until bleeding stops. (In some facilities, this is the physician's responsibility.)

(Text continues on page 502.)

TROUBLESHOOTING

Troubleshooting an IABP

When a patient has an intra-aortic balloon pump (IABP), many common problems can develop. Use this table to help you recognize and resolve such problems.

Problem	Possible causes	Interventions
High gas leak (automatic mode only)	Balloon leakage or abrasion	■ Check for blood in the tubing. ■ Stop pumping. ■ Notify the physician to remove the balloon.
	Condensation in extension tubing, volume limiter disk, or both	■ Remove condensate from the tubing and volume limiter disk. ■ Refill, autopurge, and resume pumping.
	Kink in balloon catheter or tubing	■ Check the catheter and tubing for kinks and loose connections; straighten and tighten any found. ■ Refill and resume pumping.
	Tachycardia	■ Change wean control to 1:2 or operate on "manual" mode. ■ Autopurge the balloon every 1 to 2 hours, and monitor the balloon pressure waveform closely.
	Malfunctioning or loose volume limiter disk	■ Replace or tighten the disk. ■ Refill, autopurge, and resume pumping.
	System leak	■ Perform a leak test.
Balloon line block (in automatic mode only)	Kink in balloon or catheter	■ Check the catheter and tubing for kinks and loose connections; straighten and tighten any found. ■ Refill and resume pumping.
	Balloon catheter not unfurled; sheath or balloon positioned too high	■ Notify the physician immediately to verify placement. ■ Anticipate the need for repositioning or manual inflation of the balloon.
	Condensation in tubing, volume limiter disk, or both	■ Remove condensate from the tubing and volume limiter disk. ■ Refill, autopurge, and resume pumping.
	Balloon too large for aorta	■ Decrease volume control percentage by one notch.
	Malfunctioning volume limiter disk or incorrect volume limiter disk size	■ Replace the volume limiter disk. ■ Refill, autopurge, and resume pumping.
No electrocardiogram (ECG) trigger	Inadequate signal	■ Adjust ECG gain, and change the lead or trigger mode.
	Lead disconnected	■ Replace the lead.
	Improper ECG input mode (skin or monitor) selected	■ Adjust ECG input to appropriate mode (skin or monitor).

Troubleshooting an IABP *(continued)*

PROBLEM	POSSIBLE CAUSES	INTERVENTIONS
No atrial pressure trigger	Arterial line damped	■ Flush the line.
	Arterial line open to atmosphere	■ Check connections on the arterial pressure line.
Trigger mode change	Trigger mode changed while pumping	■ Resume pumping.
Irregular heart rhythm	Patient experiencing arrhythmia, such as atrial fibrillation or ectopic beats	■ Change to R or QRS sense (if necessary to accommodate irregular rhythm). ■ Notify the physician of arrhythmia.
Erratic atrioventricular (AV) pacing	Demand for paced rhythm occurring when in AV sequential trigger mode	■ Change to pacer reject trigger or QRS sense.
Noisy ECG signal	Malfunctioning leads	■ Replace the leads. ■ Check the ECG cable.
	Electrocautery in use	■ Switch to atrial pressure trigger.
Internal trigger	Trigger mode set on internal 80 beats/minute	■ Select an alternative trigger if the patient has a heartbeat or rhythm. ■ Keep in mind that the internal trigger is used only during cardiopulmonary bypass or cardiac arrest.
Purge incomplete	OFF button pressed during autopurge; interrupted purge cycle	■ Initiate autopurging again, or initiate pumping.
High fill pressure	Malfunctioning volume limiter disk	■ Replace the volume limiter disk. ■ Refill, autopurge, and resume pumping.
	Occluded vent line or valve	■ Attempt to resume pumping. ■ If unsuccessful, notify the physician and contact the manufacturer.
No balloon drive	No volume limiter disk	■ Insert the volume limiter disk, and lock it securely in place.
	Tubing disconnected	■ Reconnect the tubing. ■ Refill, autopurge, and pump.
Incorrect timing	INFLATE and DEFLATE controls set incorrectly	■ Place the INFLATE and DEFLATE controls at set midpoints. ■ Reassess timing and readjust.
Low volume percentage	Volume control percentage not 100%	■ Assess the cause of decreased volume, and reset (if necessary).

- If the balloon was inserted surgically, the physician will close the Dacron graft and suture the insertion site. The cardiologist usually removes a percutaneous catheter.
- After balloon removal, provide wound care according to your facility's policy. Record the patient's pedal and posterior tibial pulses, and the color, temperature, and sensation of the affected limb. Enforce bed rest as appropriate (usually for 8 hours).
- Check vital signs and hemodynamic parameters every 15 minutes for 1 hour, every 30 minutes for 2 hours, and then every hour, or according to your facility's policy.

Special considerations

- Before using the IABC control system, make sure you know what the alarms and messages mean and how to respond to them.

NURSING ALERT *You must respond immediately to alarms and messages.*

- Change the dressing at the balloon insertion site every 24 hours or as needed, using strict sterile technique. Don't let povidone-iodine solution come in contact with the catheter.
- Make sure the head of the bed is elevated no more than 30 degrees.
- Watch for pump interruptions, which may result from loose ECG electrodes or leadwires, static or 60-cycle interference, catheter kinking, or improper body alignment. (See *Troubleshooting an IABP,* pages 500 and 501.)
- Make sure PTT is within normal limits before the balloon is removed *to prevent hemorrhage at insertion site.*

Complications

IABC may cause numerous complications. The most common, arterial embolism, stems from clot formation on the balloon surface. Other potential complications include extension or rupture of an aortic aneurysm, femoral or iliac artery perforation, femoral artery occlusion, and sepsis. Bleeding at the insertion site may become aggravated by pump-induced thrombocytopenia caused by platelet aggregation around the balloon.

Documentation

Document all aspects of patient assessment and management, including the patient's response to therapy. If you're responsible for the IABC device, document all routine checks, problems, and troubleshooting measures. If a technician is responsible for the IABC device, record only when and why the technician was notified as well as the result of his actions on the patient, if any. Also document any teaching of the patient, family, or close friends as well as their responses.

Selected references

American Association of Critical-Care Nurses—Standards. Available at *http://www.aacn.org/AACN/practice.nsf/Files/acstds/$file/130300StdsAcute.pdf.*

Field, M.L., et al. "Preoperative Intra Aortic Balloon Pumps in Patients Undergoing Coronary Artery Bypass Grafting," *Cochrane Database of Systematic Reviews* (1):CD004472, January 2007.

Lynn-McHale Wiegand, D.J., and Carlson, K.K., eds. *AACN Procedure Manual for Critical Care,* 5th ed. Philadelphia: W.B. Saunders Co., 2005.

Reid, M.B., and Cottrell, D. "Nursing Care of Patients Receiving Intra-aortic Balloon Counterpulsation," *Critical Care Nurse* 25(5):40-44, 46-49, October 2005.

Santa-Cruz, R.A., et al. "Aortic Counterpulsation: A Review of the Hemodynamic Effects and Indications for Use," *Catheterization and Cardiovascular Interventions* 67(1):68-77, January 2006.

Trost, J.C., and Hillis, L.D. "Intra-aortic Balloon Counterpulsation," *American Journal of Cardiology* 97(9):1391-398, May 2006.

Percutaneous transluminal coronary angioplasty

A nonsurgical approach to opening coronary vessels narrowed by arteriosclerosis, percutaneous transluminal coronary angioplasty (PTCA) uses a balloon-tipped catheter that's inserted into a narrowed coronary artery. This procedure, performed in the cardiac catheterization laboratory under local anesthesia, relieves pain due to angina and myocardial ischemia.

Cardiac catheterization usually accompanies PTCA to assess the stenosis and the efficacy of the angioplasty. Catheterization is used as a visual tool to direct the balloon-tipped catheter through the vessel's area of stenosis. As the balloon is inflated, the plaque is compressed against the vessel wall, allowing coronary blood to flow more freely. (See *Performing PTCA.*)

PTCA provides an alternative for patients who are poor surgical risks because of chronic medical problems. It's also useful for patients who have total coronary occlusion, unstable angina, and plaque buildup in several areas and for those with poor left ventricular function.

Your responsibilities in PTCA include teaching the patient and his family about the procedure and assessing for complications afterward.

Another procedure, laser-enhanced angioplasty, shows promise in vaporizing occlusions in atherosclerosis. (See *Laser-enhanced angioplasty,* page 504.)

Performing PTCA

Percutaneous transluminal coronary angioplasty (PTCA) is a procedure that opens an occluded coronary artery without opening the chest. It's performed in the cardiac catheterization laboratory after coronary angiography confirms the presence and location of the occlusion. When the occlusion is located, the physician threads a guide catheter through the patient's femoral artery and into the coronary artery under fluoroscopic guidance (as shown at right).

When the guide catheter's position at the occlusion site is confirmed by angiography, the physician carefully introduces into the catheter a double-lumen balloon that is smaller than the catheter lumen. He then directs the balloon through the lesion, where a marked pressure gradient will be obvious. The physician alternately inflates (as shown) and deflates the balloon until an angiogram verifies successful arterial dilation and the pressure gradient has decreased.

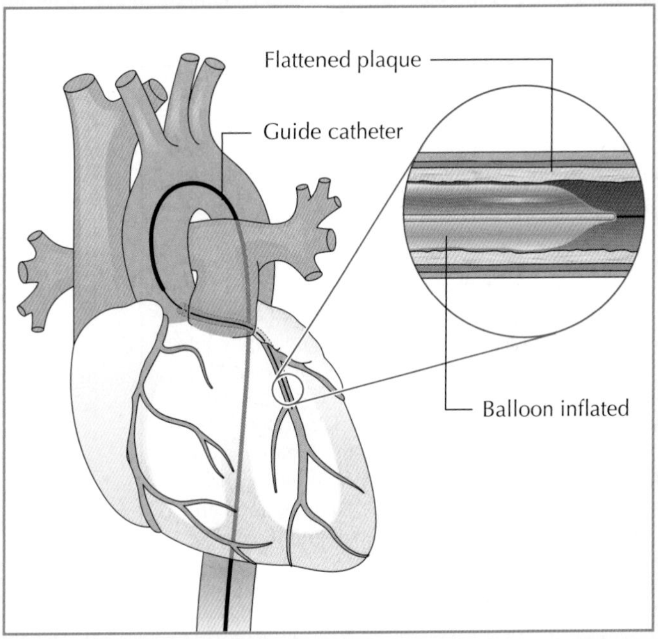

Equipment

Antimicrobial solution ▪ local anesthetic ▪ I.V. solution and tubing ▪ electrocardiogram (ECG) monitor and electrodes ▪ oxygen ▪ nasal cannula ▪ clippers ▪ sedative ▪ pulmonary artery (PA) catheter ▪ contrast medium ▪ emergency medications ▪ heparin for injection ▪ introducer kit for PTCA catheter ▪ eye protection ▪ sterile gown, gloves, and drapes ▪ optional: nitroglycerin, soft restraints.

Implementation

- Confirm the patient's identity using two patient identifiers according to your facility's policy.
- Explain the procedure to the patient and his family *to reduce the patient's fear and promote cooperation.*
- Inform the patient that the procedure lasts from 1 to 4 hours and that he may feel some discomfort from lying on a hard table for that long.
- Tell him that a catheter will be inserted into an artery or a vein in his groin and that he may feel pressure as the catheter moves along the vessel.
- Reassure him that although he'll be awake during the procedure, he'll be given a sedative. Explain that the physician or nurse may ask him how he's feeling and that he should tell them if he experiences any angina.
- Explain that the physician will inject a contrast medium *to outline the lesion's location.* Warn the patient that he may feel a hot, flushing sensation or transient nausea during the injection.

Before angioplasty

- Check the patient's history for allergies; if he has had allergic reactions to shellfish, iodine, or contrast media, notify the physician.
- Give 300 to 325 mg of aspirin at least 2 hours, preferably 4 hours, before the procedure if the patient isn't already receiving aspirin therapy. If he is receiving aspirin therapy, have the patient take 75 mg to 325 mg, as ordered, prior to the procedure *to prevent platelet aggregation.*
- Make sure the patient signs a consent form.
- Restrict food and fluids for at least 6 hours before the procedure or as ordered.
- Ensure that the results of coagulation studies, complete blood count, serum electrolyte studies, and blood typing and crossmatching are available.

Laser-enhanced angioplasty

Laser-enhanced angioplasty shows great potential for vaporizing occlusions in patients with atherosclerosis. The best results occur when the procedure is used in patients with thrombotic occlusions, but it may also be used to remove calcified plaques. New lasers that deliver energy in brief pulses have helped solve the problem of thermal or acoustic damage to local tissues. Using the pulsed beam, physicians can dispatch the blockage without destroying the vessel wall.

To perform the procedure, the physician threads a laser-containing catheter into the diseased artery. When the catheter nears the occlusion, the physician triggers the laser to emit rapid bursts. Between bursts he rotates the catheter, advancing it until the occlusion is destroyed. The procedure takes about an hour and requires only a local anesthetic. Clearing a completely occluded coronary artery requires ten 1-second bursts of laser energy, followed by balloon angioplasty. After the procedure, angiography may be used to document vessel patency.

Cardiologists have successfully used laser techniques to open totally blocked right main coronary arteries, thereby avoiding bypass surgery. They have also used combinations of direct laser energy, fiberoptics, and balloon angioplasty catheters to open totally blocked right main coronary arteries. These advances may make it possible to perform angioplasty in community hospitals in nonsurgical settings.

- Insert an I.V. line to administer the sedative and in case emergency medications are needed.
- Clip hair from the insertion site (groin or brachial area). Clean the area with antimicrobial solution.
- Give the patient a sedative, as ordered.
- Take baseline peripheral pulses in all extremities.

During angioplasty

- When the patient arrives at the cardiac catheterization laboratory, apply ECG electrodes and ensure I.V. line patency.
- Administer oxygen through a nasal cannula.
- The physician will put on a sterile gown and gloves. Open the sterile supplies and label all medications, medication containers, and other solutions on and off the sterile field.
- The physician prepares the site and injects a local anesthetic. If the patient doesn't have a PA catheter in place, the physician may insert one now.
- The physician inserts a large guide catheter into the artery. Then he threads an angioplasty catheter through the guide catheter. An angioplasty catheter is thinner and longer and has a balloon at its tip. Using a thin, flexible guide wire, he then threads the catheter up through the aorta and into the coronary artery to the area of stenosis.
- He injects a contrast medium through the angioplasty catheter and into the obstructed coronary artery *to outline the lesion's location and help assess the blockage.* He also injects heparin *to prevent the catheter from clotting,* and intracoronary nitroglycerin *to dilate coronary vessels and prevent spasm, if needed.*
- He inflates the catheter's balloon for a gradually increasing amount of time and pressure. The expanding balloon compresses the atherosclerotic plaque against the arterial wall, expanding the arterial lumen. *Because balloon inflation deprives the myocardium distal to the inflation area of blood,* the patient may experience angina at this time. If balloon inflation fails to decrease the stenosis, a larger balloon may be used.
- After angioplasty, serial angiograms help determine the effectiveness of treatment.
- The physician removes the angioplasty catheter while leaving the guide catheter in place, *in case the procedure needs to be repeated because of vessel occlusion.* The guide catheter is usually sutured at this time and is generally removed 2 to 24 hours after the procedure.

After angioplasty

- When the patient returns to the unit, he may be receiving I.V. heparin or nitroglycerin. If he is bleeding at the catheter insertion site, he may also have a sandbag on it *to prevent a hematoma.* Alternatively, manual pressure may be applied. If bleeding at the site continues, apply pressure approximately ¾" to 1¼" (2 to 3 cm) above the puncture site.
- Assess the patient's vital signs every 15 minutes for the first hour, then every 30 minutes for 4 hours, unless his condition warrants more frequent checking.
- Assess peripheral pulses distal to the catheter insertion site as well as the color, sensation, temperature, and capillary refill of the affected extremity every 15 minutes for the first hour, then every 30 minutes for 4 hours.
- Monitor ECG rhythm and arterial pressures.

NURSING ALERT Because coronary spasm may occur during or after PTCA, *monitor the patient's ECG for ST and T-wave changes, and take vital signs frequently. Coronary artery dissection may occur with no early symptoms, but it can cause restenosis of the vessel. Be alert for symp-*

toms of ischemia, which requires emergency coronary revascularization.

- Instruct the patient to remain in bed for 8 hours and to keep the affected extremity straight; if the patient is restless and moving his extremities, obtain an order to apply soft restraints, if necessary. Elevate the head of the bed 15 to 30 degrees.
- Assess the catheter site for hematoma, ecchymosis, and hemorrhage. If an area of expanding hematoma appears, mark the site and alert the physician. If bleeding occurs, locate the artery and apply manual pressure; then notify the physician.
- Administer I.V. fluids as ordered (usually 100 ml/hour) *to promote excretion of the contrast medium.* Be sure to assess for signs of fluid overload (distended neck veins, atrial and ventricular gallops, dyspnea, pulmonary congestion, tachycardia, hypertension, and hypoxemia).
- After the catheter is removed, apply direct pressure for at least 10 minutes and monitor the site often.

Special considerations

- PTCA is contraindicated in left main coronary artery disease, especially when the patient is a poor surgical risk; in patients with variant angina or critical valvular disease; and in patients with vessels that are occluded at the aortic wall orifice.
- Vascular closure devices for rapid hemostasis may be used after sheath removal. Hemostasis is achieved either by collagen induced thrombus generation (VasoSeal), a mechanical block of the puncture site and collagen induced thrombus formation (Angio-seal), generation of a thrombus (Duett), or by Perclose (nonabsorbable sutures).
- Current guidelines recommend a loading dose of clopidogrel 300 mg orally at least 6 hours before the procedure, if possible.
- Unfractionated heparin should be administered to all patients undergoing PTCA. If the patient has heparin-induced thrombocytopenia, bivalirudin or argatroban may be used.
- Devices to prevent lower extremity embolism are recommended for use during PTCA.
- CK-MB and troponin levels may be obtained if the patient is suspected of having a myocardial infarction during the PTCA or developed complications during the procedure.
- The current recommendation is to administer clopidogrel 75 mg daily after the procedure for a period of 1 to 12 months depending on the exact procedure completed. Additionally, if the patient isn't already receiving long-term aspirin therapy, aspirin 300 mg to 325 mg per day may be prescribed for 1 to 6 months, depending on the patient's condition and status. This dose is typically followed by 75 to 162 mg/day.

EQUIPMENT

Vascular stents

Two serious complications of percutaneous transluminal coronary angioplasty (PTCA) are acute vessel closure and late restenosis. To prevent these problems, physicians are performing a procedure called *stenting*. The stent currently used—the Palmaz balloon-expandable stent—consists of a stainless steel tube, the walls of which have a rectangular design. When the stent expands, each rectangle stretches to a diamond shape. The expanded stent supports the artery and helps prevent restenosis.

The stent is used in patients at risk for abrupt clotting after PTCA. Stents may also be inserted after failed PTCA to keep the patient stable until he can undergo coronary artery bypass surgery, or a stent may be used as an alternative to this surgery.

For insertion, the stent is put on a standard balloon angioplasty catheter and positioned over a guide wire (as shown below). Fluoroscopy verifies correct placement; then the stent is expanded and the catheter is removed.

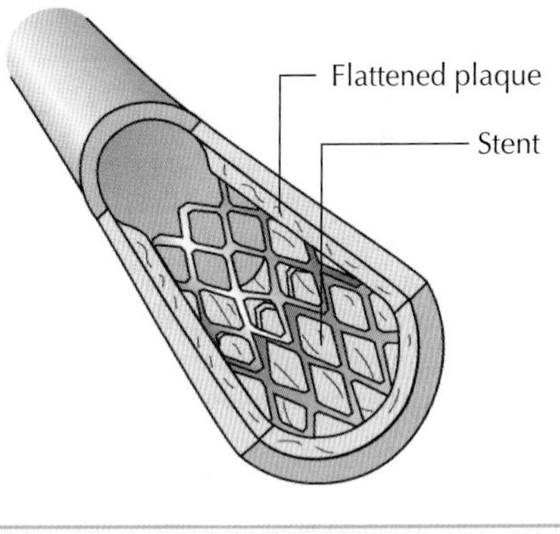

Complications

The most common complication of PTCA is prolonged angina. Others include coronary artery perforation, balloon rupture, reocclusion (necessitating a coronary artery bypass graft), MI, pericardial tamponade, hematoma, hemorrhage, reperfusion arrhythmias, and closure of the vessel. Vascular stents may be inserted to prevent vessel closure. (See *Vascular stents.*)

Documentation

Note the patient's tolerance of the procedure and his condition after it, including vital signs and the condition of the extremity distal to the insertion site. Document any complications and interventions.

SELECTED REFERENCES

Bakhai, A., et al. "Percutaneous Transluminal Coronary Angioplasty with Stents versus Coronary Artery Bypass Grafting for People with Stable Angina or Acute Coronary Syndromes," *Cochrane Database of Systematic Reviews* (1):CD004588, January 2005.

Berger, J.S., et al. "Comparison of Outcomes in Acute Myocardial Infarction Treated with Coronary Angioplasty Alone Versus Coronary Stent Implantation," *American Journal of Cardiology* 97(7):977-80, April 2006.

Chlan, L.L., et al. "Effects of Three Groin Compression Methods on Patient Discomfort, Distress, and Vascular Complications Following a Percutaneous Coronary Intervention Procedure," *Nursing Research* 54(6):391-98, November-December 2005.

Oliver, B., et al. "How Drug-eluting Stents Keep Coronary Blood Flowing," *Nursing* 35(2):36-41, February 2005.

Vlasic, W. "Nursing Care of the Client Requiring Percutaneous Coronary Intervention," *Nursing Clinics of North America* 39(4):829-44, December 2004.

BALLOON VALVULOPLASTY

Although the treatment of choice for valvular heart disease is surgery, balloon valvuloplasty is an alternative to valve replacement in patients with critical stenoses. This technique enlarges the orifice of a heart valve that has been narrowed by a congenital defect, calcification, rheumatic fever, or aging. It evolved from percutaneous transluminal coronary angioplasty and uses the same balloon-tipped catheters for dilatation.

Balloon valvuloplasty was first performed successfully on pediatric patients, then on elderly patients who had stenotic valves complicated by other medical problems such as chronic obstructive pulmonary disease. It's indicated for patients who face a high risk from surgery and for those who refuse surgery.

ELDER ALERT *Balloon valvuloplasty has proved to be more tolerable than surgery for elderly patients, especially those older than age 80.*

This procedure is performed in the cardiac catheterization laboratory under local anesthesia. The physician inserts a balloon-tipped catheter through the patient's femoral vein or artery, threads it into the heart, and repeatedly inflates it against the leaflets of the diseased valve. This increases the size of the orifice, improving valvular function and helping prevent complications from decreased cardiac output. (See *How balloon valvuloplasty works.*)

Your role includes teaching the patient and his family about valvuloplasty and monitoring the patient for potential complications.

Equipment

Antiseptic solution ▪ local anesthetic ▪ valvuloplasty or balloon-tipped catheter ▪ I.V. solution and tubing ▪ electrocardiogram (ECG) monitor and electrodes ▪ pulmonary artery (PA) catheter ▪ contrast medium ▪ oxygen ▪ sterile labels ▪ sterile marker ▪ nasal cannula ▪ sedative ▪ emergency medications ▪ clippers ▪ heparin for injection ▪ introducer kit for balloon catheter ▪ sterile gown, gloves, mask, cap, and drapes ▪ Doppler stethoscope ▪ optional: nitroglycerin.

Implementation

- Confirm the patient's identity using two patient identifiers according to your facility's policy.
- Reinforce the physician's explanation of balloon valvuloplasty, including its risks and alternatives, to the patient and his family.
- Reassure the patient that although he'll be awake during the procedure, he'll receive a sedative and local anesthetic beforehand.
- Teach the patient what to expect. For example, inform him that his groin area will be clipped and cleaned with an antiseptic; he'll feel a brief, stinging sensation when the local anesthetic is injected; and he may feel pressure as the catheter moves along the vessel. Describe the warm, flushed feeling he's likely to experience from injection of the contrast medium.
- Tell him that the procedure may last up to 4 hours and that he may feel discomfort from lying on a hard table for that long.

Before balloon valvuloplasty

- Make sure the patient has no allergies to shellfish, iodine, or contrast media and that he or a family member has signed a consent form.
- Keep the patient off food and fluids (except for medications) for at least 6 hours before balloon valvuloplasty or as ordered (usually after midnight the night before the procedure).
- Ensure that the results of routine laboratory studies and blood typing and crossmatching are available.
- Insert an I.V. line to provide access for medications.
- Take baseline peripheral pulses in all extremities.
- Clip the hair from the insertion sites; then clean the sites with antiseptic solution.
- Give the patient a sedative, as ordered.

How balloon valvuloplasty works

In balloon valvuloplasty, the physician inserts a balloon-tipped catheter through the femoral vein or artery and threads it into the heart. After locating the stenotic valve, he inflates the balloon, increasing the size of the valve opening.

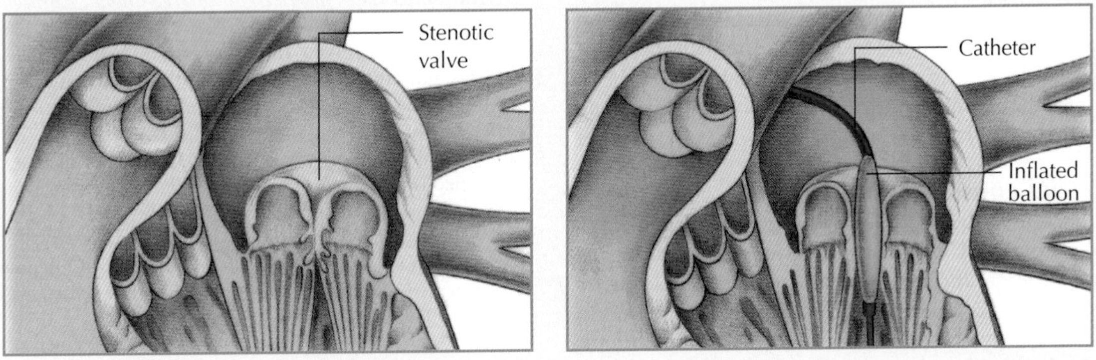

- Have the patient void.
- When the patient arrives at the cardiac catheterization laboratory, apply ECG electrodes and ensure I.V. line patency.

During balloon valvuloplasty

- Administer oxygen by nasal cannula.
- The physician will put on a sterile gown, gloves, mask, and cap and open the sterile supplies. A member of the team labels all medications, medication containers, and other solutions on and off the sterile field.
- The physician prepares and anesthetizes the catheter insertion site (usually at the femoral artery). He may insert a PA catheter if one isn't in place.
- He then inserts a large guide catheter into the site and threads a valvuloplasty or balloon-tipped catheter up into the heart.
- The physician injects a contrast medium *to visualize the heart valves and assess the stenosis.* He also injects heparin *to prevent the catheter from clotting.*
- Using low pressure, he inflates the balloon on the valvuloplasty catheter for a short time, usually 12 to 30 seconds, gradually increasing the time and pressure. If the stenosis isn't reduced, a larger balloon may be used.
- After completion of valvuloplasty, a series of angiograms is taken *to evaluate the effectiveness of the treatment.*
- The physician then sutures the guide catheter in place. He'll remove it after the effects of the heparin have worn off.

After balloon valvuloplasty

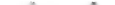

- When the patient returns to the unit, he may be receiving I.V. heparin or nitroglycerin. He may also have a sandbag over the insertion site *to prevent formation of a hematoma.*
- Monitor ECG rhythm and arterial pressures.
- Monitor the insertion site frequently for signs of hemorrhage *because exsanguination can occur rapidly.*
- *To prevent excessive hip flexion and migration of the catheter,* keep the affected leg straight and elevate the head of the bed no more than 15 degrees. If necessary, place a sheet over the affected extremity and under the unaffected extremity, then tucked on both sides *to serve as a reminder to keep the leg straight.*
- Monitor vital signs every 15 minutes for the first hour, every 30 minutes for the next 2 hours, and then hourly for the next 5 hours. If vital signs are unstable, notify the physician and continue to check them every 5 minutes.
- When you take vital signs, assess peripheral pulses distal to the catheter insertion site as well as the color, sensation, temperature, and capillary refill time of the affected extremity.
- Assess the catheter site for hematoma, ecchymosis, and hemorrhage. If hematoma expands, mark the site and alert the physician.
- Auscultate regularly for murmurs, which may indicate worsening valvular insufficiency. Notify the physician if you detect a new or worsening murmur.
- *To help the kidneys excrete the contrast medium,* provide I.V. fluids at a rate of at least 100 ml/hour. Assess the patient for signs of fluid overload: distended neck veins, atrial and ven-

tricular gallops, dyspnea, pulmonary congestion, tachycardia, hypertension, and hypoxemia. Monitor intake and output closely.

- Encourage the patient to perform deep-breathing exercises *to prevent atelectasis.* This is especially important in elderly patients.
- After the guide catheter is removed (usually 6 to 12 hours after valvuloplasty), apply direct pressure for at least 10 minutes and monitor the site frequently. Alternatively, a compression device may be used, as appropriate.
- Note the patient's tolerance of the procedure and his condition afterward.

Special considerations

- Assess the patient's vital signs constantly during the procedure, especially if it's an aortic valvuloplasty. During balloon inflation, the aortic outflow tract is completely obstructed, causing blood pressure to fall dangerously low. Ventricular ectopy is also common during balloon positioning and inflation. Start treatment for ectopy when symptoms develop or when ventricular tachycardia is sustained. Carefully assess the patient's respiratory status; *changes in rate and pattern can be the first sign of a complication such as an embolism.*
- Assess pedal pulses with a Doppler stethoscope. They'll be difficult to detect, especially if the catheter sheath remains in place. Also assess for complications: embolism, hemorrhage, chest pain, and cardiac tamponade. Using heparin and a large-bore catheter can lead to arterial hemorrhage. This complication can be reversed with protamine sulfate when the sheath is removed, or the sheath can be left in place and removed 6 to 8 hours after the heparin is discontinued.
- Chest pain can result from obstruction of blood flow during aortic valvuloplasty, so assess for symptoms of myocardial ischemia. Also be alert for signs or symptoms of cardiac tamponade (decreased or absent peripheral pulses, pale or cyanotic skin, hypotension, and paradoxical pulse), which requires emergency surgery.

Complications

Severe complications, such as myocardial infarction or calcium emboli (embolization of debris released from the calcified valve), are rare. Other complications include bleeding or hematoma at the insertion site, arrhythmias, circulatory disorders distal to the insertion site, guide wire perforation of the ventricle leading to tamponade, disruption of the valve ring, restenosis of the valve, and valvular insufficiency, which can contribute to heart failure and reduced cardiac output. Infection and an allergic reaction to the contrast medium can also occur.

Documentation

Document any complications and interventions.

SELECTED REFERENCES

Fawzy, M.E., et al. "Long-term Results of Mitral Balloon Valvuloplasty in a Series of 518 Patients and Predictors of Long-term Outcome," *Journal of Interventional Cardiology* 20(10):66-72, February 2007.

Krittayaphong, R., et al. "Improvement in Quality of Life after Percutaneous Balloon Mitral Valvulotomy in Patients with Mitral Stenosis: Does Rhythm Matter?" *Journal of Heart Valve Disease* 16(1):13-18, January 2007.

Liu, T., et al. "Prevention of Ischemic Cerebral Stroke by Percutaneous Balloon Valvuloplasty in Patients with Symptomatic Rheumatic Mitral Stenosis," *Stroke* 37(2):714, February 2006.

Ramondo, A., et al. "Relation of Patient Age to Outcome of Percutaneous Mitral Valvuloplasty," *American Journal of Cardiology* 98(11):1493-500, December 2006.

ARTERIAL AND VENOUS SHEATH REMOVAL

Endovascular procedures performed by cardiologists and vascular surgeons have dramatically increased in the past decade. Following these procedures, arterial sheaths, venous sheaths, or both may be left in place. Upon sheath removal, patient comfort may be improved and the amount of bed rest required may be shortened, thus leading to positive patient outcomes. However, sheath removal isn't without risk, and nurses must be appropriately trained.

There are many methods available to control bleeding following sheath removal, including manual compression (used alone or with a hemostasis pad), mechanical compression devices, collagen plug devices, and percutaneous suture-mediated closure devices. Manual compression can cause fatigue and injury, which can result in carpal tunnel problems for nurses. Mechanical compression techniques are effective for preventing hematoma formation; however, the prevalence of bleeding does not differ significantly for different methods of compression. If a plug-type or suture-mediated closure device is used, sheaths can be immediately removed at the end of a case, regardless of the coagulation status of the patient.

Equipment

Nonsterile gloves ▪ gown, goggles, or face shield with mask ▪ cardiac monitor ▪ indelible marker ▪ antiseptic solution ▪ sterile gauze ▪ sterile gloves ▪ suture removal kit (if the sheath is sutured in place) ▪ hypoallergenic tape ▪ linen-saver pad ▪ sterile saline (if using noninvasive hemostasis pad) ▪ transparent dressing (if using noninvasive hemostasis pad) ■ optional: mechanical hemostasis device, noninvasive hemostasis pad.

Preparation of equipment

Wash your hands and bring the equipment to the patient's bedside. Using sterile technique, open the suture removal kit and gauze packages and place them within reach. If a hemostasis pad is being used, open it using sterile technique and open the normal saline solution.

Implementation

■ Verify the order for sheath removal in the patient's chart *to assure the right procedure is being performed on the right patient at the right time.*
■ Confirm the patient's identity using two patient identifiers according to your facility's policy.

Preparing for sheath removal

■ Explain the procedure to the patient *to reduce anxiety and enhance cooperation.* Include activity restrictions, discomfort caused by pressure to the site, and signs and symptoms to report following the procedure.
■ Before sheath removal, assess for bleeding disorders and check the patient's platelet count, prothrombin time, International Normalized Ratio, partial thromboplastin time, complete blood count, and activated clotting time.
■ Obtain vital signs and check the electrocardiogram *to establish a baseline.* Check that the systolic blood pressure is less than 150 mm Hg *to facilitate hemostasis.*
■ Assess neurovascular status in the extremity distal to the sheath insertion site *to establish a baseline.*
■ Mark the pulses distal to the sheath insertion site using an indelible marker *to facilitate finding the pulses.*
■ Administer an analgesic 20 to 30 minutes before the procedure.
■ Confirm that the patient has patent I.V. access *in case emergency fluids or medications are required.*
■ Position the patient with the head of the bed flat.
■ Place the linen-saver pad underneath the affected extremity.
■ If a mechanical compression device is being used, place it under the patient before sheath removal *to reduce patient movement and the risk of bleeding after the sheath is removed.*
■ Wash your hands and put on goggles, mask, gloves, and gown.
■ Carefully remove the dressing covering the sheath insertion site.
■ Clean the insertion sites with antiseptic solution.
■ Remove nonsterile gloves and wash your hands to reduce the risk of transmission of microorganisms.
■ Put on sterile gloves.
■ Remove sutures, if present.

Sheath removal using manual or mechanical compression

■ Locate the femoral pulse proximal to the insertion site *so that compression (manual or mechanical) can be properly positioned 1 to 2 cm above the insertion site.*
■ Hold the sheath with one hand while applying manual or mechanical pressure over the femoral artery with the other hand *to reduce bleeding.*
■ Remove the sheath slowly while the patient exhales *to prevent Valsalva's maneuver* while continuing to apply pressure manually or with the mechanical device.

Sheath removal using a noninvasive hemostasis pad with manual compression

■ Moisten the pad with sterile saline *to activate the hemostatic system.*
■ Apply pressure ⅜" to ¾" (1 to 2 cm) proximal to the insertion site.
■ Apply a sterile gauze pad over the insertion site; then place the moistened pad over the gauze and apply pressure.
■ Gently remove the sheath as described above.
■ Slowly let up on applying pressure proximal to the insertion site after 3 to 4 minutes while continuing to apply pressure to the insertion site for no less than 10 minutes.
■ Apply another sterile gauze pad over the hemostasis pad and cover the site with a transparent dressing.
■ Leave the hemostasis pad in place for 24 hours.

Venous sheath removal

■ Remove the venous sheath, if present, no less than 10 minutes after removal of the arterial sheath *because pressure at the arterial site needs to be maintained for a longer time.*
■ Apply pressure over the venous and arterial sites for 10 more minutes or until bleeding has stopped.
■ If a hemostasis pad is used, follow the above directions for its use.

Follow-up care

■ Apply a sterile dressing to the arterial and venous insertion sites t*o keep the area clean and reduce the risk of infection.*
■ Assess neurovascular status, vital signs, and the insertion site in the affected limb every 15 minutes for 1 hour, then every 30 minutes for 1 hour, and then every hour for 4 hours, *to ensure adequate circulation and neurologic function.*
■ Tell the patient not to elevate the head of the bed greater than 30 degrees *to reduce the risk of disrupting hemostasis and to relieve back discomfort.*

- Instruct the patient to report any bleeding from the site, if the dressing becomes saturated, or if he has feelings of wetness and warmth on his groin or leg.
- Tell the patient to report coolness, numbness, tingling, or pain in the affected extremity.
- Keep the patient on bed rest for 2 to 6 hours, or per your facility's policy, when applying mechanical or manual pressure after arterial sheath removal *to reduce complications of bed rest and back discomfort.* Clinical studies have shown that this does not increase the risk of vascular complications.
- Keep the patient on bed rest for 1 to 4 hours, or per your facility's policy, when achieving hemostasis through percutaneous suture-mediated closure and hemostasis pads.
- Keep the patient on bed rest for no more than 4 hours, or per your facility's policy, following venous sheath removal.

Special considerations

- If the patient is obese, a second person may be required *to assist in holding back skin and abdominal folds.*
- Pressure may need to be applied for a longer period *to ensure hemostasis in the patient with hypertension.*
- Be sure to read the manufacturer's instructions and your facility's policy and procedure for correct use of mechanical compression devices. *Tissue damage can occur if the device is used incorrectly.*
- The compression time required to control bleeding depends on several factors, including the size of the sheath, whether or not the patient received heparin and antiplatelet drugs, and blood coagulation levels.

Complications

The most common complication following sheath removal is bleeding, which occurs most frequently at the femoral artery access site. Retroperitoneal bleeding may also occur. Vascular complications include hematoma, pseudoaneurysm, arteriovenous fistula formation, embolus, and thrombus. Sensory or motor impairment may occur in the affected limb. Vasovagal complications may also occur.

Documentation

Record the date, time, and name of the person removing the sheath. Include whether an arterial sheath, venous sheath, or both were removed and their locations. Record any patient and family teaching about the removal procedure and activity restrictions following sheath removal. Note the patient's level of discomfort using a 0-to-10 scale as well as the name, dose, route, and time of any analgesics given. Document that laboratory values were checked prior to sheath removal and that they were within normal limits. Record vital signs, neurovascular status, and heart rhythm before sheath removal. State whether pulses distal to the sheath insertion sites were marked. Note that the patient has a patent I.V. Include that the patient was placed in a flat position for sheath removal. Describe the condition of the sheath insertion sites, noting any redness, skin breakdown, drainage, bleeding, or hematoma formation. Note how many sutures were removed. Explain any difficulties encountered during sheath removal. Record the type of pressure or hemostasis used and how long until hemostasis was achieved. Document the frequent neurovascular, vital signs, and sheath removal site checks. Note the patient's tolerance of the procedure. Record any complications, the time and name of the person notified, orders given, nursing actions taken, and the patient's response. Include the patient's position following sheath removal and how long bed rest was maintained.

Selected references

Benson, L.M., et al. "Determining Best Practice: Comparison of Three Methods of Femoral Sheath Removal after Cardiac Interventional Procedures," *Heart Lung* 34(2):115-21, March-April 2005.

Chlan, L.L., et al. "Effects of Three Groin Compression Methods on Patient Discomfort, Distress, and Vascular Complications Following a Percutaneous Coronary Intervention Procedure," *Nursing Research* 54(6):391-98, November-December 2005.

Galli, A., and Palatnik, A. "What Is the Proper Activated Clotting Time (ACT) at Which to Remove a Femoral Sheath after PCI? What Are the Best "Protocols" for Sheath Removal?" *Critical Care Nurse* 25(2):88-95, April 2005.

Jones, T., and McCutcheon, H. "A Randomised Controlled Trial Comparing the Use of Manual Versus Mechanical Compression to Obtain Haemostasis Following Coronary Angiography," *Intensive & Critical Care Nursing* 19(1):11-20, February 2003.

Jones, T., and McCutcheon, H. "Effectiveness of Mechanical Compression Devices in Attaining Hemostasis after Femoral Sheath Removal," *American Journal of Critical Care* 11(2):155-62, March 2002.

Lynn-McHale Wiegand, D.J., and Carlson, K.K., eds. *AACN Procedure Manual for Critical Care,* 5th ed. Philadelphia: W.B. Saunders Co., 2005.

Mlekusch, W., et al. "Arterial Puncture Site Management after Percutaneous Transluminal Procedures Using a Hemostatic Wound Dressing (Clo-Sur P.A.D.) versus Conventional Manual Compression: A Randomized Controlled Trial," *Journal of Endovascular Therapy* 13(1):23-31, February 2006.

Niederstadt, J.A. "Frequency and Timing of Activated Clotting Time Levels for Sheath Removal," *Journal of Nursing Care Quality* 19(1):34-38, January-March 2004.

Tagney, J., and Lackie, D. "Bed-rest Post-femoral Arterial Sheath Removal — What Is Safe Practice? A Clinical Audit," *Nursing in Critical Care* 10(4):167-73, July-August 2005.

FEMORAL COMPRESSION

Femoral compression is used to maintain hemostasis at the puncture site following a procedure involving an arterial access site (such as cardiac catheterization or angiography). A femoral compression device is used to apply direct pressure to the arterial access site. A nylon strap is placed under the patient's buttocks and attached to the device with an inflatable plastic dome. After the dome is positioned correctly over the puncture site, it's inflated to the recommended pressure, according to the manufacturer. A physician or a specially trained nurse may apply the device.

Equipment

Femoral compression device strap ■ compression arch with dome and three-way stopcock ■ pressure inflation device ■ sterile transparent dressing ■ gloves (nonsterile and sterile) ■ protective eyewear.

Implementation

■ Confirm the patient's identity using two patient identifiers according to your facility's policy.
■ Obtain a physician's order for the femoral compression device, including the amount of pressure to be applied and the length of time the device should remain in place.
■ Explain the reason for using the device and the possible complications of the procedure. Answer any questions the patient may have.
■ Position the patient on the stretcher or bed; don't flex the involved extremity.
■ Assess the condition of the puncture site, obtain vital signs, perform neurovascular checks, and assess pain, according to your facility's policy for arterial access procedures.

Applying the femoral compression device

■ Put on nonsterile gloves and protective eyewear, and place the device strap under the patient's hips before sheath removal (in cases that warrant the use of a sheath).
■ With the assistance of another nurse, position the compression arch over the puncture site. Apply manual pressure over the dome area while the straps are secured to the arch.
■ When the dome is properly positioned over the puncture site, connect the pressure inflation device to the stopcock that's attached to the device. Turn the stopcock to the open position, and inflate the dome with the pressure inflation device to the ordered pressure. Typically, a venous sheath is removed at 20 to 40 mm Hg and an arterial sheath is removed at 60 to 80 mm Hg. Immediately after removal of the arterial sheath, inflate the device to 10 to 20 mm Hg over the systolic blood pressure. After 2 to 3 minutes, a reduction in pressure, usually a value between the patient's systolic and diastolic blood pressure, is ordered. Follow specific orders for pressure changes.
■ Assess the puncture site for proper placement of the device and for signs of bleeding or hematoma. Assess distal pulses and perform neurovascular assessments according to your facility's policy. Confirm distal pulses after any adjustments of the device.

Maintaining the device

■ When the patient is transferred to the nursing unit, assess the distal pulses, the puncture site, and placement of the device and confirm the ordered amount of pressure.
■ Check device placement, assess vital signs and the puncture site, and perform neurovascular checks every 2 hours or according to your facility's policy.
■ Deflate the device hourly and assess the puncture site for bleeding or hematoma. Assess for proper placement of the dome over the puncture site. Put on gloves and protective eyewear and reposition the compression arch and dome as necessary. Reinflate the device to the ordered pressure using the pressure inflation device.

Removing the device

■ Explain the removal procedure to the patient.
■ Put on nonsterile gloves and protective eyewear, and remove the air from the dome. Leave the dome in place at 0 mm Hg for at least 10 minutes, then loosen the straps and remove the device. Assess the puncture site for bleeding or hematoma. Apply a sterile transparent dressing according to your facility's policy.
■ Check the puncture site and distal pulses, and perform neurovascular assessments every 15 minutes for the first half hour and every 30 minutes for the next 2 hours. Your facility may require more frequent monitoring. Observe for signs of bleeding, hematoma, or infection.
■ Dispose of the device according to your facility's policy.

Special considerations

■ Advise the patient to use caution when moving in bed *to avoid malpositioning the device.* Instruct the patient not to bend the involved extremity.
■ If you note external bleeding or signs of internal bleeding, remove the device, apply manual pressure, and notify the physician.
■ Change the dressing at the puncture site every 24 to 48 hours or according to your facility's policy. (The sterile transparent dressing permits inspection of the site for bleeding, drainage, or hematoma.)

Complications

The Food and Drug Administration has issued a warning to physicians about adverse events that may occur with the use of femoral compression devices following arterial access for diagnostic and therapeutic procedures. Complications include bleeding, hematoma, retroperitoneal bleeding, and pseudoaneurysm. Other potential complications may include infection and deep vein thrombosis. Tissue damage may occur if prolonged pressure is maintained.

Documentation

Document initial application of the device, sheath removal, and the patient's tolerance of the procedure. Document vital signs, puncture site checks, distal pulses, neurovascular assessments, hourly deflation, repositioning of the device, length of time the device was in place, and removal of the device. Document patient and family teaching, complications, and interventions.

SELECTED REFERENCES

Chlan, L.L., et al. "Effects of Three Groin Compression Methods on Patient Discomfort, Distress, and Vascular Complications Following a Percutaneous Coronary Intervention Procedure," *Nursing Research* 54(6):391-98, November-December 2005.

Benson, L.M., et al. "Determining Best Practice: Comparison of Three Methods of Femoral Sheath Removal after Cardiac Interventional Procedures," *Heart Lung* 34(2):115-21, March-April 2005.

Katz, S.G., and Abando, A. "The Use of Closure Devices," *Surgical Clinics of North America* 84(5):1267-280, October 2004.

U.S. Food and Drug Administration. "Complications Related to the Use of Vascular Hemostasis Devices," October 8, 1999. Available at *www.fda.gov/cdrh/safety/vashemo.html.*

PNEUMATIC ANTISHOCK GARMENT APPLICATION AND REMOVAL

A pneumatic antishock garment (PASG; also known as *medical antishock trousers* or a *MAST suit*) consists of inflatable bladders sandwiched between double layers of fabric. When inflated, a PASG places external pressure on the lower extremities and abdomen, creating an autotransfusion effect that squeezes blood superiorly and increases blood volume to the heart, lungs, and brain by up to 30%.

A PASG is used to treat shock when systolic blood pressure falls below 80 mm Hg—or below 100 mm Hg when accompanied by signs of shock. It can control abdominal and lower extremity hemorrhage as well as help stabilize and splint pelvic and femoral fractures.

Use of a PASG is contraindicated in patients with cardiogenic shock, heart failure, pulmonary edema, tension pneumothorax, or increased intracranial pressure. The device should be used cautiously during pregnancy. A PASG must be deflated slowly, with continuous blood pressure monitoring, to prevent potentially irreversible shock from hypovolemia. It shouldn't be removed until the patient's blood volume is restored, his condition is stabilized, or he's being prepared for surgery. If necessary, the PASG can be deflated in stages in the operating room.

Equipment

PASG ▪ foot pump ▪ optional: resuscitation equipment. PASGs come in a pediatric size for patients 3½′ to 5′ (1 to 1.5 m) tall and an adult size for patients taller than 5′.

Preparation of equipment

Spread open the PASG on a smooth surface or blanket *to avoid puncturing it.* Make sure all the stopcock valves are open. Attach the foot pump.

Implementation

- Explain the procedure to the patient *to allay his fears and ensure his cooperation.*

Applying a PASG

- Take vital signs to establish baseline measurements. Assess the patient's physical condition to ensure that there are no contraindications to the use of the PASG.
- Assess the patient's injuries *to see whether he can be turned from side to side.* If he can't be turned, slide the PASG under him. If he can be turned, place the PASG next to him and logroll him onto it. You can also set up the PASG on a stretcher and place the patient on it in a supine position. (See *Applying a pneumatic antishock garment.*)
- Examine the patient for sharp objects that could injure him or the garment such as pieces of glass.
- Double-check the stopcocks to ensure they're all open *so the PASG will inflate uniformly.*
- Inflate the legs of the garment first, then the abdominal segment, to about 20 to 30 mm Hg initially.
- Monitor the patient's blood pressure and pulse rate. Continue to inflate the garment slowly while monitoring vital signs. Stop inflating when the patient's systolic blood pressure reaches the desired level, usually 100 mm Hg.
- Close all stopcocks to prevent accidental air loss.
- Monitor the patient's blood pressure, pulse rate, and respirations every 5 minutes *to determine his response to application of the PASG.* Check his pedal pulses and temperature periodically. Notify the practitioner if the circulation in the feet seems impaired.

Removing a PASG

- Before deflation, make sure I.V. lines are patent, a practitioner is in attendance, and emergency resuscitation equip-

Applying a pneumatic antishock garment

After taking the patient's baseline vital signs and explaining the treatment, prepare to apply the antishock garment. On a smooth surface, open the garment with Velcro fasteners down.

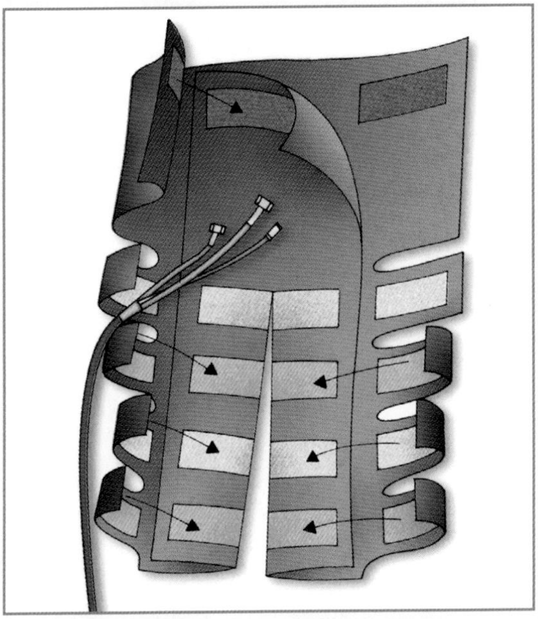

Open all stopcock valves; then attach the foot pump tubing to the valve on the pressure control unit. Can the patient be turned from side to side? If not, slide the garment under him. If he can be turned, place the garment next to him and, with assistance, move him onto it.

Before closing the garment, remove sharp objects, such as pieces of glass, stones, keys, or a buckle, that could injure the patient or tear the garment. As appropriate, pad pressure points and apply lanolin *to protect the patient's skin from irritation.*

Place the upper edge of the garment just below the patient's lowest rib. Wrap the right leg compartment around the patient's right leg. Secure the compartment by fastening all the Velcro straps from ankle to thigh.

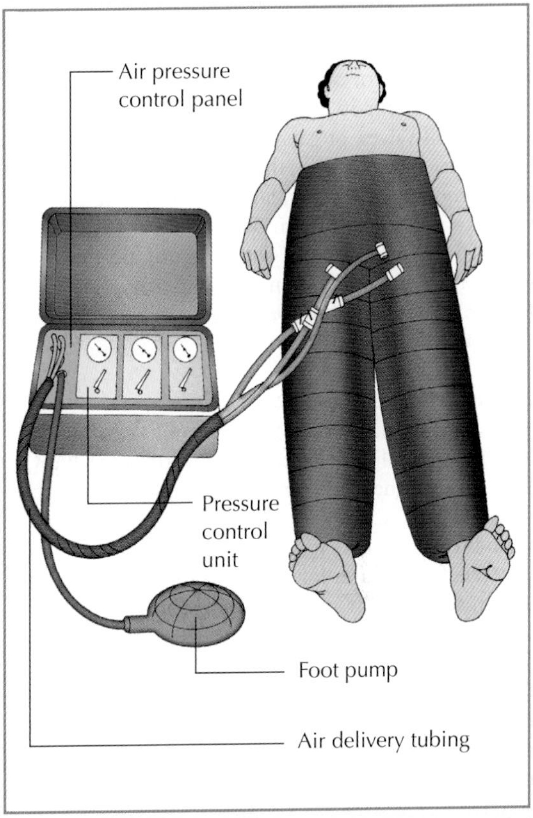

Repeat this procedure for the left leg; then wrap the abdomen. Double-check that all valves are properly positioned.

ment is immediately available. *Removing a PASG may cause the patient's blood pressure to drop rapidly.*

- Open the abdominal stopcock and start releasing small amounts of air. Closely monitor the patient's systolic blood pressure as you do this. If it drops 5 mm Hg, close the stopcock.

NURSING ALERT *Deflating the garment too quickly can allow circulating blood to rush to the abdomen or extremities, causing potentially irreversible shock.*

- If a drop in blood pressure requires you to stop deflating the PASG, increase the flow rate of I.V. solutions *to help stabilize blood pressure.*

- If blood pressure is stable, continue to deflate the PASG slowly. After deflating the abdominal section, deflate the legs simultaneously.
- When the PASG is loose enough, gently pull it off.
- Clean the PASG as required, but don't autoclave it or use solvents.

Special considerations

- In most cases, you should see a therapeutic response to treatment when the PASG is inflated to 25 mm Hg. A so-called *morbidity effect,* caused by a change in local circulation, occurs at about 50 mm Hg. Most PASGs have Velcro straps, pop-off valves, or gauges that prevent inflation beyond 104 mm Hg. Normally, the PASG shouldn't be left inflated for more than 2 hours, although it may be used for several days. A range of 25 to 50 mm Hg can usually be maintained for up to 48 hours. For prolonged use, the PASG may be inflated at a lower-than-normal pressure.
- *Because a PASG is radiolucent,* X-rays can be taken while the patient is wearing it.

Complications

Vomiting can result from compression of the abdomen. Anaerobic metabolism, which can result from the PASG's pressure being higher than the patient's systolic pressure, can lead to metabolic acidosis.

Skin breakdown may follow prolonged use. When used with severe leg fractures for long periods, tissue sloughing and necrosis caused by increased compartmental pressures have necessitated amputation.

Documentation

Record the time of application and removal and the patient's vital signs before application, during treatment, and after removal.

SELECTED REFERENCES

Hausewald, M., and Greene, E.R. "Regional Blood Flow after Pneumatic Anti-shock Garment Inflation," *Prehospital Emergency Care* 7(2):225-28, April-June 2003.

Lynn-McHale Wiegand, D.J., and Carlson, K.K., eds. *AACN Procedure Manual for Critical Care,* 5th ed. Philadelphia: W.B. Saunders Co., 2005.

Salomone, J.P., et al. "Opinions of Trauma Practitioners Regarding Prehospital Interventions for Critically Injured Patients," *Journal of Trauma* 58(3):509-15, March 2005.

8 ■ Respiratory care

INTRODUCTION

No matter where you work, you're sure to encounter patients with respiratory conditions. Such conditions may be acute or chronic and may have developed as a primary disorder or resulted from a cardiac or other disorder.

Caring for the patient with a respiratory condition will challenge your nursing skills. Not only is the patient's oxygenation compromised, but he may develop other problems as well. For instance, the patient may experience ineffective airway clearance and gas exchange, altered cardiac output, altered fluid volume, impaired thermoregulation, and decreased mobility. He may be anxious, cope ineffectively, and have an impaired ability to communicate. In addition, his nutritional status may be compromised. For such a patient, you'll need to develop an individual care plan to ensure that he achieves optimum gas exchange and physical function.

To meet your care goals, you need to have a working knowledge of the many therapies available to respiratory patients. Although many health care facilities have staff members who specialize in respiratory procedures, you still need to keep your knowledge up-to-date. That way, you'll understand the rationales behind the patient's treatment and be able to perform or assist with procedures if necessary, recognize complications, and detect the need for additional therapy. You'll also work with other members of the health care team to teach the patient and his family about equipment and procedures necessary for his care.

MONITORING

MIXED VENOUS OXYGEN SATURATION MONITORING

Mixed venous oxygen saturation monitoring uses a fiber-optic thermodilution pulmonary artery (PA) catheter to continuously monitor oxygen delivery to tissues and oxygen consumption by tissues. Monitoring of mixed venous oxygen saturation ($S\bar{v}O_2$) allows rapid detection of impaired oxygen delivery, as from decreased cardiac output, hemoglobin level, or arterial oxygen saturation. It also helps evaluate a patient's response to drug therapy, endotracheal tube suctioning, ventilator setting changes, positive end-expiratory pressure, and fraction of inspired oxygen. $S\bar{v}O_2$ usually ranges from 60% to 80%; the normal value is 75%.

Equipment

Fiber-optic PA catheter ■ co-oximeter ■ optical module and cable ■ gloves.

Preparation of equipment

Review the manufacturer's instructions for assembly and use of the fiber-optic PA catheter. Connect the optical module and cable to the monitor. Next, peel back the wrapping covering the catheter just enough to uncover the fiber-optic connector. Attach the fiber-optic connector to the optical module while allowing the rest of the catheter to remain in its sterile wrapping. Calibrate the fiber-optic catheter by following the manufacturer's instructions.

To prepare for the rest of the procedure, follow the instructions for pulmonary catheter insertion, as described in "PAP and PAWP monitoring," page 443. (See *$S\bar{v}O_2$ monitoring equipment.*)

Implementation

- Confirm the patient's identity using two patient identifiers according to your facility's policy.
- Wash your hands and put on gloves.
- Explain the procedure to the patient *to allay his fears and promote cooperation.*
- Assist with the insertion of the fiber-optic catheter just as you would for a PA catheter.
- After the catheter is inserted, confirm that the light intensity tracing on the graphic printout is within normal range *to ensure correct positioning and function of the catheter.*
- Observe the digital readout and record the $S\bar{v}O_2$ on graph paper. Repeat readings at least once each hour *to monitor and document trends.*
- Set the machine alarms 10% above and 10% below the patient's current $S\bar{v}O_2$ reading.

Recalibrating the monitor

- Draw a mixed venous blood sample from the distal port of the PA catheter. Send it to the laboratory for analysis *to compare the laboratory's $S\bar{v}O_2$ reading with that of the fiber-optic catheter.*
- If the catheter values and the laboratory values differ by more than 4%, follow the manufacturer's instructions to enter the $S\bar{v}O_2$ value obtained by the laboratory into the oximeter.
- Recalibrate the monitor every 24 hours or whenever the catheter has been disconnected from the optical module.

Special considerations

- If the patient's $S\bar{v}O_2$ drops below 60% or varies by more than 10% for 3 minutes or longer, reassess the patient. If the $S\bar{v}O_2$ doesn't return to the baseline value after nursing interventions, notify the practitioner. *A decreasing $S\bar{v}O_2$ or a value less than 60% indicates impaired oxygen delivery, as occurs in hemorrhage, hypoxia, shock, arrhythmias, or suctioning.* $S\bar{v}O_2$ may also decrease as a result of increased oxy-

EQUIPMENT

$S\bar{v}O_2$ monitoring equipment

The mixed venous oxygen saturation ($S\bar{v}O_2$) monitoring system consists of a flow-directed pulmonary artery (PA) catheter with fiber-optic filaments, an optical module, and a co-oximeter. The co-oximeter displays a continuous digital $S\bar{v}O_2$ value; the strip recorder prints a permanent record.

Catheter insertion follows the same technique as with any thermodilution flow-directed PA catheter. The distal lumen connects to an external PA pressure monitoring system; the proximal or central venous pressure lumen connects to another monitoring system or to a continuous-flow administration unit; and the optical module connects to the co-oximeter unit. As an alternative, many facilities have cardiac monitors that also monitor $S\bar{v}O_2$.

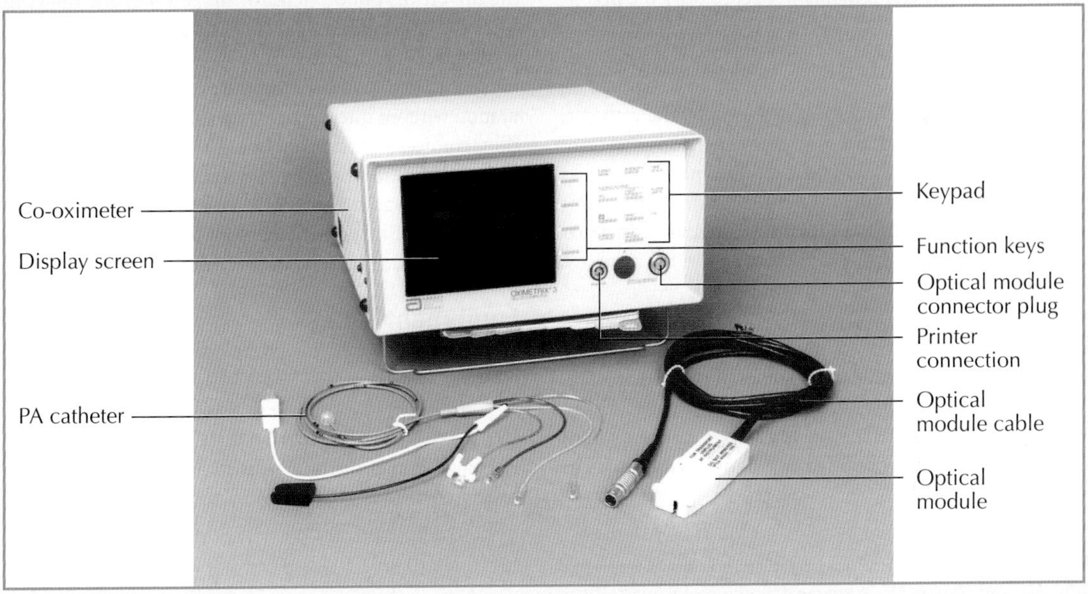

Normal $S\bar{v}O_2$ waveform

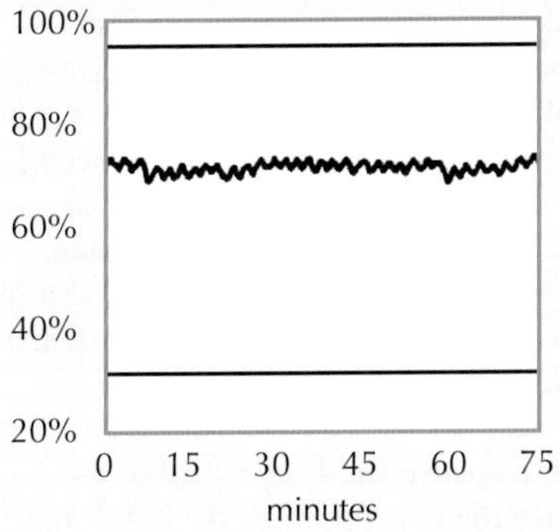

$S\bar{v}O_2$ with patient activities

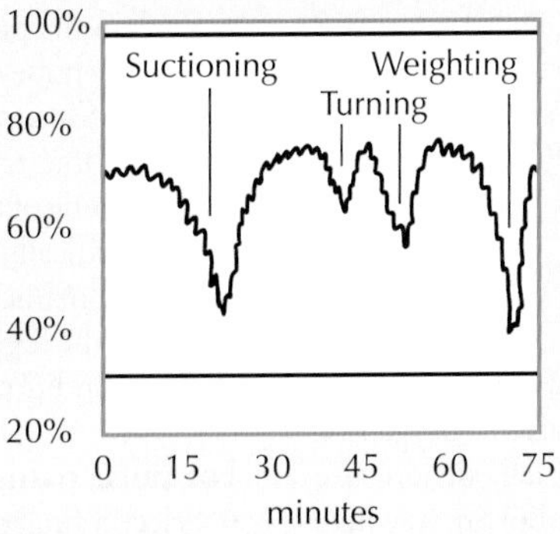

$S\bar{v}O_2$ with PEEP and FIO_2 changes

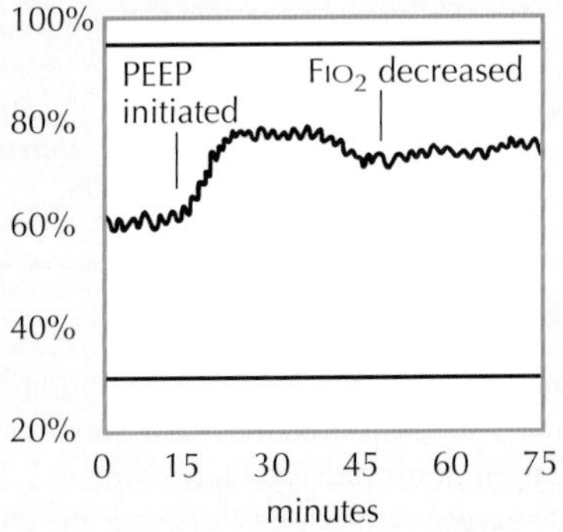

gen demand from hyperthermia, shivering, or seizures, for example.

- If the intensity of the tracing is low, make sure that all connections between the catheter and oximeter are secure and that the catheter is patent and not kinked.
- If the tracing is damped or erratic, try to aspirate blood from the catheter *to check for patency* (if allowed by your facility). If you can't aspirate blood, notify the practitioner *so that the catheter can be replaced.* Check the PA waveform *to determine whether the catheter has wedged.* If the catheter has wedged, turn the patient from side to side and instruct him to cough. If the catheter remains wedged, notify the practitioner immediately.

Complications

Thrombosis can result from local irritation by the catheter; however, a heparin flush helps prevent this complication. Thromboembolism can also occur if a thrombus breaks off and lodges in the circulatory system. Monitor the patient for signs and symptoms of infection, such as redness or drainage, at the catheter site.

Documentation

Record the $S\bar{v}O_2$ value on a flowchart, and attach a tracing as ordered. Note any significant changes in the patient's status and the results of any interventions. For comparison, note the $S\bar{v}O_2$ as measured by the fiber-optic catheter whenever a blood sample is obtained for laboratory analysis of $S\bar{v}O_2$.

SELECTED REFERENCES

Caille, V., and Squara, P. "Oxygen Uptake-to-Delivery Relationship: A Way to Assess Adequate Flow," *Critical Care* 10(Suppl 3):S4, 2006.

Lynn-McHale Wiegand, D.J., and Carlson, K.K., eds. *AACN Procedure Manual for Critical Care*, 5th ed. Philadelphia: W.B. Saunders Co., 2006.

Squara, P. "Matching Total Body Oxygen Consumption and Delivery: A Critical Objective?" *Intensive Care Medicine* 30(12):2170-179, December 2004.

PULSE OXIMETRY

Performed intermittently or continuously, oximetry is a relatively simple procedure used to monitor arterial oxygen saturation noninvasively. Pulse oximeters usually denote arterial oxygen saturation values with the symbol SpO_2, whereas invasively measured arterial oxygen saturation values are denoted by the symbol SaO_2.

The American Association for Respiratory Care has developed clinical guidelines for performing pulse oximetry. Indications for pulse oximetry include:

- monitoring the adequacy of arterial oxyhemoglobin saturation
- measuring and recording the response of arterial oxyhemoglobin saturation to therapeutic intervention or to a diagnostic procedure such as bronchoscopy
- complying with facility policy or unit protocol.

In this procedure, two diodes send red and infrared light through a pulsating arterial vascular bed such as the one in the fingertip. A photodetector slipped over the finger measures the transmitted light as it passes through the vascular bed, detects the relative amount of color absorbed by arterial blood, and calculates the exact mixed venous oxygen saturation without interference from surrounding venous blood, skin, connective tissue, or bone. Using the ear probe, oximetry works by monitoring the transmission of light waves through the vascular bed of a patient's earlobe. Results will be inaccurate if the patient's earlobe is poorly perfused, as from a low cardiac output. (See *How oximetry works.*)

Equipment

Oximeter ▪ finger or ear probe ▪ alcohol pads ▪ nail polish remover, if necessary.

Preparation of equipment

Review the manufacturer's instructions for assembly of the oximeter. Choose the appropriate place for the site you're using. Choose the appropriate probe for the site you're using.

Implementation

- Confirm the patient's identity using two patient identifiers according to your facility's policy.
- Explain the procedure to the patient.
- Validate pulse oximetry readings by comparing SpO_2 readings with SaO_2 values obtained by arterial blood gas (ABG) analysis. Obtain these two measurements simultaneously at the beginning of pulse oximetry monitoring, and then reevaluate periodically according to the patient's condition.
- If pulse oximetry readings are being monitored continuously, set the high and low alarms according to the patient's clinical condition.

For pulse oximetry using the finger probe

- Select a finger for the test. Although the index finger is commonly used, a smaller finger may be selected if the patient's fingers are too large for the equipment. Make sure the patient isn't wearing false fingernails, and remove any nail polish from the test finger. Place the transducer (photode-

EQUIPMENT

How oximetry works

The pulse oximeter allows noninvasive monitoring of the percentage of hemoglobin saturated by oxygen, or Spo_2, levels by measuring the absorption (amplitude) of light waves as they pass through areas of the body that are highly perfused by arterial blood. Oximetry also monitors pulse rate and amplitude.

Light-emitting diodes in a transducer (photodetector) attached to the patient's body (shown at right on the index finger) send red and infrared light beams through tissue. The photodetector records the relative amount of each color absorbed by arterial blood and transmits the data to a monitor, which displays the information with each heartbeat. If the Sao_2 level or pulse rate varies from preset limits, the monitor triggers visual and audible alarms.

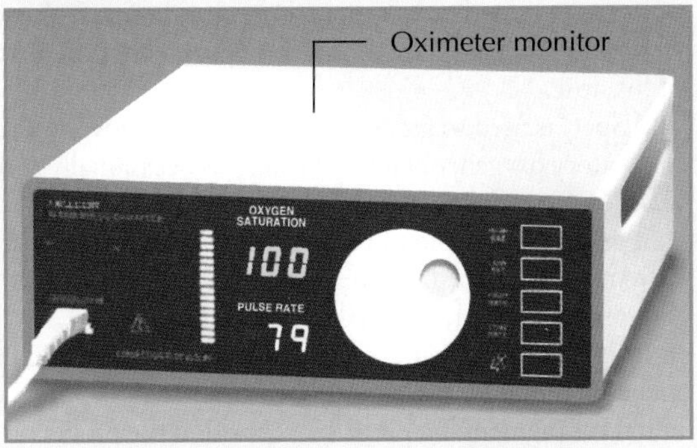

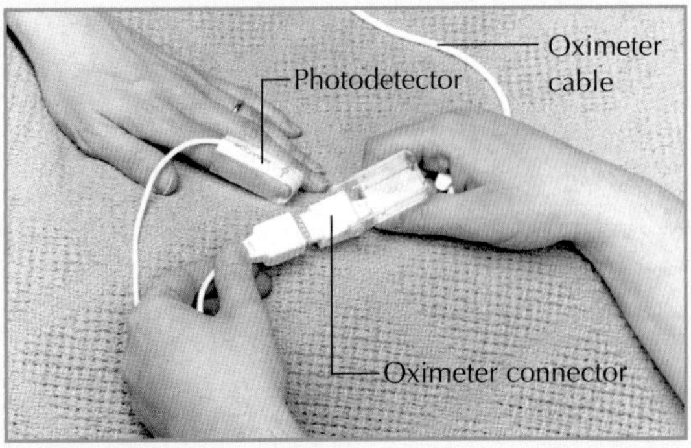

tector) probe over the patient's finger so that light beams and sensors oppose each other. If the patient has long fingernails, position the probe perpendicular to the finger, if possible, or clip the fingernail. Always position the patient's hand at heart level *to eliminate venous pulsations and to promote accurate readings.*

PEDIATRIC ALERT *If you're testing a neonate or a small infant, wrap the probe around the foot so that light beams and detectors oppose each other. For a large infant, use a probe that fits on the great toe and secure it to the foot.*

- Turn on the power switch. If the device is working properly, a beep will sound, a display will light momentarily, and the pulse searchlight will flash. The Spo_2 and pulse rate displays will show stationary zeros. After four to six heartbeats, the Spo_2 and pulse rate displays will supply information with each beat, and the pulse amplitude indicator will begin tracking the pulse.

For pulse oximetry using the ear probe

- Using an alcohol pad, massage the patient's earlobe for 10 to 20 seconds. *Mild erythema indicates adequate vascularization.*
- Following the manufacturer's instructions, attach the ear probe to the patient's earlobe or pinna. Use the ear probe stabilizer for prolonged or exercise testing. Be sure to establish good contact on the ear; *an unstable probe may set off the low-perfusion alarm.* After the probe has been attached for a few seconds, a saturation reading and pulse waveform will appear on the oximeter's screen.
- Leave the ear probe in place for 3 or more minutes until readings stabilize at the highest point, or take three separate readings and average them. Make sure you revascularize the patient's earlobe each time.
- After the procedure, remove the probe, turn off and unplug the unit, and clean the probe by gently rubbing it with an alcohol pad.

Special considerations

- The pulse rate on the pulse oximeter should correspond to the patient's actual pulse. If the rates don't correspond, the saturation reading can't be considered accurate. You should assess the patient, check the oximeter, and reposition the probe if necessary.
- Readings are typically accurate if oximetry has been performed properly; however, some factors may affect accuracy. For example, an elevated bilirubin level may falsely lower Spo_2 readings, whereas elevated carboxyhemoglobin or

TROUBLESHOOTING

Diagnosing pulse oximeter problems

To maintain a continuous display of oxygen saturation levels, you'll need to keep the monitoring site clean and dry. Make sure the skin doesn't become irritated from adhesives used to keep disposable probes in place. You may need to change the site if this happens. Disposable probes that irritate the skin can also be replaced by nondisposable models.

Another common problem with pulse oximeters is the failure of the devices to obtain a signal. If this happens, your first reaction should be to check the patient's vital signs. If they're sufficient to produce a signal, check for the following problems.

Venous pulsations

Erroneous readings may be obtained if the pulse oximeter detects venous pulsations. This may occur in patients with tricuspid regurgitation or pulmonary hypertension or if a finger probe is taped too tightly to the finger.

Poor connection

Check that the sensors are properly aligned. Make sure that wires are intact and securely fastened and that the pulse oximeter is plugged into a power source.

Inadequate or intermittent blood flow to site

Check the patient's pulse rate and capillary refill time, and take corrective action if blood flow to the site is decreased. This may mean loosening restraints, removing tight-fitting clothes, taking off a blood pressure cuff, or checking arterial and I.V. lines. If none of these interventions works, you may need to find an alternate site. Finding a site with proper circulation may also prove challenging when a patient is receiving vasoconstrictive drugs.

Equipment malfunctions

Remove the pulse oximeter from the patient, set the alarm limits according to your facility's policies, and try the instrument on yourself or another healthy person. This will tell you if the equipment is working correctly.

methemoglobin levels, such as occur in heavy smokers and urban dwellers, can cause a falsely elevated Spo_2 reading.

- Certain intravascular substances, such as lipid emulsions and dyes, can also prevent accurate readings. Other factors that may interfere with accurate results include excessive light (for example, from phototherapy, surgical lamps, direct sunlight, and excessive ambient lighting), excessive patient movement, excessive ear pigment, hypothermia, hypotension, and vasoconstriction.
- Pulse oximetry may be used to monitor Spo_2 during respiratory arrest. *Because pulse oximetry is based on perfusion,* it shouldn't be used during cardiac arrest.
- If the patient has compromised circulation in his extremities, you can place a photodetector across the bridge of his nose.
- If Spo_2 is used to guide weaning the patient from forced inspiratory oxygen, obtain ABG analysis occasionally *to correlate Spo_2 readings with Sao_2 levels.*
- If an automatic blood pressure cuff is used on the same extremity that's used for measuring Spo_2, the cuff will interfere with Spo_2 readings during inflation.
- If light is a problem, cover the probes; if patient movement is a problem, move the probe or select a different probe; and if ear pigment is a problem, reposition the probe, revascularize the site, or use a finger probe. (See *Diagnosing pulse oximeter problems.*)
- Normal Spo_2 levels for pulse oximetry are 95% to 100% for adults and 93.8% to 100% by 1 hour after birth for healthy, full-term neonates. Lower levels may indicate hypoxemia that warrants intervention. For such patients, follow your facility's policy or the practitioner's orders, which may include increasing oxygen therapy. If Sao_2 levels decrease suddenly, you may need to resuscitate the patient immediately. Notify the practitioner of any significant change in the patient's condition.
- When the Sao_2 level is greater than 80%, pulse oximetry is highly accurate in healthy people. In patients on mechanical ventilation, however, accuracy is greatly reduced when the Sao_2 level is 90% or lower.

Documentation

Document the procedure, including the date, time, procedure type, oxygen saturation, and any action taken. Chart other relevant patient assessments performed to validate the oximetry reading. Record the inspired oxygen concentration and the type of oxygen delivery device used. Also record ABG values obtained and readings in appropriate flowsheets, if indicated.

SELECTED REFERENCES

Agashe, G.S., et al. "Forehead Pulse Oximetry: Headband Use Helps Alleviate False Low Readings Likely Related to Venous Pulsation Artifact," *Anesthesiology* 105(6):1111-116, December 2006.

Allen, K. "Principles and Limitations of Pulse Oximetry in Patient Monitoring," *Nursing Times* 100(41):34-37, October 2004.

American Association for Respiratory Care. "AARC Clinical Practice Guideline: Pulse Oximetry," *Respiratory Care* 36(12):1406-409, December 1991.

Taylor, C., et al. *Fundamentals of Nursing: The Art and Science of Nursing Care*, 6th ed. Philadelphia: Lippincott Williams & Wilkins, 2008.

END-TIDAL CARBON DIOXIDE MONITORING

Monitoring of end-tidal carbon dioxide ($ETCO_2$) determines the carbon dioxide (CO_2) concentration in exhaled gas. In this technique, a photodetector measures the amount of infrared light absorbed by airway gas during inspiration and expiration. (Light absorption increases along with the CO_2 concentration.) A monitor converts these data to a CO_2 value and a corresponding waveform, or capnogram, if capnography is used. (See *How $ETCO_2$ monitoring works.* Also see *Normal CO_2 waveform*, page 522.)

$ETCO_2$ monitoring provides information about the patient's pulmonary, cardiac, and metabolic status that aids patient management and helps prevent clinical compromise. This technique has become standard during anesthesia administration and mechanical ventilation.

The sensor, which contains an infrared light source and a photodetector, is positioned at one of two sites in the monitoring setup. With a mainstream monitor, it's positioned directly at the patient's airway with an airway adapter, between the endotracheal (ET) tube and the breathing circuit tubing. With a sidestream monitor, the airway adapter is positioned at the airway (regardless of whether the patient is intubated) to allow aspiration of gas from the patient's airway back to the sensor, which lies either within or close to the monitor.

Some CO_2 detection devices provide semiquantitative indications of CO_2 concentrations, supplying an approximate range rather than a specific value for $ETCO_2$. Other devices simply indicate whether CO_2 is present during exhalation. (See *Analyzing CO_2 levels,* page 523.)

$ETCO_2$ monitoring may be used to help wean a patient with a stable acid-base balance from mechanical ventilation. It also reduces the need for frequent arterial blood gas (ABG) measurements, especially when combined with pulse oximetry. Other uses for $ETCO_2$ monitoring include assessing resuscitation efforts and identifying the return of spontaneous circulation. Because no CO_2 is exhaled when breathing stops, this technique also detects apnea.

Advanced cardiac life support guidelines recommend the confirmation of ET-tube position using clinical assessment

How $ETCO_2$ monitoring works

The optical portion of an end-tidal carbon dioxide ($ETCO_2$) monitor contains an infrared light source, a sample chamber, a special carbon dioxide (CO_2) filter, and a photodetector. The infrared light passes through the sample chamber and is absorbed in varying amounts, depending on the amount of CO_2 the patient has just exhaled. The photodetector measures CO_2 content and relays this information to the microprocessor in the monitor, which displays the CO_2 value and waveform.

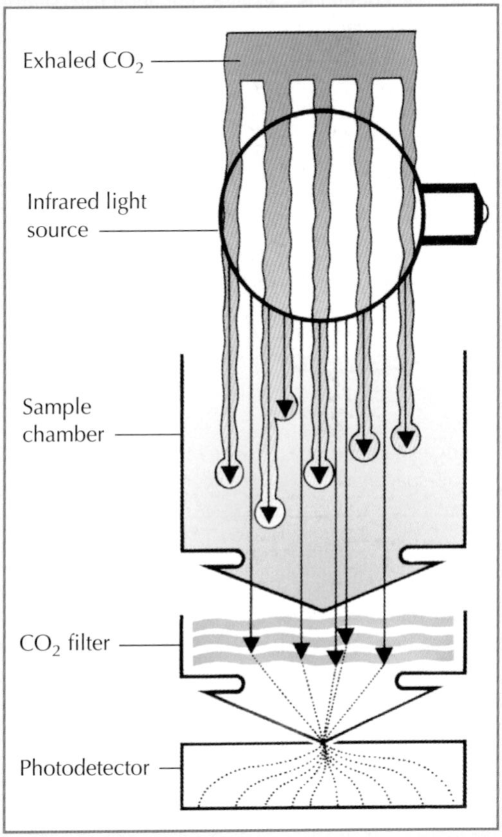

Normal CO_2 waveform

The carbon dioxide (CO_2) waveform, or capnogram, produced in end-tidal carbon dioxide ($ETCO_2$) monitoring reflects the course of CO_2 elimination during exhalation. A normal capnogram (shown below) consists of several segments, which reflect the various stages of exhalation and inhalation.

Normally, any gas eliminated from the airway during early exhalation is dead-space gas, which hasn't undergone exchange at the alveolocapillary membrane. Measurements taken during this period contain no CO_2. As exhalation continues, CO_2 concentration rises sharply and rapidly. The sensor now detects gas that has undergone exchange, producing measurable quantities of CO_2.

The final stages of alveolar emptying occur during late exhalation. During the alveolar plateau phase, CO_2 concentration rises more gradually *because alveolar emptying is more constant.*

The point at which $ETCO_2$ value is derived is the end of exhalation, when CO_2 concentration peaks. Unless an alveolar plateau is present, this value doesn't accurately estimate alveolar CO_2. During inhalation, the CO_2 concentration declines sharply to zero.

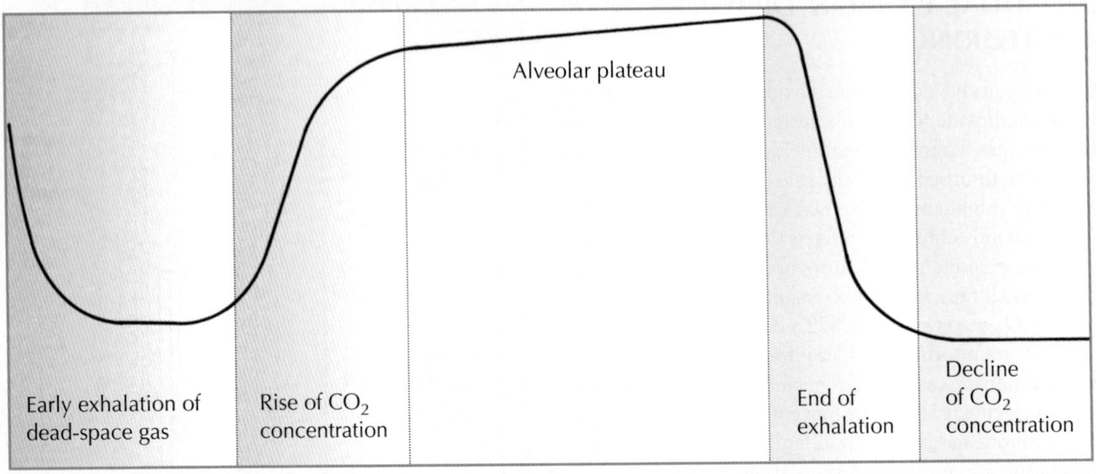

and confirmation devices, such as an $ETCO_2$ indicator or esophageal detection device. When used during ET intubation, $ETCO_2$ monitoring can avert neurologic injury and even death by confirming correct ET-tube placement and detecting accidental esophageal intubation because CO_2 isn't normally produced by the stomach.

The Society of Critical Care Medicine recommends that every intensive care unit have capnography available.

According to the American Association for Respiratory Care guidelines, capnography should be used for all patients on mechanical ventilation. Capnography is also indicated to:

- evaluate exhaled CO_2, especially $ETCO_2$, which is the maximum partial pressure of CO_2 exhaled just before the beginning of inspiration (tidal breath)
- monitor the severity of pulmonary disease and evaluate response to therapy, especially therapy intended to improve the ratio of dead space to tidal volume, matching of ventilation-perfusion ratio, and therapy intended to increase coronary blood flow
- determine that tracheal rather than esophageal intubation has taken place
- monitor the integrity of the ventilatory circuit including the artificial airway
- evaluate the efficiency of mechanical ventilatory support by determining the difference between the partial pressure of arterial CO_2 ($PaCO_2$) and the partial $PETCO_2$
- measure the volume of CO_2 elimination in order to monitor metabolic rate and alveolar ventilation
- monitor adequacy of pulmonary and coronary blood flow
- monitor inspired CO_2 when CO_2 gas is being therapeutically administered as a graphic evaluation of the ventilator-patient interface.

Ongoing $ETCO_2$ monitoring throughout intubation may also prove valuable because an ET tube may become dislodged during manipulation or patient movement or transport.

Equipment

Mainstream or sidestream CO_2 monitor ■ CO_2 sensor ■ airway adapter, as recommended by the manufacturer (a neonatal adapter may have a much smaller dead space, making it appropriate for a smaller patient) ■ gloves ■ $ETCO_2$ sensor.

Preparation of equipment

If the monitor you're using isn't self-calibrating, calibrate it as the manufacturer directs. If you're using a sidestream CO_2 monitor, be sure to replace the water trap between patients, if directed. *The trap allows humidity from exhaled gases to be condensed into an attached container.* Newer sidestream models don't require water traps.

Implementation

■ Confirm the patient's identity using two patient identifiers according to your facility's policy.
■ If the patient requires ET intubation, an $ETCO_2$ detector or monitor is usually applied immediately after the tube is inserted. If he doesn't require intubation or is already intubated and alert, explain the purpose and expected duration of monitoring. Tell an intubated patient that the monitor will painlessly measure the amount of CO_2 he exhales. Inform a nonintubated patient that the monitor will track his CO_2 concentration *to make sure his breathing is effective.*
■ Wash your hands. After turning on the monitor and calibrating it (if necessary), position the airway adapter and sensor as the manufacturer directs. For an intubated patient, position the adapter directly on the ET tube. For a nonintubated patient, place the adapter at or near the patient's airway. (An oxygen-delivery cannula may have a sample port through which gas can be aspirated for monitoring.)
■ Turn on all alarms and adjust alarm settings as appropriate for your patient. Make sure the alarm volume is loud enough to hear.

Special considerations

■ Wear gloves when handling the airway adapter *to prevent cross-contamination.* Make sure the adapter is changed with every breathing circuit and ET-tube change.
■ Place the adapter on the ET tube *to avoid contaminating exhaled gases with fresh gas flow from the ventilator.* If you're using a heat and moisture exchanger, you may be able to position the airway adapter between the exchanger and breathing circuit.

EQUIPMENT

Analyzing CO_2 levels

End-tidal carbon dioxide ($ETCO_2$) may be monitored digitally by using the cardiac monitor, or by using a color indicator device. Depending on which $ETCO_2$ detector you use, the meaning of color changes within the detector dome may differ from the analysis for the Easy Cap detector described below.
■ The rim of the Easy Cap is divided into four segments (clockwise from the top): check, a, b, and c. The check segment is solid purple, signifying the absence of carbon dioxide (CO_2).
■ The numbers in the other sections range from 0.03 to 5 and indicate the percentage of exhaled CO_2. The color should fluctuate during ventilation from purple (in section a) during inspiration to yellow (in section c) at the end of expiration. This indicates that the $ETCO_2$ levels are adequate—above 2%.
■ An end-expiratory color change from c to the b range may be the first sign of hemodynamic instability.
■ During cardiopulmonary resuscitation (CPR), an end-expiratory color change from the a or b range to the c range may mean the return of spontaneous ventilation.
■ During prolonged cardiac arrest, inadequate pulmonary perfusion leads to inadequate gas exchange. The patient exhales little or no CO_2, so the color stays in the purple range even with proper intubation. Ineffective CPR also leads to inadequate pulmonary perfusion.

Color indications on end-expiration

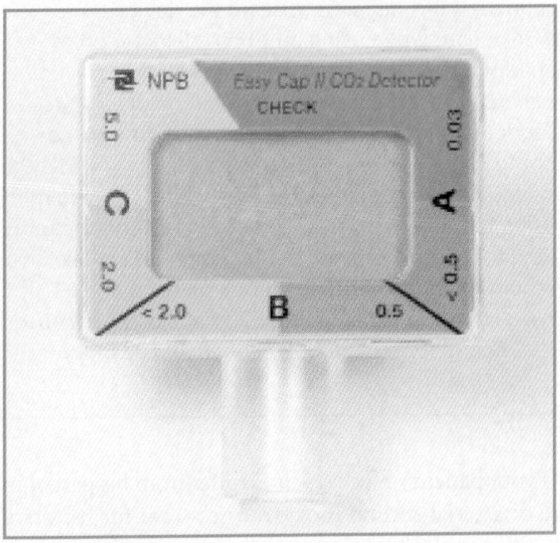

Using a disposable $ETCO_2$ detector: Some do's and don'ts

When using a disposable end-tidal carbon dioxide ($ETCO_2$) detector, check the instructions and ensure ideal working conditions for the device. Here are some additional guidelines.

Avoid high humidity, moisture, and heat

- Watch for changes indicating that the $ETCO_2$ detector's life span is decreasing—for example, sluggish color changes from breath to breath. A detector normally may be used for about 2 hours. However, using it with a ventilator that delivers high-humidity ventilation may shorten its life span to no more than 15 minutes.
- Don't use the detector with a heated humidifier or a nebulizer.
- Keep the detector protected from secretions, *which would render the device useless.* If secretions enter the dome, remove and discard the detector.
- Use a heat and moisture exchanger to protect the detector. In some detectors, this filter fits between the endotracheal (ET) tube and the detector.
- If you're using a heat and moisture exchanger, remember that it will increase your patient's breathing effort. Be alert for increased resistance and breathing difficulties, and remove the exchanger if necessary.

Take additional precautions

- Instilling epinephrine through the ET tube can damage the detector's indicator (the color may stay yellow). If this happens, discard the device.
- Take care when using an $ETCO_2$ detector on a child who weighs less than 30 lb (13.6 kg). *A small patient who rebreathes air from the dead air space (about 38 cc) will inhale too much of his own carbon dioxide.*
- Frequently spot-check the $ETCO_2$ detector you're using for effectiveness. If you must transport the patient to another area for testing or treatment, use another method to verify the tube's placement.
- Never reuse a disposable $ETCO_2$ detector *because it's intended for one-time, one-patient use only.*

- If your patient's $ETCO_2$ values differ from his partial pressure of arterial carbon dioxide, assess him for factors that can influence $ETCO_2$—especially when the differential between arterial and $ETCO_2$ values (the a-$ADCO_2$) is above normal. Such factors include decreased CO_2 production, increased CO_2 removal caused by hyperventilation, and diminished pulmonary perfusion.
- After the patient is started on $ETCO_2$ monitoring, obtain a sample for ABG analysis *to determine baseline values.* Note the difference between $ETCO_2$ and $PaCO_2$ values (a-$ADCO_2$). Typically, $ETCO_2$ levels are 1 to 6 mm Hg less than $PaCO_2$ levels. As long as a-$ADCO_2$ is normal, you can estimate the $PaCO_2$ level from the $ETCO_2$ level. Each time ABG values are obtained, note a-$ADCO_2$. If you use $ETCO_2$ values to estimate the $PaCO_2$ level, measure expired ventilation at the same time. If expired ventilation and $ETCO_2$ values are constant, the patient's a-$ADCO_2$ isn't likely to have changed. Avoid estimating the $PaCO_2$ level from the $ETCO_2$ level if the expired ventilation has changed. Alert the practitioner if the patient's a-$ADCO_2$ level is above the normal range. He may have a mismatching or shunting problem. Monitor a-$ADCO_2$ levels throughout therapy to determine the effectiveness of treatment and detect potential problems. If a-$ADCO_2$ increases, the patient may have reduced pulmonary perfusion.
- The a-$ADCO_2$ value, if correctly interpreted, provides useful information about your patient's status. For example, an increased a-$ADCO_2$ may mean that your patient has worsening dead space, especially if his tidal volume remains constant.
- Remember that $ETCO_2$ monitoring doesn't replace ABG measurements *because it doesn't assess oxygenation or blood pH.* Supplementing $ETCO_2$ monitoring with pulse oximetry may provide more complete information.
- If the CO_2 waveform is available, assess it for height, frequency, rhythm, baseline, and shape *to help evaluate gas exchange.* Make sure you know how to recognize a normal waveform and can identify any abnormal waveforms and their possible causes. If a printer is available, record and document abnormal waveforms in the patient's medical record.
- In a nonintubated patient, $ETCO_2$ values may be used to establish trends. Be aware that in a nonintubated patient, exhaled gas is more likely to mix with ambient air, and exhaled CO_2 may be diluted by fresh gas flow from the nasal cannula.
- $ETCO_2$ monitoring commonly is discontinued when the patient has been weaned effectively from mechanical ventilation or when he's no longer at risk for respiratory compromise. Carefully assess your patient's tolerance for weaning.

NURSING ALERT *After extubation, continuous $ETCO_2$ monitoring may detect the need for reintubation.*

- Disposable $ETCO_2$ detectors are available. When using a disposable $ETCO_2$ detector, always check its color under fluorescent or natural light *because the dome looks pink under incandescent light.* (See *Using a disposable ETCO_2 detector: Some do's and don'ts.*)

Complications

Inaccurate measurements—such as from poor sampling technique, calibration drift, contamination of optics with moisture or secretions, or equipment malfunction—can lead to misdiagnosis and improper treatment.

The effects of manual resuscitation or ingestion of alcohol or carbonated beverages can alter the detector's findings. Color changes detected after fewer than six ventilations can be misleading.

Documentation

Document the initial ETCO_2 value and all ventilator settings. Describe the waveform if one appears on the monitor. If the monitor has a printer, you may want to print out a sample waveform and include it in the patient's medical record.

Document ETCO_2 values at least as often as vital signs, whenever significant changes in waveform or patient status occur, and before and after weaning, respiratory, and other interventions. Periodically obtain samples for ABG analysis as the patient's condition dictates, and document the corresponding ETCO_2 values.

SELECTED REFERENCES

American Association for Respiratory Care. "AARC Clinical Practice Guideline: Capnography/Capnometry during Mechanical Ventilation," *Respiratory Care* 48(5):1321-324, May 2003.

Bair, A.E., et al. "Intubation Confirmation Techniques Associated with Unrecognized Non-tracheal Intubations by Prehospital Procedures," *Journal of Emergency Medicine* 28(4):403-407, May 2005.

Lynn-McHale Wiegand, D.J., and Carlson, K.K., eds. *AACN Procedure Manual for Critical Care*, 5th ed. Philadelphia: W.B. Saunders Co., 2006.

Zwerneman, K. "End-tidal Carbon Dioxide Monitoring: A VITAL Sign Worth Watching," *Critical Care Nursing Clinics of North America* 18(2):217-25, June 2006.

BEDSIDE SPIROMETRY

Bedside spirometry measures forced vital capacity (FVC) and forced expiratory volume (FEV), allowing calculation of other pulmonary function indices such as timed forced expiratory flow rate. Depending on the type of spirometer used, bedside spirometry can also allow direct measurement of vital capacity and tidal volume.

Bedside spirometry aids in diagnosing destructive or restrictive pulmonary dysfunction, evaluating its severity, and determining the patient's response to therapy. Allowing assessment of the relationship of flow rate to vital capacity helps distinguish between obstructive and restrictive pulmonary disease. It's also useful for evaluating preoperative anesthesia risk. Because the required breathing patterns can aggravate conditions such as bronchospasm, use of the bedside spirometer requires a review of the patient's history and close observation during testing.

Equipment

Spirometer ▪ disposable mouthpiece ▪ breathing tube, if required ▪ spirographic chart, if required ▪ chart and pen, if required ▪ optional: vital capacity predicted-values table and noseclips.

Preparation of equipment

Review the manufacturer's instructions for assembly and use of the spirometer. If necessary, firmly insert the breathing tube *to ensure a tight connection.* If the tube comes preconnected, check the seals for tightness and the tubing for leaks.

Check the operation of the recording mechanism, and insert a chart and pen if necessary. Insert the disposable mouthpiece and make sure it's tightly sealed.

Implementation

- Confirm the patient's identity using two patient identifiers according to your facility's policy.
- Explain the procedure to the patient. Emphasize that his cooperation is essential *to ensure accurate results.*
- Instruct the patient to remove or loosen any constricting clothing, such as a bra, *to prevent alteration of test results from restricted thoracic expansion and abdominal mobility.*
- Instruct the patient to void *to prevent abdominal discomfort.*
- If the patient wears dentures that fit poorly, remove them *to prevent incomplete closure of his mouth, which could allow air to leak around the mouthpiece.* If his dentures fit well, leave them in place *to promote a tight seal.*
- Plug in the spirometer, and set the baseline time.
- If desired, allow the patient to practice the required breathing with the breathing tube unhooked. After practice, replace the tube and check the seal.
- Tell the patient not to breathe through his nose. If the patient has difficulty complying, apply noseclips.
- To measure vital capacity, instruct the patient to inhale as deeply as possible, and then insert the mouthpiece so that his lips are sealed tightly around it *to prevent air leakage and ensure an accurate digital readout or spirogram recording.*

- Tell him to exhale completely. Then remove the mouthpiece *to avoid recording his next inspiration.*
- Allow the patient to rest, and repeat the procedure twice.
- To measure FEV and FVC, repeat this procedure with the chart or timer on, but instruct the patient to exhale as quickly and completely as possible. Tell him when to start, and turn on the recorder or timer at the same time.
- Allow the patient to rest, and repeat the procedure twice.
- After completing the procedure, discard the mouthpiece, remove the spirographic chart, and follow the manufacturer's instructions for cleaning and sterilizing.

Special considerations

- Don't perform pulmonary function tests immediately after a large meal *because the patient may experience abdominal discomfort.*
- Encourage the patient during the test; *this may help him to exhale more forcefully, which can be significant.* If the patient coughs during expiration, wait until coughing subsides before repeating the measurement.
- Read the vital capacity directly from the readout or spirogram chart. The vital capacity is the greatest measurement volume on complete exhalation after the deepest inhalation without forced or rapid effort. It's usually recorded in liters or milliliters. Of the three trials, accept the highest recorded exhalation volume as the vital capacity result.
- *To determine the percentage of predicted vital capacity,* first determine the patient's predicted value from the vital capacity predicted-values table; then calculate the percentage by using the following formula:

$$\frac{\text{observed vital capacity}}{\text{predicted vital capacity}} \times 100 = \%\ \text{predicted vital capacity}$$

- Read the FVC directly from the readout or spirogram chart. Although the FVC is normally approximately equal to the vital capacity, it may be reduced in obstructive disease; whereas the vital capacity remains normal. In restrictive disease, both the vital capacity and FVC may be reduced.
- *To determine the FEV for a specified time,* mark the point on the spirogram where it crosses the desired time, and draw a straight line from this point to the side of the chart, which indicates volume in liters. This measurement is usually calculated for 1, 2, and 3 seconds and reported as a percentage of vital capacity. A healthy patient will have exhaled 75%, 85%, and 95%, respectively, of his FVC. Calculate this percentage by using the following formula:

$$\frac{\text{observed forced expiratory volume}}{\text{predicted vital capacity}} \times 100 = \%\ \text{predicted vital capacity}$$

Complications

Forced exhalation can cause dizziness or light-headedness, precipitate or worsen bronchospasm, rapidly increase exhaustion (possibly to where the patient will require mechanical support), and increase air trapping in the patient with emphysema.

Documentation

Record the date and time of the procedure; the observed and calculated values, including FEV at 1, 2, and 3 seconds; complications and the nursing action taken; and the patient's tolerance of the procedure.

Selected references

Dales, R.E., et al. "Spirometry in the Primary Care Setting: Influence on Clinical Diagnosis and Management of Airflow Obstruction," *Chest* 128(4):2443-447, October 2005.

Taylor, C., et al. *Fundamentals of Nursing: The Art and Science of Nursing Care,* 5th ed. Philadelphia: Lippincott Williams & Wilkins, 2008.

Wallace, L.D., and Troy, K.E. "Office-based Spirometry for Early Detection of Obstructive Lung Disease," *Journal of the American Academy of Nurse Practitioners* 18(9):414-21, September 2006.

AIRWAY MANAGEMENT

Foreign-body airway obstruction management

Sudden airway obstruction may occur when a foreign body lodges in the throat or bronchus; when the patient aspirates blood, mucus, or vomitus; when the tongue blocks the pharynx; or when the patient experiences traumatic injury, bronchoconstriction, or bronchospasm.

An obstructed airway causes anoxia, which in turn leads to brain damage and death in 4 to 6 minutes. The Heimlich maneuver uses an upper-abdominal thrust to create diaphragmatic pressure in the static lung below the foreign body sufficient to expel the obstruction. The Heimlich maneuver is used in conscious adult patients and in children older than age 1. However, the abdominal thrust is contraindicated in pregnant women, markedly obese patients, and patients who have recently undergone abdominal surgery and in infants younger than age 1. For such patients, a chest thrust, which forces air out of the lungs to create an artificial cough, should be used.

These maneuvers are contraindicated in a patient with incomplete or partial airway obstruction or when the patient can maintain adequate ventilation to dislodge the foreign body by effective coughing. However, if the patient has poor air exchange and increased breathing difficulty, a silent cough, cyanosis, or the inability to speak or breathe, immediate action to dislodge the obstruction should be taken. (See also "Cardiopulmonary resuscitation," page 474 [for adults] and page 921 [for children].)

Implementation

Conscious adult with mild airway obstruction

- Ask the person who's coughing or using the universal distress sign (clutching the neck between the thumb and fingers) if she's choking. If she indicates that she is but can speak and cough forcefully, she has good air exchange and should be encouraged to continue to cough. Remain with the person and monitor her.

Conscious adult with severe airway obstruction

- Ask the person, "Are you choking?" If the patient nods yes and has signs of severe airway obstruction, tell her that you'll help dislodge the foreign body.
- Standing behind the patient, wrap your arms around her waist. Make a fist with one hand, and place the thumb side against her abdomen in the midline, slightly above the umbilicus and well below the xiphoid process. Then grasp your fist with the other hand (as shown below).

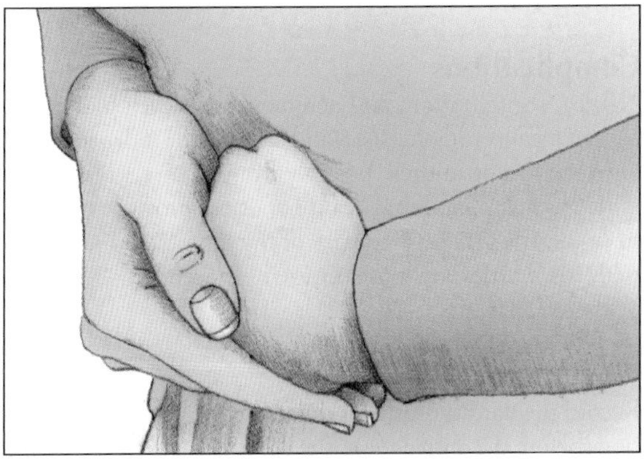

- Squeeze the patient's abdomen with quick inward and upward thrusts (as shown top of next column). Each thrust should be a separate and distinct movement; each should be forceful enough to create an artificial cough that will dislodge an obstruction.

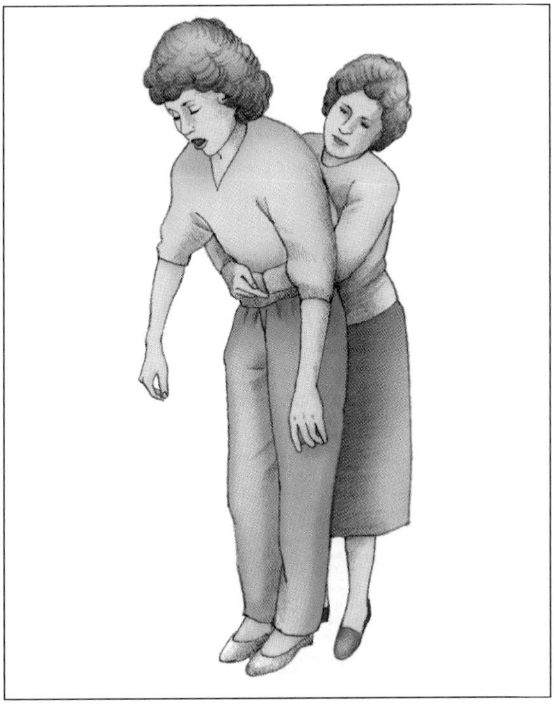

- Make sure you have a firm grasp on the patient *because she may lose consciousness and need to be lowered to the floor.* While supporting her head and neck *to prevent injury,* place the victim in a supine position and continue as described below.
- Repeat the thrusts until the foreign body is expelled or if the patient becomes unconscious. At this point, contact the emergency medical service (EMS) and follow the interventions for relieving an obstructed airway in an unconscious person.

NURSING ALERT *If the victim of an airway obstruction becomes unconscious, the lay rescuer should lower the patient to the ground and immediately contact EMS and begin cardiopulmonary resuscitation (CPR).*

Unresponsive adult

- Lower the patient to the ground and immediately contact EMS.
- Begin CPR.
- Each time the airway is opened using a head tilt-chin lift, look for an object in the patient's mouth.
- Remove the object if present.
- Attempt to ventilate the patient and follow with 30 chest compressions.

NURSING ALERT *The blind finger-sweep is no longer being taught by the American Heart Association. A finger-*

sweep should only be used when a foreign body can be seen in the mouth. Studies have shown that blind finger-sweeps may result in injury to the patient's mouth and throat or to the rescuer's fingers, and there's no evidence of its effectiveness. In addition, the tongue-jaw lift is no longer used. The patient's mouth should be opened using a head-tilt chin-lift maneuver.

For an obese or pregnant adult

- If the patient is conscious, stand behind her and place your arms under her armpits and around her chest.
- Place the thumb side of your clenched fist against the middle of the sternum, avoiding the margins of the ribs and the xiphoid process (as shown below). Grasp your fist with your other hand and perform a chest thrust with enough force to expel the foreign body. Continue until the patient expels the obstruction or loses consciousness.

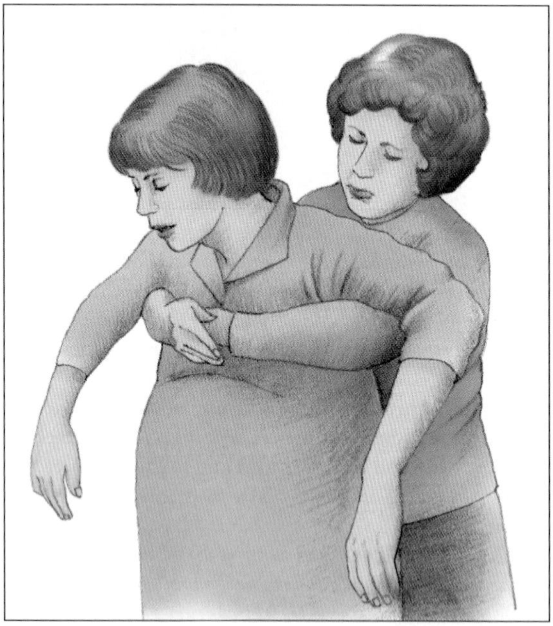

- If the patient loses consciousness, carefully lower her to the floor and place her in a supine position.
- Then follow the same steps you would use for the unresponsive adult (as described above and shown top of next column.)

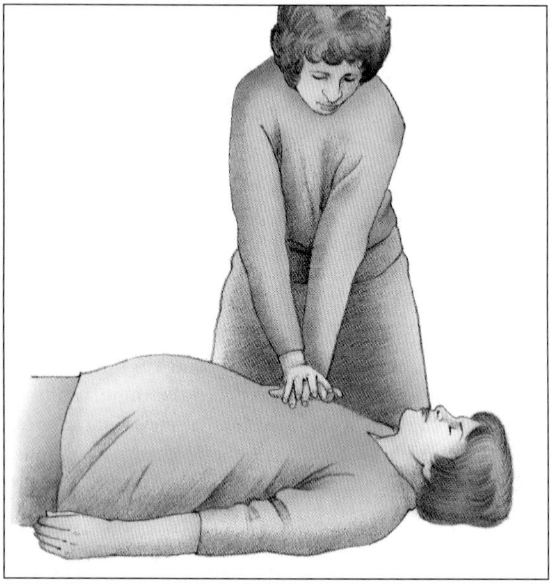

Special considerations

- If the patient vomits during abdominal thrusts, quickly wipe out her mouth with your fingers and resume the maneuver as necessary.
- Even if your efforts to clear the airway don't seem to be effective, keep trying. *As oxygen deprivation increases, smooth and skeletal muscles relax, making your maneuvers more likely to succeed.*

Complications

Nausea, regurgitation, and achiness may develop after the patient regains consciousness and can breathe independently. She may also be injured, possibly from incorrect placement of the rescuer's hands or because of osteoporosis or metastatic lesions that increase the risk of fracture. Examine the patient for injuries, such as ruptured or lacerated abdominal or thoracic viscera.

Documentation

Record the date and time of the procedure, the patient's actions before the obstruction, the approximate length of time it took to clear the airway, and the type and size of the object removed. Also, note her vital signs after the procedure, any complications that occurred and nursing actions taken, and his tolerance of the procedure. Note the time, name of the practitioner notified, any orders given, and your interventions.

Selected references

American Heart Association. "2005 American Heart Association Guidelines for Cardiopulmonary Resuscitation and Emergency Cardiovascular Care," *Circulation* 112(Suppl IV):IV-19-IV-34, December 2005.

Salati, D.S. "Responding to Foreign-body Airway Obstruction," *Nursing* 36(12 Part 1):50-51, December 2006.

Soroudi, A., et al. "Adult Foreign Body Airway Obstruction in the Prehospital Setting," *Prehospital Emergency Care* 11(1):25-29, January-March 2007.

Oropharyngeal airway insertion and care

An oropharyngeal airway, a curved rubber or plastic device, is inserted into the mouth to the posterior pharynx to establish or maintain a patent airway. In an unconscious patient, the tongue usually obstructs the posterior pharynx. The oropharyngeal airway conforms to the curvature of the palate, removing the obstruction and allowing air to pass around and through the tube. It also facilitates oropharyngeal suctioning. The oropharyngeal airway is intended for short-term use, as in the postanesthesia or postictal stage. It may be left in place longer as an airway adjunct to prevent the orally intubated patient from biting the endotracheal tube.

The oropharyngeal airway isn't the airway of choice for the patient with loose or avulsed teeth or recent oral surgery. Inserting this airway in the conscious or semiconscious patient may stimulate vomiting and laryngospasm; therefore, you'll usually insert the airway only in unconscious patients.

According to the 2005 American Heart Association guidelines for cardiopulmonary resuscitation and emergency cardiovascular care, an oropharyngeal airway should be reserved for the unconscious patient with no cough or gag reflex. The 2005 guidelines also state that the oropharyngeal airway should be inserted only by someone trained in its use.

Equipment

For inserting: Oral airway of appropriate size ▪ tongue blade ▪ padded tongue blade ▪ gloves ▪ optional: suction equipment, handheld resuscitation bag or oxygen-powered breathing device.

For cleaning: Hydrogen peroxide ▪ water ▪ basin ▪ optional: pipe cleaner.

For reflex testing: Cotton-tipped applicator.

Preparation of equipment

Select an airway of appropriate size for your patient; *an oversized airway can obstruct breathing by depressing the epiglottis into the laryngeal opening.* Usually, you'll select a small size (size 1 or 2) for an infant or child, a medium size (size 4 or 5) for the average adult, and a large size (size 6) for the large adult. Be sure to confirm the correct size of the airway by placing the airway flange beside the patient's cheek, parallel to his front teeth. If the airway is the right size, the airway curve should reach to the angle of the jaw.

Implementation

- Explain the procedure to the patient even though he may not appear to be alert. Provide privacy and put on gloves *to prevent contact with body fluids.* If the patient is wearing dentures, remove them *so they don't cause further airway obstruction.*
- Suction the patient if necessary.
- Place the patient in a supine position with his neck hyperextended if this isn't contraindicated.
- Insert the airway using the cross-finger or tongue blade technique. (See *Inserting an oral airway,* page 530.)
- Auscultate the lungs *to ensure adequate ventilation.*
- After the airway is inserted, position the patient on his side *to decrease the risk of aspiration of vomitus.*
- Perform mouth care every 2 to 4 hours as needed. Begin by holding the patient's jaws open with a padded tongue blade and gently removing the airway. Place the airway in a basin, and rinse it with hydrogen peroxide and then water. If secretions remain, use a pipe cleaner to remove them. Complete standard mouth care and reinsert the airway.
- While the airway is removed for mouth care, observe the mouth's mucous membranes *because tissue irritation or ulceration can result from prolonged airway use.*
- Frequently check the position of the airway *to ensure correct placement.*
- When the patient regains consciousness and is able to swallow, remove the airway by pulling it outward and downward, following the mouth's natural curvature. After the airway is removed, test the patient's cough and gag reflexes *to ensure that removal of the airway wasn't premature and that the patient can maintain his own airway.*
- To test for the gag reflex, use a cotton-tipped applicator to touch both sides of the posterior pharynx. To test for the cough reflex, gently touch the posterior oropharynx with the cotton-tipped applicator.

Special considerations

- Bilateral breath sounds on auscultation indicate that the airway is the proper size and in the correct position.
- Avoid taping the airway in place *because untaping it could delay airway removal, thus increasing the patient's risk of aspiration.*
- Evaluate the patient's behavior *to provide the cue for airway removal.* He's likely to gag or cough as he becomes more alert, indicating that he no longer needs the airway.

Inserting an oral airway

Unless this position is contraindicated, hyperextend the patient's head (as shown below) before using either the cross-finger or tongue blade insertion method.

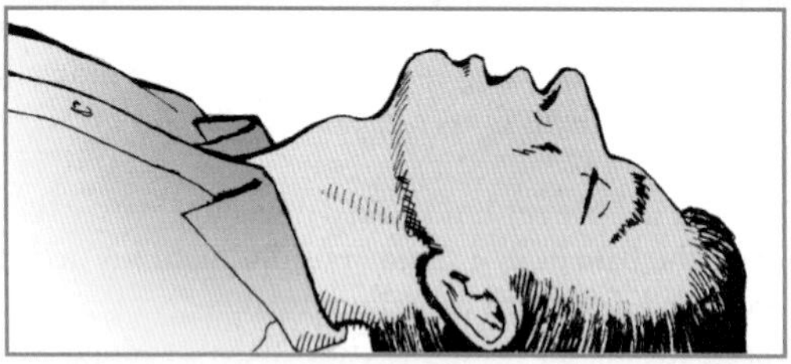

To insert an oral airway using the cross-finger method, place your thumb on the patient's lower teeth and your index finger on his upper teeth. Gently open his mouth by pushing his teeth apart (as shown below).

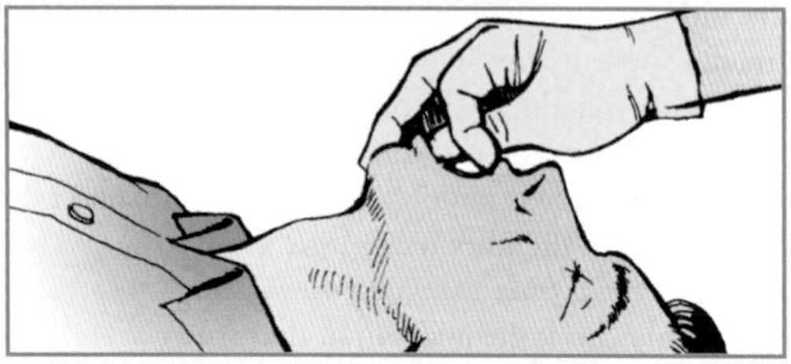

Insert the airway upside down *to avoid pushing the tongue toward the pharynx,* and slide it over the tongue toward the back of the mouth. Rotate the airway as it approaches the posterior wall of the pharynx so that it points downward (as shown below).

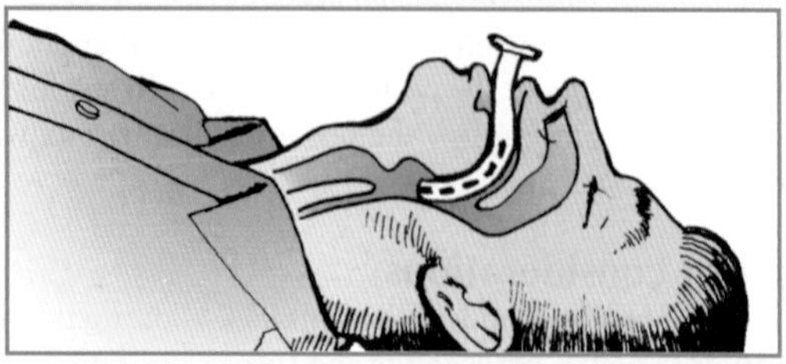

To use the tongue blade technique, open the patient's mouth and depress his tongue with the blade. Guide the airway over the back of the tongue as you did for the cross-finger technique.

Complications

Tooth damage or loss, tissue damage, and bleeding may result from insertion. If the airway is too long, it may press the epiglottis against the entrance of the larynx, producing complete airway obstruction. If the airway isn't inserted properly, it may push the tongue posteriorly, aggravating the problem of upper airway obstruction. To prevent traumatic injury, make sure the patient's lips and tongue aren't between his teeth and the airway.

Immediately after inserting the airway, check for respirations. If respirations are absent or inadequate, initiate artificial positive pressure ventilation by using a mouth-to-mask technique, a handheld resuscitation bag, or an oxygen-powered breathing device. (See "Manual ventilation," page 574.)

Documentation

Record the date and time of the airway's insertion; size of the airway; removal and cleaning of the airway; condition of mucous membranes; suctioning; adverse reactions and the nursing action taken; and the patient's tolerance of the procedure. Also document breath sounds and respiratory assessment findings.

SELECTED REFERENCES

American Heart Association. "2005 American Heart Association Guidelines for Cardiopulmonary Resuscitation and Emergency Cardiovascular Care," *Circulation* 112(Suppl IV):IV-19-IV-34, December 2005.

Dulak, S.B. "Placing an Oropharyngeal Airway," *RN* 68(2):20ac1-20ac3, February 2005.

Lynn-McHale Wiegand, D.J., and Carlson, K.K., eds. *AACN Procedure Manual for Critical Care*, 5th ed. Philadelphia: W.B. Saunders Co., 2006.

Taylor, C., et al. *Fundamentals of Nursing: The Art and Science of Nursing Care*, 5th ed. Philadelphia: Lippincott Williams & Wilkins, 2008.

Tong, J.L., and Smith, J.E. "Cardiovascular Changes Following Insertion of Oropharyngeal and Nasopharyngeal Airways," *British Journal of Anaesthesiology* 93(3):339-42, September 2004.

NASOPHARYNGEAL AIRWAY INSERTION AND CARE

Insertion of a nasopharyngeal airway — a soft rubber or latex uncuffed catheter — establishes or maintains a patent airway. This airway is the typical choice for patients who have had recent oral surgery or facial trauma and for patients with loose, cracked, or avulsed teeth. It's also used to protect the nasal mucosa from injury when the patient needs frequent nasotracheal suctioning. This type of airway may also be tolerated better than an oropharyngeal airway by a patient who isn't deeply unconscious.

According to the 2005 American Heart Association guidelines for cardiopulmonary resuscitation and emergency cardiovascular care, a nasopharyngeal airway is especially useful in patients with such conditions as clenched jaws, which prevent placement of an oral airway. It may also be used in patients with an obstructed airway to deliver ventilations with a bag-mask device. However, the guidelines warn that this type of airway should be used cautiously in patients with severe craniofacial injury. They also stress that safe use of nasopharyngeal airways requires adequate training and practice, with regular retraining.

The airway follows the curvature of the nasopharynx, passing through the nose and extending from the nostril to the posterior pharynx. The bevel-shaped pharyngeal end of the airway facilitates insertion, and its funnel-shaped nasal end helps prevent slippage.

Insertion of a nasopharyngeal airway is preferred when an oropharyngeal airway is contraindicated or fails to maintain a patent airway. A nasopharyngeal airway is contraindicated if the patient is receiving anticoagulant therapy or has a hemorrhagic disorder, sepsis, or pathologic nasopharyngeal deformity.

Equipment

For insertion: Nasopharyngeal airway of proper size ▪ tongue blade ▪ water-soluble lubricant ▪ gloves ▪ optional: suction equipment.

For cleaning: Hydrogen peroxide ▪ water ▪ basin ▪ optional: pipe cleaner.

Preparation of equipment

Measure the diameter of the patient's nostril and the distance from the tip of his nose to his earlobe. Select an airway of slightly smaller diameter than the nostril and of slightly longer length (1″ [2.5 cm]) than measured. The sizes for this type of airway are labeled according to their internal diameter.

The recommended size for a large adult is 8 to 9 mm; for a medium adult, 7 to 8 mm; and for a small adult, 6 to 7 mm. Lubricate the distal half of the airway's surface with a water-soluble lubricant *to prevent traumatic injury during insertion.*

Implementation

- Put on gloves.
- In nonemergency situations, explain the procedure to the patient.
- Lubricate the airway and properly insert it. (See *Inserting a nasopharyngeal airway,* page 532.)
- After the airway is inserted, check it regularly *to detect dislodgment or obstruction.*
- When the patient's natural airway is patent, remove the airway in one smooth motion. If the airway sticks, apply lubricant around the nasal end of the tube and around the nostril; then gently rotate the airway until it's free.

Special considerations

- When you insert the airway, remember to use a chin-lift or jaw-thrust technique *to anteriorly displace the patient's mandible.* Immediately after insertion, assess the patient's respirations. If absent or inadequate, initiate artificial positive-pressure ventilation with a mouth-to-mask technique, a handheld resuscitation bag, or an oxygen-powered breathing device.
- If the patient coughs or gags, the tube may be too long. If so, remove the airway and insert a shorter one.
- At least once every 8 hours, remove the airway to check nasal mucous membranes for irritation or ulceration.
- Clean the airway by placing it in a basin and rinsing it with hydrogen peroxide and then with water. If secretions remain, use a pipe cleaner to remove them. Reinsert the clean airway into the other nostril (if it's patent) *to avoid skin breakdown.*

Complications

Sinus infection may result from obstruction of sinus drainage. Insertion of the airway may injure the nasal mucosa and cause bleeding and possibly aspiration of blood into the trachea. Suction as necessary to remove secretions or blood. If the tube is too long, it may enter the esophagus and cause gastric distention and hypoventilation during artificial ventilation. Although semiconscious patients usually tolerate nasopharyngeal airways better than conscious patients, they may still experience laryngospasm and vomiting.

Documentation

Record the date and time of the airway's insertion; size of the airway; removal and cleaning of the airway; shifts from one nostril to the other; condition of the mucous membranes; suctioning; complications and nursing action taken; and the patient's tolerance of the procedure.

SELECTED REFERENCES

American Heart Association. "2005 American Heart Association Guidelines for Cardiopulmonary Resuscitation and Emergency Cardiovascular Care," *Circulation* 112(Suppl IV):VI-19-VI-34, December 2005.

Inserting a nasopharyngeal airway

First, hold the airway beside the patient's face *to make sure it's the proper size* (as shown below). It should be slightly smaller than the patient's nostril diameter and slightly longer than the distance from the tip of his nose to his earlobe.

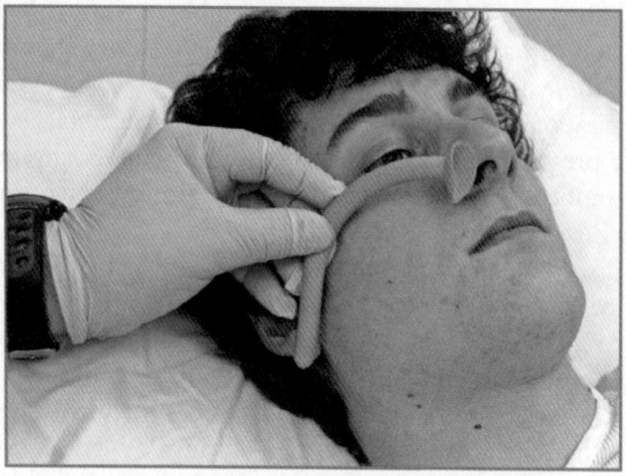

To insert the airway, hyperextend the patient's neck (unless contraindicated). Then push up the tip of his nose and pass the airway into his nostril (as shown below). Avoid pushing against any resistance *to prevent tissue trauma and airway kinking.*

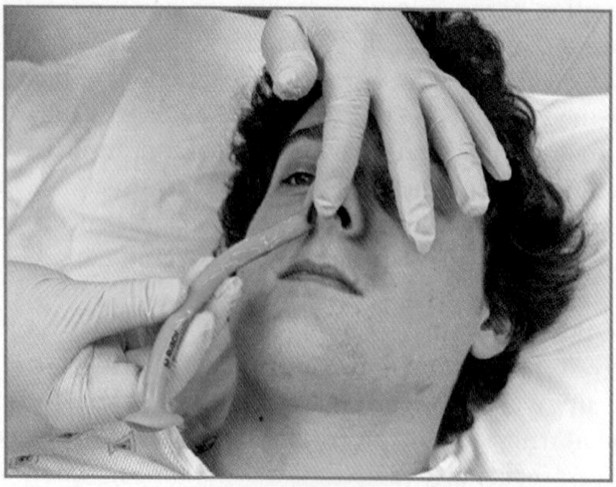

To check for correct airway placement, first close the patient's mouth. Then place your finger over the tube's opening *to detect air exchange.* Also, depress the patient's tongue with a tongue blade, and look for the airway tip behind the uvula.

Lynn-McHale Wiegand, D.J., and Carlson, K.K., eds. *AACN Procedure Manual for Critical Care*, 5th ed. Philadelphia: W.B. Saunders Co., 2006.

Taylor, C., et al. *Fundamentals of Nursing: The Art and Science of Nursing Care*, 5th ed. Philadelphia: Lippincott Williams & Wilkins, 2008.

Tong, J.L., and Smith, J.E. "Cardiovascular Changes Following Insertion of Oropharyngeal and Nasopharyngeal Airways," *British Journal of Anaesthesiology* 93(3):339-42, September 2004.

ESOPHAGEAL AIRWAY INSERTION AND REMOVAL

Esophageal airways, such as the esophageal gastric tube airway (EGTA) and the esophageal obturator airway (EOA), are used temporarily (for up to 2 hours) to maintain ventilation in comatose patients during cardiac or respiratory arrest. These devices avoid tongue obstruction, prevent air from entering the stomach, and keep stomach contents from entering the trachea. They can be inserted only after a patent airway is established. (See *Combitube.)*

Although health care providers must have special training to insert an EGTA or EOA, insertion of these airways is much simpler than endotracheal intubation. One reason is that these devices don't require visualization of the trachea or hyperextension of the neck. This makes them useful for treating patients with suspected spinal cord injuries.

Because conscious and semiconscious patients will reject an esophageal airway, these airways shouldn't be used unless the patient is unconscious and not breathing. They're also contraindicated if facial trauma prevents a snug mask fit or if the patient has an absent or weak gag reflex, has recently ingested toxic chemicals, has esophageal disease, or has taken an overdose of opioids that can be reversed by naloxone.

PEDIATRIC ALERT *Because pediatric sizes aren't currently available, esophageal airways shouldn't be used in patients younger than age 16.*

Equipment

Esophageal tube ▪ face mask #16 or #18 French nasogastric (NG) tube (for EGTA) ▪ syringe ▪ intermittent gastric suction equipment ▪ oral suction equipment ▪ goggles and gloves ▪ optional: handheld resuscitation bag, water-soluble lubricant.

Preparation of equipment

Gather the equipment. (See *Types of esophageal airways*, page 534.) Fill the face mask with air *to check for leaks.* Inflate the esophageal tube's cuff with 35 cc of air *to check for leaks;* then deflate the cuff. Connect the esophageal tube to the face mask (the lower opening on an EGTA) and listen for the tube to click *to determine proper placement.*

Implementation

- Assess the patient's condition to determine if he's an appropriate candidate for an esophageal airway.
- Put on gloves and personal protective equipment.
- Lubricate the first 1″ (2.5 cm) of the tube's distal tip with a water-soluble lubricant. With an EGTA, also lubricate the first 1″ of the NG tube's distal tip.
- If the patient's condition permits, place him in the supine position with his neck in a neutral or semiflexed position. *Hyperextension of the neck may cause the tube to enter the trachea instead of the esophagus.* Remove his dentures, if applicable.
- Insert your thumb deeply into the patient's mouth behind the base of his tongue. Place your index and middle fingers of the same hand under the patient's chin, and lift his jaw straight up.
- With your other hand, grasp the esophageal tube just below the mask in the same way you would grasp a pencil. *This promotes gentle maneuvering of the tube and reduces the risk of pharyngeal trauma.*
- Still elevating the patient's jaw with one hand, insert the tip of the esophageal tube into the patient's mouth. Gently guide the airway over the tongue into the pharynx and then into the esophagus, following the natural pharyngeal curve. No force is required for proper insertion; the tube should easily seat itself. If you encounter resistance, withdraw the tube slightly and readvance it. When the tube is fully advanced, the mask should fit snugly over the patient's mouth and nose. When this is accomplished, the cuff will lie below the level of the carina. If the cuff is above the carina, it may, when inflated, compress the posterior membranous portion of the trachea and cause tracheal obstruction.
- *Because the tube may enter the trachea,* deliver positive-pressure ventilation before inflating the cuff. Watch for the chest to rise *to confirm that the tube is in the esophagus.*
- When the tube is properly in place in the esophagus, draw 35 cc of air into the syringe, connect the syringe to the tube's cuff-inflation valve, and inflate the cuff. Avoid overinflation *because this can cause esophageal trauma.*
- If you've inserted an EGTA, insert the NG tube through the lower port on the face mask and into the esophageal tube, and advance it to the second marking so it reaches 6″ (15 cm) beyond the distal end of the esophageal tube. Suction stomach contents using intermittent gastric suction *to decompress the stomach.* This is particularly necessary after mouth-to-mouth resuscitation, *which introduces air to the stomach.* Leave the tube in place during resuscitation.

EQUIPMENT

Combitube

An alternative esophageal airway is the esophageal-tracheal combitube, which may be inserted blindly into the patient's throat. Regardless of whether the tube enters the esophagus or the trachea, openings above the entry point allow ventilation.

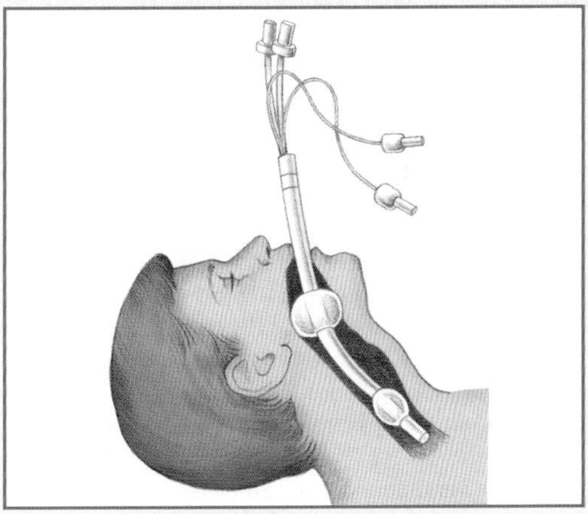

- For both airways, attach a handheld resuscitation bag or a mechanical ventilator to the face mask port (upper port) on the EGTA. Up to 100% of the fraction of inspired oxygen can be delivered this way.
- Monitor the patient *to ensure adequate ventilation.* Watch for chest movement, and suction the patient if mucus blocks the EOA tube perforations or interrupts respiration.

Removing an esophageal airway

- Assess the patient's condition *to determine if airway removal is appropriate.* The airway may be removed if respirations are spontaneous and number 16 to 20 breaths/minute. If 2 hours have elapsed since airway insertion and respirations aren't spontaneous and at the normal rate, the patient must be switched to an artificial airway that can be used for long-term ventilation such as an endotracheal (ET) tube.
- Detach the mask from the esophageal tube.
- If the patient is conscious, place him on his left side, if possible, *to avoid aspiration during removal of the esophageal tube.* If he's unconscious and requires an ET tube, insert it or assist with its insertion and inflate the cuff of the ET tube before removing the ET tube. *With the esophageal tube in place, the ET tube can be guided easily into the trachea, and*

EQUIPMENT

Types of esophageal airways

The two most commonly used types of esophageal airways are the esophageal gastric tube airway and the esophageal obturator airway. Both are described below.

Gastric tube airway

A gastric tube airway consists of an inflatable mask and an esophageal tube, as shown at right. The transparent face mask has two ports: a lower one for insertion of an esophageal tube and an upper one for ventilation, which can be maintained with a handheld resuscitation bag. The inside of the mask is soft and pliable; it molds to the patient's face and makes a tight seal, preventing air loss.

The proximal end of the esophageal tube has a one-way, nonrefluxing valve that blocks the esophagus. This valve prevents air from entering the stomach, thus reducing the risk of abdominal distention and aspiration. The distal end of the tube has an inflatable cuff that rests in the esophagus just below the tracheal bifurcation, preventing pressure on the noncartilaginous tracheal wall.

During ventilation, air is directed into the upper port in the mask and, with the esophagus blocked, enters the trachea and lungs.

Esophageal gastric tube airway

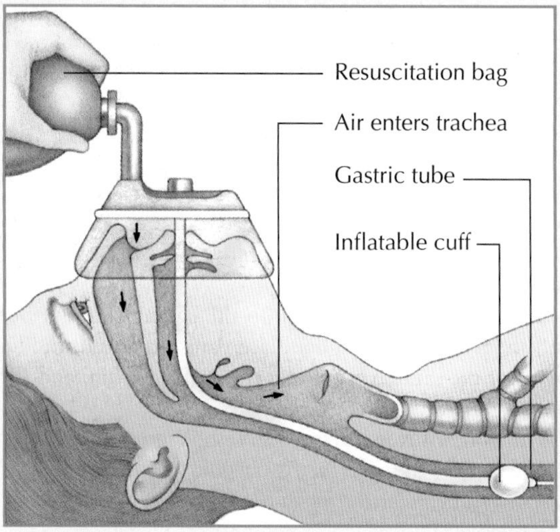

Obturator airway

An obturator airway consists of an adjustable, inflatable transparent face mask with a single port, attached by a snap lock to a blind esophageal tube. When properly inflated, the transparent mask prevents air from escaping through the nose and mouth, as shown at right.

The esophageal tube has 16 holes at its proximal end through which air or oxygen introduced into the port of the mask is transferred to the trachea. The tube's distal end is closed and circled by an inflatable cuff. When the cuff is inflated, it occludes the esophagus, preventing air from entering the stomach and acting as a barrier against vomitus and involuntary aspiration.

Esophageal obturator airway

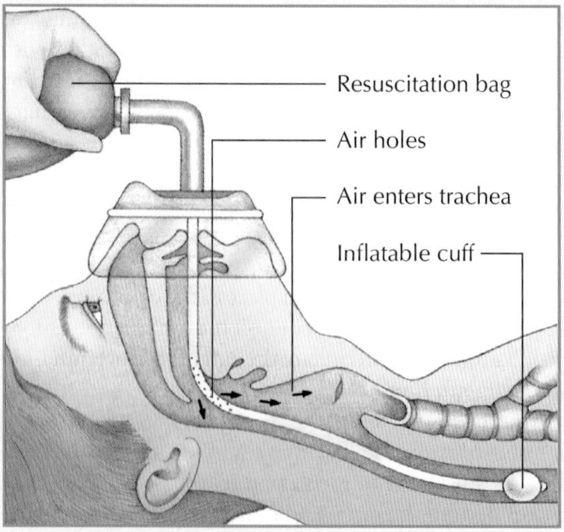

stomach contents are less likely to be aspirated when the esophageal tube is removed.

- Deflate the cuff on the esophageal tube by removing air from the inflation valve with a syringe. Don't try to remove the tube with the cuff inflated *because it may perforate the esophagus.*
- Turn the patient's head to the side, if possible, *to avoid aspiration.*
- Remove the EGTA or EOA in one swift, smooth motion, following the natural pharyngeal curve *to avoid esophageal trauma.*
- Perform oropharyngeal suctioning *to remove any residual secretions.*
- Assist the practitioner, as required, in monitoring and maintaining adequate ventilation for the patient.

Special considerations

- Store EGTAs and EOAs in the manufacturer's package until ready for use *to preserve their natural curve.*
- *To ease insertion,* you may prefer to direct the airway along the right side of the patient's mouth *because the esophagus is located to the right of and behind the trachea.* Or you may advance the tube tip upward toward the hard palate, and then invert the tip and glide it along the tongue surface and into the pharynx. *This keeps the tube centered, avoids snagging it on the sides of the throat, and eases insertion in the patient with clenched jaws.*
- Watch the unconscious patient as he regains consciousness. Explain the procedure to him, if possible, *to reduce his apprehension.* Observe also for retching; if it occurs, remove the airway immediately *because the accumulation of vomitus blocked by the airway cuff may perforate the esophagus. To help prevent complications,* don't leave the EOA in place for more than 2 hours.
- A mechanical ventilator attached to an ET or tracheostomy tube maintains more exact tidal volume than a mechanical ventilator attached to an esophageal airway.

Complications

EOAs may be inferior to endotracheal intubation in providing adequate oxygenation and ventilation. Esophageal airways may cause esophageal injuries, including rupture, and in semiconscious patients may cause laryngospasm, vomiting, and aspiration. The EOA doesn't prevent aspiration of foreign material from the mouth and pharynx into the trachea and bronchi. Tracheal occlusion can occur if the esophageal airway is inserted in the trachea.

Documentation

Record the date and time of the procedure, type of airway inserted, the patient's vital signs and level of consciousness, removal of the airway, alternative airway inserted after extubation, and complications and the nursing action taken.

Selected references

Abo, B.N., et al. "Does the Type of Out-of Hospital Airway Interfere with Other Cardiopulmonary Resuscitation Tasks?" *Resuscitation* 72(2):234-39, February 2007.

American Heart Association. "2005 American Heart Association Guidelines for Cardiopulmonary Resuscitation and Emergency Cardiovascular Care," *Circulation* 112(Suppl IV):VI-19-VI-34, December 2005.

Lynn-McHale Wiegand, D.J., and Carlson, K.K., eds. *AACN Procedure Manual for Critical Care*, 5th ed. Philadelphia: W.B. Saunders Co., 2006.

Smalley, A. "The Esophageal-Tracheal Double-Lumen Airway: Rescue for the Difficult Airway," *AANA Journal* 75(2):129-34, April 2007.

Oronasopharyngeal suction

Oronasopharyngeal suction removes secretions from the pharynx by a suction catheter inserted through the mouth or nostril. Used to maintain a patent airway, this procedure helps the patient who can't clear his airway effectively with coughing and expectoration, such as the unconscious or severely debilitated patient. The procedure should be done as often as necessary, depending on the patient's condition.

Because the catheter may inadvertently slip into the lower airway or esophagus, oronasopharyngeal suction is a sterile procedure that requires sterile equipment. However, clean technique may be used for a tonsil tip suction device. In fact, an alert patient can use a tonsil tip suction device himself to remove secretions.

Nasopharyngeal suctioning should be used with caution in patients who have nasopharyngeal bleeding or spinal fluid leakage into the nasopharyngeal area, in those who are receiving anticoagulant therapy, and in those who have blood dyscrasias because these conditions increase the risk of bleeding.

Equipment

Wall suction or portable suction apparatus unit ▪ connecting tubing ▪ water-soluble lubricant ▪ sterile normal saline solution ▪ disposable sterile container ▪ sterile suction catheter (a #10 to #16 French catheter for an adult, #8 or #10 French catheter for a child, or pediatric feeding tube for an infant) ▪ sterile gloves ▪ goggles ▪ clean gloves ▪ nasopharyngeal or oropharyngeal airway (optional for frequent suctioning) ▪ overbed table ▪ waterproof trash bag ▪ towel ▪ optional: tongue blade, tonsil tip suction device.

A commercially prepared kit contains a sterile catheter, disposable container, and sterile gloves.

Preparation of equipment

Before beginning, check your facility's policy to determine whether a practitioner's order is required for oropharyngeal suctioning. Also, review the patient's blood gas and oxygen saturation values, and check vital signs. Evaluate the patient's ability to cough and deep-breathe *to determine his ability to move secretions up the tracheobronchial tree.* Check his history for a deviated septum, nasal polyps, nasal obstruction, traumatic injury, epistaxis, or mucosal swelling.

If no contraindications exist, gather and place the suction equipment on the patient's overbed table or bedside stand. Position the table or stand on your preferred side of the bed *to facilitate suctioning.* Connect the tubing to the suctioning unit. Date and then open the bottle of normal saline solution. Open the waterproof trash bag.

Implementation

- Confirm the patient's identity using two patient identifiers according to your facility's policy.
- Explain the procedure to the patient even if he's unresponsive. Inform him that suctioning may stimulate transient coughing or gagging, but tell him that coughing helps to mobilize secretions. If he has been suctioned before, just summarize the reasons for the procedure. Reassure him throughout the procedure *to minimize anxiety and fear, which can increase oxygen consumption.* Also, ask which nostril is more patent.
- Wash your hands. Put on personal protective equipment, as appropriate.
- Place the patient in semi-Fowler's or high Fowler's position, if tolerated, *to promote lung expansion and effective coughing.* Consider increasing supplemental oxygen, as per your facility's protocol, prior to suctioning. If the patient is unconscious, position him on his side facing you *to help drainage of secretions.*
- Place a towel across the patient's chest.
- Turn on the suction from the wall or portable unit, and set the pressure according to your facility's policy. The pressure is usually set between 100 and 150 mm Hg; *higher pressures cause excessive trauma without enhancing secretion removal.* Occlude the end of the connecting tubing *to check suction pressure.*
- Using strict sterile technique, open the suction catheter kit or the packages containing the sterile catheter, disposable container, and gloves. Put on the gloves; consider your dominant hand sterile and your nondominant hand nonsterile. Using your nondominant hand, pour the sterile saline into the sterile container.
- With your nondominant hand, place a small amount of water-soluble lubricant on the sterile area. The lubricant is used *to facilitate passage of the catheter during nasopharyngeal suctioning.*
- Pick up the catheter with your dominant (sterile) hand, and attach it to the connecting tubing (as shown below). Use your nondominant hand to control the suction valve while your dominant hand manipulates the catheter.

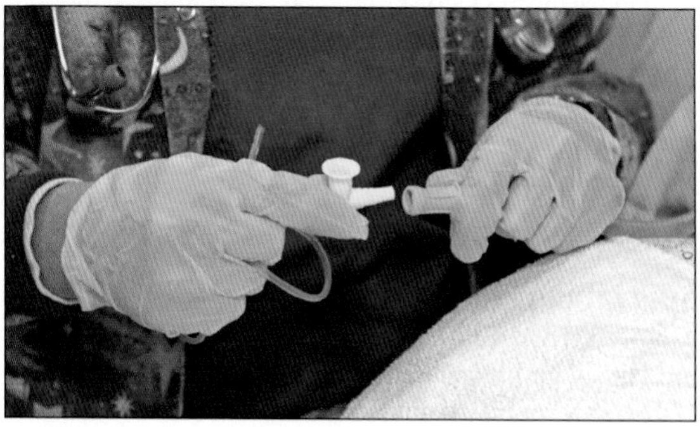

- Dip the catheter into the sterile saline *to moisten the inside of the catheter* (as shown below).

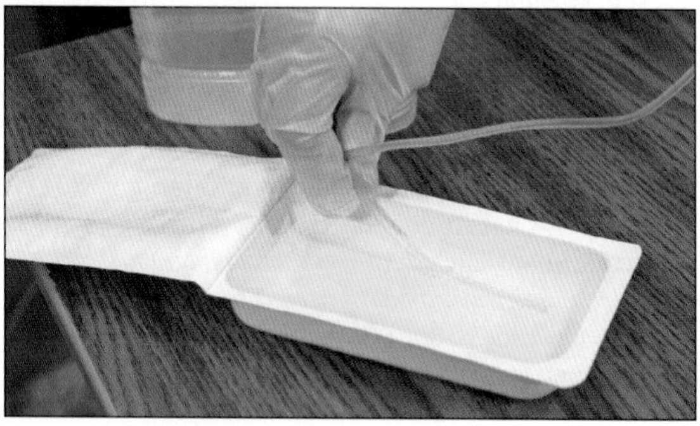

- Instruct the patient to cough and breathe slowly and deeply several times before beginning suction. Coughing helps loosen secretions and may decrease the amount of suctioning necessary, while deep breathing helps minimize or prevent hypoxia. (See *Airway clearance tips.*)

For nasal insertion

- Raise the tip of the patient's nose with your nondominant hand *to straighten the passageway and facilitate insertion of the catheter.* Without applying suction, gently insert the suction catheter into the patient's nares (as shown top of next page). Roll the catheter between your fingers *to help it advance through the turbinates.* Continue to advance the catheter approximately 5″ to 6″ (12.5 to 15 cm) until you reach the pool of secretions or the patient begins to cough.

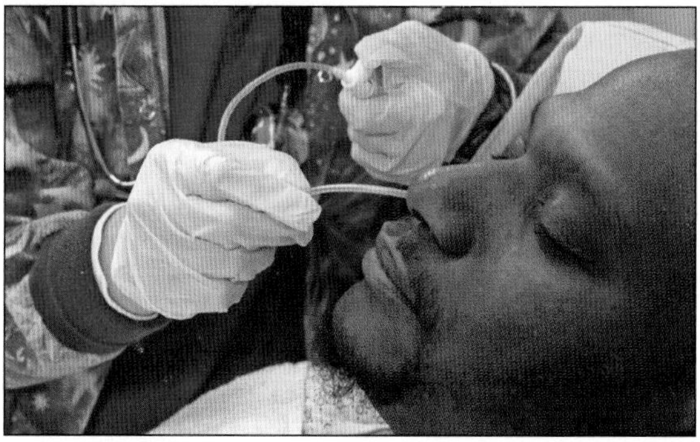

For oral insertion

■ Without applying suction, gently insert the catheter into the patient's mouth. Advance it 3″ to 4″ (7.5 to 10 cm) along the side of the patient's mouth until you reach the pool of secretions or the patient begins to cough. Suction both sides of the patient's mouth and pharyngeal area.
■ Using intermittent suction, withdraw the catheter from either the mouth or the nose with a continuous rotating motion *to minimize invagination of the mucosa into the catheter's tip and side ports.* Apply suction for only 10 to 15 seconds at a time *to minimize tissue trauma.*
■ Between passes, wrap the catheter around your dominant hand *to prevent contamination.*
■ If secretions are thick, clear the lumen of the catheter by dipping it in water and applying suction.
■ Repeat the procedure for up to 3 times until gurgling or bubbling sounds stop and respirations are quiet. Allow 30 seconds to 1 minute between attempts *to allow reoxygenation and reventilation.*
■ Flush the connecting tubing with normal saline solution.
■ After completing suctioning, pull off your sterile glove over the coiled catheter, and discard it and the nonsterile glove along with the container of saline.
■ Replace the used items *so they're ready for the next suctioning,* and wash your hands.

Special considerations

■ If the patient has no history of nasal problems, alternate suctioning between nostrils *to minimize traumatic injury.* If repeated oronasopharyngeal suctioning is required, the use of a nasopharyngeal or oropharyngeal airway will help with catheter insertion, reduce traumatic injury, and promote a patent airway. *To facilitate catheter insertion for oropharyngeal* suctioning, depress the patient's tongue with a tongue blade, or ask another nurse to do so. *This helps you to visualize the back of the throat and also prevents the patient from biting the catheter.*

Airway clearance tips

Deep breathing and coughing are vital for removing secretions from the lungs. Other techniques used to help clear the airways include diaphragmatic breathing and forced expiration. Here's how to teach these techniques to your patients.

Diaphragmatic breathing

First, tell the patient to lie supine, with his head elevated 15 to 20 degrees on a pillow. Tell him to place one hand on his abdomen and then inhale *so that he can feel his abdomen rise.* Explain that this is known as "breathing with the diaphragm."

Next, instruct the patient to exhale slowly through his nose — or, better yet, through pursed lips — while letting his abdomen collapse. Explain that this action decreases his respiratory rate and increases his tidal volume.

Suggest that the patient perform this exercise for 30 minutes several times per day. After he becomes accustomed to the position and has learned to breathe using his diaphragm, he may apply abdominal weights of 8.8 to 11 lb (4 to 5 kg). The weights enhance the movement of the diaphragm toward the head during expiration.

To enhance the effectiveness of exercise, the patient may also manually compress the lower costal margins, perform straight leg lifts, and coordinate the breathing technique with a physical activity such as walking.

Forced expiration

Explain to the patient that forced expiration (also known as *huff coughing*) helps clear secretions while causing less traumatic injury than does a cough. To perform the technique, tell the patient to forcefully expire without closing his glottis, starting with a mid- to low-lung volume. Tell him to follow this expiration with a period of diaphragmatic breathing and relaxation.

Inform the patient that if his secretions are in the central airways, he may have to use a more forceful expiration or a cough to clear them.

■ If the patient has excessive oral secretions, consider using a tonsil tip catheter *because this allows the patient to remove oral secretions independently.*
■ Let the patient rest after suctioning while you continue to observe him. Auscultate breath sounds *to determine effectiveness of procedure.* The frequency and duration of suc-

tioning depends on the patient's tolerance for the procedure and on any complications.

Home care

Oronasopharyngeal suctioning may be performed in the home using a portable suction machine. Under these circumstances, suctioning is a clean rather than a sterile procedure. Properly cleaned catheters can be reused, putting less financial strain on patients.

Catheters should be cleaned by first washing them in water with a detergent, followed by one of the following: a 60-minute soak in a solution of vinegar and water with an acetic acid content of 1.25% or greater; quaternary ammonium compound; gluteraldehyde or boiling water when possible. The catheters should then be rinsed with normal saline solution or tap water.

Whether the patient requires disposable or reusable suction equipment, you should make sure the patient and his caregivers have received proper teaching and support.

Complications

Increased dyspnea caused by hypoxia and anxiety may result from this procedure. Hypoxia can result because oxygen from the oronasopharynx is removed with the secretions. The amount of oxygen removed varies, depending upon the duration of the suctioning, suction flow and pressure, the size of the catheter in relation to the size of the patient's airway, and his physical condition.

In addition, bloody aspirate can result from prolonged or traumatic suctioning. Water-soluble lubricant can help to minimize traumatic injury.

Documentation

Record the date, time, reason for suctioning, and technique used; amount, color, consistency, and odor (if any) of the secretions; the patient's respiratory status before and after the procedure; complications and the nursing action taken; and the patient's tolerance for the procedure.

Selected references

American Association for Respiratory Care. "AARC Clinical Practice Guideline: Nasotracheal Suctioning," *Respiratory Care* 49(9):1080-1084, September 2004.

Cason, C.L., et al. "Nurses' Implementation of Guidelines for Ventilator-associated Pneumonia for the Centers for Disease Control and Prevention," *American Journal of Critical Care* 16(1):28-36, January 2007.

Centers for Disease Control and Prevention. "Guidelines for the Prevention of Health-care Associated Bacterial Pneumonia," *MMWR* 53(RR-3):3-10, March 2004.

Grap, M.J., and Munro, C.L. "Preventing Ventilator-associated Pneumonia: Evidence-based Care," *Critical Care Nursing Clinics of North America* 16(3):349-58, September 2004.

Lynn-McHale Wiegand, D.J., and Carlson, K.K., eds. *AACN Procedure Manual for Critical Care*, 5th ed. Philadelphia: W.B. Saunders Co., 2006.

Taylor, C., et al. *Fundamentals of Nursing: The Art and Science of Nursing Care*, 5th ed. Philadelphia: Lippincott Williams & Wilkins, 2008.

Endotracheal intubation

Endotracheal (ET) intubation involves the oral or nasal insertion of a flexible tube through the larynx into the trachea for the purposes of controlling the airway and mechanically ventilating the patient. Performed by a practitioner, anesthetist, respiratory therapist, or nurse educated in the procedure, ET intubation usually occurs in emergencies, such as cardiopulmonary arrest or in diseases such as epiglottitis. However, intubation may also occur under more controlled circumstances such as just before surgery. In such instances, ET intubation requires patient teaching and preparation.

The 2005 International Consensus Conference on Cardiopulmonary Resuscitation and Emergency Cardiovascular Care Science provides recommendations on the skill level needed to intubate, methods of confirming ET tube placement, and alternatives to intubation.

The guidelines recommend that only health care workers with adequate training and experience or frequent retraining should perform ET intubation. If a health care worker isn't authorized to perform ET intubation, alternative measures, such as a laryngeal mask airway or an esophageal-tracheal Combitube, may be used. These alternatives are less likely to cause aspiration than the use of a bag-mask.

Advantages of the procedure are that it establishes and maintains a patent airway, protects against aspiration by sealing off the trachea from the digestive tract, permits removal of tracheobronchial secretions in patients who can't cough effectively, and provides a route for mechanical ventilation. Disadvantages are that it bypasses normal respiratory defenses against infection, reduces cough effectiveness, and prevents verbal communication.

Oral ET intubation is contraindicated in patients with severe airway trauma or obstruction that won't permit safe passage of an endotracheal tube. It may also be contraindicated in cervical spine injury because the need for complete immobilization makes ET intubation difficult.

Equipment

Two ET tubes (one spare) in appropriate size ▪ 10-ml syringe ▪ stethoscope ▪ gloves ▪ lighted laryngoscope with a handle and blades of various sizes, curved and straight ▪ sedative ▪ local anesthetic spray ▪ mucosal vasoconstricting agent (for nasal intubation) ▪ overbed or other table ▪ water-soluble lubricant ▪ adhesive or other strong tape or commercial tube holder ▪ compound benzoin tincture ▪ goggles ▪ oral airway or bite block (for oral intubation) ▪ suction equipment ▪ handheld resuscitation bag with sterile swivel adapter ▪ humidified oxygen source ▪ carbon dioxide detector ▪ optional: prepackaged intubation tray, stylet.

Preparation of equipment

Quickly gather the individual supplies or use a prepackaged intubation tray, which will contain most of the necessary supplies. First, select an ET tube of the appropriate size—typically, 2.5 to 5.5 mm, uncuffed, for children and 6 to 10 mm, cuffed, for adults. The typical size of an oral tube is 7 to 8 mm for women and 8 to 9 mm for men. Select a slightly smaller tube for nasal intubation.

Check the light in the laryngoscope by snapping the appropriate-sized blade into place; if the bulb doesn't light, replace the batteries or the laryngoscope (whichever will be quicker).

Using sterile technique, open the package containing the ET tube and, if desired, open the other supplies on an overbed table. Pour the sterile water into the basin. Then, *to ease insertion,* you may lubricate the first 1″ (2.5 cm) of the distal end of the ET tube with the water-soluble lubricant, using sterile technique. Do this by squeezing the lubricant directly on the tube. Use only water-soluble lubricant *because it can be absorbed by mucous membranes.*

Next, attach the syringe to the port on the tube's exterior pilot cuff. Slowly inflate the cuff, observing for uniform inflation. Then use the syringe to deflate the cuff.

A stylet may be used on oral intubations *to stiffen the tube.* The entire stylet may be lubricated. Insert the stylet into the tube so that its distal tip lies about ½″ (1.3 cm) *inside* the distal end of the tube. Make sure the stylet doesn't protrude from the tube *to avoid vocal cord trauma.* Prepare the humidified oxygen source and the suction equipment for immediate use. If the patient is in bed, remove the headboard *to provide easier access.*

Implementation

- Administer sedatives, as ordered, *to induce amnesia or analgesia and help calm and relax the conscious patient.* Remove dentures and bridgework, if present.
- Hyperventilate with 100% oxygen using a handheld resuscitation bag; continue until the tube is inserted *to prevent hypoxia.*
- Place the patient supine in the sniffing position so that his mouth, pharynx, and trachea are extended. For a blind intubation, place the patient's head and neck in a neutral position.
- Put on gloves and personal protective equipment.
- For oral intubation, a local anesthetic (such as lidocaine) may be sprayed deep into the posterior pharynx *to diminish the gag reflex and reduce patient discomfort.* For nasal intubation, spray a local anesthetic and a mucosal vasoconstrictor into the nasal passages *to anesthetize the nasal turbinates and reduce the chance of bleeding.*
- If necessary, suction the patient's pharynx just before tube insertion *to improve visualization of the patient's pharynx and vocal cords.*
- Time each intubation attempt, limiting attempts to less than 30 seconds *to prevent hypoxia.* Hyperventilate the patient between attempts if necessary.

Intubation with direct visualization

- Stand at the head of the patient's bed. Using your right hand, hold the patient's mouth open by crossing your index finger over your thumb, placing your thumb on the patient's upper teeth and your index finger on his lower teeth. *This technique provides greater leverage.*
- Grasp the laryngoscope handle in your left hand, and gently slide the blade into the right side of the patient's mouth. Center the blade, and push the patient's tongue to the left. Hold the patient's lower lip away from his teeth *to prevent the lip from being traumatized.*
- Advance the blade *to expose the epiglottis.* When using a straight blade, insert the tip under the epiglottis; when using a curved blade, insert the tip between the base of the tongue and the epiglottis.
- Lift the laryngoscope handle upward and away from your body at a 45-degree angle *to reveal the vocal cords.* Avoid pivoting the laryngoscope against the patient's teeth *to avoid damaging them.*
- If desired, have an assistant apply pressure to the cricoid ring *to occlude the esophagus and minimize gastric regurgitation.*
- When performing an oral intubation, insert the ET tube into the right side of the patient's mouth. When performing a nasotracheal intubation, insert the ET tube through the nostril and into the pharynx.
- Guide the tube into the vertical openings of the larynx between the vocal cords, being careful not to mistake the horizontal opening of the esophagus for the larynx. If the vocal cords are closed because of a spasm, wait a few seconds for them to relax; then gently guide the tube past them *to avoid traumatic injury.*
- Advance the tube until the cuff disappears beyond the vocal cords. Avoid advancing the tube farther *to avoid occluding a major bronchus and precipitating lung collapse.*

■ Holding the ET tube in place, quickly remove the stylet, if present.

Blind nasotracheal intubation

■ Pass the ET tube along the floor of the nasal cavity. If necessary, use gentle force to pass the tube through the nasopharynx and into the pharynx.

■ Listen and feel for air movement through the tube as it's advanced *to ensure that the tube is properly place in the airway.*

■ Slip the tube between the vocal cords when the patient inhales *because the vocal cords separate on inhalation.*

■ When the tube is past the vocal cords, the breath sounds should become louder. If, at any time during tube advancement, breath sounds disappear, withdraw the tube until they reappear.

After intubation

■ Remove the laryngoscope. If the patient was intubated orally, insert an oral airway or a bite block *to prevent the patient from obstructing airflow or puncturing the tube with his teeth.*

■ Inflate the tube's cuff with 5 to 10 cc of air until you feel resistance. When the patient is mechanically ventilated, you'll use the minimal-leak technique or the minimal occlusive volume technique to establish correct inflation of the cuff. (For instructions, see "Tracheal cuff–pressure measurement," page 550.)

■ Confirm ET tube placement by listening for bilateral breath sounds, observing chest expansion, and using techniques, such as capnography or capnometry.

■ The 2005 American Heart Association guidelines recommend confirming ET tube placement using techniques other than physical examination, such as esophageal detector devices, qualitative end-tidal carbon dioxide indicators, and capnographic and capnometric devices. Be aware that devices that rely on exhaled carbon dioxide may not be accurate in patients in cardiac arrest *because of reduced lung perfusion* and in patients with large amounts of dead space in the lungs such as a patient with a large pulmonary embolus. Other methods that complement nonphysical examination techniques include observing for bilateral chest expansion, auscultating for bilateral breath sounds or an absence of abdominal sounds, feeling for warm exhalations, and observing for condensation in the ET tube.

■ If you don't hear any breath sounds, auscultate over the stomach while ventilating with the resuscitation bag. *Stomach distention, belching, or a gurgling sound indicates esophageal intubation.* Immediately deflate the cuff and remove the tube. After reoxygenating the patient *to prevent hypoxia,* repeat insertion using a sterile tube *to prevent contamination of the trachea.*

■ Auscultate bilaterally *to exclude the possibility of endobronchial intubation.* If you fail to hear breath sounds on both sides of the chest, you may have inserted the tube into one of the mainstem bronchi (usually the right one *because of its wider angle at the bifurcation*); such insertion occludes the other bronchus and lung and results in atelectasis on the obstructed side. Or the tube may be resting on the carina, resulting in dry secretions that obstruct both bronchi. (The patient's coughing and fighting the ventilator will alert you to the problem.) *To correct these situations,* deflate the cuff, withdraw the tube 1 to 2 mm, auscultate for bilateral breath sounds, and reinflate the cuff.

■ When you've confirmed correct tube placement, administer oxygen or initiate mechanical ventilation, and suction, if indicated.

■ *To secure tube position,* apply compound benzoin tincture to each cheek and let it dry. Tape the tube firmly with adhesive or other strong tape or use a commercial tube holder. (See *Methods to secure an ET tube.*)

■ Clearly note the centimeter marking on the tube where it exits the patient's mouth or nose. *By periodically monitoring this mark, you can detect tube displacement.*

■ Make sure a chest X-ray is taken *to verify tube position.*

■ Place a swivel adapter between the tube and the humidified oxygen source *to allow for intermittent suctioning and to reduce tube tension.*

■ Place the patient on his side with his head in a comfortable position *to avoid tube kinking and airway obstruction.*

■ Auscultate both sides of the chest, and watch chest movement as indicated by the patient's condition *to ensure correct tube placement and full lung ventilation.* Provide frequent oral care to the orally intubated patient, and position the ET tube *to prevent formation of pressure ulcers and avoid excessive pressure on the sides of the mouth.* Provide frequent nasal and oral care to the nasally intubated patient *to prevent formation of pressure ulcers and drying of oral mucous membranes.*

■ Suction secretions through the ET tube as the patient's condition indicates *to clear secretions and prevent mucus plugs from obstructing the tube.*

Special considerations

■ Orotracheal intubation is preferred in emergencies *because insertion is easier and faster than it is with nasotracheal intubation.* However, maintaining exact tube placement is more difficult, and the tube must be well secured *to avoid kinking and prevent bronchial obstruction or accidental extubation.* Orotracheal intubation is also poorly tolerated by the conscious patient because it stimulates salivation, coughing, and retching.

Methods to secure an ET tube

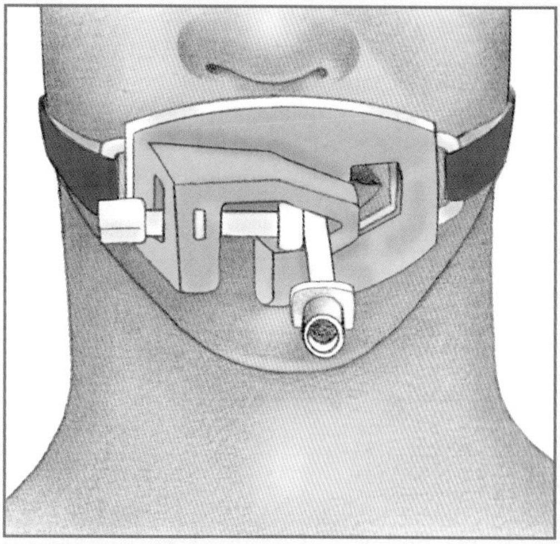

An endotracheal (ET) tube should be secured with a tracheal tube holder for either the adult or infant patient, as recommended by the American Heart Association and American Pediatric Association. Alternatively, the tube may be taped in place to prevent dislodgment.

Before securing an ET tube in place, make sure the patient's face is clean, dry, and free of beard stubble. If possible, suction his mouth and dry the tube just before taping. Check the reference mark on the tube *to ensure correct placement.* After securing, always check for bilateral breath sounds *to ensure that the tube hasn't been displaced by manipulation.*

To secure the tube, use one of the following methods.

Method 1

ET tube holders are available that help secure a tracheal tube in place. Made of hard plastic or of softer materials, the tube holder is a convenient way to secure an ET tube in place. The tube holder is available in adult and pediatric sizes, and some models may come with bite blocks attached. The strap is placed around the patient's neck and secured around the tube with Velcro fasteners. *Because each model is different,* check with the manufacturer's guidelines for correct placement and care.

(continued)

- Nasotracheal intubation is preferred for elective insertion when the patient is capable of spontaneous ventilation for a short period. Blind intubation is typically used in conscious patients who risk imminent respiratory arrest or who have cervical spinal injury.
- Although nasotracheal intubation is more comfortable than oral intubation, it's also more difficult to perform. *Because the tube passes blindly through the nasal cavity,* the procedure causes greater tissue trauma, increases the risk of infection by nasal bacteria introduced into the trachea, and risks pressure necrosis of the nasal mucosa. However, exact tube placement is easier, and the risk of dislodgment is lower. The cuff on the ET tube maintains a closed system that permits positive-pressure ventilation and protects the airway from aspiration of secretions and gastric contents.
- Although low-pressure cuffs have significantly reduced the incidence of tracheal erosion and necrosis caused by cuff pressure on the tracheal wall, overinflation of a low-pressure cuff can negate the benefit. Use the minimal-leak technique to avoid these complications. Inflating the cuff a bit more to make a complete seal with the least amount of air is the next most desirable method.
- Always record the volume of air needed to inflate the cuff. A gradual increase in this volume indicates tracheal dilatation or erosion. A sudden increase in volume indicates rupture of the cuff and requires immediate reintubation if the patient is being ventilated or if he requires continuous cuff inflation to maintain a high concentration of delivered oxygen. When the cuff has been inflated, measure its pressure at least every 8 hours *to avoid overinflation.* Normal cuff pressure is about 18 mm Hg.
- When neither method of endotracheal intubation is possible, consider the alternative of retrograde intubation. (See *Retrograde intubation: An alternative form of airway maintenance,* page 544.)

Complications

Endotracheal intubation can result in apnea caused by reflex breath-holding or interruption of oxygen delivery; bronchospasm; aspiration of blood, secretions, or gastric contents; tooth damage or loss; and injury to the lips, mouth, pharynx, or vocal cords. It can also result in laryngeal edema and erosion and in tracheal stenosis, erosion, and necro-

(Text continues on page 544.)

Methods to secure an ET tube *(continued)*

Method 2

Cut two 2″ (5-cm) strips and two 15″ (38.1-cm) strips of 1″ cloth adhesive tape. Then cut a 13″ (33-cm) slit in one end of each 15″ strip (as shown below). (Some facilities require the tape to encircle the patient's head; check your facility's policy and procedure manual.)

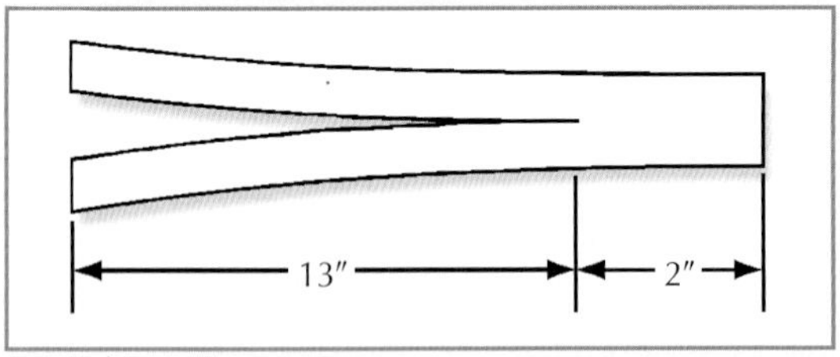

Apply compound benzoin tincture to the patient's cheeks. Place the 2″ strips on his cheeks, creating a new surface on which to anchor the tape securing the tube. When frequent retaping is necessary, this helps preserve the patient's skin integrity. If the patient's skin is excoriated or at risk, you can use a transparent semipermeable dressing to protect the skin.

Apply the benzoin tincture to the tape on the patient's face and to the part of the tube where you'll be applying the tape. On the side of the mouth where the tube will be anchored, place the unslit end of the long tape on top of the tape on the patient's cheek.

Wrap the top half of the tape around the tube twice, pulling the tape tightly around the tube. Then, directing the tape over the patient's upper lip, place the end of the tape on his other cheek. Cut off any excess tape. Use the lower half of the tape to secure an oral airway, if necessary (as shown above right).

Or twist the lower half of the tape around the tube twice, and attach it to the original cheek (as shown top of next column). *Taping in opposite directions places equal traction on the tube.*

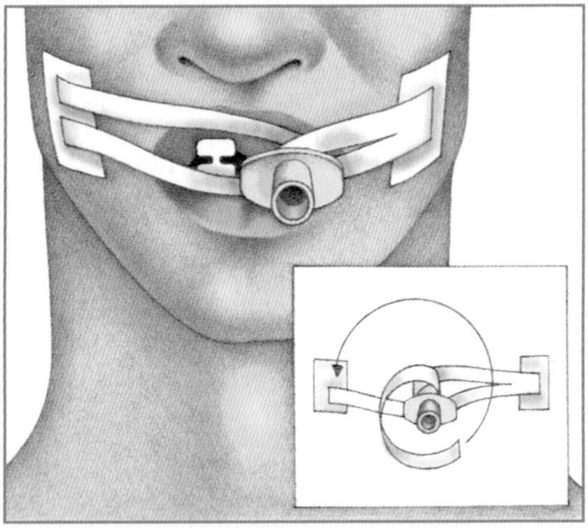

If you've taped in an oral airway or are concerned about the tube's stability, apply the other 15″ strip of tape in the same manner, starting on the other side of the patient's face (as shown below). If the tape around the tube is too bulky, use only the upper part of the tape and cut off the lower part. If the patient has copious oral secretions, seal the tape by cutting a 1″ piece of paper tape, coating it with benzoin tincture, and placing the paper tape over the adhesive tape.

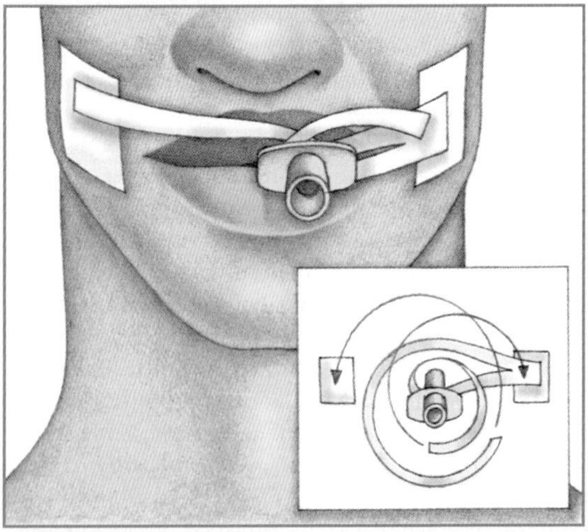

Methods to secure an ET tube *(continued)*

Method 3

Cut one piece of 1″ cloth adhesive tape long enough to wrap around the patient's head and overlap in front. Then cut an 8″ (20.3-cm) piece of tape and center it on the longer piece, sticky sides together. Next, cut a 5″ (12.7-cm) slit in each end of the longer tape (as shown below).

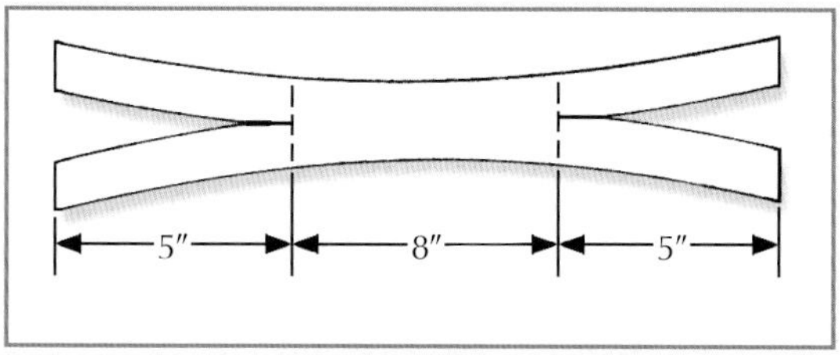

Apply benzoin tincture to the patient's cheeks, under his nose, and under his lower lip. Don't spray benzoin directly on his face *because the vapors can be irritating if inhaled and can also harm the eyes.*

Place the top half of one end of the tape under the patient's nose, and wrap the lower half around the ET tube. Place the lower half of the other end of the tape along his lower lip, and wrap the top half around the tube (as shown below).

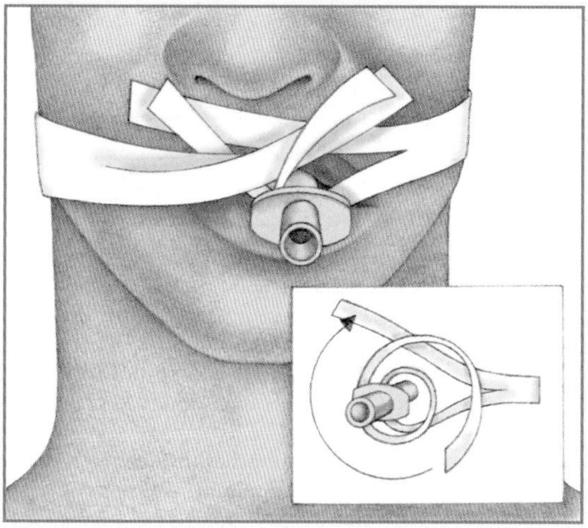

Method 4

Cut a tracheostomy tie in two pieces, one a few inches longer than the other, and cut two 6″ (15.2-cm) pieces of 1″ cloth adhesive tape. Then cut a 2″ slit in one end of both pieces of tape. Fold back the other end of the tape ½″ (1.3 cm) so that the sticky sides are together, and cut a small hole in it (as shown below).

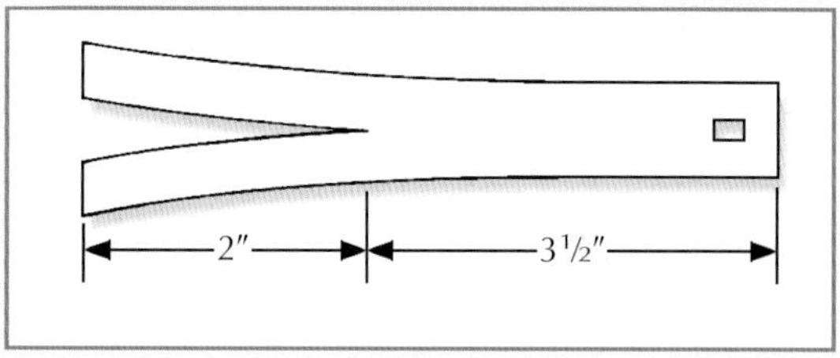

Apply benzoin tincture to the part of the ET tube that will be taped. Wrap the split ends of each piece of tape around the tube, one piece on each side. Overlap the tape to secure it.

Apply the free ends of the tape to both sides of the patient's face. Then insert tracheostomy ties through the holes in the tape and knot the ties (as shown below).

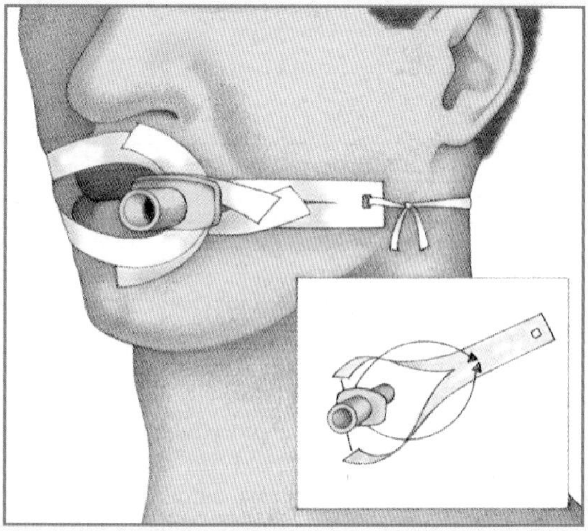

Bring the longer tie behind the patient's neck. *Knotting the ties on the side prevents the patient from lying on the knot and developing a pressure ulcer.*

Retrograde intubation: An alternative form of airway maintenance

When a patient's airway can't be secured using conventional oral or nasal intubation, retrograde intubation should be considered. In this technique, a wire is inserted through the trachea and out the mouth and is then used to guide the insertion of an endotracheal (ET) tube (as shown below).

The procedure has numerous advantages: It requires little or no head movement, it's less invasive than cricothyrotomy or tracheotomy and doesn't leave a permanent scar, and it doesn't require direct visualization of the vocal cords. However, only physicians, nurses, and paramedics who've been specially trained may perform retrograde intubation.

Retrograde intubation is contraindicated in patients with complete airway obstruction, a thyroid tumor, an enlarged thyroid gland that overlies the cricothyroid ligament, or coagulopathy and in those whose mouths can't open wide enough to allow the guide wire to be retrieved. Possible complications include minor bleeding and hematoma formation at the puncture site, subcutaneous emphysema, hoarseness, and bleeding into the trachea.

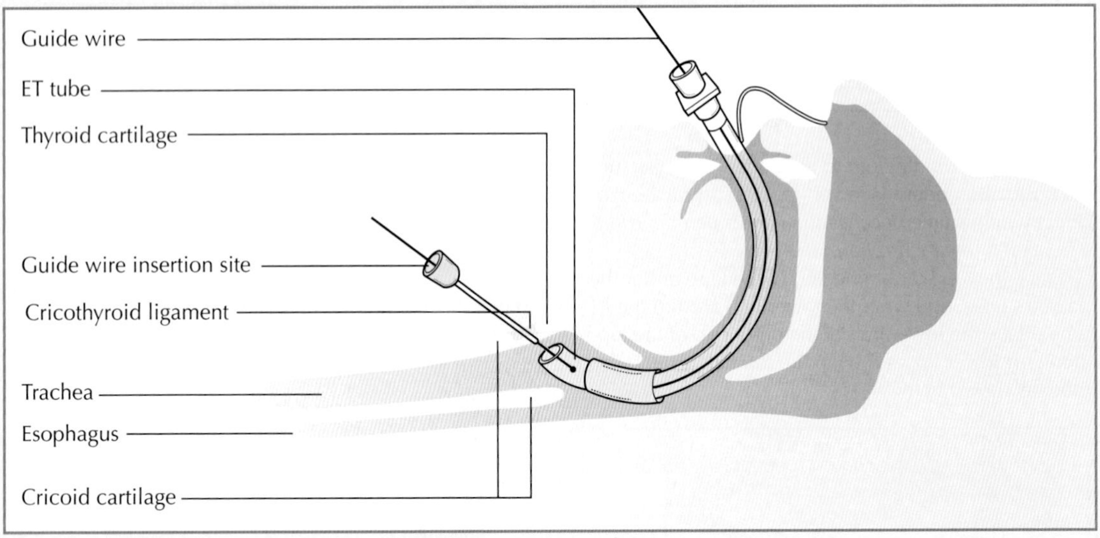

sis. Nasotracheal intubation can result in nasal bleeding, laceration, sinusitis, and otitis media.

Documentation

Record the date and time of the procedure; its indication and success or failure; tube type and size; cuff size and location in centimeters at the lip area, amount of inflation, and inflation technique; administration of medication; initiation of supplemental oxygen or ventilation therapy; results of chest auscultation and results of the chest X-ray; complications and interventions; and the patient's reaction to the procedure.

SELECTED REFERENCES

American Heart Association. "2005 AHA Guidelines for Cardiopulmonary Resuscitation and Emergency Cardiovascular Care: International Consensus on Science," *Circulation* 112(22 Suppl): IV-1-IV-211, November 2005.

Lynn-McHale Wiegand, D.J., and Carlson, K.K., eds. *AACN Procedure Manual for Critical Care,* 5th ed. Philadelphia: W.B. Saunders Co., 2005.

Weitzel, N., et al. "Blind Nasotracheal Intubation for Patients with Penetrating Neck Trauma," *Journal of Trauma* 56(5):1097-101, May 2004.

Werner, S.L., et al. "Pilot Study to Evaluate the Accuracy of Ultrasonography in Confirming Endotracheal Tube Placement," *Annals of Emergency Medicine* 49(1):75-80, January 2007.

ENDOTRACHEAL TUBE CARE

The intubated patient requires meticulous care to ensure airway patency and prevent complications until he can maintain independent ventilation. This care includes frequent assessment of airway status, maintenance of proper cuff pressure to prevent tissue ischemia and necrosis, repositioning of the tube to avoid traumatic manipulation, and constant monitoring for complications. Endotracheal (ET) tubes are repositioned for patient comfort or if a chest X-ray shows improper placement. Move the tube from one side of the mouth to the other to prevent pressure ulcers.

Equipment

For maintaining the airway: Stethoscope ▪ suction equipment ▪ gloves.

For repositioning the tube: 10-ml syringe ▪ compound benzoin tincture ▪ stethoscope ▪ adhesive or hypoallergenic tape or commercial tube holder ▪ suction equipment ▪ sedative or 2% lidocaine ▪ gloves ▪ handheld resuscitation bag with mask (in case of accidental extubation).

For removing the tube: 10-ml syringe ▪ suction equipment ▪ supplemental oxygen source with mask ▪ cool-mist large-volume nebulizer ▪ handheld resuscitation bag with mask ▪ gloves ▪ equipment for reintubation.

Preparation of equipment

For repositioning the ET tube: Assemble all equipment at the patient's bedside. Using sterile technique, set up the suction equipment.

For removing the ET tube: Assemble all equipment at the patient's bedside. Set up the suction and supplemental oxygen equipment. Have all equipment ready for emergency reintubation.

Implementation

- Confirm the patient's identity using two patient identifiers according to your facility's policy.
- Explain the procedure to the patient even if he doesn't appear to be alert.
- Provide privacy, wash your hands thoroughly, and put on gloves.

Maintaining airway patency

- Auscultate the patient's lungs regularly and at any sign of respiratory distress. If you detect an obstructed airway, determine the cause and treat it accordingly. If secretions are obstructing the lumen of the tube, suction the secretions from the tube. (See "Tracheal suction," page 561)
- If the ET tube has slipped from the trachea into the right or left mainstem bronchus, breath sounds will be absent over one lung. Obtain a chest X-ray as ordered *to verify tube placement* and, if necessary, carefully reposition the tube.

Repositioning the ET tube

- Get help from a respiratory therapist or another nurse *to prevent accidental extubation during the procedure if the patient coughs.*
- Hyperoxygenate the patient, then suction the patient's trachea through the ET tube to remove any secretions, *which can cause the patient to cough during the procedure. Coughing increases the risk of trauma and tube dislodgment.* Then suction the patient's pharynx *to remove any secretions that may have accumulated above the tube cuff. This helps to prevent aspiration of secretions during cuff deflation.*
- *To prevent traumatic manipulation of the tube,* instruct the assisting nurse to hold it as you carefully untape the tube or unfasten the commercial tube holder. When freeing the tube, locate a landmark such as a number on the tube or measure the distance from the patient's mouth to the top of the tube *so that you have a reference point when moving the tube.*
- Next, deflate the cuff by attaching a 10-ml syringe to the pilot balloon port and aspirating air until you meet resistance and the pilot balloon deflates. Deflate the cuff before moving the tube *because the cuff forms a seal within the trachea and movement of an inflated cuff can damage the tracheal wall and vocal cords.*
- Reposition the tube as necessary, noting new landmarks or measuring the length. Then immediately reinflate the cuff. To do this, instruct the patient to inhale, and slowly inflate the cuff using a 10-ml syringe attached to the pilot balloon port. As you do this, use your stethoscope to auscultate the patient's neck *to determine the presence of an air leak.* When air leakage ceases, stop cuff inflation and, while still auscultating the patient's neck, aspirate a small amount of air until you detect a slight leak. *This creates a minimal air leak, which indicates that the cuff is inflated at the lowest pressure possible to create an adequate seal.* If the patient is being mechanically ventilated, aspirate to create a minimal air leak during the inspiratory phase of respiration *because the positive pressure of the ventilator during inspiration will create a larger leak around the cuff.* Note the number of cubic centimeters of air required to achieve a minimal air leak.
- Measure cuff pressure, and compare the reading with previous pressure readings *to prevent overinflation.* Then use benzoin and tape to secure the tube in place, or refasten the commercial tube holder.
- Make sure the patient is comfortable and the airway patent. Properly clean or dispose of equipment.
- When the cuff is inflated, measure its pressure at least every 8 hours to avoid overinflation. (See "Tracheal cuff–pressure measurement," page 550.)

■ Auscultate the lungs to ensure bilateral breath sounds.

Removing the ET tube

■ When you're authorized to remove the tube, obtain another nurse's assistance *to prevent traumatic manipulation of the tube when it's untaped or unfastened.*

■ Elevate the head of the patient's bed to approximately 90 degrees.

■ Suction the patient's oropharynx and nasopharynx *to remove any accumulated secretions and to help prevent aspiration of secretions when the cuff is deflated.*

■ Using a handheld resuscitation bag or the mechanical ventilator, give the patient several deep breaths through the ET tube *to hyperinflate his lungs and increase his oxygen reserve.*

■ Attach a 10-ml syringe to the pilot balloon port, and aspirate air until you meet resistance and the pilot balloon deflates. If you fail to detect an air leak around the deflated cuff, notify the practitioner immediately and don't proceed with extubation. *Absence of an air leak may indicate marked tracheal edema, which can result in total airway obstruction if the ET tube is removed.*

■ If you detect the proper air leak, untape or unfasten the ET tube while the assisting nurse stabilizes the tube.

■ Insert a sterile suction catheter through the ET tube. Then apply suction and ask the patient to take a deep breath and to open his mouth fully and pretend to cry out. *This causes abduction of the vocal cords and reduces the risk of laryngeal trauma during withdrawal of the tube.*

■ Simultaneously remove the ET tube and the suction catheter in one smooth, outward and downward motion, following the natural curve of the patient's mouth. *Suctioning during extubation removes secretions retained at the end of the tube and prevents aspiration.*

■ Give the patient supplemental oxygen. For maximum humidity, use a cool-mist, large-volume nebulizer *to help decrease airway irritation, patient discomfort, and laryngeal edema.*

■ Encourage the patient to cough and deep-breathe. Remind him that a sore throat and hoarseness are to be expected and will gradually subside.

■ Make sure the patient is comfortable and the airway is patent. Clean or dispose of equipment.

■ After extubation, auscultate the patient's lungs frequently and watch for signs of respiratory distress. Be especially alert for stridor or other evidence of upper airway obstruction. If ordered, draw an arterial sample for blood gas analysis.

Special considerations

■ When repositioning an ET tube, be especially careful in patients with highly sensitive airways. Sedation or direct instillation of 2% lidocaine to numb the airway may be indicated in such patients. *Because the lidocaine is absorbed systemically,* you must have a practitioner's order to use it.

■ After extubation of a patient who has been intubated for an extended time, keep reintubation supplies readily available for at least 12 hours or until you're sure he can tolerate extubation.

■ Never extubate a patient unless someone skilled at intubation is readily available.

■ If you inadvertently cut the pilot balloon on the cuff, immediately call the person responsible for intubation in your facility, who will remove the damaged ET tube and replace it with one that's intact. Don't remove the tube *because a tube with an air leak is better than no airway.*

Complications

Traumatic injury to the larynx or trachea may result from tube manipulation, accidental extubation, or tube slippage into the right bronchus. Ventilatory failure and airway obstruction, due to laryngospasm or marked tracheal edema, are the gravest possible complications of extubation.

Documentation

After tube repositioning, record the date and time of the procedure, reason for repositioning (such as malpositioning shown by chest X-ray), new tube position, total amount of air in the cuff after the procedure, complications and interventions, and the patient's tolerance of the procedure. Document the physical findings and nonphysical examination to confirm tube placement.

After extubation, record the date and time of extubation, presence or absence of stridor or other signs of upper airway edema, type of supplemental oxygen administered, complications and required subsequent therapy, and the patient's tolerance of the procedure.

SELECTED REFERENCES

Akca, O. "Endotracheal Tube Cuff Leak: Can Optimum Management of Cuff Pressure Prevent Pneumonia?" *Critical Care Medicine* 35(6):1624-626, June 2007.

American Heart Association. "2005 AHA Guidelines for Cardiopulmonary Resuscitation and Emergency Cardiovascular Care: International Consensus on Science," *Circulation* 112(22 Suppl):IV-1-IV-211, November 2005.

Birkett, K.M., et al. "Reporting Unplanned Extubation," *Intensive and Critical Care Nursing* 21(2):65-75, April 2005.

Centers for Disease Control and Prevention. "Guidelines for Preventing Health-care-associated Pneumonia, 2003: Recommendations of CDC and the Healthcare Infection Control Practices Advisory Committee," *MMWR* 53(RR-3):1-36, March 2004.

Chao, D.C., and Scheinhorn, D.J. "Determining the Best Threshold of Rapid Shallow Breathing Index in a Therapist-Implemented Patient-Specific Weaning Protocol," *Respiratory Care* 52(2):159-65, February 2007.

"Evidence-Based Guidelines for Weaning and Discontinuing Ventilatory Support: A Collective Task Force Facilitated by the American College of Chest Physicians, the American Association for Respiratory Care, and the American College of Critical Care Medicine," *Respiratory Care* 47(1):69-90, January 2002.

Frutos-Vivar, F., et al. "Risk Factors for Extubation Failure in Patients Following a Successful Spontaneous Breathing Trial," *Chest* 130(6):1664-671, December 2006.

Lynn-McHale Wiegand, D.J., and Carlson, K.K., eds. *AACN Procedure Manual for Critical Care,* 5th ed. Philadelphia: W.B. Saunders Co., 2005.

Vollman, K. "Oral Hygiene in the Intubated Patient," *Critical Care Nurse* 26(4):54, August 2006.

LARYNGEAL MASK AIRWAY INSERTION

The laryngeal mask airway (LMA) is used to establish and maintain a patent airway in the unconscious patient. It is used extensively in the operating room by anesthesia personnel and is also appropriate for emergency airway and ventilatory support when endotracheal intubation is not immediately possible. The laryngeal mask airway may also be used in place of a face mask during adult, pediatric, and neonatal resuscitation.

The LMA consists of a semi-rigid tube attached to a silicone mask. The mask is placed into the patient's mouth and advanced blindly until it rests above the larynx. The patient may then breathe spontaneously or be assisted with moderate positive pressure ventilation.

The LMA doesn't protect the patient from regurgitation and aspiration; therefore, it should be used in patients with full stomachs only in emergency situations where intubation isn't possible, or if ventilation by face mask is ineffective. In addition, the LMA should only be inserted into the patient who has lost protective cough and gag reflexes. The LMA should also be used cautiously in the patient with delayed gastric emptying due to the risk of regurgitation.

There are a number of different types of LMAs available. Those most common types used outside of the operating room include the reusable type, which must be cleaned and sterilized between uses; or the disposable (single patient use) type. In addition, an intubating LMA is available and may be used to initially provide a patent airway and then facilitate endotracheal intubation.

Equipment

Appropriately sized LMA based on patient's weight (reusable, disposable, or intubating) (see *LMA specifications,* page 548) ▪ syringe of appropriate size for inflating cuff ▪ water-soluble lubricant ▪ nonsterile gloves and other personal protective equipment ▪ oxygen equipment ▪ tape or device to secure tube ▪ bag-valve or mouth-to-mask device ▪ bite block ▪ stethoscope ▪ suction equipment ▪ pulse oximetry, if available ▪ capnometer, if available.

Preparation of equipment

While the equipment is being prepared, ventilate and oxygenate the patient with a bag-valve or mouth-to-mouth mask device, if necessary. Remove the LMA from its package and visually inspect it for discoloration, cracks, or kinks in the tube; also make sure it's the right size. Inspect the airway opening and check that the aperture bars are intact. Manually tighten the connector, if needed. Test the patency of the cuff by first withdrawing all air and then overinflating it with air injected through the pilot balloon. While inflated, visually inspect the cuff for symmetry, then deflate the cuff. Don't use the LMA if it's leaking air or asymmetry of the cuff is noted when inflated. Assemble suction equipment and check that it's working properly.

Implementation

- If this is a planned procedure, verify the order in the patient's medical record.
- Confirm the patient's identity using two patient identifiers according to your facility's policy.
- Assess the patient's level of consciousness *because the LMA shouldn't be inserted into a patient who may resist insertion.*
- Wash your hands.
- Put on gloves and personal protective equipment.
- Teach the family about the procedure, as the patient's condition allows, *to provide them with information and reduce anxiety.*
- Lubricate the posterior surface of the LMA, using a water-soluble lubricant, *to ease insertion.* Avoid getting the lubricant on the anterior surface of the cuff *because this increases the risk of it being aspirated.*
- Place the patient in the supine position with a folded towel or blanket under the head to flex the neck and extend the head (the "sniffing position") *to ease insertion of the LMA.*
- Stand behind the patient's head and place the nondominant hand under the patient's head, lifting the head slightly and keeping upward pressure.
- Hold the LMA in the dominant hand like a pencil, with the index finger placed at the junction of the mask and the tube. The lumen of the LMA should be facing up, with the

EQUIPMENT

LMA specifications

The following chart will help guide you in choosing the right size laryngeal mask airway (LMA) for your patient.

Size	Patient weight	Maximal cuff inflation volume	Overinflation volume for cuff test
1	Up to 5 kg	4 ml	8 ml
1½	5 to 10 kg	7 ml	10 ml
2	10 to 20 kg	10 ml	15 ml
2½	20 to 30 kg	14 ml	21 ml
3	30 to 50 kg	20 ml	30 ml
4	50 to 70 kg	30 ml	45 ml
5	70 to 100 kg	40 ml	60 ml
6	Greater than 100 kg	50 ml	75 ml

lubricated posterior surface facing the floor. (See *Inserting the LMA.*)

■ Flex the wrist fully so that the tip of the LMA points toward the patient's head and down and insert the tip of the LMA into the patient's mouth.

■ Press the posterior surface of the LMA against the hard palate and advance it into the oropharynx. *By applying pressure up against the hard palate, the LMA will advance to the proper position.*

■ Use the middle finger to open the patient's jaw and check that the cuff is compressed against the hard palate. If the cuff isn't flattened against the hard palate, remove the LMA and insert it again.

■ While maintaining pressure on the LMA so that it stays pressed against the hard palate, extend the index finger fully while continuing to advance the LMA until resistance is met. The LMA should now be in the correct position.

■ Remove the nondominant hand from under the patient's head, and use it to hold the LMA in place while removing the index finger. *This keeps the LMA in place while the index finger of the dominant hand is removed from the patient's mouth.*

■ Without holding the LMA, use the syringe to inflate the cuff to an intracuff pressure of about 60 cm H_2O. Only one-half the maximum inflation volume is required to make a seal. Don't overinflate the cuff. *Inflating the cuff without holding the tube allows it to settle itself into the correct position during cuff inflation.*

■ Check the mouth to make sure the cuff isn't visible, and observe for minor outward movement of the tube and minor neck bulging in the area of the cricothyroid, *indicating proper tube placement and cuff inflation.*

■ Verify correct placement by auscultation of bilateral breath sounds using a stethoscope, and by monitoring through pulse oximetry or capnography, if available.

■ Use a bag-valve device connected to an oxygen source, if indicated, to gently deliver ventilations using a peak airway pressure less than 20 cm H_2O and a tidal volume of 8 ml/kg of body weight or less. *Using low pressure ventilations avoids exceeding cuff pressure and reduces the risk of forcing air into the stomach.*

■ Insert a bite block *to keep the patient from biting on the tube causing it to become occluded or move out of proper position.*

■ Tape the LMA and bite block securely to the patient's face or use a commercial device to secure the tube.

Special considerations

■ If there's a risk that the patient may have neck trauma, insert the LMA with the patient's neck in a neutral position.

■ Introducers from the manufacturer may be available to assist with insertion. In that case, the introducer is used in place of the index finger. The introducer maintains contact between the posterior aspect of the tube and the patient's hard palate, and should be used according to the manufacturer's instructions.

■ Never use extreme force when inserting a LMA.

■ If there's any concern about the final placement of the LMA, the device should be removed and repositioned.

■ Avoid use of the LMA in patients who need high pressures for ventilation as the LMA has a low pressure seal, which may be ineffective when used with these high pressures.

Inserting the LMA

Use the following steps to correctly insert an LMA.

Hold the laryngeal mask airway (LMA) with your dominant hand, using the index finger and thumb to grasp the tube behind the cuff.

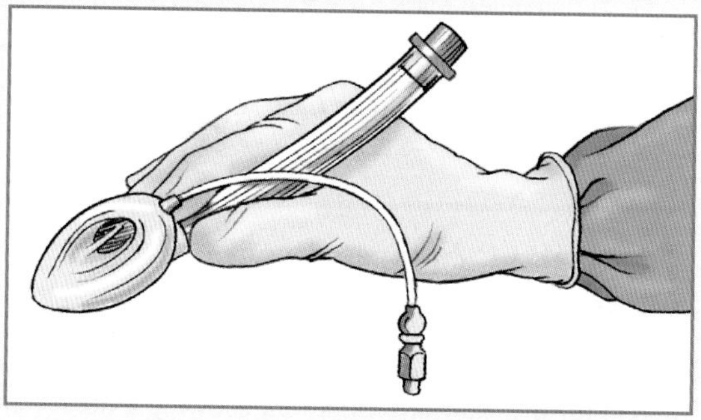

Then extend the patient's head while flexing the neck and flatten the LMA against the patient's hard palate. Use your middle finger to gently press down on the patient's jaw.

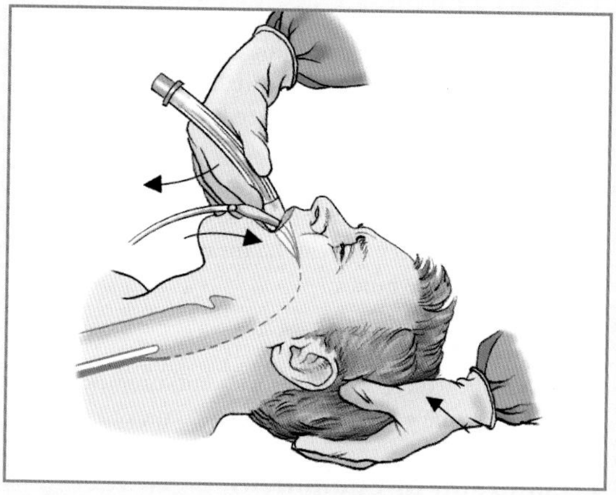

Use your index finger to insert the LMA, while following the hard and soft palates.

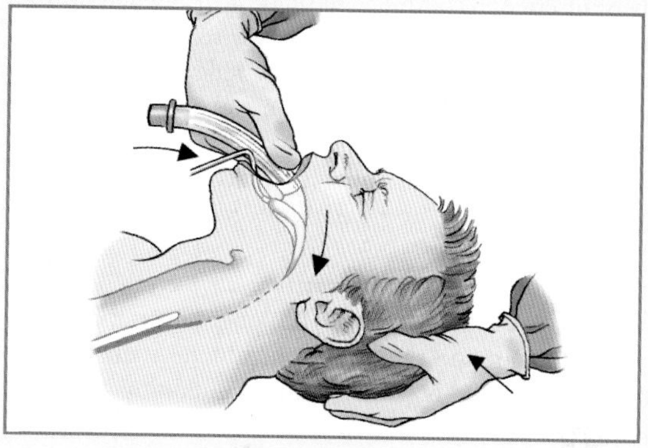

Continue to gently advance the LMA until you feel resistance at the hypopharynx.

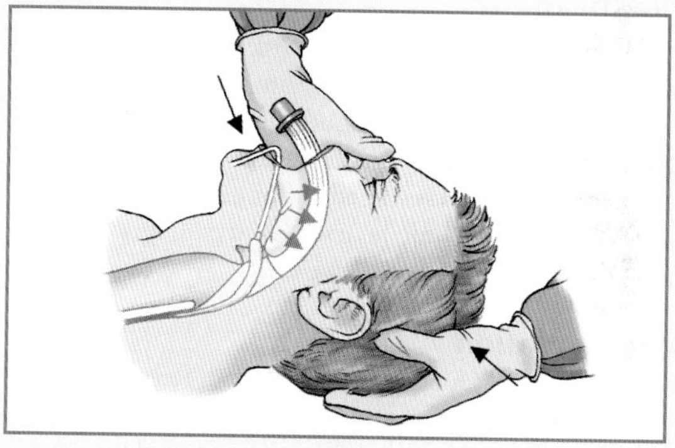

After the LMA is in place, gently remove your index finger while you place gentle pressure on the patient's jaw with your opposite hand. After your index finger is removed, remove both hands.

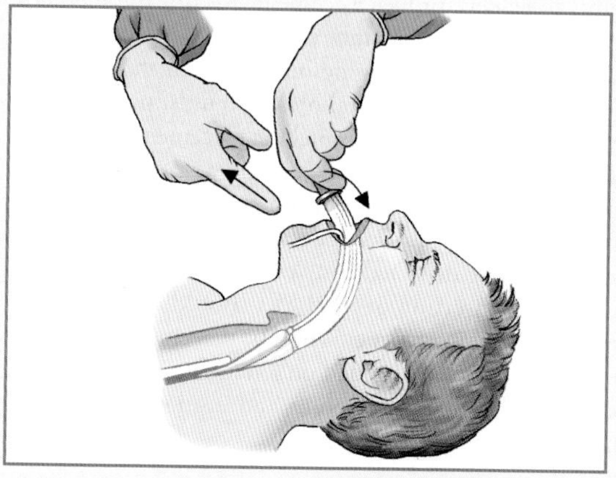

■ Insertion of an LMA in a patient with intact or partially intact airway reflexes may result in coughing, gagging, regurgitation, or laryngospasm. Therefore, an LMA should only be inserted in controlled settings, such as when the patient is under anesthesia; in emergency settings, in which the patient has lost protective airway reflexes; or in situations where endotracheal intubation isn't readily available or possible.
■ Monitor the patient's respiratory status continually *to ensure proper ventilation, oxygenation, and tube placement while the LMA is in place.*
■ Assess for an air leak *that may indicate the LMA isn't in correct position.* If the patient has prolonged expirations and oval swelling around the cricoid membrane is absent, remove the LMA and reinsert it while maintaining adequate ventilations to the patient.
■ If the patient vomits, turn the patient to the side *to allow for drainage of contents and suction the airway.*

Complications

Aspiration of stomach contents is a risk as the LMA doesn't protect the airway. Use of excessive force during insertion can result in trauma to the mouth, teeth, or pharynx, including lacerations, bleeding, or edema. Use of excessive air to inflate the cuff can result in edema or nerve damage. Other complications include hoarseness, dysphagia, stridor, dysarthria, and dysphonia.

Documentation

Document why LMA insertion was needed. Record method of ventilating and oxygenating the patient while preparing for LMA insertion. Note that the cuff was tested for patency and the device was visually inspected with no irregularities noted. Record the date, time, and name of the person performing the procedure. Include the size of the LMA, volume of air used to inflate the cuff, and the number of attempts to achieve proper placement. Record the methods used to determine proper tube placement, such as visual inspection, minor neck bulging in the area of the cricothyroid, auscultation of bilateral breath sounds, pulse oximetry, or capnometer readings. Include placement of the bite block and how the bite block and tube were secured. Document whether the patient is breathing spontaneously or receiving assisted or controlled ventilations. Include the amount of oxygen being delivered. Any evidence of trauma to the airway from insertion of the LMA should also be documented. Frequent assessments of tube placement and respiratory status may be recorded on a frequent patient assessment sheet. Include any teaching and support given to the family.

SELECTED REFERENCES

Baillard, C., et al. "Noninvasive Ventilation Improves Preoxygenation Before Intubation of Hypoxic Patients," *American Journal of Respiratory and Critical Care Medicine* 174(2):171-77, July 2006.

Chmielewski, C., and Snyder-Clickett, S. "The Use of the Laryngeal Mask Airway with Mechanical Positive Pressure Ventilation," *AANA Journal* 72(5):347-51, October 2004.

Jevon, P. "Laryngeal Mask Airway," *Nursing Times* 102(36):28-29, September 2006.

Lynn-McHale Wiegand, D.J., and Carlson, K.K., eds. *AACN Procedure Manual for Critical Care,* 5th ed. Philadelphia: W.B. Saunders Co., 2005.

TRACHEAL CUFF–PRESSURE MEASUREMENT

An endotracheal (ET) or tracheostomy cuff provides a closed system for mechanical ventilation, allowing a desired tidal volume to be delivered to the patient's lungs. To function properly, the cuff must exert enough pressure on the tracheal wall to seal the airway without compromising the blood supply to the tracheal mucosa.

The ideal pressure (known as *minimal occlusive volume*) is the lowest amount needed to seal the airway. Many authorities recommend maintaining a cuff pressure lower than venous perfusion pressure — usually 20 to 25 cm H_2O. (More than 25 cm H_2O may exceed venous perfusion pressure.) Actual cuff pressure will vary with each patient. To keep pressure within safe limits, measure minimal occlusive volume at least once each shift or as directed by your facility's policy. Cuff pressure can be measured by a respiratory therapist or by the nurse.

Equipment

10-ml syringe ■ three-way stopcock ■ cuff pressure manometer ■ stethoscope ■ suction equipment ■ gloves.

Preparation of equipment

Assemble all equipment at the patient's bedside. If measuring with a blood pressure manometer, attach the syringe to one stopcock port; then attach the tubing from the manometer to another port of the stopcock. Turn off the stopcock port where you'll be connecting the pilot balloon cuff *so that air can't escape from the cuff.* Use the syringe to instill air into the manometer tubing until the pressure reading reaches 10 mm Hg. *This will prevent sudden cuff deflation when you open the stopcock to the cuff and the manometer.*

Implementation

■ Confirm the patient's identity using two patient identifiers according to your facility's policy.
■ Explain the procedure to the patient.
■ Put on gloves and suction the ET or tracheostomy tube and the patient's oropharynx *to remove accumulated secretions above the cuff.*
■ Attach the cuff pressure manometer to the pilot balloon port.
■ Place the diaphragm of the stethoscope over the trachea, and listen for an air leak (as shown below). Keep in mind that a smooth, hollow sound indicates a sealed airway; a loud, gurgling sound indicates an air leak.

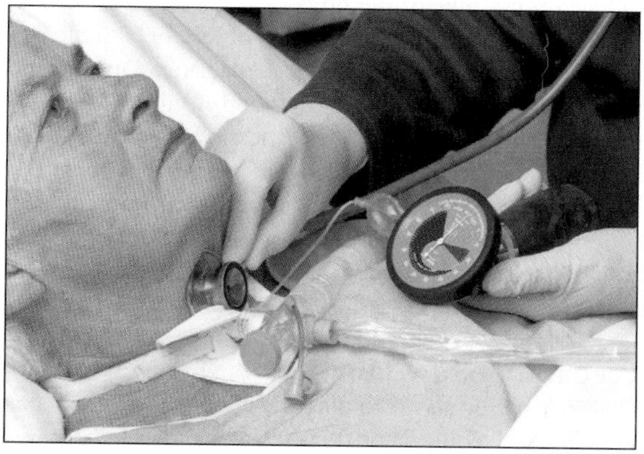

■ If you don't hear an air leak, press the red button under the dial of the cuff pressure manometer to slowly release air from the balloon on the tracheal tube (as shown below). Auscultate for an air leak.

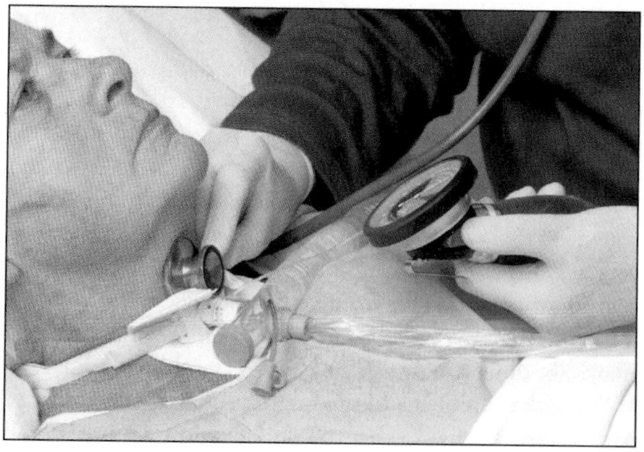

■ As soon as you hear an air leak, release the red button and gently squeeze the handle of the cuff pressure manometer to inflate the cuff (as shown top of next column). Continue to add air to the cuff until you no longer hear an air leak.

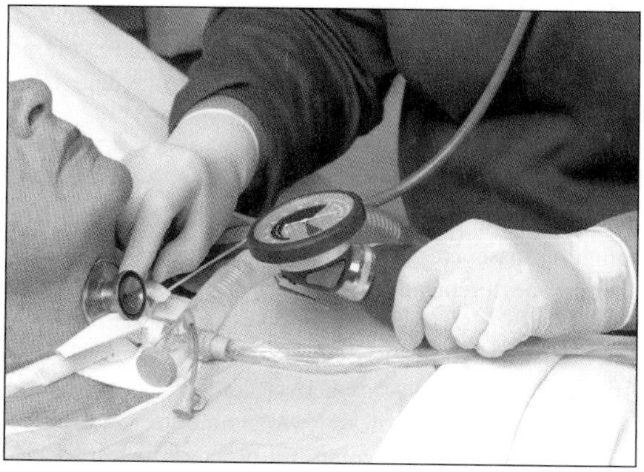

■ When the air leak ceases, read the dial on the cuff pressure manometer (as shown below). This is the minimal pressure required to effectively occlude the trachea around the tracheal tube. In many cases, this pressure will fall within the green area (20 to 25 cm H_2O) on the manometer dial.

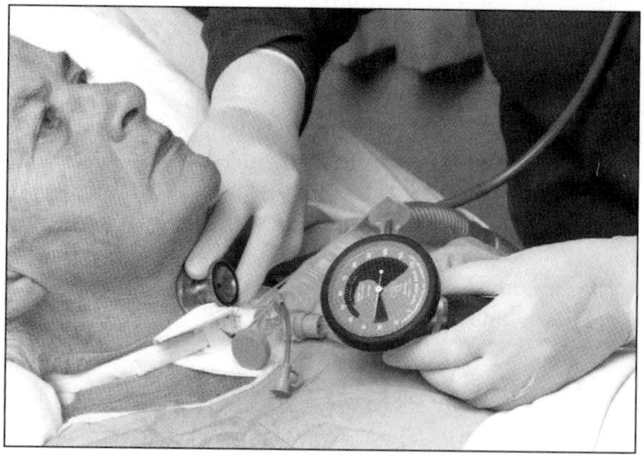

■ Disconnect the cuff pressure manometer from the pilot balloon port. Document the pressure value.

Special considerations

■ Measure cuff pressure at least every 8 hours *to avoid overinflation.*
■ Keep in mind that some patients require less pressure, whereas others — for example, those with tracheal malacia (an abnormal softening of the tracheal tissue) — require more pressure. Maintaining the cuff pressure at the lowest possible level will minimize cuff-related problems.
■ When measuring cuff pressure, keep the connection between the measuring device and the pilot balloon port tight *to avoid an air leak that could compromise cuff pressure.* If you're using a stopcock, don't leave the manometer in the OFF position *because air will leak from the cuff if the syringe accidentally comes off.* Also, note the volume of air needed to

inflate the cuff. A gradual increase in this volume indicates tracheal dilation or erosion. A sudden increase in volume indicates rupture of the cuff and requires immediate reintubation if the patient is being ventilated.

Complications

Aspiration of upper airway secretions, underventilation, or coughing spasms may occur if a leak is created during cuff pressure measurement.

Documentation

After cuff pressure measurement, record the date and time of the procedure, cuff pressure, total amount of air in the cuff after the procedure, complications and the nursing action taken, and the patient's tolerance of the procedure.

SELECTED REFERENCES

Akca, O. "Endotracheal Tube Cuff Leak: Can Optimum Management of Cuff Pressure Prevent Pneumonia?" *Critical Care Medicine* 35(6):1624-626, June 2007.

Galinski, M., et al. "Intracuff Pressures of Endotracheal Tubes in the Management of Airway Emergencies: The Need for Pressure Monitoring," *Annals of Emergency Medicine* 47(6):545-47, June 2006.

Lynn-McHale Wiegand, D.J., and Carlson, K.K., eds. *AACN Procedure Manual for Critical Care*, 5th ed. Philadelphia: W.B. Saunders Co., 2006.

Young, P.J., et al. "A Low-volume, Low-pressure Tracheal Tube Cuff Reduces Pulmonary Aspiration," *Critical Care Medicine* 34(3):632-39, March 2006.

TRACHEOTOMY

A tracheotomy involves the surgical creation of an external opening—called a *tracheostomy*—into the trachea and insertion of an indwelling tube to maintain the airway's patency. If all other attempts to establish an airway have failed, a practitioner may perform a tracheotomy at a patient's bedside. This procedure may be necessary when an airway obstruction results from laryngeal edema, foreign body obstruction, or a tumor. An emergency tracheotomy may also be performed when endotracheal intubation is contraindicated.

Use of a cuffed tracheostomy tube provides and maintains a patent airway, prevents the unconscious or paralyzed patient from aspirating food or secretions, allows removal of tracheobronchial secretions from the patient unable to cough, replaces an endotracheal tube, and permits the use of positive-pressure ventilation.

When laryngectomy accompanies a tracheostomy, the physician may insert a laryngectomy tube—a shorter version of a tracheostomy tube. In addition, the patient's trachea is sutured to the skin surface. Consequently, with a laryngectomy, accidental tube expulsion doesn't precipitate immediate closure of the tracheal opening. When healing occurs, the patient has a permanent neck stoma through which respiration takes place.

Although tracheostomy tubes come in plastic and metal, plastic tubes are much more commonly used because they have a universal adapter for respiratory support equipment, such as a mechanical ventilator, and a cuff to allow positive-pressure ventilation.

Equipment

Tracheostomy tube of the proper size (usually #13 to #38 French or #00 to #9 Jackson) with obturator ▪ sterile tracheotomy tray (usually contains tracheal dilator, vein retractor, hemostats, and clamps) ▪ sutures and needles ▪ 4″ × 4″ gauze pads ▪ sterile drapes, gloves, mask, and gown ▪ sterile bowls ▪ stethoscope ▪ dressing ▪ pillow ▪ tracheostomy ties ▪ suction apparatus and tubing ▪ alcohol pad ▪ antiseptic solution ▪ sterile water ▪ 5-ml syringe with 22G needle ▪ local anesthetic such as lidocaine ▪ oxygen therapy device ▪ oxygen source ▪ syringe.

Preparation of equipment

Have one person stay with the patient while another obtains the necessary equipment. Wash your hands; then, maintaining sterile technique, open the tray. Take the tracheostomy tube from its container, and place it on the sterile field. If necessary, set up the suction equipment, and make sure it works. When the physician opens the sterile bowls, pour in the antiseptic solution.

Implementation

- Confirm the patient's identity using two patient identifiers according to your facility's policy.
- Sedate the patient, as ordered, *to decrease his pain and anxiety.*
- Explain the procedure to the patient even if he's unresponsive.
- Assess his condition and provide privacy. Maintain ventilation until the tracheotomy is performed.
- Before the physician begins, place a pillow under the patient's shoulders and neck and hyperextend his neck.
- Wipe the top of the local anesthetic vial with an alcohol pad. Invert the vial so that the physician can withdraw the anesthetic using the 22G needle attached to the 5-ml syringe.
- The physician will put on a sterile gown, gloves, and mask.
- Help the physician with the tube insertion, as needed. (See *Assisting with a tracheotomy*.)

Assisting with a tracheotomy

To perform a tracheotomy, the physician will first clean the area from the chin to the nipples with antiseptic solution. Next, he'll place sterile drapes on the patient and locate the area for the incision—usually 1 to 2 cm below the cricoid cartilage. Then he'll inject a local anesthetic.

He'll make a horizontal or vertical incision in the skin. *(A vertical incision helps avoid arteries, veins, and nerves on the lateral borders of the trachea.)* Then he'll dissect subcutaneous fat and muscle and move the muscle aside with vein retractors to locate the tracheal rings. He'll make an incision between the second and third tracheal rings (as shown top right) and use hemostats to control bleeding.

He'll inject a local anesthetic into the tracheal lumen *to suppress the cough reflex,* and then he'll create a stoma in the trachea. When this is done, carefully apply suction *to remove blood and secretions that may obstruct the airway or be aspirated into the lungs.* The physician then inserts the tracheostomy tube and obturator into the stoma (as shown middle right). After inserting the tube, he'll remove the obturator.

Apply a sterile tracheostomy dressing, and anchor the tube with tracheostomy ties (as shown below right). Check for air movement through the tube and auscultate the lungs to *ensure proper placement.*

An alternative approach

In another approach, the physician inserts the tracheostomy tube percutaneously at the bedside. Using either a series of dilators or a pair of forceps, he creates a stoma for tube insertion. Unlike the surgical technique, this method dilates rather than cuts the tissue structures.

After the skin is prepared and anesthetized, the physician makes a 1-cm midline incision. When the stoma reaches the desired size, the physician inserts the tracheostomy tube. When the tube is in place, inflate the cuff, secure the tube, and check the patient's breath sounds. Next, obtain a portable chest X-ray.

Incision site

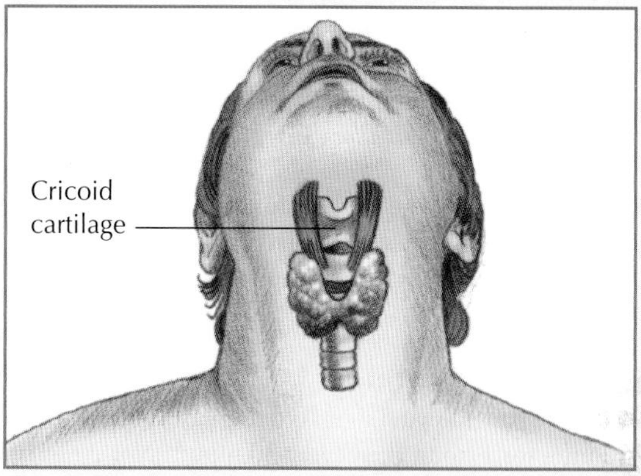

Tube insertion

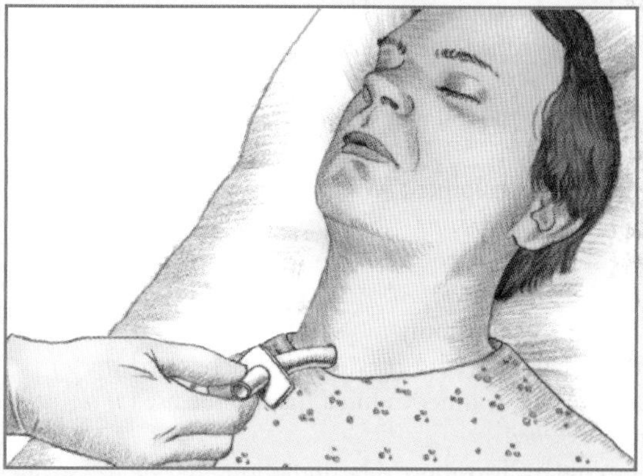

Sterile dressing

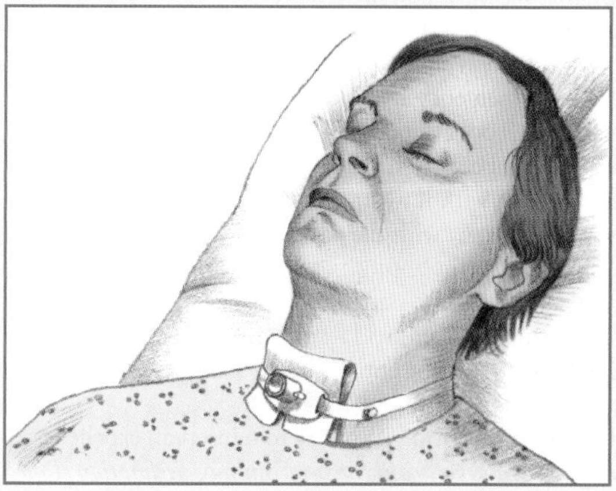

- When the tube is in position, attach it to the appropriate oxygen therapy device.
- Inject air into the distal cuff port *to inflate the cuff.*
- The physician will suture the corners of the incision.
- Put on sterile gloves.
- Apply the sterile tracheostomy dressing under the tracheostomy tube flange. Place the tracheostomy ties through the openings of the tube flanges, and tie them on the side of the patient's neck. *This allows easy access and prevents pressure necrosis at the back of the neck.*
- Clean or dispose of the used equipment according to policy. Replenish all supplies, as needed.
- Make sure a chest X-ray is ordered *to confirm tube placement.*

Special considerations

- Assess the patient's vital signs and respiratory status every 15 minutes for 1 hour, then every 30 minutes for 2 hours, and then every 2 hours until his condition is stable.
- Monitor the patient carefully for signs of infection. Ideally, the tracheotomy should be performed using sterile technique, as described. However, in an emergency, this may not be possible.
- Make sure the following equipment is always at the patient's bedside:
  - suctioning equipment *because the patient may need his airway cleared at any time*
  - the sterile obturator used to insert the tracheostomy tube *in case the tube is expelled*
  - a sterile tracheostomy tube and obturator (the same size as the one used) *in case the tube must be replaced quickly*
  - a spare, sterile inner cannula that can be used *if the cannula is expelled*
  - a sterile tracheostomy tube and obturator one size smaller than the one used, *which may be needed if the tube is expelled and the trachea begins to close*
  - a sterile tracheal dilator or sterile hemostats *to maintain an open airway before inserting a new tracheostomy tube.*
- Review emergency first-aid measures, and always follow your facility's policy concerning an expelled or blocked tracheostomy tube. When a blocked tube can't be cleared by suctioning or withdrawing the inner cannula, policy may require you to stay with the patient while someone else calls the physician or the appropriate code. You should continue trying to ventilate the patient with whatever method works —for example, a handheld resuscitation bag. Don't remove the tracheostomy tube entirely; *doing so may close the airway completely.*
- Use extreme caution if you try to reinsert an expelled tracheostomy tube *to avoid tracheal trauma, perforation, compression, and asphyxiation.*

Complications

A tracheotomy can cause an airway obstruction (from improper tube placement), hemorrhage, edema, a perforated esophagus, subcutaneous or mediastinal emphysema, aspiration of secretions, tracheal necrosis (from cuff pressure), infection, or lacerations of arteries, veins, or nerves.

Documentation

Record the reason for the procedure, the date and time it took place, and the patient's respiratory status before and after the procedure. Include complications that occurred during the procedure, the amount of cuff pressure, and the respiratory therapy initiated after the procedure. Also, note the patient's response to respiratory therapy.

SELECTED REFERENCES

Barquist, E.S., et al. "Tracheostomy in Ventilator-dependent Trauma Patients: A Prospective, Randomized Intention-to-treat Study," *Journal of Trauma* 60(1):90-97, January 2006.

Beiderlinden, M, et al. "Risk Factors Associated with Bleeding During and After Percutaneous Dilational Tracheostomy," *Anaesthesia* 62(4):342-46, April 2007.

Lynn-McHale Wiegand, D.J., and Carlson, K.K., eds. *AACN Procedure Manual for Critical Care*, 5th ed. Philadelphia: W.B. Saunders Co., 2006.

Miller, C.D. "Difficult Airway Society Guidelines," *Anaesthesia* 59(12):1246-247, December 2004.

Silvester, W., et al. "Percutaneous versus Surgical Tracheostomy: A Randomized Controlled Study with Long-term Follow-up," *Critical Care Medicine* 34(8):2145-152, August 2006.

TRACHEOSTOMY CARE

Whether a tracheotomy is performed in an emergency situation or after careful preparation, as a permanent measure or as temporary therapy, tracheostomy care has identical goals: to ensure airway patency by keeping the tube free of mucus buildup, to maintain mucous membrane and skin integrity, to prevent infection, and to provide psychological support.

The patient may have one of three types of tracheostomy tube—uncuffed, cuffed, or fenestrated. Tube selection depends on the patient's condition and the practitioner's preference. (See *Types of tracheostomy tubes.*)

An *uncuffed tube,* which may be plastic or metal, allows air to flow freely around the tracheostomy tube and through the larynx, thus reducing the risk of tracheal damage. A *cuffed tube,* made of plastic, is disposable. A plastic *fenestrated tube* permits speech through the upper airway when the external opening is capped and the cuff is deflated. It also allows easy removal of the inner cannula for cleaning. However, a fenestrated tube may become occluded.

If the patient is on a ventilator, a tube with an inflated cuff must be used to seal the space between the trachea and the tube so that air moves through the tube to the lungs. The patient who's breathing normally on his own may need the cuff inflated when he takes nutrition orally.

Tracheostomy care should be performed using aseptic technique until the stoma has healed to prevent infection. For recently performed tracheotomies — less than 7 days postoperatively — or unhealed tracheostomies, the site should be assessed at least every 4 hours and the stoma should be cleaned and redressed every 8 hours. Tracheostomy care should be performed at least every shift on a healed tracheostomy. Sterile gloves should be worn for all manipulations at the tracheostomy site. After the stoma has healed, clean gloves may be substituted for sterile ones.

Provide safety measures for the patient, such as admitting him to a room close to the nurses' station, keeping an emergency tracheostomy tray on the unit, and a label at the nurses' station near the call unit if the patient can't speak.

Keep with the patient at all times (especially when traveling for tests), an emergency replacement tracheostomy tube of the present size and one size smaller, a curved hemostat or tracheal dilator/obturator for the current tube, and a large-bore suction catheter and suction machine. Make sure that the areas to which the patient may travel (such as X-ray) have working suction equipment.

Equipment

For sterile stoma and outer-cannula care: Waterproof trash bag ▪ two sterile solution containers ▪ normal saline solution ▪ hydrogen peroxide ▪ sterile cotton-tipped applicators ▪ sterile 4″ × 4″ gauze pads ▪ sterile gloves ▪ prepackaged sterile tracheostomy dressing (or 4″ × 4″ gauze pad) ▪ equipment and supplies for suctioning and for mouth care ▪ water-soluble lubricant or topical antibiotic cream ▪ materials, as needed, for cuff procedures and for changing tracheostomy ties (see below).

For sterile inner-cannula care: All of the preceding equipment plus a prepackaged commercial tracheostomy-care set, or sterile forceps ▪ sterile nylon brush ▪ sterile 6″ (15.2-cm) pipe cleaners ▪ clean gloves ▪ a third sterile solution container ▪ disposable temporary inner cannula.

For changing tracheostomy ties: 30″ (76.2-cm) length of tracheostomy twill tape ▪ bandage scissors ▪ sterile gloves ▪ hemostat.

For emergency tracheostomy tube replacement: Sterile tracheal dilator or sterile hemostat ▪ sterile obturator that fits the tracheostomy tube in use ▪ two extra sterile tracheostomy tube and obturator in appropriate size ▪ suction equipment and supplies.

EQUIPMENT

Types of tracheostomy tubes

There are advantages and disadvantages to cuffed and uncuffed tracheostomy tubes. Cuffed tubes (shown below) help seal that area between the tube and trachea, decreasing the patient's risk of aspiration. However, if the cuff pressure isn't regularly monitored, it may erode the trachea. Also, if the cuff is inflated, the patient can't talk and needs an alternate means of communication.

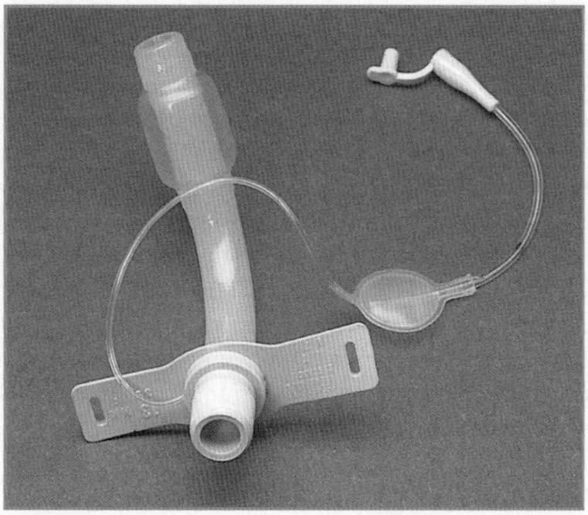

Uncuffed tubes (shown below) allow the patient to eat and talk. However, this type of tube can't be used in a patient who's receiving mechanical ventilation because oxygen may escape from around the tube.

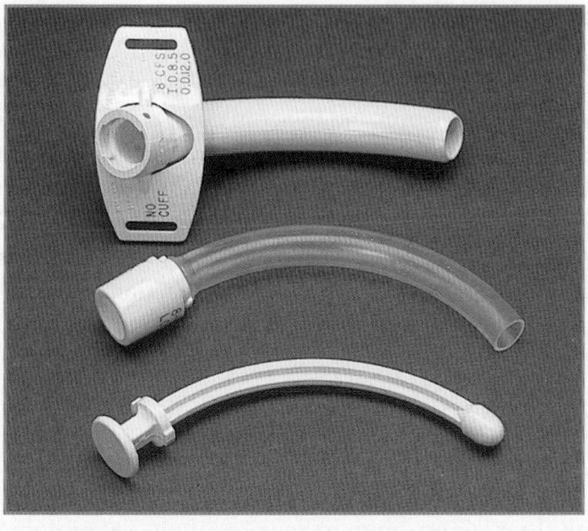

Keep these supplies in full view in the patient's room at all times for easy access in case of emergency. Consider taping an emergency sterile tracheostomy tube in a sterile wrapper to the head of the bed for easy access in an emergency.

For cuff procedures: 5- or 10-ml syringe ■ padded hemostat ■ stethoscope.

Preparation of equipment

Wash your hands, and assemble all equipment and supplies in the patient's room. Check the expiration date on each sterile package, and inspect the package for tears. Open the waterproof trash bag, and place it next to you *so that you can avoid reaching across the sterile field or the patient's stoma when discarding soiled items.*

Establish a sterile field near the patient's bed (usually on the overbed table), and place equipment and supplies on it. Pour normal saline solution, hydrogen peroxide, or a mixture of equal parts of both solutions into one of the sterile solution containers; then pour normal saline solution into the second sterile container for rinsing. For inner-cannula care, you may use a third sterile solution container to hold the gauze pads and cotton-tipped applicators saturated with cleaning solution. If you'll be replacing the disposable inner cannula, open the package containing the new inner cannula while maintaining sterile technique. Obtain or prepare new tracheostomy ties, if indicated.

Implementation

- Confirm the patient's identity using two patient identifiers according to your facility's policy.
- Assess the patient's condition *to determine his need for care.*
- Explain the procedure to the patient even if he's unresponsive. Provide privacy.
- Place the patient in semi-Fowler's position (unless it's contraindicated) *to decrease abdominal pressure on the diaphragm and promote lung expansion.*
- Remove any humidification or ventilation device.
- If the patient is being mechanically ventilated, administer hyperoxygenation and hyperinflation using the ventilator settings. If he's breathing on his own, evaluate the need for preoxygenation and instruct him to take deep breaths.
- Using sterile technique, suction the entire length of the tracheostomy tube *to clear the airway of any secretions that may hinder oxygenation.* (See "Tracheal suction," page 561.)
- Reconnect the patient to the humidifier or ventilator, if necessary.

Cleaning a stoma and outer cannula

- Put on sterile gloves.
- With your dominant hand, saturate a sterile gauze pad with the cleaning solution. Squeeze out the excess liquid *to prevent accidental aspiration.* Then wipe the patient's neck under the tracheostomy tube flanges and twill tapes.
- Saturate a second pad, and wipe until the skin around the tracheostomy is cleaned. Use more pads or cotton-tipped applicators to clean the stoma site and the tube's flanges. Wipe only once with each pad, and then discard it *to prevent contamination of a clean area with a soiled pad.*
- Rinse debris and peroxide (if used) with one or more sterile 4″ × 4″ gauze pads dampened in normal saline solution. Dry the area thoroughly with additional sterile gauze pads; then apply a new sterile tracheostomy dressing.
- Remove and discard your gloves.

Cleaning a nondisposable inner cannula

- Put on sterile gloves.
- Using your nondominant hand, remove and discard the patient's tracheostomy dressing. Then, with the same hand, disconnect the ventilator or humidification device, and unlock the tracheostomy tube's inner cannula by rotating it counterclockwise (as shown below). Place the inner cannula in the container of hydrogen peroxide.

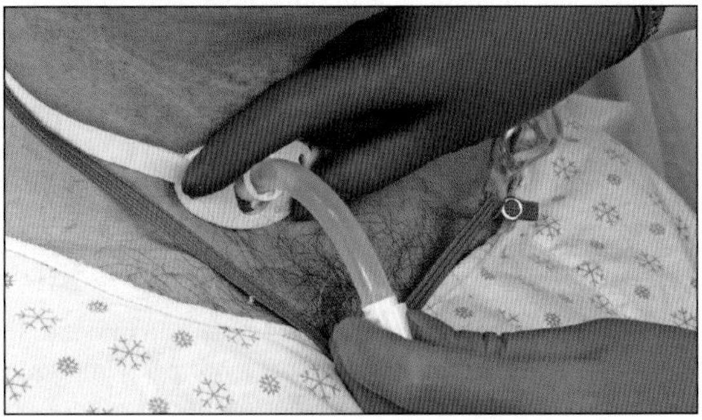

- Working quickly, use your dominant hand to scrub the cannula with the sterile nylon brush (as shown below). If the brush doesn't slide easily into the cannula, use a sterile pipe cleaner.

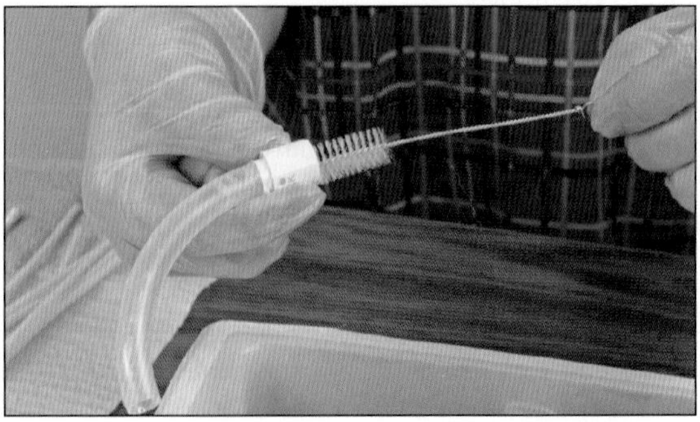

■ Immerse the cannula in the container of normal saline solution (as shown below), and agitate it for about 10 seconds *to rinse it thoroughly.*

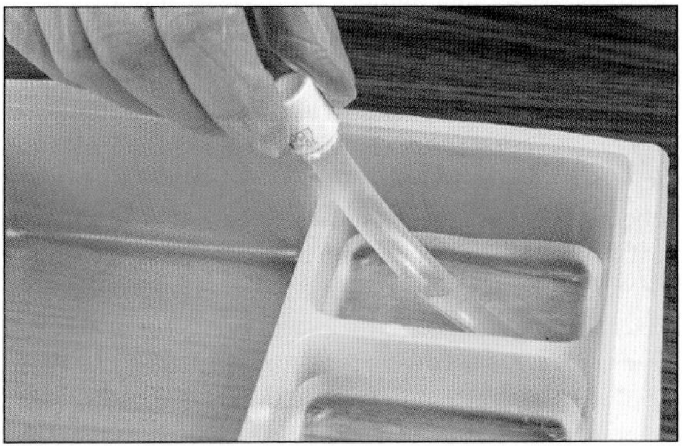

■ Inspect the cannula for cleanliness. Repeat the cleaning process if necessary. If it's clean, tap it gently against the inside edge of the sterile container *to remove excess liquid and prevent aspiration.* Don't dry the outer surface *because a thin film of moisture acts as a lubricant during insertion.*

■ Reinsert the inner cannula into the patient's tracheostomy tube (as shown below). Lock it in place and then gently pull on it *to make sure it's positioned securely.* Reconnect the mechanical ventilator. Apply a new sterile tracheostomy dressing.

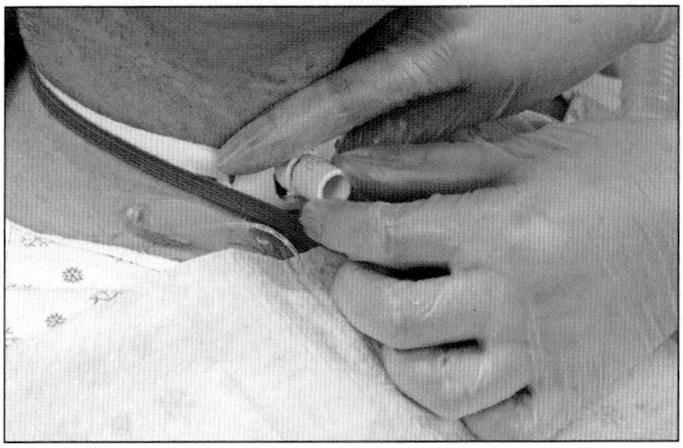

■ If the patient can't tolerate being disconnected from the ventilator for the time it takes to clean the inner cannula, replace the existing inner cannula with a clean one and reattach the mechanical ventilator. Then clean the cannula just removed from the patient, and store it in a sterile container the next time.

Caring for a disposable inner cannula

■ Put on clean gloves.

■ Using your dominant hand, remove the patient's inner cannula. After evaluating the secretions in the cannula, discard it properly.

■ Pick up the new inner cannula, touching only the outer locking portion. Insert the cannula into the tracheostomy and, following the manufacturer's instructions, lock it securely.

Changing tracheostomy ties

■ Change the ties as necessary and when soiled after the first change by the surgeon.

■ Obtain assistance from another nurse or a respiratory therapist *because of the risk of accidental tube expulsion during this procedure.* Patient movement or coughing can dislodge the tube.

■ Wash your hands thoroughly, and put on sterile gloves.

■ If you aren't using commercially packaged tracheostomy ties, prepare new ties from a 30″ (76.2-cm) length of twill tape by folding one end back 1″ (2.5 cm) on itself. Then, with the bandage scissors, cut a ½″ (1.3-cm) slit down the center of the tape from the folded edge.

■ Prepare the other end of the tape the same way.

■ Hold both ends together and, using scissors, cut the resulting circle of tape so that one piece is approximately 10″ (25 cm) long and the other is about 20″ (51 cm) long.

■ Help the patient into semi-Fowler's position if possible.

■ After your assistant puts on gloves, instruct her to hold the tracheostomy tube in place *to prevent its expulsion during replacement of the ties.* If you must perform the procedure without assistance, fasten the clean ties in place before removing the old ties *to prevent tube expulsion.*

■ With the assistant's gloved fingers holding the tracheostomy tube in place, cut the soiled tracheostomy ties with the bandage scissors or untie them and discard the ties. Be careful not to cut the tube of the pilot balloon.

■ Thread the slit end of one new tie a short distance through the eye of one tracheostomy tube flange from the underside; use the hemostat, if needed, to pull the tie through. Then thread the other end of the tie completely through the slit end, and pull it taut so it loops firmly through the flange. *This avoids knots that can cause throat discomfort, tissue irritation, pressure, and necrosis at the patient's throat.*

■ Fasten the second tie to the opposite flange in the same manner.

■ Instruct the patient to flex his neck while you bring the ties around to the side, and tie them together with a square knot. *Flexion produces the same neck circumference as coughing and helps prevent an overly tight tie.* Instruct your assistant to place one finger under the tapes as you tie them *to ensure that they're tight enough to avoid slippage but loose enough to prevent choking or jugular vein constriction. Placing the closure on the side allows easy access and prevents pressure necrosis at the back of the neck when the patient is recumbent.*

■ After securing the ties, cut off the excess tape with the scissors and instruct your assistant to release the tracheostomy tube.
■ Make sure the patient is comfortable and can reach the call button easily.
■ Check tracheostomy-tie tension often on patients with traumatic injury, radical neck dissection, or cardiac failure *because neck diameter can increase from swelling and cause constriction;* also check neonatal or restless patients frequently *because ties can loosen and cause tube dislodgment.*

Concluding tracheostomy care

■ Replace any humidification device.
■ Provide oral care, as needed, *because the oral cavity can become dry and malodorous or develop sores from encrusted secretions.*
■ Observe soiled dressings and any suctioned secretions for amount, color, consistency, and odor.
■ Properly clean or dispose of all equipment, supplies, solutions, and trash according to policy.
■ Take off and discard your gloves.
■ Make sure all necessary supplies are readily available at the bedside.
■ Repeat the procedure at least once every 8 hours or as needed. Change the dressing as often as necessary regardless of whether you also perform the entire cleaning procedure *because a wet dressing with exudate or secretions predisposes the patient to skin excoriation, breakdown, and infection.*

Deflating and inflating a tracheostomy cuff

■ Read the cuff manufacturer's instructions *because cuff types and procedures vary widely.*
■ Assess the patient's condition, explain the procedure to him, and reassure him. Wash your hands thoroughly.
■ Help the patient into semi-Fowler's position, if possible, or place him in a supine position so secretions above the cuff site will be pushed up into his mouth if he's receiving positive-pressure ventilation.
■ Suction the oropharyngeal cavity *to prevent pooled secretions from descending into the trachea after cuff deflation.*
■ Release the padded hemostat clamping the cuff inflation tubing, if a hemostat is present.
■ Insert a 5- or 10-ml syringe into the cuff pilot balloon, and slowly withdraw all air from the cuff. Leave the syringe attached to the tubing for later reinflation of the cuff. *Slow deflation allows positive lung pressure to push secretions upward from the bronchi. Cuff deflation may also stimulate the patient's cough reflex, producing additional secretions.*
■ Remove any ventilation device. Suction the lower airway through any existing tube *to remove all secretions.* Then reconnect the patient to the ventilation device.
■ While the cuff is deflated, observe the patient for adequate ventilation, and suction as necessary. If the patient has difficulty breathing, reinflate the cuff immediately by depressing the syringe plunger very slowly. Inject the least amount of air necessary to achieve an adequate tracheal seal.
■ When inflating the cuff, you may use the minimal-leak technique or the minimal occlusive volume technique *to help gauge the proper inflation point.* (For more information, see "Endotracheal intubation," page 538, and "Endotracheal tube care," page 545.)
■ If you're inflating the cuff using cuff pressure measurement, be careful not to exceed 25 mm Hg. If pressure exceeds 25 mm Hg, notify the practitioner *because you may need to change to a larger size tube, use higher inflation pressures, or permit a larger air leak.* Recommended cuff pressure is about 18 mm Hg.
■ After you've inflated the cuff, if the tubing doesn't have a one-way valve at the end, clamp the inflation line with a padded hemostat (*to protect the tubing*), and remove the syringe.
■ Check for a minimal-leak cuff seal. You shouldn't feel air coming from the patient's mouth, nose, or tracheostomy site, and a conscious patient shouldn't be able to speak.
■ Be alert for air leaks from the cuff itself. Suspect a leak if injection of air fails to inflate the cuff or increase cuff pressure, if you're unable to inject the amount of air you withdrew, if the patient can speak, if ventilation fails to maintain adequate respiratory movement with pressures or volumes previously considered adequate, or if air escapes during the ventilator's inspiratory cycle.
■ Note the exact amount of air used to inflate the cuff *to detect tracheal malacia if more air is consistently needed.*
■ Make sure the patient is comfortable and can easily reach the call button and communication aids.
■ Properly clean or dispose of all equipment, supplies, and trash according to your facility's policy.
■ Replenish any used supplies, and make sure all necessary emergency supplies are at the bedside.

Special considerations

■ Keep appropriate equipment at the patient's bedside for immediate use in an emergency. (For a list, see "Tracheotomy," page 552.)
■ Consult the practitioner about first-aid measures you can use for your tracheostomy patient should an emergency occur. Follow your facility's policy regarding procedure if a tracheostomy tube is expelled or if the outer cannula becomes blocked. If the patient's breathing is obstructed — for example, when the tube is blocked with mucus that can't be removed by suctioning or by withdrawing the inner cannula — call the appropriate code, and provide manual resusci-

tation with a handheld resuscitation bag or reconnect the patient to the ventilator. Don't remove the tracheostomy tube entirely *because this may allow the airway to close completely.* Use extreme caution when attempting to reinsert an expelled tracheostomy tube *because of the risk of tracheal trauma, perforation, compression, and asphyxiation.* Reassure the patient until the physician arrives (usually a minute or less in this type of code or emergency).

- Refrain from changing tracheostomy ties unnecessarily during the immediate postoperative period before the stoma track is well formed (usually 4 days) *to avoid accidental dislodgment and expulsion of the tube.* Unless secretions or drainage is a problem, ties can be changed once per day.
- Refrain from changing a single-cannula tracheostomy tube or the outer cannula of a double-cannula tube. *Because of the risk of tracheal complications,* the physician usually changes the cannula, with the frequency of change depending on the patient's condition.
- If the patient's neck or stoma is excoriated or infected, apply a water-soluble lubricant or topical antibiotic cream as ordered. Remember not to use a powder or an oil-based substance on or around a stoma *because aspiration can cause infection and abscess.*
- Replace all equipment, including solutions, regularly according to policy *to reduce the risk of nosocomial infections.*

Home care

If the patient is being discharged with a tracheostomy, start self-care teaching as soon as he's receptive. Teach the patient how to change and clean the tube. If he's being discharged with suction equipment (a few patients are), make sure he and his family feel knowledgeable and comfortable about using this equipment.

Complications

Complications that can occur within the first 48 hours after tracheostomy tube insertion include:

- hemorrhage at the operative site, causing aspiration of blood
- bleeding or edema in tracheal tissue, causing airway obstruction
- aspiration of secretions; introduction of air into the pleural cavity, causing pneumothorax
- hypoxia or acidosis, triggering cardiac arrest
- introduction of air into surrounding tissues, causing subcutaneous emphysema.

Secretions collecting under dressings and twill tape can encourage skin excoriation and infection. Hardened mucus or a slipped cuff can occlude the cannula opening and obstruct the airway. Tube displacement can stimulate the cough reflex if the tip rests on the carina, or it can cause blood vessel erosion and hemorrhage. Just the presence of the tube or cuff pressure can produce tracheal erosion and necrosis.

Documentation

Record the date and time of the procedure; type of procedure; the amount, consistency, color, and odor of secretions; stoma and skin condition; the patient's respiratory status before, during, and after the procedure; change of the tracheostomy tube by the physician; the duration of any cuff deflation; the amount of any cuff inflation; and cuff pressure readings and specific body position. Note complications and the nursing action taken; patient or family teaching and their comprehension and progress; and the patient's tolerance of the treatment.

SELECTED REFERENCES

Crimslick, J.T., et al. "Standardizing Adult Tracheostomy Tube Styles: What is the Clinical and Cost-effective Impact?" *Dimensions of Critical Care Nursing* 25(1):35-43, January-February 2006.

Dhand, R., and Johnson, J.C. "Care of the Chronic Tracheostomy," *Respiratory Care* 51(9):984-1001, September 2006.

Dodek, P., et al. "Evidence-based Clinical Practice Guideline for the Prevention of Ventilator-associated Pneumonia," *Annals of Internal Medicine* 141(4):305-13, August 2004.

Feber, T. "Tracheostomy Care for Community Nurses: Basic Principles," *British Journal of Community Nursing* 11(5):186,188-90, 192-93, May 2006.

Lynn-McHale Wiegand, D.J., and Carlson, K.K., eds. *AACN Procedure Manual for Critical Care*, 5th ed. Philadelphia: W.B. Saunders Co., 2006.

Russel, C. "Providing the Nurse with a Guide to Tracheostomy Care and Management," *British Journal of Nursing* 14(8):428-33, April-May 2005.

Taylor, C., et al. *Fundamentals of Nursing: The Art and Science of Nursing Care*, 5th ed. Philadelphia: Lippincott Williams & Wilkins, 2008.

TRACHEOSTOMY AND VENTILATOR SPEAKING VALVE

Patients with a tracheostomy tube can't speak because the cuffed tracheostomy tube that directs air into the lungs on inspiration expels air through the tracheostomy tube rather than the vocal cords, mouth, and nose. Therefore, providing a means of nonverbal communication for such patients is crucial for their physical and emotional well-being as well as that of family members and hospital personnel.

Traditional methods of communication have included writing, lip-reading, alphabet boards, and gestures. However, there's a positive-closure, one-way speaking valve that's now available. The Passy-Muir Tracheostomy and Ventilator Speaking Valve (PMV) opens upon inspiration to allow the patient to inspire through the tracheostomy tube. It closes after inspiration, redirecting the exhaled air around the tube, through the vocal cords, and out the mouth, thus allowing the patient to speak. Short- and long-term adult, pediatric, and infant tracheostomy and ventilator-dependent patient may benefit from the use of a PMV. PMV use is contraindicated in patients with severe tracheal or laryngeal stenosis, laryngectomy, or excessive oral secretions and in patients who are unconscious or at risk for gross aspiration.

To function safely, the tracheostomy cuff must be completely deflated to enable the patient to exhale, or the tracheostomy tube must be cuffless. For maximum airflow around the tube, the tube should be no larger than two-thirds the size of the tracheal lumen.

The PMV 005 is most commonly used by nonventilated tracheostomy patients, but it can be used by ventilator patients with rubber, nondisposable ventilator tubing. The PMV 007 fits easily into the ventilator tubing used by medically ventilated tracheostomy patients. Both valves fit the 15-mm hub of adult, pediatric, and neonatal tracheostomy tubes and can be used by patients either on or off the ventilator.

Two other PMV valves include the PMV 2000 and the PMV 2001. Both of these valves are low-profile and low-resistance, feature the positive closure design, and can be used on or off the ventilator. The PMV 2000 is clear in color and is used more readily in the home care setting because it's less noticeable. The PMV 2001 is a bright purple color and is used more often in a health care facility because the color is more noticeable. These valves also include safety ties that prevent valve loss if the patient inadvertently coughs the PMV out of the tracheostomy tube. A PMV O_2 adapter is available for use with the PMV 2000 series speaking valves. This adapter allows improved mobility and comfort for patients who require a tracheostomy tube, speaking valve, and low-flow supplemental oxygen.

Equipment

Appropriately sized PMV ▪ gloves ▪ suction equipment ▪ 10-ml luer-lock syringe ▪ instruction booklet.

Implementation

- Confirm the patient's identity using two patient identifiers according to your facility's policy.
- Elevate the head of the patient's bed about 45 degrees.
- The tracheostomy cuff must be completely deflated before valve is placed.
- Put on gloves and deflate the cuff slowly *so he can get used to using his upper airways again.* Attach a 10-ml syringe to the tracheostomy tube's pilot balloon and remove the air until air can no longer be extracted and a vacuum is created (as shown below).

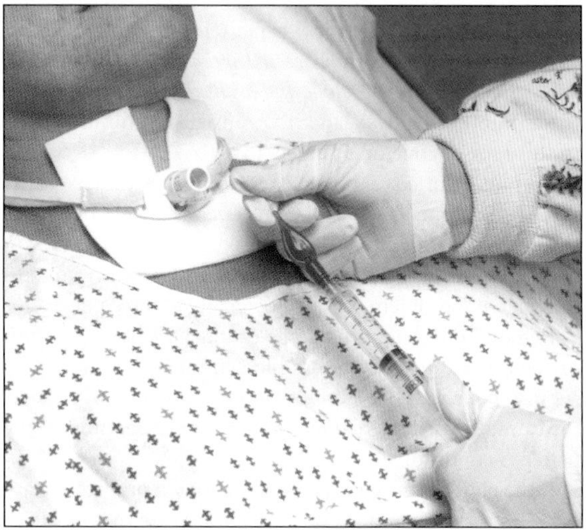

- Suction the trachea and oral cavity, as needed.
- Hold the valve between your fingers. For a patient who isn't ventilator-dependent, attach the valve to the hub of the existing tracheostomy hub with a quarter-turn twist (as shown below).

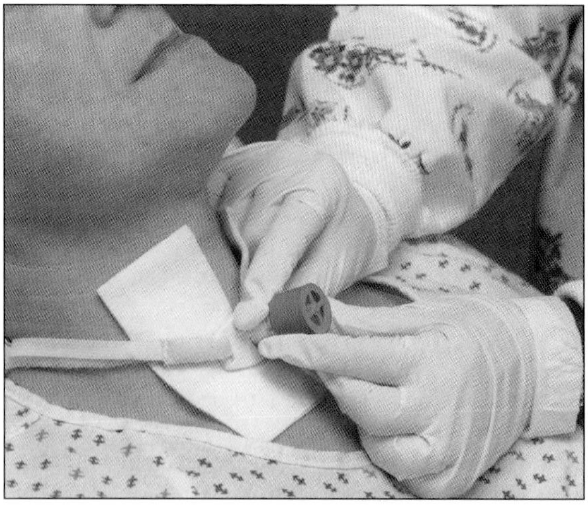

- After the valve is in place, encourage the patient to relax and concentrate on exhaling through his mouth and nose. Have him count aloud to 10, or speak, as he becomes comfortable breathing with the valve in place. The speech-language pathologist can facilitate voice production and speech.
- The aqua-colored PMV 007 is more convenient for ventilator-dependent patients *because it's tapered to fit into dis-*

posable ventilator tubing. Insert the PMV into the end of the wide-mouth, short-flex tubing (as shown below).

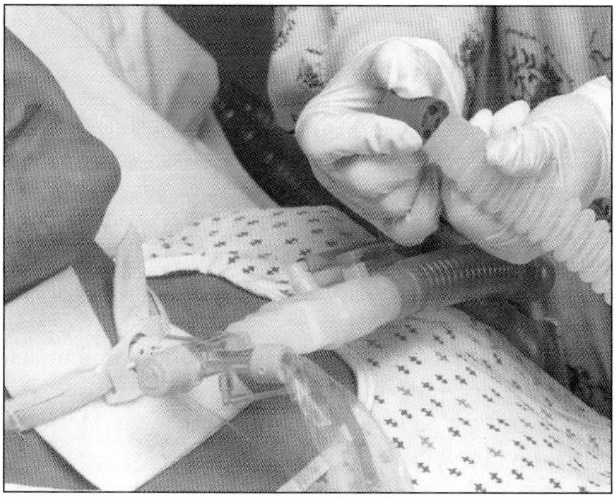

■ Connect the other end of the short-flex tubing to the ventilator tubing. Then attach the PMV (connected to the short-flex tubing) and the ventilator tubing to the closed-suction system (as shown below).

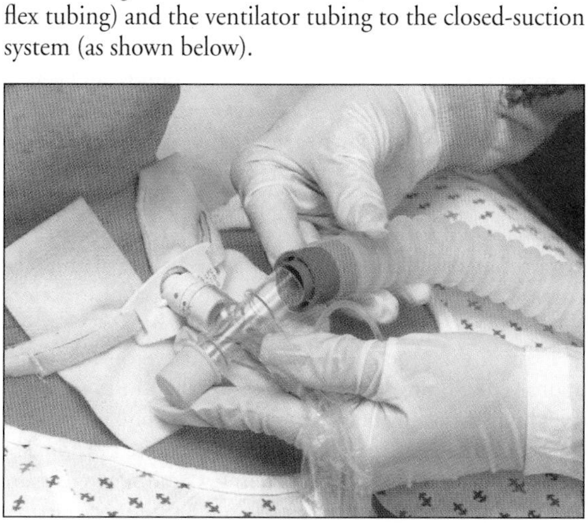

■ The PMV can also be attached between the swivel adapter and the short-flex tubing and ventilator tubing.
■ Post cuff-deflation warning signs in the room and label the tracheostomy pilot balloon *to remind health care providers to reinflate the pilot balloon after removing the PMV.*
■ Gently twist the PMV to remove it; restore the original setup, then return ventilator settings to original levels and reinflate the pilot balloon cuff. Always remember to reinflate the tracheostomy cuff after removing the PMV.

Special considerations

■ *For maximum airflow around the tube,* the tube shouldn't be larger than two-thirds the size of the tracheal lumen.

NURSING ALERT *Don't place the PMV on the tracheostomy tube before deflating the cuff* because the patient won't be able to breathe.

■ The nurse and respiratory therapist are responsible for monitoring the patient's response to the PMV by evaluating blood pressure, heart rate, and respiratory status.
■ Make sure that the patient is involved in the decision to use the ventilator speaking valve; make sure he understands how it functions and what to expect.
■ If he's anxious, especially during cuff deflation, he may be unwilling to use the valve; provide emotional support.
■ If he can't tolerate the valve initially; troubleshoot to determine the cause.
■ To correct, try repositioning the patient, using a smaller tracheostomy tube, changing to a cuffless tube, or correcting airway obstruction. Some patients have to build tolerance, wearing the valve a few minutes at a time at first.
■ If repeated trials fail, the speech-language pathologist should assess the patient for other communication options.

NURSING ALERT *Remove the PMV if the patient shows signs of distress, including significant change in blood pressure or heart rate, increased respiratory rate, dyspnea, diaphoresis, anxiety, uncontrollable coughing, or arterial oxygen saturation less than 90%. Reassess the patient before trying the valve again.*

Patient teaching

■ Explain the procedure to the patient. Provide written instructions, as needed.

Documentation

Note the patient's response to the procedure. Record how long the PMV has been in place. Document respiratory and hemodynamic status and secretion management, and note the patient's ability to vocalize.

SELECTED REFERENCES

Hess, D.R. "Facilitating Speech in the Patient with a Tracheostomy," *Respiratory Care* 50(4):519-25, April 2005.
Hull, E.M., et al. "Tracheostomy Speaking Valves for Children: Tolerance and Clinical Benefit," *Pediatric Rehabilitation* 8(3):214-19, July-September 2005.

TRACHEAL SUCTION

Tracheal suction involves the removal of secretions from the trachea or bronchi by means of a catheter inserted through the mouth or nose, a tracheal stoma, a tracheostomy tube, or an endotracheal (ET) tube. Besides removing secretions, tracheal suctioning also stimulates the cough reflex. This procedure helps maintain a patent airway to promote optimal exchange of oxygen and carbon dioxide and to prevent pneumonia that results from pooling of secretions. Performed as frequently as the patient's condition warrants, tracheal suction calls for strict sterile technique.

According to American Association for Respiratory Care (AARC) guidelines, the need to remove accumulated pulmonary secretions is evidenced by one of the following:

- breath sounds that are coarse or "noisy" on auscultation, such as gurgling, rhonchi, or diminished breath sounds
- increased peak inspiratory pressures during volume-controlled ventilation or decreased tidal volume during pressure-controlled ventilation
- patient's inability to generate an effective spontaneous cough
- visible secretions in the airway
- suspected aspiration of gastric or upper airway secretions
- clinically apparent increased work of breathing
- deterioration of arterial blood gas values
- restlessness
- feelings of secretions in the chest (tactile fremitus)
- chest X-ray that shows atelectasis or consolidation.

According to AARC guidelines, before suctioning the patient, hyperoxygenate him with 100% oxygen for at least 30 seconds. Sterile technique should be employed. The duration of each suctioning should be approximately 10 to 15 seconds. Suction pressure should be set as low as possible and yet effectively clear secretions. Following suctioning, the patient should be hyperoxygenated again for 1 minute or longer by the same technique used to preoxygenate the patient.

Tracheal suction is only one component of bronchial hygiene. Encourage the patient to clear his airways by coughing and teach him proper coughing techniques. Push adequate hydration to facilitate removal of secretions. Perform suctioning only when necessary and when other methods of removing secretions haven't been effective. Indeed, suctioning shouldn't be performed as a routine procedure. Assess the patient for clinical signs that suctioning is necessary, such as coarse breath sounds on auscultation, noisy respirations, prolonged expiratory breath sounds, and increased or decreased heart rate, respiratory rate, or blood pressure.

Equipment

Oxygen source (mechanical ventilator, wall or portable unit, and handheld resuscitation bag with a mask, 15-mm adapter, or a positive end-expiratory pressure valve, if indicated) ▪ wall or portable suction apparatus with tubing ▪ collection container ▪ connecting tube ▪ suction catheter kit or a sterile suction catheter, one sterile glove, one clean glove, and a disposable sterile solution container ▪ 1-L bottle of sterile water or normal saline solution ▪ sterile water-soluble lubricant (for nasal insertion) ▪ syringe for deflating cuff of ET or tracheostomy tube ▪ waterproof trash bag ▪ goggles and face mask or face shield ▪ optional: sterile towel.

Preparation of equipment

Choose a suction catheter of appropriate size. The diameter should be no larger than half the inside diameter of the tracheostomy or ET tube *to minimize hypoxia during suctioning.* (A #12 or #14 French catheter may be used for an 8-mm or larger tube.) Place the suction apparatus on the patient's overbed table or bedside stand. Position the table or stand on your preferred side of the bed *to facilitate suctioning.*

Attach the collection container to the suction unit and the connecting tube to the collection container. Label and date the normal saline solution or sterile water. Open the waterproof trash bag.

Implementation

- Confirm the patient's identity using two patient identifiers according to your facility's policy.
- Before suctioning, determine whether your facility requires a practitioner's order and obtain one, if necessary.
- Assess the patient's vital signs, breath sounds, and general appearance *to establish a baseline for comparison after suctioning.* Review the patient's arterial blood gas values and oxygen saturation levels if they're available. Evaluate the patient's ability to cough and deep-breathe *because this will help move secretions up the tracheobronchial tree.* If you'll be performing nasotracheal suctioning, check the patient's history for a deviated septum, nasal polyps, nasal obstruction, nasal trauma, epistaxis, or mucosal swelling.
- Explain the procedure to the patient even if he's unresponsive. Tell him that suctioning usually causes transient coughing or gagging but that coughing is helpful for removal of secretions. If the patient has been suctioned previously, summarize the reasons for suctioning. Continue to reassure the patient throughout the procedure *to minimize anxiety, promote relaxation, and decrease oxygen demand.*
- Unless contraindicated, place the patient in semi-Fowler's or high Fowler's position *to promote lung expansion and productive coughing.*
- Wash your hands. Put on personal protective equipment, as appropriate.
- Remove the top from the normal saline solution or water bottle.
- Open the package containing the sterile solution container.
- Using strict sterile technique, open the suction catheter kit, and put on the gloves. If using individual supplies, open the suction catheter and the gloves, placing the nonsterile

glove on your nondominant hand and then the sterile glove on your dominant hand.
- Using your nondominant (nonsterile) hand, pour the normal saline solution or sterile water into the solution container.
- Place a small amount of water-soluble lubricant on the sterile area. Lubricant may be used to facilitate passage of the catheter during nasotracheal suctioning.
- Place a sterile towel over the patient's chest, if desired, *to provide an additional sterile area.*
- Using your dominant (sterile) hand, remove the catheter from its wrapper. Keep it coiled *so it can't touch a nonsterile object.* Using your other hand to manipulate the connecting tubing, attach the catheter to the tubing (as shown below).

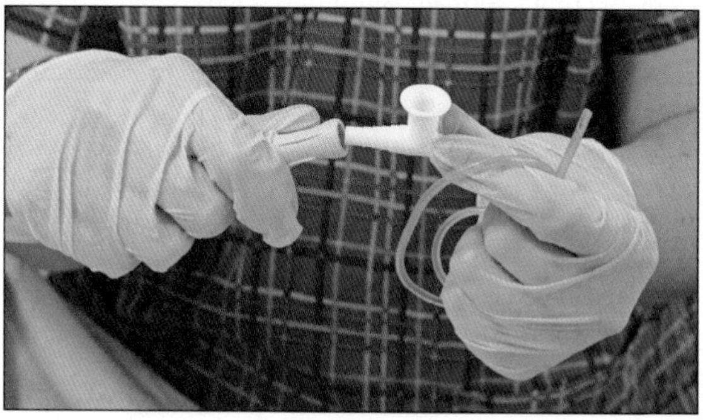

- Using your nondominant hand, set the suction pressure according to facility policy. Typically, pressure may be set between 100 and 150 mm Hg. *Higher pressures don't enhance secretion removal and may cause traumatic injury.* Occlude the suction port *to assess suction pressure.*
- Dip the catheter tip in the saline solution (as shown below) *to lubricate the outside of the catheter and reduce tissue trauma during insertion.*

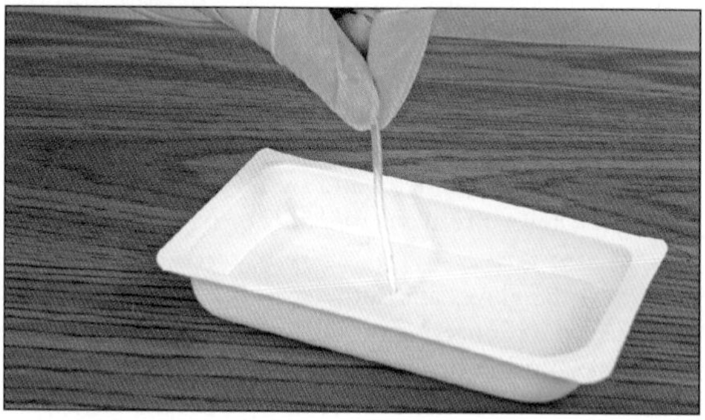

- With the catheter tip in the sterile solution, occlude the control valve with the thumb of your nondominant hand (as shown top of next column). Suction a small amount of solution through the catheter *to lubricate the inside of the catheter, thus facilitating passage of secretions through it.*

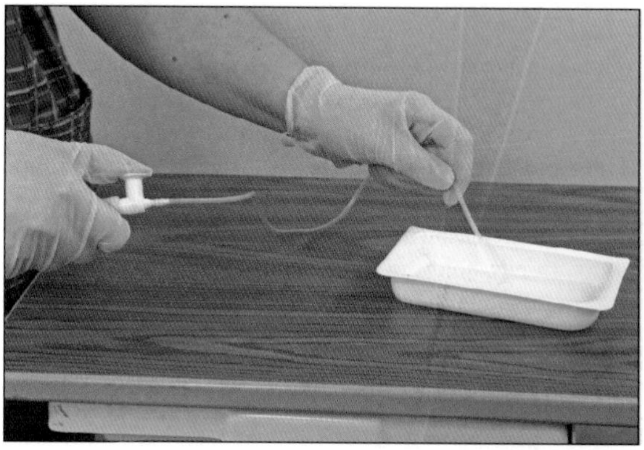

- For nasal insertion of the catheter, lubricate the tip of the catheter with the sterile, water-soluble lubricant *to reduce tissue trauma during insertion.*
- If the patient isn't intubated or is intubated but isn't receiving supplemental oxygen or aerosol, instruct him to take three to six deep breaths *to help minimize or prevent hypoxia during suctioning.*
- If the patient isn't intubated but is receiving oxygen, evaluate his need for preoxygenation. If indicated, instruct him to take three to six deep breaths while using his supplemental oxygen. (If needed, the patient may continue to receive supplemental oxygen during suctioning by leaving his nasal cannula in one nostril or by keeping the oxygen mask over his mouth.)
- If the patient is being mechanically ventilated, preoxygenate him *to minimize hypoxia after suctioning.* Use the ventilator (rather than a handheld resuscitation bag) to hyperoxygenate and hyperinflate the lungs before suctioning. Be aware that providing hyperoxygenation on some ventilators requires a washout time of up to 2 minutes *to ensure a higher oxygen concentration to travel through the tubing and reach the patient.* Newer models may be able to provide increased oxygen concentrations to the patient in less time.
- To preoxygenate using the ventilator, first adjust the fraction of inspired oxygen (FIO_2) and tidal volume according to your facility's policy and patient need. Next, either use the sigh mode or manually deliver three to six breaths. If you have an assistant for the procedure, the assistant can manage the patient's oxygen needs while you perform the suctioning.

Nasotracheal insertion in a nonintubated patient
- Disconnect the oxygen from the patient, if applicable.

■ Using your nondominant hand, raise the tip of the patient's nose *to straighten the passageway and facilitate insertion of the catheter.*
■ Insert the catheter into the patient's nostril while gently rolling it between your fingers *to help it advance through the turbinates.*
■ As the patient inhales, quickly advance the catheter as far as possible. *To avoid oxygen loss and tissue trauma,* don't apply suction during insertion.
■ If the patient coughs as the catheter passes through the larynx, briefly hold the catheter still, and then resume advancement when the patient inhales.

Insertion in an intubated patient
■ If you're using a closed system, see *Closed tracheal suctioning.*
■ Using your nonsterile hand, disconnect the patient from the ventilator.
■ Using your sterile hand, gently insert the suction catheter into the artificial airway (as shown below). Advance the catheter, without applying suction, until you meet resistance. If the patient coughs, pause briefly and then resume advancement.

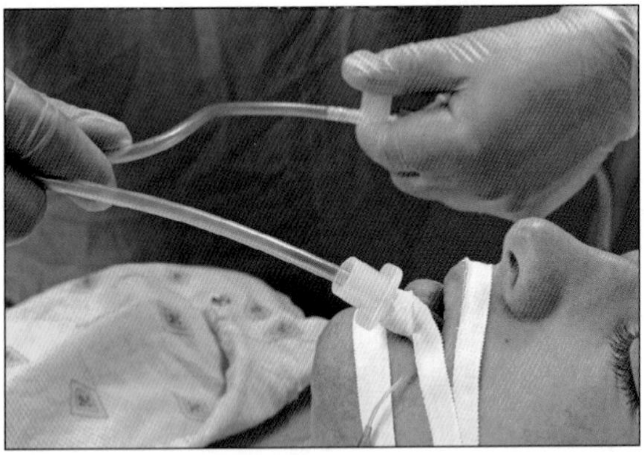

Suctioning the patient
■ After inserting the catheter, apply suction intermittently by removing and replacing the thumb of your nondominant hand over the control valve. Simultaneously use your dominant hand to withdraw the catheter as you roll it between your thumb and forefinger. *This rotating motion prevents the catheter from pulling tissue into the tube as it exits, thus avoiding tissue trauma.*
■ Never suction more than 10 to 15 seconds at a time *to prevent hypoxia.* Don't pass the catheter more than twice *to reduce trauma to the tracheal mucosa.*
■ If the patient is intubated, use your nondominant hand to stabilize the tip of the ET tube as you withdraw the catheter *to prevent mucous membrane irritation or accidental extubation.*
■ If applicable, resume oxygen delivery by reconnecting the source of oxygen or ventilation and hyperoxygenating the patient's lungs before continuing *to prevent or relieve hypoxia.*
■ Observe the patient, and allow him to rest for a few minutes before the next suctioning. The timing of each suctioning and the length of each rest period depend on his tolerance of the procedure and the absence of complications. *To enhance secretion removal,* encourage the patient to cough between suctioning attempts.
■ Observe the secretions. If they're thick, clear the catheter periodically by dipping the tip in the saline solution and applying suction. Normally, sputum is watery and tends to be sticky. Tenacious or thick sputum usually indicates dehydration. Watch for color variations. White or translucent color is normal; discolored secretions (yellow, green) may indicate infection; brown usually indicates old blood; red indicates fresh blood. When sputum contains blood, note whether it is streaked or well mixed. Also, indicate how often blood appeared.
■ If the patient's heart rate and rhythm are being monitored, observe for arrhythmias. If they occur, stop suctioning and ventilate the patient.
■ Patients who can't mobilize secretions effectively may need to perform tracheal suctioning after discharge. (See *Tracheal suctioning at home,* page 566.)

After suctioning
■ After suctioning, hyperoxygenate the patient being maintained on a ventilator by using the ventilator's sigh mode, as described earlier.
■ Readjust the FIO_2 and, for ventilated patients, the tidal volume to the ordered settings.
■ After suctioning the lower airway, assess the patient's need for upper airway suctioning. If the cuff of the ET or tracheostomy tube is inflated, suction the upper airway before deflating the cuff with a syringe. (See "Oronasopharyngeal suction," page 535, and "Endotracheal tube care," page 545.) Always change the catheter and sterile glove before resuctioning the lower airway *to avoid introducing microorganisms into the lower airway.*
■ Discard the gloves and catheter in the waterproof trash bag. Clear the connecting tubing by aspirating the remaining saline solution or water. Discard and replace suction equipment and supplies according to your facility's policy. Wash your hands.
■ Auscultate the lungs bilaterally and take vital signs, if indicated, *to assess the procedure's effectiveness.* Note the patient's skin color, breathing pattern, and respiratory rate.

Closed tracheal suctioning

The closed tracheal suction system can ease removal of secretions and reduce patient complications. Consisting of a sterile suction catheter in a clear plastic sleeve, the system permits the patient to remain connected to the ventilator during suctioning. As a result, the patient can maintain the tidal volume, oxygen concentration, and positive end-expiratory pressure delivered by the ventilator while being suctioned. In turn, this reduces the occurrence of suction-induced hypoxemia.

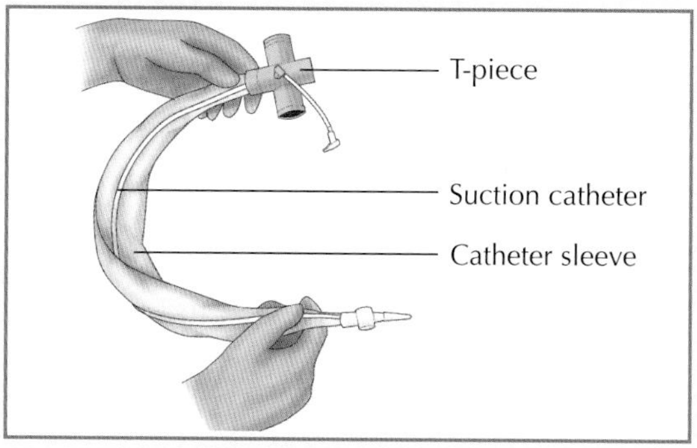

Another advantage of this system is a reduced risk of infection, even when the same catheter is used many times. Because the catheter remains in a protective sleeve, gloves aren't required, but are still recommended. The caregiver doesn't need to touch the catheter and the ventilator circuit remains closed.

Implementation

To perform the procedure, gather a closed suction control valve, a T-piece to connect the artificial airway to the ventilator breathing circuit, and a catheter sleeve that encloses the catheter and has connections at each end for the control valve and the T-piece. Put on personal protective equipment, if you haven't already done so. Then follow these steps:

- Remove the closed suction system from its wrapping. Attach the control valve to the connecting tubing.
- Depress the thumb suction control valve, and keep it depressed while setting the suction pressure to the desired level.
- Connect the T-piece to the ventilator breathing circuit, making sure that the irrigation port is closed; then connect the T-piece to the patient's endotracheal or tracheostomy tube.
- Hyperoxygenate the patient using the ventilator.
- With one hand keeping the T-piece parallel to the patient's chin, use the thumb and index finger of the other hand to advance the catheter through the tube and into the patient's tracheobronchial tree (as shown below). It may be necessary to gently retract the catheter sleeve as you advance the catheter.

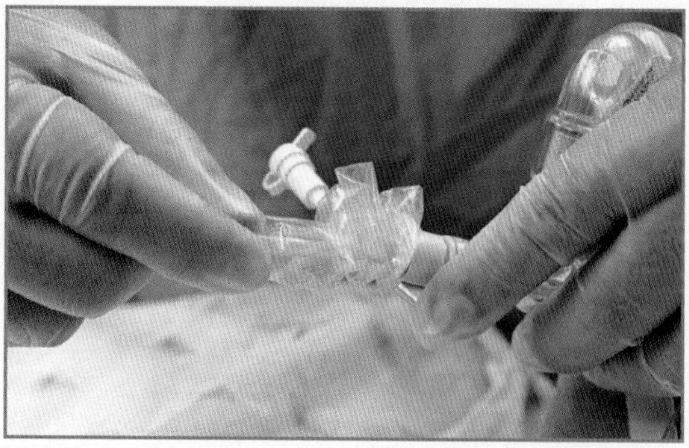

- While continuing to hold the T-piece and control valve, apply intermittent suction and withdraw the catheter until it reaches its fully extended length in the sleeve (as shown below). Repeat the procedure, as necessary.

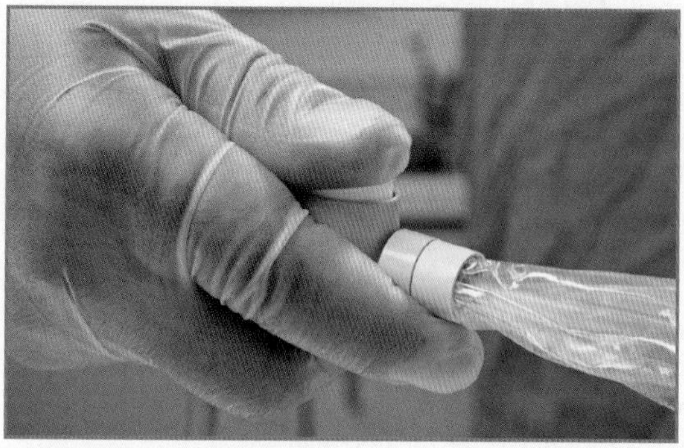

- After you've finished suctioning, flush the catheter by maintaining suction while slowly introducing normal saline solution or sterile water into the irrigation port.
- Place the thumb control valve in the off position.
- Dispose of and replace the suction equipment and supplies according to your facility's policy.
- Remove your gloves and wash your hands.
- Change the closed suction system every 24 hours *to minimize the risk of infection.*

HOMECARE

Tracheal suctioning at home

If a patient can't mobilize secretions effectively by coughing, he may have to perform tracheal suctioning at home using either clean or sterile technique. Most patients use clean technique, which consists of thorough hand washing and possibly wearing a clean glove. However, a patient with poor hand-washing technique, recurrent respiratory infections, or a compromised immune system or one who has had recent surgery may need to use sterile technique.

Clean technique

Because the cost of disposable catheters can be prohibitive, many patients reuse disposable catheters, but the practice remains controversial. If the catheter has thick secretions adhering to it, the patient may clean it with Control III—a quaternary compound.

An alternative to disposable catheters is to use nondisposable, red rubber catheters. Consult your facility's policy regarding the care and cleaning of suction catheters in the home setting.

Supplies needed

Obviously, the supplies needed will vary with the technique used. If the patient will be using clean technique, he'll need suction catheter kits (or clean gloves, suction catheters, and basin) and distilled water. If he'll be using sterile technique, everything will need to be sterile: the suction catheters, gloves, basin, and water (or normal saline solution).

The type of suction machine necessary will depend on the patient's needs. You'll need to evaluate the amount of suction the machine provides, how easy it is to clean, how much it costs, the volume of the collection bottles, and whether the machine has an overflow safety device *to prevent secretions from entering the compressor.* You'll also need to determine whether the patient needs a machine that operates on batteries and, if so, how long the batteries will last and whether and how they can be recharged.

Nursing goals

Before discharge, the patient and his family should demonstrate the suctioning procedure. They also need to recognize the indications for suctioning, the signs and symptoms of infection, the importance of adequate hydration, and when to use adjunct therapy, such as aerosol therapy, chest physiotherapy, oxygen therapy, or a handheld resuscitation bag. At discharge, arrange for a home health care provider and a durable medical equipment vendor to follow up with the patient.

Special considerations

- Raising the patient's nose into the sniffing position helps align the larynx and pharynx and may facilitate passing the catheter during nasotracheal suctioning. If the patient's condition permits, have an assistant extend the patient's head and neck above his shoulders. The patient's lower jaw may need to be moved up and forward. If the patient is responsive, ask him to stick out his tongue *so he won't be able to swallow the catheter during insertion.*
- During suctioning, the catheter typically is advanced as far as the mainstem bronchi. However, *because of tracheobronchial anatomy,* the catheter tends to enter the right mainstem bronchi instead of the left. Using an angled catheter (such as a coudé) may help you guide the catheter into the left mainstem bronchus. Rotating the patient's head to the right seems to have a limited effect.
- In addition to the closed tracheal method, oxygen insufflation offers a new approach to suctioning. This method uses a double-lumen catheter that allows oxygen insufflation during the suctioning procedure.
- Don't allow the collection container on the suction machine to become more than three-quarters full *to keep from damaging the machine.*

Complications

Because oxygen is removed along with secretions, the patient may experience hypoxemia and dyspnea. Anxiety may alter respiratory patterns. Cardiac arrhythmias can result from hypoxia and stimulation of the vagus nerve in the tracheobronchial tree. Tracheal or bronchial trauma can result from traumatic or prolonged suctioning.

Patients with compromised cardiovascular or pulmonary status are at risk for hypoxemia, arrhythmias, hypertension, or hypotension. Patients with a history of nasopharyngeal bleeding, those who are taking anticoagulants, those who have undergone a tracheostomy recently, and those who have a blood dyscrasia are at increased risk for bleeding as a result of suctioning. Use caution when suctioning patients who have increased intracranial pressure *because suction may further increase pressure.*

If the patient experiences laryngospasm or bronchospasm (rare complications) during suctioning, disconnect the suction catheter from the connecting tubing and allow the catheter to act as an airway. Discuss with the patient's practitioner the use of bronchodilators or lidocaine *to reduce the risk of this complication.*

Documentation

Record the date and time of the procedure; the technique used; the reason for suctioning; the amount, color, consistency, and odor (if any) of the secretions; complications and the nursing action taken; and pertinent data regarding the patient's subjective response to the procedure. Also chart preprocedure and postprocedure breath sounds and vital signs.

SELECTED REFERENCES

American Association for Respiratory Care. "AARC Clinical Practice Guideline: Endotracheal Suctioning of Mechanically Ventilated Adults and Children with Artificial Airways," *Respiratory Care* 38(5):500-504, May 1993.

American Association for Respiratory Care. "AARC Clinical Practice Guideline: Suctioning of the Patient in the Home," *Respiratory Care* 44(1):99-104, January 1999.

The Joanna Briggs Institute. "Best Practice: Tracheal Suctioning of Adults with an Artificial Airway," 4(4):106, 2000. Available at: *www.joannabriggs.edu.au/bpmenu/html*

Lorente, L., et al. "Tracheal Suction by Closed System Without Daily Change versus Open System," *Intensive Care Medicine* 32(4):538-44, April 2006.

Lorente, L., et al. "Ventilator-associated Pneumonia Using a Closed versus an Open Tracheal Suction System," *Critical Care Medicine* 33(1):115-19, January 2005.

Lynn-McHale Wiegand, D.J., and Carlson, K.K., eds. *AACN Procedure Manual for Critical Care*, 5th ed. Philadelphia: W.B. Saunders Co., 2006.

Shah, S., et al. "An In Vitro Evaluation of the Effectiveness of Endotracheal Suction Catheters," *Chest* 128(5):3699-704, November 2005.

Taylor, C., et al. *Fundamentals of Nursing: The Art and Science of Nursing Care*, 5th ed. Philadelphia: Lippincott Williams & Wilkins, 2008.

CRICOTHYROTOMY

When endotracheal intubation or a tracheotomy can't be performed quickly to establish an airway, an emergency cricothyrotomy may be necessary. Performed rarely, cricothyrotomy involves puncturing the trachea through the cricothyroid membrane. (See *Performing an emergency cricothyrotomy,* page 568.)

Usually, your role will be to assist a physician with this procedure. Ideally, cricothyrotomy is performed using sterile technique but, in an emergency, this may not be possible.

Equipment

Have one person stay with the patient while another collects the necessary equipment.

For scalpel or needle cricothyrotomy: Sterile gloves ■ goggles ■ antiseptic solution ■ sterile 4″ × 4″ gauze pads ■ dilator ■ tape ■ oxygen source.

For scalpel cricothyrotomy: Scalpel ■ #6 or smaller tracheostomy tube (if available) ■ handheld resuscitation bag or T tube and wide-bore oxygen tubing.

For needle cricothyrotomy: 14G (or larger) through-the-needle or over-the-needle catheter ■ 10-ml syringe ■ tape ■ I.V. extension tubing ■ hand-operated release valve or pressure-regulating adjustment valve.

Implementation

- Put on sterile gloves and goggles.
- The patient's neck is hyperextended to expose the area of the incision site.
- Hold the patient's head in the correct position while the surgeon performs the procedure.

Special considerations

- Immediately after the procedure, check for bleeding at the insertion site, subcutaneous emphysema or inadequate ventilation, and tracheal or vocal cord damage.

PEDIATRIC ALERT *Scalpel cricothyrotomy isn't recommended for children younger than age 12* because it could damage the cricoid cartilage — the only circumferential support to the upper trachea.

Complications

Hemorrhage, perforation of the thyroid or esophagus, and subcutaneous or mediastinal emphysema may occur from this procedure. Infection may also occur several days after the procedure.

Documentation

Your documentation of the procedure should include the date, time, and circumstances requiring the procedure and the patient's vital signs. Note whether the patient initiated spontaneous respirations after the procedure.

Record how much and by what method oxygen was delivered. Also document procedures that were performed after the airway was established — for example, endotracheal intubation or tracheostomy.

Performing an emergency cricothyrotomy

To perform this procedure, the surgeon puts on sterile gloves and cleans the patient's neck with a gauze pad soaked in antiseptic solution. *To reduce the risk of contamination,* he uses a circular motion, working outward from the incision site. Personal protective equipment (gown, gloves, mask, eye protectors) should be worn by all involved in the procedure, as appropriate.

- The surgeon locates the precise insertion site by sliding the thumb and fingers down to the thyroid gland. The outer borders are located when the space between his fingers and thumb widens.
- The surgeon will move his finger across the center of the gland, over the anterior edge of the cricoid ring.

Using a scalpel

- A horizontal incision less than ½″ (1.3 cm) long is made in the cricothyroid membrane just above the cricoid ring.

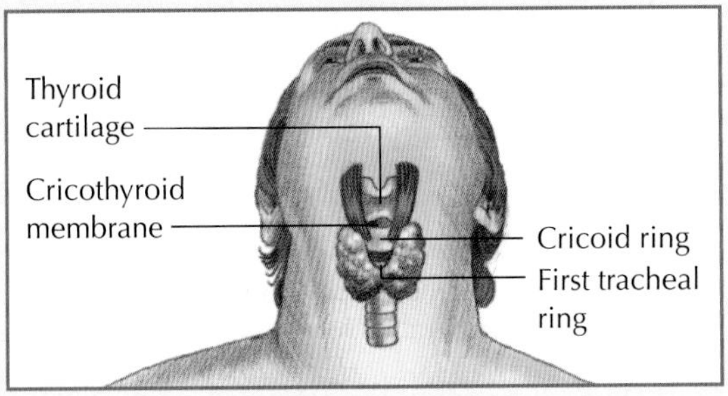

- A dilator is inserted *to prevent tissue from closing around the incision.* If a dilator isn't available, the handle of the scalpel is inserted and rotated 90 degrees (as shown below).

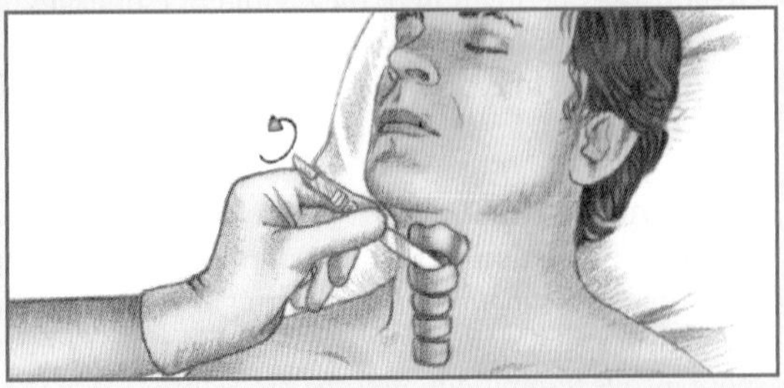

- A #6 or smaller tracheostomy tube is inserted and secured *to maintain a patent airway.* If a tracheostomy tube isn't available, the dilator or scalpel handle is taped in place until a tracheostomy tube is available.
- If the patient can breathe spontaneously, assist by attaching a humidified oxygen source to the tracheostomy tube with a T tube; if he can't, attach a handheld resuscitation bag. You'll need to inflate the cuff of the tracheostomy tube with a syringe *to provide positive-pressure ventilation.*
- Auscultate bilaterally for breath sounds, and take the patient's vital signs.
- Dispose of the gloves and other personal protective gear properly and wash your hands.

Using a needle

- A 10-ml syringe is attached to a 14G (or larger) through-the-needle or over-the-needle catheter. The catheter is inserted into the cricothyroid membrane just above the cricoid ring.
- The catheter is directed downward to the trachea at a 45-degree angle (as shown below) *to avoid damaging the vocal cords.* Negative pressure is maintained by pulling back the syringe plunger as the catheter is advanced. The catheter has entered the trachea when air enters the syringe.

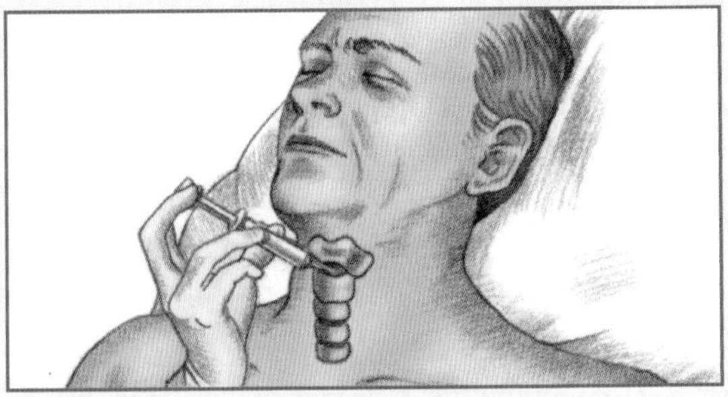

- When the catheter reaches the trachea, it's advanced and the needle and syringe are removed. Assist in taping the catheter in place.
- Attach the catheter hub to one end of the I.V. extension tubing. At the other end, attach a hand-operated release valve or a pressure-regulating adjustment valve. Connect the entire assembly to an oxygen source.
- Press the release valve to introduce oxygen into the trachea and inflate the lungs. When you can see that they're inflated, release the valve *to allow passive exhalation.* Adjust the pressure-regulating valve to the minimum pressure needed for adequate lung inflation.
- Auscultate bilaterally for breath sounds, and take the patient's vital signs.
- Dispose of the gloves properly and wash your hands.

SELECTED REFERENCES

Lynn-McHale Wiegand, D.J., and Carlson, K.K., eds. *AACN Procedure Manual for Critical Care*, 5th ed. Philadelphia: W.B. Saunders Co., 2006.

Price, R.J. "Surgical Cricothyroidotomy Technique," *Anesthesiology* 103(3):667-68, September 2005.

Scrase, I., and Woollard, M. "Needle vs. Surgical Cricothyroidotomy: A Shortcut to Effective Ventilation," *Anaesthesia* 61(10):962-74, October 2006.

OTHER TREATMENTS

OXYGEN ADMINISTRATION

A patient will need oxygen therapy when hypoxemia results from a respiratory or cardiac emergency or an increase in metabolic function.

In a *respiratory emergency,* oxygen administration enables the patient to reduce his ventilatory effort. When conditions such as atelectasis or adult respiratory distress syndrome impair diffusion, or when lung volumes are decreased from alveolar hypoventilation, this procedure boosts alveolar oxygen levels.

In a *cardiac emergency,* oxygen therapy helps meet the increased myocardial workload as the heart tries to compensate for hypoxemia. Oxygen administration is particularly important for a patient whose myocardium is already compromised—perhaps from a myocardial infarction (MI) or cardiac arrhythmia.

When *metabolic demand* is high (in cases of massive trauma, burns, or high fever, for instance) oxygen administration supplies the body with enough oxygen to meet its cellular needs. This procedure also increases oxygenation in the patient with a reduced blood oxygen-carrying capacity, perhaps from carbon monoxide poisoning or sickle cell crisis.

The American Association for Respiratory Care recommends careful monitoring of the patient receiving oxygen therapy. Clinical assessment should include examination of the pulmonary, cardiac, and neurologic systems. At the beginning of oxygen therapy, oxygen saturation and tension should be measured. These parameters should also be measured again within 8 to 12 hours of initiating therapy with a fraction of inspired oxygen greater than or equal to 0.4. The parameters also should be measured within 2 hours of starting therapy for a patient with a primary diagnosis of chronic obstructive pulmonary disease and within 72 hours in a patient with a myocardial infarction. Oxygen saturation and tension should be measured in neonates within 1 hour of birth.

The adequacy of oxygen therapy is determined by arterial blood gas (ABG) analysis, oximetry monitoring, and clinical examinations. The patient's disease, physical condition, and age will help determine the most appropriate method of administration.

Equipment

The equipment needed depends on the type of delivery system ordered. (See *Guide to oxygen delivery systems,* pages 570 to 573.) Equipment includes selections from the following list: oxygen source (wall unit, cylinder, liquid tank, or concentrator) ■ flowmeter ■ adapter, if using a wall unit, or a pressure-reduction gauge, if using a cylinder ■ sterile humidity bottle and adapter ■ sterile distilled water ■ OXYGEN PRECAUTION sign ■ appropriate oxygen delivery system (a nasal cannula, simple mask, or nonrebreather mask for low-flow and variable oxygen concentrations; a Venturi mask, aerosol mask, T tube, tracheostomy collar, tent, or oxygen hood for high-flow and specific oxygen concentrations) ■ small-diameter and large-diameter connection tubing ■ flashlight (for nasal cannula) ■ water-soluble lubricant ■ gauze pads and tape (for oxygen masks) ■ jet adapter for Venturi mask (if adding humidity) ■ gloves ■ stethoscope ■ sphygmomanometer ■ optional: oxygen analyzer.

Preparation of equipment

Although a respiratory therapist typically is responsible for setting up, maintaining, and managing the equipment, you'll need a working knowledge of the oxygen system being used.

Check the oxygen outlet port *to verify flow.* Pinch the tubing near the prongs and listen for a higher pitched sound caused by the increased pressure.

Implementation

- Gather the appropriate equipment.
- Confirm the patient's identity using two patient identifiers according to your facility's policy.
- Obtain a baseline assessment including vital signs, lung sounds, and a physical assessment. In an emergency situation, verify that he has an open airway before administering oxygen.
- Explain the procedure to the patient, and let him know why he needs oxygen *to ensure his cooperation.*
- Check the patient's room *to make sure it's safe for oxygen administration.* Whenever possible, replace electrical devices with nonelectrical ones and post a NO SMOKING sign in the patient's room.

PEDIATRIC ALERT *If the patient is a child and is in an oxygen tent, remove all toys that may produce a spark.* Oxygen supports combustion, and the smallest spark can cause a fire.

- Place an OXYGEN PRECAUTION sign over the patient's bed and on the door to his room.

(Text continues on page 573.)

EQUIPMENT

Guide to oxygen delivery systems

Patients may receive oxygen through one of several administration systems. Each has its own benefits, drawbacks, and indications for use. The advantages and disadvantages of each system are compared below.

Nasal cannula

Oxygen is delivered through plastic cannulas in the patient's nostrils.

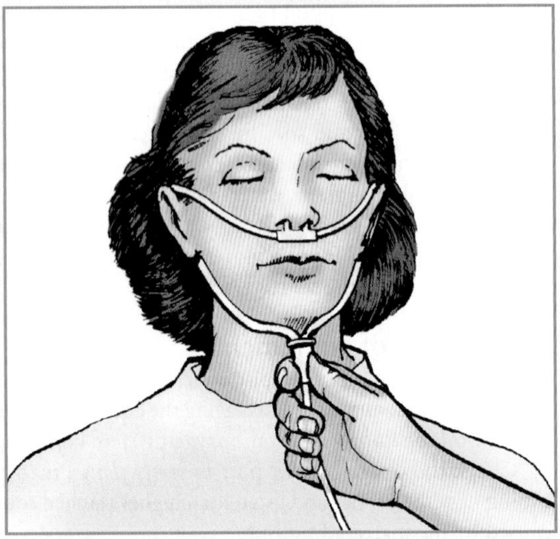

Advantages: Safe and simple; comfortable and easily tolerated; nasal prongs can be shaped to fit any face; effective for low oxygen concentrations; allows movement, eating, and talking; inexpensive and disposable.

Disadvantages: Can't deliver concentrations higher than 40%; can't be used in complete nasal obstruction; may cause headaches or dry mucous membranes; can dislodge easily.

Administration guidelines: Ensure the patency of the patient's nostrils with a flashlight. If patent, hook the cannula tubing behind the patient's ears and under the chin. Slide the adjuster upward under the chin to secure the tubing. If using an elastic strap to secure the cannula, position it over the ears and around the back of the head. Avoid applying it too tightly, *which can result in excess pressure on facial structures as well as cannula occlusion*. With a nasal cannula, oral breathers achieve the same oxygen delivery as nasal breathers. Oxygen can be administered without humidification at flow less than or equal to 4 L/minute.

Simple mask

Oxygen flows through an entry port at the bottom of the mask and exits through large holes on the sides of the mask.

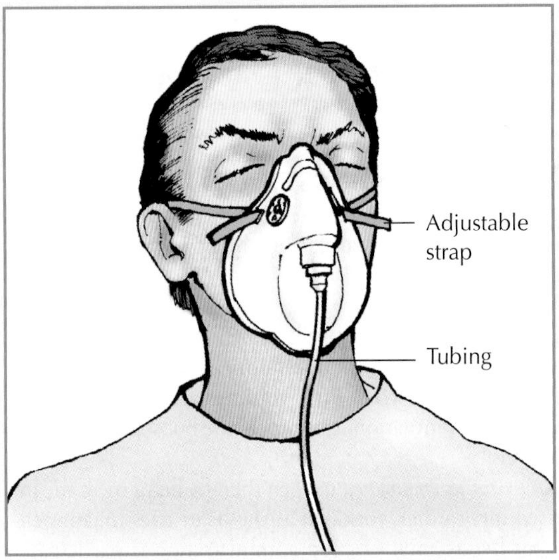

Advantages: Can deliver concentrations of 35% to 50%.

Disadvantages: Hot and confining; may irritate patient's skin; tight seal, which may cause discomfort, is required for higher oxygen concentration; interferes with talking and eating; impractical for long-term therapy because of imprecision.

Administration guidelines: Select the mask size that offers the best fit. Place the mask over the patient's nose, mouth, and chin, and mold the flexible metal edge to the bridge of the nose. Adjust the elastic band around the head to hold the mask firmly but comfortably over the cheeks, chin, and bridge of the nose. For elderly or cachectic patients with sunken cheeks, tape gauze pads to the mask over the cheek area to try to create an airtight seal. *Without this seal, room air dilutes the oxygen, preventing delivery of the prescribed concentration.* A minimum of 5 L/minute is required in all masks to flush expired carbon dioxide from the mask so that the patient doesn't rebreathe it.

Guide to oxygen delivery systems *(continued)*

Nonrebreather mask

On inhalation, the one-way inspiratory valve opens, directing oxygen from a reservoir bag into the mask. On exhalation, gas exits the mask through the one-way expiratory valves and enters the atmosphere. The patient breathes air only from the bag.

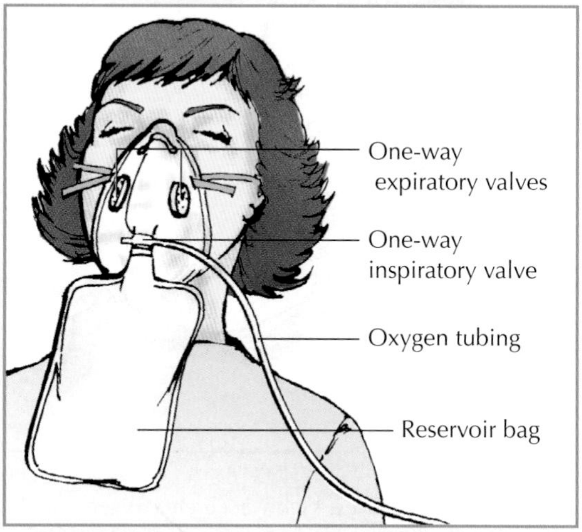

Advantages: Delivers the highest possible oxygen concentration (60% to 80%) short of intubation and mechanical ventilation; effective for short-term therapy; doesn't dry mucous membranes; can be converted to a partial rebreather mask, if necessary, by removing the one-way valve.

Disadvantages: Requires a tight seal, which may be difficult to maintain and may cause discomfort; may irritate the patient's skin; interferes with talking and eating; impractical for long-term therapy.

Administration guidelines: Follow procedures listed for the simple mask. Make sure that the mask fits very snugly and that the one-way valves are secure and functioning. *Because the mask excludes room air,* a valve malfunction could cause carbon dioxide buildup and suffocate an unconscious patient. If the reservoir bag collapses more than slightly during inspiration, raise the flow rate until you see only a slight deflation. *Marked or complete deflation indicates an insufficient flow rate.* Keep the reservoir bag from twisting or kinking. Ensure free expansion by making sure the bag lies outside the patient's gown and bedcovers.

CPAP mask

This system allows the spontaneously breathing patient to receive continuous positive airway pressure (CPAP) with or without an artificial airway.

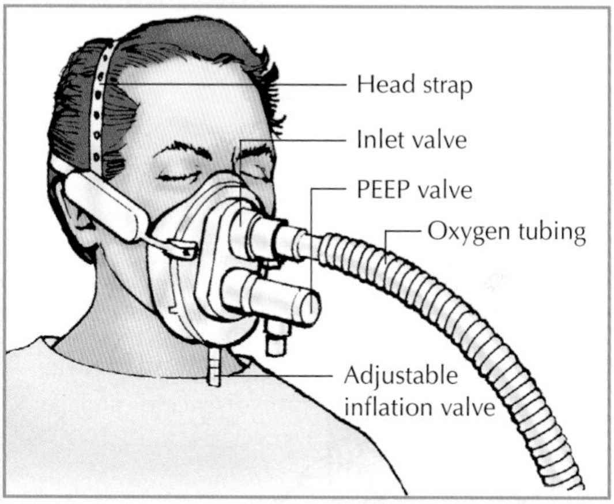

Advantages: Noninvasively improves arterial oxygenation by increasing functional residual capacity; allows the patient to avoid intubation; allows the patient to talk and cough without interrupting positive pressure.

Disadvantages: Requires a tight fit, which may cause discomfort; interferes with eating and talking; heightened risk of aspiration if the patient vomits; increased risk of pneumothorax, diminished cardiac output, and gastric distention; generally contraindicated in patients with chronic obstructive pulmonary disease, bullous lung disease, low cardiac output, or tension pneumothorax.

Administration guidelines: Place one strap behind the patient's head and the other strap over his head *to ensure a snug fit.* Attach one latex strap to the connector prong on one side of the mask. Then use one hand to position the mask on the patient's face while using the other hand to connect the strap to the other side of the mask. After the mask is applied, assess the patient's respiratory, circulatory, and GI function every hour. Watch for signs of pneumothorax, decreased cardiac output, a drop in blood pressure, and gastric distention.

(continued)

Guide to oxygen delivery systems *(continued)*

Transtracheal oxygen

The patient receives oxygen through a catheter inserted into the base of his neck in a simple outpatient procedure.

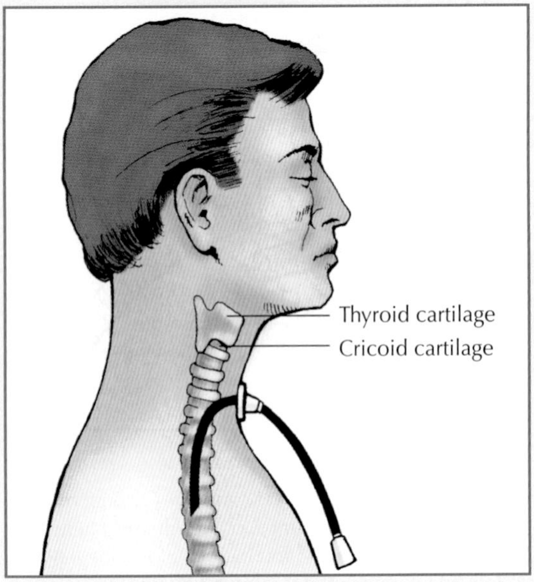

Advantages: Supplies oxygen to the lungs throughout the respiratory cycle; provides continuous oxygen without hindering mobility; doesn't interfere with eating or talking; doesn't dry mucous membranes; catheter can easily be concealed by a shirt or scarf.

Disadvantages: Not suitable for use in patients at risk for bleeding or those with severe bronchospasm, uncompensated respiratory acidosis, pleural herniation into the base of the neck, or high corticosteroid dosages.

Administration guidelines: After insertion, obtain a chest X-ray *to confirm placement.* Monitor the patient for bleeding, respiratory distress, pneumothorax, pain, coughing, or hoarseness. Don't use the catheter for about 1 week following insertion *to decrease the risk of subcutaneous emphysema.*

Venturi mask

The mask is connected to a Venturi device, which mixes a specific volume of air and oxygen.

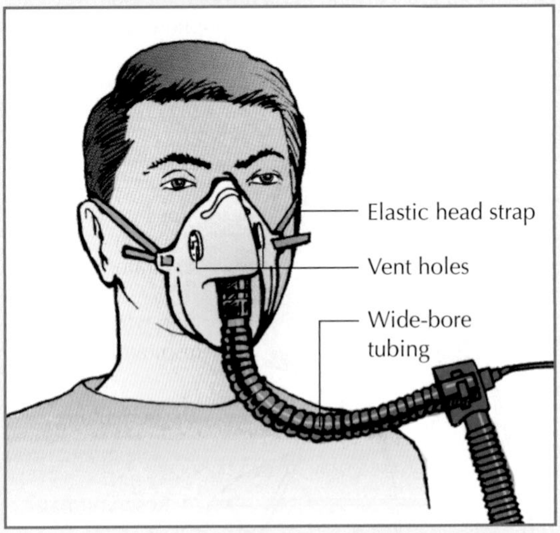

Advantages: Delivers highly accurate oxygen concentration despite the patient's respiratory pattern because the same amount of air is always entrained; dilute jets can be changed or dial turned to change oxygen concentration; doesn't dry mucous membranes; humidity or aerosol can be added.

Disadvantages: Confining and may irritate skin; oxygen concentration may be altered if mask fits loosely, tubing kinks, oxygen intake ports become blocked, flow is insufficient, or the patient is hyperpneic; interferes with eating and talking; condensate may collect and drip on the patient if humidification is used.

Administration guidelines: Make sure that the oxygen flow rate is set at the amount specified on each mask and that the Venturi valve is set for the desired fraction of inspired oxygen.

Guide to oxygen delivery systems *(continued)*

Aerosols

A face mask, hood, tent, or tracheostomy tube or collar is connected to wide-bore tubing that receives aerosolized oxygen from a jet nebulizer. The jet nebulizer, which is attached near the oxygen source, adjusts air entrainment in a manner similar to the Venturi device.

Advantages: Administers high humidity; gas can be heated (when delivered through artificial airway) or cooled (when delivered through a tent).

Disadvantages: Condensate collected in the tracheostomy collar or T tube may drain into the tracheostomy; the weight of the T tube can put stress on the tracheostomy tube.

Administration guidelines: Guidelines vary with the type of nebulizer used: ultrasonic, large-volume, small-volume, and in-line types. When using a high-output nebulizer, watch for signs of overhydration, pulmonary edema, crackles, and electrolyte imbalance.

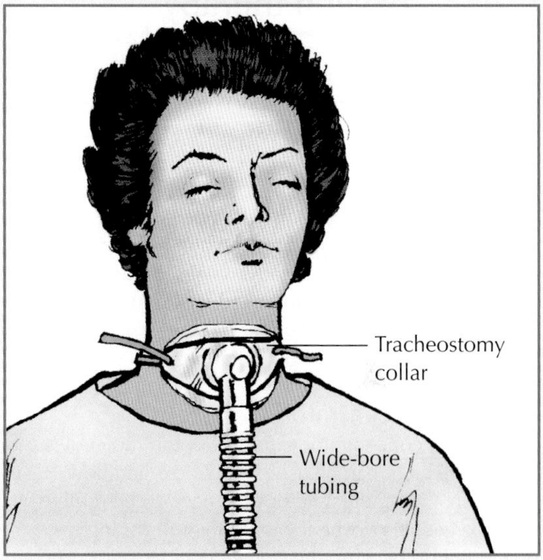

- Help place the oxygen delivery device on the patient. Make sure it fits properly and is stable. Pad any pressure areas *to prevent skin breakdown.*
- Monitor the patient's response to oxygen therapy. Check his ABG values during initial adjustments of oxygen flow. When the patient is stabilized, you may use pulse oximetry to monitor trends. Check the patient frequently for signs of hypoxia, such as decreased level of consciousness, increased heart rate, arrhythmias, restlessness, perspiration, dyspnea, use of accessory muscles, yawning or flared nostrils, cyanosis, and cool, clammy skin. Obtain vital signs, as needed.
- Observe the patient's skin integrity *to prevent skin breakdown on pressure points from the oxygen delivery device.* Wipe moisture or perspiration from the patient's face and from the mask as needed.

Special considerations

NURSING ALERT *Never administer oxygen by nasal cannula at more than 2 L/minute to a patient with chronic lung disease unless you have a specific order to do so.* That's because some patients with chronic lung disease become dependent on a state of hypercapnia and hypoxia to stimulate their respirations, and supplemental oxygen could cause them to stop breathing. *However, long-term oxygen therapy of 12 to 17 hours daily may help patients with chronic lung disease sleep better, survive longer, and experience a reduced incidence of pulmonary hypertension.*

- When monitoring a patient's response to a change in oxygen flow, check the pulse oximetry monitor or measure ABG values 20 to 30 minutes after adjusting the flow. In the interim, monitor the patient closely for any adverse response to the change in oxygen flow.
- If the patient will be receiving oxygen at a concentration above 60% for more than 24 hours, watch carefully for signs of oxygen toxicity.
- *Prolonged high concentrations of oxygen can cause lung injury.* Surfactant activity may be impaired and increased capillary congestion, edema, interstitial space thickening, and fibrotic changes may occur. The patient may experience symptoms of tracheobronchial irritation, such as coughing and substernal discomfort.
- Remind the patient to cough and deep-breathe frequently *to prevent atelectasis. To prevent the development of serious lung damage,* measure ABG values repeatedly to determine whether high oxygen concentrations are still necessary.

Home care

Before discharging a patient who will receive oxygen therapy at home, make sure you're familiar with the types of oxygen therapy, the kinds of services that are available, and the service schedules offered by local home suppliers. Together

HOME CARE

Types of home oxygen therapy

Oxygen therapy can be administered at home using an oxygen tank, an oxygen concentrator, or liquid oxygen.

Oxygen tank

Commonly used for patients who need oxygen on a standby basis or who need a ventilator at home, the oxygen tank has several disadvantages, including its cumbersome design and the need for frequent refills. *Because oxygen is stored under high pressure,* the oxygen tank also poses a potential hazard.

Oxygen concentrator

The oxygen concentrator extracts oxygen molecules from room air. It can be used for low oxygen flow (less than 4 L/minute) and doesn't need to be refilled with oxygen. However, it won't function during a power failure *because the oxygen concentrator runs on electricity.*

Liquid oxygen

The liquid oxygen option is commonly used by patients who are oxygen-dependent but still mobile. It includes a large liquid reservoir for home use. When the patient wants to leave the house, he fills a portable unit worn over the shoulder; this supplies oxygen for up to 3 hours, depending on the liter flow.

with the practitioner and the patient, choose the device that's best suited to the patient. (See *Types of home oxygen therapy.*)

If the patient will be receiving transtracheal oxygen therapy, teach him how to properly clean and care for the catheter. Advise him to keep the skin surrounding the insertion site clean and dry *to prevent infection.*

No matter which device the patient uses, you'll need to evaluate his and his family's ability and motivation to administer oxygen therapy at home. Make sure they understand the reason the patient is receiving oxygen and the safety issues involved in oxygen administration. Teach them how to properly use and clean the equipment and supplies.

If the patient will be discharged with oxygen for the first time, make sure his health insurance covers home oxygen. If it doesn't, find out what criteria he must meet to obtain coverage. Without a third-party payer, he may not be able to afford home oxygen therapy.

Documentation

Record the date and time of oxygen administration; the type of delivery device used; the oxygen flow rate; the patient's vital signs, skin color, respiratory effort, and breath sounds; the patient's response before and after initiation of therapy; and patient or family teaching provided.

Selected references

Lynn-McHale Wiegand, D.J., and Carlson, K.K., eds. *AACN Procedure Manual for Critical Care*, 5th ed. Philadelphia: W.B. Saunders Co., 2006.

O'Reilly, P., et al. "Long-term Continuous Oxygen Treatment in Chronic Obstructive Pulmonary Disease: Proper Use, Benefits, and Unresolved Issues," *Current Opinions in Pulmonary Medicine* 13(2):120-24, March 2007.

Slessarev, M. "Efficiency of Oxygen Administration: Sequential Gas Delivery versus Flow into a Cone Methods," *Critical Care Medicine* 34(3):829-34, March 2006.

Taylor, C., et al. *Fundamentals of Nursing: The Art and Science of Nursing Care*, 5th ed. Philadelphia: Lippincott Williams & Wilkins, 2008.

Wettstein, R.B., et al. "Delivered Oxygen Concentrations Using Low-Flow and High-Flow Cannulas," *Respiratory Care* 50(5):604-609, May 2005.

Manual ventilation

A handheld resuscitation bag is an inflatable device that can be attached to a face mask or directly to an endotracheal (ET) or tracheostomy tube to allow manual delivery of oxygen or room air to the lungs of a patient who can't breathe by himself. Usually used in an emergency, manual ventilation can also be performed while the patient is disconnected temporarily from a mechanical ventilator, such as during a tubing change, during transport, or before suctioning. In such instances, use of the handheld resuscitation bag maintains ventilation. Oxygen administration with a resuscitation bag can help improve a compromised cardiorespiratory system.

The American Heart Association has established guidelines for using manual ventilation with a handheld resuscitation bag. Basic life support providers should perform manual bag-mask ventilation until advanced cardiac life support providers arrive to provide alternate airway ventilation measures. If tracheal intubation isn't the best option for the patient, such ventilation methods as the laryngeal mask airway or the esophageal-tracheal Combitube can be used. These alternative measures to ventilation are less likely to result in aspiration of stomach contents. The best method of airway management varies based on the health care provider's experience, emergency medical service or health care system characteristics, and the patient's condition.

Equipment

Handheld resuscitation bag ■ mask, if needed ■ oxygen source (wall unit or tank) ■ oxygen tubing ■ nipple adapter attached to oxygen flowmeter ■ gloves ■ goggles ■ suction apparatus and tubing, as needed ■ oral airway, if needed ■ optional: oxygen reservoir, positive end-expiratory pressure (PEEP) valve. (See *Using a PEEP valve.*)

Preparation of equipment

The typical bag-mask device used for positive-pressure ventilation has a self-inflating bag with a nonrebreathing valve connected to the face mask. Unless the patient is intubated or has a tracheostomy, select a mask that fits snugly over the mouth and nose. Attach the mask to the resuscitation bag.

If oxygen is readily available, connect the handheld resuscitation bag to the oxygen. Attach one end of the oxygen tubing to the bottom of the bag and the other end to the nipple adapter on the flowmeter of the oxygen source.

Adjust the oxygen to a minimal flow rate of 10 to 12 L/minute and oxygen greater than 40%. Ideally, an oxygen reservoir should be used. This device attaches to an adapter on the bottom of the bag and delivers 100% oxygen.

Implementation

■ Put on gloves and other personal protective equipment.
■ Before using the handheld resuscitation bag, check the patient's upper airway for foreign objects. If present, remove them *because this alone may restore spontaneous respirations in some instances. Also, foreign matter or secretions can obstruct the airway and impede resuscitation efforts.* Suction the patient *to remove any secretions that may obstruct the airway.* If necessary, insert an oropharyngeal or nasopharyngeal airway *to maintain airway patency.* If the patient has a tracheostomy or ET tube in place, suction the tube.
■ If appropriate, remove the bed's headboard and stand at the head of the bed *to help keep the patient's neck extended and to free space at the side of the bed for other activities such as cardiopulmonary resuscitation.*
■ Tilt the patient's head backward, if not contraindicated, and pull his jaw forward to move the tongue away from the base of the pharynx and prevent obstruction of the airway. (See *Using a handheld resuscitation bag and mask*, page 576.)
■ Keeping your nondominant hand on the patient's mask, exert downward pressure *to seal the mask against his face.* For an adult patient, use your dominant hand to compress the bag to give 8 to 10 breaths/minute.
■ Depress the 1-L bag by about one-half to two-thirds of its volume or a 2-L bag about one-third of its volume to deliver a tidal volume sufficient to achieve a visible chest rise.
■ Deliver each breath over 1 second. Allow the patient to exhale before giving another ventilation.

Using a PEEP valve

Add positive end-expiratory pressure (PEEP) to manual ventilation by attaching a PEEP valve to the resuscitation bag. This may improve oxygenation if the patient hasn't responded to increased fraction of inspired oxygen levels. Always use a PEEP valve to manually ventilate a patient who has been receiving PEEP on the ventilator.

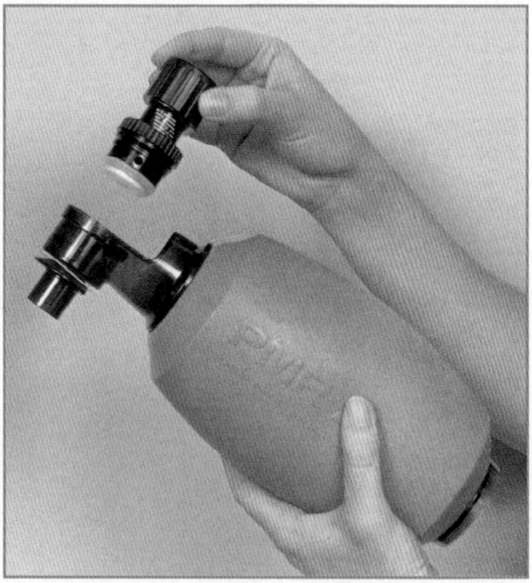

PEDIATRIC ALERT *For infants and children, deliver 20 breaths/minute, or one compression of the bag every 3 to 5 seconds. Use a pediatric handheld resuscitation bag with a volume of at least 450 to 500 ml.*

■ Deliver breaths with the patient's own inspiratory effort, if it's present. Don't attempt to deliver a breath as the patient exhales.
■ Observe the patient's chest *to ensure that it rises and falls with each compression.* If ventilation fails to occur, check the fit of the mask and the patency of the patient's airway; if necessary, reposition his head and ensure patency with an oral airway.

Special considerations

■ Avoid neck hyperextension if the patient has a possible cervical injury; instead, use the jaw-thrust technique to open the airway.

Using a handheld resuscitation bag and mask

Bag-mask resuscitation by one rescuer

1. Circle the edges of the mask with the index and first finger of one hand while lifting the jaw with the other fingers. Make sure that there's a tight seal. Use the other hand to compress the bag. Make sure that the chest rises with each breath.

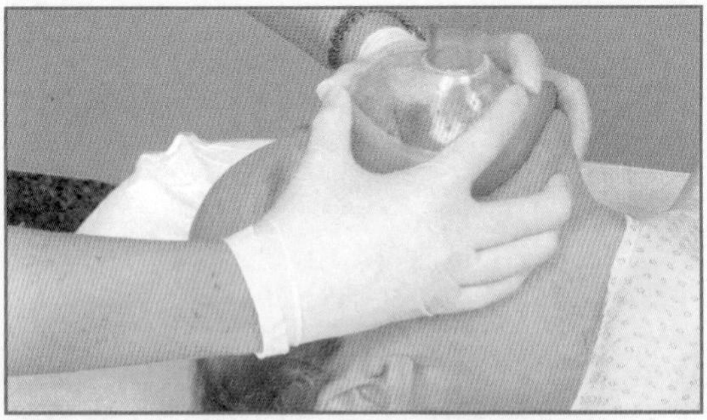

2. Make sure that the patient's mouth remains open underneath the mask. Attach the bag to the mask and to the tubing leading to the oxygen source.

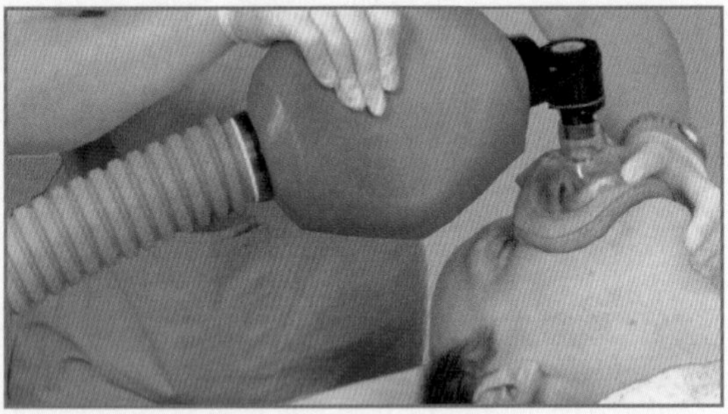

3. Alternatively, if the patient has a tracheostomy or endotracheal tube in place, remove the mask from the bag and attach the handheld resuscitation bag directly to the tube.

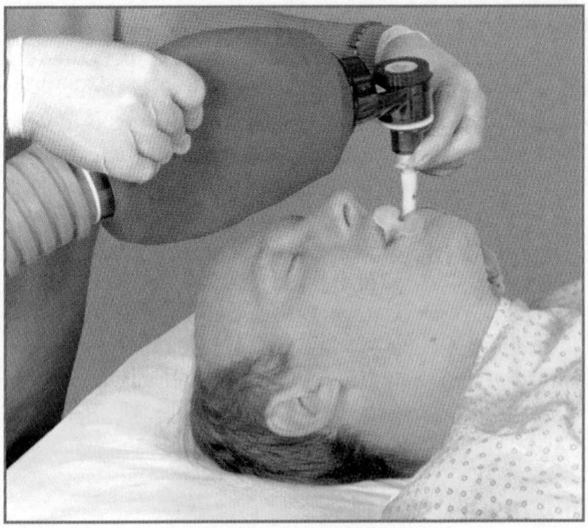

Bag-mask resuscitation by two rescuers

One rescuer stands at the victim's head and uses the thumb and the first finger of both hands to completely seal the edges of the mask. The other fingers lift the jaw and extend the victim's neck. The second rescuer squeezes the bag over 1 second until the chest rises.

■ If you need both hands to keep the patient's mask in place and maintain hyperextension, use the lower part of your arm to compress the bag against your side.

■ Observe for vomiting through the clear part of the mask. If vomiting occurs, stop the procedure immediately, lift the mask, turn the patient to his side, wipe and suction the vomitus, and resume resuscitation.

■ Underventilation commonly occurs because the handheld resuscitation bag is difficult to keep positioned tightly on the patient's face while ensuring an open airway. Furthermore, the volume of air delivered to the patient varies with the type of bag used and the hand size of the person compressing the bag. An adult with a small or medium-sized hand may not consistently deliver 1 L of air. *For these reasons,* have someone assist with the procedure, if possible.

Complications

Aspiration of vomitus can result in pneumonia, and gastric distention may result from air forced into the patient's stomach.

Documentation

In an emergency, record the date and time of the procedure; manual ventilation efforts; complications and the nursing action taken; and the patient's response to treatment, according to your facility's protocol for respiratory arrest.

In a nonemergency situation, record the date and time of the procedure, reason and length of time the patient was disconnected from mechanical ventilation and received manual ventilation, complications and the nursing action taken, and the patient's tolerance of the procedure.

SELECTED REFERENCES

American Heart Association. "2005 AHA Guidelines for Cardiopulmonary Resuscitation and Emergency Cardiovascular Care: International Consensus on Science," *Circulation* 112(22 Suppl):IV-1-IV-211, November 2005.

Aufderheude, T.P., et al. "Death by Hyperventilation: A Common and Life-threatening Problem During Cardiopulmonary Resuscitation" *Critical Care Medicine* 32(9suppl):S345-51, September 2004.

Lynn-McHale Wiegand, D.J., and Carlson, K.K., eds. *AACN Procedure Manual for Critical Care*, 5th ed. Philadelphia: W.B. Saunders Co., 2006.

Turki, M. "Peak Pressures During Manual Ventilation," *Respiratory Care* 50(3):340-44, March 2005.

MECHANICAL VENTILATION

A mechanical ventilator moves air in and out of a patient's lungs. Although the equipment serves to ventilate a patient, it doesn't ensure adequate gas exchange. Mechanical ventilators may use either positive or negative pressure to ventilate patients.

Positive-pressure ventilators exert a positive pressure on the airway, which causes inspiration while increasing tidal volume (V_T). The inspiratory cycles of these ventilators may vary in volume, pressure, or time. For example, a volume-cycled ventilator — the type used most commonly — delivers a preset volume of air each time, regardless of the amount of lung resistance. A pressure-cycled ventilator generates flow until the machine reaches a preset pressure regardless of the volume delivered or the time required to achieve the pressure. A time-cycled ventilator generates flow for a preset amount of time. A high-frequency ventilator uses high respiratory rates and low V_T to maintain alveolar ventilation.

Negative-pressure ventilators act by creating negative pressure, which pulls the thorax outward and allows air to flow into the lungs. Examples of such ventilators are the iron lung, the cuirass (chest shell), and the body wrap. Negative-pressure ventilators are used mainly to treat neuromuscular disorders, such as Guillain-Barré syndrome, myasthenia gravis, and poliomyelitis.

Other indications for ventilator use include central nervous system disorders, such as cerebral hemorrhage and spinal cord transsection, adult respiratory distress syndrome, pulmonary edema, chronic obstructive pulmonary disease, flail chest, and acute hypoventilation.

Equipment

Oxygen source ▪ air source that can supply 50 psi ▪ mechanical ventilator ▪ humidifier ▪ ventilator circuit tubing, connectors, and adapters ▪ condensation collection trap ▪ spirometer, respirometer, or electronic device to measure flow and volume ▪ in-line thermometer ▪ gloves ▪ handheld resuscitation bag with reservoir ▪ suction equipment ▪ sterile distilled water ▪ equipment for arterial blood gas (ABG) analysis ▪ soft restraints, if indicated ▪ optional: oximeter, capnography device.

Preparation of equipment

In most facilities, respiratory therapists assume responsibility for setting up the ventilator. If necessary, check the manufacturer's instructions for setting it up. In most cases, you'll need to add sterile distilled water to the humidifier and connect the ventilator to the appropriate gas source.

Plug the ventilator into the electrical outlet, and turn it on. Adjust the settings on the ventilator, as ordered. (See *Mechanical ventilation glossary,* page 578.) Make sure the ventilator's alarms are set as ordered and that the humidifier is filled with sterile distilled water.

Implementation

- Verify the practitioner's order for ventilator support. If the patient isn't already intubated, prepare him for intubation. (See "Endotracheal intubation," page 538.)
- When possible, explain the procedure to the patient and his family *to help reduce anxiety and fear.* Assure the patient and his family that staff members are nearby to provide care.
- Perform a complete physical assessment, and draw blood for ABG analysis *to establish a baseline.*
- Make sure the patient is being adequately oxygenated.
- Suction the patient, if necessary.
- Put on gloves if you haven't already done so. Connect the endotracheal tube to the ventilator. Observe for chest expansion, and auscultate for bilateral breath sounds *to verify that the patient is being ventilated.*
- Monitor the patient's ABG values after the initial ventilator setup (usually 20 to 30 minutes), after changes in ventilator settings, and as the patient's clinical condition indicates *to determine whether the patient is being adequately ventilated and to avoid oxygen toxicity.* Be prepared to adjust ventilator settings based on ABG analysis.
- Check the ventilator tubing frequently for condensation, *which can cause resistance to airflow and which may also be aspirated by the patient.* As needed, drain the condensate into a collection trap or briefly disconnect the patient from the

Mechanical ventilation glossary

Although a respiratory therapist usually monitors ventilator settings based on the practitioner's order, you should understand all of the following terms.

Assist-control mode: The ventilator delivers a preset rate; however, the patient can initiate additional breaths, which trigger the ventilator to deliver the preset tidal volume (V_T) at positive pressure.

Continuous positive airway pressure (CPAP): A setting that prompts the ventilator to deliver positive pressure to the airway throughout the respiratory cycle. It works only on patients who can breathe spontaneously.

Control mode: The ventilator delivers a preset V_T at a fixed rate regardless of whether the patient is breathing spontaneously.

Fraction of inspired oxygen (FIO_2): The amount of oxygen delivered to the patient by the ventilator. The dial or digital display on the ventilator that sets this percentage is labeled by the term oxygen concentration or oxygen percentage.

Inspiratory-expiratory (I:E) ratio: This ratio compares the duration of inspiration to the duration of expiration. The I:E ratio of normal, spontaneous breathing is 1:2, meaning that expiration is twice as long as inspiration.

Inspiratory flow rate (IFR): The IFR denotes the V_T delivered within a certain time. Its value can range from 20 to 120 L/minute.

Minute ventilation or minute volume (V_E): This measurement results from the multiplication of respiratory rate and V_T.

Peak inspiratory pressure (PIP): Measured by the pressure manometer on the ventilator, peak inspiratory pressure reflects the amount of pressure required to deliver a preset V_T.

Positive end-expiratory pressure (PEEP): In this mode, the ventilator is triggered to apply positive pressure at the end of each expiration to increase the area for oxygen exchange by helping to inflate and keep open collapsed alveoli.

Pressure support ventilation (PSV): This mode allows the ventilator to apply a preset amount of positive pressure when the patient inspires spontaneously. PSV increases V_T while decreasing the patient's breathing workload.

Respiratory rate: The number of breaths per minute delivered by the ventilator; also called *frequency.*

Sensitivity setting: A setting that determines the amount of effort the patient must exert to trigger the inspiratory cycle.

Sigh volume: A ventilator-delivered breath that's 1½ times as large as the patient's tidal volume.

Synchronized intermittent mandatory ventilation (SIMV): The ventilator delivers a preset number of breaths at a specific V_T. The patient may supplement these mechanical ventilations with his own breaths, in which case the V_T and rate are determined by his own inspiratory ability.

Tidal volume (V_T): V_T refers to the volume of air delivered to the patient with each cycle, usually 8 to 12 cc/kg.

ventilator (ventilating him with a handheld resuscitation bag if necessary), and empty the water into a receptacle. Don't drain the condensate into the humidifier *because the condensate may be contaminated with the patient's secretions.* Also, avoid accidental drainage of condensation into the patient's airway.

- Inspect the humidification device regularly and remove condensate, as needed. Inspect heat and moisture exchangers, and replace if secretions contaminate the insert of filter. Note humidifier settings. The heated humidifier should be set to deliver an inspired gas temperature of 91.4° F (33° C) plus or minus 3.6° F (2° C) and should provide a minimum of 30 mg/L of water vapor with routine use to an intubated patient.
- If you're using a heated humidifier, monitor the inspired air temperature as close to the patient's airway as possible. The inspiratory gas shouldn't be greater than 98.6° F (37° C) at the opening of the airway. Check that the high temperature alarm is set no higher than 98.6° F and no lower than 86° F (30° C). Observe the amount and consistency of the patient's secretions. If the secretions are copious or increasingly tenacious when a heat and moisture exchanger is used, a heated humidifier should be used instead.
- Check the in-line thermometer to make sure the temperature of the air delivered to the patient is close to body temperature.
- When monitoring the patient's vital signs, count spontaneous breaths as well as ventilator-delivered breaths.
- Change, clean, or dispose of the ventilator tubing and equipment according to your facility's policy *to reduce the risk of bacterial contamination.*

Weaning from the ventilator

Successful weaning from the ventilator depends on the patient's ability to breathe on his own. This means that he must have a spontaneous respiratory effort that can keep him ventilated, a stable cardiovascular system, and sufficient respiratory muscle strength and level of consciousness to sustain spontaneous breathing. The patient should meet some or all of the following criteria.

Readiness criteria

- Arterial oxygen saturation ($Sa{O_2}$) greater than 92% on fraction of inspired oxygen less than or equal to 40%, positive end-expiratory pressure less than or equal to 5 cm H_2O
- Hemodynamically stable, adequately resuscitated, and doesn't require vasoactive support
- Serum electrolyte levels and pH within normal range
- Hematocrit greater than 25%
- Core body temperature greater than 96.8° F (36° C) and less than 102.2° F (39° C)
- Pain adequately managed
- Successful withdrawal of a neuromuscular blocker
- Arterial blood gas values within normal limits or at patient's baseline

Weaning intervention (long term—more than 72 hours)

- Transfer to pressure-support ventilation (PSV) mode and adjust support level to maintain patient's respiratory rate at less than 35 breaths/minute.
- Observe for 30 minutes for signs of early failure, such as:
  - sustained respiratory rate greater than 35 breaths/minute
  - $Sa{O_2}$ less than 89%
  - tidal volume less than or equal to 5 ml/kg
  - sustained minute ventilation greater than 200 ml/kg/minute
  - evidence of respiratory or hemodynamic distress: labored respiratory pattern, increased diaphoresis or anxiety or both, sustained heart rate greater than 20% higher or lower than baseline, systolic blood pressure greater than 180 mm Hg or less than 90 mm Hg higher.
- If tolerated, continue trial for 2 hours, then return patient to "rest" settings by adding ventilator breaths or increasing PSV to achieve a total respiratory rate of less than 20 breaths/minute.
- After 2 hours of rest, repeat trial for 2 to 4 hours at same PSV level as previous trial. If the patient exceeds the tolerance criteria, stop the trial and return to "rest" settings. In this case, the next trial should be performed at a higher support level than the failed trial.
- Record the results after each weaning episode, including specific parameters and the time frame if failure was observed.
- The goal is to increase trial lengths and reduce the PSV level needed in increments.
- With each successful trial, the PSV level may be decreased by 2 to 4 cm H_2O, the time interval may be increased by 1 to 2 hours, or both while keeping the patient within tolerable parameters.
- Ensure nocturnal ventilation at "rest" settings (with a respiratory rate of less than 20 breaths/minute) for at least 6 hours each night until the patient's weaning trials demonstrate readiness to discontinue support.

- When ordered, begin to wean the patient from the ventilator. (See *Weaning from the ventilator.*)

Special considerations

- Provide emotional support to the patient during all phases of mechanical ventilation *to reduce his anxiety and promote successful treatment.* Even if the patient is unresponsive, continue to explain all procedures and treatments to him.
- Make sure the ventilator alarms are on at all times. *These alarms alert the nursing staff to potentially hazardous conditions and changes in patient status.* If an alarm sounds and the problem can't be identified easily, disconnect the patient from the ventilator and use a handheld resuscitation bag to ventilate him. (See *Responding to ventilator alarms,* page 580.)
- Unless contraindicated, turn the patient from side to side every 1 to 2 hours *to facilitate lung expansion and removal of secretions.* Perform active or passive range-of-motion exercises for all extremities *to reduce the hazards of immobility.* If the patient's condition permits, position him upright at regular intervals *to increase lung expansion.* When moving the patient or the ventilator tubing, be careful to prevent condensation in the tubing from flowing into the lungs *because aspiration of this contaminated moisture can cause infection.* Provide care for the patient's artificial airway as needed.

TROUBLESHOOTING

Responding to ventilator alarms

SIGNAL	POSSIBLE CAUSE	NURSING INTERVENTIONS
Low-pressure alarm	■ Tube disconnected from ventilator	■ Reconnect the tube to the ventilator.
	■ Endotracheal (ET) tube displaced above vocal cords or tracheostomy tube extubated	■ Check tube placement and reposition, if needed. If extubation or displacement has occurred, ventilate the patient manually and call the practitioner immediately.
	■ Leaking tidal volume from low cuff pressure (from an underinflated or ruptured cuff or a leak in the cuff or one-way valve)	■ Listen for a whooshing sound around the tube, indicating an air leak. If you hear one, check cuff pressure. If you can't maintain pressure, call the practitioner; a new tube may need to be inserted.
	■ Ventilator malfunction	■ Disconnect the patient from the ventilator and ventilate him manually if necessary. Obtain another ventilator.
	■ Leak in ventilator circuitry (from loose connection or hole in tubing, loss of temperature-sensitive device, or cracked humidification jar)	■ Make sure all connections are intact. Check for holes or leaks in the tubing and replace, if necessary. Check the humidification jar and replace if cracked.
High-pressure alarm	■ Increased airway pressure or decreased lung compliance caused by worsening disease	■ Auscultate the lungs for evidence of increasing lung consolidation, barotrauma, or wheezing. Call the practitioner, if indicated.
	■ Patient biting on oral ET tube	■ Insert a bite block, if needed. ■ Consider pain medication or sedation, if appropriate.
	■ Secretions in airway	■ Look for secretions in the airway. To remove them, suction the patient or have him cough.
	■ Condensate in large-bore tubing	■ Check tubing for condensate and remove any fluid.
	■ Intubation of right mainstem bronchus	■ Auscultate the lungs for evidence of diminished or absent breath sounds in the left lung fields. ■ Check tube position. If it has slipped, call the practitioner; the tube may need to be repositioned.
	■ Patient coughing, gagging, or attempting to talk	■ If the patient fights the ventilator, the practitioner may order a sedative or neuromuscular blocking agent.
	■ Chest wall resistance	■ Reposition the patient to see if doing so improves chest expansion. If repositioning doesn't help, administer the prescribed analgesic.
	■ Failure of high-pressure relief valve	■ Have faulty equipment replaced.
	■ Bronchospasm	■ Assess the patient for the cause. Report to the practitioner, and treat, as ordered.

- Assess the patient's peripheral circulation, and monitor his urine output for signs of decreased cardiac output. Watch for signs and symptoms of fluid volume excess or dehydration.
- Place the call light within the patient's reach, and establish a method of communication such as a communication board *because intubation and mechanical ventilation impair the patient's ability to speak.* An artificial airway may help the patient to speak by *allowing air to pass through his vocal cords.*
- Administer a sedative or neuromuscular blocking agent as ordered *to relax the patient or eliminate spontaneous breathing efforts that can interfere with the ventilator's action.* Remember that the patient receiving a neuromuscular blocking drug requires close observation *because of his inability to breathe or communicate.*
- If the patient is receiving a neuromuscular blocking agent, make sure he also receives a sedative. *Neuromuscular blocking agents cause paralysis without altering the patient's level of consciousness.* Reassure the patient and his family that the paralysis is temporary. Also make sure emergency equipment is readily available in case the ventilator malfunctions or the patient is extubated accidentally. Continue to explain all procedures to the patient, and take additional steps to ensure his safety, such as raising the side rails of his bed while turning him and covering and lubricating his eyes.
- Make sure that the patient gets adequate rest and sleep *because fatigue can delay weaning from the ventilator.* Provide subdued lighting, safely muffle equipment noises, and restrict staff access to the area *to promote quiet during rest periods.*
- When weaning the patient, continue to observe for signs of hypoxia. Schedule weaning to fit comfortably and realistically with the patient's daily regimen. Avoid scheduling sessions after meals, baths, or lengthy therapeutic or diagnostic procedures. Have the patient help you set up the schedule *to give him some sense of control over a frightening procedure.* As the patient's tolerance for weaning increases, help him sit up out of bed *to improve his breathing and sense of well-being.* Suggest diversionary activities *to take his mind off breathing.*

Home care

If the patient will be discharged on a ventilator, evaluate the family's or the caregiver's ability and motivation to provide such care. Well before discharge, develop a teaching plan that will address the patient's needs. For example, teaching should include information about ventilator care and settings, artificial airway care, suctioning, respiratory therapy, communication, nutrition, therapeutic exercise, the signs and symptoms of infection, and ways to troubleshoot minor equipment malfunctions.

Also evaluate the patient's need for adaptive equipment, such as a hospital bed, wheelchair or walker with a ventilator tray, patient lift, and bedside commode. Determine whether the patient needs to travel; if so, select appropriate portable and backup equipment.

Before discharge, have the patient's caregiver demonstrate his ability to use the equipment. At discharge, contact a durable medical equipment vendor and a home health nurse to follow up with the patient. Also, refer the patient to community resources, if available.

Complications

Mechanical ventilation can cause tension pneumothorax, decreased cardiac output, oxygen toxicity, fluid volume excess caused by humidification, infection, and such GI complications as distention or bleeding from stress ulcers.

Documentation

Document the date and time of initiation of mechanical ventilation. Name the type of ventilator used for the patient, and note its settings. Describe the patient's subjective and objective response to mechanical ventilation, including vital signs, breath sounds, use of accessory muscles, intake and output, and weight. List any complications and nursing actions taken. Record all pertinent laboratory data, including ABG analysis results and oxygen saturation levels.

During weaning, record the date and time of each session, the weaning method, and baseline and subsequent vital signs, oxygen saturation levels, and ABG values. Again describe the patient's subjective and objective responses, including level of consciousness, respiratory effort, arrhythmias, skin color, and need for suctioning.

List all complications and nursing actions taken. If the patient was receiving pressure support ventilation (PSV) or using a T-piece or tracheostomy collar, note the duration of spontaneous breathing and the patient's ability to maintain the weaning schedule. If using intermittent mandatory ventilation, with or without PSV, record the control breath rate, the time of each breath reduction, and the rate of spontaneous respirations.

SELECTED REFERENCES

American Association for Respiratory Care. "AARC Clinical Practice Guideline: Humidification During Mechanical Ventilation," *Respiratory Care* 37(8):887-90, August 1992.

American Association for Respiratory Care. "AARC Evidence-Based Clinical Practice Guideline: Care of the Ventilator Circuit and Its Relation to Ventilator-associated Pneumonia," *Respiratory Care* 48(9):869-79, September 2003.

Chao, D.C., and Scheinhorn, D.J. "Determining the Best Threshold of Rapid Shallow Breathing Index in a Therapist-implemented Patient-specific Weaning Protocol," *Respiratory Care* 52(2):159-65, February 2007.

Happ, M.B., et al. "Family Presence and Surveillance During Weaning from Prolonged Ventilation," *Heart and Lung* 36(1):47-57, January-February 2007.

Kress, J.P., and Hall, J.B. "Sedation in the Mechanically Ventilated Patient," *Critical Care Medicine* 34(10):2541-546, October 2006.

Kress, J.P., et al. "Daily Sedative Interruption in Mechanically Ventilated Patients at Risk for Coronary Artery Disease," *Critical Care Medicine* 35(2):365-71, February 2007.

Lynn-McHale Wiegand, D.J., and Carlson, K.K., eds. *AACN Procedure Manual for Critical Care*, 5th ed. Philadelphia: W.B. Saunders Co., 2006.

Rose, L., and Ed, A. "Advanced Modes of Mechanical Ventilation: Implications for Practice," *AACN Advanced Critical Care* 17(2):145-58, April-June 2006.

Tablan, O.C., et al. CDC Healthcare Infection Control Practices Advisory Committee. "Guidelines for Preventing Healthcare-associated Pneumonia, 2003: Recommendations of CDC and the Healthcare Infection Control Practices Advisory Committee," *MMWR* 53(RR-3):1-36, March 2004.

CONTINUOUS POSITIVE AIRWAY PRESSURE

Continuous positive airway pressure (CPAP) is used to provide low flow pressure into the airways to help hold the airway open, mobilize secretions, and treat atelectasis—all of which eases the work of breathing. Nonintubated patients receive CPAP through a high flow generating system and its use may eliminate the need for intubation. CPAP is also commonly used to treat chronic obstructive sleep apnea as it prevents the palate and tongue from collapsing and obstructing the airways. Many patients are started on CPAP in the hospital, and then continue CPAP use at home. CPAP has traditionally been administered through a face mask, but newer, more comfortable methods include the face pillow and nasal mask.

It may also be administered to an intubated patient through a ventilator setting.

CPAP is contraindicated in patients with chronic obstructive lung disease, bullous lung disease, low cardiac output, or tension pneumothorax due to the increase in thoracic pressure.

Equipment

Nasal mask, nasal pillows, or face mask properly sized ▪ permanent marker ▪ CPAP machine ▪ oxygen delivery tubing ▪ washcloth ▪ water ▪ optional: oxygen source, oxygen tubing, pulse oximetry.

Preparation of equipment

Set up the CPAP machine according to manufacturer's instructions. Position the CPAP machine so the tubing easily reaches the patient and plug in the machine. Don't plug the CPAP machine into an outlet with another plug in it, and don't use an extension cord to reach the outlet. Connect the oxygen delivery tubing to the air outlet valve on the CPAP unit, if ordered.

Implementation

- Check the practitioner's order.
- Confirm the patient's identity using two patient identifiers according to your facility's policy.
- Explain the procedure to the patient *to decrease anxiety and increase compliance.*
- Wash your hands and use personal protective equipment, as appropriate, *to prevent bacterial contamination.*
- Have the patient wash his face with the washcloth and water *to remove facial oils and help achieve a better fit.*
- Check the face mask, nasal mask, or nasal pillow to make sure the cushion isn't hard or broken. If it is, replace it.

Nasal mask

- Place the nasal mask so the longer straps are located at the top of the mask (as shown below).

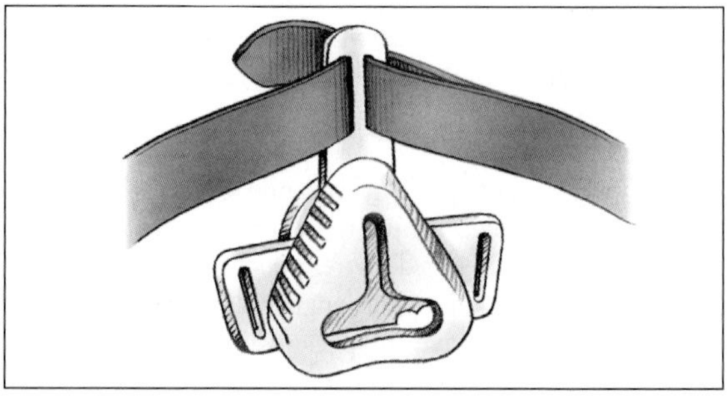

- Make sure that the Velcro is facing away from you and thread the four tabs through the slots on the sides and top of the mask (as shown below).

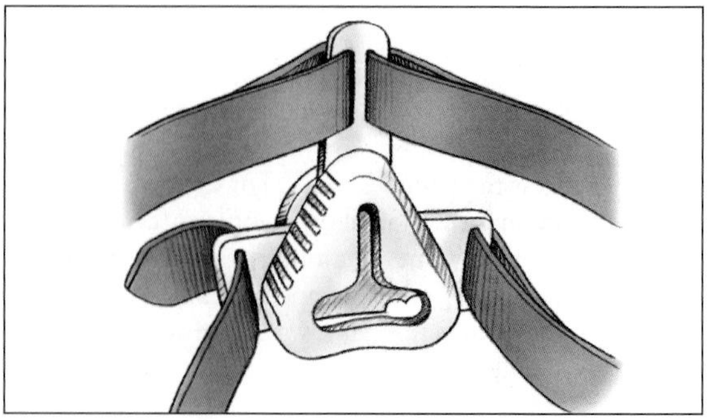

■ Pull the straps through the slots and fasten them using the Velcro.
■ Place the mask over the patient's nose and position the headgear over the patient's head (as shown below).

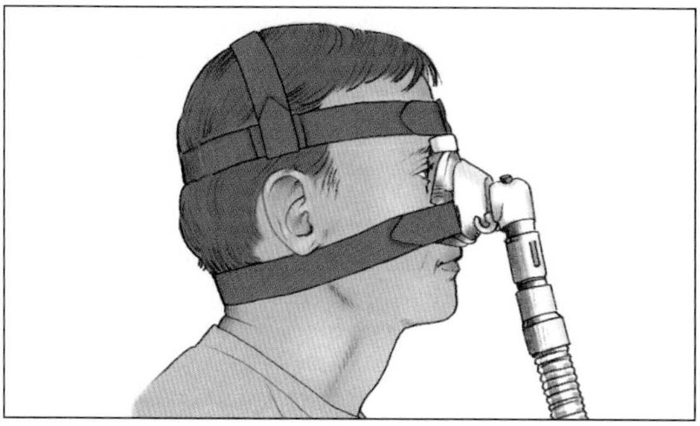

■ Gradually tighten all the straps on the mask until a seal is obtained. The mask doesn't have to be very tight to fit correctly—it just has to have a seal.
■ Use the permanent marker to mark the straps with the final position *to eliminate having to fit the mask each time the patient wears it.*

Nasal pillow

■ Insert the nasal pillows into the shell making sure they fit correctly and that there's no air leaking around them (as shown below).

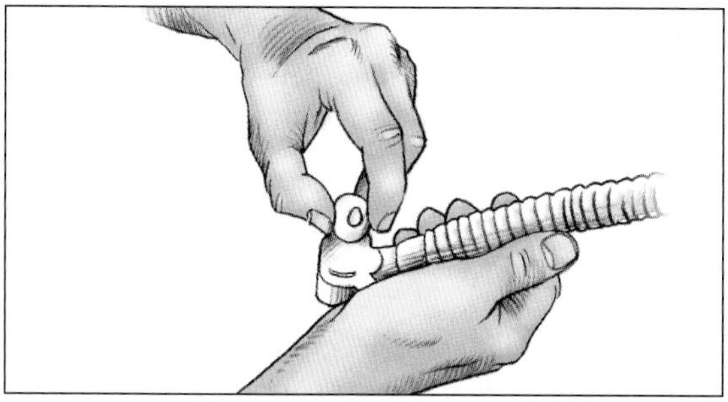

■ Place the headgear around the patient's head and use the Velcro straps to achieve the proper fit. Once the straps are in the correct place, remove the headgear without undoing the straps.
■ Attach the nasal pillow to the headgear by wrapping the Velcro around the tubing, leaving room for rotation (as shown top of next column).

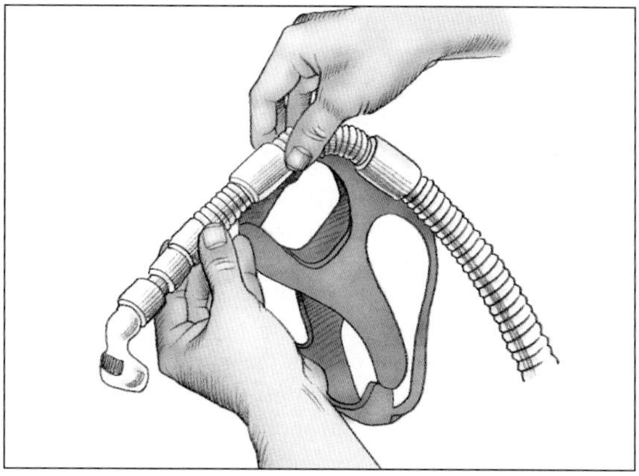

■ Place the completely assembled headgear back on the patient and position the nasal pillows comfortably.
■ Attach the shell strap across the shell and adjust the tension of the strap until there's a seal in both nostrils (as shown below).

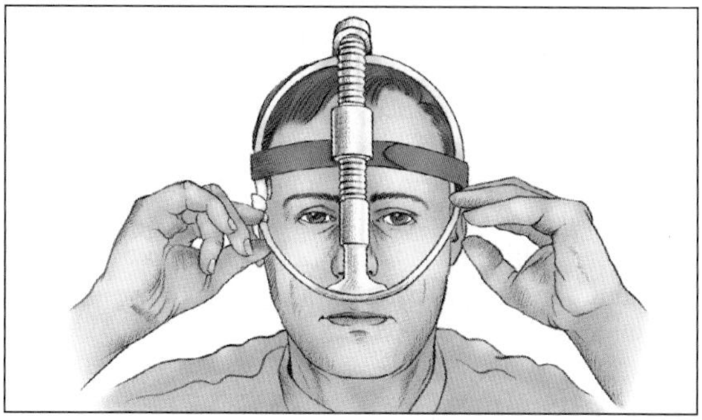

■ Be careful not to block the exhalation port on the backside of the shell.

Face mask

■ Hold the mask against the patient's face and position the headgear over his head.
■ Using the Velcro straps, adjust the straps as with the nasal mask until there are no leaks present (as shown below).

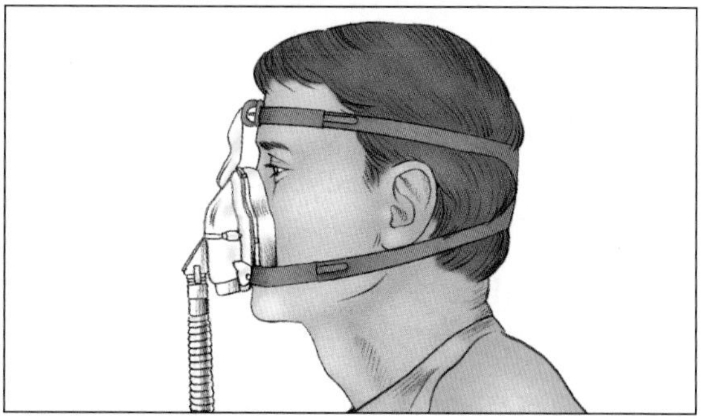

■ Connect the flexible tubing to the mask and turn on the airflow.

Administering CPAP

■ After the administration device is correctly fitted on the patient, turn on the pressure generator.
■ Turn on the CPAP unit before turning on the oxygen flow to the ordered level.
■ If ordered, monitor the patient's pulse oximetry during the treatment.
■ When the treatment is over, in the morning or upon discontinuation of the order, turn off the pressure generator and remove the headgear and appliance from the patient.
■ Clean the equipment according to facility policy and store properly.

Special considerations

■ If the mask isn't properly fitted, the patient may complain of dry or sore eyes. If this is the case, remove the mask and headgear and readjust them to minimize leaks.
■ The patient may need to use a humidifier with the CPAP unit if he complains of a runny nose, or dryness or burning in his nose and throat. Discuss this with the practitioner and obtain an order for humidification.
■ Always make sure there's air coming out of the unit when the power is turned on.
■ *Because CPAP via a mask can cause nausea and vomiting,* it shouldn't be used in a patient who's unresponsive or at risk for aspiration.

Patient teaching

■ Teach the patient how to use the machine at home, including fitting the mask and care of the equipment.
■ Make sure the patient has the name and phone number of the company that will be supplying the machine and a contact number for him to ask questions.

Complications

The majority of complications come from ill-fitting masks, such as dry eyes, runny or dry nose, or burning in the throat or nose. Some patients may be allergic to the mask or develop skin irritation from the contact of the mask to their face. If this happens, apply a barrier between the mask and the skin. Other complications include nosebleeds, abdominal bloating, headaches, and nightmares. CPAP may also potentially cause decreased cardiac output due to increased intrathoracic pressure.

Documentation

Document the CPAP settings, the length of time the patient was on the CPAP, how the patient tolerated the CPAP, and if there were any complications. Record patient teaching.

SELECTED REFERENCES

American Association for Respiratory Care. "AARC Clinical Practice Guideline: Pulse Oximetry," *Respiratory Care* 36(12):1406-409, December 1991.

American Association for Respiratory Care. "AARC Clinical Practice Guideline: Use of Positive Airway Pressure Adjuncts to Bronchial Hygiene Therapy," *Respiratory Care* 28(5):516-21, May 1993.

Collop, N. "The Effect of Obstructive Sleep Apnea on Chronic Medical Disorders," *Cleveland Clinic Journal of Medicine* 74(1):72-78, January 2007.

Davidhizar, R.E., and Hart, A.N. "Living with a CPAP Machine," *Journal of Practical Nursing* 55(3):20-22, Fall 2005.

Dikerson, S.S., and Kennedy, M.C. "CPAP Devices: Encouraging Patients with Sleep Apnea," *Rehabilitation Nurse* 31(3):114-22, May-June 2006.

Kaneko, Y. "Cardiovascular Effects of Continuous Positive Airway Pressure in Patients with Heart Failure and Obstructive Sleep Apnea," *New England Journal of Medicine* 348(13):1233-241, March 2003.

Mador, M.J., et al. "Effect of Heated Humidification on Compliance and Quality of Life in Patients with Sleep Apnea Using Nasal Continuous Positive Airway Pressure," *Chest* 126(4):2151-158, October 2005.

INCENTIVE SPIROMETRY

Incentive spirometry involves using a breathing device to help the patient achieve maximal ventilation. The device measures respiratory flow or respiratory volume and induces the patient to take a deep breath and hold it for several seconds. This deep breath increases lung volume, boosts alveolar inflation, and promotes venous return. This exercise also establishes alveolar hyperinflation for a longer time than is possible with a normal deep breath, thus preventing and reversing the alveolar collapse that causes atelectasis and pneumonitis.

The American Association for Respiratory Care guidelines recommend the use of an incentive spirometer for conditions predisposing to the development of pulmonary atelectasis, such as:

■ upper abdominal surgery
■ thoracic surgery
■ surgery in patients with chronic obstructive pulmonary disease
■ restrictive lung defect associated with quadriplegia or a dysfunctional diaphragm.

Five to 10 breaths are suggested per session every hour while awake (approximately 100 breaths per day).

Devices used for incentive spirometry provide a visual incentive to breathe deeply. Some are activated when the patient inhales a certain volume of air; the device then estimates the amount of air inhaled. Others contain plastic floats, which rise according to the amount of air the patient pulls through the device when he inhales.

Patients at low risk for developing atelectasis may use a flow incentive spirometer. Patients at high risk may need a volume incentive spirometer, which measures lung inflation more precisely.

Incentive spirometry benefits the patient on prolonged bed rest, especially the postoperative patient who may regain his normal respiratory pattern slowly due to such predisposing factors as abdominal or thoracic surgery, advanced age, inactivity, obesity, smoking, and decreased ability to cough effectively and expel lung secretions.

Equipment

Flow or volume incentive spirometer, as indicated, with sterile disposable tube and mouthpiece ■ stethoscope ■ watch. The tube and mouthpiece are sterile on first use and clean on subsequent uses.

Preparation of equipment

Assemble the ordered equipment at the patient's bedside. Read the manufacturer's instructions for spirometer setup and operation.

Remove the sterile flow tube and mouthpiece from the package, and attach them to the device. Set the flow rate or volume goal as determined by the practitioner and based on the patient's preoperative performance. Turn on the machine, if necessary.

Implementation

■ Confirm the patient's identity using two patient identifiers according to your facility's policy.
■ Assess the patient's condition.
■ Explain the procedure to the patient, making sure that she understands the importance of performing incentive spirometry regularly *to maintain alveolar inflation.*
■ Wash your hands.
■ Help the patient into a comfortable sitting or semi-Fowler's position *to promote optimal lung expansion.* If you're using a flow incentive spirometer and the patient is unable to assume or maintain this position, she can perform the procedure in any position as long as the device remains upright. *Tilting a flow incentive spirometer decreases the required patient effort and reduces the exercise's effectiveness.*
■ Auscultate the patient's lungs to provide a baseline for comparison with posttreatment auscultation.
■ Instruct the patient to insert the mouthpiece and close her lips tightly around it *because a weak seal may alter flow or volume readings.*
■ Instruct the patient to exhale normally and then inhale as slowly and as deeply as possible. If she has difficulty with this step, tell her to suck as she would through a straw but more slowly (as shown below). Ask the patient to retain the entire volume of air she inhaled for 3 seconds or, if you're using a device with a light indicator, until the light turns off. *This deep breath creates sustained transpulmonary pressure near the end of inspiration and is sometimes called a sustained maximal inspiration.*

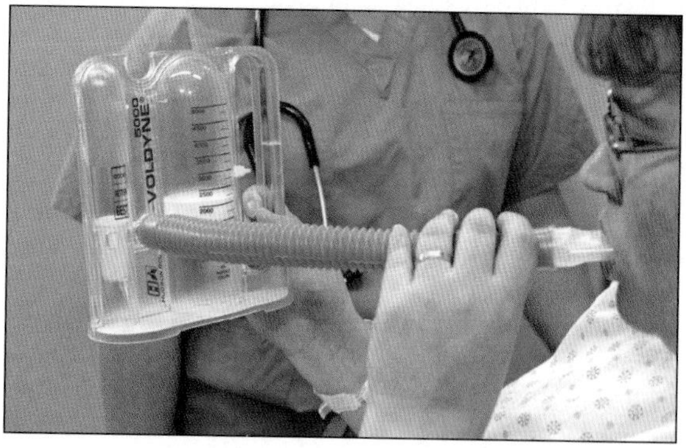

■ Tell the patient to remove the mouthpiece and exhale normally. Allow her to relax and take several normal breaths before attempting another breath with the spirometer. Repeat this sequence 5 to 10 times during every waking hour. Note tidal volumes.
■ Evaluate the patient's ability to cough effectively, and encourage her to cough after each effort *because deep lung inflation may loosen secretions and facilitate their removal.* Observe any expectorated secretions.
■ Auscultate the patient's lungs and compare findings with the first auscultation.
■ Instruct the patient to remove the mouthpiece. Wash the device in warm water and shake it dry. Avoid immersing the spirometer itself *because this enhances bacterial growth and impairs the internal filter's effectiveness in preventing inhalation of extraneous material.*
■ Place the mouthpiece in a plastic storage bag between exercises, and label it and the spirometer, if applicable, with the patient's name *to avoid inadvertent use by another patient.*

Special considerations

■ If the patient is scheduled for surgery, make a preoperative assessment of her respiratory pattern and capability *to ensure the development of appropriate postoperative goals.* Teach the patient how to use the spirometer before surgery *so that she can concentrate on your instructions and practice the exercise.* A preoperative evaluation will also help in establishing a postoperative therapeutic goal.
■ Avoid exercising at mealtime *to prevent nausea.* If the patient has difficulty breathing only through her mouth, provide a noseclip *to fully measure each breath.* Provide paper

and a pencil *so the patient can note exercise times.* Exercise frequency varies with condition and ability.

- Immediately after surgery, monitor the exercise frequently *to ensure compliance and assess achievement.*
- Adaptions for the spirometer are available to allow for use with a tracheal stoma.
- Premedicate the patient, as needed, *for comfort and to improve effort.*

Documentation

Record any preoperative teaching you provided. Document preoperative flow or volume levels, the date and time of the procedure, the type of spirometer, the flow or volume levels achieved, and the number of breaths taken. Also, note the patient's condition before and after the procedure, her tolerance of the procedure, and the results of both auscultations.

If you've used a flow incentive spirometer, compute the volume by multiplying the setting by the duration that the patient kept the ball (or balls) suspended, as follows. If the patient suspended the ball for 3 seconds at a setting of 500 cc during each of 10 breaths, multiply 500 cc by 3 seconds and then record this total (1,500 cc) and the number of breaths as follows: 1,500 cc × 10 breaths. If you've used a volume incentive spirometer, take the volume reading directly from the spirometer. For example, record 1,000 cc × 5 breaths.

SELECTED REFERENCES

American Association for Respiratory Care. "AARC Clinical Practice Guideline: Incentive Spirometry," *Respiratory Care* 36(12):1402-405, December 1991.

Harton, S.C., et al. "Frequency and Predictors of Return to Incentive Spirometry Volume Baseline after Cardiac Surgery," *Progress in Cardiovascular Nursing* 22(1):7-12, Winter 2007.

Pasquina, P., et al. "Respiratory Therapy to Prevent Pulmonary Complications after Abdominal Surgery: A Systematic Review," *Chest* 130(6):1887-899, December 2006.

Taylor, C., et al. *Fundamentals of Nursing: The Art and Science of Nursing Care*, 5th ed. Philadelphia: Lippincott Williams & Wilkins, 2008.

INTERMITTENT POSITIVE-PRESSURE BREATHING

Intermittent positive-pressure breathing (IPPB) delivers room air or oxygen into the lungs at a pressure higher than atmospheric pressure. This delivery ceases when pressure in the mouth or in the breathing circuit tube increases to a predetermined airway pressure.

IPPB was formerly the mainstay of pulmonary therapy, with its proponents claiming that the device delivered aerosolized medications deeper into the lungs, decreased the work of breathing, and assisted in the mobilization of secretions. Studies now show that IPPB has no clinical benefit over handheld nebulizers. However, it continues to be used.

Typically, personnel from the respiratory therapy department deliver these treatments.

Equipment

IPPB machine ▪ breathing circuit tubing ▪ other necessary tubing (usually one or two sections) ▪ mouthpiece or mask ▪ noseclips, if necessary ▪ source of pressurized gas at 50 psi, if necessary ▪ oxygen, if desired ▪ prescribed medication and normal saline solution ▪ sphygmomanometer ▪ stethoscope ▪ facial tissues and waste bag, or specimen cup ▪ warm, soapy water ▪ optional: suction equipment.

Preparation of equipment

Contact a respiratory therapist or follow the manufacturer's instructions to set up the equipment properly.

Implementation

- Confirm the practitioner's order.
- Confirm the patient's identity using two patient identifiers according to your facility's policy.
- Explain the procedure to the patient *to ensure his cooperation.* Tell him to sit erect in a chair, if possible, *to allow for optimal lung expansion.* Otherwise, place him in semi-Fowler's position. Wash your hands.
- Take baseline blood pressure and heart rate, especially if a bronchodilator will be administered, and listen to breath sounds for posttreatment comparisons.
- Instill the ordered medication into the nebulizer cup and turn on the IPPB machine to the appropriate settings.
- Instruct the patient to breathe deeply and slowly through his mouth as if sucking on a straw. Encourage the patient to let the machine do the work.
- During treatment, instruct the patient to hold his breath for a few seconds after full inspiration *to allow for greater distribution of gas and medication.* Then instruct him to exhale normally.
- During treatment, take the patient's blood pressure and heart rate. *IPPB treatment increases intrathoracic pressure and may temporarily decrease cardiac output and venous return, resulting in tachycardia, hypotension, or headache.* Monitoring also detects reactions to the bronchodilator. If you find a sudden change in blood pressure or an increase in heart rate of 20 beats/minute or more, stop the treatment and notify the practitioner.

IPPB teaching tips

Before your patient is discharged, teach him the following important points about intermittent positive-pressure breathing (IPPB):

- If he'll be continuing IPPB treatments at home, have him demonstrate the proper setup, use, and cleaning of the equipment before discharge. Tell him that he shouldn't change the pressure settings without checking with his practitioner.
- Suggest that the patient avoid using IPPB immediately before or after a meal *because of possible nausea and reduced lung expansion.*
- Instruct him to discontinue treatment and call his practitioner if he experiences dizziness.

- If the patient is tolerating the treatment, continue until the medication in the nebulizer is exhausted, which is usually about 10 minutes.
- After treatment, or as needed, have the patient expectorate into tissues or a specimen cup, or suction him, as necessary. Listen to his breath sounds, and compare them to the pretreatment assessment.
- Shake excess moisture from the nebulizer and the mouthpiece or mask. After 24 hours of use, either discard the equipment or clean it with warm, soapy water. Then remove the equipment, rinse in warm water, and air-dry. When it's dry, store it in a clean plastic bag.

Special considerations

- If possible, avoid administering IPPB treatment immediately before or after a meal because the treatment may induce nausea and because a full stomach reduces lung expansion.
- Never give IPPB treatment without medication or sterile saline in the nebulizer *because this could dry the patient's airways and make secretions more difficult to mobilize.* If the purpose of treatment is to mobilize secretions, use a specimen cup to measure the secretions obtained.
- If the patient wears dentures, leave them in place *to ensure a proper seal,* but remove them if they slide out of position. If the patient has an artificial airway, use a special adapter such as mechanical ventilation tubing to give IPPB treatments. When using a mask to administer treatments, allow the patient frequent rest periods, and observe for gastric distention *because this is more likely to occur with a mask.*
- If the patient's blood pressure is stable during the initial treatment, you may not need to check it during subsequent treatments unless he has a history of cardiovascular disease, hypotension, or sensitivity to a drug delivered in the treatment.
- If the patient will be using IPPB at home, provide appropriate patient teaching. (See *IPPB teaching tips.*)

Complications

Gastric insufflation may result from swallowed air and occurs more commonly with a mask than with a mouthpiece. Dizziness can result from hyperventilation. The work of breathing can be increased, especially if the patient is uncomfortable with or frightened by the machine. Decreased blood pressure can result from decreased venous return, especially in the patient with hypovolemia or cardiovascular disease. Increased intracranial pressure can result from impeded venous return from the brain. Spontaneous pneumothorax may result from increased intrathoracic pressure; this complication is rare but is most likely to occur in patients with emphysematous blebs.

Documentation

Record the date, time, and duration of treatment; medication administered; pressure used; vital signs; breath sounds before and after treatment; amount of sputum produced; complications and nursing actions taken; and the patient's tolerance of the procedure.

SELECTED REFERENCES

American Association of Respiratory Care. "AARC Clinical Practice Guideline: Selection of Aerosol Delivery Device," *Respiratory Care* 37(8):891-97, August 2002.

American Association for Respiratory Care. "AARC Clinical Practice Guideline: Intermittent Positive Pressure Breathing," *Respiratory Care* 48(5):540-46, May 2003.

Keenan, S.P., et al. "Noninvasive Positive-pressure Ventilation for Postextubation Respiratory Distress: A Randomized Control Trial," *JAMA* 287(24):3238-244, June 2002.

HUMIDIFIER THERAPY

Humidifiers, which deliver a maximum amount of water vapor without producing particulate water, are used to prevent drying and irritation of the upper airway in conditions

EQUIPMENT

Comparing humidifiers

Type	Description and uses	Advantages	Disadvantages
Bedside 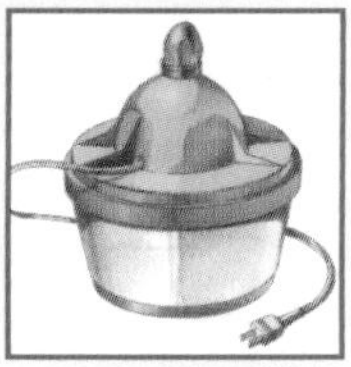	■ Spinning disk splashes water against baffle, creating small drops and increasing evaporation; motor disperses mist to directly humidify room air	■ May be used with all oxygen masks and nasal cannulas ■ Easy to operate ■ Inexpensive	■ Produces humidity inefficiently ■ Can't be used for patients with bypassed upper airway ■ May harbor bacteria and molds
Heated vaporizer 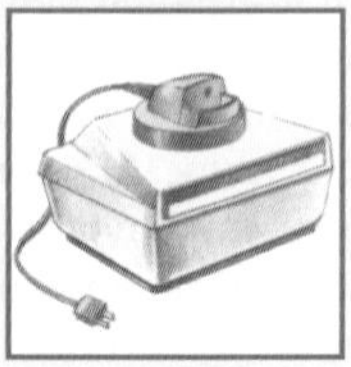	■ Provides direct humidification to room air by heating the water in the reservoir	■ May be used with all oxygen masks and nasal cannulas ■ Easy to operate ■ Inexpensive	■ Can't guarantee the amount of humidity delivered ■ Risk of burn injury if the machine is knocked over
Diffusion head 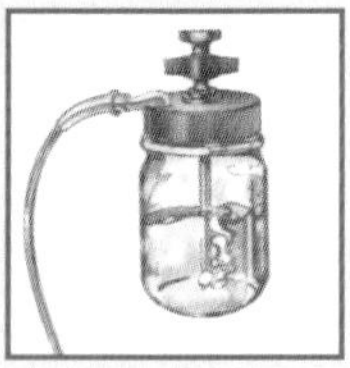	■ In-line humidifier most commonly used with low-flow oxygen delivery systems; gas flows through porous diffuser in reservoir to increase gas-liquid interface; provides humidification to patients using a nasal cannula or oxygen mask (except the Venturi mask)	■ Easy to use ■ Inexpensive	■ Provides only 20% to 30% humidity at body temperature ■ Can't be used for a patient with bypassed upper airway
Cascade bubble diffusion 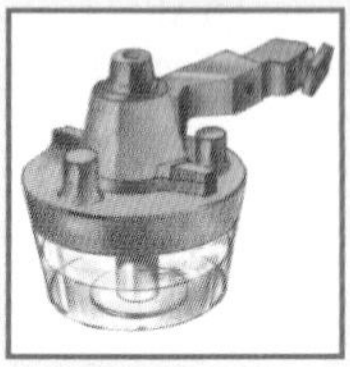	■ Gas forced through plastic grid in reservoir of warmed water to create fine bubbles; commonly used in patients receiving mechanical ventilation or continuous positive airway pressure therapy	■ Delivers 100% humidity at body temperature ■ Most effective of all evaporative humidifiers	■ If correct water level isn't maintained, mucosa can become irritated

such as croup, in which the upper airway is inflamed, or when secretions are particularly thick and tenacious.

Some humidifiers heat the water vapor, which raises the moisture-carrying capacity of gas and thus increases the amount of humidity delivered to the patient. Room humidifiers add humidity to an entire room, whereas humidifiers added to gas lines humidify only the air being delivered to the patient. (See *Comparing humidifiers.*)

Equipment

Humidifier or vaporizer ■ bottled distilled water, or tap water if the unit has a demineralizing capability ■ container for waste water ■ flowmeter ■ oxygen source, if needed ■ disinfectant.

Preparation of equipment

For a bedside humidifier: Open the reservoir and add sterile distilled water to the fill line; then close the reservoir. Keep all room windows and doors closed tightly *to maintain adequate humidification.* Plug the unit into the electrical outlet.

For a heated vaporizer: Remove the top and fill the reservoir to the fill line with tap water. Replace the top securely. Place the vaporizer about 4′ (1.2 m) from the patient, directing the steam toward but not directly onto the patient. Place the unit in a spot where it can't be overturned *to avoid hot water burns.* This is especially important if children will be in the room.

Plug the unit into an electrical outlet. Steam should soon rise from the unit into the air. Close all windows and doors *to maintain adequate humidification.*

For a diffusion head humidifier: Unscrew the humidifier reservoir, and add sterile distilled water to the appropriate level. (If using a disposable unit, screw the cap with the extension onto the top of the unit.) Then screw the reservoir back onto the humidifier, and attach the flowmeter to the oxygen source.

Screw the humidifier onto the flowmeter until the seal is tight. Then set the flowmeter at a rate of 2 L/minute and check for gentle bubbling. Next, check the positive-pressure release valve by occluding the end valve on the humidifier. The pressure should back up into the humidifier, signaled by a high-pitched whistle. If this doesn't occur, tighten all connections and try again.

For a cascade bubble diffusion humidifier: Unscrew the cascade reservoir and add sterile distilled water to the fill line. Screw the top back onto the reservoir. Plug in the heater unit, and set the temperature between 95° F (35° C) and 100.4° F (38° C).

Implementation

- Check to make sure the humidifier or vaporizer has been prepared properly.
- Confirm the patient's identity using two patient identifiers according to your facility's policy.

For a bedside humidifier

- Direct the humidifier unit's nozzle away from the patient's face (but toward the patient) for effective treatment. Check for a fine mist emission from the nozzle, *which indicates proper operation.*
- Check the unit every 4 hours for proper operation and the water level every 8 hours. When refilling, unplug the unit, discard any old water, wipe with a disinfectant, rinse the reservoir container, and refill with sterile distilled water, as necessary.
- Keep the unit cleaned and refilled with sterile water *to reduce the risk of bacterial growth.* Replace the unit every 7 days, and send used units for proper decontamination.

For a heated vaporizer

- Check the unit every 4 hours for proper functioning.
- If steam production seems insufficient, unplug the unit, discard the water, and refill with half distilled water and half tap water, or clean the unit well.
- Check the water level in the unit every 8 hours. To refill, unplug the unit, discard any old water, wipe with a disinfectant, rinse the reservoir container, and refill with tap water, as necessary.

For a diffusion head humidifier

- Attach the oxygen delivery device to the humidifier and then to the patient. Then adjust the flowmeter to the appropriate oxygen flow rate.
- Check the reservoir every 4 hours. If the water level drops too low, empty the remaining water, rinse the jar, and refill it with sterile water. (As the reservoir water level decreases, the evaporation of water in the gas decreases, reducing humidification of the delivered gas.)
- Change the humidification system regularly *to prevent bacterial growth and invasion.*
- Periodically assess the patient's sputum; *sputum that's too thick can hinder mobilization and expectoration.* If this occurs, the patient requires a device that can provide higher humidity.

For a cascade bubble diffusion humidifier

- Assess the temperature of the inspired gas near the patient's airway every 2 hours when used in critical care and every 4 hours when used in general patient care. If the cascade becomes too hot, drain the water and replace it. *Overheated water vapor can cause respiratory tract burns.*
- Check the reservoir's water level every 2 to 4 hours, and fill as necessary. If the water level falls below the minimum water level mark, humidity will decrease to that of room air.
- Be alert for condensation buildup in the tubing, which can result from the high humidification produced by the cascade.
- Check the tubing frequently and empty the condensate as necessary *so it can't drain into the patient's respiratory tract, encourage growth of microorganisms, or obstruct dependent sections of tubing.* To do so, disconnect the tubing, drain the condensate into a container, and dispose of it properly. Never drain the condensate into the humidification system.
- Change the cascade regularly according to your facility's policy.

Special considerations

- *Because it creates a humidity level comparable to that of ambient air,* the diffusion head humidifier is used only for oxygen flow rates greater than 4 L/minute.
- *Because the bedside humidifier doesn't deliver a precise amount of humidification,* assess the patient regularly *to determine the effectiveness of therapy.* Ask him if he has noticed any improvement, and evaluate his sputum.
- Like the bedside humidifier, the heated vaporizer doesn't deliver a precise amount of humidification, so assess the patient regularly by asking if he's feeling better and by examining his sputum.
- Keep in mind that a humidifier, if not kept clean, can cause or aggravate respiratory problems, especially for people allergic to molds. Refer to your facility's policy for changing and disposing of humidification equipment.

Home care

Make sure the patient and his family understand the reason for using a humidifier and know how to use the equipment. Give them specific written guidelines concerning all aspects of home care.

Instruct the patient using a bedside humidifier at home to fill it with plain tap water and to periodically use sterile distilled water *to prevent mineral buildup.* Also, tell him to run white vinegar through the unit *to help clean it, prevent bacterial buildup, and dissolve deposits.*

Tell the patient using a heated vaporizer unit to rinse it with bleach and water every 5 days. Also tell him to run white vinegar through it *to help clean it, prevent bacterial buildup, and dissolve deposits.*

Complications

Cascade humidifiers can cause aspiration of tubal condensation and, if the air is heated, can cause pulmonary burns. Humidifiers, if contaminated, can cause infection.

Documentation

Record the date and time when humidification began and was discontinued; the type of humidifier; the flow rate (of a gas system); thermometer readings (if heated); complications and the nursing action taken; and the patient's reaction to humidification.

SELECTED REFERENCES

American Association for Respiratory Care. "AARC Clinical Practice Guideline: Humidification During Mechanical Ventilation," *Respiratory Care* 37(8):887-90, August 1992.

American Association for Respiratory Care. "AARC Evidence-based Clinical Practice Guideline: Care of the Ventilator Circuit and Its Relation to Ventilator-associated Pneumonia," *Respiratory Care* 48(9):869-79, September 2003.

Branson, R.D. "Humidification of Respired Gases During Mechanical Ventilation: Mechanical Considerations," *Respiratory Care Clinics of North America* 12(2):253-61, June 2006.

Ebell, M.H. "Humidified Air for Croup?" *American Family Practitioner* 75(1):50, January 2007.

Niel-Weise, B.S., et al. "Humidification Policies for Mechanically Ventilated Intensive Care Patients and Prevention of Ventilator-associated Pneumonia: A Systematic Review of Randomized Controlled Trials," *Journal of Hospital Infection* 65(4):285-91, April 2007.

Scolnik, D., et al. "Controlled Delivery of High vs. Low Humidity vs. Mist Therapy for Croup in Emergency Departments: A Randomized Controlled Trial," *JAMA* 295(11):1274-280, March 2006.

Simasek, M., and Blandio, D.A. "Treatment of the Common Cold," *American Family Practitioner* 75(4):515-20, February 2007.

Taylor, C., et al. *Fundamentals of Nursing: The Art and Science of Nursing Care,* 5th ed. Philadelphia: Lippincott Williams & Wilkins, 2008.

NEBULIZER THERAPY

An established component of respiratory care, nebulizer therapy aids bronchial hygiene by restoring and maintaining mucous blanket continuity; hydrating dried, retained secretions; promoting expectoration of secretions; humidifying inspired oxygen; and delivering medications. The therapy may be administered through nebulizers that have a large or small volume, are ultrasonic, or are placed inside ventilator tubing.

Ultrasonic nebulizers are electrically driven and use high-frequency vibrations to break up surface water into particles. The resultant dense mist can penetrate smaller airways and is useful for hydrating secretions and inducing a cough. Large-volume nebulizers are used to provide humidity for an artificial airway such as a tracheostomy, and small-volume nebulizers are used to deliver medications such as bronchodilators. In-line nebulizers are used to deliver medications to patients who are being mechanically ventilated. In this case, the nebulizer is placed in the inspiratory side of the ventilatory circuit as close to the endotracheal tube as possible.

Equipment

For an ultrasonic nebulizer: Ultrasonic gas-delivery device ▪ large-bore oxygen tubing ▪ nebulizer couplet compartment.

For a large-volume nebulizer (such as a Venturi jet): Pressurized gas source ▪ flowmeter ▪ large-bore oxygen tubing ▪ nebulizer bottle ▪ sterile distilled water ▪ in-line thermometer (if using heater).

For a small-volume nebulizer (such as a mini-nebulizer): Pressurized gas source ■ flowmeter ■ oxygen tubing ■ nebulizer cup ■ mouthpiece or mask ■ normal saline solution or sterile water ■ prescribed medication.

For an in-line nebulizer: Pressurized gas source ■ flowmeter ■ nebulizer cup ■ normal saline solution ■ prescribed medication.

Preparation of equipment

For an ultrasonic nebulizer: Fill the couplet compartment on the nebulizer to the level indicated.

For a large-volume nebulizer: Fill the water chamber to the indicated level with sterile distilled water. Avoid using saline solution *to prevent corrosion.* Add a heating device, if ordered, and place a thermometer in-line between the outlet port and the patient, as close to the patient as possible, *to monitor the actual temperature of the inhaled gas and to avoid burning the patient.* If the unit will supply oxygen, analyze the flow at the patient's end of the tubing *to ensure delivery of the prescribed oxygen percentage.*

For a small-volume nebulizer: Draw up the prescribed medication, inject it into the nebulizer cup, and add the prescribed amount of saline solution or water. Attach the mouthpiece, mask, or other gas-delivery device.

For an in-line nebulizer: Draw up the medication and diluent, remove the nebulizer cup, quickly inject the medication, and then replace the cup. If using an intermittent positive-pressure breathing machine, attach the mouthpiece and mask to the machine. (For more information, see "Intermittent positive-pressure breathing," page 586.)

Implementation

- Confirm the patient's identity using two patient identifiers according to your facility's policy.
- Explain the procedure to the patient, and wash your hands.
- Take the patient's vital signs, and auscultate his lung fields *to establish a baseline.* If possible, place the patient in a sitting or high Fowler's position *to encourage full lung expansion and promote aerosol dispersion.* Encourage the patient to take slow, even breaths during the treatment.

For an ultrasonic nebulizer

- Before beginning, administer an inhaled bronchodilator (metered-dose inhaler or small-volume nebulizer) *to prevent bronchospasm.*
- Turn on the machine, and check the outflow port to ensure proper misting.
- Check the patient frequently during the procedure *to observe for adverse reactions.* Watch for labored respirations *because ultrasonic nebulizer therapy may hydrate retained secretions and obstruct airways.* Take the patient's vital signs, and auscultate his lung fields.
- Encourage the patient to cough and expectorate, or suction, as needed.

For a large-volume nebulizer

- Attach the delivery device to the patient.
- Encourage the patient to cough and expectorate, or suction, as needed.
- Check the water level in the nebulizer at frequent intervals and refill or replace as indicated. When refilling a reusable container, discard the old water *to prevent infection from bacterial or fungal growth,* and refill the container to the indicator line with sterile distilled water.
- Change the nebulizer unit and tubing according to your facility's policy *to prevent bacterial contamination.*
- If the nebulizer is heated, tell the patient to report warmth, discomfort, or hot tubing *because these may indicate a heater malfunction.* Use the in-line thermometer to monitor the temperature of the gas the patient is inhaling. If you turn off the flow for more than 5 minutes, unplug the heater *to avoid overheating the water and burning the patient when the aerosol is resumed.*

For a small-volume nebulizer

- After attaching the flowmeter to the gas source, attach the nebulizer to the flowmeter and then adjust the flow to at least 10 L/minute but no more than 14 L/minute (as shown below) *to ensure adequate functioning while preventing excess venting.*

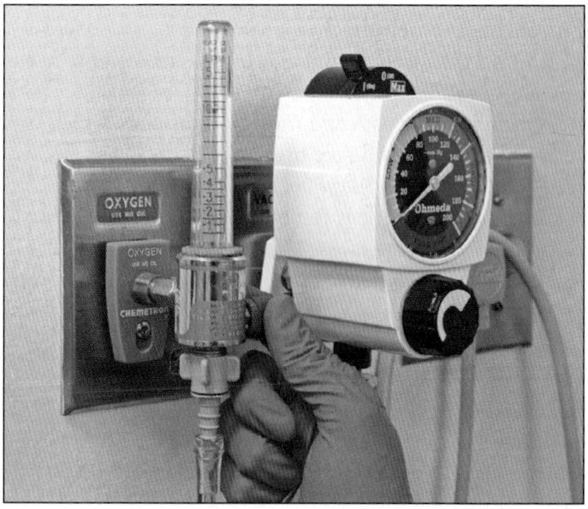

- Check the outflow port to ensure adequate misting.
- Assist the patient with the mouthpiece or mask. Instruct the patient to grasp the mouthpiece securely with his teeth

and lips (as shown below). The patient should inhale slowly through his mouth and hold each breath for 5 to 10 seconds before exhaling through his mouth.

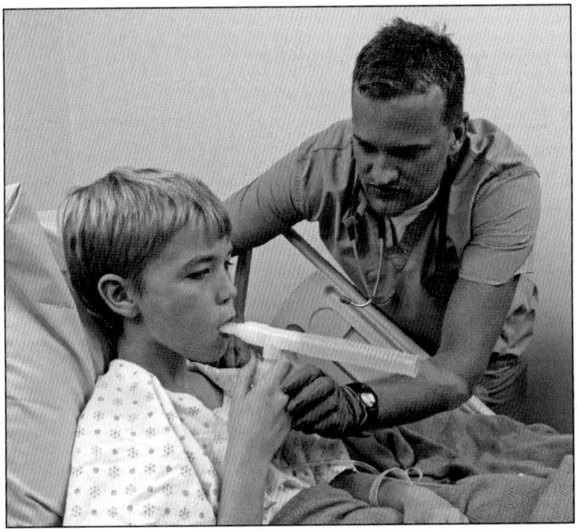

- Remain with the patient during the treatment, which lasts 15 to 20 minutes, and take his vital signs *to detect any adverse reaction to the medication.*
- Encourage the patient to cough and expectorate, or suction, as necessary.
- Change the nebulizer cup and tubing according to your facility's policy *to prevent bacterial contamination.*

For an in-line nebulizer

- Turn on the machine and check the outflow port *to ensure proper misting.*
- Remain with the patient during the treatment, which lasts 15 to 20 minutes, and take his vital signs *to detect any adverse reaction to the medication.*
- Encourage the patient to cough, and suction excess secretions, as necessary.
- Auscultate the patient's lungs *to evaluate the effectiveness of therapy.*

Special considerations

- When using high-output nebulizers, such as an ultrasonic nebulizer on pediatric patients or patients with a delicate fluid balance, be alert for signs of overhydration (exhibited by unexplained weight gain occurring over several days after the beginning of therapy), pulmonary edema, crackles, and electrolyte imbalance.
- If oxygen is being delivered concomitantly, the fraction of inspired oxygen (FIO_2) may be diluted if the flow isn't adequate. Therefore, if the mist disappears when the patient inhales, increase the gas flow.

Complications

Nebulized particulates can irritate the mucosa in some patients and cause bronchospasm and dyspnea. Other complications include airway burns (when heating elements are used), infection from contaminated equipment (although rare), and adverse reactions from medications.

Documentation

Record the date, time, and duration of therapy; type and amount of medication; FIO_2 or oxygen flow, if administered; baseline and subsequent vital signs and breath sounds; and the patient's response to treatment.

SELECTED REFERENCES

American Association for Respiratory Care. "AARC Clinical Practice Guideline: Bland Aerosol Administration—2003 Revision & Update," *Respiratory Care* 48(5):529-33, May 2003.

Bayat, M., and Cook, A.M. "Intrapulmonary Administration of Medications," *Journal of Neuroscience Nursing* 36(4):231-35, August 2004.

Dolovich, M.B., et al. "Device Selection and Outcomes of Aerosol Therapy: Evidence-based Guidelines: American College of Chest Practitioners/American College of Asthma, Allergy, and Immunology," *Chest* 127(1):335-71, January 2005.

Geller, D.E. "Comparing Clinical Features of Nebulizer, Metered-dose Inhaler and Dry Powder Inhaler," *Respiratory Care* 50(10):1313-321, October 2005.

CHEST PHYSIOTHERAPY

Chest physiotherapy includes postural drainage, chest percussion and vibration, and coughing and deep-breathing exercises. Together, these techniques mobilize and eliminate secretions, reexpand lung tissue, and promote efficient use of respiratory muscles. Of critical importance to the bedridden patient, chest physiotherapy helps prevent or treat atelectasis and may also help prevent pneumonia, two respiratory complications that can seriously impede recovery.

Postural drainage performed in conjunction with percussion and vibration encourages peripheral pulmonary secretions to empty by gravity into the major bronchi or trachea and is accomplished by sequential repositioning of the patient. Usually, secretions drain best with the patient positioned so that the bronchi are perpendicular to the floor. Lower and middle lobe bronchi usually empty best with the patient in the head-down position; upper lobe bronchi, in the head-up position. (See *Positioning a patient for postural drainage.*)

Percussing the chest with cupped hands mechanically dislodges thick, tenacious secretions from the bronchial walls. Some specialty beds have a percussion therapy option, which

Positioning a patient for postural drainage

The following illustrations show the various postural drainage positions and the areas of the lungs affected by each.

Lower lobes: Posterior basal segments

Elevate the foot of the bed 30 degrees. Have the patient lie prone with his head lowered. Position pillows under his chest and abdomen. Percuss his lower ribs on both sides of his spine.

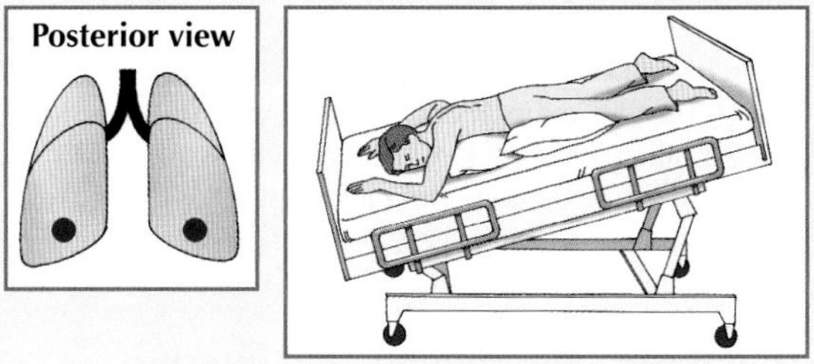

Lower lobes: Lateral basal segments

Elevate the foot of the bed 30 degrees. Instruct the patient to lie on his abdomen with his head lowered and his upper leg flexed over a pillow for support. Then have him rotate a quarter turn upward. Percuss his lower ribs on the uppermost portion of his lateral chest wall.

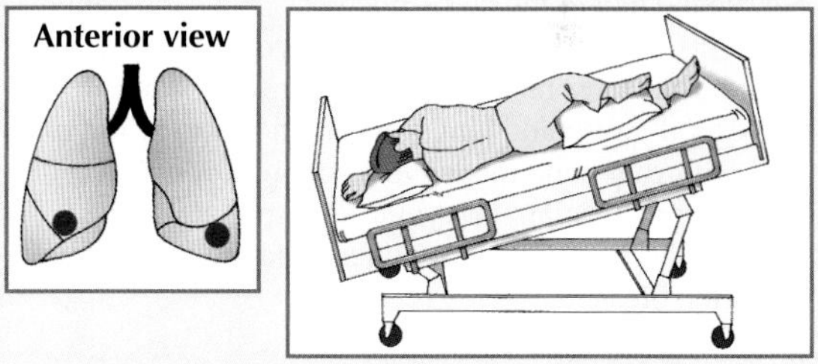

Lower lobes: Anterior basal segments

Elevate the foot of the bed 30 degrees. Instruct the patient to lie on his side with his head lowered. Then place pillows as shown. Percuss with a slightly cupped hand over his lower ribs just beneath the axilla. If an acutely ill patient has trouble breathing in this position, adjust the bed to an angle he can tolerate. Then begin percussion.

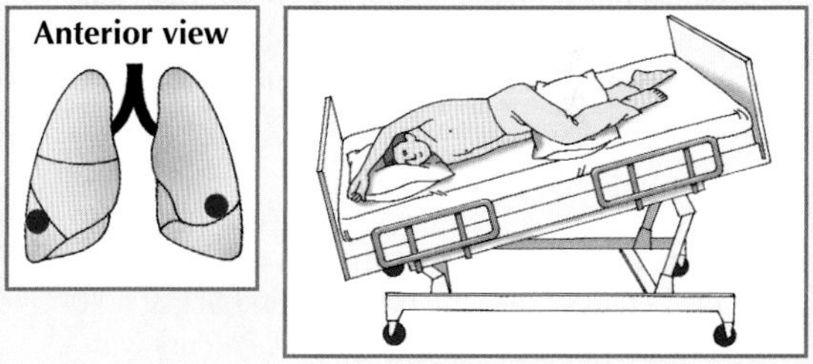

Lower lobes: Superior segments

With the bed flat, have the patient lie on his abdomen. Place two pillows under his hips. Percuss on both sides of his spine at the lower tip of his scapulae.

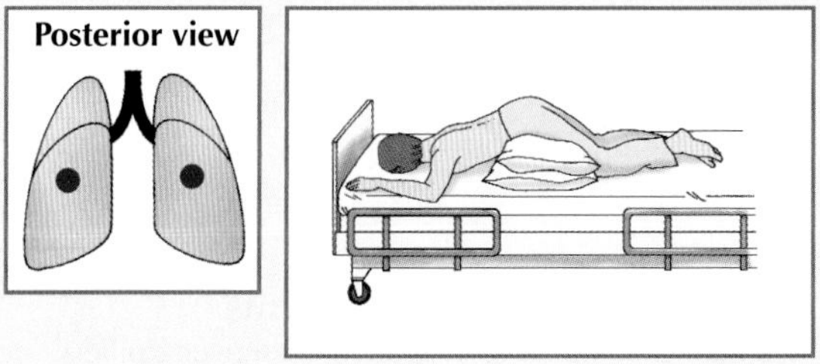

(continued)

Positioning a patient for postural drainage *(continued)*

Right middle lobe: Medial and lateral segments

Elevate the foot of the bed 15 degrees. Have the patient lie on his left side with his head down and his knees flexed. Then have him rotate a quarter turn backward. Place a pillow beneath him. Percuss with your hand moderately cupped over the right nipple. For a woman, cup your hand so that its heel is under the armpit and your fingers extend forward beneath the breast.

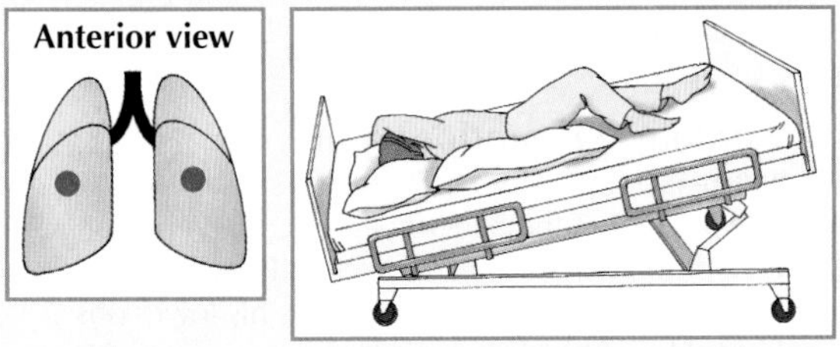

Left upper lobe: Superior and inferior segments, lingular portion

Elevate the foot of the bed 15 degrees. Have the patient lie on his right side with his head down and knees flexed. Then have him rotate a quarter turn backward. Place a pillow behind him, from shoulders to hips. Percuss with your hand moderately cupped over his left nipple. For a woman, cup your hand so that its heel is beneath the armpit and your fingers extend forward beneath the breast.

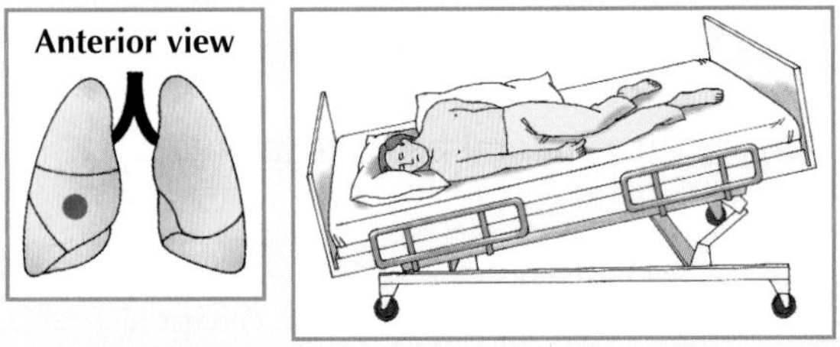

Upper lobes: Anterior segments

Make sure the bed is flat. Have the patient lie on his back with a pillow folded under his knees. Then have him rotate slightly away from the side being drained. Percuss between his clavicle and nipple.

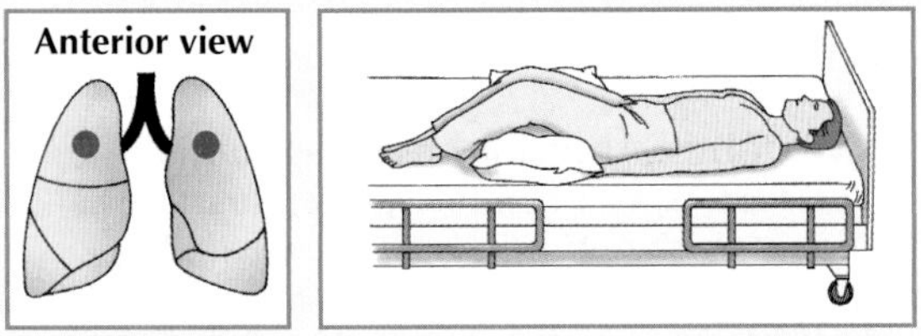

Upper lobes: Apical segments

Keep the bed flat. Have the patient lean back at a 30-degree angle against you and a pillow. Percuss with a cupped hand between his clavicles and the top of each scapula.

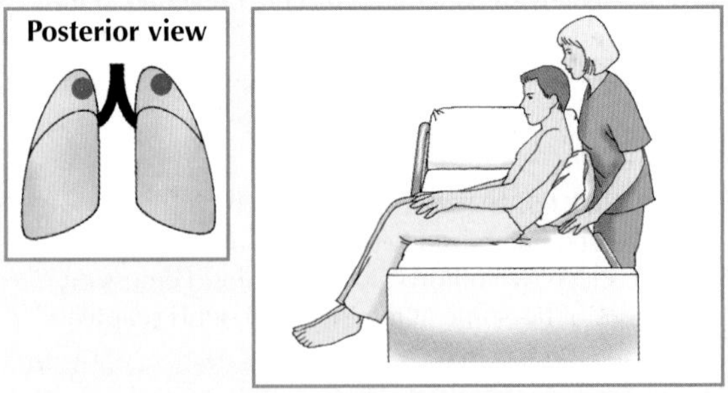

Upper lobes: Posterior segments

Keep the bed flat. Have the patient lean over a pillow at a 30-degree angle. Percuss and clap his upper back on each side.

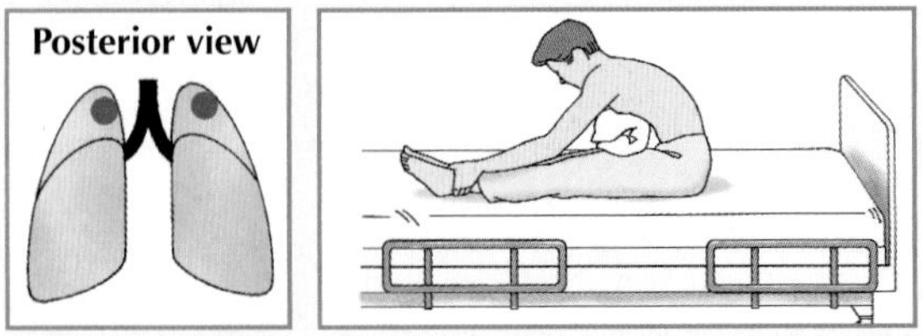

may be used in select patients. Vibration can be used with percussion or as an alternative to it in a patient who's frail, in pain, or recovering from thoracic surgery or trauma.

Candidates for chest physiotherapy include patients who expectorate large amounts of sputum, such as those with bronchiectasis and cystic fibrosis. The procedure hasn't proved effective in treating patients with status asthmaticus, lobar pneumonia, or acute exacerbations of chronic bronchitis when the patient has scant secretions and is being mechanically ventilated. Chest physiotherapy has little value for treating patients with stable, chronic bronchitis.

In critical care patients, including those on mechanical ventilation, postural drainage therapy (PDT) should be performed every 4 to 6 hours, as indicated. The PDT order should be reevaluated at least every 48 hours, based on assessments from individual treatments. In spontaneously breathing patients, PDT frequentcy should be determined by assessing the patient's response to therapy. Acute care patient orders should be reevaluated, based on patient response to therapy, at least every 72 hours or with a change in the patient's status.

Contraindications may include active pulmonary bleeding with hemoptysis and the immediate posthemorrhage stage, fractured ribs or an unstable chest wall, lung contusions, pulmonary tuberculosis, untreated pneumothorax, acute asthma or bronchospasm, lung abscess or tumor, bony metastasis, head injury, and recent myocardial infarction.

Equipment

Stethoscope ▪ pillows ▪ tilt or postural drainage table (if available) or adjustable hospital bed ▪ emesis basin ▪ facial tissues ▪ suction equipment ▪ equipment for oral care ▪ trash bag ▪ optional: sterile specimen container, mechanical ventilator, supplemental oxygen.

Preparation of equipment

Gather the equipment at the patient's bedside. Set up suction equipment and test its function.

Implementation

- Confirm the patient's identity using two patient identifiers according to your facility's policy.
- Explain the procedure to the patient, provide privacy, and wash your hands.
- Auscultate the patient's lungs to determine baseline respiratory status.
- Position the patient, as ordered. In generalized disease, drainage usually begins with the lower lobes, continues with the middle lobes, and ends with the upper lobes. In localized disease, drainage begins with the affected lobes and then proceeds to the other lobes *to avoid spreading the disease to uninvolved areas.*
- Instruct the patient to remain in each position for 3 to 15 minutes. During this time, perform percussion and vibration, as ordered. (See *Performing percussion and vibration,* page 596.)
- After postural drainage, percussion, or vibration, instruct the patient to cough *to remove loosened secretions.* First, tell him to inhale deeply through his nose and then exhale in three short huffs. Then have him inhale deeply again and cough through a slightly open mouth. Three consecutive coughs are highly effective. An effective cough sounds deep, low, and hollow; an ineffective one, high-pitched. Have the patient perform exercises for about 1 minute and then rest for 2 minutes. Gradually progress to a 10-minute exercise period four times daily.
- Provide oral hygiene because secretions may have a foul taste or a stale odor.
- Auscultate the patient's lungs to evaluate the effectiveness of therapy.

Special considerations

- For optimal effectiveness and safety, modify chest physiotherapy according to the patient's condition. For example, initiate or increase the flow of supplemental oxygen, if indicated. Also, suction the patient who has an ineffective cough reflex. If the patient tires quickly during therapy, shorten the sessions *because fatigue leads to shallow respirations and increased hypoxia.*
- Maintain adequate hydration in the patient receiving chest physiotherapy *to prevent mucus dehydration and promote easier mobilization.* Avoid performing postural drainage immediately before or within 1½ hours after meals *to avoid nausea, vomiting, and aspiration of food or vomitus.*
- *Because chest percussion can induce bronchospasm,* any adjunct treatment (for example, intermittent positive-pressure breathing, aerosol, or nebulizer therapy) should precede chest physiotherapy.
- Refrain from percussing over the spine, liver, kidneys, or spleen *to avoid injury to the spine or internal organs.* Also avoid performing percussion on bare skin or the female patient's breasts. Percuss over soft clothing (but not over buttons, snaps, or zippers), or place a thin towel over the chest wall. Remember to remove jewelry that might scratch or bruise the patient.
- Explain coughing and deep-breathing exercises preoperatively *so that the patient can practice them when he's pain-free and better able to concentrate.* Postoperatively, splint the patient's incision using your hands or, if possible, teach the patient to splint it himself *to minimize pain during coughing.*
- Try to schedule the last session just before bedtime *to help maximize the patient's oxygenation while he's sleeping.*

Performing percussion and vibration

To perform percussion, instruct the patient to breathe slowly and deeply, using the diaphragm, *to promote relaxation.* Hold your hands in a cupped shape, with fingers flexed and thumbs pressed tightly against your index fingers. Percuss each segment for 1 to 2 minutes by alternating your hands against the patient in a rhythmic manner. Listen for a hollow sound on percussion *to verify correct performance of the technique.*

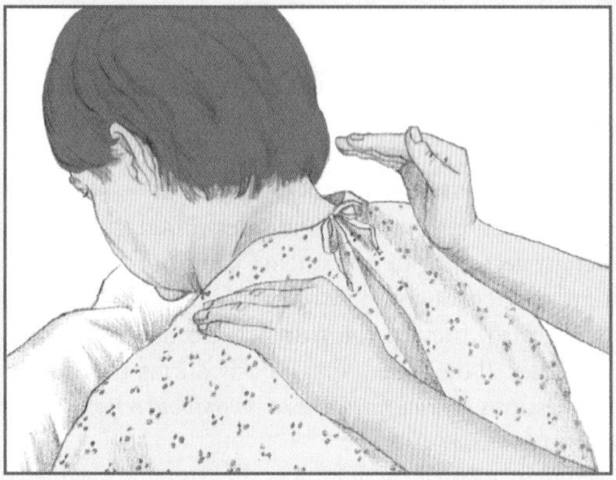

To perform vibration, ask the patient to inhale deeply and then exhale slowly through pursed lips. During exhalation, firmly press your fingers and the palms of your hands against the chest wall. Tense the muscles of your arms and shoulders in an isometric contraction *to send fine vibrations through the chest wall.* Vibrate during five exhalations over each chest segment.

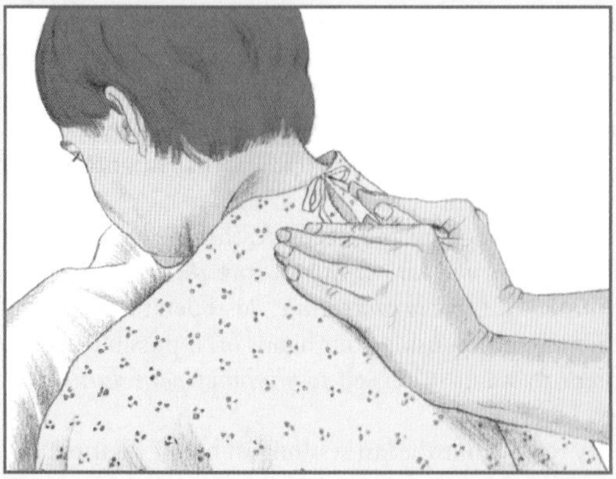

Complications

During postural drainage in head-down positions, pressure on the diaphragm by abdominal contents can impair respiratory excursion and lead to hypoxia or postural hypotension. The head-down position may also lead to increased intracranial pressure, which precludes the use of chest physiotherapy in a patient with acute neurologic impairment. Vigorous percussion or vibration can cause rib fracture, especially in a patient with osteoporosis. In an emphysematous patient with blebs, coughing could lead to pneumothorax.

Documentation

Record the date and time of chest physiotherapy; positions for secretion drainage and length of time each is maintained; chest segments percussed or vibrated; color, amount, odor, and viscosity of secretions produced and the presence of any blood; complications and nursing actions taken; and the patient's tolerance of treatment.

SELECTED REFERENCES

McCarven, B., et al. "Vibration and its Effects on the Respiratory System," *Australian Journal of Physiotherapy* 52(1):39-43, 2005.

McCool, F.D., et al. "Non-pharmacological Airway Clearance Therapies: AACP Evidence-based Clinical Practice Guidelines," *Chest* 129(1 suppl):2505-595, January 2006.

Pruitt, B., et al. "Clearing Away Pulmonary Secretions," *Nursing* 35(7):36-41, July 2005.

Taylor, C., et al. *Fundamentals of Nursing: The Art and Science of Nursing Care*, 5th ed. Philadelphia: Lippincott Williams & Wilkins, 2008.

PRONE POSITIONING

Prone positioning is a therapeutic maneuver to improve oxygenation and pulmonary mechanics in patients with acute lung injury or acute respiratory distress syndrome (ARDS). Also known as *proning,* the procedure involves physically turning a patient from a supine position (on the back) to a facedown position (prone position). This positioning may improve oxygenation in patients by shifting blood flow to regions of the lung that are better ventilated. With the appropriate equipment, prone positioning may also facilitate better movement of the diaphragm by allowing the abdomen to expand more fully.

The criteria for prone positioning frequently include:

- acute onset of respiratory failure
- hypoxemia, specifically a Pa_{O_2}/F_{IO_2} ratio of 300 or less for acute lung injury or a Pa_{O_2}/F_{IO_2} ratio of 200 or less for ARDS

■ radiological evidence of diffuse bilateral pulmonary infiltrates.

The physical challenges of proning have been a traditional barrier to its use. However, equipment innovations (such as a lightweight, cushioned frame that straps to the front of the patient before turning) have helped to minimize the risks associated with moving patients and maintaining them in the prone position for several hours at a time.

Prone positioning is usually performed for 6 or more hours per day, for as long as 10 days, until the requirement for a high concentration of inspired oxygen resolves. Aside from early intervention, factors predictive of patients' responses aren't consistent among studies, and patients' initial responses aren't always predictive of their subsequent responses. Patients with extrapulmonary ARDS (such as ARDS due to multiple trauma) appear to respond consistently to prone positioning. Although research has demonstrated improved oxygenation with proning, it's unclear whether the survival rate is increased.

The procedure is indicated to support mechanically ventilated patients with ARDS, who require high concentrations of inspired oxygen. Prone positioning may correct severe hypoxemia and help maintain adequate oxygenation (Po_2 greater than 60%) while avoiding ventilator-induced lung injury.

Prone positioning is contraindicated in patients whose heads can't be supported in a facedown position, or those who are unable to tolerate a head-down position. Relative contraindications include:

■ increased intracranial pressure
■ unstable spine, chest, or pelvis
■ unstable bone fractures
■ left ventricular failure (nonpulmonary respiratory failure)
■ shock
■ abdominal compartment syndrome or abdominal surgery
■ patients who are extremely obese (more than 300 lb [136 kg])
■ pregnancy.

Hemodynamically unstable patients (systolic blood pressure less than 90 mm Hg) despite aggressive fluid resuscitation and vasopressors should be thoroughly evaluated before being placed in the prone position.

Equipment

Vollman Prone Positioner (HillRom), or other prone positioning device ■ gloves ■ personal protective equipment, as appropriate ■ draw sheet ■ small towel ■ small pillow or rolled towel ■ suction equipment, as needed ■ oral care supplies ■ eye lubricant.

Preparation of equipment

Clean the positioner according to your facility's policy between positioning turns and when discontinuing prone positioning.

Implementation

■ Confirm the patient's identity using two patient identifiers according to your facility's policy.
■ Assess the patient's hemodynamic status *to determine whether the patient will be able to tolerate the prone position.*
■ Assess the patient's neurologic status prior to prone positioning. Generally, the patient will be heavily sedated. Although agitation isn't a contraindication for proning, it must be managed effectively.
■ Determine whether the patient's size and weight will allow turning him on a generally narrow critical care bed. Consider obtaining a wider specialty bed, if needed.

Before turning the patient

■ Explain the purpose and procedure of prone positioning to the patient and his family.
■ Wash your hands, and put on gloves or other protective wear, as appropriate.
■ Provide eye care, including lubrication and horizontal taping of the patient's eyelids, if indicated.
■ Make sure the patient's tongue is inside his mouth; if edematous or protruding, insert a bite block.
■ Secure the patient's endotracheal (ET) tube or tracheotomy tube *to prevent dislodgment.*
■ Perform anterior body wound care and dressing changes.
■ Empty ileostomy or colostomy drainage bags.
■ Remove anterior chest wall electrocardiogram monitoring leads, while ensuring ability to monitor the patient's cardiac rate and rhythm. These leads will be repositioned onto the patient's back once he's prone.
■ Make sure that the brake of the bed is engaged. Attach the surface of the prone positioner to the bed frame, as recommended by the manufacturer.
■ Position staff appropriately; a minimum of three people is required: one on either side of the bed and one at the head of the bed.

NURSING ALERT *The staff member at the head of the bed is responsible for monitoring the ET tube and mechanical ventilator tubing.*

■ Adjust all patient tubing and invasive monitoring lines *to prevent dislodgment, kinking, disconnection, or contact with the patient's body during the turning procedure and while the patient remains in the prone position* (as shown top of next page).

NURSING ALERT *Place all lines inserted in the upper torso over the right or left shoulder, with the exception of chest tubes, which are placed at the foot of the bed. All lines inserted in the lower torso are positioned at the foot of the bed.*

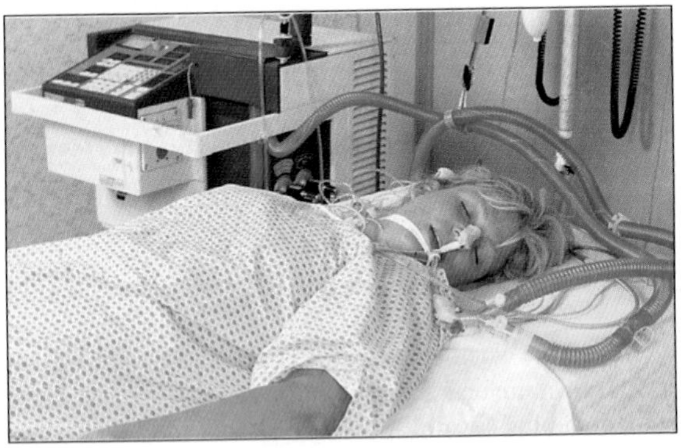

■ Turn the patient's face away from the ventilator, placing the ET tubing on the side of the patient's face that's turned away from the ventilator. Loop the remaining tubing above the patient's head *to prevent disconnection of the ventilator tubing or kinking of the ET tube during proning.*
■ Place the straps of the prone positioner under the patient's head, chest, and pelvic area.
■ Attach the prone-positioning device to the patient by placing the frame on top of the patient.
■ Position the nonmovable chest piece, which acts as a marker for the proper device placement, so that it's resting between the patient's clavicles and sixth ribs.

NURSING ALERT *If the patient has a short neck or limited neck range of motion (ROM), align the chest piece lower, at the third intercostal space; move both headpieces up to the top of the frame so that only the forehead is supported by the head cushion and the chin is suspended* to reduce the risk of skin breakdown.

■ Adjust the pelvic piece of the device so that it rests ½" (1.3 cm) above the iliac crest.

NURSING ALERT *Evaluate the distance between the chest and pelvic pieces to ensure suspension of the abdomen, while preventing bowing of the patient's back.*

■ Adjust the chin and forehead pieces of the device so that facial support is provided in either a facedown or side-lying position without interfering with the ET tube.
■ Secure the positioning device to the patient, by fastening all the soft adjustable straps on one side before tightening them on the opposite side (as shown top of next column). Once secured, lift the positioner *to ensure a secure fit.*

NURSING ALERT *To help ensure a secure fit, look for cushion compression. If the frame isn't tightly secured, shear and friction injuries to the chest and pelvic area may occur.*

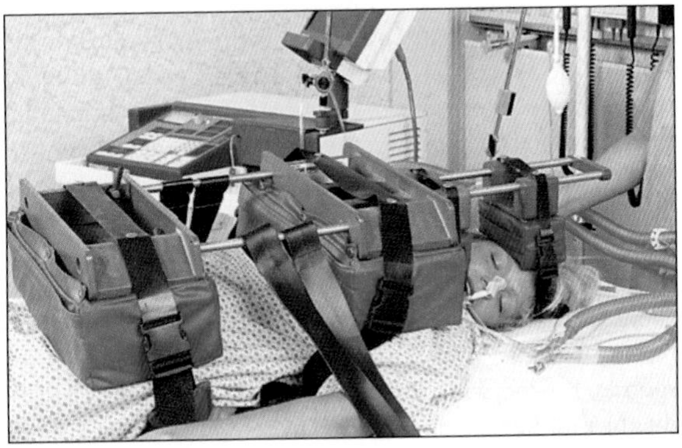

Turning the patient

■ Lower the side rails of the bed, and move the patient to the edge of the bed farthest away from the ventilator by using a draw sheet. The person closest to the patient maintains body contact with the bed at all times, serving as a side rail.
■ Tuck the straps attached to the steel bar closest to the center of the bed underneath the patient. Then tuck the patient's arm and hand that are resting in the center of the bed under the buttocks. Cross the leg closest to the edge of the bed over the opposite leg at the ankle, *which will help with forward motion when the turning process begins.*

NURSING ALERT *If the patient's arm can't be straightened to tuck under his buttocks, tuck his arm into the open space between the chest and pelvic pads.*

■ Turn the patient toward the ventilator at a 45-degree angle.

NURSING ALERT *Always turn the patient in the direction of the mechanical ventilator.*

■ The person on the side of the bed with the ventilator grasps the upper steel bar. The person on the other side of the bed grasps the lower steel bar or turning straps of the device.
■ Lift the patient by the frame into the prone position on the count of three.
■ Gently move the patient's tucked arm and hand *so they're parallel to his body and comfortable* (as shown on next page).

NURSING ALERT *To prevent placing stress on the shoulder capsule, don't extend the patient's arm to a 90-degree angle.*

■ Loosen the straps if the patient is clinically stable.

NURSING ALERT *Keeping the straps securely fastened in an unstable patient allows for rapid supine repositioning in an emergency.*

■ Support the patient's feet with a pillow or towel roll *to provide correct flexion while in the prone position.*

NURSING ALERT *Pad the patient's elbows* **to prevent ulnar nerve compression.**

■ Monitor the patient's response to proning using vital signs, pulse oximetry, and mixed venous oxygen saturation. The patient's vital signs should return to normal within 10 minutes of being placed prone. During the initial proning, arterial blood gases should be obtained within 30 minutes of proning and within 30 minutes prior to returning the patient to the supine position.

■ Reposition the patient's head hourly while in the prone position *to prevent facial breakdown.* As one person lifts the patient's head, the second person moves the headpieces to provide head support in a different position.

■ Provide ROM to shoulders, arms, and legs every 2 hours.

■ Give oral care and suction the patient, as needed.

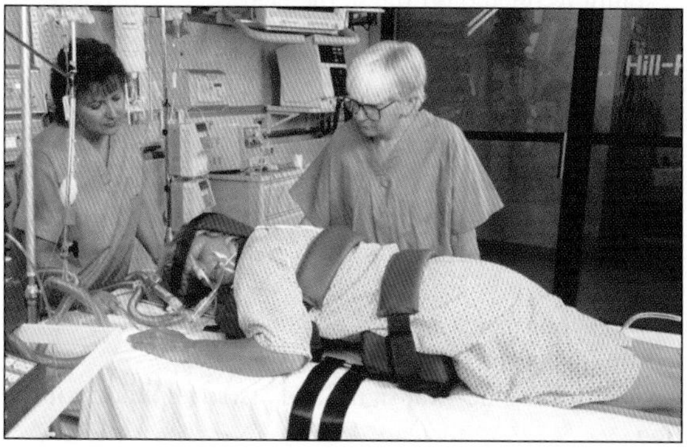

Returning the patient to the supine position

■ Securely fasten positioning device straps.

■ Remove the posterior chest electrocardiogram leads while ensuring the ability to monitor the patient's rate and rhythm. The leads will be replaced on the patient's chest once he's in the supine position.

■ Position the patient on the edge of the bed closest to the ventilator.

■ Adjust all patient tubing and monitoring lines to prevent dislodgment.

■ Position a staff member on each side of the bed and one at the head.

■ Straighten the patient's arms and rest them on either side. Cross the leg closest to the edge of the bed over the opposite leg.

■ Using the steel bars of the device, turn the patient to a 45-degree angle away from the ventilator, and then roll him to the supine position.

■ Position the patient's arms parallel to his body.

■ Unfasten the positioning device, and remove it from the patient.

Special considerations

■ A practitioner's order is usually required before prone positioning of a critically ill patient.

■ The procedure requires special training and established guidelines to ensure patient safety.

■ Not all patients with ARDS respond favorably to prone positioning, and the benefit sometimes decreases over time. The patient may not have an immediate positive response to the prone position. Maximum response may take up to 6 hours.

■ Patients may require increased sedation during proning.

■ The prone-positioning schedule is generally determined by the patient's ability to maintain improvements in PaO_2 while in the prone position.

■ *To reduce the risk of aspirating gastric contents during the turning procedure,* turn off the tube feedings one hour before turning the patient. The feeding can be safely restarted once the patient is positioned.

■ Use capnography, if possible, to verify correct endotracheal tube placement during proning.

■ Reposition the patient every 4 to 6 hours *to prevent pressure-related injury.*

■ Discontinue the procedure when the patient no longer demonstrates improved oxygenation with the position change.

NURSING ALERT ***Lateral rotation therapy is strongly recommended with prone positioning.***

Complications

Potential complications of prone positioning include:

■ inadvertent ET extubation
■ airway obstruction
■ decreased oxygen saturation
■ apical atelectasis
■ obstructed chest tube
■ pressure injuries on the weight-bearing parts of the body, including the knees and chest
■ hemodynamic instability
■ dislodgment of central venous access
■ transient arrhythmias
■ reversible dependent edema of the face (forehead, eyelids, conjunctiva, lips, and tongue) and anterior chest wall
■ contractures
■ enteral feeding intolerance
■ aspiration of enteral feeding when repositioned
■ corneal ulceration.

NURSING ALERT *Critically ill patients with active intra-abdominal processes, regardless of position, are at risk for sepsis and septic shock.*

Documentation

Document the patient's response to therapy, ability to tolerate the turning procedure, length of time in the position, and positioning schedule. Also document monitoring, complications, and interventions.

SELECTED REFERENCES

deLeon, D.G., and Spieglern, P. "The Role of Prone Positions in the Management of Hypoxemic Acute Respiratory Failure," *Clinical Pulmonary Medicine* 12(2):128-29, March 2005.

Essat, Z. "Prone Positioning in Patients with Acute Respiratory Distress Syndrome," *Nursing Standard* 20(9):52-55, November 2005.

Lynn-McHale Wiegand, D.J., and Carlson, K.K., eds. *AACN Procedure Manual for Critical Care*, 5th ed. Philadelphia: W.B. Saunders Co., 2006.

Thomas, P.J., et al. "Positioning Practices for Ventilated Intensive Care Patients: Current Practice, Indications and Contraindications," *Australian Critical Care* 19(4):122-26, 128, 130-32, November 2006.

Vollman, K.M. "Prone Positioning in the Patient who has Acute Respiratory Distress Syndrome: The Art and Science," *Critical Care Nursing Clinic of North America* 16(3):319-36, September 2004.

THORACENTESIS

Thoracentesis involves the aspiration of fluid or air from the pleural space. It relieves pulmonary compression and respiratory distress by removing accumulated air or fluid that results from injury or such conditions as tuberculosis, cancer, or heart failure. It also provides a specimen of pleural fluid or tissue for analysis and allows instillation of chemotherapeutic agents or other medications into the pleural space. Thoracentesis is contraindicated in patients with bleeding disorders. Thoracentesis should be used cautiously in patients who are uncooperative, have uncontrolled coughing, an uncertain pleural fluid location, one functional lung, or who are on positive end-expiratory pressure ventilation.

Equipment

Most hospitals use a prepackaged thoracentesis tray that typically includes the following: sterile gloves ▪ sterile drapes ▪ antiseptic solution ▪ 1% or 2% lidocaine ▪ 5-ml syringe with 21G and 25G needles for anesthetic injection ▪ 17G thoracentesis needle for aspiration or Teflon catheter ▪ 50-ml syringe ▪ three-way stopcock and tubing ▪ sterile specimen containers ▪ sterile hemostat ▪ sterile 4" × 4" gauze pads.

You'll also need the following: occlusive dressing ▪ sphygmomanometer ▪ gloves ▪ stethoscope ▪ laboratory request slips ▪ drainage bottles ▪ optional: sterile marker, sterile label, clippers, biopsy needle, prescribed sedative with 3-ml syringe and 21G needle, drainage bottles if the physician expects a large amount of drainage.

Preparation of equipment

Assemble all equipment at the patient's bedside or in the treatment area. Check the expiration date on each sterile package, and inspect for tears. Prepare the necessary laboratory request form. Make sure the patient has signed an appropriate consent form. Note drug allergies, especially to the local anesthetic. Have the patient's chest X-rays available. Label all medications, medication containers, and other solutions on and off the sterile field.

Implementation

- Confirm the patient's identity using two patient identifiers according to your facility's policy.
- Explain the procedure to the patient. Inform him that he may feel some discomfort and a sensation of pressure during the needle insertion. Provide privacy and emotional support.
- Wash your hands and put on gloves.
- Administer the prescribed sedative.
- Obtain baseline vital signs, and assess respiratory function.
- Position the patient. Make sure he's firmly supported and comfortable. (See *Positioning for thoracentesis.*)
- Remind the patient not to cough, breathe deeply, or move suddenly during the procedure *to avoid puncture of the visceral pleura or lung.* If the patient coughs, the physician will briefly halt the procedure and withdraw the needle slightly *to prevent puncture.*
- Expose the patient's entire chest or back, as appropriate.
- Clip the aspiration site, if needed.
- Wash your hands again before touching the sterile equipment. Then using sterile technique, open the thoracentesis tray and assist the physician, as necessary, in disinfecting the site.
- If an ampule of local anesthetic isn't included in the sterile tray and a multidose vial of local anesthetic is to be used, assist the physician by wiping the rubber stopper with an alcohol pad and holding the inverted vial while the physician withdraws the anesthetic solution.
- After draping the patient and injecting the anesthetic, the physician attaches a three-way stopcock with tubing to the

aspirating needle and turns the stopcock *to prevent air from entering the pleural space through the needle.*

- Attach the other end of the tubing to the drainage bottle.
- The physician then inserts the needle into the pleural space and attaches a 50-ml syringe to the needle's stopcock. A hemostat may be used *to hold the needle in place and prevent pleural tear or lung puncture.* As an alternative, the physician may introduce a Teflon catheter into the needle, remove the needle, and attach a stopcock and syringe or drainage tubing to the catheter *to reduce the risk of pleural puncture by the needle.*
- Support the patient verbally throughout the procedure, and keep him informed of each step. Assess him for signs of anxiety, and provide reassurance, as necessary.
- Check vital signs regularly during the procedure. Continually observe the patient for such signs of distress as pallor, vertigo, faintness, weak and rapid pulse, decreased blood pressure, dyspnea, tachypnea, diaphoresis, chest pain, blood-tinged mucus, and excessive coughing. Alert the physician if such signs develop *because they may indicate complications, such as hypovolemic shock or tension pneumothorax.*
- Put on gloves and assist the physician, as necessary, in specimen collection, fluid drainage, and dressing the site.
- After the physician withdraws the needle or catheter, apply pressure to the puncture site, using a sterile 4″ × 4″ gauze pad. Then apply a new sterile gauze pad, and secure it with an occlusive dressing.
- Place the patient in a comfortable position, take his vital signs, and assess his respiratory status.
- Label the specimens properly, and send them to the laboratory.
- Discard disposable equipment. Clean nondisposable items, and return them for sterilization.
- Check the patient's vital signs and the dressing for drainage every 15 minutes for 1 hour. Then continue to assess the patient's vital signs and respiratory status, as indicated by his condition.
- A chest X-ray is usually done afterward *to check for pneumothorax.*

Special considerations

- To prevent pulmonary edema and hypovolemic shock after thoracentesis, fluid is removed slowly, and no more than 1,000 ml of fluid is removed during the first 30 minutes. Removing the fluid increases the negative intrapleural pressure, which can lead to edema if the lung doesn't reexpand to fill the space.
- Pleuritic or shoulder pain may indicate pleural irritation by the needle point.

Positioning for thoracentesis

The choice of the position may vary. Usually the patient is sitting upright and leaning forward. If the patient is sitting on the edge of the bed, support his legs and have him lean forward and rest his head and arms on a pillow on the over-bed table. If the patient can't sit, turn him on the unaffected side with the arm of the affected side raised comfortably above his head. The head of the bed may be elevated 30 to 45 degrees unless contraindicated. Recumbent thoracentesis may be performed with ultrasound guidance. *Proper positioning stretches the chest or back and allows easier access to the intercostal spaces.*

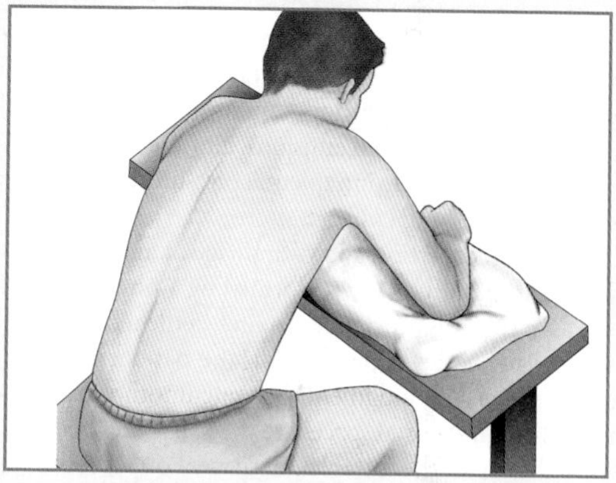

Complications

Pneumothorax (possibly leading to mediastinal shift and requiring chest tube insertion) can occur if the needle punctures the lung and air enters the pleural cavity. Hemoptysis may also occur if the lung is punctured. Pyogenic infection can result from contamination during the procedure. Hemothorax may result if the thoracentesis needle punctures one of the intercostal vessels. Other potential difficulties include pain, cough, anxiety, dry taps, subcutaneous hematoma, and vasovagal syncope.

Documentation

Record the date and time of thoracentesis; location of the puncture site; volume and description (color, viscosity, odor) of the fluid withdrawn; specimens sent to the laboratory; vital signs and respiratory assessment before, during, and after the procedure; postprocedural tests such as a chest X-ray; complications and the nursing action taken; and the patient's reaction to the procedure.

SELECTED REFERENCES

Aeony, Y., et al. "Thoracentesis Without Ultrasound Guidance: Infrequent Complications When Performed by an Experienced Pulmonologist," *Journal of Bronchology* 12(4):200-202, October 2005.

Feller-Kopman, D., et al. "The Relationship of Pleural Pressure to Symptom Development During Therapeutic Thoracentesis," *Chest* 129(6):1556-560, June 2006.

Lynn-McHale Wiegand, D.J., and Carlson, K.K., eds. *AACN Procedure Manual for Critical Care*, 5th ed. Philadelphia: W.B. Saunders Co., 2006.

Rushing, J. "Assisting with Thoracentesis," *Nursing* 36(12 pt 1):18, December 2006.

CHEST TUBE INSERTION

The pleural space normally contains a thin layer of lubricating fluid that allows the viscera and parietal pleura to move without friction during respiration. An excess of fluid (hemothorax or pleural effusion), air (pneumothorax), or both in this space alters intrapleural pressure and causes partial or complete lung collapse.

Chest tube insertion allows drainage of air or fluid from the pleural space. Usually performed by a physician with a nurse assisting, this procedure requires sterile technique. The insertion site varies depending on the patient's condition and the physician's judgment. For pneumothorax, the second to third intercostal spaces are the usual sites because air rises to the top of the intrapleural space. For hemothorax or pleural effusion, the fourth to sixth intercostal spaces are common sites because fluid settles to the lower levels of the intrapleural space. For removal of air and fluid, a chest tube is inserted into a high and a low site.

After insertion, one or more chest tubes are connected to a thoracic drainage system that removes air, fluid, or both from the pleural space and prevents backflow into that space, thus promoting lung reexpansion. (See "Thoracic drainage," page 604.)

Equipment

Two pairs of sterile gloves ▪ sterile drape ▪ vial of 1% lidocaine ▪ antiseptic solution ▪ 10-ml syringe ▪ alcohol pad ▪ 22G 1″ needle ▪ 25G ⅜″ needle ▪ sterile scalpel (usually with #11 blade) ▪ two rubber-tipped clamps for each chest tube inserted ▪ sterile 4″ × 4″ gauze pads ▪ two sterile 4″ × 4″ drain dressings ▪ 3″ or 4″ sturdy, elastic tape ▪ 1″ adhesive tape for connections ▪ chest tube of appropriate size (#16 to #20 French catheter for air or serous fluid; #28 to #40 French catheter for blood, pus, or thick fluid), with or without a trocar ▪ sterile Kelly clamp ▪ suture material (usually 2-0 silk with cutting needle) ▪ thoracic drainage system with tubing ▪ sterile Y-connector (for two chest tubes on the same side) ▪ petroleum gauze ▪ sterile water.

Prepackaged sterile chest tube trays are commercially available and usually contain most of the equipment needed.

Preparation of equipment

Check the expiration date on the sterile packages, and inspect for tears. Then assemble all equipment in the patient's room, and set up the thoracic drainage system. Label all medications, medication containers, and other solutions on and off the sterile field. Place the thoracic drainage system next to the patient's bed below chest level *to facilitate drainage.*

Implementation

- Confirm the patient's identity using two patient identifiers according to your facility's policy.
- In a nonemergency situation, make sure the patient has signed the appropriate consent form.
- Explain the procedure to the patient, provide privacy, and wash your hands.
- Record baseline vital signs and respiratory assessment.
- Position the patient appropriately. If he has a *pneumothorax,* place him in high Fowler's, semi-Fowler's, or the supine position. The physician will insert the tube in the anterior chest at the midclavicular line in the second to third intercostal space. If the patient has a *hemothorax,* have him lean over the overbed table or straddle a chair with his arms dangling over the back. The physician will insert the tube in the fourth to sixth intercostal space at the midaxillary line. For either pneumothorax or hemothorax, the patient may lie on his unaffected side with arms extended over his head.
- When you've positioned the patient properly, place the chest tube tray on the overbed table. Open it using sterile technique.
- The physician puts on sterile gloves and prepares the insertion site by cleaning the area with antiseptic solution.
- Wipe the rubber stopper of the lidocaine vial with an alcohol pad. Then invert the bottle, and hold it for the physician to withdraw the anesthetic.
- Immediately after the drainage system is connected, instruct the patient to take a deep breath, hold it momentarily, and slowly exhale *to assist drainage of the pleural space and lung reexpansion.*
- After the physician anesthetizes the site, he makes a small incision and inserts the chest tube. Next, he either immediately connects the chest tube to the thoracic drainage system or momentarily clamps the tube close to the patient's chest until he can connect it to the drainage system. He may then secure the tube to the skin with a suture.

■ As the physician is inserting the chest tube, reassure the patient and assist the physician, as necessary.
■ Open the packages containing the petroleum gauze, 4″ × 4″drain dressings, and gauze pads, and put on sterile gloves. Then place the petroleum gauze and two 4″ × 4″ drain dressings around the insertion site, one from the top and the other from the bottom. Place several 4″ × 4″gauze pads on top of the drain dressings. Tape the dressings, covering them completely *to form an occlusive dressing.*
■ Securely tape the chest tube to the patient's chest distal to the insertion site *to help prevent accidental tube dislodgment.*
■ Securely tape the junction of the chest tube and the drainage tube *to prevent their separation.*
■ Check the status of the drainage tubing. Be sure the tubing remains at the level of the patient and no dependent loops are present.
■ A portable chest X-ray is then done *to check tube position.*
■ Take the patient's vital signs every 15 minutes for 1 hour, then as his condition indicates. Auscultate his lungs at least every 4 hours following the procedure *to assess air exchange in the affected lung.* Diminished or absent breath sounds indicate that the lung hasn't reexpanded.
■ Monitor and record the drainage in the drainage collection chamber. (See "Thoracic drainage," page 604.)

Special considerations

■ Remember that routine changing of the chest tube isn't recommended *because of the risk of tension pneumothorax.*
■ During patient transport, keep the thoracic drainage system below chest level. Don't clamp the chest tube or tip the drainage system during transport.
■ If the chest tube comes out, cover the site immediately with 4″ × 4″ gauze pads and tape them in place. Stay with the patient, and monitor his vital signs every 10 minutes. Observe him for signs of tension pneumothorax (hypotension, distended jugular veins, absent or decreased breath sounds, tracheal shift, hypoxemia, weak and rapid pulse, dyspnea, tachypnea, diaphoresis, and chest pain). Have another staff member notify the physician, and gather the equipment needed to reinsert the tube.
■ Place the rubber-tipped clamps at the bedside. If a drainage bottle breaks, a commercial system cracks, or a tube disconnects, clamp the chest tube momentarily as close to the insertion site as possible. *Because no air or liquid can escape from the pleural space while the tube is clamped,* observe the patient closely for signs of tension pneumothorax while the clamp is in place. Instead of clamping the tube, you can submerge the distal end of the tube in a container of normal saline solution to create a temporary water seal while you replace the drainage system. Check your facility's policy manual for the proper procedure.

Documentation

Record the date and time of chest tube insertion, the insertion site, drainage system used, presence of drainage and bubbling, vital signs and auscultation findings, complications, and the nursing action taken.

SELECTED REFERENCES

Allibone, L. "Principles for Inserting and Managing Chest Drains," *Nursing Times* 101(42):45-49, October 2005.
Carroll, P. "Keeping Up with Mobile Chest Drains," *RN* 68(10):26-31, October 2005.
Coughlin, A.M., and Parchinsky, C. "Go with the Flow of Chest Tube Therapy," *Nursing* 36(3):36-41, March 2006.
Lynn-McHale Wiegand, D.J., and Carlson, K.K., eds. *AACN Procedure Manual for Critical Care*, 5th ed. Philadelphia: W.B. Saunders Co., 2006.
Roman, M., and Mercado, D. "Review of Chest Tube Use," *Medsurg Nursing* 15(1):41-43, February 2006.

CHEST TUBE REMOVAL

After the patient's lung has reexpanded and any drainage has been controlled, the practitioner may order the tube to be clamped or suction discontinued, with the tube left to water seal for several hours prior to removal of the chest tube to assess patient tolerance. This allows time to observe the patient for signs and symptoms of respiratory distress — an indication that air or fluid remains trapped in the pleural space. The practitioner may also order a chest X-ray prior to removal. A chest tube is usually removed within 7 days of insertion to prevent infection along the tube tract. In many cases, the practitioner will remove the chest tube, but in some states, specially trained nurses may remove the tube.

Equipment:

Clean gloves ■ personal protective equipment ■ sterile gloves ■ suture removal kit ■ sterile forceps ■ linen-saver pad ■ petroleum gauze ■ sterile 4″ × 4″ gauze ■ tape.

Implementation

■ Check the physician's orders for preparing the patient for chest tube removal, and clamp or discontinue suction to the chest tube, as ordered.
■ Gather appropriate equipment.
■ Confirm the patient's identity using two patient identifiers according to your facility's policy.
■ Explain the procedure to the patient to ensure his cooperation and decrease anxiety.

- Premedicate the patient, as ordered.
- Provide privacy and wash your hands.
- Obtain vital signs and respiratory assessment.
- Place the patient in semi-Fowlers' position or on his unaffected side.
- Place a linen-saver pad under the affected side *to protect the linen from drainage and to provide a place to put the chest tube after removal.*
- Put on clean gloves and remove the chest tube dressings, being careful not to dislodge the chest tube prematurely. Discard soiled dressings.
- Put on sterile gloves, hold the chest tube in place with sterile forceps, and cut the suture anchoring the tube.
- Make sure the chest tube is securely clamped, and then instruct the patient to perform Valsalva's maneuver by exhaling fully and bearing down. *Valsalva's maneuver effectively increases intrathoracic pressure and prevents air from entering the pleural space during removal.*
- Hold an airtight dressing, usually petroleum gauze, so that you can cover the insertion site with it immediately after removing the tube. After removing the tube and covering the insertion site, cover it with gauze and secure the dressing with tape. Be sure to cover the dressing completely with tape *to make it as airtight as possible.*
- Dispose of the chest tube, soiled gloves, and equipment according to your facility's policy.
- Take vital signs, as ordered, and assess the depth and quality of the patient's respirations. Assess the patient carefully for signs and symptoms of pneumothorax, subcutaneous emphysema, or infection.
- Obtain chest X-ray postprocedure, as ordered.
- Position the patient for comfort and encourage coughing and deep breathing.

Special considerations

- If the chest tube comes out accidentally, cover the site immediately with gauze pads and tape them in place. Stay with the patient, and monitor his vital signs every 10 minutes. Observe him for signs and symptoms of tension pneumothorax (hypotension, distended jugular veins, absent or decreased breath sounds, tracheal shift, hypoxemia, weak and rapid pulse, dyspnea, tachypnea, diaphoresis, and chest pain). Have another staff member notify the physician, and gather equipment needed to reinsert the tube.
- Assess the chest tube site and dressing for drainage and redress, as ordered or by facility protocol.
- Monitor the patient's respiratory status and report changes to the practitioner.

Documentation

Record preparation procedures, patient respiratory status, premedication and effectiveness, date and time of chest tube removal, and patient's tolerance of procedure. Document site condition, any complications and nursing actions taken, and patient teaching provided.

Selected references

Bruce, E.A., et al. "Chest Drain Removal Pain and Its Management: A Literature Review," *Journal of Clinical Nursing* 15(2):145-54, February 2006.

Dulak, S.B. "Hands-on Help. Removing Chest Tubes," *RN* 68(8):28ac1-28ac4, August 2005.

Higgins, D. "Removal of Chest Drains," *Nursing Times* 102(13):26-27, March-April 2006.

Lynn-McHale Wiegand, D.J., and Carlson, K.K., eds. *AACN Procedure Manual for Critical Care*, 5th ed. Philadelphia: W.B. Saunders Co., 2006.

Puntillo, K., and Ley, S.J. "Appropriately Timed Analgesics Control Pain Due to Chest Tube Removal," *American Journal of Critical Care* 13(4):292-301, July 2004.

Roman, M., and Mercado, D. "Review of Chest Tube Use," *Medsurg Nursing* 15(1):41-43, February 2006.

Thoracic drainage

Thoracic drainage uses gravity and possibly suction to restore negative pressure and remove any material that collects in the pleural cavity. A self-contained, disposable system combines drainage collection, a water seal, and suction into a single unit. (See *Disposable drainage systems.*)

Specifically, thoracic drainage may be ordered to remove accumulated air, fluids (blood, pus, chyle, serous fluids, gastric juices), or solids (blood clots) from the pleural cavity; to restore negative pressure in the pleural cavity; or to reexpand a partially or totally collapsed lung.

Equipment

Thoracic drainage system (Pleur-evac, Argyle, Ohio, or Thora-Klex system, which can function as gravity draining systems or be connected to suction to enhance chest drainage) with tubing and connector ▪ sterile water ▪ adhesive tape ▪ two rubber-tipped Kelly clamps ▪ sterile 50-ml catheter-tip syringe ▪ suction source, if ordered.

Preparation of equipment

Check the practitioner's order *to determine the type of drainage system to be used and specific procedural details.* If appropriate, request the drainage system and suction system from the central supply department. Collect the appropriate equipment, and take it to the patient's bedside.

Disposable drainage systems

Commercially prepared disposable drainage systems combine drainage collection, water seal, and suction control in one unit (as shown below). These systems ensure patient safety with positive- and negative-pressure relief valves and have a prominent air-leak indicator. Some systems produce no bubbling sound.

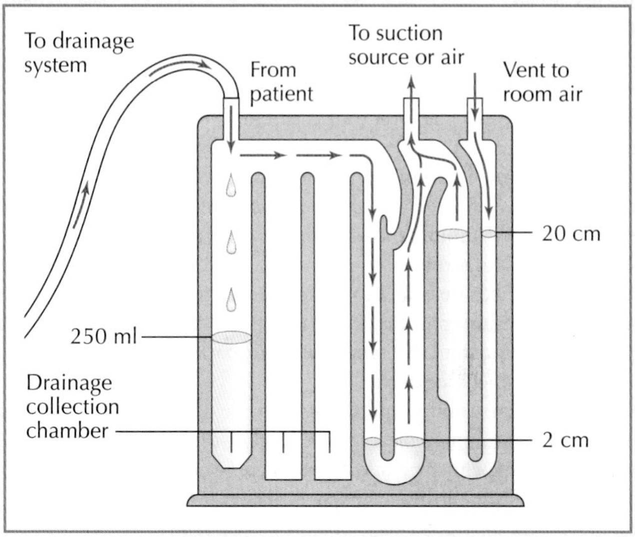

Implementation

- Confirm the patient's identity using two patient identifiers according to your facility's policy.
- Explain the procedure to the patient, and wash your hands.
- Maintain sterile technique throughout the entire procedure and whenever you make changes in the system or alter any of the *connections to avoid introducing pathogens into the pleural space.*

Setting up a disposable system

- Open the packaged system, and place it on the floor in the rack supplied by the manufacturer *to avoid accidentally knocking it over or dislodging the components.* After the system is prepared, it may be hung from the side of the patient's bed.
- Remove the plastic connector from the short tube that's attached to the water-seal chamber. Using a 50-ml catheter-tip syringe, instill sterile water into the water-seal chamber until it reaches the 2-cm mark or the mark specified by the manufacturer. Replace the plastic connector.
- If suction is ordered, remove the cap (also called the *muffler* or *atmosphere vent cover*) on the suction-control chamber *to open the vent.* Next, instill sterile water until it reaches the 20-cm mark or the ordered level, and recap the suction-control chamber.
- Using the long tube, connect the patient's chest tube to the closed drainage collection chamber. Secure the connection with tape.
- Connect the short tube on the drainage system to the suction source, and turn on the suction. Gentle bubbling should begin in the suction chamber, *indicating that the correct suction level has been reached.*

Managing closed-chest underwater seal drainage

- Repeatedly note the character, consistency, and amount of drainage in the drainage collection chamber.
- Mark the drainage level in the drainage collection chamber by noting the time and date at the drainage level on the chamber every 8 hours (or more often if there's a large amount of drainage).
- Check the water level in the water-seal chamber every 8 hours. If necessary, carefully add sterile water until the level reaches the 2-cm mark indicated on the water-seal chamber of the commercial system.
- Check for fluctuation in the water-seal chamber as the patient breathes. Normal fluctuations of 2″ to 4″ (5 to 10 cm) reflect pressure changes in the pleural space during respiration. *To check for fluctuation when a suction system is being used,* momentarily disconnect the suction system so the air vent is opened, and observe for fluctuation.
- Check for intermittent bubbling in the water-seal chamber. This occurs normally when the system is removing air

from the pleural cavity. If bubbling isn't readily apparent during quiet breathing, have the patient take a deep breath or cough. Absence of bubbling indicates that the pleural space has sealed.

- Check the water level in the suction-control chamber. Detach the chamber or bottle from the suction source; when bubbling ceases, observe the water level. If necessary, add sterile water to bring the level to the 20-cm line or as ordered.
- Check for gentle bubbling in the suction control chamber *because it indicates that the proper suction level has been reached.* Vigorous bubbling in this chamber increases the rate of water evaporation.
- Periodically check that the air vent in the system is working properly. Occlusion of the air vent results in a buildup of pressure in the system that could cause the patient to develop a tension pneumothorax.
- Coil the system's tubing, and secure it to the edge of the bed. Be sure the tubing remains at the level of the patient. Avoid creating dependent loops, kinks, or pressure on the tubing. Avoid lifting the drainage system above the patient's chest *because fluid may flow back into the pleural space.*
- Be sure to keep two rubber-tipped clamps at the bedside to clamp the chest tube *if system cracks or to locate an air leak in the system.*
- Encourage the patient to cough frequently and breathe deeply *to help drain the pleural space and expand the lungs.*
- Tell him to sit upright *for optimal lung expansion* and to splint the insertion site while coughing *to minimize pain.*
- Check the rate and quality of the patient's respirations, and auscultate his lungs periodically *to assess air exchange in the affected lung.* Diminished or absent breath sounds may indicate that the lung hasn't reexpanded.
- Tell the patient to report breathing difficulty immediately. Notify the practitioner immediately if the patient develops cyanosis, rapid or shallow breathing, subcutaneous emphysema, chest pain, or excessive bleeding.

NURSING ALERT *Some facilities permit milking of tubing when clots are visible. This is a controversial procedure because it creates increased intrapleural pressure, so be sure to check your facility's policy. If permitted, gently milk the tubing in the direction of the drainage chamber when clots are visible.*

- Check the chest tube dressing at least every 8 hours. Palpate the area surrounding the dressing for crepitus or subcutaneous emphysema, *which indicates that air is leaking into the subcutaneous tissue surrounding the insertion site.* Change the dressing if necessary or according to your facility's policy.
- Encourage active or passive range-of-motion (ROM) exercises for the patient's arm or the affected side if he has been splinting the arm. Usually, the thoracotomy patient will splint his arm *to decrease his discomfort.*
- Give ordered pain medication, as needed, for comfort and to help with deep-breathing, coughing, and ROM exercises.
- Remind the ambulatory patient to keep the drainage system below chest level and to be careful not to disconnect the tubing *to maintain the water seal.* With a suction system, the patient must stay within range of the length of tubing attached to a wall outlet or portable pump.

Special considerations

- Instruct staff and visitors to avoid touching the equipment *to prevent complications from separated connections.*
- If excessive continuous bubbling is present in the water-seal chamber, especially if suction is being used, rule out a leak in the drainage system. Try to locate the leak by clamping the tube momentarily at various points along its length. Begin clamping at the tube's proximal end, and work down toward the drainage system, paying special attention to the seal around the connections. If a connection is loose, push it back together and tape it securely. *The bubbling will stop when a clamp is placed between the air leak and the water seal.* If you clamp along the tube's entire length and the bubbling doesn't stop, the drainage unit may be cracked and need replacement.
- If the drainage collection chamber fills, replace it. To do this, double-clamp the tube close to the insertion site (use two clamps facing in opposite directions), exchange the system, remove the clamps, and retape the bottle connection.

NURSING ALERT *Never leave the tubes clamped for more than a minute* **to prevent a tension pneumothorax, which may occur when clamping stops air and fluid from escaping.**

- If the system cracks, clamp the chest tube momentarily with the two rubber-tipped clamps at the bedside (placed there at the time of tube insertion). Place the clamps close to each other near the insertion site; they should face in opposite directions *to provide a more complete seal.* Observe the patient for altered respirations while the tube is clamped. Then replace the damaged equipment. (Prepare the new unit before clamping the tube.)
- Instead of clamping the tube, you can submerge the distal end of the tube in a container of normal saline solution *to create a temporary water seal while you replace the bottle.* Check your facility's policy for the proper procedure.

Complications

Tension pneumothorax may result from excessive accumulation of air, drainage, or both and eventually may exert pressure on the heart and aorta, causing a precipitous fall in cardiac output.

Documentation

Record the date and time thoracic drainage began, type of system used, amount of suction applied to the pleural cavity, presence or absence of bubbling or fluctuation in the water-seal chamber, initial amount and type of drainage, and the patient's respiratory status.

At the end of each shift record the frequency of system inspection; how frequently chest tubes were milked; amount, color, and consistency of drainage; presence or absence of bubbling or fluctuation in the water-seal chamber; the patient's respiratory status; condition of the chest dressings; pain medication, if given; and complications and the nursing action taken.

SELECTED REFERENCES

Carroll, P. "Keeping Up with Mobile Chest Drains," *RN* 68(10):26-31, October 2005.

Coughlin, A.M., and Parchinsky, C. "Go with the Flow of Chest Tube Therapy," *Nursing* 36(3):36-41, March 2006.

Lynn-McHale Wiegand, D.J., and Carlson, K.K., eds. *AACN Procedure Manual for Critical Care*, 5th ed. Philadelphia: W.B. Saunders Co., 2006.

Roman, M., and Mercado, D. "Review of Chest Tube Use," *Medsurg Nursing* 15(1):41-43, February 2006.

LATEX ALLERGY PROTOCOL

Latex—a natural product of the rubber tree—is used in many products in the health care field as well as other areas. With the increased use of latex in barrier protection and medical equipment, more and more nurses and patients are becoming hypersensitive to it. Certain groups of people are at increased risk for developing latex allergy. These groups include people who have had or will undergo multiple surgical procedures (especially those with a history of spina bifida), health care workers (especially those in the emergency department and operating room), workers who manufacture latex and latex-containing products, and people with a genetic predisposition to latex allergy.

People who are allergic to certain "cross-reactive" foods, including avocados, bananas, chestnuts, cherries, grapes, kiwis, passion fruit, tomatoes, and peaches, may also be allergic to latex. Exposure to latex elicits an allergic response similar to the one elicited by these foods.

For people with latex allergy, latex becomes a hazard when the protein in latex comes in direct contact with mucous membranes or is inhaled, which happens when powdered latex surgical gloves are used. People with asthma are at greater risk for developing worsening symptoms from airborne latex.

Latex allergy screening questionnaire

To determine whether the patient has a latex sensitivity or allergy, ask the following screening questions:

Allergies

- Do you have a history of hay fever, asthma, eczema, allergies, or rashes? If so, what type of reaction do you have?
- Have you experienced an allergic reaction, local sensitivity, or itching following exposure to latex products, such as balloons or condoms?
- Do you have shortness of breath or wheezing after blowing up balloons or after a dental visit? Do you have itching in or around your mouth after eating a banana?
- If you experience shortness of breath or wheezing when blowing up latex balloons, describe your reaction.
- Are you allergic to any foods, especially bananas, avocados, kiwi, or chestnuts? If so, describe your reaction.

Occupation

- What's your occupation?
- Are you exposed to latex in your occupation?
- Do you experience a reaction to latex products at work? If so, describe your reaction.
- If you've had a rash on your hands develop after wearing latex gloves, how long after putting on the gloves did it take for the rash to develop?
- What did the rash look like?

Personal history

- Do you have any congenital abnormalities? If yes, explain.
- Have you ever had itching, swelling, hives, cough, shortness of breath, or other allergic symptoms during or after using condoms or diaphragms or following a vaginal or rectal examination?

Surgical history

- Have you had previous surgical procedures? Did you experience associated complications? If so, describe them.
- Have you had previous dental procedures? Did complications result? If so, describe them.
- Do you have spina bifida or a urinary tract problem that requires surgery or catheterization?

Creating a latex-free environment

- Ask all patients about latex sensitivity. Use a screening questionnaire *to determine latex sensitivity.*
- Teach the patient to treat the latex allergy the same as a food or drug allergy by informing all future health care providers about his allergy.
- Include information about latex allergy on the patient's identification bracelet. Make sure that the information is also noted on the front of the patient's chart and in the facility's database.
- Post a LATEX ALLERGY sign in the patient's room.
- Implement and disseminate latex allergy protocols and lists of nonlatex substitutes that can be used to care for the patient.
- Remove all latex-containing products that may come in contact with the patient.
- Use tubing made of polyvinyl chloride.
- Check adhesives and tapes, including electrocardiogram electrodes and dressing supplies, for latex content.
- Have a special latex-free crash cart outside the room at all times during the patient's hospitalization.
- Notify central supply and pharmacy that the patient has a latex allergy *so that latex contact is eliminated from drugs and other materials prepared for the patient.*
- Notify dietary staff of relevant food allergies and instruct them to avoid handling the patient's food with powdered latex gloves.

The diagnosis of latex allergy is based on the patient's history and physical examination. Laboratory testing should be performed to confirm or eliminate the diagnosis. Skin testing can be done, but the AlaSTAT test, Hycor assay, and the Pharmacia CAP test are the only U.S. Food and Drug Administration-approved blood tests available. Some laboratories may also choose to perform an enzyme-linked immunosorbent assay.

Latex allergy can produce a myriad of symptoms, including generalized itching (on the hands and arms, for example); itchy, watery, or burning eyes; sneezing and coughing (hay fever–type symptoms); rash; hives; bronchial asthma, scratchy throat, or difficulty breathing; edema of the face, hands, or neck; and anaphylaxis.

To help identify people at risk for latex allergy, ask latex allergy–specific questions during the health history. (See *Latex allergy screening questionaire,* page 607.) If the patient's history reveals latex sensitivity, the practitioner assigns him to one of three categories based on the extent of his sensitization. Group 1 includes patients who have a history of anaphylaxis or a systemic reaction when exposed to a natural latex product. Group 2 patients have a clear history of an allergic reaction of a nonsystemic type. Group 3 patients don't have a previous history of latex hypersensitivity but are designated as "high risk" because of an associated medical condition, occupation, or "crossover" allergy.

If you determine that your patient has a sensitivity to latex, make sure he doesn't come in contact with latex *because such contact could result in a life-threatening hypersensitivity reaction.* Also, be sure to record the patient's allergies in his permanent medical record. Creating a latex-safe environment is the only way to safeguard your patient. (See *Creating a latex-free environment.*) Hypoallergenic latex gloves contain significant amounts of latex allergens and shouldn't be worn in the vicinity of someone who's allergic to latex. Many health care facilities now designate "latex-free" equipment, which is usually kept on a cart that can be moved into the patient's room.

The National Institute of Occupational Safety and Health has published an advisory document on natural latex rubber in the workplace. It recommends that nonlatex gloves be used for all activities that aren't likely to involve contact with infectious materials (for example, food preparation, routine housekeeping, and maintenance).

Equipment

Latex allergy patient identification wristband ■ latex-free equipment cart with necessary supplies, including room contents ■ anaphylaxis kit ■ optional: LATEX ALLERGY sign.

Preparation of equipment

After you've determined that the patient has a latex allergy or is sensitive to latex, arrange for him to be placed in a private room. If that isn't possible, make the room latex-free, even if the roommate hasn't been designated as hypersensitive to latex. *This prevents the spread of airborne particles from latex products used on the other patient.*

Implementation

- Assess for possible latex allergy in all patients being admitted to the delivery room or short procedure unit or having a surgical procedure.

Anesthesia induction and latex allergy

Latex allergy can cause signs and symptoms in both conscious and anesthetized patients.

Causes of intraoperative reaction	Signs and symptoms in conscious patient	Signs and symptoms in anesthetized patient
▪ Latex contact with mucous membrane ▪ Latex contact with intraperitoneal serosal lining ▪ Inhalation of airborne latex particles during anesthesia ▪ Injection of antibiotics and anesthetic agents through latex ports	▪ Abdominal cramping ▪ Anxiety ▪ Bronchoconstriction ▪ Diarrhea ▪ Feeling of faintness ▪ Generalized pruritus ▪ Itchy eyes ▪ Nausea ▪ Shortness of breath ▪ Swelling of soft tissue (hands, face, tongue) ▪ Vomiting ▪ Wheezing	▪ Bronchospasm ▪ Cardiopulmonary arrest ▪ Facial edema ▪ Flushing ▪ Hypotension ▪ Laryngeal edema ▪ Tachycardia ▪ Urticaria ▪ Wheezing

For all patients in groups 1 and 2

▪ If the patient has a confirmed latex allergy, bring a cart with nonlatex supplies into his room.

▪ Document on the patient's chart (according to your facility's policy) that the patient has a latex allergy. If policy requires that the patient wear a latex allergy identification bracelet, place it on the patient.

▪ If the patient will be receiving anesthesia, make sure LATEX ALLERGY is clearly visible on the front of his chart. (See *Anesthesia induction and latex allergy*.) Notify the circulating nurse in the surgical unit, the postanesthesia care unit nurses, and any other team members that the patient has a latex allergy.

▪ If the patient must be transported to another area of the hospital, make sure the nonlatex cart accompanies him and that all health care workers who come in contact with him are wearing nonlatex gloves. The patient may need to wear a mask with cloth ties when leaving his room *to protect him from inhaling airborne latex particles.*

▪ If the patient will have an I.V. line, make sure I.V. access is accomplished using all nonlatex products. Post a LATEX ALLERGY sign on the I.V. tubing *to prevent access of the line using latex products.*

▪ If latex tubing must be used, flush I.V. tubing with 50 ml of I.V. solution *because of latex ports in the I.V. tubing.*

▪ Place a warning label on I.V. bags that reads "Do not use latex injection ports."

▪ Use a nonlatex tourniquet. If none are available, use a latex tourniquet over clothing.

▪ Remove the vial stopper to mix and draw up medications.

▪ Use nonlatex oxygen administration equipment. Remove the elastic, and tie equipment on with gauze.

▪ Wrap your stethoscope with a nonlatex product *to protect the patient from latex contact.*

▪ Wrap Tegaderm over the patient's finger or use a nonlatex glove before using pulse oximetry.

▪ Use nonlatex syringes when administering medication through a syringe.

▪ If the patient has an allergic reaction to latex, you must act immediately. (See *Managing a latex allergy reaction,* page 610.)

Special considerations

▪ Remember that signs and symptoms of latex allergy usually occur within 30 minutes of anesthesia induction. However, the time of onset can range from 10 minutes to several hours.

▪ Don't forget that, as a health care worker, you're in a position to develop a latex hypersensitivity. If you suspect that you're sensitive to latex, contact the employee health services department concerning facility protocol for latex-sensitive

Managing a latex allergy reaction

If you determine that your patient is having an allergic reaction to a latex product, act immediately. Make sure that you perform emergency interventions using latex-free equipment. If the latex product that caused the reaction is known, remove it and perform the following measures:

- If the allergic reaction develops during medication administration or a procedure, stop the medication or procedure immediately.
- Assess airway, breathing, and circulation.
- Administer 100% oxygen with continuous pulse oximetry.
- Start I.V. volume expanders with lactated Ringer's solution or normal saline solution.
- Administer epinephrine according to the patient's symptoms.
- Administer famotidine, as ordered.
- If bronchospasm is evident, treat it with nebulized albuterol, as ordered.
- Secondary treatment for latex allergy reaction is aimed at treating the swelling and tissue reaction to the latex as well as breaking the chain of events associated with the allergic reaction. It includes:
  –diphenhydramine
  –methylprednisolone
  –famotidine.
- Document the event and the exact cause (if known). If latex particles have entered the I.V. line, insert a new I.V. line with a new catheter, new tubing, and new infusion attachments as soon as possible.

employees. Use nonlatex products whenever possible *to help reduce your exposure to latex.* If you must wear latex gloves, the powder-free variety is recommended because when powdered gloves are used, the natural rubber latex proteins attach to the cornstarch powder particles and become airborne with glove donning and removal.

- Don't assume that if something doesn't look like rubber it isn't latex. Latex can be found in a wide variety of equipment, including electrocardiograph leads, oral and nasal airway tubing, tourniquets, nerve stimulation pads, temperature strips, and blood pressure cuffs.

Documentation

Document the results of latex allergy screening, the date and time of screening, and notification of staff of the patient's status. Document placement of signs and warning labels.

Selected references

Centers for Disease Control and Prevention. National Institute for Occupational Safety and Health. "Latex Allergy: A Prevention Guide," Department of Health and Human Services (NIOSH). Publication No. 98-113. Available at: *www.cdc.gov/niosh/latexfs.html*

Lenehan, G.P. "Latex Allergies: Separating Fact from Fiction," *Nursing* Suppl:12-17, February 2004.

Noble, K.A. "The Patient with Latex Allergy," *Journal of Perianesthesia Nursing* 20(4):285-88, August 2005.

Smith, K., et al. "What You Should Know About Latex Allergy," *The Nurse Practitioner* 29(12):24, December 2004.

9 ■ Neurologic care

INTRODUCTION

A neurologic examination provides a record of vital information regarding the patient's neurologic function. Its purpose is to determine the presence of nervous system dysfunction. A skilled examiner knows the proper technique for testing function and is familiar with the expected normal responses to testing. Precise nursing skills and a meticulous attention to detail are indispensable in preserving and restoring optimal nervous system function.

NEUROLOGIC ASSESSMENT AND EXAMINATION

A neurologic physical examination may be conducted by the practitioner. For nursing purposes, this examination is used to determine whether nervous system dysfunction is present and to determine the patient's responses to actual or potential health problems precipitated by the dysfunction. The neurologic examination is typically preceded by a physical examination and history. It should be conducted in a systematic, hierarchical approach from the highest level of function (cerebral cortex) to the lowest (reflexes) and should include a review of the patient's mental state; cranial nerve, motor, and sensory systems; and cerebellar function and reflexes.

The first step in a neurologic examination is to assess neurologic vital signs, starting with the patient's level of consciousness and orientation level. Many patients with neurologic disorders experience changes in perception—from confusion to psychosis. Unaddressed, such disorientation further impairs the patient's ability to participate in recovery. Recognizing this will help you intervene properly.

To record or track assessment findings, use special flowcharts or neurologic assessment forms. In common use at most health care facilities, these charts and forms separate and grade components of a neurologic assessment, assisting the nurse and other caregivers to quickly recognize changes in neurologic status and to plan subsequent patient care.

Respiratory assessment constitutes an important part of an overall neurologic assessment. That is because patients with neurologic damage—especially those with traumatic brain or spinal cord injuries—are at considerable risk for respiratory complications. These injuries may depress the respiratory control center and paralyze the muscles used for breathing. As a result, brain tissue, which is especially sensitive to blood oxygen levels, can quickly be damaged by inadequate oxygenation.

Thorough respiratory care goes hand in hand with neurologic care. Frequent position changes, chest physiotherapy, and tracheal suctioning are typical interventions. Additional techniques for preventing complications and promoting comfort include pain management and maintaining a quiet, stress-free environment.

Rehabilitation

Neurologic rehabilitation begins on admission and touches all aspects of daily care. Because neurologic impairment can alter every area of function, the patient's identity may change. Consequently, rehabilitation procedures must address the psychosocial and physiologic changes associated with the patient's condition—a task that requires enormous time and patience.

The success of rehabilitation efforts may hinge largely on the patient's ability to adapt to significant—even profound—changes. A few of the factors that influence this ability to adapt include the patient's age, the deficit itself, and available support systems. Another ingredient needed for effective rehabilitation is sensitive and skilled nursing care. Such care can dramatically improve the patient's prospects for positive adaptation and recovery.

MONITORING

NEUROLOGIC ASSESSMENT

Neurologic assessment supplements the routine measurement of temperature, pulse rate, and respirations by evaluating the patient's level of consciousness (LOC), pupillary activity, and orientation to person, place, and date. They provide a simple, indispensable tool for quickly checking the patient's neurologic status.

If the patient's condition and circumstances of admission allow, the first neurologic assessment should occur at the time of admission to establish a baseline. The frequency and extent of the neurologic assessment will depend on the stability of the patient and the underlying condition. For a stable patient who's doing well, an assessment may be ordered every 4 to 8 hours. For an unstable patient, it may be ordered as frequently as every 5 minutes to monitor changes and the need for intervention.

LOC, a measure of environmental and self-awareness, reflects cortical function and usually provides the first sign of central nervous system deterioration. Changes in pupillary activity (pupil size, shape, equality, and response to light) may signal increased intracranial pressure (ICP) associated with a space-occupying lesion caused by an increase of fluid or tissue in the associated area. Evaluating muscle strength

Using the Glasgow Coma Scale

The Glasgow Coma Scale provides a standard reference for assessing or monitoring level of consciousness in a patient with a suspected or confirmed brain injury. This scale measures three responses to stimuli—eye opening response, motor response, and verbal response—and assigns a number to each of the possible responses within these categories.

A score of 3 is the lowest, and 15 is the highest. A score of 7 or less indicates coma. The Glasgow scale is commonly used in the emergency department, at the scene of an accident, and for evaluation of the hospitalized patient.

CHARACTERISTIC	RESPONSE	SCORE
Eye opening response	■ Spontaneous	4
	■ To verbal command	3
	■ To pain	2
	■ No response	1
Best motor response	■ Obeys commands	6
	■ To painful stimuli	
	– Localizes pain; pushes stimulus away	5
	– Flexes and withdraws	4
	– Abnormal flexion	3
	– Extension	2
	– No response	1
Best verbal response (Arouse the patient with painful stimuli if necessary.)	■ Oriented and converses	5
	■ Disoriented and converses	4
	■ Uses inappropriate words	3
	■ Makes incomprehensible sounds	2
	■ No response	1
		Total: 3 to 15

and tone, reflexes, and posture also may help identify nervous system damage.

Finally, changes in vital signs alone don't indicate possible neurologic compromise. Alterations in LOC or papillary changes are the early signs that indicate neurologic problems. Therefore, any changes in vital signs should be evaluated in light of a complete neurologic assessment. Because vital signs are controlled at the medullary level, changes noted after the deterioration of neurologic status are too late, and irreversible neurologic damage should be suspected.

Equipment

Penlight ■ thermometer ■ sterile cotton ball or cotton-tipped applicator ■ stethoscope ■ sphygmomanometer ■ pupil size chart ■ pencil or pen.

Implementation

■ Confirm the patient's identity using two patient identifiers according to your facility's policy.

■ Explain the procedure to the patient even if he's unresponsive. Then wash your hands and provide privacy.

Assessing LOC and orientation

■ Assess the patient's LOC by evaluating his responses. Use standard methods such as the Glasgow Coma Scale and the Rancho Los Amigos Cognitive Scale. (See *Using the Glasgow Coma Scale*. See also *Using the Rancho Los Amigos Cognitive Scale,* page 614.)

■ Begin by measuring the patient's response to verbal, light tactile (touch), and painful (nail bed pressure) stimuli. First, ask the patient his full name. If he responds appropriately, assess his orientation to person, place, and date. Ask him

Using the Rancho Los Amigos Cognitive Scale

Widely used to classify brain-injured patients according to their behavior, the Rancho Los Amigos Cognitive Scale describes phases of recovery—from coma to dependent functioning—on a scale of I (unresponsive) to VIII (purposeful, appropriate, alert, and oriented). This scale is useful in assessing patients who have posttraumatic amnesia.

LEVEL	RESPONSE	CHARACTERISTIC
I	None	The patient is unresponsive to any stimulus.
II	Generalized	The patient makes limited, inconsistent, nonpurposeful responses, often to pain only.
III	Localized	The patient can localize and withdraw from painful stimuli, can make purposeful responses and focus on presented objects, and may follow simple commands but inconsistently and in a delayed manner.
IV	Confused and agitated	The patient is alert but agitated, confused, disoriented, and aggressive. He can't perform self-care and has no awareness of present events. Bizarre behavior is likely; agitation appears related to internal confusion.
V	Confused and inappropriate	The patient is alert and responds to commands but is easily distracted and can't concentrate on tasks or learn new information. He becomes agitated in response to external stimuli, and his behavior and speech are inappropriate. His memory is severely impaired, and he can't carry over learning from one situation to another.
VI	Confused and appropriate	The patient has some awareness of himself and others but is inconsistently oriented. He can follow simple directions consistently with cueing and can relearn some old skills such as activities of daily living (ADLs), but he continues to have serious memory problems (especially with short-term memory).
VII	Automatic and appropriate	The patient is consistently oriented, with little or no confusion, but frequently appears robotlike when performing daily routines. His awareness of himself and his interaction with his environment increase, but he lacks insight, judgment, problem-solving skills, and the ability to plan realistically.
VIII	Purposeful and appropriate	The patient is alert and oriented, recalls and integrates past events, learns new activities, and performs ADLs independently; however, deficits in stress tolerance, judgment, and abstract reasoning persist. He may function in society at a reduced level.

where he is and then what day, season, and year it is. (Expect disorientation to affect the sense of date first, then time, place, caregivers and, finally, self.) When he responds verbally, assess the quality of speech *to determine if it is clear and concise.* Rambling responses indicate difficulty with thought processing and organization.

- Assess the patient's ability to understand and follow one-step commands that require a motor response. For example, ask him to open and close his eyes or stick out his tongue.

Identifying warning postures

Decorticate and decerebrate postures are ominous signs of central nervous system deterioration.

Decorticate (abnormal flexion)

In the decorticate posture, the patient's arms are adducted and flexed, with the wrists and fingers flexed on the chest. The legs may be stiffly extended and internally rotated, with plantar flexion of the feet.

The decorticate posture may indicate a lesion of the frontal lobe, internal capsule, or cerebral peduncles.

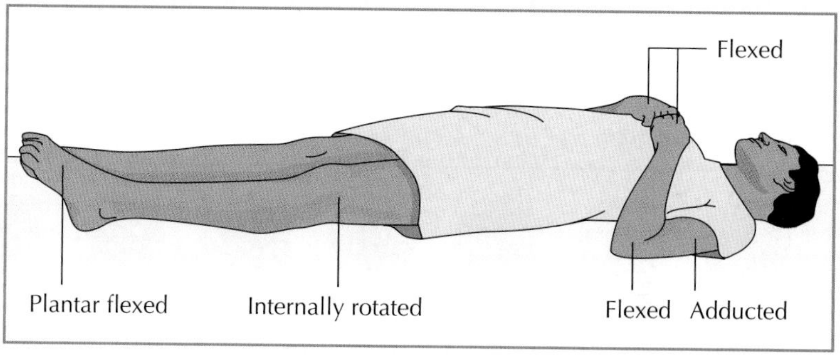

Decerebrate (extension)

In the decerebrate posture, the patient's arms are adducted and extended with the wrists pronated and the fingers flexed. One or both of the legs may be stiffly extended, with plantar flexion of the feet.

The decerebrate posture may indicate lesions of the upper brain stem.

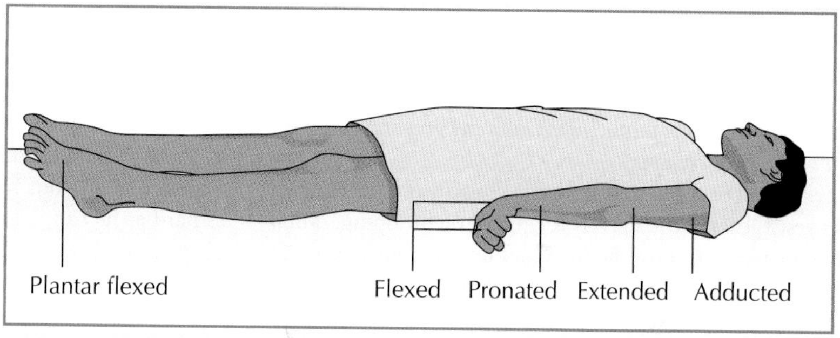

Note whether the patient can maintain his LOC. If you must gently shake him to keep him focused on your verbal commands, he may have sustained neurologic compromise.

- If the patient doesn't respond to commands, apply a painful stimulus. With moderate pressure, squeeze the nail beds on fingers and toes, and note his response. Check motor responses bilaterally *to rule out monoplegia (paralysis of a single area) and hemiplegia (paralysis of one side of the body).*

A patient's response to painful stimuli should be described as one of the following: localization—the patient withdraws from the pain, attempts to push away the painful stimulus, and can localize where the pain originates; withdrawal—the patient moves slightly, but makes no attempt to push the painful stimulus away; or unresponsive—the patient doesn't react to the application of painful stimulus (commonly seen in patients in a deep coma).

NURSING ALERT *If decorticate or decerebrate posturing develops in response to stimuli, notify the practitioner immediately. (See* Identifying warning postures.*)*

Examining pupils and eye movement

- Ask the patient to open his eyes. If he doesn't respond, gently lift his upper eyelids. Inspect each pupil for size and shape, and compare the two for equality. *To evaluate pupil size more precisely,* use a chart showing the various pupil sizes (in increments of 1 mm, with the normal diameter ranging from 2 to 6 mm). (See *Testing the pupils,* page 616.) Remember, pupil size varies considerably, and some patients have normally unequal pupils (anisocoria). Also check whether the pupils are positioned in, or deviate from, the midline.
- Test the patient's direct light response. First, darken the room. Then hold each eyelid open in turn. Swing the penlight from the patient's ear toward the midline of the face. Shine the light directly into the eye. Normally, the pupil constricts immediately. When you remove the penlight, the pupil should dilate immediately. Wait about 20 seconds before testing the other pupil *to allow it to recover from reflex stimulation.*

Testing the pupils

Slightly darken the room. Then test the pupils for direct response (reaction of the pupil you're testing) and consensual response (reaction of the opposite pupil) by holding a penlight about 20″ (51 cm) from the patient's eyes, directing the light at the eye from the side.

Next, test accommodation by placing your finger about 4″ (10 cm) from the bridge of the patient's nose. Ask him to look at a fixed object in the distance and then to look at your finger. His eyes should converge, and his pupils should constrict.

Grading pupil size

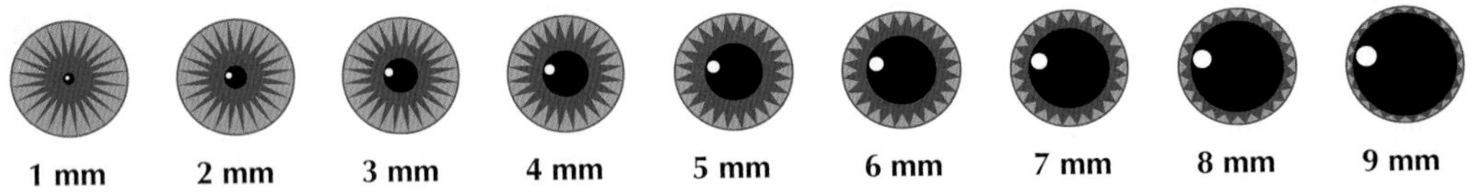

- Now test consensual light response. Hold both eyelids open, but shine the light into one eye only. Watch for constriction in the other pupil, *which indicates proper nerve function of the optic chiasm.*
- Brighten the room and have the conscious patient open his eyes. Observe the eyelids for ptosis or drooping. Then check extraocular movements. Hold up one finger, and ask the patient to follow it with his eyes alone. As you move the finger up, down, laterally, and obliquely, see if the patient's eyes track together to follow your finger (conjugate gaze). Watch for involuntary jerking or oscillating eye movements either laterally or vertically upon moving eyes (nystagmus).
- Check the patient's accommodation-convergency reflex. Hold up one finger midline to the patient's face and several feet away. Have the patient focus on your finger. Gradually move your finger toward his nose while he focuses on your finger. *This should cause his eyes to converge and both pupils to constrict equally.*
- If the patient is comatose, test the corneal reflex by touching a wisp of cotton ball to the cornea. This normally causes an immediate blink reflex. Repeat for the other eye.
- If the patient is unconscious, test the oculocephalic (doll's eye) reflex. Hold the patient's eyelids open. Then quickly but gently turn his head to one side and then the other. If the patient's eyes move in the opposite direction from the side to which you turn the head, the reflex is intact.

NURSING ALERT *Never test the doll's eye reflex on an awake, alert patient or if you know or suspect that the patient has a cervical spine injury.*

Evaluating motor function

- Identify the patient's strength on a scale of 0 to 5, with 0 being no muscle strength and 5 being full muscle strength.
- If the patient is conscious, test his grip strength in both hands. Extend your hands, ask him to squeeze your fingers as hard as he can, and compare the strength of each hand. Grip strength is usually slightly stronger in the dominant hand.
- Test arm strength by having the patient close his eyes and hold his arms straight out in front of him with the palms up for 20 to 30 seconds. See if either arm drifts downward or pronates (pronator drift), *indicating muscle weakness.*
- Test leg strength by having the patient raise his legs, one at a time, against gentle downward pressure from your hand. Gently push down on each leg at the midpoint of the thigh *to evaluate muscle strength.*
- Flex and extend the extremities on both sides *to evaluate muscle tone.*
- Test the plantar reflex in all patients. To do so, stroke the lateral aspect of the sole of the patient's foot with your thumbnail or another moderately sharp object. Normally, this elicits flexion of all toes. Watch for a positive Babinski's sign—dorsiflexion of the great toe with fanning of the other toes—*which indicates an upper motor neuron lesion.*

PEDIATRIC ALERT *A positive Babinski's sign is normal in patients younger than age 2.*

Completing the neurologic examination

Take the patient's temperature, pulse rate, respiratory rate, and blood pressure. His pulse pressure—the difference between systolic pressure and diastolic pressure—is especially important *because widening pulse pressure can indicate increasing ICP.*

Special considerations

NURSING ALERT *If a previously stable patient suddenly develops a change in neurologic or routine vital signs, further assess his condition, and notify the practitioner immediately.* A change in the LOC is one of the earliest changes that may occur with increased ICP. Changes in pulse and blood pressure also occur, but are generally seen late in the course of increasing ICP. Other vital sign changes include widening pulse pressure, increase in systolic blood pressure, and bradycardia. Cushing's triad, also called *Cushing's sign,* is a late sign indicating brain stem dysfunction. Vital signs associated with Cushing's triad include hypertension (usually with widened pulse pressure), bradycardia, and abnormal or irregular respiratory patterns.

Documentation

Baseline data require detailed documentation; subsequent notes can be brief unless the patient's condition changes. Record the patient's LOC and orientation, pupillary activity, motor function, and routine vital signs as your facility's policy directs.

To save time while keeping complete records, you may be allowed to use abbreviations. However, use only commonly understood abbreviations and terms *to avoid misinterpretation.* Examples include the following:

- A + O × 3 = alert and oriented to person, place, and date
- PERRLA = pupils equal, round, reactive to light and accommodation
- PERRL = pupils equal, round, reactive to light
- EOMI = extraocular movements intact.

Also describe the patient's behavior—for example, "difficult to arouse by gentle shaking," "sleepy," or "unresponsive to painful stimuli."

Selected references

American Association of Neuroscience Nurses. *Core Curriculum for Neuroscience Nursing,* 4th ed. Philadelphia: W.B. Saunders Co., 2004.

Fairley, D., and Pearce, A. "Assessment of Consciousness: Part One," *Nursing Times* 102(4):26-27, January 2006.

Fairley, D., and Pearce, A. "Assessment of Consciousness: Part Two," *Nursing Times* 102(5):26-27, January 2006.

Iacono, L.A., and Lyones, K.A. "Making GCS as Easy as 1, 2, 3, 4, 5, 6," *Journal of Trauma Nursing* 12(3):77-81, July-September 2005.

Lynn-McHale Wiegand, D.J., and Carlson, K.K., eds. *AACN Procedure Manual for Critical Care,* 5th ed. Philadelphia: W.B. Saunders Co., 2005.

Morgan, A. "Neurological Assessment," *Nursing Standard* 20(14-16):67, December-January 2006.

Intracranial pressure monitoring

Intracranial pressure (ICP) monitoring measures pressure exerted by the brain, blood, and cerebrospinal fluid (CSF) against the inside of the skull. Normal ICP is 0 to 15 mm Hg, with the ICP threshold of 20 to 25 mm Hg as the highest acceptable limit before instituting treatment. Indications for monitoring ICP include head trauma with bleeding or edema, overproduction or insufficient absorption of CSF (hydrocephalus), cerebral hemorrhage, and space-occupying brain lesions. ICP monitoring can detect elevated ICP early, before clinical danger signs develop. Prompt intervention can then help avert or diminish neurologic damage caused by cerebral hypoxia and shifts of brain mass.

The four basic ICP monitoring systems are intraventricular catheter, subarachnoid bolt, epidural or subdural sensor, and intraparenchymal monitoring. (See *Understanding ICP monitoring systems,* pages 618 and 619.)

Regardless of which system is used, the procedure is typically performed by a neurosurgeon in the operating room, emergency department, or intensive care unit (ICU). Insertion of an ICP monitoring device requires sterile technique to reduce the risk of central nervous system (CNS) infection. Setting up equipment for the monitoring systems also requires strict asepsis.

Equipment

Monitoring unit and transducers, as ordered ▪ 16 to 20 sterile 4″ × 4″ gauze pads ▪ linen-saver pads ▪ clippers ▪ sterile drapes ▪ antiseptic solution ▪ sterile gown ▪ surgical mask ▪ two pairs of sterile gloves ▪ sedation, as needed ▪ sterile dressing ▪ one roll of 4″ roller gauze, as needed ▪ sterile marker ▪ sterile labels ▪ optional: yardstick, I.V. pole.

Preparation of equipment

Monitoring units and setup protocols are varied and complex and differ among health care facilities. Check your facility's guidelines for your particular unit.

Various types of preassembled ICP monitoring units are also available, each with its own setup protocols. These units are designed to reduce the risk of infection by eliminating the need for multiple stopcocks, manometers, and transducer dome assemblies. When preparing the equipment, label all medications, medication containers, and other solutions on and off the sterile field.

EQUIPMENT

Understanding ICP monitoring systems

Intracranial pressure (ICP) can be monitored using one of four systems.

Intraventricular catheter monitoring

In intraventricular catheter monitoring, which monitors ICP directly, the physician inserts a small polyethylene or silicone rubber catheter into the lateral ventricle through a burr hole.

Although this method measures ICP most accurately and drains cerebrospinal fluid (CSF), it carries the greatest risk of infection. This is the only type of ICP monitoring that allows evaluation of brain compliance and drainage of significant amounts of CSF.

Contraindications usually include stenotic cerebral ventricles, cerebral aneurysms in the path of catheter placement, and suspected vascular lesions.

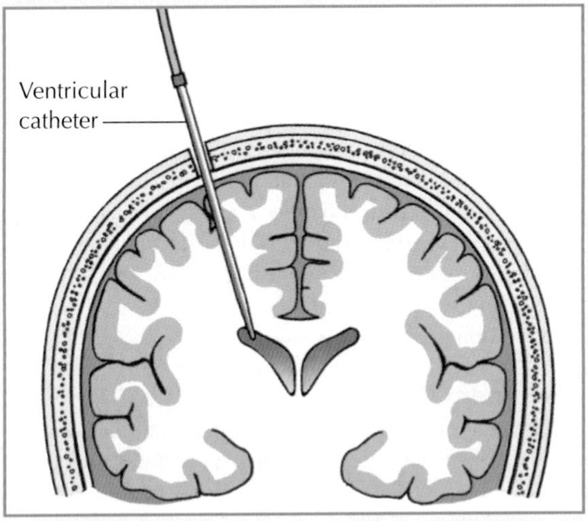

Subarachnoid bolt monitoring

Subarachnoid bolt monitoring involves insertion of a special bolt into the subarachnoid space through a twist-drill burr hole that's positioned in the front of the skull behind the hairline.

Placing the bolt is easier than placing an intraventricular catheter, especially if a computed tomography scan reveals that the cerebrum has shifted or the ventricles have collapsed. This type of ICP monitoring also carries less risk of infection and parenchymal damage *because the bolt doesn't penetrate the cerebrum.*

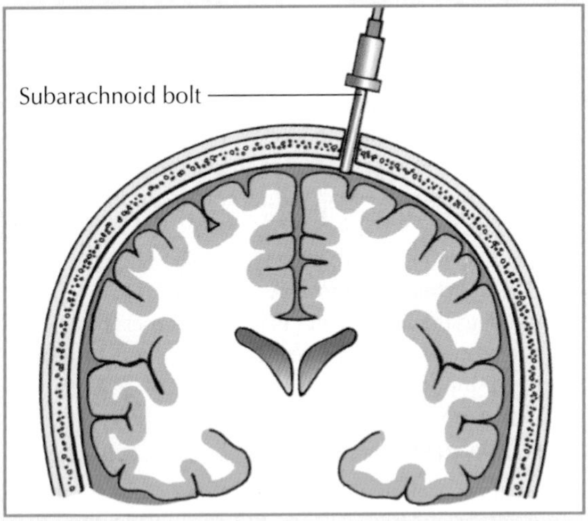

Implementation

■ Confirm the patient's identity using two patient identifiers according to your facility's policy.

■ Explain the procedure to the patient or his family. Make sure the patient or a responsible family member has signed a consent form.

■ Determine whether the patient is allergic to iodine preparations.

■ Provide privacy if the procedure is being done in an open emergency department or ICU. Wash your hands.

■ Obtain baseline routine and neurologic vital signs *to aid in prompt detection of decompensation during the procedure.*

■ Place the patient in the supine position, and elevate the head of the bed 30 degrees (or as ordered). Document the number of bed crank rotations, or hang a yardstick on an

Epidural or subdural sensor monitoring

ICP can also be monitored from the epidural or subdural space. For epidural monitoring, a fiber-optic sensor is inserted into the epidural space through a burr hole. This system's main drawback is its questionable accuracy *because ICP isn't being measured directly from a CSF-filled space.*

For subdural monitoring, a fiber-optic transducer-tipped catheter is tunneled through a burr hole, and its tip is placed on brain tissue under the dura mater. The main drawback to this method is its inability to drain CSF.

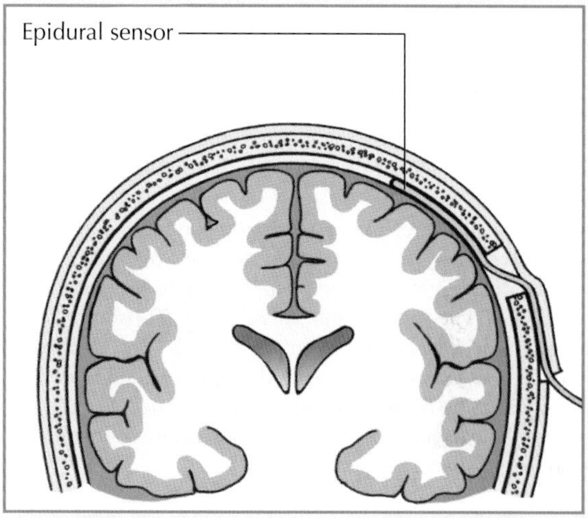

Intraparenchymal monitoring

In intraparenchymal monitoring, the physician inserts a catheter through a small subarachnoid bolt and, after puncturing the dura, advances the catheter a few centimeters into the brain's white matter. There is no need to balance or calibrate the equipment after insertion.

Although this method doesn't provide direct access to CSF, measurements are accurate *because brain tissue pressures correlate well with ventricular pressures.* Intraparenchymal monitoring may be used to obtain ICP measurements in patients with compressed or dislocated ventricles.

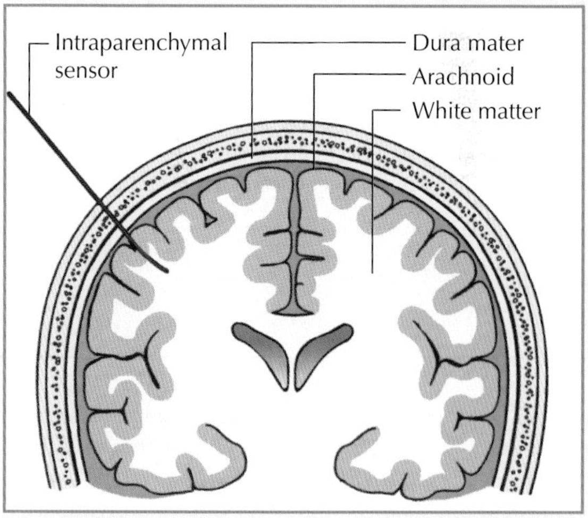

I.V. pole and mark the exact elevation. If possible, lock the bed controls once the bed is in position at the ordered height.

- Place linen-saver pads under the patient's head.
- Clip his hair at the insertion site, as indicated by the physician, *to decrease the risk of infection.* Carefully fold and remove the linen-saver pads *to avoid spilling loose hair onto the bed.* The neurosurgeon will drape the patient with sterile drapes and scrub the insertion site for 2 minutes with antiseptic solution with the nurse's assistance.
- The physician puts on the sterile gown, mask, and sterile gloves. He then opens the interior wrap of the sterile supply tray and proceeds with insertion of the catheter or bolt.
- *To facilitate placement of the device,* hold the patient's head in your hands or attach a long strip of 4″ roller gauze to one side rail, and bring it across the patient's forehead to the op-

EQUIPMENT

Setting up an ICP monitoring system

To set up an intracranial pressure (ICP) monitoring system, follow these steps.

- Begin by opening a sterile towel. On the sterile field, place a 20-ml luer-lock syringe, an 18G needle, a 250-ml bag filled with normal saline solution (with outer wrapper removed), and a disposable transducer.
- Put on sterile gloves and gown as per your facility's policy, and fill the 20-ml syringe with normal saline solution from the I.V. bag.
- Remove the injection cap from the patient line and attach the syringe. Turn the system stopcock off to the short end of the patient line, and flush through to the drip chamber (as shown at right). Allow a few drops to flow through the flow chamber (the manometer), the tubing, and the one-way valve into the drainage bag. (Fill the tubing and the manometer slowly *to minimize air bubbles.* If any air bubbles surface, be sure to force them from the system.)

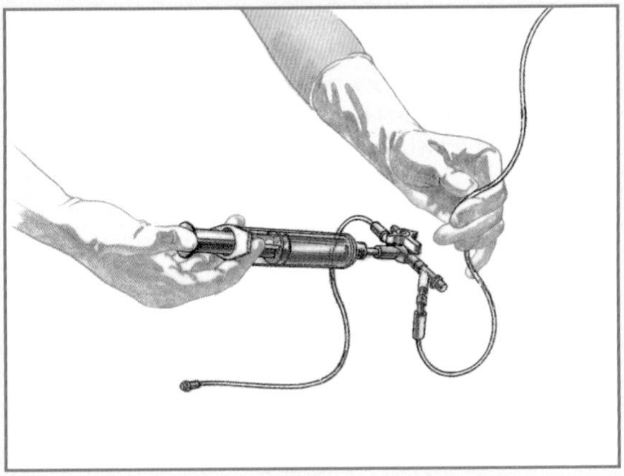

- Attach the manometer to the I.V. pole at the head of the bed.
- Slide the drip chamber onto the manometer, and align the chamber to the zero point (as shown at right), which should be at the inner canthus of the patient's eye.
- Next, connect the transducer to the monitor.
- Put on a clean pair of sterile gloves.
- Keeping one hand sterile, turn off the stopcock to the patient.

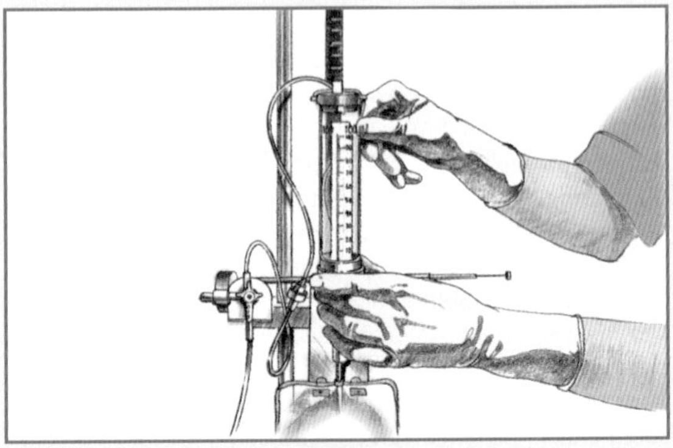

posite rail. Reassure the conscious patient, or administer reversible, quick-acting sedation *to help ease his anxiety.* Talk to him frequently *to assess his level of consciousness (LOC) and detect signs of deterioration.* Watch for cardiac arrhythmias and abnormal respiratory patterns.

- After insertion, apply antiseptic solution and a sterile dressing to the site. If not done by the physician, connect the catheter to the appropriate monitoring device, depending on the system used. (See *Setting up an ICP monitoring system.*)
- If the physician has set up a drainage system, attach the drip chamber to the headboard or bedside I.V. pole, as ordered.

NURSING ALERT *Positioning the drip chamber too high may raise ICP; positioning it too low may cause excessive CSF drainage.*

- Inspect the insertion site at least every 4 hours (or according to your facility's policy) for redness, swelling, and drainage. Clean the site, reapply antiseptic solution, and apply a dry sterile dressing according to your facility's policy.
- Assess the patient's clinical status, and take routine and neurologic vital signs hourly or as ordered. Make sure you've obtained orders for pressure parameters from the physician.
- Calculate cerebral perfusion pressure (CPP) hourly; use the equation: CPP = MAP – ICP (MAP refers to mean arterial pressure). If the CPP isn't within the specific parameters, notify the practitioner.

■ Align the zero point with the center line of the patient's head, level with the middle of the ear (as shown at right).
■ Lower the flow chamber to zero, and turn off the stopcock to the dead-end cap. With a clean hand, balance the system according to the monitor guidelines.

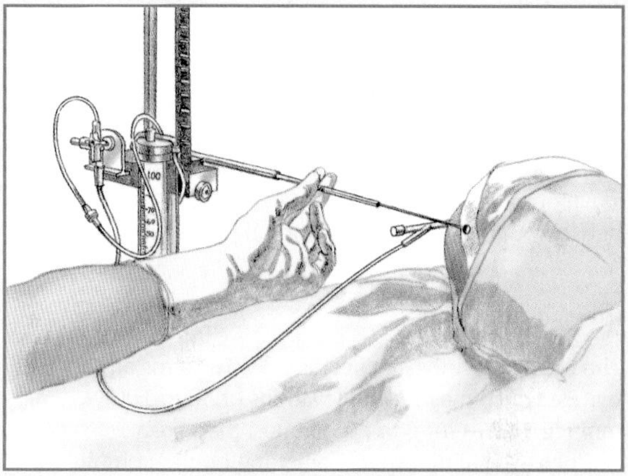

■ Turn off the system stopcock to drainage, and raise the flow chamber to the ordered height (as shown at right).
■ Return the stopcock to the ordered position, and observe the monitor for the return of the ICP patterns.

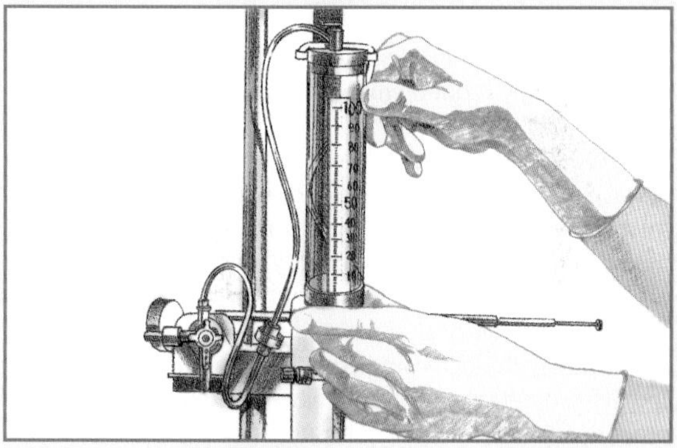

■ Observe digital ICP readings and waves. Remember, the trend revealed by multiple readings is more significant than any single reading. (See *Interpreting ICP waveforms,* page 622.) If you observe continually elevated ICP readings, note how long they're sustained. If they last several minutes, notify the practitioner immediately. Finally, record and describe any CSF drainage for color, amount, and consistency.

Special considerations

PEDIATRIC ALERT *In infants, ICP monitoring can be performed without penetrating the scalp. In this external method, a photoelectric transducer with a pressure-sensitive membrane is taped to the anterior fontanel. The transducer responds to pressure at the site and transmits readings to a bedside monitor and recording system. The external method is restricted to infants* because pressure readings can be obtained only at fontanels, the incompletely ossified areas of the skull.

■ Osmotic diuretic agents such as mannitol reduce cerebral edema *by shrinking intracranial contents.* Given by I.V. drip or bolus, mannitol draws water from tissues into plasma; it doesn't cross the blood-brain barrier. Monitor serum electrolyte levels and osmolality readings closely *because the patient may become dehydrated very quickly.* Be aware that a rebound increase in ICP may occur. (See *Nursing management of increased ICP,* page 623.)

■ *To avoid rebound increased ICP,* 50 ml of albumin may be given with the mannitol bolus. Note, however, that you'll see a residual rise in ICP before it decreases. If your patient

Interpreting ICP waveforms

Three waveforms—A, B, and C—are used to monitor intracranial pressure (ICP). A waves are an ominous sign of intracranial decompensation and poor compliance. B waves correlate with changes in respiration, and C waves correlate with changes in arterial pressure.

Normal waveform

A normal ICP waveform typically shows a steep upward systolic slope followed by a downward diastolic slope with a dicrotic notch. In most cases, this waveform occurs continuously and indicates an ICP between 0 and 15 mm Hg—normal pressure.

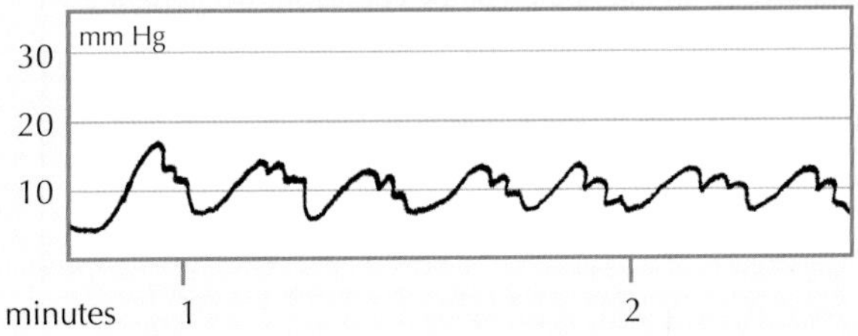

A waves

The most clinically significant ICP waveforms are A waves, which may reach elevations of 50 to 100 mm Hg, persist for 5 to 20 minutes, then drop sharply—signaling exhaustion of the brain's compliance mechanisms. A waves signify a reduction in cerebral perfusion pressure with ensuing hypoxia and decompensation. *Because A waves are an ominous sign,* they require emergency treatment.

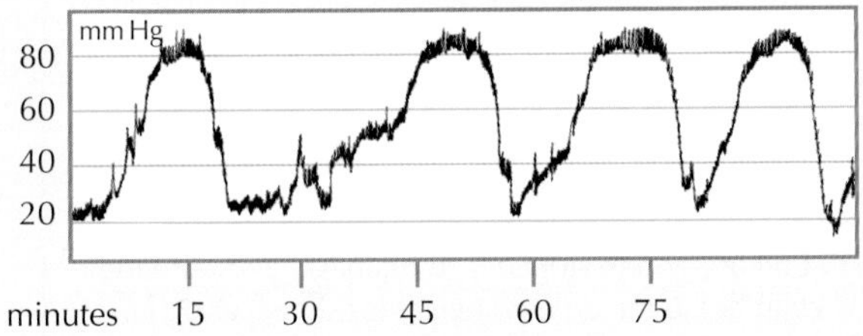

B waves

B waves, which appear sharp and rhythmic with a sawtooth pattern, occur every ½ to 2 minutes and may reach elevations of 50 mm Hg. The clinical significance of B waves isn't clear, but the waves correlate with respiratory changes and may occur more frequently with decreasing compensation. *Because B waves sometimes precede A waves,* notify the practitioner if B waves occur frequently.

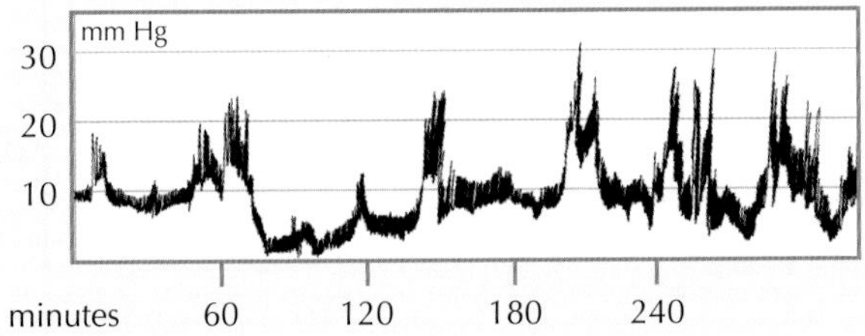

C waves

C waves are rapid and rhythmic, but not sharp and last 1 to 2 minutes with an ICP of 20 to 50 mm Hg. Clinically insignificant, they may fluctuate with respirations or systemic blood pressure changes.

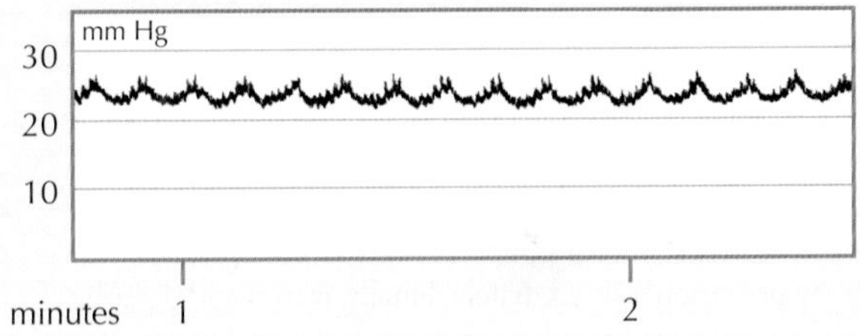

Waveform showing equipment problem

A waveform such as the one shown at right signals a problem with the transducer or monitor. Check for line obstruction and determine whether the transducer needs rebalancing. If the patient has a low ICP reading, this may be a normal wave.

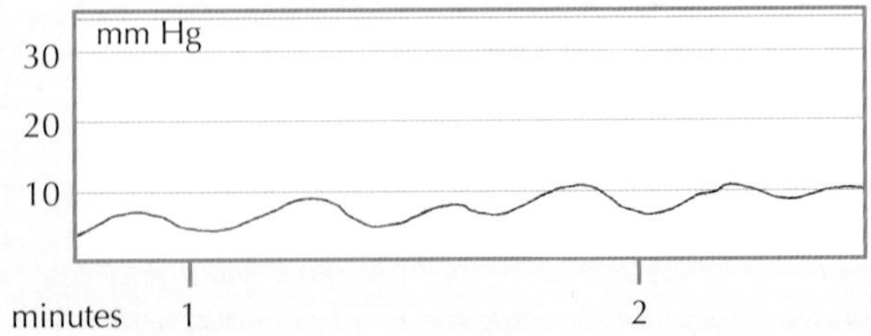

Nursing management of increased ICP

By performing nursing care gently, slowly, and cautiously, you can help manage—or even significantly reduce—increased intracranial pressure (ICP). If possible, urge your patient to participate in his own care. Here are some steps you can take to manage increased ICP:

- Plan your care to include rest periods between activities *to allow the patient's ICP to return to baseline, thus avoiding lengthy and cumulative pressure elevations.*
- Try to speak to the patient before attempting any procedures, even if he appears comatose. Touch him on an arm or leg first before touching him in a more personal area, such as the face or chest. This is especially important if the patient doesn't know you or if he's confused or sedated.
- Suction the patient for 10 seconds or less when needed to remove secretions and maintain airway patency. Avoid depriving him of oxygen for long periods while suctioning, and always hyperventilate the patient with oxygen after the procedure. Monitor his heart rate while suctioning. If multiple catheter passes are needed to clear secretions, hyperventilate the patient between them *to bring ICP as close to baseline as possible.*
- *To promote venous drainage,* keep the patient's head in the midline position, even when he's positioned on his side. Avoid flexing the neck or hip more than 90 degrees, and keep the head of the bed elevated 30 to 45 degrees.
- *To avoid increasing intrathoracic pressure, which raises ICP,* discourage Valsalva's maneuver and isometric muscle contractions. *To avoid isometric contractions,* distract the patient when giving him painful injections (by asking him to wiggle his toes and by massaging the area before injection to relax the muscle), and have him concentrate on breathing through difficult procedures such as bed-to-stretcher transfers. *To keep the patient from holding his breath when moving around in bed,* tell him to relax as much as possible during position changes. If necessary, administer a stool softener *to help prevent constipation and unnecessary straining during defecation.* Make sure trach ties and cervical collars are loose enough *to avoid compression of the jugular veins.*
- If the patient is heavily sedated, monitor his respiratory rate and blood gas levels. Depressed respirations will compromise ventilations and oxygen exchange. Maintaining adequate respiratory rate and volume will help reduce ICP.
- If you're in a specialty unit, you may be able to hyperventilate the patient *to counter sustained ICP elevations.* This procedure is one of the best ways to reduce high ICP at bedside for short periods. Consult your facility's procedure manual.

has heart failure or severe renal dysfunction, monitor for problems in adapting to the increased intravascular volumes.

- Monitor intake and output carefully to confirm normovolemia and to ensure adequate MAP *to assure good CPP.* The patient may be on a fluid restriction of 1,200 to 1,500 ml/day *to help prevent cerebral edema from worsening.*
- A barbiturate-induced coma depresses the reticular activating system and reduces the brain's metabolic demand. Reduced demand for oxygen and energy reduces cerebral blood flow, thereby lowering ICP.
- Hyperventilation with oxygen from a handheld resuscitation bag or ventilator helps rid the patient of excess carbon dioxide, thereby constricting cerebral vessels and reducing cerebral blood volume and ICP. However, only normal brain tissues respond *because blood vessels in damaged areas have reduced vasoconstrictive ability.* Hyperventilation should only be done in an acute situation *to decrease ICP until other measures can be instituted.*

NURSING ALERT ***Hyperventilation with a handheld resuscitation bag or a ventilator should be performed with care* because hyperventilation can cause ischemia.**

- Before tracheal suctioning, hyperventilate the patient with 100% oxygen as ordered. Apply suction for a maximum of 10 seconds. Avoid inducing hypoxia *because this condition greatly increases cerebral blood flow.*
- *Because fever raises brain metabolism, which increases cerebral blood flow,* fever reduction (achieved by administering acetaminophen, sponge baths, or a hypothermia blanket) also helps to reduce ICP. However, rebound increases in ICP and brain edema may occur if rapid rewarming takes place after hypothermia or if cooling measures induce shivering.
- Withdrawal of CSF through the drainage system reduces CSF volume and thus reduces ICP. Although less commonly used, surgical removal of a skull-bone flap provides room for the swollen brain to expand. If this procedure is performed, prevent direct trauma to the exposed tissue, keep

the site clean and dry *to prevent infection,* and maintain sterile technique when changing the dressing.

Complications

CNS infection, the most common hazard of ICP monitoring, can result from contamination of the equipment setup or of the insertion site.

NURSING ALERT *Be especially cautious when positioning the ventriculostomy; if the drip chamber is too high, it may raise ICP; if it's too low, it may cause excessive CSF drainage. Such loss can rapidly decompress the cranial contents and damage bridging cortical veins,* leading to hematoma formation. Decompression can also lead to rupture of existing hematomas or aneurysms, causing hemorrhage.

Watch for signs of impending increased ICP or overt decompensation: pupillary dilation (unilateral or bilateral); decreased pupillary response to light; decreasing LOC; rising systolic blood pressure and widening pulse pressure; bradycardia; slowed, irregular respirations; and, in late decompensation, decerebrate posturing.

Documentation

Record the date and time of the insertion procedure, dressing appearance, and the patient's response. Note the insertion site and the type of monitoring system used. Change the dressing according to your facility's policy. Record ICP digital readings and waveforms and CPP hourly in your notes, on a flowchart, or directly on readout strips, depending on your facility's policy. Document any factors that may affect ICP (for example, drug administration, stressful procedures, or sleep).

Record routine and neurologic vital signs hourly—or more frequently if the patient's condition warrants—and describe the patient's clinical status. Note the amount, character, and frequency of any CSF drainage (for example, "between 6 p.m. and 7 p.m., 15 ml of blood-tinged CSF"). Record the ICP reading in response to drainage.

Selected references

American Association of Neuroscience Nurses. *Core Curriculum for Neuroscience Nursing,* 4th ed. Philadelphia: W.B. Saunders Co., 2004.

Cremer, O.L., et al. "Need for Intracranial Pressure Monitoring Following Severe Traumatic Brain Injury," *Critical Care Medicine* 34(5):1583-84, May 2006.

Kuo, J.R., et al. "Intraoperative Applications of Intracranial Pressure Monitoring in Patients with Severe Head Injury," *Journal of Clinical Neuroscience* 12(2):218-23, February 2006.

Lynn-McHale Wiegand, D.J., and Carlson, K.K., eds. *AACN Procedure Manual for Critical Care,* 5th ed. Philadelphia: W.B. Saunders Co., 2005.

March, K. "Intracranial Pressure Monitoring: Why Monitor?" *AACN Clinical Issues* 16(4):456-75, October-December 2005.

Jugular venous oxygen saturation monitoring

Jugular venous oxygen saturation ($Sjvo_2$) monitoring measures the venous oxygenation saturation of blood as it leaves the brain, reflecting the oxygen saturation of blood after cerebral perfusion has taken place. After comparing $Sjvo_2$ with the arterial venous oxygenation, you can determine whether blood flow to the brain matches the brain's metabolic demand.

$Sjvo_2$ monitoring is often used with other types of cerebral hemodynamic monitoring—such as intracranial pressure (ICP) monitoring—to provide detailed information regarding pressure and perfusion states during treatment. Treatment regimens can be titrated to enhance pressure and perfusion.

The normal range for $Sjvo_2$ is from 55% to 70%. Values higher than 70% indicate hyperperfusion, whereas values between 40% and 54% indicate relative hypoperfusion. Values lower than 40% indicate ischemia.

Data from monitoring can also be used to calculate:

- cerebral extraction of oxygen ($Ceo_2 = Sao_2$ [arterial oxygen saturation] – $Sjvo_2$)
- cerebral arterial oxygen content ($Cao_2 = 1.34 \times Hb$ [hemoglobin] $\times Sao_2 - 0.0031 \times Pao_2$ [partial pressure of arterial oxygen])
- global cerebral oxygen extraction ratio ($o_2ER = Sao_2 - Sjvo_2/Sao_2$) and jugular venous oxygen content saturation ($Cjvo_2 = 1.34 \times Hb \times Sjvo_2 + 0.0031 \times Pjvo_2$ [jugular bulb venous oxygen tension])
- arteriovenous jugular oxygen content ($AvjDo_2 = Cao_2 - Cjvo_2$), which help determine cerebral oxygen use, metabolic demand, and adequacy of oxygen delivery.

Monitoring of $Sjvo_2$ allows the nurse to maximize the balance between cerebral perfusion, oxygenation, and metabolism. Criteria for $Sjvo_2$ monitoring include any neurologic injury where ischemia is a threat and may include intra-operative monitoring, subarachnoid hemorrhage, and post-acute head injury with increased ICP.

Equipment

Insertion of $Sjvo_2$ monitoring catheter

Sterile towels ▪ sterile drapes ▪ surgical caps ▪ gowns ▪ sterile gloves ▪ masks ▪ antiseptic solution ▪ central venous catheter insertion kit ▪ 1% or 2% lidocaine without epinephrine ▪ 5- or 10-ml syringe, with an 18G and 23G needle ▪ #5 French percutaneous introducer ▪ #4 French fiber-optic $Sjvo_2$ catheter ▪ oximetric monitor with cable ▪ 500 ml normal saline solution (heparinized or nonheparinized, according to your facility's policy) ■ pressure tubing with continuous flush device ■ pressure bag or device ■ sterile occlusive dressing ■ sterile marker ■ sterile labels.

Removal of $Sjvo_2$ monitoring catheter

Sterile gloves ■ suture removal set ■ sterile hemostat ■ sterile scissors ■ antiseptic solution ■ sterile occlusive dressing.

Preparation of equipment

■ Using sterile technique, prime the pressure tubing system, removing all air bubbles and maintaining sterility of system for insertion.
■ Follow the manufacturer's instructions for calibration of the catheter before insertion.

Implementation

Insertion of $Sjvo_2$ monitoring catheter

■ Confirm the patient's identity using two patient identifiers according to your facility's policy.
■ Explain the procedure to the patient and provide privacy.
■ Wash your hands and put on sterile gloves.
■ Position the patient with his head elevated at 30 to 45 degrees and his neck in a neutral position. Document baseline ICP.
■ Turn the patient's head laterally, away from the site chosen for catheter insertion. Note and document any change in ICP.
■ Put on new sterile gloves. Using sterile technique, open and prepare the central venous pressure insertion tray, and add a #5 French sterile introducer, and a #4 French fiberoptic $Sjvo_2$ catheter. Label all medications, medication containers, and other solutions on and off the sterile field.
■ Scrub the insertion site with an antiseptic solution.
■ Position the sterile drapes over the upper thorax and neck, exposing only the insertion site.
■ Assist the physician during insertion, as needed.
■ Monitor neurologic status, vital signs, ICP, and pain during insertion.
■ After the line is in place, attach the pressure tubing and confirm patency of both jugular catheter lumens by aspirating and flushing.
■ Clean the insertion site with antiseptic solution, and apply the sterile occlusive dressing.
■ Obtain a lateral cervical spine or lateral skull X-ray *to confirm catheter placement at the level of the jugular bulb.*

NURSING ALERT *Optimum placement of the $Sjvo_2$ catheter tip is at the level of the jugular bulb of the internal jugular vein. The tip of the catheter should be viewed at the upper border of the second cervical vertebra.*

■ Draw a jugular venous blood gas sample, and perform calibration according to the manufacturer's guidelines.

NURSING ALERT *In vivo calibration is necessary to ensure reliability of the data.*

Monitoring and care

■ Assess neurologic status, vital signs, and ICP immediately after insertion.

NURSING ALERT Because the catheter in the jugular bulb can inhibit venous outflow, *a sustained ICP more than 5 mm Hg over preinsertion baseline may be an indication for catheter removal.*

■ Record baseline parameters for continuously monitored $Sjvo_2$. Calculate $AvjDo_2$, Ceo_2, and o_2ER as a baseline.
■ Assess for a change in ICP *because increased ICP is a frequent cause of desaturation in patients with brain injury.*

NURSING ALERT *Repeated patterns of desaturation have been shown to be predictors of poor outcomes in patients with severe head injury.*

NURSING ALERT *Desaturation is an emergency requiring immediate intervention to restore cerebral blood flow and oxygen delivery. (See* Common causes of desaturation, *page 626.)*

■ Continuously monitor $Sjvo_2$.
■ Verify accuracy of the reading by drawing $Sjvo_2$ every 8 to 12 hours. The blood sample reading should be within 4% of monitor.

NURSING ALERT *Significant change in readings following sampling can signify errors related to aspiration of blood. Avoid errors by aspirating blood slowly during sampling procedure (1 ml/minute).*

■ Record $Sjvo_2$ and ICP values and note trends. Assess ICP in relation to $Sjvo_2$. Notify the practitioner of any deviation from the trend.
■ Maintain a safe environment during monitoring *to prevent accidental dislodgement of the catheter.*
■ Change the dressing using sterile technique if it becomes soiled or loosened and as indicated by your facility's policy for central line redressing.
■ Change the I.V. solution and tubing for the catheter according to your facility's policy for central lines.
■ *To prevent catheter coiling,* identify rhythmic fluctuations in $Sjvo_2$ trends. Obtain a lateral cervical spine or lateral skull X-ray *to assess position of the catheter in the external jugular vein (compare to X-ray done on insertion).* If coiling is confirmed, consider replacing the catheter.

NURSING ALERT *Rhythmic fluctuations of trends that are unrelated to changes in ICP, CPP (cerebral perfusion pressure), or systemic blood pressure signify coiling of the catheter.*

Common causes of desaturation

You may encounter periods of desaturation and need to be prepared to take action. This table lists more common causes of desaturation and appropriate interventions.

CAUSE	NURSING INTERVENTIONS
Systemic hypoxemia (one of the most common causes of cerebral hypoxia)	If the oxygen saturation is less than 90%, increase the oxygen percentage or fraction of inspired oxygen, and adjust the ventilator settings as ordered.
Anemia (hemoglobin less than 90 g/L)	Report abnormal results to the practitioner, and administer a blood transfusion if ordered.
Systemic hypotension (mean blood pressure less than 70 mm Hg)	Report abnormal results to the practitioner, and administer a fluid challenge or vasopressors if ordered.
Increased intracranial pressure (ICP over 20 mm Hg)	Elevate the head of the bed 30 degrees, decrease external stimuli, administer osmotic diuretics such as mannitol, and adjust the ventilator settings to produce mild hyperventilation ($Paco_2$ [partial pressure of arterial carbon dioxide] 30 to 35 mm Hg). Other measures may include drainage of cerebrospinal fluid and methods to reduce cerebral oxygen demand, such as sedation, neuromuscular blockade, or barbiturate coma.

Removing an $Sjvo_2$ monitoring catheter

- Explain the procedure to the patient and provide privacy.
- Wash your hands and prepare the equipment.
- Deactivate alarms.
- Turn stopcocks off, position the patient properly, monitor vital signs, put on sterile gloves, and assist the physician with catheter removal as needed.
- Apply direct pressure to the site until there are no signs of active bleeding.
- Put on new sterile gloves. Apply antiseptic solution and the sterile occlusive dressing to the catheter site.
- Assess the site for signs of bleeding every 15 minutes for 1 hour, then every 30 minutes for 1 hour, and then 1 hour later.

Special considerations

- Use sedation or analgesia, as indicated, *to maintain the monitor and enhance CPP.*
- Perform in vivo calibration with jugular blood gas sample as recommended by the monitor manufacturer (usually performed each shift).
- Replace an $Sjvo_2$ catheter with low light intensity. Check the fiber-optic catheter for obstruction or occlusion. Aspirate the catheter until blood can be freely sampled and normal light intensity is displayed. If you can't aspirate a blood sample, the catheter needs to be replaced.

NURSING ALERT *Low light intensity may indicate catheter occlusion or damage to the fiber optics.*

- For an $Sjvo_2$ catheter with high light intensity, adjust the patient's head *to ensure neutral neck position.*

NURSING ALERT *High light intensity indicates a vessel-wall artifact—usually encountered during repositioning of the patient.*

Complications

Complications associated with $Svjo_2$ monitoring are similar to complications that can occur with any central line, the most common being line sepsis. Other risks include:

- pneumothorax
- carotid artery puncture
- internal jugular thrombosis
- excessive bleeding.

In rare instances, the catheter can also cause impaired cerebral venous drainage and increased ICP.

Documentation

Document difficulties encountered during insertion, depth (in centimeters) of the catheter, patient tolerance of the procedure, and the ICP reading during insertion. Record the baseline $SjvO_2$ reading and initial CeO_2 and $AvjDO_2$ calculations.

Record $SjvO_2$ and ICP hourly. Record CeO_2, $AvjDO_2$, and O_2ER when indicated. Document your assessment of the insertion site, expected and unexpected outcomes, interventions taken, and patient and family education provided.

SELECTED REFERENCES

American Association of Neuroscience Nurses. *Core Curriculum for Neuroscience Nursing,* 4th ed. Philadelphia: W.B. Saunders Co., 2004.

Dunn, I.F., et al. "Neuromonitoring in Neurological Critical Care," *Neurocritical Care* 4(1):83-92, 2006.

Lynn-McHale Wiegand, D.J., and Carlson, K.K., eds. *AACN Procedure Manual for Critical Care,* 5th ed. Philadelphia: W.B. Saunders Co., 2005.

Stevens, W.J. "Multimodal Monitoring: Head Injury Management Using $SjvO_2$ and LICOX," *Journal of Neuroscience Nursing* 36(6):332-39, December 2004.

Tobias, J.D. "Cerebral Oxygenation Monitoring: Near-Infrared Spectroscopy," *Expert Review of Medical Devices* 3(2):235-43, March 2006.

CEREBRAL BLOOD FLOW MONITORING

Traditionally, caregivers have estimated cerebral blood flow (CBF) in neurologically compromised patients by calculating cerebral perfusion pressure. However, modern technology permits continuous regional blood flow monitoring at the bedside.

A sensor placed on the cerebral cortex calculates CBF in the capillary bed by thermal diffusion. Thermistors within the sensor detect the temperature differential between two metallic plates—one heated, one neutral. This differential is inversely proportional to CBF: As the differential decreases, CBF increases—and vice versa. CBF monitoring reveals the effects of interventions on it. This monitoring technique yields important information about the effects of interventions on CBF. It also yields continuous real-time values for CBF, which are essential in conditions in which compromised blood flow may put the patient at risk, such as ischemia and infarction.

CBF monitoring is indicated whenever CBF alterations are anticipated. It's used most commonly in patients with subarachnoid hemorrhage (in which a vasospasm may restrict blood flow), trauma associated with high intracranial pressure, or vascular tumors.

EQUIPMENT

CBF monitoring system

To monitor cerebral blood flow (CBF) at the patient's bedside, you may use a monitor such as the one shown below. This monitor has a digital display; some also display waveforms. The CBF sensor, placed in the cerebral cortex, measures blood flow continuously.

Bedside CBF monitor

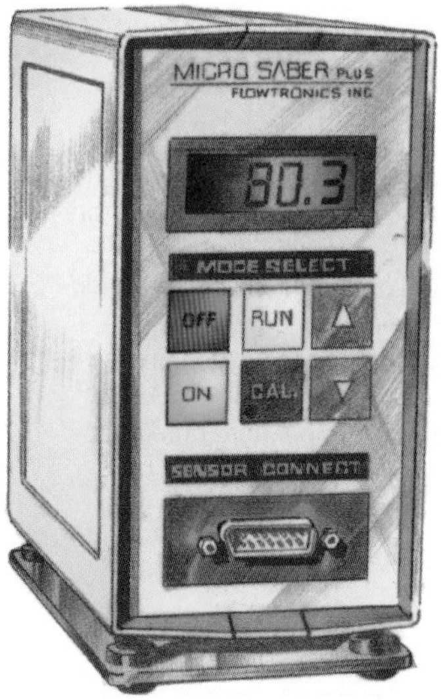

Equipment

CBF monitoring requires a special sensor that attaches to a computer data system or to a small analog monitor that operates on a battery for patient transport. (See *CBF monitoring system.*)

For site care: Sterile 4″ × 4″ gauze pads ▪ clean gloves ▪ sterile gloves ▪ antiseptic solution ▪ tape.

For removing sensor: Sterile suture removal tray ▪ 1″ adhesive tape ▪ sterile 4″ × 4″ gauze pads ▪ clean gloves ▪ sterile gloves ▪ suture material.

Preparation of equipment

Depending on the type of system you're using, you may need to verify that a battery has been inserted in the monitor to

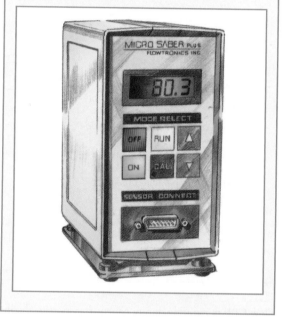

Inserting a CBF sensor

Typically, the surgeon inserts a cerebral blood flow (CBF) sensor during a craniotomy. He tunnels the sensor toward the craniotomy site and then carefully inserts the metallic plates of the thermistor to make sure that they continuously contact the surface of the cerebral cortex. After closing the dura and replacing the bone flap, he closes the scalp.

Insertion site

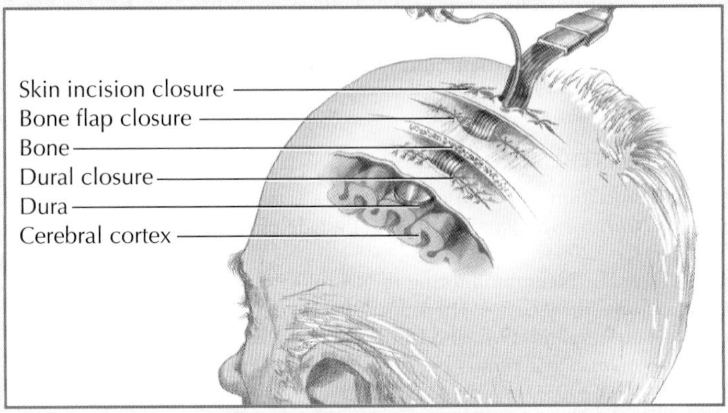

The sensor uses thermistors housed inside it to measure CBF. The thermistors consist of two metallic plates—one heated and one neutral. The sensor detects the temperature difference between the two plates. This difference is inversely proportional to CBF. As CBF increases, the temperature difference decreases—and vice versa.

Sensor

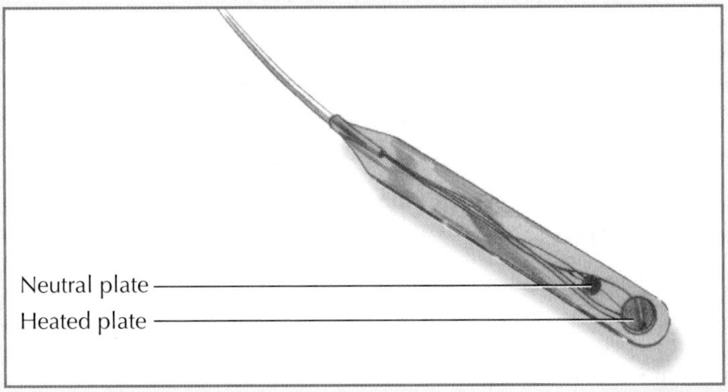

allow CBF monitoring during patient transport to the intensive care unit.

First, assemble the following equipment at the bedside: a monitor and a sensor cable with an attached sensor. Attach the distal end of the sensor cable (from the patient's head) to the SENSOR CONNECT port on the monitor. When the sensor cable is securely in place, press the ON key to activate the monitor.

Next, calibrate the system by pressing the CAL key. You should see the red light appear on the CAL button. Ideally, you'll begin by calibrating the sensor to 00.0 by pressing the directional arrows. Readouts of plus or minus 0.1 are also acceptable.

Implementation

- Make sure the patient or a family member is fully informed about the procedures involved in CBF monitoring, and obtain a signed consent form. If the patient will need CBF monitoring after surgery, advise him that a sensor will be in place for about 3 days. Tell the patient that the insertion site will be covered with a dry, sterile dressing. Mention that the sensor may be removed at the bedside.
- The surgeon typically inserts the sensor in the operating room during or following a craniotomy. (Occasionally, he may insert it through a burr hole.) He implants the sensor far from major blood vessels and verifies that the metallic plates have good contact with the brain surface. (See *Inserting a CBF sensor.*)
- Press the RUN key to display the CBF reading. Observe the monitor's digital display, and document the baseline value.
- Record the CBF hourly. Be sure to watch for trends, and correlate values with the patient's clinical status. Be aware that stimulation or activity may cause a 10% increase or de-

crease in CBF. If you detect a 20% increase or decrease, suspect poor contact between the sensor and the cerebral cortex.

Caring for the insertion site

- Wash your hands. Put on clean gloves, and remove the dressing from the sensor insertion site.
- Observe the site for cerebrospinal fluid (CSF) leakage, a potential complication. Then remove and discard your gloves.
- Next, put on sterile gloves. Using sterile technique, clean the insertion site with a gauze pad soaked in antiseptic solution. Clean the site, starting at the center and working outward in a circular pattern.
- Using a new gauze pad soaked with antiseptic solution, clean the exposed part of the sensor from the insertion site to the end of the sensor.
- Next, place sterile 4″ × 4″ gauze pads over the insertion site to completely cover it. Tape all edges securely *to create an occlusive dressing.*

Removing the sensor

- Usually, the CBF sensor remains in place for about 3 days when used for postoperative monitoring.
- Explain the procedure to the patient; then wash your hands. Put on clean gloves, remove the dressing, and dispose of the gloves and dressing properly.
- Open the suture removal tray and the package of suture material. The surgeon removes the anchoring sutures and then gently removes the sensor from the insertion site.
- After the surgeon closes the wound with stitches, put on sterile gloves, apply a folded gauze pad to the site, and tape it in place. Observe the condition of the site, including any leakage.

Special considerations

- CBF fluctuates with the brain's metabolic demands, ranging from 60 to 90 ml/100 g/minute normally. However, the patient's neurologic condition dictates the acceptable range. For instance, in a patient in a coma, CBF may be half the normal value; in a patient in a barbiturate-induced coma with burst suppression on the EEG, CBF may be as low as 10 ml/100 g/minute. Vasospasm secondary to subarachnoid hemorrhage may result in CBF below 40 ml/100 g/ minute. In an awake patient, CBF above 90 ml/100 g/minute may indicate hyperemia.
- If you suspect poor contact between the sensor and the cerebral cortex, turn the patient toward the side of the sensor or gently wiggle the catheter back and forth (using a sterile-gloved hand). *To determine whether these maneuvers have improved contact between the sensor and the cortex,* observe the CBF value on the monitor as you perform them.
- If your patient has low CBF but no neurologic symptoms that indicate ischemia, suspect a fluid layer (a small hematoma) between the sensor and the cortex.
- As with intracranial pressure monitoring, CBF monitoring may lead to infection. Administer prophylactic antibiotics, as ordered, and maintain a sterile dressing around the insertion site. CSF leakage, another potential complication, may occur at the sensor insertion site. *To prevent leakage,* the surgeon usually places an additional suture at the site.
- *To reduce the risk of infection,* change the dressing at the insertion site daily using sterile technique.

Complications

The most common complication of CBF monitoring is infection. CSF leakage at the insertion may also occur.

Documentation

Document cleaning of the site, appearance of the site, and dressing changes. After sensor removal, document any leakage from the site.

SELECTED REFERENCES

Albano, C., et al. "Innovations in the Management of Cerebral Injuries," *Critical Care Nursing Quarterly* 28(2):135-49, April-June 2005.

American Association of Neuroscience Nurses. *Core Curriculum for Neuroscience Nursing,* 4th ed. Philadelphia: W.B. Saunders Co., 2004.

Kirkness, C.J. "Cerebral Blood Flow Monitoring in Clinical Practice," *AACN Clinical Issues* 16(4):472-87, October-December 2005.

Lynn-McHale Wiegand, D.J., and Carlson, K.K., eds. *AACN Procedure Manual for Critical Care,* 5th ed. Philadelphia: W.B. Saunders Co., 2005.

TRANSCRANIAL DOPPLER MONITORING

Transcranial Doppler ultrasonography is a noninvasive, low-risk method of monitoring and assessing blood flow in the intracranial vessels, specifically the circle of Willis. This procedure is used at the patient's bedside in the intensive care unit to monitor patients who have experienced cerebrovascular disorders, such as stroke, head trauma, or subarachnoid hemorrhage. It can help detect intracranial stenosis, vasospasm, and arteriovenous malformations as well as assess collateral pathways. Because it has the advantage of monitoring a continuous waveform, it can be used in intraoperative monitoring of cerebral circulation and in tracking a patient's blood-flow velocity and trends.

The transcranial Doppler unit transmits pulses of high-frequency ultrasound, which are then reflected back to the transducer by the red blood cells moving in the vessel being monitored. This information is then processed by the instrument into an audible signal and a velocity waveform, which is displayed on the monitor. The displayed waveform is actually a moving graph of blood flow velocities with TIME displayed along the horizontal axis, VELOCITY displayed along the vertical axis, and AMPLITUDE represented by various colors or intensities within the waveform. The heart's contractions speed up the movement of blood cells during systole and slow it down during diastole, resulting in a waveform that varies in velocity over the cardiac cycle.

The major benefits of transcranial Doppler monitoring are that it provides instantaneous, real-time information about cerebral blood flow (CBF) and that it's noninvasive and painless for the patient. Also, the unit itself is portable and easy to use. The major disadvantage is that it relies on the ability of ultrasound waves to penetrate thin areas of the cranium; this is difficult if the patient has thickening of the temporal bone, which increases with age.

The transcranial Doppler unit should always be used with its power set at the lowest level needed to provide an adequate waveform. This procedure requires specialized training to ensure accurate vessel identification and correct interpretation of the signals.

Equipment

Transcranial Doppler unit ▪ transducer with an attachment system ▪ terry cloth headband ▪ ultrasonic coupling gel ▪ marker ▪ tissues.

Implementation

- Confirm the patient's identity using two patient identifiers according to your facility's policy.
- Explain the procedure to the patient, and answer any questions he has about the procedure as thoroughly as possible.
- Place him in the proper position—usually the supine position.
- Turn the Doppler unit on and observe as it performs a self-test. The screen should show six parameters: PEAK (CM/S), MEAN (CM/S), DEPTH (M/M), DELTA (%), EMBOLI (AGR), and PI+.
- Enter the patient's name and identification number in the appropriate place on the Doppler unit. Depending on the unit you're using, you may need to enter additional information, such as the patient's diagnosis or the practitioner's name.
- Indicate the vessel that you wish to monitor (usually the right or left middle cerebral artery [MCA]). You'll also need to set the approximate depth of the vessel within the skull (50 mm for the MCA).
- Next, use the keypad to increase the power level to 100% *to initially locate the signal.* You can later decrease the level, as needed, depending on the thickness of the patient's skull.
- Examine the temporal region of the patient's head, and mentally identify the three windows of the transtemporal access route: posterior, middle, and anterior (as shown below).

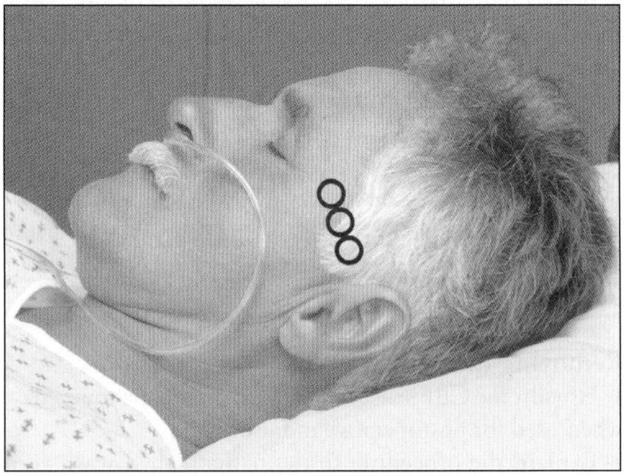

- Apply a generous amount of ultrasonic gel at the level of the temporal bone between the tragus of the ear and the end of the eyebrow, over the area of the three windows.
- Next, place the transducer on the posterior window. Angle the transducer slightly in an anterior direction, and slowly move it in a narrow circle. This movement is commonly called the "flashlighting" technique. As you hold the transducer at an angle and perform flashlighting, also begin to very slowly move the transducer forward across the temporal area. As you do this, listen for the audible signal with the highest pitch. This sound corresponds to the highest velocity signal, which corresponds to the signal of the vessel you are assessing. You can also use headphones *to let you better evaluate the audible signal and provide patient privacy.*
- After you've located the highest-pitched signal, use a marker to draw a circle around the transducer head on the patient's temple (as shown top of next page). Note the angle of the transducer *so that you can duplicate it after the transducer attachment system is in place.*

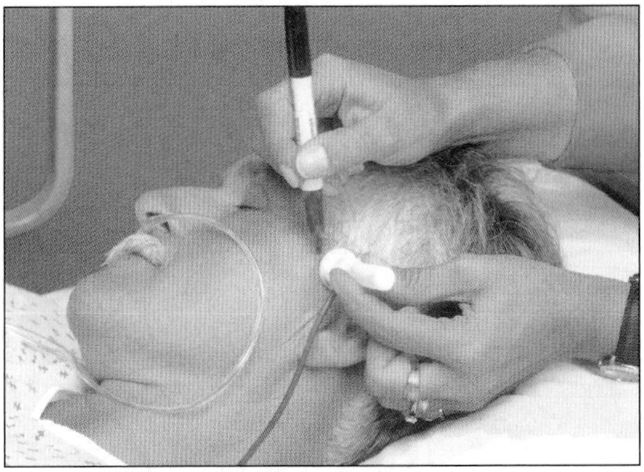

■ Next, place the transducer system on the patient. To do this, first place the plate of the transducer attachment system over the patient's temporal area; match the circular opening in the plate exactly with the circle drawn on the patient's head. Then, holding the plate in place, encircle the patient's head with the straps attached to the system. Finally, tighten the straps *so that the transducer attachment system will stay in place on the patient's head.*

■ Fill the circular opening in the plate with the ultrasonic gel.

■ Place the transducer in the gel-filled opening in the attachment system plate. Using the plastic screws provided, loosely secure the two plates together. *This will hold the transducer in place but allow it to rotate for the best angle.*

■ Adjust the position and angle of the transducer until you again hear the highest-pitched audible signal. When you hear this signal, look at the waveform on the monitor screen. You should see a clear waveform with a bright white line (called an envelope) at the upper edge of the waveform. The envelope exactly follows the contours of the waveform itself.

■ If the envelope doesn't follow the waveform's contours, adjust the GAIN setting. If the signal is wrapping around the screen, use the SCALE key to increase the scale and the BASELINE key to drop the baseline.

■ When you've determined that you have the strongest, highest-pitched signal and the best waveform, lock the transducer in place by tightening the plastic screws (as shown top of next column). The tightened plates will hold the transducer at the angle you've chosen. Disconnect the transducer handle.

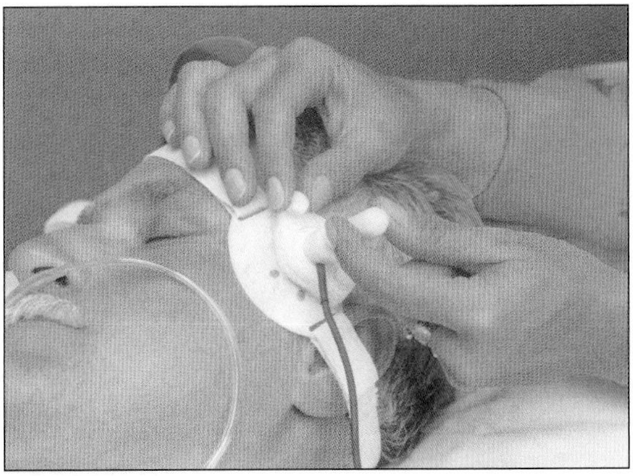

■ Place a wide terry cloth headband over the transducer attachment system, and secure it around the patient's head *to provide additional stability for the transducer.*

■ Look at the monitor screen. You should be able to see a waveform and read the numeric values of the peak, mean velocities, and pulsatility index (PI+) above the displayed waveform. The shape of the waveform reveals more information. (See *Comparing velocity waveforms,* page 632.)

Special considerations

■ Velocity changes in the transcranial Doppler signal correlate with changes in CBF. The parameter that most clearly reflects this change is the mean velocity. First, establish a baseline for the mean velocity. Then, as the patient's velocity increases or decreases, the value (%) will change negatively or positively from the baseline.

NURSING ALERT *In extreme situations, such as when blood flow is reduced by a severely restricted vessel, transcranial Doppler monitoring results may not correlate with the degree of vasospasm.*

■ Emboli appear as high-intensity transients that occur randomly during the cardiac cycle. Emboli make a distinctive "clicking," "chirping," or "plunking" sound. You can set up an emboli counter to count either the total number of emboli aggregates or the number of embolic events per minute.

■ Various screens can be stored on the system's hard drive and can be recalled or printed.

■ Before using the transcranial Doppler system, be sure to remove turban head dressings or thick dressings over the test site.

Documentation

Record the date and the time that the monitoring began and which artery is being monitored. Document any patient teaching as well as the patient's tolerance of the procedure.

Comparing velocity waveforms

A normal transcranial Doppler signal is usually characterized by mean velocities that fall within the normal reported values. Additional information can be gathered by evaluating the shape of the velocity waveform.

Effect of significant proximal vessel obstruction

A delayed systolic upstroke can be seen in a waveform when significant proximal vessel obstruction is present.

Normal

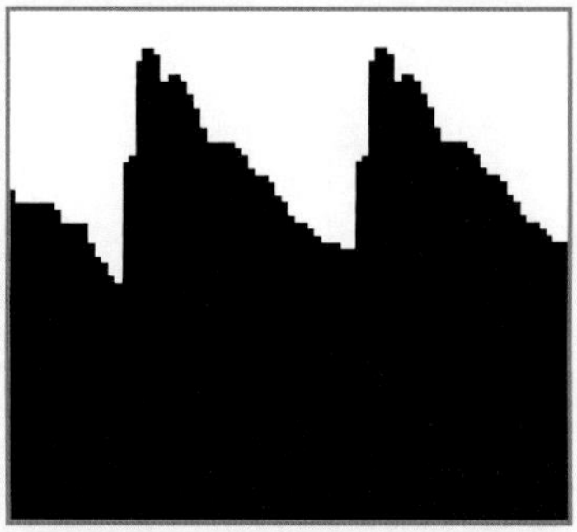

Proximal vessel obstruction

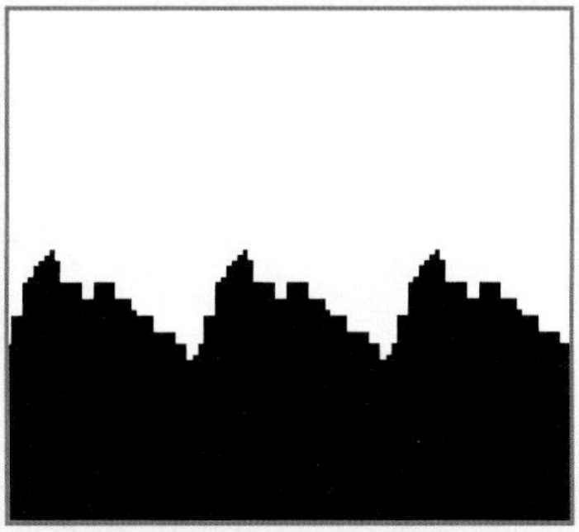

Effect of increased cerebrovascular resistance

Changes in cerebrovascular resistance, such as those that occur with increased intracranial pressure, cause a decrease in diastolic flow.

Normal

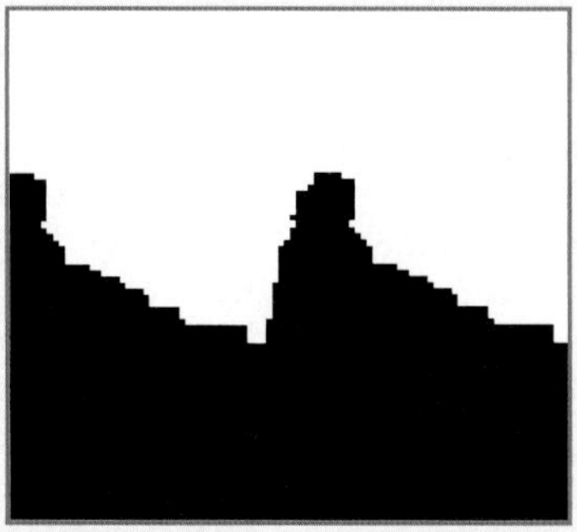

Increased resistance

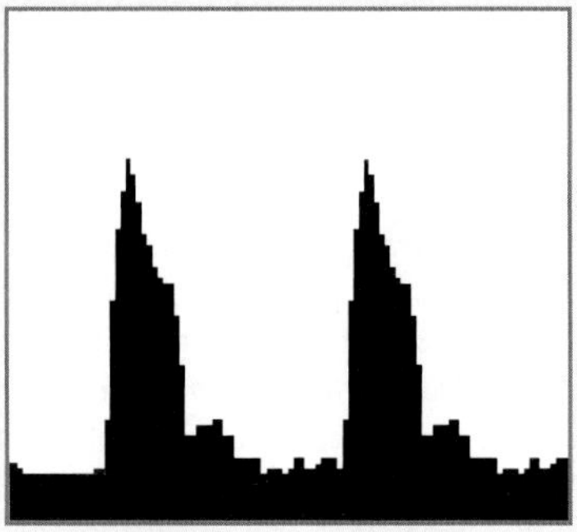

Selected references

Demchuk, A.M, et al. "Transcranial Doppler in Acute Stroke," *Neuroimaging Clinics of North America* 15(3):473-80, August 2005.

Evans, D.H. "Embolus Differentiation Using Multifrequency Transcranial Doppler," *Stroke* 37(7):1641, July 2006.

Lynn-McHale Wiegand, D.J., and Carlson, K.K., eds. *AACN Procedure Manual for Critical Care,* 5th ed. Philadelphia: W.B. Saunders Co., 2005.

White, H., and Venkatesh, B. "Applications of Transcranial Doppler in the ICU: A Review," *Intensive Care Medicine* 32(7):981-94, July 2006.

Bispectral index monitoring

Bispectral index monitoring involves the use of an electronic device that converts EEG waves into a number. This number, statistically derived based on raw EEG data, indicates the depth or level of a patient's sedation and provides a direct measure of the effects of sedatives and anesthetics on the brain. Rather than relying on subjective assessments and vital signs, bispectral index monitoring provides objective, reliable data on which to base care, thus minimizing the risks of oversedation and undersedation.

The bispectral index monitor is attached to a sensor applied to the patient's forehead. The sensor obtains information about the patient's electrical brain activity and translates this information into a number from 0 (indicating no brain activity) to 100 (indicating a patient who is awake and alert). In the intensive care unit, monitoring is used to assess sedation when the patient is receiving mechanical ventilation or neuromuscular blockers or during barbiturate coma or bedside procedures.

EQUIPMENT

Bispectral index monitoring

Bispectral index monitoring consists of a monitor and cable connected to a sensor applied to the patient's forehead (as shown below).

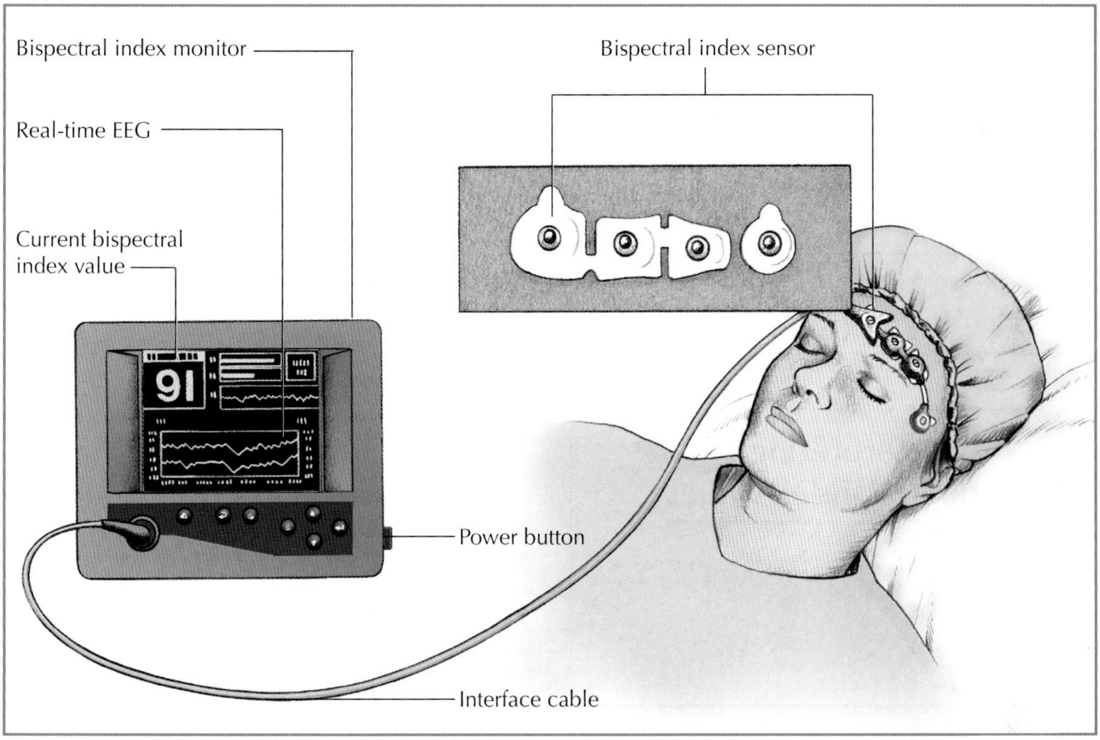

Equipment

Bispectral index monitor and cable ▪ bispectral index sensor ▪ alcohol swabs ▪ soap and water.

Preparation of equipment

Place the bispectral index monitor close to the patient's bed, and plug the power cord into the wall outlet.

Implementation

▪ Confirm the patient's identity using two patient identifiers according to your facility's policy.
▪ Explain the procedure and rationale to the patient and family. (See *Bispectral index monitoring*.)
▪ Provide privacy. Wash your hands and follow standard precautions.
▪ Clean the patient's forehead with soap and water and allow it to dry. If necessary, wipe the forehead with an alcohol swab *to ensure that the skin is oil-free.* Allow the alcohol to dry.
▪ Open the sensor package, and apply the sensor to the patient's forehead. Position the circle labeled "1" midline—approximately 1½" (about 4 cm) above the bridge of the nose.
▪ Position the circle labeled "3" on the right or left temple area, at the level of the outer canthus of the eye, between the corner of the eye and the patient's hairline.
▪ Ensure that the circle labeled "4" and the line below it are parallel to the eye on the appropriate side.
▪ Apply gentle, firm pressure around the edges of the sensor, including the areas in between the numbered circles, *to ensure proper adhesion.*

TROUBLESHOOTING

Sensor problems

When initiating bispectral index monitoring, be aware that the monitor may display messages that indicate a problem. This chart highlights these messages and offers possible solutions.

Message	Possible solutions
High impedance message	Check sensor adhesion; reapply firm pressure to each of the numbered circles on the sensor for 5 seconds each; if message continues, check the connection between the sensor and the monitor; if necessary, apply a new sensor.
Noise message	Remove possible pressure on the sensor; investigate possible electrical interference from equipment.
Lead-off message	Check sensor for electrode displacement or lifting; reapply with firm pressure, or if necessary, apply a new sensor.

Interpreting bispectral index values

Use the following guidelines to interpret your patient's bispectral index value.

Bispectral index		
100	Awake	
80	Light/moderate sedation	Light hypnotic state
70	Deep sedation (low probability of explicit recall)	Light hypnotic state
60	General anesthesia (low probability of consciousness)	Moderate hypnotic state
40	Deep hypnotic state	
0	Flat-line EEG	

- Press firmly on each of the numbered circles for approximately 5 seconds *to ensure that the electrodes adhere to the skin.*
- Connect the sensor to the interface cable and monitor.
- Turn on the monitor.
- Watch the monitor for information related to impedance (electrical resistance) testing.

NURSING ALERT *Be aware that for the monitor to display a reading, impedance values must be below a specified threshold. If not, be prepared to troubleshoot sensor problems. (See* Sensor problems.*)*

- Select a smoothing rate (the time during which data is analyzed for calculation of the bispectral index; usually 15 or 30 seconds) using the "advance set up" button based on your facility's policy. Read and record the bispectral index value.

Special considerations

- Always evaluate bispectral index value in light of other patient assessment findings—don't rely on bispectral index value alone. (See *Interpreting bispectral index values.*)
- Keep in mind that movement may occur with low bispectral index values. Be alert for possible artifact that could falsely elevate bispectral index values.

NURSING ALERT *Bispectral index values may be elevated due to muscle shivering, tightening, or twitching, or the use of mechanical devices either with the patient or in close proximity to the patient, bispectral index monitor, or sensor. Interpret the bispectral index value cautiously in these situations.*

- Anticipate the need to adjust the dosage of sedation based on the patient's bispectral index value.

NURSING ALERT *Keep in mind that a decrease in stimulation, increased sedation, recent administration of a neuromuscular blocking agent or analgesia, or hypothermia may decrease bispectral index, thus indicating the need for a decrease in sedative agents. Pain may cause an elevated bispectral index, indicating a need for an increase in sedation.*

- Check the sensor site according to the facility's policy. Change the sensor every 24 hours.

Documentation

Document initiation of bispectral index monitoring, including baseline bispectral index value and location of sensor. Record assessment findings in conjunction with bispectral index value *to provide a clear overall picture of patient's condition.*

Record any increases or decreases in bispectral index values, along with actions instituted based on values and any changes in sedative agents administered.

SELECTED REFERENCES

Bader, M.K., et al. "Refractory Increased Intracranial Pressure in Severe Traumatic Brain Injury: Barbiturate Coma and Bispectral Index Monitoring," *AACN Clinical Issues* 16(4):526-41, October-December 2005.

Leblanc, J.M., et al. "Role of the Bispectral Index in Sedation Monitoring in the ICU," *Annals of Pharmacotherapy* 40(3):490-500, March 2006.

Luebbehusen, M. "Technology Today: Bispectral Index Monitoring," *RN* 68(9):50-54, September 2005.

Olson, D.M., and Krebbs, L.M. "Use Bispectral Index to Gauge Consciousness," *Nursing* 34(7):53, July 2004.

PERIPHERAL NERVE STIMULATION

Peripheral nerve stimulation assesses and monitors the depth of neuromuscular blockade in patients receiving neuromuscular-blocking drugs, which are administered to produce paralysis. Neuromuscular-blocking drugs may be given to facilitate breathing and mechanical ventilation in patients with severe lung injury; assist with the treatment of severe muscle spasms in the patient with seizures, tetanus, and drug overdose; and help in the management of increased intracranial pressure in patients with head injury.

A peripheral nerve stimulator (PNS) is used to evaluate the level of neuromuscular blockade and determine the lowest therapeutic dose of the neuromuscular-blocking drug needed to produce paralysis. The PNS works by stimulating a peripheral nerve with a series of brief electrical pulses to produce a muscle response or twitch.

The "train-of-four" (TOF) is the most commonly used method for monitoring neuromuscular blockade. Using this method, a series of four electrical impulses are delivered to a particular peripheral nerve. If four twitches occur, then 75% or less of the receptors are blocked. Three twitches occur when 80% of the receptors are blocked. One or two twitches correspond to 85% to 90% neuromuscular blockade. After the neuromuscular blockade drug is administered, it's titrated so that each set of four electrical impulses produces one or two muscle twitches.

Equipment

Peripheral nerve stimulator ▪ two electrode gel patches ▪ two lead wires ▪ optional: scissors.

Implementation

- Confirm the patient's identity using two patient identifiers according to your facility's policy.
- Explain the reasons for neuromuscular blockade and peripheral nerve stimulation to the patient and family *to increase their understanding and reduce anxiety.*
- Wash your hands thoroughly.
- Select a site for electrode placement that is accessible and without edema, wounds, catheters, or dressings *to ensure optimum placement of electrodes.*
- If the patient has excessive hair where an electrode is to be placed, clip the hair with scissors *to improve contact of the pad with the skin.*

Ulnar nerve stimulation

- Clean and dry the patient's arm where the electrodes are to be placed *to reduce skin resistance.*
- Place the patient's arm in a relaxed position with the palm up so that the ulnar nerve is easily accessible.
- Place one electrode over the ulnar nerve at the crease of the wrist and the other electrode 1 to 2 cm away in the groove of the carpi ulnaris tendon (as shown below) *to ensure stimulation of the ulnar nerve.*

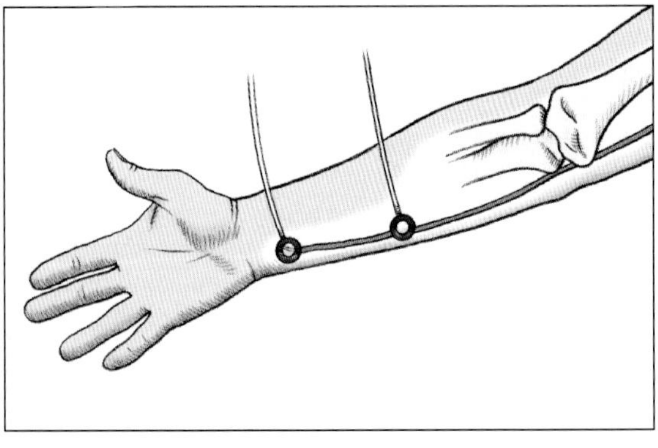

- Attach the lead wires to the PNS.

■ Connect the black lead (negative) to the electrode nearest the wrist and the red lead (positive) to the electrode on the forearm.
■ Switch the PNS on and choose a low milliampere (mA)—commonly 10 mA to 20 mA—*because higher current can cause overstimulation of the nerve and rhythmic nerve firing.*
■ Press the TOF button to initiate the four impulses and count the number of twitches the stimulation produces. Visually count the number of thumb adductions or twitches while lightly feeling for twitches. Don't count finger movement that's caused by muscle stimulation.
■ Turn off the PNS.

Facial nerve stimulation
■ Clean and dry the patient's face where the electrodes are to be placed *to reduce skin resistance.*
■ Place one electrode near the outer canthus of the eye and a second electrode 2 cm below and at the level of the tragus of the ear (as shown below).

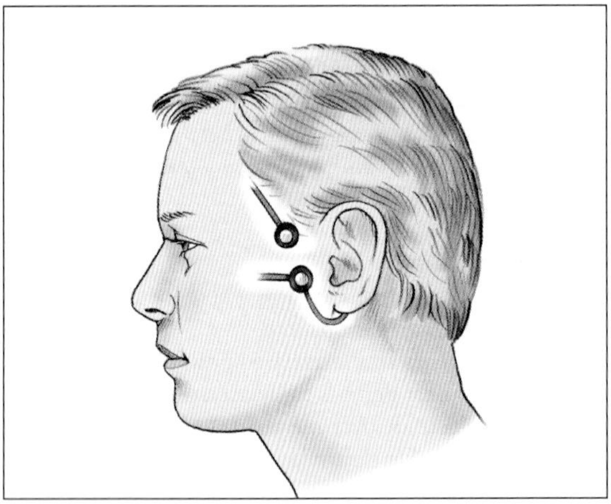

■ Attach the lead wires to the PNS, and connect the black lead (negative) to the electrode nearest the tragus and the red lead (positive) to the electrode near the outer canthus of the eye.
■ Switch the PNS on and choose a low milliampere (mA)—commonly 10 mA to 20 mA—*because higher current can cause overstimulation of the nerve and rhythmic nerve firing.*
■ Press the TOF button to initiate the four impulses and count the eyebrow twitches that the stimulation produces. Visually count the number of twitches while lightly feeling for twitches.
■ Turn off the PNS.

Posterior tibial nerve stimulation
■ Clean and dry the patient's foot where the electrodes are to be placed *to reduce skin resistance.*
■ Place one electrode 2 cm behind the medial malleolus and a second electrode 2 cm above the first electrode (as shown below).

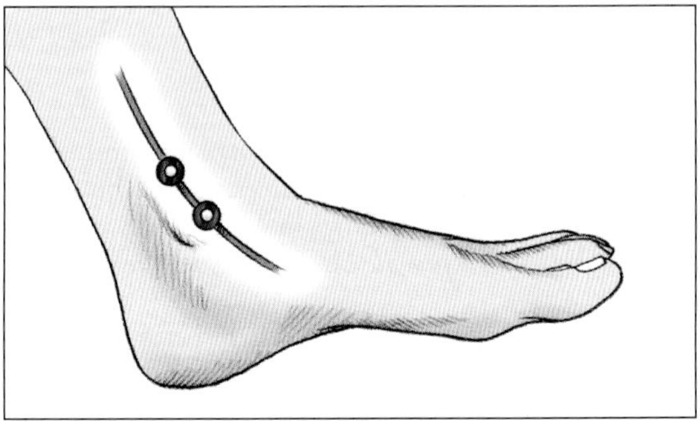

■ Attach the lead wires to the PNS.
■ Connect the black lead (negative) to the electrode behind the medial malleolus and the red lead (positive) to the electrode above the first.
■ Switch the PNS on and choose a low milliampere (mA)—commonly 10 mA to 20 mA—*because higher current can cause overstimulation of the nerve and rhythmic nerve firing.*
■ Press the TOF button to initiate the four impulses. Note plantar flexion of the great toe and count the number of twitches that the stimulation produces.
■ Turn off the PNS.

Establishing supramaximal stimulation
■ *To determine the baseline amplitude setting for a patient who has not received neuromuscular blockade,* set the amplitude to 10mA and press the TOF button to initiate the stimulus. *This determines the intensity where further increases in current no longer boost the intensity of the four twitches.*
■ Note the number of twitches produced.
■ Increase the amplitude 10 mA at a time until four muscle twitches are produced by the TOF. *This establishes the amount of current that should be used for peripheral nerve stimulation and enhances the reliability of testing.*

Establishing TOF following neuromuscular blockade
■ Determine the TOF 10 to 15 minutes following a bolus dose or any change in neuromuscular drug administration *to assess the level of neuromuscular blockade.*
■ If more than one or two twitches are observed, determine whether this level of neuromuscular blockade is acceptable for the patient's condition.

■ If a higher level of neuromuscular blockade is needed, increase the amount of neuromuscular drug being administered, as ordered or according to your facility's policy, and test the TOF again in 10 to 15 minutes.

Ongoing care

■ Perform respiratory, cardiovascular, and neurologic assessments before any increase in the level of neuromuscular blockade.
■ Perform neurovascular checks hourly.
■ Change electrodes daily or more frequently if they become loose or the gel has dried out *to ensure optimum conduction.*
■ Assess the skin under the electrodes for signs of irritation or breakdown, *which could impede conduction.*
■ Reevaluate the level of neuromuscular blockade every 4 to 8 hours, as ordered or according to your facility's policy, once the patient is stable and an adequate level of neuromuscular blockade is reached.

Special considerations

■ *Because neuromuscular blocking drugs don't produce amnesia, sedation, or analgesia,* sedative and analgesic drugs should always be administered before giving a neuromuscular blocking drug.
■ When the neuromuscular blockade infusion is discontinued, check the TOF. Four out of four muscle twitches should be present before discontinuing mechanical ventilation.
■ If the patient has hemiplegia, hemiparesis, or peripheral neuropathy (due to diabetes), the motor response to PNS may not be as pronounced, which may cause the nurse to mistakenly believe that a higher dose of neuromuscular-blocking drugs is needed. With hemiplegia and hemiparesis, place the electrodes on the unaffected limb, if possible.
■ Check the site of electrode placement carefully *because incorrect placement can lead to muscle, rather than nerve, stimulation.*
■ Note that a higher current may be needed to elicit a response in the patient with diabetes due to peripheral neuropathy.
■ If no twitches are elicited at a level that previously elicited a response, troubleshoot the PNS before increasing the level of neuromuscular blockade. Check the polarity of the leads, battery charge, electrode contact with the skin, condition of electrode gel pads, and lead wire connections.

Complications

Excessive neuromuscular blockade can cause protracted paralysis and muscle weakness. During TOF testing, the patient may experience mild discomfort, but moderate to severe discomfort shouldn't occur. Skin irritation and breakdown can occur under the electrode pads. Cardiac arrhythmias can result if the PNS lead wires come in contact with an external pacing catheter or lead wires.

Documentation

Record the date and time of the assessment. Record the initial TOF assessment, amplitude used, and dose of neuromuscular blockade drug being administered. Document each subsequent TOF assessment on the appropriate flow sheet as a ratio of twitches per four stimulations (for example, 0/4, 1/4, 2/4, 3/4, 4/4). Note the current used as well as any bolus doses or changes in the rate of infusion of the neuromuscular-blocking drug. Record the respiratory, cardiovascular, and neurologic assessments on a frequent assessment form. Note any adverse effects of neuromuscular blockade, the time and name of the practitioner notified, orders given, nursing interventions performed, and the patient's response. Include any patient and family teaching.

SELECTED REFERENCES

Ballard, N., et al. "Patients' Recollections of Therapeutic Paralysis in the Intensive Care Unit," *American Journal of Critical Care* 15(1):86-94, January 2006.
Jones, S.K. "An Algorithm for Train-of-Four Monitoring in Patients Receiving Continuous Neuromuscular Blocking Agents," *Dimensions of Critical Care Nursing* 22(2):50-57, March-April 2003.
Loyola, R., Dreher, H.M. "Management of Pharmacologically Induced Neuromuscular Blockade Using Peripheral Nerve Stimulation," *Dimensions of Critical Care Nursing* 22(4):157-64, July-August 2003.
Lynn-McHale Wiegand, D.J., and Carlson, K.K., eds. *AACN Procedure Manual for Critical Care*, 5th ed. Philadelphia: W.B. Saunders Co., 2005.

TREATMENTS

CEREBROSPINAL FLUID DRAINAGE

Cerebrospinal fluid (CSF) drainage aims to reduce CSF pressure to the desired level and then to maintain it at that level. Fluid is withdrawn from the lateral ventricle (ventriculostomy). Ventricular drainage is used to reduce increased intracranial pressure (ICP). External CSF drainage is used most commonly to manage increased ICP and to facilitate spinal or cerebral dural healing after traumatic injury or surgery. In either case, CSF is drained by a catheter or a ventriculostomy tube in a sterile, closed drainage collection system.

CSF drainage

Cerebrospinal fluid (CSF) drainage aims to control intracranial pressure (ICP) during treatment for traumatic injury or other conditions that cause a rise in ICP.

For a ventricular drain, the physician makes a burr hole in the patient's skull and inserts the catheter into the ventricle. The distal end of the catheter is connected to a closed drainage system.

The ventricular system is usually attached to this drainage system to permit drainage of CSF if needed.

Closed drainage system

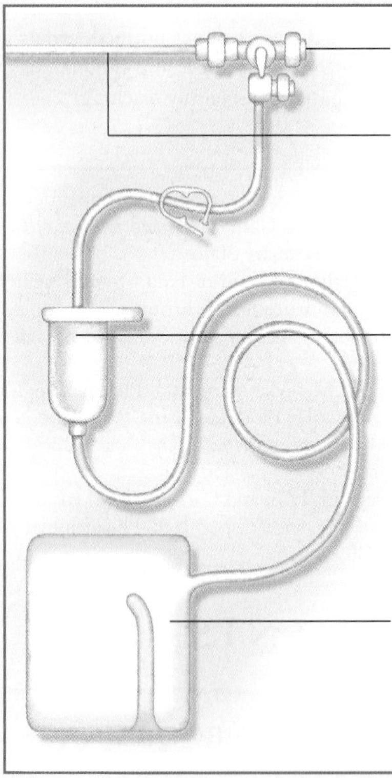

Other therapeutic uses include ICP monitoring via the ventriculostomy; direct instillation of medications, contrast media, or air for diagnostic radiology; and aspiration of CSF for laboratory analysis.

To place the ventricular drain, the physician inserts a ventricular catheter through a burr hole in the patient's skull. Usually, this is done in the operating room, with the patient receiving a general anesthetic. (See *CSF drainage*.)

Equipment

Overbed table ▪ sterile gloves ▪ antiseptic solution ▪ sterile fenestrated drape ▪ 3-ml syringe for local anesthetic ▪ 25G ¾" needle for injecting anesthetic ▪ local anesthetic (usually 1% lidocaine) ▪ sterile gauze ▪ clippers, if needed ▪ #5 French whistle-tip catheter or ventriculostomy tube ▪ external drainage set (includes drainage tubing and sterile collection bag) ▪ suture material ▪ sterile dressing ▪ paper tape ▪ I.V. pole ▪ ventriculostomy tray and twist drill ▪ sterile marker ▪ sterile labels ▪ optional: pain medication.

Preparation of equipment

Open all equipment using sterile technique. Check all packaging for breaks in seals and for expiration dates. Label all medications, medication containers, and other solutions on and off the sterile field.

Implementation

- Confirm the patient's identity using two patient identifiers according to your facility's policy.
- Consent should be obtained by the physician from the patient or a responsible family member and should be documented according to your facility's policy.
- Wash your hands thoroughly.
- Perform a baseline neurologic assessment, including vital signs, *to help detect alterations or signs of deterioration.*
- Administer any pain medications or sedation as ordered.

Inserting a ventricular drain

- Place the patient in the supine position.
- Place the equipment tray on the overbed table, and unwrap the tray.
- Adjust the height of the bed *so that the physician can perform the procedure comfortably.*
- Illuminate the area of the catheter insertion site.
- The physician will clean the insertion site, administer a local anesthetic, and clip the hair from the area of the insertion site. He'll put on sterile gloves and drape the insertion site.
- To insert the drain, the physician will request a ventriculostomy tray with a twist drill. After completing the ventriculostomy, he'll connect the drainage system and suture the ventriculostomy in place. Then he'll cover the insertion site with a sterile dressing.
- After the physician places the catheter, connect it to the external drainage system tubing. Secure connection points with tape or a connector. Place the collection system, including drip chamber and collection bag, on an I.V. pole.

Monitoring CSF drainage

- Maintain a continuous hourly output of CSF by raising or lowering the drainage system drip chamber. *To maintain CSF outflow,* the drip chamber should be slightly lower than or at the level of the lumbar drain insertion site. Sometimes you may need to carefully raise or lower the drip chamber *to increase or decrease CSF flow.* For ventricular drains, ensure that the flow chamber of the ICP monitoring setup remains positioned as ordered. You should also correlate changes in ICP to the drainage.
- To drain CSF as ordered, put on gloves, and then turn the main stopcock on to drainage. *This allows CSF to collect in the graduated flow chamber.* Document the time and the amount of CSF obtained. Then turn the stopcock off to drainage. To drain the CSF from this chamber into the drainage bag, release the clamp below the flow chamber. Never empty the drainage bag. Instead, replace it when it's full using sterile technique.
- Check the dressing frequently for drainage, *which could indicate CSF leakage.*
- Check the tubing for patency by watching the CSF drops in the drip chamber.
- Observe CSF for color, clarity, amount, blood, and sediment. CSF specimens for laboratory analysis should be obtained from the collection port attached to the tubing, not from the collection bag.
- Change the collection bag when it's full or every 24 hours according to your facility's policy.

Special considerations

- Maintaining a continual hourly output of CSF is essential *to prevent overdrainage or underdrainage.* Underdrainage or lack of CSF may reflect kinked tubing, catheter displacement, or a drip chamber placed higher than the catheter insertion site. Overdrainage can occur if the drip chamber is placed too far below the catheter insertion site.
- Raising or lowering the head of the bed can affect the CSF flow rate. When changing the patient's position, reposition the drip chamber.
- Patients may experience a chronic headache during continuous CSF drainage. Assess for signs of hemorrhage, which may include headache. Reassure the patient that this isn't unusual; administer analgesics, as appropriate.
- For ventricular drains, make sure ICP waveforms are being monitored at all times.
- Follow strict sterile technique when connecting tubing, flushing, or taking samples from the drainage system and during dressing changes.

Complications

Signs of excessive CSF drainage include headache, tachycardia, diaphoresis, and nausea. Acute overdrainage may result in collapsed ventricles, tonsillar herniation, and medullary compression.

NURSING ALERT *If drainage accumulates too rapidly, clamp the system, notify the physician immediately, and perform a complete neurologic assessment because this constitutes a potential neurosurgical emergency.*

Cessation of drainage may indicate clot formation. If you can't quickly identify the cause of the obstruction, notify the physician. If drainage is blocked, the patient may develop signs of increased ICP.

Infection may cause meningitis. To prevent this, administer antibiotics, as ordered. Maintain a sterile closed system and a dry, sterile dressing over the site.

Documentation

Record the date and time of the insertion procedure and the patient's response. Record routine vital signs and neurologic assessment findings at least every 4 hours.

Document the color, clarity, and amount of CSF at least every 8 hours or according to your facility's policy. Record hourly and 24-hour CSF output, and describe the condition of the dressing.

SELECTED REFERENCES

American Association of Neuroscience Nurses. *Core Curriculum for Neuroscience Nursing,* 4th ed. Philadelphia: W.B. Saunders Co., 2004.

Bota, D.P., et al. "Ventriculostomy-related Infections in Critically Ill Patients: A 6-year Experience," *Journal of Neurosurgery* 103(3):468-72, September 2005.

Hickey, J.V. *The Clinical Practice of Neurological and Neurosurgical Nursing,* 5th ed. Philadelphia: Lippincott Williams & Wilkins, 2003.

Lo, C.H., et al. "External Ventricular Drain Infections are Independent of Drain Durations: An Argument against Elective Revision," *Journal of Neurosurgery* 106(3):378-83, March 2007.

Lynn-McHale Weigand, D.J., and Carlson, K.K., eds. *AACN Procedure Manual for Critical Care,* 5th ed. Philadelphia: W.B. Saunders Co., 2005.

HALO-VEST TRACTION

Halo-vest traction immobilizes the head and neck after traumatic injury to the cervical vertebrae, the most common of all spinal injuries. This procedure, which can prevent further injury to the spinal cord, is performed by a neurosurgeon or an orthopedic surgeon, with nursing assistance, in the emergency department, at the patient's bedside, or in the operating room after surgical reduction of vertebral injuries. The halo-vest traction device consists of a metal ring that fits over the patient's head and metal bars that connect the ring to a plastic vest that distributes the weight of the entire apparatus around the chest. (See *Comparing halo-vest traction devices.*)

When in place, halo-vest traction allows the patient greater mobility than does traction with skull tongs. It also carries less risk of infection because it doesn't require skin incisions and drill holes to position skull pins.

Equipment

Halo-vest traction unit ▪ halo ring ▪ cervical collar or sandbags (if needed) ▪ plastic vest ▪ board or padded headrest ▪ tape measure ▪ halo ring conversion chart ▪ clippers ▪ 4″ × 4″ gauze pads ▪ antiseptic solution ▪ sterile gloves ▪ Allen wrench ▪ four positioning pins ▪ multiple-dose vial of 1% lidocaine ▪ alcohol pads ▪ 3-ml syringe ▪ 25G needle ▪ five sterile skull pins (one more than needed) ▪ torque screwdriver ▪ sheepskin liners ▪ clean gloves ▪ cotton-tipped applicators ▪ medicated powder or cornstarch ▪ normal saline solution ▪ optional: pain medication (such as an analgesic).

Most facilities supply packaged halo-vest traction units that include software (jacket and sheepskin liners), hardware (halo, head pins, upright bars, and screws), and tools (torque screwdriver, two conventional wrenches, Allen wrench, and screws and bolts). These units don't include sterile gloves, antiseptic solution, sterile drapes, cervical collars, or equipment for local anesthetic injection.

Preparation of equipment

Obtain a halo-vest traction unit with halo rings and plastic vests in several sizes. Vest sizes are based on the patient's head and chest measurements. Check the expiration date of the prepackaged tray, and check the outside covering for damage *to ensure the sterility of the contents.* Then assemble the equipment at the patient's bedside.

Implementation

- Check the support that was applied to the patient's neck on the way to the hospital. If necessary, apply the cervical collar immediately or immobilize the head and neck with sandbags. Keep the cervical collar or sandbags in place until the halo is applied. This support will then be carefully removed *to facilitate application of the vest. Because the patient is likely to be frightened,* try to reassure him.
- Remove the headboard and any furniture at the head of the bed *to provide ample working space.*

NURSING ALERT *Never put the patient's head on a pillow before applying the halo* **to avoid further injury to the spinal cord.**

- Elevate the bed to a working level that gives the physician easy access to the front and back of the halo unit.
- Stand at the head of the bed, and see if the patient's chin lines up with his midsternum, *indicating proper alignment.* If ordered, support the patient's head in your hands and gently rotate the neck into alignment without flexing or extending it.

Assisting with halo application

- Ask another nurse to help you with the procedure.
- Explain the procedure to the patient, wash your hands, and provide privacy.
- Have the assisting nurse hold the patient's head and neck stable while the physician removes the cervical collar or sandbags. Maintain this support until the halo is secure, while you assist with pin insertion.
- The physician measures the patient's head with a tape measure and refers to the halo ring conversion chart to determine the correct ring size. (The ring should clear the head by ⅔″ [1.7 cm] and fit ⅓″ [1 cm] above the bridge of the nose.)
- The physician selects four pin sites: ½″ above the lateral one-third of each eyebrow and ½″ above the top of each ear in the occipital area. He also takes into account the degree and type of correction needed to provide proper cervical alignment.
- Trim the hair at the pin sites with clippers *to facilitate subsequent care and help prevent infection.* Then use 4″ × 4″ gauze pads soaked in antiseptic solution to clean the sites.
- Open the halo-vest unit using sterile technique *to avoid contamination.* The physician puts on the sterile gloves and removes the halo and the Allen wrench. He then places the halo over the patient's head and inserts the four positioning pins *to hold the halo in place temporarily.*
- Help the physician prepare the anesthetic. First, clean the injection port of the multiple-dose vial of lidocaine with the alcohol pad. Then, invert the vial so the physician can insert a 25G needle attached to the 3-ml syringe and withdraw the anesthetic.
- The physician injects the anesthetic at the four pin sites. He may change needles on the syringe after each injection.
- The physician removes four of the five skull pins from the sterile setup and firmly screws in each pin at a 90-degree angle to the skull. When the pins are in place, he removes the positioning pins. He then tightens the skull pins with the torque screwdriver.

EQUIPMENT

Comparing halo-vest traction devices

TYPE	DESCRIPTION	ADVANTAGES
Low profile (standard)	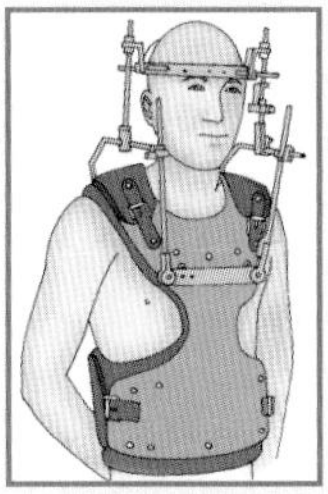 ■ Traction and compression are produced by threaded support rods on either side of the halo ring. ■ Flexion and extension are obtained by moving the swivel arm to an anterior or posterior position, depending on the location of the skull pins.	■ Immobilizes cervical spine fractures while allowing patient mobility ■ Facilitates surgery of the cervical spine and permits flexion and extension ■ Allows airway intubation without losing skeletal traction ■ Facilitates necessary alignment by an adjustment at the junction of the threaded support rods and horizontal frame
Mark II (type of low profile)	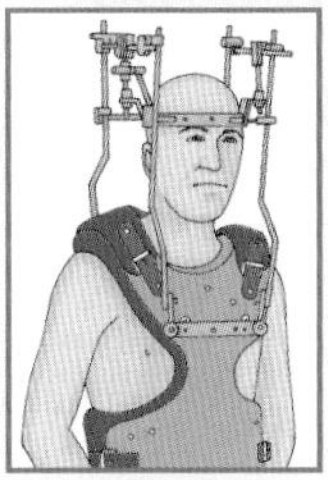 ■ Traction and compression are produced by threaded support rods on either side of the halo ring. ■ Flexion and extension are obtained by swivel clamps, which allow the bars to intersect and hold at any angle.	■ Enables the physician to assemble the metal framework quicker ■ Allows unobstructed access for anteroposterior and lateral X-rays of the cervical spine ■ Allows the patient to wear his usual clothing because uprights are shaped closer to the body
Mark III (update of Mark II)	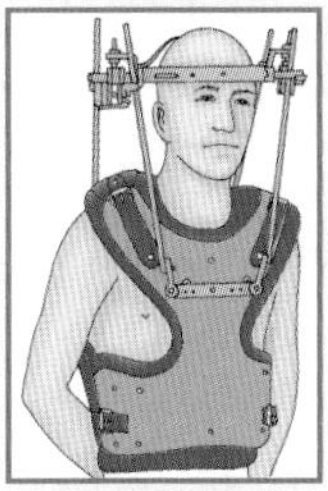 ■ Traction and compression are produced by threaded support rods on either side of the halo ring. ■ Flexion and extension are accommodated by a serrated split articulation coupling attached to the halo ring, which can be adjusted in 4-degree increments.	■ Simplifies application while promoting patient comfort ■ Eliminates shoulder pressure and discomfort by using a flexible padded strap instead of the vest's solid plastic shoulder ■ Accommodates the tall patient with modified hardware and shorter uprights and allows unobstructed access for medial and lateral X-rays
Trippi-Wells tongs	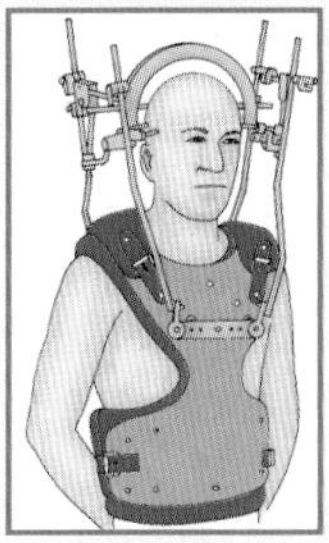 ■ Traction is produced by four pins that compress the skull. ■ Flexion and extension are obtained by adjusting the midline vertical plate.	■ Applies tensile force to the neck or spine while allowing patient mobility ■ Makes it possible to change from mobile to stationary traction without interrupting traction ■ Adjusts to three planes for mobile and stationary traction ■ Allows unobstructed access for medial and lateral X-rays

Applying the vest

■ After the physician measures the patient's chest and abdomen, he selects a vest of appropriate size.

■ Place the sheepskin liners inside the front and back of the vest *to make it more comfortable to wear and to help prevent pressure ulcers.*

■ Help the physician carefully raise the patient while the other nurse supports the head and neck. Slide the back of the vest under the patient and gently lay him down. The physician then fastens the front of the vest on the patient's chest using Velcro straps.

- The physician attaches the metal bars to the halo and vest and tightens each bolt in turn *to avoid tightening any single bolt completely, causing maladjusted tension.* When halo-vest traction is in place, X-rays should be taken immediately *to check the depth of the skull pins and verify proper alignment.*

Caring for the patient

- Take routine and neurologic vital signs at least every 2 hours for 24 hours (preferably every hour for 48 hours) and then every 4 hours until stable. (See *Performing a head-to-toe assessment,* pages 34 to 45.)

NURSING ALERT *Notify the physician immediately if you observe any loss of motor function or any decreased sensation from baseline* because these findings could indicate spinal cord trauma.

- Put on gloves. Gently clean the pin sites every 4 hours with cotton-tipped applicators. Rinse the sites with normal saline solution *to remove any excess cleaning solution.* Then clean the pin sites with antiseptic solution. *Meticulous pin-site care prevents infection and removes debris that might block drainage and lead to abscess formation.* Watch for signs of infection—a loose pin, swelling or redness, purulent drainage, pain at the site—and notify the physician if these signs develop.
- The physician retightens the skull pins with the torque screwdriver 24 and 48 hours after the halo is applied. If the patient complains of a headache after the pins are tightened, obtain an order for an analgesic. If pain occurs with jaw movement or any movement of the head or neck, notify the physician immediately *because this may indicate that pins have slipped onto the thin temporal plate.*
- Examine the halo-vest unit every shift *to make sure that everything is secure and that the patient's head is centered within the halo.* If the vest fits correctly, you should be able to insert one or two fingers under the jacket at the shoulder and chest when the patient is lying supine.
- Wash the patient's chest and back daily. First, place the patient on his back. Loosen the bottom Velcro straps *so you can get to the chest and back.* Then, reaching under the vest, wash and dry the skin. Check for tender, reddened areas or pressure spots that may develop into ulcers. If necessary, use a hair dryer to dry damp sheepskin *because moisture predisposes the skin to pressure ulcer formation.* Lightly dust the skin with medicated powder or cornstarch *to prevent itching.* If itching persists, check to see if the patient is allergic to sheepskin and if any drug he's taking might cause a skin rash. If your facility's policy allows, change the vest lining as necessary.
- Turn the patient on his side (less than 45 degrees) to wash his back. Then close the vest.
- Be careful not to put any stress on the apparatus, *which could knock it out of alignment and lead to subluxation of the cervical spine.*

Special considerations

NURSING ALERT *Keep two conventional wrenches available at all times; they may be taped to the patient's halo vest on the chest area. In case of cardiac arrest, use them to remove the distal anterior bolts. Pull the two upright bars outward. Unfasten the Velcro straps, and remove the front of the vest. Use the sturdy back of the vest as a board for cardiopulmonary resuscitation (CPR). Some vests have a hinged front to raise the breast plate for CPR. Know the type of vest your patient has. To prevent subluxating the cervical injury, start CPR with the jaw thrust maneuver, which avoids hyperextension of the neck. Pull the patient's mandible forward while maintaining proper head and neck alignment. This pulls the tongue forward to open the airway.*

- Never lift the patient up by the vertical bars. *This could strain or tear the skin at the pin sites or misalign the traction.*
- *To prevent falls,* walk with the ambulatory patient. Remember, he'll have difficulty seeing objects at or near his feet, and the weight of the halo-vest unit (about 10 lb [4.5 kg]) may throw him off balance. If the patient is in a wheelchair, lower the leg rests *to prevent the chair from tipping backward.*
- *Because the vest limits chest expansion,* routinely assess pulmonary function, especially in a patient with pulmonary disease.

Home care

Teach the patient to turn slowly—in small increments—*to avoid losing his balance.* Remind him to avoid bending forward *because the extra weight of the halo apparatus could cause him to fall.* Teach him to bend at the knees rather than the waist.

Have a physical therapist teach the patient how to use assistive devices to extend his reach and to help him put on socks and shoes. Suggest that he wear shirts that button in front and that are larger than usual *to accommodate the halo-vest.*

Most important, teach the patient about pin-site care and about shampooing and hair care.

Complications

Manipulating the patient's neck during application of halo-vest traction may cause subluxation of the spinal cord, or it could push a bone fragment into the spinal cord, possibly compressing the cord and causing paralysis below the break.

Inaccurate positioning of the skull pins can lead to a puncture of the skull and dura mater, causing a loss of cerebrospinal fluid and a serious central nervous system infection. Nonsterile technique during application of the halo or inadequate pin-site care can also lead to infection at the pin sites. Pressure ulcers can develop if the vest fits poorly or chafes the skin.

Documentation

Record the date and time that the halo-vest traction was applied. Also note the length of the procedure and the patient's response. After application, record routine and neurologic vital signs. Document pin-site care and note any signs of infection.

SELECTED REFERENCES

American Association of Neuroscience Nurses. *Core Curriculum for Neuroscience Nursing,* 4th ed. Philadelphia: W.B. Saunders Co., 2004.

Holmes, S.B., and Brown, S.J. "Skeletal Pin Site Care: National Association of Orthopaedic Nurses Guidelines for Orthopaedic Nursing," *Orthopedic Nursing* 24(2):99-107, March-April 2005.

Lynn-McHale Weigand, D.J., and Carlson, K.K., eds. *AACN Procedure Manual for Critical Care,* 5th ed. Philadelphia: W.B. Saunders Co., 2005.

Patterson, M.M. "Multicenter Pin Care Study," *Orthopedic Nursing* 24(5):349-60, September-October 2005.

PAIN MANAGEMENT

Pain is defined as the sensory and emotional experience associated with actual or potential tissue damage. Thus, pain includes not only the perception of an uncomfortable stimulus, but also the response to that perception. It's important to remember that the patient's self-report of pain is the most reliable indicator of the existence of pain. When a patient feels severe pain, he seeks medical help because he believes the pain signals a serious problem. This perception produces anxiety, which, in turn, increases the pain. To assess and manage pain properly, the nurse must depend on the patient's subjective description in addition to objective tools.

In health care, the practitioner's role is to identify and treat the cause of pain, and prescribe medications and other interventions to relieve pain, whereas nurses have traditionally been responsible for assessing and managing a patient's pain.

According to Joint Commission standards, health care facilities are required to develop policies and procedures for pain control, which include developing policies and procedures supporting the appropriate use of analgesics and other pain control therapies. Health care providers are expected to be knowledgeable about pain assessment and management. The new standards also state that:

- pain should be assessed on admission and regularly reassessed
- patients should be informed of relevant providers in pain assessment and management
- patients and their families should be educated regarding their roles in pain management as well as the potential limitations and adverse effects of pain treatments
- pain assessment should include personal, cultural, spiritual, and ethnic beliefs
- patients will be involved in making care decisions
- routine and as needed analgesics are to be administered.

Several interventions can be used to manage pain. These include analgesic administration, emotional support, comfort measures, and complementary and attenuated therapies such as cognitive techniques to distract the patient. Severe pain usually requires an opioid analgesic. Invasive measures, such as epidural analgesia or patient-controlled analgesia (PCA), may also be required.

Equipment

Pain assessment tool or scale ▪ oral hygiene supplies ▪ water ▪ nonopioid analgesic (such as acetaminophen or aspirin) ▪ optional: PCA device, mild opioid (such as oxycodone or codeine), strong opioid (such as morphine or hydromorphone).

Implementation

- Confirm the patient's identity using two patient identifiers according to your facility's policy.
- Explain to the patient how pain medications work together with other pain management therapies *to provide relief.* Also explain that management aims to keep pain at a low level *to permit optimal bodily function.*
- Assess the patient's pain by asking key questions and noting his response to the pain. For instance, ask him to describe its duration, severity, and location. Look for physiologic or behavioral clues to the pain's severity. (See *How to assess pain,* page 644.)
- Develop nursing diagnoses. Appropriate nursing diagnostic categories include pain (acute, chronic), anxiety, activity intolerance, fear, risk for injury, deficient knowledge, and powerlessness.
- Work with the patient to develop a nursing care plan using interventions appropriate to the patient's lifestyle. These may include prescribed medications, emotional support, comfort measures, complementary and alternative therapies such as cognitive techniques, and education about pain and its management. Emphasize the importance of maintaining

How to assess pain

To assess pain properly, you'll need to consider the patient's description and your observations of the patient's physical and behavioral responses. Start by asking the following series of key questions (bearing in mind that the patient's responses will be shaped by his prior experiences, self-image, and beliefs about his condition):

- Where is the pain located? How long does it last? How often does it occur?
- Can you describe the pain?
- What brings the pain on?
- What relieves the pain or makes it worse?

Ask the patient to rank his pain on a scale of 0 to 10, with 0 denoting lack of pain and 10 denoting the worst pain. *This helps the patient verbally evaluate pain therapies.*

Observe the patient's behavioral and physiologic responses to pain. Physiologic responses may be sympathetic or parasympathetic.

Behavioral responses

Behavioral responses include altered body position, moaning, sighing, grimacing, withdrawal, crying, restlessness, muscle twitching, irritability, and immobility.

Sympathetic responses

Sympathetic responses are commonly associated with mild to moderate pain and include pallor, elevated blood pressure, dilated pupils, skeletal muscle tension, dyspnea, tachycardia, and diaphoresis.

Parasympathetic responses

Parasympathetic responses are commonly associated with severe, deep pain and include pallor, decreased blood pressure, bradycardia, nausea and vomiting, weakness, dizziness, and loss of consciousness.

Assess pain at least every 2 hours and during rest, during activity, and through the night when pain is usually heightened. Keep in mind that the ability to sleep doesn't indicate absence of pain.

good bowel habits, respiratory function, and mobility *because pain may exacerbate any problems in these areas.*

- Implement your care plan. *Because individuals respond to pain differently,* you'll find that what works for one person may not work for another.

Giving medications

- If the patient is allowed oral intake, begin with a nonopioid analgesic, such as acetaminophen or aspirin, every 4 to 6 hours, as ordered.
- If the patient needs more relief than a nonopioid analgesic provides, you may give a mild opioid (such as oxycodone or codeine) as ordered.
- If the patient needs still more pain relief, you may administer a strong opioid (such as morphine or hydromorphone) as prescribed. Administer oral medications if possible. Check the appropriate drug information for each medication given.
- If ordered, teach the patient how to use a PCA device. *Such a device can help the patient manage his pain and decrease his anxiety.*

Providing emotional support

- Show your concern by spending time talking with the patient. *Because of his pain and his inability to manage it,* the patient may be anxious and frustrated. *Such feelings can worsen his pain.*

Performing comfort measures

- Periodically reposition the patient *to reduce muscle spasms and tension and to relieve pressure on bony prominences.* Increasing the angle of the bed can reduce pull on an abdominal incision, diminishing pain. If appropriate, elevate a limb *to reduce swelling, inflammation, and pain.*
- Splinting or supporting abdominal and chest incisions with a pillow when coughing or changing position will help decrease pain.
- Apply cold compresses, as appropriate, *to decrease discomfort.*
- Give the patient a back massage *to help relax tense muscles.*
- Perform passive range-of-motion exercises *to prevent stiffness and further loss of mobility, relax tense muscles, and provide comfort.*
- Provide oral hygiene. Keep a fresh water glass or cup at the bedside *because many pain medications tend to dry the mouth.*
- Wash the patient's face and hands.

Using complementary and alternative therapies

- Help the patient enhance the effect of analgesics by using such techniques as distraction, guided imagery, deep breathing, and relaxation. You can easily use these "mind-over-pain" techniques at the bedside. Choose the method the patient prefers. If possible, start these techniques when the patient feels little or no pain. If he feels persistent pain,

Visual pain rating

You can evaluate pain in a nonverbal manner for pediatric patients age 3 and older and for adults with language difficulties. One instrument is the Wong-Baker FACES pain rating scale shown below left, and another uses two simple faces, such as the ones shown below right. Ask the patient to choose the face that describes how he's feeling—either happy because he has no pain, or sad because he has some or a lot of pain. Alternatively, to pinpoint varying levels of pain, you can ask the patient to draw a face.

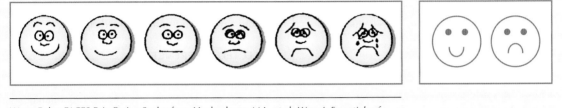

Wong-Baker FACES Pain Rating Scales from Hockenberry, M.J., et al. *Wong's Essentials of Pediatric Nursing*, 7th ed. St. Louis: Mosby, Inc., 2005. Reprinted with permission.

begin with short, simple exercises. Before beginning, dim the lights, remove the patient's restrictive clothing, and eliminate noise from the environment.

– For *distraction,* have the patient recall a pleasant experience or focus his attention on an enjoyable activity. For instance, he can use music as a distraction by turning on the radio when the pain begins. Have him close his eyes and concentrate on listening, raising or lowering the volume as his pain increases or subsides. Note, however, that distraction is usually most helpful in relieving pain lasting for brief episodes or for painful procedures of short duration.

– For *guided imagery,* help the patient concentrate on a peaceful, pleasant image, such as a walk on the beach. Encourage him to concentrate on the details of the image he has selected by asking about its sight, sound, smell, taste, and touch. *The positive emotions evoked by this exercise minimize pain.*

– For *deep breathing,* have the patient stare at an object and then slowly inhale and exhale as he counts aloud *to maintain a comfortable rate and rhythm.* Have him concentrate on the rise and fall of his abdomen. Encourage him to feel more and more weightless with each breath while he concentrates on the rhythm of his breathing or on any restful image.

– For *muscle relaxation,* have the patient focus on a particular muscle group. Then ask him to tense the muscles and note the sensation. After 5 to 7 seconds, tell him to relax the muscles and concentrate on the relaxed state. Have him note the difference between the tense and relaxed states. After he tenses and relaxes one muscle group, have him proceed to another and another, until he's covered his entire body.

Special considerations

- Evaluate your patient's response to pain management. If he's still in pain, reassess him and alter your care plan as appropriate.
- Culture and beliefs affect behavioral responses to pain and treatment preferences. Patient expectations regarding pain relief need to be taken into account when developing the care plan for pain management.

ELDER ALERT ***Pain shouldn't be considered a normal part of the aging process. Provide pain relief for the elderly patient using pharmacologic and nonpharmacologic approaches. Remember, safety is a special concern, especially the risk for falls due to impaired mobility from pain and from adverse effects from opioids.***

ELDER ALERT ***It's important to identify age-related factors that affect assessment and pain management in elderly patients. Because of adverse effects, certain medications, such as meperidine and propoxyphene, should be avoided.***

PEDIATRIC ALERT *Remember, children experience pain just as adults do, but developmental factors make pain assessment in children more difficult. Neonates and young children have difficulty expressing pain verbally, and it's important to look for behavioral cues (such as crying, facial grimacing, or eye closing). Pain tools, such as the Wong/Baker Faces Pain Rating Scale, are available to assess pain in children. (See* Visual pain rating.*)*

- Patients receiving opioid analgesics may be at risk for developing tolerance, dependence, or addiction. Patients with acute pain may have a smaller risk of dependence or addiction than patients with chronic pain.

Uses of TENS

Transcutaneous electrical nerve stimulation (TENS), which must be prescribed by a physician, is most successful if administered and taught to the patient by a therapist skilled in its use. TENS has been used for temporary relief of acute pain, such as postoperative pain, and for ongoing relief of chronic pain such as that associated with sciatica.

Types of pain that respond to TENS include:
- arthritis pain
- bone fracture pain
- bursitis pain
- cancer-related pain
- lower back pain
- musculoskeletal pain
- myofascial pain
- pain from neuralgias and neuropathies
- phantom limb pain
- whiplash pain.

- If a patient receiving an opioid analgesic experiences abstinence syndrome when the drug is withdrawn abruptly, suspect physical dependence. The signs and symptoms include anxiety, irritability, chills and hot flashes, excessive salivation and tearing, rhinorrhea, sweating, nausea, vomiting, and seizures. These signs and symptoms are likely to begin in 6 to 12 hours and peak in 24 to 72 hours. *To reduce the risk of dependence,* discontinue an opioid by decreasing the dose gradually each day. You may switch to an oral opioid and decrease its dose gradually.
- If a patient becomes addicted, his behavior will be characterized by compulsive drug use and a craving for the drug to experience effects other than pain relief. A patient demonstrating such behavior usually has a preexisting problem that's exacerbated by the opioid use. Discuss the addicted patient's problem with supportive personnel, and make appropriate referrals to experts.
- During periods of intense pain, the patient's ability to concentrate diminishes. If the patient is in severe pain, help him select a cognitive technique that's simple to use. After he selects a technique, encourage him to use it consistently.

Complications

The most common adverse effects of analgesics include respiratory depression (the most serious), sedation, constipation, nausea, and vomiting.

Documentation

Document each step of the nursing process. Describe the subjective information you elicited from the patient, using his own words. Note the location, quality, and duration of the pain as well as any precipitating factors.

Record your nursing diagnoses, including the pain relief method selected. Use a flow sheet to document pain assessment findings. Summarize your interventions and the patient's response. If the patient's pain wasn't relieved, note alternative treatments to consider the next time pain occurs. Record any complications of drug therapy.

Selected references

Assessment and Management of Acute Pain. Bloomington, Minn.: Institute for Clinical Systems Improvement, March 2006.

Assessment and Management of Chronic Pain. Bloomington, Minn.: Institute for Clinical Systems Improvement, November 2005.

Comprehensive Accreditation Manual for Hospitals: Pain Management Standards. Chicago: The Joint Commission, 2007.

D'Arcy, Y. "Managing Pain in a Patient Who's Drug Dependent," *Nursing* 37(3):37-41, March 2007.

Lewandowski, W., et al. "Changes in the Meaning of Pain with the Use of Guided Imagery," *Pain Management Nursing* 6(2):58-67, June 2005.

Plaisance, L. "Is Your Patient's Cancer Pain under Control?" *Nursing* 35(5)52-55, May 2005.

Transcutaneous electrical nerve stimulation

Transcutaneous electrical nerve stimulation (TENS) is based on the gate control theory of pain, which proposes that painful impulses pass through a "gate" in the brain. TENS is performed with a portable, battery-powered device that transmits painless electrical current to peripheral nerves or directly to a painful area over relatively large nerve fibers. This treatment effectively alters the patient's perception of pain by blocking painful stimuli traveling over smaller fibers.

Used for postoperative patients and those with chronic pain, TENS reduces the need for analgesic drugs and may allow the patient to resume normal activities. Typically, a course of TENS treatments lasts 3 to 5 days. Some conditions such as phantom limb pain may require continuous stimulation; other conditions such as a painful arthritic joint require shorter periods (3 to 4 hours). (See *Uses of TENS.*) TENS is contraindicated for patients with cardiac pacemakers because it can interfere with pacemaker function. The procedure is also contraindicated for pregnant patients because its effect on the fetus is unknown. It's also contraindicated in patients with dementia. TENS should be used cautiously in all patients with cardiac disorders. TENS

EQUIPMENT

Positioning TENS electrodes

In transcutaneous electrical nerve stimulation (TENS), electrodes placed around peripheral nerves (or an incisional site) transmit mild electrical pulses to the brain. The current is thought to block pain impulses. The patient can influence the level and frequency of his pain relief by adjusting the controls on the device.

Typically, electrode placement varies even though patients may have similar complaints. Electrodes can be placed in several ways:

- to cover the painful area or surround it, as with muscle tenderness or spasm or painful joints
- to "capture" the painful area between electrodes, as with incisional pain.

In peripheral nerve injury, electrodes should be placed proximal to the injury (between the brain and the injury site) *to avoid increasing pain.* Placing electrodes in a hypersensitive area also increases pain. In an area lacking sensation, electrodes should be placed on adjacent dermatomes.

These illustrations show combinations of electrode placement (red squares) and areas of nerve stimulation (shaded pink) for lower back and leg pain.

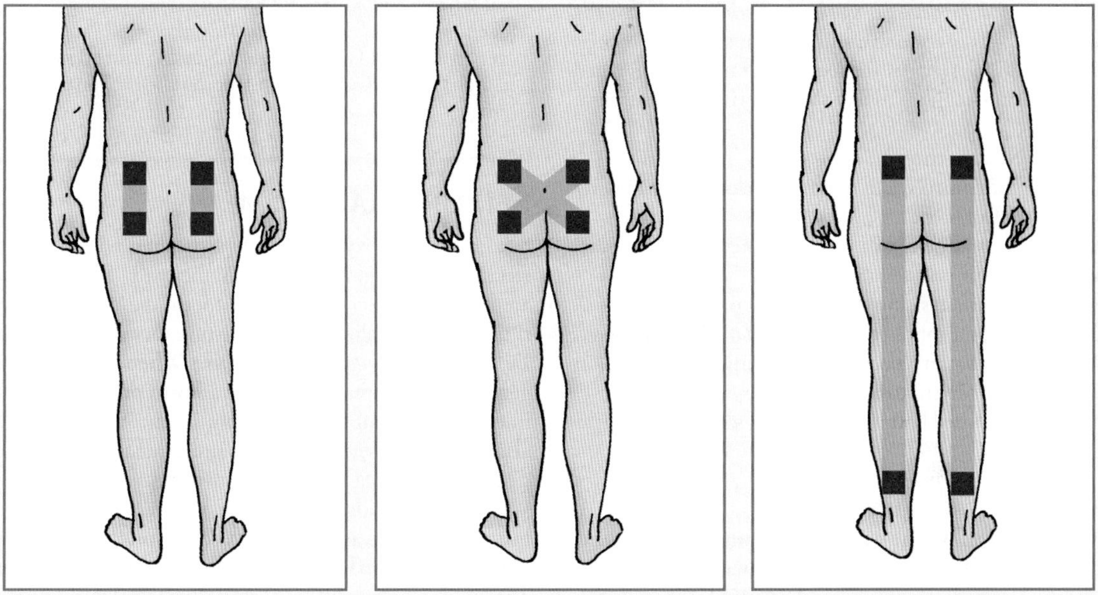

electrodes shouldn't be placed on the head or neck of patients with vascular disorders or seizure disorders.

Equipment

TENS device ▪ alcohol pads ▪ pre-gelled electrodes ▪ warm water and soap ▪ lead wires ▪ charged battery pack ▪ battery recharger ▪ adhesive patch or hypoallergenic tape.

Commercial TENS kits are available. They include the stimulator, lead wires, electrodes, spare battery pack, battery recharger and, occasionally, an adhesive patch.

Preparation of equipment

Before beginning the procedure, always test the battery pack *to make sure it's fully charged.*

Implementation

- Confirm the patient's identity using two patient identifiers according to your facility's policy.
- Wash your hands and provide privacy. If the patient has never seen a TENS unit, show him the device and explain the procedure.

Before TENS treatment

- With an alcohol pad, thoroughly clean and dry the skin where the electrode will be applied.
- Place the ordered number of electrodes on the proper skin area, leaving at least 2″ (5 cm) between them. (See *Positioning TENS electrodes.*) Then secure them with the adhe-

sive patch or hypoallergenic tape. Tape all sides evenly *so that the electrodes are firmly attached to the skin.*

- Plug the pin connectors into the electrode sockets. *To protect the cords,* hold the connectors—not the cords themselves—during insertion.
- Turn the channel controls to the OFF position or as recommended in the operator's manual.
- Plug the lead wires into the jacks in the control box.
- Turn the amplitude and rate dials slowly as the manual directs. (The patient should feel a tingling sensation.) Then adjust the controls on this device to the prescribed settings or to settings that are most comfortable. Most patients select stimulation frequencies of 60 to 100 Hz.
- Attach the TENS control box to part of the patient's clothing, such as a belt, pocket, or bra.
- *To make sure the device is working effectively,* monitor the patient for signs of excessive stimulation, such as muscular twitches, and for signs of inadequate stimulation, signaled by the patient's inability to feel any mild tingling sensation.

After TENS treatment

- Turn off the controls, and unplug the electrode lead wires from the control box.
- If another treatment will be given soon, leave the electrodes in place; if not, remove them.
- Clean the patient's skin with alcohol pads. (Don't soak the electrodes in alcohol *because it will damage the rubber.*)
- Remove the battery pack from the unit, and replace it with a charged battery pack.
- Recharge the used battery pack *so that it's always ready for use.*

Special considerations

- If you must move the electrodes during the procedure, turn off the controls first. Follow the practitioner's orders regarding electrode placement and control settings. *Incorrect placement of the electrodes will result in inappropriate pain control. Setting the controls too high can cause pain; setting them too low will fail to relieve pain.*

NURSING ALERT ***Never place the electrodes near the patient's eyes or over the nerves that innervate the carotid sinus or laryngeal or pharyngeal muscles*** **to avoid interference with critical nerve function.**

- If TENS is used continuously for postoperative pain, remove the electrodes at least daily *to check for skin irritation, provide skin care, and to rotate sites of electrode placement.*
- If appropriate, let the patient study the operator's manual. Teach him how to place the electrodes properly and how to take care of the TENS unit.

Documentation

On the patient's medical record and the nursing care plan, record the electrode sites and the control settings. Document the patient's tolerance to treatment. Evaluate pain control, and record the location of pain and the rate of the patient's pain using a pain scale.

SELECTED REFERENCES

American Association of Neuroscience Nurses. *Core Curriculum for Neuroscience Nursing,* 4th ed. Philadelphia: W.B. Saunders Co., 2004.

Hickey, J.V. *The Clinical Practice of Neurologic and Neurosurgical Nursing,* 5th ed. Philadelphia: Lippincott Williams & Wilkins, 2003.

"How the TENS Pain Control Unit Works." Available at *www.vitalityweb.com/backstore/TENSpain.htm.*

McLennon, S.M. *Persistent Pain Management.* Iowa City: University of Iowa Gerontological Nursing Interventions Research Center, Research Translation and Dissemination Core, August 2005.

SEIZURE MANAGEMENT

Seizures are paroxysmal events associated with abnormal electrical discharges of neurons in the brain. Partial seizures are usually unilateral, involving a localized or focal area of the brain. Generalized seizures involve the entire brain. (See *Differentiating among seizure types.*) When a patient has a generalized seizure, nursing care aims to protect him from injury and prevent serious complications. Appropriate care also includes observation of seizure characteristics to help determine the area of the brain involved.

Patients considered at risk for seizures are those with a history of seizures and those with conditions that predispose them to seizures. These conditions include metabolic abnormalities, such as hypocalcemia, hypoglycemia, and pyridoxine deficiency; brain tumors or other space-occupying lesions; infections, such as meningitis, encephalitis, and brain abscess; traumatic injury, especially if the dura mater was penetrated; ingestion of toxins, such as mercury, lead, or carbon monoxide; genetic abnormalities, such as tuberous sclerosis and phenylketonuria; perinatal injuries; and stroke. Patients at risk for seizures need precautionary measures to help prevent injury if a seizure occurs. (See *Precautions for generalized seizures,* page 650.)

Most major seizures (generalized or tonic-clonic) last only 1 to 2 minutes and demand little of the person observing the seizure. All that's needed is to let the seizure run its course, to ensure that the patient is in no physical danger, and to maintain a patent airway. However, a patient with status epilepticus, in which he experiences repeated seizures with-

Differentiating among seizure types

The hallmark of epilepsy is recurring seizures, which can be classified as partial or generalized. Some patients may be affected by more than one type of seizure.

Partial seizures (focal, local seizures)

Arising from a localized area in the brain, partial seizures cause specific symptoms. Categories of partial seizures include simple partial seizures (consciousness is intact), complex partial seizures (some loss of consciousness occurs), and partial seizures in which seizure activity may be spread to the entire brain, thereby causing a generalized seizure.

Simple partial seizures

A simple partial seizure can be present in several ways depending upon the focal point of the seizure in the brain.

- Motor symptoms (jerking of the thumb or the cheek)
- Somatosensory symptoms (visual, vestibular, gustatory, olfactory or auditory hallucinations or sensations)
- Autonomic symptoms (such as tachycardia, sweating, pupillary dilation)
- Psychic symptoms (which rarely occur without some changes in consciousness such as feelings of déjà vu or dreamy states).

Complex partial seizures

Consciousness becomes impaired with a complex partial seizure. This type of seizure begins as a simple partial seizure in which the consciousness isn't impaired and evolves to an impairment of consciousness. The same symptoms that present during a simple partial seizure are still seen as the seizure develops into a complex partial seizure.

Partial seizures evolving to generalized tonic-clonic seizures

A partial seizure can be either a simple partial or a complex partial seizure that progresses to a generalized seizure. An aura may precede the progression. Loss of consciousness occurs immediately or within 1 to 2 minutes of the start of the progression.

Generalized seizures (convulsive or nonconvulsive)

As the term suggests, generalized seizures cause a general electrical abnormality within the brain. They include several distinct types.

Absence (petit mal) seizures

An absence seizure occurs commonly in children, but it may also affect adults. It usually begins with a brief change in the level of consciousness, indicated by blinking or rolling of the eyes, or a blank stare, and slight mouth movements. Typically, the seizure lasts 1 to 10 seconds. The impairment is so brief that the patient (or parent) is sometimes unaware of it. If not properly treated, these seizures can recur as often as 100 times per day and may result in learning difficulties.

Myoclonic seizures

A myoclonic seizure is marked by brief bilateral muscular jerks of the body extremities. They may occur in a rhythmic manner and may be accompanied by brief loss of consciousness.

Generalized tonic-clonic (grand mal) seizures

Typically, a generalized tonic-clonic seizure begins with a loud cry, precipitated by air rushing from the lungs through the vocal cords. The patient falls to the ground, losing consciousness. The body stiffens (tonic phase) and then alternates between episodes of muscle spasm and relaxation (clonic phase). Tongue biting, incontinence, labored breathing, apnea, and subsequent cyanosis may also occur. The seizure stops in 2 to 5 minutes, when abnormal electrical conduction of the neurons is completed. The patient then regains consciousness but is somewhat confused and may have difficulty talking. If he can talk, he may complain of drowsiness, fatigue, headache, muscle soreness, and arm or leg weakness. He may fall into a deep sleep after the seizure.

Atonic seizures (drop attacks)

Characterized by a general loss of postural tone and a temporary loss of consciousness, an atonic seizure occurs in young children. It's sometimes called a "drop attack" because it causes the child to fall.

Precautions for generalized seizures

By taking appropriate precautions, you can help protect a patient from injury, aspiration, and airway obstruction should he have a seizure. Plan your precautions using information obtained from the patient's history. What kind of seizure has the patient previously had? Is he aware of exacerbating factors? Sleep deprivation, missed doses of anticonvulsants, and even upper respiratory infections can increase seizure frequency in some people who've had seizures. Was his previous seizure an acute episode, or did it result from a chronic condition?

Gather the equipment

Based on answers provided in the patient's history, you can tailor your precautions to his needs. Start by gathering the appropriate equipment, including a hospital bed with full-length side rails, commercial side rail pads or six bath blankets (four for a crib), adhesive tape, an oral airway, and oral or nasal suction equipment.

Bedside preparations

Carry out the precautions you think appropriate for the patient. Remember that a patient with preexisting seizures who's being admitted for a change in medication, treatment of an infection, or detoxification may have an increased risk of seizures.

- Explain the reasons for the precautions to the patient.
- *To protect the patient's limbs, head, and feet from injury if he has a seizure while in bed,* cover the side rails, headboard, and footboard with side rail pads or bath blankets. If you use blankets, keep them in place with adhesive tape. Keep the side rails raised while the patient is in bed *to prevent falls.* Keep the bed in a low position *to minimize any injuries that may occur if the patient climbs over the rails.*
- Place an airway at the patient's bedside, or tape it to the wall above the bed according to your facility's protocol. Keep suction equipment, oxygen, a mask, and a handheld resuscitation bag nearby *in case you need to establish a patent airway.* Explain to the patient how the airway will be used.
- If the patient has frequent or prolonged seizures, prepare an I.V. saline lock *to facilitate administration of emergency medications.*

out regaining consciousness, requires immediate medical intervention.

Equipment

Oral airway ▪ suction equipment ▪ side rail pads ▪ additional equipment: I.V. line, normal saline solution, oxygen, endotracheal tube, intubation equipment.

Implementation

- If you are with a patient when he experiences an aura, help him into bed, raise the side rails, and adjust the bed flat. If he's away from his room, lower him to the floor and place a pillow, blanket, or other soft material under his head *to keep it from hitting the floor.*
- Provide privacy, if possible.
- When you have a patient in the hospital who has a known seizure history, maintain I.V. access or a saline lock so that if he does have a seizure, there's I.V. access *to administer medications.*
- Stay with the patient during the seizure, and be ready to intervene if complications such as airway obstruction develop. If necessary, have another staff member obtain the appropriate equipment and notify the practitioner of the obstruction.
- Depending on your facility's policy, if the patient is in the beginning of the tonic phase of the seizure, you may insert an oral airway into his mouth *so that his tongue doesn't block his airway.* If an oral airway isn't available, don't try to hold his mouth open or place your hands inside *because you may be bitten.* After the patient's jaw becomes rigid, don't force the airway into place *because you could break his teeth or cause another injury.* Turn the patient to his side *to allow secretions to drain and the tongue to fall forward.* Never force any objects into the patient's mouth unless his airway is compromised.
- Move hard or sharp objects out of the patient's way, and loosen his clothing.
- Don't forcibly restrain the patient or restrict his movements during the seizure *because the force of the patient's movements against restraints could cause muscle strain or even joint dislocation.*
- Continually assess the patient during the seizure. Observe the earliest symptom, such as head or eye deviation as well as how the seizure progresses, what form it takes, and how long it lasts. *Your description may help determine the seizure's type and cause.*
- If this is the patient's first seizure, notify the practitioner immediately. If the patient has had seizures before, notify the practitioner only if the seizure activity is prolonged or if the patient fails to regain consciousness. (See *Understanding status epilepticus.*)

- If ordered, establish an I.V. line and infuse normal saline solution at a keep-vein-open rate.
- If the seizure is prolonged and the patient becomes hypoxemic, administer oxygen as ordered. Some patients may require endotracheal intubation.
- For a patient known to be diabetic, administer 50 ml of dextrose 50% in water by I.V. push as ordered. For a patient known to be an alcoholic, a 100-mg bolus of thiamine may be ordered to stop the seizure.
- After the seizure, turn the patient on his side and apply suction if necessary *to facilitate drainage of secretions and maintain a patent airway.* Insert an oral airway, if needed.
- Check for injuries.
- Reorient and reassure the patient, as necessary.
- When the patient is comfortable and safe, document what happened during the seizure.
- After the seizure, monitor vital signs and mental status every 15 to 20 minutes for 2 hours.
- Ask the patient about his aura and activities preceding the seizure. *The type of aura (auditory, visual, olfactory, gustatory, or somatic) helps pinpoint the site in the brain where the seizure originated.*

Understanding status epilepticus

A continuous seizure state unless interrupted by emergency interventions, status epilepticus can occur in all seizure types. The most life-threatening example is *generalized tonic-clonic status epilepticus*, a continuous generalized tonic-clonic seizure without intervening return of consciousness.

Status epilepticus, always an emergency, is accompanied by respiratory distress. It can result from abrupt withdrawal of anticonvulsant medications, hypoxic or metabolic encephalopathy, acute head trauma, or septicemia secondary to encephalitis or meningitis.

Emergency treatment of status epilepticus usually consists of diazepam, lorazepam, fosphenytoin, or phenobarbital; dextrose 50% I.V. (when seizures are secondary to hypoglycemia); and thiamine I.V. (in the presence of chronic alcoholism or withdrawal).

Special considerations

- *Because a seizure commonly indicates an underlying disorder,* a complete diagnostic workup will be ordered if the cause of the seizure isn't evident.

Complications

The patient who experiences a seizure may experience an injury, respiratory difficulty, and decreased mental capability. Common injuries include scrapes and bruises suffered when the patient hits objects during the seizure and traumatic injury to the tongue caused by biting. If you suspect a serious injury, such as a fracture or deep laceration, notify the practitioner and arrange for appropriate evaluation and treatment.

Changes in respiratory function may include aspiration, airway obstruction, and hypoxemia. After the seizure, complete a respiratory assessment and notify the practitioner if you suspect a problem. Expect most patients to experience a postictal period of decreased mental status lasting 30 minutes to 24 hours. Reassure the patient that this doesn't indicate incipient brain damage.

Documentation

Document that the patient requires seizure precautions, and record all precautions taken. Record the date and the time the seizure began as well as its duration and any precipitating factors. Identify any sensation that may be considered an aura. If the seizure was preceded by an aura, have the patient describe what he experienced.

Record any involuntary behavior that occurred at the onset, such as lip smacking, chewing movements, or hand and eye movements. Describe where the movement began and the parts of the body involved. Note any progression or pattern to the activity. Document whether the patient's eyes deviated to one side and whether the pupils changed in size, shape, equality, or reaction to light. Note if the patient's teeth were clenched or open. Record any incontinence, vomiting, or salivation that occurred during the seizure.

Note the patient's response to the seizure. Was he aware of what happened? Did he fall into a deep sleep following the seizure? Was he upset or ashamed? Document any medications given, any complications experienced during the seizure, and any interventions performed. Finally, record the patient's postseizure mental status.

SELECTED REFERENCES

ACEP Clinical Policies Committee; Clinical Policies Subcommittee on Seizures. "Clinical Policy: Critical Issues in the Evaluation and Management of Adult Patients Presenting to the Emergency Department with Seizures," *Annals of Emergency Medicine* 43(5):605-25, May 2004.

Armon, K., and Baumer, J.H. "Evidence-Based Guideline for Post-Seizure Management," *Archives of Diseases in Childhood* 89(11):1077, November 2004.

Cincinnati Prehospital Stroke Scale

This scale identifies a high percentage of acute strokes in patients by focusing on three physical findings.

Facial droop

Ask the patient to smile or show his teeth.

- Normal—both sides of the patient's face move equally
- Abnormal—one side of the face doesn't move or move as well as the other side

Arm drift

Ask the patient to close his eyes and extend his arms out in front of him for 10 seconds.

- Normal—both arms move the same or not at all
- Abnormal—one arm doesn't move, or one arm drifts compared with the other

Abnormal speech

Ask the patient to repeat the sentence "You can't teach an old dog new tricks."

- Normal—the patient can say the sentence with no slurring and uses the correct words
- Abnormal—words are slurred, the patient can't speak, or he uses the wrong words

If the patient experiences any one of the three abnormal physical findings, the probability that he's had a stroke is 72%.

Lynn-McHale Wiegand, D.J., and Carlson, K.K. eds. *AACN Procedure Manual for Critical Care,* 5th ed. Philadelphia: W.B. Saunders Co., 2005.

Taylor, C., et al. *Fundamentals of Nursing: The Art and Science of Nursing Care,* 6th ed. Philadelphia: Lippincott Williams & Wilkins, 2008.

Stroke management

A stroke is a sudden impairment of cerebral circulation in one or more of the blood vessels supplying the brain. A stroke interrupts or diminishes oxygen supply and commonly causes serious damage or necrosis in brain tissues. The sooner circulation returns to normal after a stroke, the better chances are for complete recovery. However, about one-half of those who survive a stroke remain permanently disabled and experience a recurrence within weeks, months, or years.

The major causes of stroke are thrombosis, embolism, and hemorrhage. Thrombosis is the most common cause in middle-age and elderly people, who have a higher incidence of atherosclerosis, diabetes, and hypertension. Thrombosis causes ischemia in brain tissue supplied by the affected vessel as well as congestion and edema; the latter may produce more clinical adverse effects than the thrombosis itself, but these symptoms subside with the edema.

Embolism, the second most common cause of stroke, is an occlusion of a blood vessel caused by a fragmented clot, a tumor, fat, bacteria, or air. It can occur at any age, especially among patients with a history of rheumatic heart disease, endocarditis, posttraumatic valvular disease, or myocardial fibrillation and other cardiac arrhythmias. It can also occur after open-heart surgery.

Hemorrhagic stroke results from chronic hypertension or aneurysms, which cause sudden rupture of a cerebral artery, thereby diminishing blood supply to the area served by the artery. In addition, blood accumulates deep within the brain, further compressing neural tissue and causing even greater damage.

Early treatment of a stroke relies heavily on early recognition and detection of signs and symptoms of a stroke and prompt activation of the emergency medical service (EMS) system. Stroke and transient ischemic shock can be correctly identified in three of four people using the Cincinnati Prehospital Stroke Scale. Nurses and physicians can evaluate the patient using this scale in less than 1 minute. (See *Cincinnati Prehospital Stroke Scale.*)

EMS providers should establish the precise time and onset of stroke signs and symptoms. The time of onset must be obtained to evaluate the patient for fibrinolytic therapy. Early notification of emergency department personnel enables them to prepare for the arrival of a stroke patient and shortens the time required to determine whether the patient has indications for acute stroke therapy.

Implementation

- During the acute phase, focus efforts on survival needs and prevention of further complications. Emergency department personnel should assess a patient suspected of having a stroke within 10 minutes. (See *Algorithm for suspected stroke.*)

Algorithm for suspected stroke

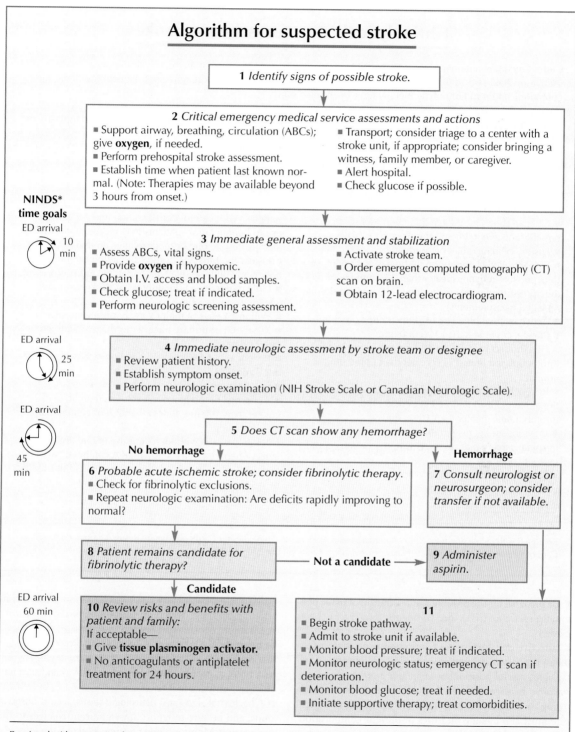

1 *Identify signs of possible stroke.*

2 *Critical emergency medical service assessments and actions*
- Support airway, breathing, circulation (ABCs); give **oxygen**, if needed.
- Perform prehospital stroke assessment.
- Establish time when patient last known normal. (Note: Therapies may be available beyond 3 hours from onset.)
- Transport; consider triage to a center with a stroke unit, if appropriate; consider bringing a witness, family member, or caregiver.
- Alert hospital.
- Check glucose if possible.

NINDS* time goals

ED arrival 10 min

3 *Immediate general assessment and stabilization*
- Assess ABCs, vital signs.
- Provide **oxygen** if hypoxemic.
- Obtain I.V. access and blood samples.
- Check glucose; treat if indicated.
- Perform neurologic screening assessment.
- Activate stroke team.
- Order emergent computed tomography (CT) scan on brain.
- Obtain 12-lead electrocardiogram.

ED arrival 25 min

4 *Immediate neurologic assessment by stroke team or designee*
- Review patient history.
- Establish symptom onset.
- Perform neurologic examination (NIH Stroke Scale or Canadian Neurologic Scale).

ED arrival 45 min

5 *Does CT scan show any hemorrhage?*

No hemorrhage

6 *Probable acute ischemic stroke; consider fibrinolytic therapy.*
- Check for fibrinolytic exclusions.
- Repeat neurologic examination: Are deficits rapidly improving to normal?

Hemorrhage

7 *Consult neurologist or neurosurgeon; consider transfer if not available.*

8 *Patient remains candidate for fibrinolytic therapy?*

Not a candidate → **9** *Administer aspirin.*

Candidate

ED arrival 60 min

10 *Review risks and benefits with patient and family:*
If acceptable—
- Give **tissue plasminogen activator.**
- No anticoagulants or antiplatelet treatment for 24 hours.

11
- Begin stroke pathway.
- Admit to stroke unit if available.
- Monitor blood pressure; treat if indicated.
- Monitor neurologic status; emergency CT scan if deterioration.
- Monitor blood glucose; treat if needed.
- Initiate supportive therapy; treat comorbidities.

Fibrinolytic therapy for ischemic stroke

Current recommendations of the American Heart Association (AHA) state that the tissue plasminogen activator (tPA) (Activase) should be administered to carefully selected patients, with strict adherence to treatment protocols, after contraindications to fibrinolytic therapy have been ruled out.

Contraindications

AHA guidelines contraindicate fibrinolytic therapy in a patient with any of the following factors:

- Evidence of intracranial bleeding on pretreatment noncontrast computed tomography (CT) scan
- Suspicion of a subarachnoid hemorrhage despite normal findings on CT scan
- CT scan shows multilobal infarction (denser than one-third of cerebral hemisphere)
- History of intracranial hemorrhage
- Uncontrolled hypertension (at time of treatment, systolic pressure remains greater than 185 mm Hg or diastolic pressure remains greater than 110 mm Hg despite repeated measurements)
- Active internal bleeding or acute trauma (fracture)
- Platelet count less than 100,000 mm^3
- Heparin received within 48 hours resulting in partial thromboplastin time (PTT) greater than upper limit of normal
- Recent use of an anticoagulant and elevated International Normalized Ration (INR) greater than 1.7 or prothrombin time greater than 15 seconds
- Previous stroke, head trauma, or intracranial or intraspinal surgery that occurred within 3 months of the current condition
- Arterial puncture at a noncompressible site within past 7 days
- History of arteriovenous malformation, neoplasm, or aneurysm
- Witnessed seizure at onset of stroke

Relative contraindications and precautions

Recent experience suggests that under some circumstances—with careful consideration and weighing of risk-to-benefit ratio—patients may receive fibrinolytic therapy despite one or more relative contraindications. Consider the pros and cons of tPA administration carefully if any of these relative contraindications is present:

- Only minor or rapidly improving stroke symptoms (clearing spontaneously)
- Within 14 days of major surgery or serious trauma
- Recent GI or urinary tract hemorrhage (within previous 21 days)
- Recent acute myocardial infarction (MI) (within previous 3 months)
- Post-MI pericarditis
- Abnormal blood glucose level (less than 50 or greater than 400 mg/dl [less than 2.8 or greater than 22.2 mmol/L])

Note: In patients without recent use of oral anticoagulants or heparin, treatment with tPA can be initiated before availability of coagulation study results but should be discontinued if the INR is greater than 1.7 or the PTT is elevated by local laboratory standards.

- Be prepared for the possible administration of tissue plasminogen activator (tPA). (See *Fibrinolytic therapy for ischemic stroke.*)
- Effective care emphasizes continuing neurologic assessment, support of respiration, continuous monitoring of vital signs, careful positioning *to prevent aspiration and contractures,* management of GI problems, and careful monitoring of fluid, electrolyte, and nutritional status. Patient care must also include measures to prevent complications such as infection.
- Maintain a patent airway and oxygenation. Loosen constricting clothing. Watch for ballooning of the cheek with respiration. *The side that balloons is usually the side affected by the stroke.* If the patient is unconscious, keep him in a lateral position *to allow secretions to drain naturally,* or suction secretions, as needed. Insert an artificial airway and start mechanical ventilation, if necessary.
- Check vital signs and neurologic status, record observations, and be sure to report any significant changes to the practitioner. Monitor blood pressure, level of consciousness, pupillary changes, motor function (voluntary and involun-

tary), sensory function, speech, skin color, temperature, and signs of increased intracranial pressure (ICP), nuchal rigidity, or flaccidity.

- Maintain fluid and electrolyte balance. If the patient can take liquids orally, offer them as often as fluid limitations permit. Administer I.V. fluids as ordered. Never give too much I.V. fluid too fast *because doing so can increase ICP.*
- Offer the urinal or bedpan every 2 hours. If the patient is incontinent, he may need an indwelling catheter, but this should be avoided, if possible, *because indwelling catheters increase risk of infection.*
- Check for gag reflex before offering small oral feedings of semisolid foods. Place the food tray within the patient's visual field *because loss of peripheral vision is common.* If oral feedings aren't possible, insert a nasogastric tube.
- Be alert for signs that the patient is straining during elimination *because this also raises ICP.* Modify diet and administer stool softeners and laxatives as ordered.
- Provide meticulous mouth care. Clean and irrigate the patient's mouth to remove food particles. Care for his dentures, as needed.
- Provide meticulous eye care. Remove secretions with a cotton ball and sterile normal saline solution. Instill eye drops, as ordered. Patch the patient's affected eye if he can't close his lid.
- Maintain correct body alignment and positioning. Use high-topped sneakers *to prevent footdrop and contracture,* and convoluted foam, flotation, sheepskin, or pulsating mattresses *to prevent pressure ulcers.* Elevate affected limbs *to control dependent edema.*
- *To prevent pneumonia,* turn the patient at least every 2 hours.
- Assist the patient with exercise. Perform range-of-motion exercises for the affected and unaffected sides. Teach and encourage the patient to use his unaffected side and to exercise his affected side.
- Give medications, as ordered, and watch for and report adverse effects.
- Establish and maintain communication with the patient. If he's aphasic, set up a simple method of communicating basic needs. Phrase your questions so he can answer using this system. Repeat yourself quietly and calmly and use gestures, if necessary, to help him understand.
- Provide psychological support. Set realistic short-term goals. Involve the patient's family in his care when possible, and explain his deficits and strengths.

Special considerations

- Remember that if a stroke is impending, blood pressure rises suddenly, pulse is rapid and bounding, and the patient may complain of a headache.
- If surgery is scheduled, provide preoperative teaching. Make sure the patient and his family understand the surgery and its possible adverse effects.

Home care

Teach the patient and his family about the disorder. Explain the diagnostic tests, treatments, and rehabilitation he'll have to undergo.

Review ways to decrease the risk of future stroke, such as smoking cessation, maintenance of ideal weight with prescribed diet, control of diabetes and hypertension and minimization of stress, and avoidance of prolonged bed rest.

Teach the patient and his family about the schedule, dosage actions, and adverse effects of prescribed drugs. Make sure the patient taking aspirin realizes that he can't substitute acetaminophen for aspirin.

Review signs and symptoms of impending stroke, and advise the patient to seek prompt treatment if signs occur.

Documentation

Document the patient's vital signs and neurologic assessment findings on a special flowchart. If the patient was started on tPA, be sure to record date, time, and patient reaction to the medication as well as any patient teaching you performed.

SELECTED REFERENCES

American Heart Association. "2005 AHA Guidelines for Cardiopulmonary Resuscitation and Emergency Cardiovascular Care. Part 9: Adult Stroke," *Circulation* 112(Suppl 22):IV-111-IV-120, November 2005.

Hickey, J.V. *The Clinical Practice of Neurological and Neurosurgical Nursing,* 5th ed. Philadelphia: Lippincott Williams & Wilkins, 2003.

Lawson, C. "Best Practice in Management of Patients with Acute Stroke," *Nursing Times* 102(34):28-30, August 2006.

Lynn-McHale Wiegand, D.J., and Carlson, K.K., eds. *AACN Procedure Manual for Critical Care,* 5th ed. Philadelphia: W.B. Saunders Co., 2005.

10 ■ Gastrointestinal care

INTRODUCTION

GI conditions affect just about everyone at one time or another. These conditions, so intimately tied to psychological health and stability, range from simple changes in bowel habits to life-threatening disorders requiring major surgery and radical lifestyle changes.

Patient care for GI conditions also varies widely. For example, the patient with simple constipation may need only brief teaching about diet and exercise. However, the patient with colorectal cancer may need ongoing nursing care ranging from encouragement and support during the diagnostic workup to meticulous colostomy care during recovery.

Your role in GI procedures

Therapeutic GI procedures reflect the wide spectrum of systemic abnormalities. They may involve feeding a patient through a tube, teaching a patient how to use a gastrostomy feeding button, or minimizing a patient's anxiety before abdominal surgery or his discomfort after it.

To carry out responsibilities like these successfully, you need to address both the emotional and the physical needs of the patient. Decisions, such as where to place an incision or which type of colostomy to use, have important emotional implications for the patient. Your knowledge of anatomy and physiology as well as your familiarity with surgical procedures will influence your care plan and, ultimately, how the patient responds.

Patients undergoing certain GI procedures, especially those that are uncomfortable or embarrassing, require considerable emotional support. Helping such patients maintain their sense of dignity, while at the same time eliciting their cooperation, requires a skillful blend of compassion and judgment.

For many GI procedures, you'll need to work cooperatively with other staff members, including the pharmacist, physicians, laboratory personnel, diagnostic technicians, dietitians, and the case manager.

NASAL AND ORAL ACCESS

NASOGASTRIC TUBE INSERTION AND REMOVAL

Usually inserted to decompress the stomach, a nasogastric (NG) tube can prevent vomiting after major surgery. An NG tube is typically in place for 48 to 72 hours after surgery, by which time peristalsis usually resumes. It may remain in place for shorter or longer periods, however, depending on its use.

The NG tube has other diagnostic and therapeutic applications, especially in assessing and treating upper GI bleeding, collecting gastric contents for analysis, performing gastric lavage, aspirating gastric secretions, and administering medications and nutrients.

Inserting an NG tube requires close observation of the patient and verification of proper placement. Removing the tube requires careful handling to prevent injury or aspiration. The tube must be inserted with extra care in pregnant patients and in those with an increased risk of complications. For example, the practitioner will order an NG tube for a patient with aortic aneurysm, myocardial infarction, gastric hemorrhage, or esophageal varices only if he believes that the benefits outweigh the risks of intubation.

Most NG tubes have a radiopaque marker or strip at the distal end so that the tube's position can be verified by X-ray studies. If the position can't be confirmed, the practitioner may order fluoroscopy to verify placement.

The most common NG tubes are the Levin tube, which has one lumen, and the Salem sump tube, which has two lumens, one for suction and drainage and a smaller one for ventilation. Air flows through the vent lumen continuously. This protects the delicate gastric mucosa by preventing a vacuum from forming should the tube adhere to the stomach lining. (See *Types of NG tubes.*)

Equipment

For inserting an NG tube: Tube (usually #12, #14, #16, or #18 French for a normal adult) ▪ towel or linen-saver pad ▪ facial tissues ▪ emesis basin ▪ penlight ▪ 1″ or 2″ hypoallergenic tape ▪ gloves ▪ water-soluble lubricant ▪ cup or glass of water with straw (if appropriate) ▪ pH test strip ▪ tongue blade ▪ catheter-tip or bulb syringe or irrigation set ▪ safety pin ▪ ordered suction equipment ▪ alcohol pad, if needed ▪ optional: ice, warm water, rubber band.

For removing an NG tube: Gloves ▪ catheter-tip syringe ▪ normal saline solution ▪ towel or linen-saver pad ▪ adhesive remover ▪ mouth care supplies.

Preparation of equipment

Inspect the NG tube for defects, such as rough edges or partially closed lumens. Then check the tube's patency by flushing it with water. *To ease insertion,* increase a stiff tube's flexibility by coiling it around your gloved fingers for a few seconds or by dipping it into warm water. Stiffen a limp rubber tube by briefly chilling it in ice.

EQUIPMENT

Types of NG tubes

The practitioner will choose the type and diameter of nasogastric (NG) tube that best suits the patient's needs, including lavage, aspiration, enteral therapy, or stomach decompression. Choices may include the Levin and Salem sump tubes.

Levin tube

The Levin tube is a rubber or plastic tube that has a single lumen, a length of 42″ to 50″ (106.5 to 127 cm), and holes at the tip and along the side.

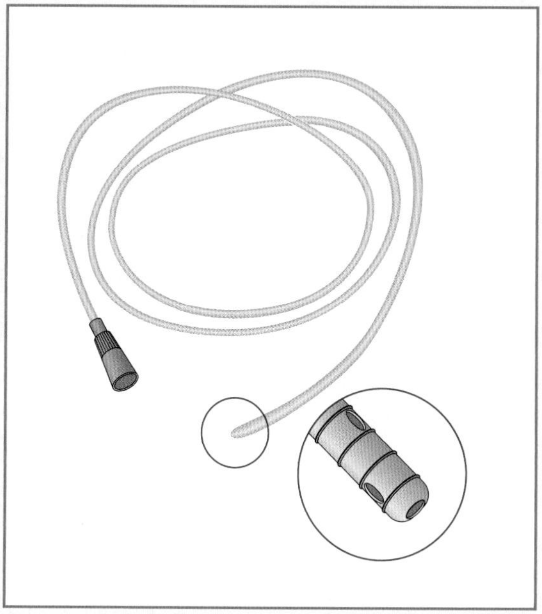

Salem sump tube

A Salem sump tube is a double-lumen tube that is made of clear plastic and has a blue sump port (pigtail) that allows atmospheric air to enter the patient's stomach. Thus, the tube floats freely and doesn't adhere to or damage gastric mucosa. The larger port of this 48″ (122-cm) tube serves as the main suction conduit. The tube has openings at 45, 55, 65, and 75 cm as well as a radiopaque line to verify placement.

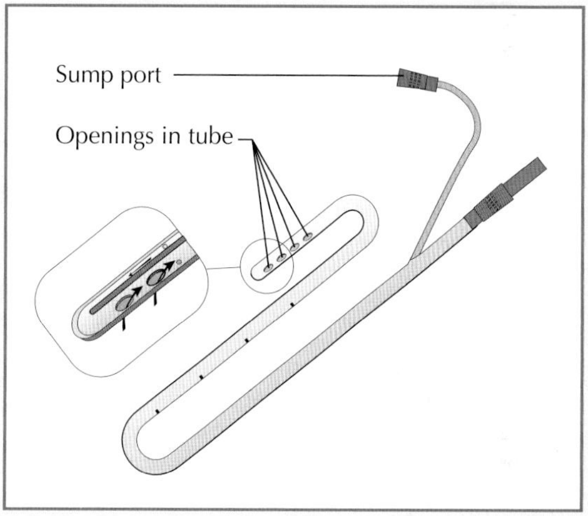

Levin tube illustration courtesy of National Catheter Co., Argyle, N.Y.

Implementation

- Whether you're inserting or removing an NG tube, be sure to provide privacy, wash your hands, and put on gloves before inserting the tube. Check the practitioner's order to determine the type of tube that should be inserted.

Inserting an NG tube

- Confirm the patient's identity using two patient identifiers according to your facility's policy.
- Explain the procedure to the patient *to ease anxiety and promote cooperation.* Inform her that she may experience some nasal discomfort, that she may gag, and that her eyes may water. Emphasize that swallowing will ease the tube's advancement.
- Agree on a signal that the patient can use if she wants you to stop briefly during the procedure.
- Gather and prepare all necessary equipment.
- Help the patient into high Fowler's position unless contraindicated.
- Stand at the patient's right side if you're right-handed or at her left side if you're left-handed *to ease insertion.*
- Drape the towel or linen-saver pad over the patient's chest *to protect her gown and bed linens from spills.*
- Have the patient gently blow her nose *to clear her nostrils.*
- Place the facial tissues and emesis basin well within the patient's reach.
- Help the patient face forward with her neck in a neutral position.

■ *To determine how long the NG tube must be to reach the stomach,* hold the end of the tube at the tip of the patient's nose. Extend the tube to the patient's earlobe and then down to the xiphoid process (as shown below).

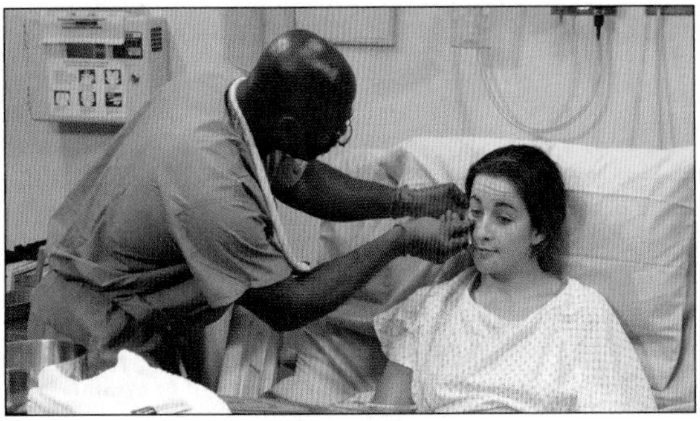

■ Mark this distance on the tubing with the tape. (Average measurements for an adult range from 22″ to 26″ [56 to 66 cm].) It may be necessary to add 2″ (5 cm) to this measurement in tall individuals *to ensure entry into the stomach.*
■ *To determine which nostril will allow easier access,* use a penlight and inspect for a deviated septum or other abnormalities. Ask the patient if she ever had nasal surgery or a nasal injury. Assess airflow in both nostrils by occluding one nostril at a time while the patient breathes through her nose. Choose the nostril with the better airflow. If the patient is able to respond, ask whether she has had an NG tube placed previously. If so, ask which nostril is better for insertion.
■ Lubricate the first 3″ (7.6 cm) of the tube with a water-soluble gel *to minimize injury to the nasal passages. Using a water-soluble lubricant prevents lipoid pneumonia,* which may result from aspiration of an oil-based lubricant or from accidental slippage of the tube into the trachea.
■ Instruct the patient to hold her head straight and upright.
■ Grasp the tube with the end pointing downward, curve it if necessary, and carefully insert it into the more patent nostril (as shown below).

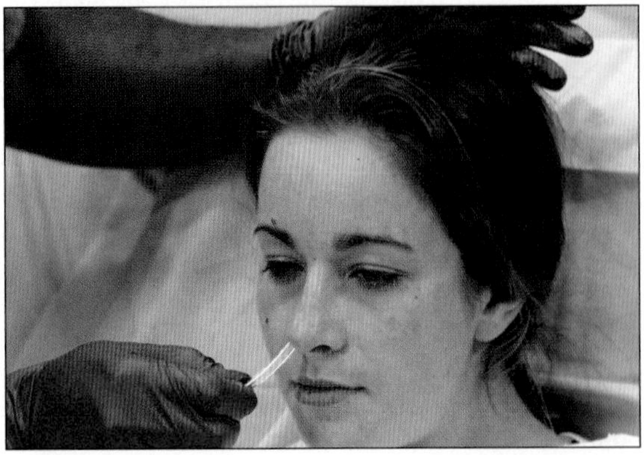

■ Aim the tube downward and toward the ear closer to the chosen nostril. Advance it slowly *to avoid pressure on the turbinates and resultant pain and bleeding.*
■ When the tube reaches the nasopharynx, you'll feel resistance. Instruct the patient to lower her head slightly *to close the trachea and open the esophagus.* Then rotate the tube 180 degrees toward the opposite nostril *to redirect it so that the tube won't enter the patient's mouth.*
■ Unless contraindicated, offer the patient a cup or glass of water with a straw. Direct her to sip and swallow as you slowly advance the tube (as shown below). *This helps the tube pass to the esophagus.* (If you aren't using water, ask the patient to swallow.)

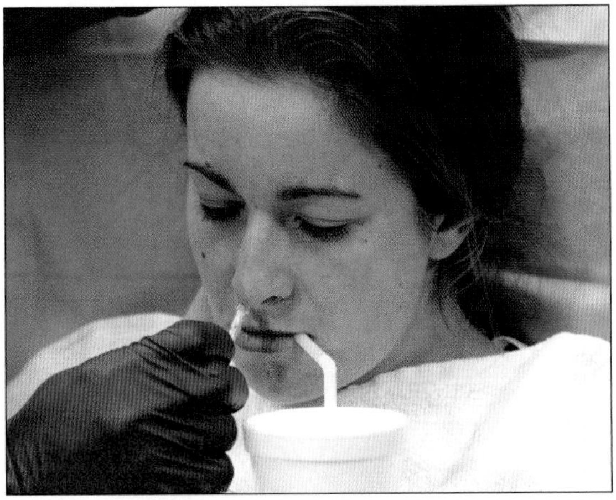

Ensuring proper tube placement

■ Use a tongue blade and penlight to examine the patient's mouth and throat for signs of a coiled section of tubing (especially in an unconscious patient). *Coiling indicates an obstruction.*
■ Keep an emesis basin and facial tissues readily available for the patient.
■ As you carefully advance the tube and the patient swallows, watch for respiratory distress signs, *which may mean the tube is in the bronchus and must be removed immediately.*
■ Stop advancing the tube when the tape mark reaches the patient's nostril.
■ Attach a catheter-tip or bulb syringe to the tube and try to aspirate stomach contents (as shown top of next page). If you don't obtain stomach contents, position the patient on her left side to move the contents into the stomach's greater curvature, and aspirate again.

NURSING ALERT *When confirming tube placement, never place the tube's end in a container of water. If the tube should be malpositioned in the trachea, the patient may aspirate water. Water without bubbles doesn't confirm proper* *placement. Instead, the tube may be coiled in the trachea or the esophagus.*

■ Examine the aspirate and place a small amount on the pH test strip. Probability of gastric placement is increased if the aspirate has a typical gastric fluid appearance (grassy-green, clear and colorless with mucus shreds, or brown) and the pH is less than or equal to 5.0.

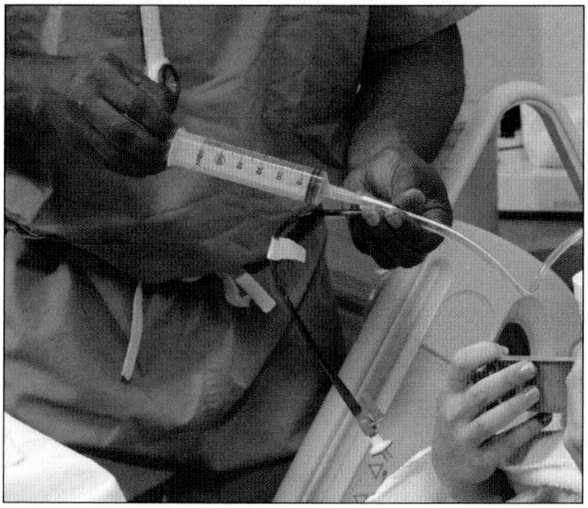

■ Ideally, proper tube placement should be confirmed by X-ray.

■ Secure the NG tube to the patient's nose with hypoallergenic tape (or other designated tube holder). If the patient's skin is oily, wipe the bridge of the nose with an alcohol pad and allow to dry. You will need about 4″ (10 cm) of 1″ tape. Split one end of the tape up the center about 1½″ (3.8 cm). Make tabs on the split ends (by folding sticky sides together). Stick the uncut tape end on the patient's nose so that the split in the tape starts about ½″ (1.3 cm) to 1½″ from the tip of her nose. Crisscross the tabbed ends around the tube (as shown below). Then apply another piece of tape over the bridge of the nose to secure the tube.

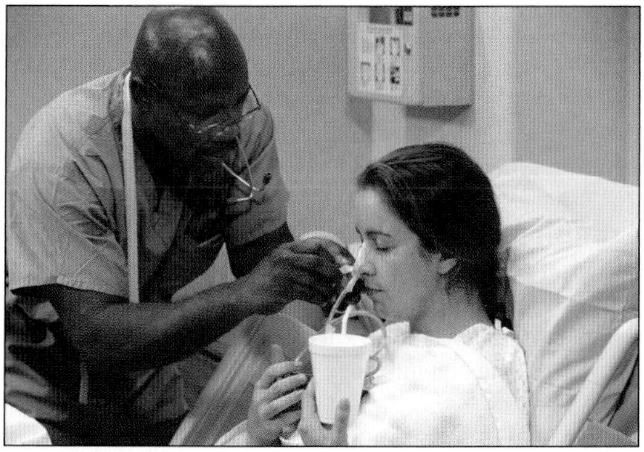

■ Alternatively, stabilize the tube with a prepackaged product that secures and cushions it at the nose.

■ *To reduce discomfort from the weight of the tube,* tie a slipknot around the tube with a rubber band, and then secure the rubber band to the patient's gown with a safety pin, or wrap another piece of tape around the end of the tube and leave a tab. Then fasten the tape tab to the patient's gown.

■ Attach the tube to suction equipment if ordered, and set the designated suction pressure.

■ Provide frequent nose and mouth care while the tube is in place.

Removing an NG tube

■ Explain the procedure to the patient, informing her that it may cause some nasal discomfort and sneezing or gagging.

■ Assess bowel function by auscultating for peristalsis or flatus.

■ Help the patient into semi-Fowler's position. Then drape a towel or linen-saver pad across her chest (as shown below) *to protect her gown and bed linens from spills.*

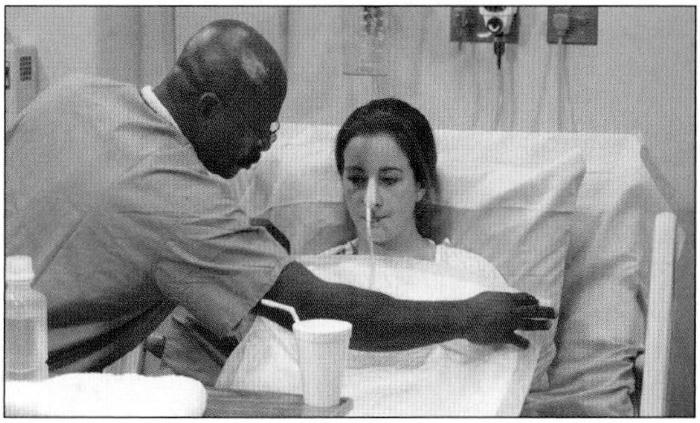

■ Wash your hands and put on gloves.

■ Using a catheter-tip syringe, flush the tube with 10 ml of air or normal saline solution (as shown below) *to ensure that the tube doesn't contain stomach contents that could irritate tissues during tube removal.*

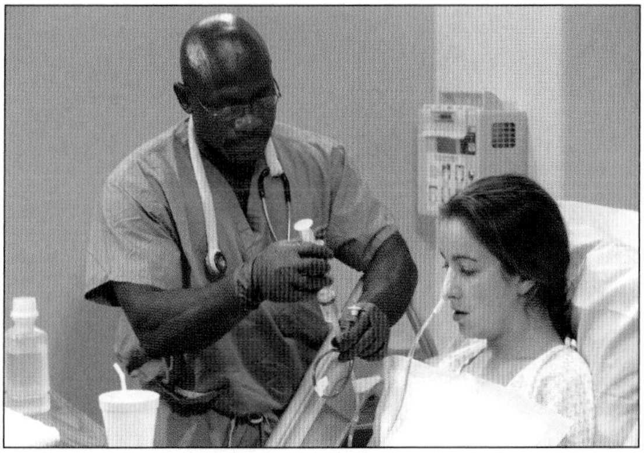

HOME CARE

Using an NG tube at home

If your patient will need to have a nasogastric (NG) tube in place at home—for short-term feeding or gastric decompression, for example—find out who will insert the tube. If the patient will have a home care nurse, identify her and, if possible, tell the patient when to expect her.

If the patient or a family member will perform the procedure, you'll need to provide additional instruction and supervision. Use this checklist to prepare your teaching topics:

- how and where to obtain equipment needed for home intubation
- how to insert the tube
- verifying tube placement by aspirating stomach contents
- correcting tube misplacement
- preparing formula for tube feeding
- how to store formula if appropriate
- administering formula through the tube
- how to remove and dispose of an NG tube
- how to clean and store a reusable NG tube
- how to use the NG tube for gastric decompression if appropriate
- how to set up and operate suctioning equipment
- troubleshooting suctioning equipment
- how to perform mouth care and other hygienic procedures.

- Untape the tube from the patient's nose, and then unpin it from her gown.
- Clamp the tube by folding it in your hand (as shown below).

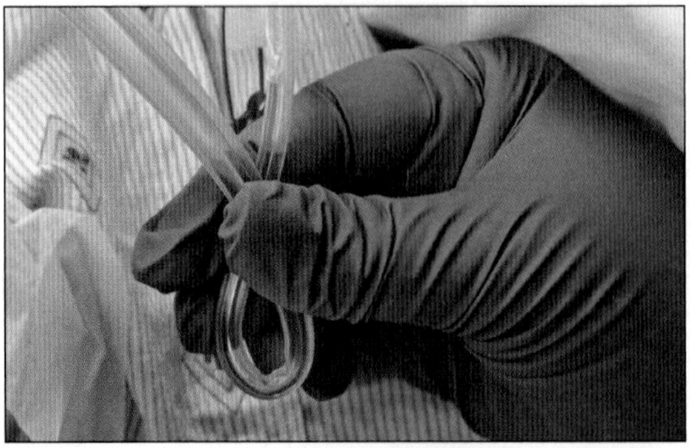

- Ask the patient to hold her breath *to close the epiglottis.* Then withdraw the tube gently and steadily. (When the distal end of the tube reaches the nasopharynx, you can pull it quickly.)
- When possible, immediately cover and remove the tube *because its sight and odor may nauseate the patient.*
- Assist the patient with thorough mouth care, and clean the tape residue from her nose with adhesive remover.
- For the next 48 hours, monitor the patient for signs of GI dysfunction, including nausea, vomiting, abdominal distention, and food intolerance. GI dysfunction may necessitate reinsertion of the tube.

Special considerations

- If the patient has a deviated septum or other nasal condition that prevents nasal insertion, pass the tube orally after removing any dentures, if necessary. Sliding the tube over the tongue, proceed as you would for nasal insertion.
- When using the oral route, remember to coil the end of the tube around your hand. *This helps curve and direct the tube downward at the pharynx.*
- If your patient is unconscious, tilt her chin toward her chest *to close the trachea.* Then advance the tube between respirations *to ensure that it doesn't enter the trachea.*
- While advancing the tube in an unconscious patient (or in a patient who can't swallow), stroke the patient's neck *to encourage the swallowing reflex and facilitate passage down the esophagus.*
- While advancing the tube, observe for signs that it has entered the trachea, such as choking or breathing difficulties in a conscious patient and cyanosis in an unconscious patient or a patient without a cough reflex. If these signs occur, remove the tube immediately. Allow the patient time to rest; then try to reinsert the tube.
- After tube placement, vomiting suggests tubal obstruction or incorrect position. Assess immediately to determine the cause.

Home care

An NG tube may be inserted or removed at home. Indications for insertion include gastric decompression and short-term feeding. A home care nurse or the patient may insert the tube, deliver the feeding, and remove the tube. (See *Using an NG tube at home.*)

Complications

Potential complications of prolonged intubation with an NG tube include skin erosion at the nostril, sinusitis, esophagitis, esophagotracheal fistula, gastric ulceration, and pulmonary and oral infection. Additional complications that may result from suction include electrolyte imbalances and dehydration.

Documentation

Record the type and size of the NG tube and the date, time, and route of insertion. Also note the type and amount of suction, if used, and describe the drainage, including the amount, color, character, consistency, and odor. Note the patient's tolerance of the procedure. Include in your notes any signs and symptoms signaling complications, such as nausea, vomiting, and abdominal distention. Document subsequent irrigation procedures and continuing problems after irrigation.

When you remove the tube, be sure to record the date and time. Describe the color, consistency, and amount of gastric drainage. Note any unusual events following NG removal, such as nausea, vomiting, abdominal distention, and food intolerance. Again, note the patient's tolerance of the procedure.

SELECTED REFERENCES

Higgins, D. "Nasogastric Tube Insertion," *Nursing Times* 101(37):28-29, September 2005.

Jones, A.P., et al. "Insertion of a Nasogastric Tube under Direct Vision," *Anaesthesia* 61(3):305, March 2006.

Khair, J. "Guidelines for Testing the Placing of Nasogastric Tubes," *Nursing Times* 101(20):26-27, May 2006.

May, S. "Testing Nasogastric Tube Positioning in the Critically Ill: Exploring the Evidence," *British Journal of Nursing* 16(7):414-18, April 2007.

Metheney, N., et al. "Effectiveness of pH Measurements in Predicting Feeding Tube Placement. An Update," *Nursing Research* 42(6):324-31, June 1993.

Metheney, N., et al. "Visual Characteristics of Aspirates from Feeding Tubes as a Method for Predicting Tube Location," *Nursing Research* 43(5):282-87, May 1994.

Metheney, N., and Titer, M. "Assessing Placement of Feeding Tubes," *AJN* 101(5):36-45, May 2001.

Taylor, C., et al. *Fundamentals of Nursing: The Art and Science of Nursing Care*, 6th ed. Philadelphia: Lippincott Williams & Wilkins, 2008.

NASOGASTRIC TUBE CARE

Providing effective nasogastric (NG) tube care requires meticulous monitoring of the patient and the equipment. Monitoring the patient involves checking drainage from the NG tube and assessing GI function. Monitoring the equipment involves verifying correct tube placement and irrigating the tube to ensure patency and to prevent mucosal damage.

Specific care measures vary only slightly for most of the commonly used NG tubes: the single-lumen Levin tube and the double-lumen Salem sump tube.

Equipment

Irrigant (usually normal saline solution) ■ irrigant container ■ 60-ml catheter-tip syringe or bulb syringe ■ suction equipment ■ sponge-tipped swabs or toothbrush and toothpaste ■ petroleum jelly ■ ½″ or 1″ hypoallergenic tape ■ water-soluble lubricant ■ gloves ■ pH test strip ■ linen-saver pad ■ optional: emesis basin.

Preparation of equipment

Make sure suction equipment works properly. (See *Common gastric suction devices,* page 664.) When using a Salem sump tube with suction, connect the larger, primary lumen (for drainage and suction) to suction equipment and select appropriate setting, as ordered (usually low constant suction). If the practitioner doesn't specify the setting, follow manufacturer's directions. A Levin tube usually calls for intermittent low suction.

Implementation

- Confirm the patient's identity using two patient identifiers according to your facility's policy.
- Explain the procedure and provide privacy.
- Wash your hands and put on gloves.

Irrigating an NG tube

- Review the irrigation schedule (usually every 4 hours) if the practitioner orders this procedure.
- Assess tube placement by looking for discrepancies in tube markings or by measuring the external tube length and comparing it with the length documented in the chart. Have the patient open his mouth so that you can check to see if the tube is coiled.
- Aspirate stomach contents *to check correct positioning and to prevent the patient from aspirating the irrigant.*
- Examine the aspirate and place a small amount on the pH test strip. Probability of gastric placement is increased if the aspirate has a typical gastric fluid appearance (grassy-green, clear and colorless with mucus shreds, or brown) and pH is less than or equal to 5.0.
- Measure the amount of irrigant in the bulb syringe or in the 60-ml catheter-tip syringe (usually 10 to 20 ml) *to maintain an accurate intake and output record.*
- When using suction, unclamp and disconnect the tube from the suction equipment while holding it over a linen-saver pad or an emesis basin *to collect any drainage.*
- Slowly instill the irrigant into the NG tube. (When irrigating the Salem sump tube, you may instill small amounts

EQUIPMENT

Common gastric suction devices

A variety of wall-mounted suction devices are available for applying negative pressure to nasogastric (NG) and other drainage tubes. Two common types are shown here.

Portable suction machine

In the portable suction machine, a vacuum created intermittently by an electric pump draws gastric contents up the NG tube and into the collecting bottle.

Stationary suction machine

A stationary wall-unit apparatus can provide intermittent or continuous suction. On-off switches and variable power settings let you set and adjust the suction force on either machine.

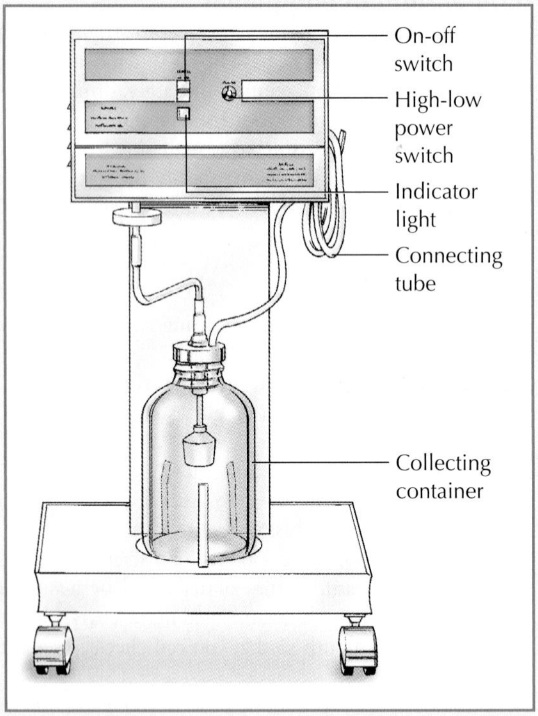

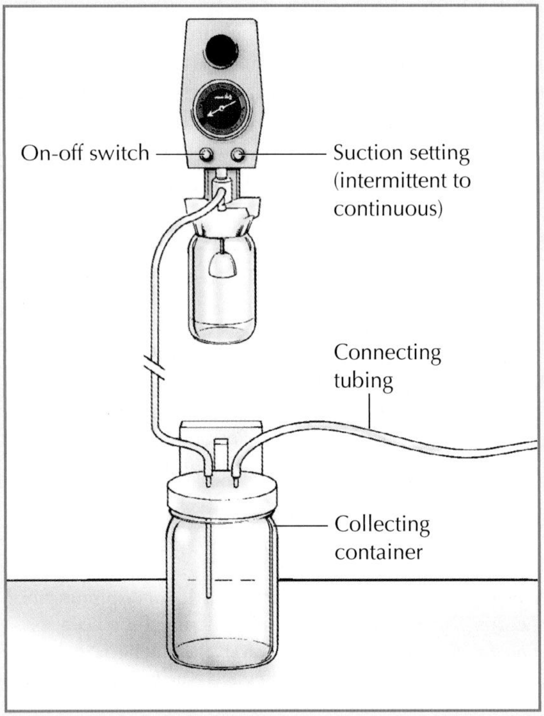

of solution into the vent lumen without interrupting suction; however, you should instill greater amounts into the larger, primary lumen.)

- Gently aspirate solution with a bulb syringe or 60-ml catheter-tip syringe or connect the tube to suction equipment, as ordered. *Gentle aspiration prevents excessive pressure on a suture line and on delicate gastric mucosa.* Report bleeding.
- Reconnect the tube to suction after completing irrigation.

Instilling a solution through an NG tube

- If the practitioner orders instillation, inject the solution, and don't aspirate it. Note the amount of instilled solution as "intake" on the intake and output record.
- Reattach the tube to suction, as ordered.
- After attaching the Salem sump tube's primary lumen to suction, instill 10 to 20 cc of air into the vent lumen *to verify patency.* Listen for a soft hiss in the vent. If you don't hear this sound, suspect a clogged tube; recheck patency by instilling 10 ml of normal saline solution and 10 to 20 cc of air in the vent.

Monitoring patient comfort and condition

■ Provide mouth care once a shift, or as needed. Depending on the patient's condition, use sponge-tipped swabs to clean his teeth or assist him to brush them with toothbrush and toothpaste. Coat the patient's lips with petroleum jelly *to prevent dryness from mouth breathing.*

■ Change the tape securing the tube as needed or at least daily. Clean the skin, apply fresh tape, and dab water-soluble lubricant on the nostrils, as needed.

■ Regularly check the tape that secures the tube *because sweat and nasal secretions may loosen the tape.*

■ Assess bowel sounds regularly (every 4 to 8 hours) *to verify GI function.*

■ Measure the drainage amount and update the intake and output record every 8 hours. Be alert for electrolyte imbalances with excessive gastric output.

■ Inspect gastric drainage and note its color, consistency, odor, and amount. Normal gastric secretions have no color or appear yellow-green from bile and have a mucoid consistency. Immediately report any drainage with a coffee-bean color; *this may indicate bleeding.* If you suspect that the drainage contains blood, use a screening test (such as Hematest) for occult blood according to your facility's policy.

Special considerations

■ Irrigate the NG tube with 30 ml of irrigant before and after instilling medication. (See "Nasogastric tube drug administration," page 295.) Clamp the tube and wait about 30 minutes, or as ordered, after instillation before reconnecting the suction equipment *to allow sufficient time for the medication to be absorbed.*

■ When no drainage appears, check the suction equipment for proper function. Then, holding the NG tube over a linen-saver pad or an emesis basin, separate the tube and the suction source. Check the suction equipment by placing the suction tubing in an irrigant container. If the apparatus draws the water, check the NG tube for proper function. Be sure to note the amount of water drawn into the suction container on the intake and output record.

■ A dysfunctional NG tube may be clogged or incorrectly positioned. Attempt to irrigate the tube, reposition the patient, or rotate and reposition the tube. However, if the tube was inserted during surgery, avoid this maneuver *to ensure that the movement doesn't interfere with gastric or esophageal sutures.* Notify the practitioner.

■ If you can ambulate the patient and interrupt suction, disconnect the NG tube from the suction equipment. Clamp the tube *to prevent stomach contents from draining out of the tube.*

■ If the patient has a Salem sump tube, watch for gastric reflux in the vent lumen when pressure in the stomach exceeds atmospheric pressure. This problem may result from a clogged primary lumen or from a suction system that is set up improperly. Assess the suction equipment for proper functioning. Then irrigate the NG tube and instill 30 cc of air into the vent tube *to maintain patency.* Don't attempt to stop reflux by clamping the vent tube. Unless contraindicated, elevate the patient's torso more than 30 degrees, and keep the vent tube above his midline *to prevent a siphoning effect.*

Complications

Epigastric pain and vomiting may result from a clogged or improperly placed tube. Any NG tube—the Levin tube in particular—can move and aggravate esophagitis, ulcers, or esophageal varices, causing hemorrhage. Perforation may result from aggressive intubation. Dehydration and electrolyte imbalances may result from removing body fluids and electrolytes by suctioning. Pain, swelling, and salivary dysfunction may signal parotitis, which occurs in dehydrated, debilitated patients. Intubation can cause nasal skin breakdown and discomfort and increased mucous secretions. Aspiration pneumonia may result from gastric reflux. Vigorous suction may damage the gastric mucosa and cause significant bleeding, possibly interfering with endoscopic assessment and diagnosis.

Documentation

Regularly record tube placement confirmation (usually every 4 to 8 hours). Keep a precise record of fluid intake and output, including the instilled irrigant in fluid input. Track the irrigation schedule and note the actual time of each irrigation. Describe drainage color, consistency, odor, and amount. Also note tape change times and condition of the nares.

SELECTED REFERENCES

Best, C. "Caring for the Patient with a Nasogastric Tube," *Nursing Standard* 20(3):59-65, September-October 2005.

McKay, L. "Nasogastric Intubation," *Nursing Standard* 20(24):63, February 2006.

Metheney, N., et al. "Effectiveness of pH Measurements in Predicting Feeding Tube Placement: An Update," *Nursing Research* 42(6):324-31, June 1993.

Richardson, D.S., et al. "An Evidence-Based Approach to Nasogastric Tube Management: Special Considerations," *Journal of Pediatric Nursing* 21(5):388-93, October 2006.

Taylor, C., et al. *Fundamentals of Nursing: The Art and Science of Nursing Care,* 6th ed. Philadelphia: Lippincott Williams & Wilkins, 2008.

Is iced lavage effective?

Most experts question the effectiveness of using an iced irrigant for gastric lavage to treat GI bleeding. Here's why.

Iced irrigating solutions stimulate the vagus nerve, which triggers increased hydrochloric acid secretion. In turn, this stimulates gastric motility, which can irritate the bleeding site.

Some physicians prefer using unchilled normal saline solution (which may prevent rapid electrolyte loss) or even water if the patient must avoid sodium. They point out that no research exists to support the use of an iced irrigant to stop acute GI bleeding.

Gastric lavage

After recent poisoning or a drug overdose, especially in patients who have central nervous system depression or an inadequate gag reflex, gastric lavage flushes the stomach and removes ingested substances through a gastric lavage tube. The procedure is also used to empty the stomach in preparation for endoscopic examination. For patients with gastric or esophageal bleeding, lavage with tepid or iced water or normal saline solution may be used to stop bleeding. However, some controversy exists over the effectiveness of iced lavage for this purpose. (See *Is iced lavage effective?*) Indeed, according to the American Academy of Clinical Toxicology, gastric lavage shouldn't be used routinely in the management of poisoned patients. In experimental studies, the amount of marker removed by gastric lavage was highly variable and diminished with time, indicating that the method doesn't improve clinical outcome. In fact, it's believed that in many cases, gastric lavage may cause or increase morbidity. Gastric lavage shouldn't be used unless the patient has ingested a life-threatening amount of the poison and lavage can occur within 60 minutes of ingestion. Even in this situation, however, clinical improvement hasn't been proved in controlled studies.

Gastric lavage can be continuous or intermittent. Typically, this procedure is done in the emergency department or intensive care unit by a physician, gastroenterologist, or nurse; a wide-bore lavage tube is almost always inserted by a gastroenterologist.

Gastric lavage is contraindicated after ingestion of a corrosive substance (such as lye, ammonia, or mineral acids) because the lavage tube may perforate the already compromised esophagus.

Correct lavage tube placement is essential for patient safety because accidental misplacement (in the lungs, for example) followed by lavage can be fatal. Other complications of gastric lavage include bradyarrhythmias and aspiration of gastric fluids.

Equipment

Lavage setup (two graduated containers for drainage, three pieces of large-lumen rubber tubing, Y connector, and a clamp or hemostat) ▪ 2 to 3 L of normal saline solution or tap water, or appropriate antidote, as ordered ▪ I.V. pole ▪ basin of ice, if ordered ▪ Ewald tube or any large-lumen gastric tube, typically #36 to #40 French (see *Using wide-bore gastric tubes*) ▪ water-soluble lubricant or anesthetic ointment ▪ stethoscope ▪ 1½" hypoallergenic tape ▪ 50-ml bulb or catheter-tip syringe ▪ gloves ▪ face shield ▪ linen-saver pad or towel ▪ Yankauer or tonsil-tip suction device ▪ suction apparatus ▪ calibrated container ▪ pH strip ▪ labeled specimen container ▪ laboratory request form ▪ optional: patient restraints, charcoal tablets, norepinephrine.

A prepackaged, syringe-type irrigation kit may be used for intermittent lavage. For poisoning or a drug overdose, however, the continuous lavage setup may be more appropriate to use *because it's a faster and more effective means of diluting and removing the harmful substance.*

Preparation of equipment

Set up the lavage equipment. (See *Preparing for gastric lavage*, page 668.) If iced lavage is ordered, chill the desired irrigant (water or normal saline solution) in a basin of ice. Lubricate the end of the lavage tube with the water-soluble lubricant or anesthetic ointment.

Implementation

- Explain the procedure to the patient, provide privacy, and wash your hands.
- Put on gloves and a face shield.
- Drape the towel or linen-saver pad over the patient's chest *to protect him from spills.*
- If the patient wears dentures, remove them.
- The physician inserts the lavage tube nasally and advances it slowly and gently *because forceful insertion may injure tissues and cause epistaxis.* He checks the tube's placement by injecting about 30 cc of air into the tube with the bulb syringe and then auscultating the patient's abdomen with a stethoscope. If the tube is in place, he'll hear the sound of air entering the stomach.
- *Because the patient may vomit when the lavage tube reaches the posterior pharynx during insertion,* be prepared to suction the airway immediately with either a Yankauer or a tonsil-tip suction device.

EQUIPMENT

Using wide-bore gastric tubes

If you need to deliver a large volume of fluid rapidly through a gastric tube (when irrigating the stomach of a patient with profuse gastric bleeding or poisoning, for example), a wide-bore gastric tube usually serves best. Typically inserted orally, these tubes remain in place only long enough to complete the lavage and evacuate stomach contents.

Ewald tube

In an emergency, using a single-lumen tube with several openings at the distal end, such as an Ewald tube, allows you to aspirate large amounts of gastric contents quickly.

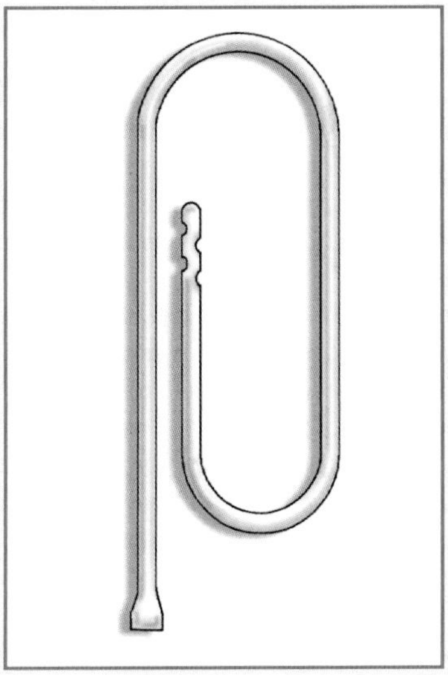

Levacuator tube

A Levacuator tube has two lumens. Use the larger lumen for evacuating gastric contents; the smaller, for instilling an irrigant.

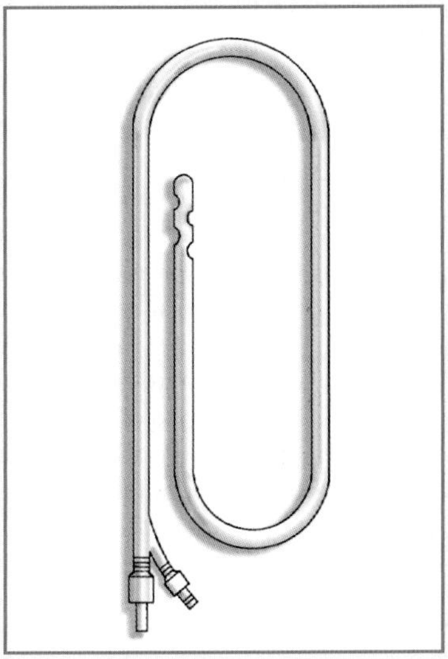

Edlich tube

An Edlich tube is a single-lumen tube that has four openings near the closed distal tip. A funnel or syringe may be connected at the proximal end. Like the Ewald tube, the Edlich tube lets you withdraw large quantities of gastric contents quickly.

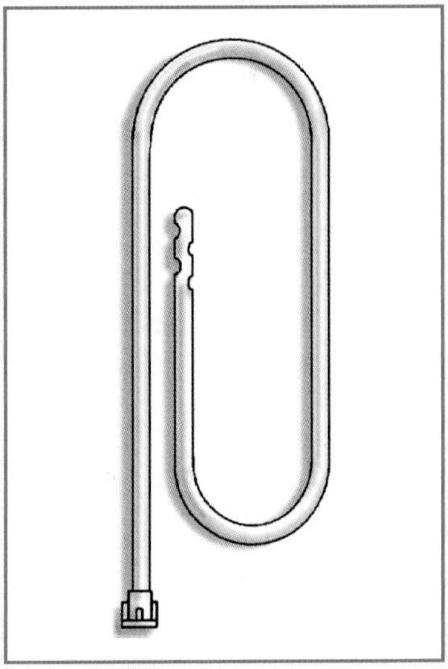

- When the lavage tube passes the posterior pharynx, help the patient into Trendelenburg's position and turn him toward his left side in a three-quarter prone posture. *This position minimizes passage of gastric contents into the duodenum and may prevent the patient from aspirating vomitus.*
- After securing the lavage tube nasally or orally and making sure the irrigant inflow tube on the lavage setup is clamped, connect the unattached end of this tube to the lavage tube. Check tube placement by injecting air into the tube while listening over the stomach or by testing the pH of the aspirate. Allow the stomach contents to empty into the drainage container before instilling any irrigant. *This confirms proper tube placement and decreases the risk of overfilling the stomach with irrigant and inducing vomiting.* If you're using a syringe irrigation set, aspirate stomach contents with a 50-ml bulb or catheter-tip syringe before instilling the irrigant.
- When you confirm proper tube placement, begin gastric lavage by instilling about 250 ml of irrigant *to assess the patient's tolerance and prevent vomiting.* Water or normal saline solution should be used, preferably warmed to 68.4° F (20.2°F) *to avoid the risk of hypothermia.*
- Clamp the inflow tube and unclamp the outflow tube *to allow the irrigant to flow out.* If you're using the syringe irrigation kit, aspirate the irrigant with the syringe and empty it into a calibrated container. Measure the outflow amount to make sure it equals at least the amount of irrigant you instilled. *This prevents accidental stomach distention and vom-*

EQUIPMENT

Preparing for gastric lavage

Prepare the gastric lavage setup as follows:

- Connect one of the three pieces of large-lumen tubing to the irrigant container.
- Insert the stem of the Y connector in the other end of the tubing.
- Connect the remaining two pieces of tubing to the free ends of the Y connector.
- Place the unattached end of one of the tubes into one of the drainage containers. (Later, you'll connect the other piece of tubing to the patient's gastric tube.)
- Clamp the tube leading to the irrigant.
- Suspend the entire setup from the I.V. pole, hanging the irrigant container at the highest level.

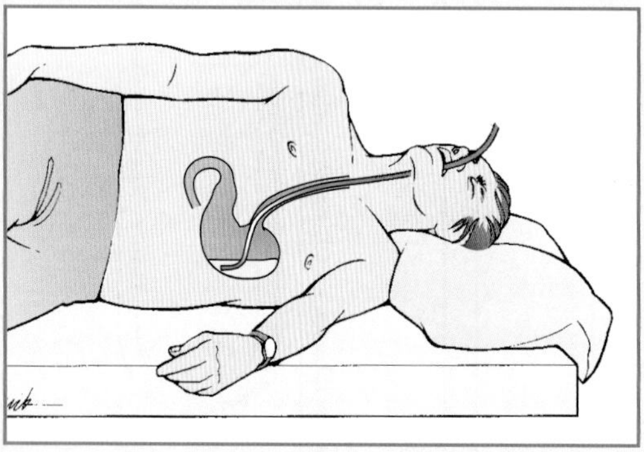

iting. If the drainage amount falls significantly short of the instilled amount, reposition the tube until sufficient solution flows out. Gently massage the abdomen over the stomach *to promote outflow.*

- Repeat the inflow-outflow cycle until returned fluids appear clear. *This signals that the stomach no longer holds harmful substances or that bleeding has stopped.*
- Assess the patient's vital signs, urine output, and level of consciousness (LOC) every 15 minutes. Notify the physician of any changes.
- If ordered, remove the lavage tube.

Special considerations

- *To control GI bleeding,* the physician may order continuous irrigation of the stomach with an irrigant and a vasoconstrictor, such as norepinephrine. After the stomach absorbs norepinephrine, the portal system delivers the drug directly to the liver, where it's metabolized. *This prevents the drug from circulating systemically and initiating a hypertensive response.* Or the physician may direct you to clamp the outflow tube for a prescribed period after instilling the irrigant and the vasoconstrictive medication and before withdrawing it. *This allows the mucosa time to absorb the drug.*
- Never leave a patient alone during gastric lavage. Observe continuously for any changes in LOC, and monitor vital signs frequently *because the natural vagal response to intubation can depress the patient's heart rate.*
- If you need to restrain the patient, secure restraints on the same side of the bed or stretcher *so you can free them quickly without moving to the other side of the bed.* Don't restrain the patient in a "spread eagle" position; *this position would keep him immobile and put him at risk for aspirating vomitus.*
- Remember also to keep tracheal suctioning equipment nearby and watch closely for airway obstruction caused by vomiting or excess oral secretions. Throughout gastric lavage, you may need to suction the oral cavity frequently *to ensure an open airway and prevent aspiration.* For the same reasons, and if he doesn't exhibit an adequate gag reflex, the patient may require an endotracheal tube before the procedure.
- When aspirating the stomach for ingested poisons or drugs, save the contents in a labeled container to send to the laboratory for analysis. If ordered, after lavage to remove poisons or drugs, mix charcoal tablets with the irrigant (water or normal saline solution), and administer the mixture through the NG tube. *The charcoal will absorb remaining toxic substances.* The tube may be clamped temporarily, allowed to drain via gravity, attached to intermittent suction, or removed.
- When performing gastric lavage to stop bleeding, keep precise intake and output records *to determine the amount of bleeding.* When large volumes of fluid are instilled and withdrawn, serum electrolyte and arterial blood gas levels may be measured during or at the end of lavage.

Complications

Vomiting and subsequent aspiration, the most common complication of gastric lavage, occurs more often in a groggy patient. Bradyarrhythmias also may occur. After iced lavage especially, the patient's body temperature may drop, thereby triggering cardiac arrhythmias.

Documentation

Record the date and time of lavage, the size and type of NG tube used, the volume and type of irrigant, and the amount of drained gastric contents. Document this information on the intake and output record sheet, and include your observations, including the color and consistency of drainage. Also keep precise records of the patient's vital signs and LOC, any drugs instilled through the tube, the time the tube was removed, and how well the patient tolerated the procedure.

SELECTED REFERENCES

American Academy of Clinical Toxicology, European Association of Poison Centres and Clinical Toxicologists. "Position Paper: Gastric Lavage," *Journal of Toxicology, Clinical Toxicology* 42(7):933-43, 2004.

Heard, K. "Gastrointestinal Decontamination," *Medical Clinics of North America* 89(6):1067-78, November 2005.

Lynn-McHale Wiegand, D.J., and Carlson, K.K., eds. *AACN Procedure Manual for Critical Care,* 5th ed. Philadelphia: W.B. Saunders Co., 2005.

FEEDING TUBE INSERTION AND REMOVAL

Inserting a feeding tube nasally or orally into the stomach or duodenum allows a patient who can't or won't eat to receive nourishment. The feeding tube also permits administration of supplemental feedings to a patient who has very high nutritional requirements, such as an unconscious patient or one with extensive burns. Typically, a feeding tube is inserted by a nurse as ordered. The preferred feeding tube route is nasal, but the oral route may be used for patients with such conditions as a deviated septum or a head or nose injury.

The practitioner may order duodenal feeding when the patient can't tolerate gastric feeding or when he expects gastric feeding to produce aspiration. Absence of bowel sounds or possible intestinal obstruction contraindicates using a feeding tube.

Feeding tubes differ somewhat from standard nasogastric tubes. Made of silicone, rubber, or polyurethane, feeding tubes have small diameters and great flexibility. This reduces oropharyngeal irritation, necrosis from pressure on the tracheoesophageal wall, distal esophageal irritation, and discomfort from swallowing. To facilitate passage, some feeding tubes are weighted with tungsten, and some need a guide wire to keep them from curling in the back of the throat.

These small-bore tubes usually have radiopaque markings and a water-activated coating, which provides a lubricated surface.

Equipment

For insertion: Feeding tube (#6 to #18 French, with or without guide wire) ▪ linen-saver pad ▪ gloves ▪ hypoallergenic tape ▪ water-soluble lubricant ▪ cotton-tipped applicators ▪ skin preparation (such as tincture of benzoin) ▪ facial tissues ▪ penlight ▪ small cup of water with straw, or ice chips ▪ emesis basin ▪ 60-ml syringe ▪ pH test strip.

During use: Mouthwash or normal saline solution ▪ toothbrush.

For removal: Linen-saver pad or towel ▪ bulb syringe.

Preparation of equipment

Have the proper size tube available. Usually, the practitioner orders the smallest-bore tube that will allow free passage of the liquid feeding formula. Read the instructions on the tubing package carefully *because tube characteristics vary according to the manufacturer.* (For example, some tubes have marks at the appropriate lengths for gastric, duodenal, and jejunal insertion.)

Examine the tube to make sure it's free of defects, such as cracks or rough or sharp edges. Next, run water through the tube. *This checks for patency, activates the coating, and facilitates removal of the guide.*

Implementation

- Confirm the patient's identity using two patient identifiers according to your facility's policy.
- Explain the procedure to the patient and show him the tube *so that he knows what to expect and can cooperate more fully.*
- Provide privacy. Wash your hands and put on gloves.
- Assist the patient into semi-Fowler's or high Fowler's position.
- Place a linen-saver pad across the patient's chest *to protect him from spills.*
- *To determine the tube length needed to reach the stomach,* first extend the distal end of the tube from the tip of the patient's nose to his earlobe. Coil this portion of the tube around your fingers *so the end will remain curved until you insert it.* Then extend the uncoiled portion from the earlobe to the xiphoid process. Use a small piece of hypoallergenic tape to mark the total length of the two portions.

Inserting the tube nasally

- Using the penlight, assess nasal patency. Inspect nasal passages for a deviated septum, polyps, or other obstructions. Occlude one nostril, then the other, *to determine which has the better airflow.* Assess the patient's history of nasal injury or surgery.
- Lubricate the curved tip of the tube (and the feeding tube guide, if appropriate) with a small amount of water-soluble lubricant *to ease insertion and prevent tissue injury.*
- Ask the patient to hold the emesis basin and facial tissues in case he needs them.

■ To advance the tube, insert the curved, lubricated tip into the more patent nostril and direct it along the nasal passage toward the ear on the same side. When it passes the nasopharyngeal junction, turn the tube 180 degrees *to aim it downward into the esophagus.* Tell the patient to lower his chin to his chest *to close the trachea.* Then give him a small cup of water with a straw or ice chips. Direct him to sip the water or suck on the ice and swallow frequently. *This will ease the tube's passage.* Advance the tube as he swallows.

Inserting the tube orally

■ Have the patient lower his chin *to close his trachea,* and ask him to open his mouth.

■ Place the tip of the tube at the back of the patient's tongue, give water, and instruct the patient to swallow, as above. Remind him to avoid clamping his teeth down on the tube. Advance the tube as he swallows.

Positioning the tube

■ Keep passing the tube until the tape marking the appropriate length reaches the patient's nostril or lips. Tube placement should be confirmed by X-ray.

■ After confirming proper tube placement, remove the tape marking the tube length.

■ Tape the tube to the patient's nose and remove the guide wire.

■ *To advance the tube to the duodenum,* especially a tungsten-weighted tube, position the patient on his right side. *This lets gravity assist tube passage through the pylorus.* Move the tube forward 2″ to 3″ (5 to 7.5 cm) hourly until X-ray studies confirm duodenal placement. (An X-ray must confirm placement before feeding begins *because duodenal feeding can cause nausea and vomiting if accidentally delivered to the stomach.*)

■ Apply a skin preparation to the patient's cheek before securing the tube with tape. *This helps the tube adhere to the skin and also prevents irritation.*

■ Tape the tube securely to the patient's cheek *to avoid excessive pressure on his nostrils.*

Removing the tube

■ Protect the patient's chest with a linen-saver pad or towel.

■ Flush the tube with air, clamp or pinch it *to prevent fluid aspiration during withdrawal,* and withdraw it gently but quickly.

■ Promptly cover and discard the used tube.

Special considerations

■ Check gastric residual contents before each feeding. Feeding should be held if residual volumes are greater than 200 ml on two successive assessments. Successful aspiration also confirms correct tube placement before feeding by testing the pH of the gastric aspirate. Attach the syringe to the tube and gently aspirate stomach contents. Examine the aspirate and place a small amount on the pH test strip. Probability of gastric placement is increased if the aspirate has a typical gastric fluid appearance (grassy-green, clear and colorless with mucus shreds, or brown) and pH is less than or equal to 5.0.

■ Flush the feeding tube every 4 hours with 20 to 30 ml of normal saline solution or warm water *to maintain patency.* Retape the tube at least daily, and as needed. Alternate taping the tube toward the inner and outer side of the nose *to avoid constant pressure on the same nasal area.* Inspect the skin for redness and breakdown.

■ Provide nasal hygiene daily using the cotton-tipped applicators and water-soluble lubricant *to remove crusted secretions.* Also help the patient brush his teeth, gums, and tongue with mouthwash or a saline solution at least twice daily.

■ If the patient can't swallow the feeding tube, use a guide wire *to aid insertion.*

■ Precise feeding-tube placement is especially important *because small-bore feeding tubes may slide into the trachea without causing immediate signs or symptoms of respiratory distress, such as coughing, choking, gasping, or cyanosis.* However, the patient will usually cough if the tube enters the larynx. To be sure that the tube clears the larynx, ask the patient to speak. If he can't, the tube is in the larynx. Withdraw the tube at once and reinsert.

■ If you meet resistance during aspiration, stop the procedure *because resistance may result simply from the tube lying against the stomach wall.* If the tube coils above the stomach, you won't be able to aspirate stomach contents. To rectify this, change the patient's position or withdraw the tube a few inches, readvance it, and try to aspirate again. If the tube was inserted with a guide wire, don't use the guide wire to reposition the tube. The practitioner may do so, using fluoroscopic guidance.

Home care

If your patient will use a feeding tube at home, make appropriate home care nursing referrals, and teach the patient and caregivers how to use and care for a feeding tube. Teach them how to obtain equipment, insert and remove the tube, prepare and store feeding formula, and solve problems with tube position and patency.

Complications

Prolonged intubation may lead to skin erosion at the nostril, sinusitis, esophagitis, esophagotracheal fistula, gastric ulceration, and pulmonary and oral infection.

Documentation

For tube insertion, record the date, time, tube type and size, insertion site, area of placement, and confirmation of proper placement. Also record the name of the person performing the procedure. For tube removal, record the date and time and the patient's tolerance of the procedure.

SELECTED REFERENCES

Guenter, P., and Silkroski, M. *Tube Feeding: Practical Guidelines and Nursing Protocols.* Gaithersburg, Md.: Aspen Pubs., Inc., 2001.

Lynn-McHale Wiegand, D.J., and Carlson, K.K., eds. *AACN Procedure Manual for Critical Care,* 5th ed. Philadelphia: W.B. Saunders Co., 2005.

Metheney, N.A., and Titer, M. "Assessing Placement of Feeding Tubes," *AJN* 101(5):36-45, May 2001.

Metheney, N.A., et al. "Indicators of Tubesite during Feedings," *Journal of Neuroscience Nursing* 37(6):320-25, December 2005.

Reising, D.L., and Neal, R.S. "Enteral Tube Flushing: What You Think Are the Best Practices May Not Be," *AJN* 105(3):58-63, March 2005.

Taylor, C., et al. *Fundamentals of Nursing: The Art and Science of Nursing Care,* 6th ed. Philadelphia: Lippincott Williams & Wilkins, 2008.

TUBE FEEDINGS

Tube feedings involve delivery of a liquid feeding formula directly to the stomach (known as *gastric gavage*), duodenum, or jejunum. Gastric gavage typically is indicated for a patient who can't eat normally because of dysphagia or oral or esophageal obstruction or injury. Gastric feedings also may be given to an unconscious or intubated patient or to a patient recovering from GI tract surgery who can't ingest food orally.

According to the American Gastroenterological Association, nutrition support should be initiated after 1 to 2 weeks without nutrient intake. Enteral feeding is preferable to parenteral therapy provided there are no contraindications, access can be safely attained, and oral intake isn't possible. For short-term (less than 30-day) feeding, nasogastric (NG) or nasoenteric tubes are preferable to gastrostomy or jejunostomy tubes. Tube feeding is contraindicated in patients who have no bowel sounds or a suspected intestinal obstruction.

Duodenal or jejunal feedings decrease the risk of aspiration because the formula bypasses the pylorus. Jejunal feedings result in reduced pancreatic stimulation; thus, the patient may require an elemental diet.

Patients usually receive gastric feedings on an intermittent schedule. For duodenal or jejunal feedings, however, most patients seem to better tolerate a continuous slow drip.

Liquid nutrient solutions come in various formulas for administration through a nasogastric tube, small-bore feeding tube, gastrostomy or jejunostomy tube, percutaneous endoscopic gastrostomy or jejunostomy tube, or gastrostomy feeding button. (For more information, see "Transabdominal tube feeding and care," page 690.)

Equipment

For gastric feedings: Feeding formula ▪ graduated container ▪ 120 ml of water ▪ gavage bag with tubing and flow regulator clamp ▪ towel or linen-saver pad, if needed ▪ 60-ml syringe ▪ pH test strip ▪ optional: infusion pump, tubing set (for continuous administration), adapter to connect gavage tubing to feeding tube.

For duodenal or jejunal feedings: Feeding formula ▪ enteral administration set containing a gavage container, drip chamber, roller clamp or flow regulator, and tube connector ▪ I.V. pole ▪ 60-ml syringe with adapter tip ▪ water ▪ optional: pump administration set (for an enteral infusion pump), Y connector.

For nasal and oral care: Cotton-tipped applicators ▪ water-soluble lubricant ▪ sponge-tipped swabs ▪ petroleum jelly.

A bulb syringe or large catheter-tip syringe may be substituted for a gavage bag after the patient demonstrates tolerance for a gravity drip infusion. The practitioner may order an infusion pump *to ensure accurate delivery of the prescribed formula.*

Preparation of equipment

Be sure to refrigerate formulas prepared in the dietary department or pharmacy. Refrigerate commercial formulas only after opening them. Check the date on all formula containers. Discard expired commercial formula. Use powdered formula within 24 hours of mixing. Always shake the container well *to mix the solution thoroughly.*

Allow the formula to warm to room temperature before administration. *Cold formula can increase the chance of diarrhea.* Never warm it over direct heat or in a microwave *because heat may curdle the formula or change its chemical composition. Also, hot formula may injure the patient.*

Pour 60 ml of water into the graduated container. After closing the flow clamp on the administration set, pour the appropriate amount of formula into the gavage bag. Hang no more than a 4- to 6-hour supply at one time *to prevent bacterial growth.*

Open the flow clamp on the administration set to remove air from the lines. *This keeps air from entering the patient's stomach and causing distention and discomfort.*

Implementation

- Confirm the patient's identity using two patient identifiers according to your facility's policy.
- Provide privacy and wash your hands.
- Inform the patient that he'll receive nourishment through the tube, and explain the procedure to him. If possible, give him a schedule of subsequent feedings.
- If the patient has a nasal or oral tube, cover his chest with a towel or linen-saver pad *to protect him and the bed linens from spills.*
- Assess the patient's abdomen for bowel sounds and distention.

Delivering a gastric feeding

- *To limit the risk of aspiration and reflux,* raise the head of the patient's bed 30 to 45 degrees during feeding and for 1 hour after feeding. Use intermittent or continuous feeding regimens rather than the rapid bolus method.
- Check placement of the feeding tube *to be sure it hasn't slipped out since the last feeding.*

NURSING ALERT *Never give a tube feeding until you're sure the tube is properly positioned in the patient's stomach.* **Administering a feeding through a misplaced tube can cause formula to enter the patient's lungs.**

- *To check tube patency and position,* remove the cap or plug from the feeding tube, and use the syringe to aspirate stomach contents (as shown below). Examine the aspirate and place a small amount on the pH test strip. The probability of gastric placement is increased if the aspirate has a gastric fluid appearance (grassy-green, clear and colorless with mucus shreds, or brown) and a pH less than or equal to 5.0.

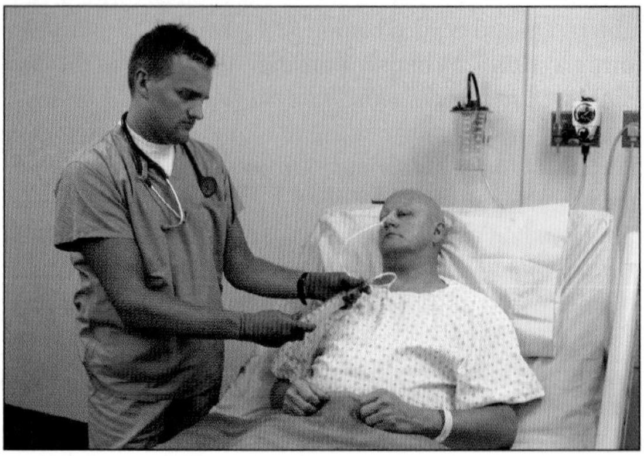

- If there's no gastric secretion return, the tube may be in the esophagus. You'll need to advance the tube and recheck placement before continuing.
- *To assess gastric emptying,* aspirate and measure residual gastric contents. Hold feedings if residual volume is greater then the predetermined amount specified in the practitioner's order (usually 50 to 100 ml). Reinstill any aspirate obtained. The guidelines by the American Society for Parenteral and Enteral Nutrition specify that feedings should be held if residual is greater than 200 ml on two successive assessments.
- Connect the gavage bag tubing to the feeding tube. Depending on the type of tube used, you may need to use an adapter to connect the two (as shown below).

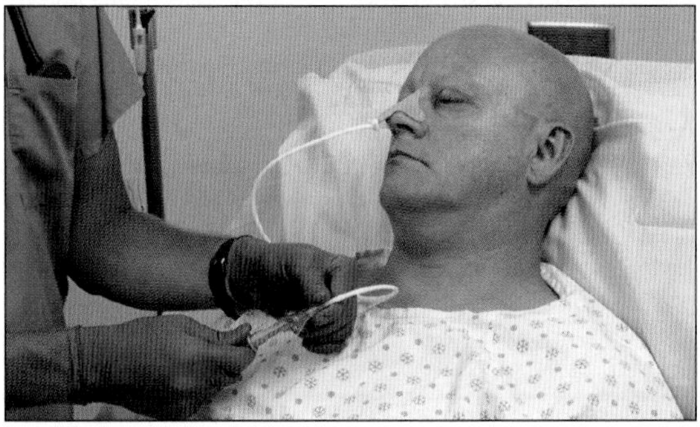

- If you're using a bulb or catheter-tip syringe, remove the bulb or plunger and attach the syringe to the pinched-off feeding tube (as shown below) *to prevent excess air from entering the patient's stomach, causing distention.* If you're using an infusion pump, thread the tube from the formula container through the pump according to the manufacturer's directions. Purge the tubing of air and attach it to the feeding tube.

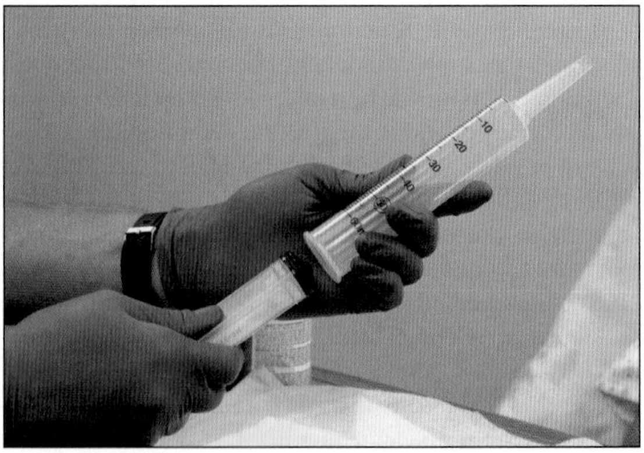

■ Open the regulator clamp on the gavage bag tubing, and adjust the flow rate appropriately. When using a bulb syringe, fill the syringe with formula and release the feeding tube *to allow formula to flow through it.* The height at which you hold the syringe will determine the flow rate. When the syringe is three-quarters empty, pour more formula into it (as shown below).

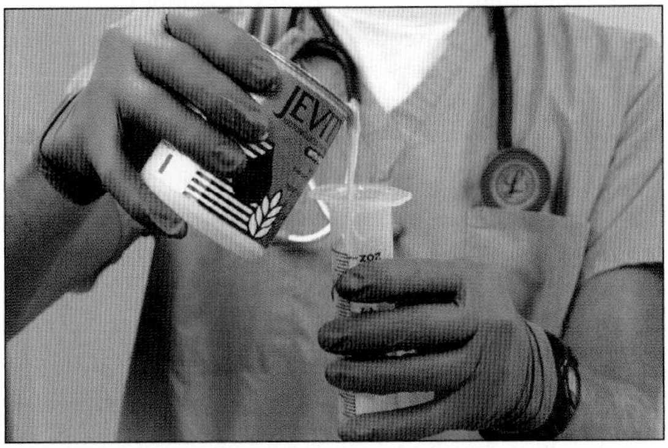

■ *To prevent air from entering the tube and the patient's stomach,* never allow the syringe to empty completely. If you're using an infusion pump, set the flow rate according to the manufacturer's directions. Always administer a tube feeding slowly—typically 200 to 350 ml over 15 to 30 minutes, depending on the patient's tolerance and the practitioner's order—*to prevent sudden stomach distention, which can cause nausea, vomiting, cramps, or diarrhea.*

■ After administering the appropriate amount of formula, flush the tubing by adding about 60 ml of water to the gavage bag or bulb syringe, or manually flush it using a barrel syringe (as shown below). *This maintains the tube's patency by removing excess formula, which could occlude the tube.*

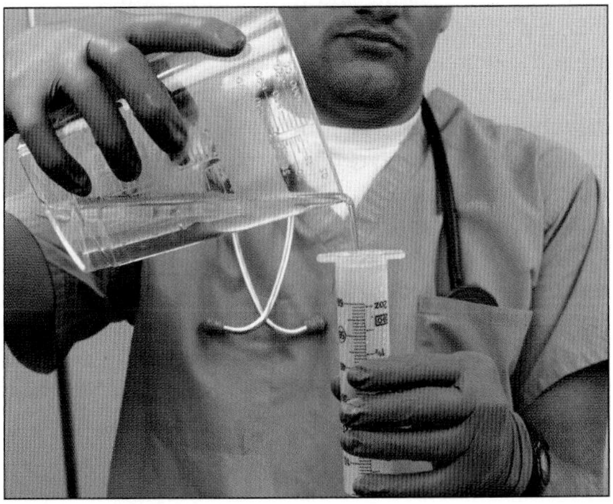

■ If you're administering a continuous feeding, flush the feeding tube every 4 hours *to help prevent tube occlusion.* Monitor gastric emptying every 4 hours.

■ To discontinue gastric feeding (depending on the equipment you're using), close the regulator clamp on the gavage bag tubing, disconnect the syringe from the feeding tube, or turn off the infusion pump.

■ Cover the end of the feeding tube with its plug or cap *to prevent leakage and contamination of the tube.*

■ Leave the patient in semi-Fowler's or high Fowler's position for at least 1 hour.

■ Rinse all reusable equipment with warm water. Dry it and store it in a convenient place for the next feeding. Change equipment every 24 hours or according to your facility's policy.

Delivering a duodenal or jejunal feeding

■ Elevate the head of the bed and place the patient in low Fowler's position.

■ Open the enteral administration set and hang the gavage container on the I.V. pole.

■ If you're using a nasoduodenal tube, measure its length *to check tube placement.* Remember that you may not get any residual when you aspirate the tube.

■ Open the flow clamp and regulate the flow to the desired rate. To regulate the rate using a volumetric infusion pump, follow the manufacturer's directions for setting up the equipment. Most patients receive small amounts initially, with volumes increasing gradually once tolerance is established.

■ Flush the tube every 4 hours with water *to maintain patency and provide hydration.* A needle catheter jejunostomy tube may require flushing every 2 hours *to prevent formula buildup inside the tube.* A Y connector may be useful for frequent flushing. Attach the continuous feeding to the main port and use the side port for flushes.

■ Change equipment every 24 hours or according to your facility's policy.

Special considerations

■ If the feeding solution doesn't initially flow through a bulb syringe, attach the bulb and squeeze it gently to start the flow. Then remove the bulb. Never use the bulb to force the formula through the tube.

■ If the patient becomes nauseated or vomits, stop the feeding immediately. *The patient may vomit if the stomach becomes distended from overfeeding or delayed gastric emptying.*

■ *To reduce oropharyngeal discomfort from the tube,* allow the patient to brush his teeth or care for his dentures regularly, and encourage frequent gargling. If the patient is unconscious, administer oral care with sponge-tipped swabs every 4 hours. Use petroleum jelly on dry, cracked lips. (*Note:* Dry mucous membranes may indicate dehydration, which requires increased fluid intake.) Clean the patient's nostrils with cotton-tipped applicators, apply lubricant along the mucosa, and assess the skin for signs of breakdown.

- During continuous feedings, assess the patient frequently for abdominal distention. Flush the tubing by adding about 50 ml of water to the gavage bag or bulb syringe. *This maintains the tube's patency by removing excess formula, which could occlude the tube.*
- If the patient develops diarrhea, administer small, frequent, less concentrated feedings, or administer bolus feedings over a longer time. Also, make sure the formula isn't cold and that proper storage and sanitation practices have been followed. The loose stools associated with tube feedings make extra perineal and skin care necessary. Changing to a formula with more fiber may eliminate liquid stools.
- If the patient becomes constipated, the practitioner may increase the fruit, vegetable, or sugar content of the formula. Assess the patient's hydration status *because dehydration may produce constipation.* Increase fluid intake as necessary. If the condition persists, administer an appropriate drug or enema, as ordered.
- Drugs can be administered through the feeding tube. Except for enteric-coated drugs or sustained-release medications, crush tablets or open and dilute capsules in water before administering them. Be sure to flush the tubing afterward *to ensure full instillation of medication.* Keep in mind that some drugs may change the osmolarity of the feeding formula and cause diarrhea.
- Small-bore feeding tubes may kink, making instillation impossible. If you suspect this problem, try changing the patient's position, or withdraw the tube a few inches and restart. Never use a guide wire to reposition the tube.
- Constantly monitor the flow rate of a blended or high-residue formula *to determine if the formula is clogging the tubing as it settles. To prevent such clogging,* squeeze the bag frequently to agitate the solution.
- Collect blood samples, as ordered. *Glycosuria, hyperglycemia, and diuresis can indicate an excessive carbohydrate level, leading to hyperosmotic dehydration, which may be fatal.* Monitor blood glucose levels *to assess glucose tolerance.* (A patient with a serum glucose level of less than 170 mg/dl is considered stable.) Also monitor serum levels of electrolytes, blood urea nitrogen, and glucose as well as serum osmolality and other pertinent findings *to determine the patient's response to therapy and to assess his hydration status.*
- Check the flow rate hourly *to ensure correct infusion.* (With an improvised administration set, use a time tape to record the rate *because it's difficult to get precise readings from an irrigation container or enema bag.*)
- For duodenal or jejunal feeding, most patients tolerate a continuous drip better than bolus feedings. *Bolus feedings can cause such complications as hyperglycemia, glycosuria, and diarrhea.*
- Until the patient acquires a tolerance for the formula, you may need to dilute it to half or three-quarters strength to start, and increase it gradually. Patients under stress or who are receiving steroids may experience a pseudodiabetic state. Assess such patients frequently *to determine the need for insulin.*

Home care

Patient education for home tube feeding includes instructions on an infusion control device *to maintain accuracy,* use of the syringe or bag and tubing, care of the tube and insertion site, and formula-mixing. Formula may be mixed in an electric blender according to package directions. Formula not used within 24 hours must be discarded. If the formula must hang for more than 8 hours, advise the patient to use a gavage or pump administration set with an ice pouch *to decrease the incidence of bacterial growth.* Tell him to use a new bag daily.

Teach family members signs and symptoms to report to the practitioner or home care nurse as well as measures to take in an emergency.

Complications

Erosion of esophageal, tracheal, nasal, and oropharyngeal mucosa can result if tubes are left in place for a long time. If possible, use smaller-lumen tubes *to prevent such irritation.* Check your facility's policy regarding the frequency of changing feeding tubes *to prevent complications.* (See *Managing tube feeding problems.*)

Using the gastric route, frequent or large-volume feedings can cause bloating and retention. Dehydration, diarrhea, and vomiting can cause metabolic disturbances. Cramping and abdominal distention usually indicate intolerance.

Using the duodenal or jejunal route, clogging of the feeding tube is common. The patient may experience metabolic, fluid, and electrolyte abnormalities including hyperglycemia, hyperosmolar dehydration, coma, edema, hypernatremia, and essential fatty acid deficiency.

The patient may also experience dumping syndrome, in which a large amount of hyperosmotic solution in the duodenum causes excessive diffusion of fluid through the semipermeable membrane and results in diarrhea. In a patient with low serum albumin levels, these symptoms may result from low oncotic pressure in the duodenal mucosa.

Managing tube feeding problems

COMPLICATION	NURSING INTERVENTIONS
Aspiration of gastric secretions	■ Discontinue feeding immediately. ■ Perform tracheal suction of aspirated contents, if possible. ■ Notify the practitioner. Prophylactic antibiotics and chest physiotherapy may be ordered. ■ Check tube placement before feeding *to prevent complication.*
Tube obstruction	■ Flush the tube with warm water. If necessary, replace the tube. ■ Flush the tube with 50 ml of water after each feeding *to remove excess sticky formula, which could occlude the tube.* ■ When possible, use liquid forms of medications. Otherwise, and if not contraindicated, crush well.
Oral, nasal, or pharyngeal irritation or necrosis	■ Provide frequent oral hygiene using mouthwash or sponge-tipped swabs. Use petroleum jelly on cracked lips. ■ Change the tube's position. If necessary, replace the tube.
Vomiting, bloating, diarrhea, or cramps	■ Reduce the flow rate. ■ Verify tube placement. ■ Administer metoclopramide *to increase GI motility.* ■ Warm the formula to *prevent GI distress.* ■ For 30 minutes after feeding, position the patient on his right side with his head elevated *to facilitate gastric emptying.* ■ Notify the practitioner. *He may want to reduce the amount of formula being given during each feeding.*
Constipation	■ Provide additional fluids if the patient can tolerate them. ■ Have the patient participate in an exercise program, if possible. ■ Administer a bulk-forming laxative. ■ Review medications. Discontinue medications that have a tendency to cause constipation. ■ Increase fruit, vegetable, or sugar content of the feeding.
Electrolyte imbalance	■ Monitor serum electrolyte levels. ■ Notify the practitioner. *He may want to adjust the formula content to correct the deficiency.*
Hyperglycemia	■ Monitor blood glucose levels. ■ Notify the practitioner of elevated levels. ■ Administer insulin, if ordered. ■ The practitioner may adjust the sugar content of the formula.

Documentation

On the intake and output sheet, record the date, volume of formula, and volume of water. In your notes, document abdominal assessment findings (including tube exit site, if appropriate), amount of residual gastric contents, tube patency, and verification of tube placement; amount, type, and time of feeding. Discuss the patient's tolerance of the feeding, including nausea, vomiting, cramping, diarrhea, and distention.

Note the result of blood tests, hydration status, and any drugs given through the tube. Include the date and time of administration set changes, oral and nasal hygiene, and results of specimen collections.

EQUIPMENT

Common types of nasoenteric-decompression tubes

The type of nasoenteric-decompression tube chosen for your patient will depend on the size of the patient and his nostrils, the estimated duration of intubation, and the reason for the procedure. For example, to remove viscous material from the patient's intestinal tract, the physician may select a tube with a wide bore and a single lumen.

Whichever tube you use, you'll need to provide good mouth care and check the patient's nostrils often for signs of irritation. If you see any signs of irritation, retape the tube *so that it doesn't cause tension,* and then lubricate the nostril. Or check with the physician to see if the tube can be inserted through the other nostril.

Most tubes are impregnated with a radiopaque mark *so that placement can easily be confirmed by X-ray or other imaging technique.*

Tubes such as the pre-weighted Andersen Miller-Abbot type intestinal tube (shown below) have a tungsten-weighted inflatable latex balloon tip designed for temporary management of mechanical obstruction in the small or large intestines.

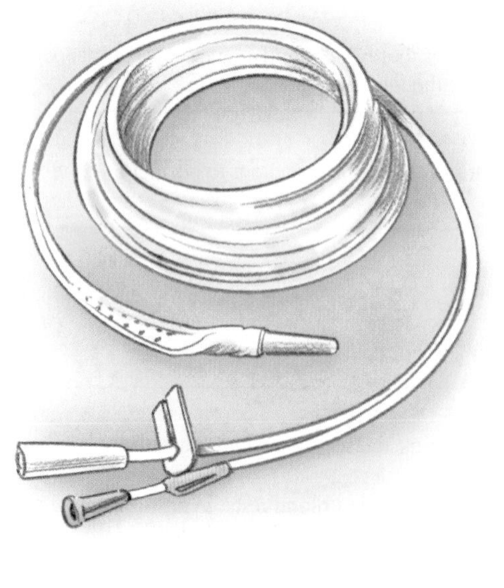

SELECTED REFERENCES

American Society for Parenteral and Enteral Nutrition. "Access for Administration of Nutrition Support," *Journal of Parenteral Enteral Nutrition* 26(Suppl 1):33SA-41SA, January-February 2002. Available at *www.guideline.gov.*

Bowman, A., et al. "Implementation of an Evidence-Based Feeding Protocol and Aspiration Risk Reduction Algorithm," *Critical Care Nursing Quarterly* 28(4):324-33, October-December 2005.

Ellett, M.L. "Important Facts about Intestinal Feeding Tube Placement," *Gastroenterology Nursing* 29(2):112-24, March-April 2006.

Guenter, P., and Silkroski, M. *Tube Feeding: Practical Guidelines and Nursing Protocols.* Gaithersburg, Md.: Aspen Pubs., Inc., 2001.

Metheny, N.A. "Preventing Respiratory Complications of Tube Feedings: Evidence-Based Practice," *American Journal of Critical Care* 15(4):360-69, July 2006.

Metheny, N.A., et al. "Indicators of Tubesite during Feedings," *Journal of Neuroscience Nursing* 37(6):320-25, December 2005.

Taylor, C., et al. *Fundamentals of Nursing: The Art and Science of Nursing Care,* 6th ed. Philadelphia: Lippincott Williams & Wilkins, 2008.

NASOENTERIC-DECOMPRESSION TUBE INSERTION AND REMOVAL

The nasoenteric-decompression tube is inserted nasally and advanced beyond the stomach into the intestinal tract. It's used to aspirate intestinal contents for analysis and to treat intestinal obstruction. The tube may also help to prevent nausea, vomiting, and abdominal distention after GI surgery. A physician will usually insert or remove a nasoenteric-decompression tube, but sometimes, a nurse will remove it.

The nasoenteric-decompression tube may have a pre-weighted tip and a balloon at one end of the tube that holds air or water to stimulate peristalsis and facilitate the tube's passage through the pylorus and into the intestinal tract. (See *Common types of nasoenteric-decompression tubes.*)

Equipment

Sterile 10-ml syringe ■ nasoenteric-decompression tube ■ container of water ■ 5 to 10 ml of water, as ordered ■ suction-decompression equipment ■ gloves ■ towel or linen-saver pad ■ water-soluble lubricant ■ 4″ × 4″ gauze pad ■ ½″ hypoallergenic tape ■ bulb syringe or 60-ml catheter-tip syringe ■ rubber band ■ safety pin ■ specimen container ■ basin of ice or warm water ■ penlight ■ waterproof marking pen ■ glass of water with straw ■ optional: ice chips, local anesthetic.

Preparation of equipment

Stiffen a flaccid tube by chilling it in a basin of ice *to facilitate insertion.* To make a stiff tube flexible, dip it into warm water.

Air or water is added to the balloon either before or after insertion of the tube, depending on the type of tube used. Follow the manufacturer's recommendations.

Set up suction-decompression equipment, if ordered, and make sure it works properly.

Implementation

- Confirm the patient's identity using two patient identifiers according to your facility's policy.
- Explain the procedure to the patient, forewarning him that he may experience some discomfort. Provide privacy and adequate lighting.
- Wash your hands and put on gloves.
- Position the patient as the physician specifies, usually in semi-Fowler's or high Fowler's position. You may also need to help the patient hold his neck in a hyperextended position.
- Protect the patient's chest with a linen-saver pad or towel.
- Agree with the patient on a signal that can be used to stop the insertion briefly if necessary.

Assisting with insertion

- The physician assesses the patency of the patient's nostrils. *To evaluate which nostril has better airflow in a conscious patient,* he holds one nostril closed and then the other as the patient breathes. In an unconscious patient, he examines each nostril with a penlight *to check for polyps, a deviated septum, or other obstruction.*
- *To decide how far the tube must be inserted to reach the stomach,* the physician places the tube's distal end at the tip of the patient's nose and then extends the tube to the earlobe and down to the xiphoid process. He either marks the tube with a waterproof marking pen or holds it at this point.
- The physician applies water-soluble lubricant to the first few inches of the tube *to reduce friction and tissue trauma and to facilitate insertion.*
- If the balloon already contains water, the physician holds it so the fluid runs to the bottom. Then he pinches the balloon closed *to retain the fluid as the insertion begins.*
- Tell the patient to breathe through his mouth or to pant as the balloon enters his nostril. After the balloon begins its descent, the physician releases his grip on it, allowing the weight of the fluid or the pre-weighted tip to pull the tube into the nasopharynx. When the tube reaches the nasopharynx, the physician instructs the patient to lower his chin and to swallow. In some cases, the patient may sip water through a straw *to facilitate swallowing as the tube advances,* but not after the tube reaches the trachea. *This prevents injury from aspiration.* The physician continues to advance the tube slowly *to prevent it from curling or kinking in the stomach.*
- *To confirm the tube's passage into the stomach,* the physician aspirates stomach contents with a bulb syringe.
- *To keep the tube out of the patient's eyes and to help avoid undue skin irritation,* fold a 4″ × 4″ gauze pad in half and tape it to the patient's forehead with the fold directed toward the patient's nose. The physician can slide the tube through this sling, leaving enough slack for the tube to advance.
- Position the patient as directed *to help advance the tube.* He'll typically lie on his right side until the tube clears the pylorus (about 2 hours). The physician will confirm passage by X-ray.
- After the tube clears the pylorus, the physician may direct you to advance it 2″ to 3″ (5 to 7.6 cm) every hour and to reposition the patient until the premeasured mark reaches the patient's nostril. Gravity and peristalsis will help advance the tube. (Notify the physician if you can't advance the tube.)
- Keep the remaining premeasured length of tube well lubricated *to ease passage and prevent irritation.*
- Don't tape the tube while it advances to the premeasured mark unless the physician asks you to do so.
- After the tube progresses the necessary distance, the physician will order an X-ray *to confirm tube positioning.* When the tube is in place, secure the external tubing with tape *to help prevent further progression.*
- Loop a rubber band around the tube and pin the rubber band to the patient's gown with a safety pin.
- If ordered, attach the tube to suction.

Removing the tube

- Assist the patient into semi-Fowler's or high Fowler's position. Drape a linen-saver pad or towel across the patient's chest.
- Wash your hands and put on gloves.
- Clamp the tube and disconnect it from the suction. *This prevents the patient from aspirating any gastric contents that leak from the tube during withdrawal.*
- If your patient has a tube with an inflated balloon tip, attach a 10-ml syringe to the balloon port and withdraw the air or water.
- Slowly withdraw between 6″ and 8″ (15 and 20 cm) of the tube. Wait 10 minutes and withdraw another 6″ to 8″. Wait another 10 minutes. Continue this procedure until the tube reaches the patient's esophagus (with 18″ [45 cm] of the tube remaining inside the patient). At this point, you can gently withdraw the tube completely.

Special considerations

■ For a double- or triple-lumen tube, note which lumen accommodates balloon inflation and which accommodates drainage.

■ Apply a local anesthetic, if ordered, to the nostril or the back of the throat *to dull sensations and the gag reflex for intubation.* Letting the patient gargle with a liquid anesthetic or holding ice chips in his mouth for a few minutes serves the same purpose.

Complications

Nasoenteric-decompression tubes may cause reflux esophagitis, nasal or oral inflammation, and nasal, laryngeal, or esophageal ulceration.

Documentation

Record the date and time the nasoenteric-decompression tube was inserted and by whom. Note the patient's tolerance of the procedure; the type of tube used; the suction type and amount; and the color, amount, and consistency of drainage. Also note the date, time, and name of the person removing the tube and the patient's tolerance of the removal procedure.

Selected references

Smeltzer, S.C., et al. *Brunner & Suddarth's Textbook of Medical-Surgical Nursing,* 11th ed. Philadelphia: Lippincott Williams & Wilkins, 2008.

Nasoenteric-decompression tube care

The patient with a nasoenteric-decompression tube needs special care and continuous monitoring to ensure tube patency, to maintain suction and bowel decompression, and to detect such complications as fluid-electrolyte imbalances related to aspiration of intestinal contents. Precise intake and output records are an integral part of the patient's care. Frequent mouth and nose care is also essential to provide comfort and to prevent skin breakdown. Finally, a patient with a nasoenteric-decompression tube will need encouragement and support during insertion and removal of the tube and while the tube is in place.

Equipment

Suction apparatus with intermittent suction capability (stationary or portable unit) ■ container of water ■ intake and output record sheets ■ mouthwash and water mixture ■ sponge-tipped swabs ■ petroleum jelly or water-soluble lubricant ■ cotton-tipped applicators ■ safety pin ■ tape or rubber band ■ disposable irrigation set ■ irrigant ■ optional: throat comfort measures, such as gargle, viscous lidocaine, throat lozenges, ice collar, sour hard candy, or gum.

Preparation of equipment

Assemble the suction apparatus and set up the suction unit. If indicated, test the unit by turning it on and placing the end of the suction tubing in a container of water. If the tubing draws in water, the unit works.

Implementation

■ Confirm the patient's identity using two patient identifiers according to your facility's policy.

■ Explain to the patient and his family the purpose of the procedure. Answer questions clearly and thoroughly *to ease anxiety and enhance cooperation.*

■ After tube insertion, have the patient lie quietly on his right side for about 2 hours *to promote the tube's passage.* After the tube advances past the pylorus, his activity level may increase, as ordered.

■ After the tube advances to the desired position, coil the excess external tubing and secure it to the patient's gown or bed linens with a safety pin attached to tape or a rubber band looped around it. *This prevents kinks in the tubing, which would interrupt suction.* Once in the desired location, the tube may be taped to the patient's face.

■ Maintain slack in the tubing *so the patient can move comfortably and safely in bed.* Show him how far he can move without dislodging the tube.

■ After securing the tube, connect it to the tubing on the suction machine *to begin decompression.*

■ Check the suction machine at least every 2 hours *to confirm proper functioning and to ensure tube patency and bowel decompression.* Excessive negative pressure may draw the mucosa into the tube openings, impair the suction's effectiveness, and injure the mucosa. By using intermittent suction, you may avoid these problems. *To check functioning in an intermittent suction unit,* look for drainage in the connecting tube and dripping into the collecting container. Empty the container every 8 hours and measure the contents.

■ After decompression and before extubation, as ordered, provide a clear-to-full liquid diet *to assess bowel function.*

■ Record intake and output accurately *to monitor fluid balance.* If you irrigate the tube, its length may prohibit aspiration of the irrigant, so record the amount of instilled irrigant as "intake." Typically, normal saline solution supersedes water as the preferred irrigant *because water, which is hypotonic, may increase electrolyte loss through osmotic action, especially if you irrigate the tube often.*

TROUBLESHOOTING

Clearing a nasoenteric-decompression tube obstruction

If your patient's nasoenteric-decompression tube appears to be obstructed, notify the physician right away. He may order the following measures to restore patency quickly and efficiently:

- First, disconnect the tube from the suction source and irrigate with normal saline solution. Use gravity flow to help clear the obstruction unless ordered otherwise.
- If irrigation doesn't reestablish patency, the tube may be obstructed by its position against the gastric mucosa. To rectify this, tug slightly on the tube to move it away from the mucosa.
- If gentle tugging doesn't restore patency, the tube may be kinked and may need additional manipulation. Before proceeding, though, take these precautions:
  - Never reposition or irrigate a nasoenteric-decompression tube (without a physician's order) in a patient who has had GI surgery.
  - Avoid manipulating a tube in a patient who had the tube inserted during surgery *because doing so may disturb new sutures.*
  - Don't try to reposition a tube in a patient who was difficult to intubate (because of an esophageal stricture, for example).

- Observe the patient for signs and symptoms of disorders related to suctioning and intubation. Signs and symptoms of dehydration, a fluid-volume deficit, or a fluid-electrolyte imbalance include dry skin and mucous membranes, decreased urine output, lethargy, exhaustion, and fever.
- Watch for signs and symptoms of pneumonia related to the patient's inability to clear his pharynx or cough effectively with a tube in place. Be alert for fever, chest pain, tachypnea or labored breathing, and diminished breath sounds over the affected area.
- Observe drainage characteristics: color, amount, consistency, odor, and any unusual changes.
- Provide mouth care frequently (at least every 4 hours) *to increase the patient's comfort and promote a healthy oral cavity. If the tube remains in place for several days, mouth breathing will leave the lips, tongue, and other tissues dry and cracked.*
- Encourage the patient to brush his teeth or rinse his mouth with the mouthwash and water mixture.
- Lubricate the patient's lips with either sponge-tipped swabs or petroleum jelly applied with a cotton-tipped applicator.
- At least every 4 hours, gently clean and lubricate the patient's external nostrils with either petroleum jelly or water-soluble lubricant on a cotton-tipped applicator *to prevent skin breakdown.*
- Watch for peristalsis to resume, signaled by bowel sounds, passage of flatus, decreased abdominal distention, and possibly, a spontaneous bowel movement. *These signs may require tube removal.*

Special considerations

- If the suction machine works improperly, replace it immediately. If the machine works properly but no drainage accumulates in the collection container, suspect an obstruction in the tube.
- As ordered, irrigate the tube with the irrigation set to clear the obstruction. (See *Clearing a nasoenteric-decompression tube obstruction.*)
- If your patient is ambulatory and his tube connects to a portable suction unit, he may move short distances while connected to the unit. Or, if feasible and ordered, the tube can be disconnected and clamped briefly while he moves around.
- If the tubing irritates the patient's throat or makes him hoarse, offer relief with mouthwash, gargles, viscous lidocaine, throat lozenges, an ice collar, sour hard candy, or gum, as appropriate.
- Make sure the tube isn't pressing on the nostril *to prevent skin breakdown.*
- If the tip of the balloon falls below the ileocecal valve (confirmed by X-ray), the tube can't be removed nasally. It has to be advanced and removed through the anus.
- If the balloon at the end of the tube protrudes from the anus, notify the physician. Most likely, the tube can be disconnected from suction, the proximal end severed, and the remaining tube removed gradually through the anus either manually or by peristalsis.

Complications

Potential complications include fluid-volume deficit, electrolyte imbalance, and pneumonia.

Documentation

Record the frequency and type of mouth and nose care provided. Describe the therapeutic effect, if any. Document in your notes the amount, color, consistency, and odor of the drainage obtained each time you empty the collection container.

Record the amount of drainage on the intake and output sheet. Always document the amount of any irrigant or other fluid introduced through the tube or taken orally by the patient.

If the suction machine malfunctions, note the length of time it wasn't functioning and the nursing action taken. Document the amount and character of any vomitus. Also note the patient's tolerance of the tube's insertion and removal.

SELECTED REFERENCES

Burlacu, C.L., et al. "Continuous Gastric Decompression for Postoperative Nausea and Vomiting after Coronary Revascularization Surgery," *Anesthesia and Analgesia* 100(2):321-26, February 2005.

Lynn-McHale Wiegand, D.J., and Carlson, K.K., eds. *AACN Procedure Manual for Critical Care,* 5th ed. Philadelphia: W.B. Saunders Co., 2005.

Nelson, B., et al. "Systematic Review of Prophylactic Nasogastric Decompression after Abdominal Operations," *British Journal of Surgery* 92(6):673-80, June 2005.

ESOPHAGEAL TUBE INSERTION AND REMOVAL

Used to control hemorrhage from esophageal or gastric varices, an esophageal tube is inserted nasally or orally and advanced into the esophagus or stomach. Ordinarily, a physician inserts and removes the tube. In an emergency situation, a nurse may remove it.

Once the tube is in place, a gastric balloon secured at the end of the tube can be inflated and drawn tightly against the cardia of the stomach. The inflated balloon secures the tube and exerts pressure on the cardia. The pressure, in turn, controls the bleeding varices.

Most tubes also contain an esophageal balloon to control esophageal bleeding. (*See Types of esophageal tubes.*) Usually, gastric or esophageal balloons are deflated after 24 hours. If the balloon remains inflated longer than 24 hours, pressure necrosis may develop and cause further hemorrhage or perforation.

Other procedures to control bleeding include irrigation with tepid or iced saline solution and drug therapy with a vasopressor. Used with the esophageal tube, these procedures provide effective, temporary control of acute variceal hemorrhage.

Equipment

Esophageal tube ▪ nasogastric (NG) tube (if using a Sengstaken-Blakemore tube) ▪ two suction sources ▪ basin of ice ▪ irrigation set ▪ 2 L of normal saline solution ▪ two 60-ml syringes ▪ water-soluble lubricant ▪ ½″ or 1″ adhesive tape ▪ stethoscope ▪ foam nose guard ▪ four rubber-shod clamps (two clamps and two plastic plugs for a Minnesota tube) ▪ anesthetic spray (as ordered) ▪ traction equipment (football helmet or a basic frame with traction rope, pulleys, and a 1-lb [0.5-kg] weight) ▪ mercury aneroid manometer ▪ Y-connector tube (for Sengstaken-Blakemore or Linton tube) ▪ cup of water with straw ▪ scissors ▪ gloves ▪ gown ▪ waterproof marking pen ▪ goggles ▪ sphygmomanometer.

Preparation of equipment

Keep the traction helmet at the bedside or attach traction equipment to the bed so that either is readily available after tube insertion. Place the suction machines nearby and plug them in. Open the irrigation set and fill the container with normal saline solution. Place all equipment within reach.

Test the balloons on the esophageal tube for air leaks by inflating them and submerging them in the basin of water. *If no bubbles appear in the water, the balloons are intact.* Remove them from the water and deflate them. Clamp the tube lumens, *so that the balloons stay deflated during insertion.*

To prepare the Minnesota tube, connect the mercury manometer to the gastric pressure monitoring port. Note the pressure when the balloon fills with 100, 200, 300, 400, and 500 cc of air.

Check the aspiration lumens for patency, and make sure they're labeled according to their purpose. If they aren't identified, label them carefully with the marking pen.

Chill the tube in a basin of ice. *This will stiffen it and facilitate insertion.*

Implementation

- Confirm the patient's identity using two patient identifiers according to your facility's policy.
- Explain the procedure and its purpose to the patient, and provide privacy.
- Wash your hands, and put on gloves, gown, and goggles *to protect yourself from splashing blood.*
- Assist the patient into semi-Fowler's position, and turn him slightly toward his left side. *This position promotes stomach emptying and helps prevent aspiration.*
- Explain that the physician will inspect the patient's nostrils (for patency).
- *To determine the length of tubing needed,* hold the balloon at the patient's xiphoid process and then, extend the tube to

EQUIPMENT

Types of esophageal tubes

When working with patients who have an esophageal tube, remember the advantages of the most common types.

Sengstaken-Blakemore tube

A Sengstaken-Blakemore tube is a triple-lumen, double-balloon tube that has a gastric aspiration port, which allows you to obtain drainage from below the gastric balloon and also to instill medication.

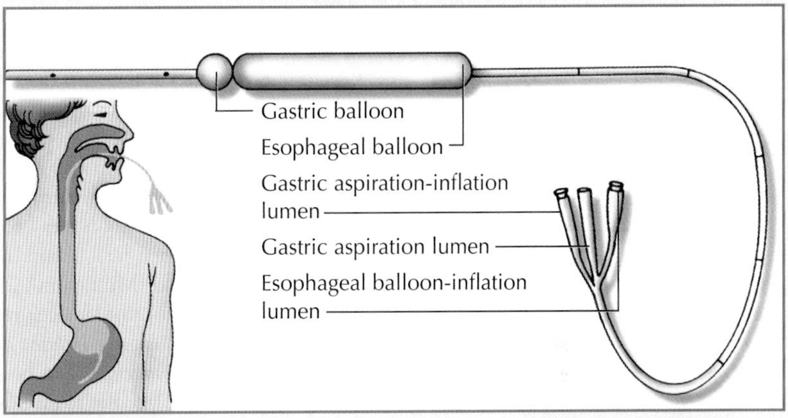

Linton tube

A Linton tube is a triple-lumen, single-balloon tube that has a port for gastric aspiration and one for esophageal aspiration. Additionally, the Linton tube reduces the risk of esophageal necrosis *because it doesn't have an esophageal balloon.*

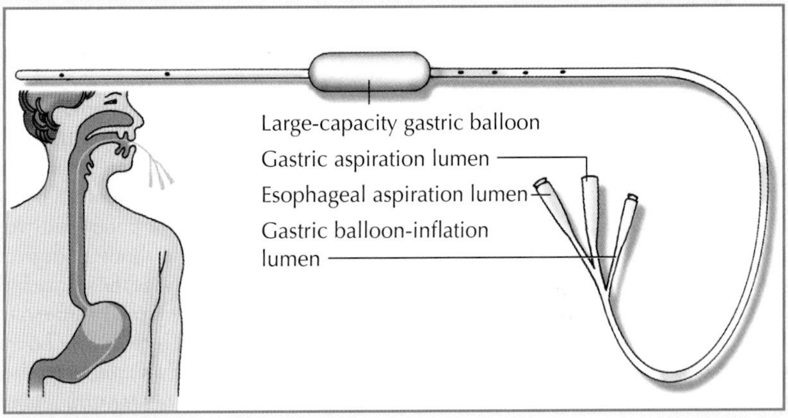

Minnesota esophagogastric tamponade tube

A Minnesota esophagogastric tamponade tube is an esophageal tube that has four lumens and two balloons. The device provides pressure-monitoring ports for both balloons without the need for Y connectors. One port is used for gastric suction, the other for esophageal suction.

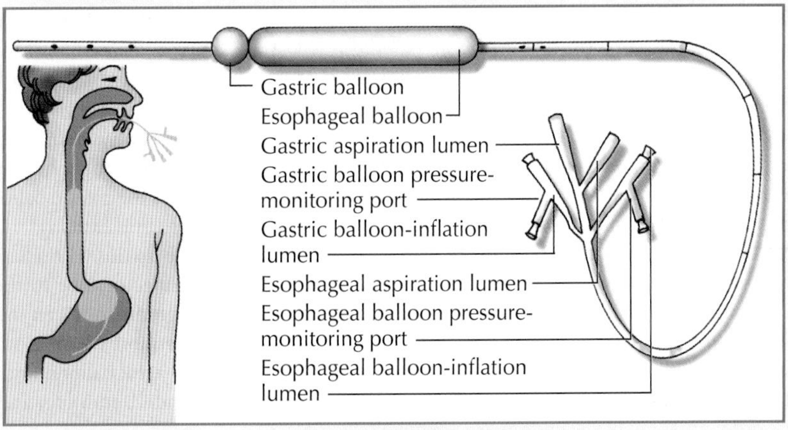

Securing an esophageal tube

To reduce the risk of the gastric balloon's slipping down or away from the cardia of the stomach, secure an esophageal tube to a football helmet. Tape the tube to the face guard, as shown, and fasten the chin strap.

To remove the tube quickly, unfasten the chin strap and pull the helmet slightly forward. Cut the tape and the gastric balloon and esophageal balloon lumens. Be sure to hold onto the tube near the patient's nostril.

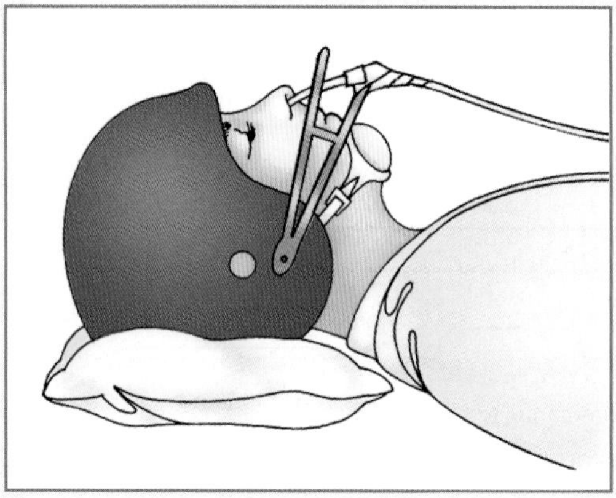

the patient's ear and forward to his nose. Using a waterproof pen, mark this point on the tubing.

- Inform the patient that the physician will spray his throat (posterior pharynx) and nostril with an anesthetic *to minimize discomfort and gagging during intubation.*
- After lubricating the tip of the tube with water-soluble lubricant *to reduce friction and facilitate insertion,* the physician will pass the tube through the more patent nostril. As he does, he'll direct the patient to tilt his chin toward his chest and to swallow when he senses the tip of the tube in the back of his throat. *Swallowing helps to advance the tube into the esophagus and prevents intubation of the trachea.* (If the physician introduces the tube orally, he'll direct the patient to swallow immediately.) As the patient swallows, the physician quickly advances the tube at least 1½" (3.8 cm) beyond the previously marked point on the tube.
- *To confirm tube placement,* the physician will aspirate stomach contents through the gastric port. He'll also auscultate the stomach with a stethoscope as he injects air. After partially inflating the gastric balloon with 50 to 100 cc of air, he'll order an X-ray of the abdomen *to confirm correct placement of the balloon.* Before fully inflating the balloon, he'll use the 60-ml syringe to irrigate the stomach with normal saline solution and empty the stomach as completely as possible. *This helps the patient avoid regurgitating gastric contents when the balloon inflates.*
- After confirming tube placement, the physician will fully inflate the gastric balloon (250 to 500 cc of air for a Sengstaken-Blakemore tube; 700 to 800 cc of air for a Linton tube) and clamp the tube. If he's using a Minnesota tube, he'll connect the pressure-monitoring port for the gastric balloon lumen to the mercury manometer and then inflate the balloon in 100-cc increments until it fills with up to 500 cc of air. As he introduces the air, he'll monitor the intragastric balloon pressure *to make sure the balloon stays inflated.* Then he'll clamp the ports. For the Sengstaken-Blakemore or Minnesota tube, the physician will gently pull on the tube until he feels resistance, *which indicates that the gastric balloon is inflated and exerting pressure on the cardia of the stomach.* When he senses that the balloon is engaged, he'll place the foam nose guard around the area where the tube emerges from the nostril.
- Be ready to tape the nose guard in place around the tube. *This helps to minimize pressure on the nostril from the traction and decreases the risk of necrosis.*
- With the nose guard secured, traction can be applied to the tube with a traction rope and a 1-lb weight (0.5 kg), or the tube can be pulled gently and taped tightly to the face guard of a football helmet. (See *Securing an esophageal tube.*)
- With pulley-and-weight traction, lower the head of the bed to about 25 degrees *to produce countertraction.*
- Lavage the stomach through the gastric aspiration lumen with normal saline solution (iced or tepid) until the return fluid is clear. *The vasoconstriction thus achieved stops the hemorrhage; the lavage empties the stomach. Any blood detected later in the gastric aspirate indicates that bleeding remains uncontrolled.*
- Attach one of the suction sources to the gastric aspiration lumen. *This empties the stomach, helps prevent nausea and possible vomiting, and allows continuous observation of the gastric contents for blood.*
- If the physician inserted a Sengstaken-Blakemore or a Minnesota tube, he'll inflate the esophageal balloon as he inflates the gastric balloon *to compress the esophageal varices and control bleeding.*

To do this with a Sengstaken-Blakemore tube, attach the Y-connector tube to the esophageal lumen. Then attach a sphygmomanometer inflation bulb to one end of the Y-connector and the manometer to the other end. Inflate the esophageal balloon until the pressure gauge ranges between 30 and 40 mm Hg, and clamp the tube.

To do this with a Minnesota tube, attach the mercury manometer directly to the esophageal pressure-monitoring outlet. Then, using the 60-ml syringe and pushing the air slowly into the esophageal balloon port, inflate the balloon until the pressure gauge ranges from 35 to 45 mm Hg.

- Set up esophageal suction *to prevent accumulation of secretions that may cause vomiting and pulmonary aspiration.* This is important *because swallowed secretions can't pass into the stomach if the patient has an inflated esophageal balloon in place.* If the patient has a Linton or a Minnesota tube, attach the suction source to the esophageal aspiration port. If the patient has a Sengstaken-Blakemore tube, advance an NG tube through the other nostril into the esophagus to the point where the esophageal balloon begins, and attach the suction source, as ordered.

Removing the tube

- The physician will deflate the esophageal balloon by aspirating the air with a syringe. (He may order the esophageal balloon to be deflated at 5-mm Hg increments every 30 minutes for several hours.) Then if bleeding doesn't recur, he'll remove the traction from the gastric tube and deflate the gastric balloon (also by aspiration). The gastric balloon is always deflated just before removing the tube *to prevent the balloon from riding up into the esophagus or pharynx and obstructing the airway or, possibly, causing asphyxia or rupture.*
- After disconnecting all suction tubes, the physician will gently remove the esophageal tube. If he feels resistance, he'll aspirate the balloons again. (To remove a Minnesota tube, he'll grasp it near the patient's nostril and cut across all four lumens approximately 3" [7.5 cm] below that point. *This ensures deflation of all balloons.*)
- After the tube has been removed, assist the patient with mouth care.

Special considerations

- If the patient appears cyanotic or if other signs of airway obstruction develop during tube placement, remove the tube immediately *because it may have entered the trachea instead of the esophagus.* After intubation, keep scissors taped to the head of the bed. If respiratory distress occurs, cut across all lumens while holding the tube at the nares, and remove the tube quickly.
- Unless contraindicated, the patient can sip water through a straw during intubation *to facilitate tube advancement.*
- Keep in mind that the intraesophageal balloon pressure varies with respirations and esophageal contractions. Baseline pressure is the important pressure.
- The balloon on the Linton tube should stay inflated no longer than 24 hours *because necrosis of the cardia may result.* Usually, the physician removes the tube only after a trial period (lasting at least 12 hours) with the esophageal balloon deflated or with the gastric balloon tension released from the cardia *to check for rebleeding.* In some facilities, the physician may deflate the esophageal balloon for 5 to 10 minutes every hour *to temporarily relieve pressure on the esophageal mucosa.*

Complications

Erosion and perforation of the esophagus and gastric mucosa may result from the tension placed on these areas by the balloons during traction. Esophageal rupture may result if the gastric balloon accidentally inflates in the esophagus. Acute airway occlusion may result if the balloon dislodges and moves upward into the trachea. Other erosions, nasal tissue necrosis, and aspiration of oral secretions may also complicate the patient's condition.

Documentation

Record the date and time of insertion and removal, the type of tube used, and the name of the physician who performed the procedure. Also document the intraesophageal balloon pressure (for Sengstaken-Blakemore and Minnesota tubes), intragastric balloon pressure (for Minnesota tube), or amount of air injected (for Sengstaken-Blakemore and Linton tubes). Also record the amount of fluid used for gastric irrigation and the color, consistency, and amount of gastric returns, both before and after lavage.

SELECTED REFERENCES

Greenwald, B. "The Minnesota Tube; Its Use and Care in Bleeding Esophageal and Gastric Varices," *Gastroenterology Nursing* 27(5):212-17, September-October 2004.

Greenwald, B. "Two Devices That Facilitate the Use of the Minnesota Tube," *Gastroenterology Nursing* 27(6):268-70, November-December 2004.

Lynn-McHale Wiegand, D.J., and Carlson, K.K., eds. *AACN Procedure Manual for Critical Care,* 5th ed. Philadelphia: W.B. Saunders Co., 2005.

Zaman, A. "Current Management of Esophageal Varices," *Current Treatment Options in Gastroenterology* 6(6):499-507, December 2003.

ESOPHAGEAL TUBE CARE

Although the physician inserts an esophageal tube, the nurse cares for the patient during and after intubation. Typically, the patient is in the intensive care unit for close observation and constant care. The environment may help to increase the patient's tolerance for the procedure and may help to control bleeding. Sedatives may be contraindicated, especially for a patient with portal systemic encephalopathy.

Most important, the patient who has an esophageal tube in place to control variceal bleeding (typically from portal hypertension) must be observed closely for esophageal rupture because varices weaken the esophagus. Additionally, possible traumatic injury from intubation or esophageal balloon inflation increases the chance of rupture. Emergency surgery is usually performed if a rupture occurs, but the operation has a low success rate.

Equipment

Manometer ▪ two 2-L bottles of normal saline solution ▪ irrigation set ▪ water-soluble lubricant ▪ several cotton-tipped applicators ▪ mouth-care equipment ▪ nasopharyngeal suction apparatus ▪ several #12 French suction catheters ▪ intake and output record sheets ▪ gloves ▪ goggles ▪ sedatives ▪ traction weights or football helmet ▪ scissors.

Implementation

- Confirm the patient's identity using two patient identifiers according to your facility's policy.
- *To ease the patient's anxiety,* explain the care that you'll give.
- Provide privacy. Wash your hands and put on gloves and goggles.
- Monitor the patient's vital signs every 5 minutes to 1 hour, as ordered. *A change in vital signs may signal complications or recurrent bleeding.*
- If the patient has a Sengstaken-Blakemore or Minnesota tube, check the pressure gauge on the manometer every hour *to detect any leaks in the esophageal balloon and to verify the set pressure.*
- Maintain drainage and suction on gastric and esophageal aspiration ports as ordered. *This is important because fluid accumulating in the stomach may cause the patient to regurgitate the tube, and fluid accumulating in the esophagus may lead to vomiting and aspiration.*
- Irrigate the gastric aspiration port, as ordered, using the irrigation set and normal saline solution. *Frequent irrigation keeps the tube from clogging. Obstruction in the tube can lead to regurgitation of the tube and vomiting.*
- *To prevent pressure ulcers,* clean the patient's nostrils, and apply water-soluble lubricant frequently. Use warm water to loosen crusted nasal secretions before applying the lubricant with cotton-tipped applicators. Make sure the tube isn't pressing against the nostril.
- Provide mouth care often *to rid the patient's mouth of foul-tasting matter and to relieve dryness from mouth breathing.*
- Use #12 French catheters to provide gentle oral suctioning, if necessary, *to help remove secretions.*
- Offer emotional support. Keep the patient as quiet as possible, and administer sedatives, if ordered.
- Make sure the traction weights hang from the foot of the bed at all times. Never rest them on the bed. Instruct housekeepers and other coworkers not to move the weights *because reduced traction may change the position of the tube.*
- Elevate the head of the bed about 25 degrees *to ensure countertraction for the weights.*
- Keep the patient on complete bed rest *because exertion, such as coughing or straining, increases intra-abdominal pressure, which may trigger further bleeding.*
- Keep the patient in semi-Fowler's position *to reduce blood flow into the portal system and to prevent reflux into the esophagus.*
- Monitor intake and output, as ordered.

Special considerations

- Observe the patient carefully for esophageal rupture indicated by signs and symptoms of shock, increased respiratory difficulties, and increased bleeding. Tape scissors to the head of the bed *so you can cut the tube quickly to deflate the balloons if asphyxia develops.* When performing this emergency intervention, hold the tube firmly close to the nostril before cutting.
- If using traction, be sure to release the tension before deflating any balloons. If weights and pulleys supply traction, remove the weights. If a football helmet supplies traction, untape the esophageal tube from the face guard before deflating the balloons. *Deflating the balloon under tension triggers a rapid release of the entire tube from the nose, which may injure mucous membranes, initiate recurrent bleeding, and obstruct the airway.*
- If the physician orders an X-ray study to check the tube's position or to view the chest, lift the patient in the direction of the pulley, and then place the X-ray film behind his back. Never roll him from side to side *because pressure exerted on the tube in this way may shift the tube's position.* Similarly, lift the patient to make the bed or to assist him with the bedpan.

Complications

Esophageal rupture, the most life-threatening complication associated with esophageal balloon tamponade, can occur at any time but is most likely to occur during intubation or inflation of the esophageal balloon. Asphyxia may result if the balloon moves up the esophagus and blocks the airway. Aspiration of pooled esophageal secretions may also complicate this procedure.

Documentation

Read the manometer hourly, and record the esophageal pressures. Note when the balloons are deflated and by whom. Document vital signs, the condition of the patient's nostrils, routine care, and any drugs administered. Also note the color, consistency, and amount of gastric returns.

Record any signs and symptoms of complications and the nursing actions taken. Document gastric port and nasogastric tube irrigations. Maintain accurate intake and output records.

Selected references

Greenwald, B. "The Minnesota Tube: Its Use and Care in Bleeding Esophageal and Gastric Varices," *Gastroenterology Nursing* 27(5):212-17, September-October 2004.

Lynn-McHale Wiegand, D.J., and Carlson, K.K., eds. *AACN Procedure Manual for Critical Care,* 5th ed. Philadelphia: W.B. Saunders Co., 2005.

Vogel, S.B., et al. "Esophageal Perforation in Adults: Aggressive/Conservative Treatment Lowers Morbidity and Mortality," *Annals of Surgery* 241(6):1016-21, June 2005.

RECTAL ACCESS

Rectal tube insertion and removal

Whether GI hypomotility simply slows the normal release of gas and feces or results in paralytic ileus, inserting a rectal tube may relieve the discomfort of distention and flatus. Decreased motility may result from various medical or surgical conditions, certain medications (such as atropine), or even swallowed air. Conditions that contraindicate using a rectal tube include recent rectal or prostatic surgery, recent myocardial infarction, and diseases of the rectal mucosa.

Equipment

Stethoscope ■ linen-saver pads ■ drape ■ water-soluble lubricant ■ commercial kit or #22 to #34 French rectal tube of soft rubber or plastic ■ container (emesis basin, plastic bag, or water bottle with vent) ■ tape ■ gloves.

Implementation

■ Confirm the patient's identity using two patient identifiers according to your facility's policy.
■ Bring all equipment to the patient's bedside, provide privacy, and wash your hands.
■ Explain the procedure and encourage the patient to relax.
■ Check for abdominal distention. Using the stethoscope, auscultate for bowel sounds.
■ Place the linen-saver pads under the patient's buttocks *to absorb any drainage that may leak from the tube.*
■ Position the patient in the left-lateral Sims' position *to facilitate rectal tube insertion.*
■ Put on gloves.
■ Drape the patient's exposed buttocks.
■ Lubricate the rectal tube tip with water-soluble lubricant *to ease insertion and prevent rectal irritation.*
■ Lift the patient's right buttock *to expose the anus.*
■ Insert the rectal tube tip into the anus, advancing the tube 2″ to 4″ (5 to 10 cm) into the rectum. Direct the tube toward the umbilicus along the anatomic course of the large intestine(as shown below).

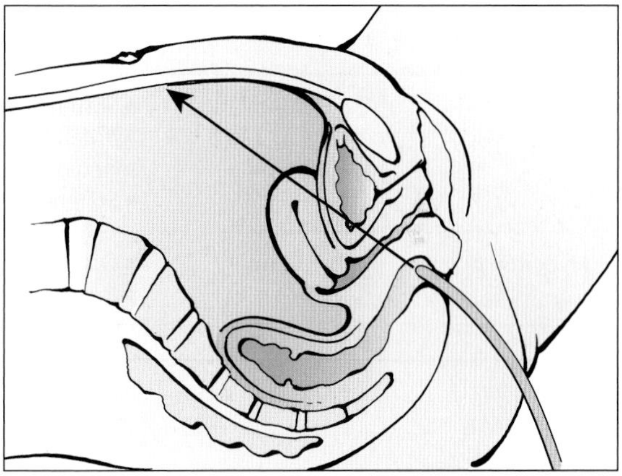

■ As you insert the tube, tell the patient to breathe slowly and deeply, or suggest that he bear down as he would for a bowel movement *to relax the anal sphincter and ease insertion.*
■ Using tape, secure the rectal tube to the buttocks. Then attach the tube to the container *to collect possible leakage.*
■ Remove the tube after 15 to 20 minutes. If the patient reports continued discomfort or if gas wasn't expelled, you can repeat the procedure in 2 to 3 hours if ordered.
■ Clean the patient, and replace soiled linens and the linen-saver pad. Make sure the patient feels as comfortable as possible. Again, check for abdominal distention and listen for bowel sounds.
■ If you will reuse the equipment, clean it and store it in the bedside cabinet; otherwise discard the tube.

Special considerations

■ Inform the patient about each step and reassure him throughout the procedure *to encourage cooperation and promote relaxation.*
■ Fastening a plastic bag (like a balloon) to the external end of the tube lets you observe gas expulsion. Leaving a rectal tube in place indefinitely does little to promote peristalsis, can reduce sphincter responsiveness, and may lead to per-

Commonly used enema solutions

SOLUTION	AMOUNT	ACTION	TIME TO TAKE EFFECT	ADVERSE EFFECTS
Tap water (hypotonic)	500 to 1,000 ml	■ Distends intestine ■ Increases peristalsis ■ Softens stool	15 minutes	Fluid and electrolyte imbalance, water intoxication
Normal saline (isotonic)	500 to 1,000 ml	■ Distends intestine ■ Increases peristalsis ■ Softens stool	15 minutes	Fluid and electrolyte imbalance, sodium retention
Soap	500-1,000 ml (concentrate at 3 to 5 ml/1,000 ml)	■ Distends intestine ■ Irritates intestinal mucosa ■ Softens stool	10 to 15 minutes	Rectal mucosa irritation or damage
Hypertonic	70 to 130 ml	■ Distends intestine ■ Irritates intestinal mucosa	5 to 10 minutes	Sodium retention
Oil (mineral, olive, or cottonseed oil)	150 to 200 ml	■ Lubricates stool and intestinal mucosa	30 minutes	Rectal mucosa irritation

manent sphincter damage or pressure necrosis of the mucosa.

■ Repeat insertion periodically *to stimulate GI activity.* If the tube fails to relieve distention, notify the practitioner.

Documentation

Record the date and time that you insert the tube. Write down the amount, color, and consistency of any evacuated matter. Describe the patient's abdomen—hard, distended, soft, or drumlike on percussion. Note bowel sounds before and after insertion.

SELECTED REFERENCES

Azpiroz, F., and Malagelada, J.R. "Abdominal Bloating," *Gastroenterology* 129(3):1060-78, September 2005.

Craven, R.F., and Hirnle, C.J. *Fundamentals of Nursing: Human Health and Function,* 5th ed. Philadelphia: Lippincott Williams & Wilkins, 2006.

Taylor, C., et al. *Fundamentals of Nursing: The Art and Science of Nursing,* 6th ed. Philadelphia: Lippincott Williams & Wilkins, 2008.

ENEMA ADMINISTRATION

Enema administration involves instilling a solution into the rectum and colon. In a retention enema, the patient holds the solution within the rectum or colon for 30 minutes to 1 hour. In a cleansing enema, the patient expels the solution almost completely within 15 minutes. Both types of enema stimulate peristalsis by mechanically distending the colon and stimulating rectal wall nerves.

Enemas are used to clean the lower bowel in preparation for diagnostic or surgical procedures, to relieve distention and promote expulsion of flatus, to lubricate the rectum and colon, and to soften hardened stool for removal. They're contraindicated, however, after recent colon or rectal surgery or myocardial infarction, and in a patient with an acute abdominal condition of unknown origin, such as suspected appendicitis. They should be administered cautiously to a patient with an arrhythmia.

Equipment

Prescribed solution ■ bath (utility) thermometer ■ enema administration bag with attached rectal tube and clamp ■ I.V.

pole ▪ gloves ▪ linen-saver pads ▪ bath blanket ▪ two bedpans with covers, or bedside commode ▪ water-soluble lubricant ▪ toilet tissue ▪ stethoscope ▪ plastic bag for equipment ▪ water ▪ gown ▪ washcloth ▪ soap and water ▪ if observing enteric precautions: plastic trash bags, labels ▪ optional (for patients who can't retain the solution): plastic rectal tube guard, indwelling urinary catheter, or rectal catheter with 30-ml balloon and syringe.

Prepackaged disposable enema sets are available, as are small-volume enema solutions in both irrigating and retention types and in pediatric sizes.

Preparation of equipment

Prepare the prescribed type and amount of solution, as indicated. (See *Commonly used enema solutions.*) The standard volume of an irrigating enema is 750 to 1,000 ml for an adult.

PEDIATRIC ALERT *Standard irrigating enema volumes for pediatric patients are 500 to 750 ml for a school-age child; 250 to 500 ml for a toddler or preschooler; and 250 ml or less for an infant.*

Because some ingredients may be mucosal irritants, make sure the proportions are correct and the agents are thoroughly mixed *to avoid localized irritation.* Warm the solution *to reduce patient discomfort.* Administer an adult's enema at 105° to 110° F (40.6° to 43° C).

PEDIATRIC ALERT *Administer a child's enema at 100° F (37.8° C)* to avoid burning rectal tissues.

Clamp the tubing and fill the solution bag with the prescribed solution. Unclamp the tubing, flush the solution through the tubing, and then reclamp it. *Flushing detects leaks and removes air that could cause discomfort if introduced into the colon.*

Hang the solution container on the I.V. pole and take all supplies to the patient's room. If you're using an indwelling urinary catheter or rectal catheter, fill the syringe with 30 ml of water.

Implementation

- Confirm the patient's identity using two patient identifiers according to your facility's policy.
- Check the practitioner's order and assess the patient's condition.
- Assess the patient, paying special attention to his abdomen. Be sure to auscultate for bowel sounds; *a cleansing enema will increase peristalsis.*
- Provide privacy and explain the procedure. If you're administering an enema to a child, familiarize him with the equipment and allow a parent or another relative to remain with him during the procedure *to provide reassurance.*
- Ask the patient if he's had previous difficulty retaining an enema *to determine whether you need to use a rectal tube guard or a catheter.*
- Wash your hands.
- Assist the patient, as necessary, in putting on a hospital gown. *The gown makes enema administration easier, and the patient worries less about soiling it.*
- Assist the patient into the left-lateral Sims' position. *This will facilitate the solution's flow by gravity into the descending colon.* If contraindicated or if the patient reports discomfort, reposition him on his back or right side.
- Put on gloves.
- Place linen-saver pads under the patient's buttocks *to prevent soiling the linens.* Replace the top bed linens with a bath blanket *to provide privacy and warmth.*
- Have a bedpan or commode nearby for the patient to use. If the patient may use the bathroom, make sure it will be available when the patient needs it. Have toilet tissue within the patient's reach.
- Lubricate the distal tip of the rectal catheter with water-soluble lubricant *to facilitate rectal insertion and reduce irritation.*
- Separate the patient's buttocks and touch the anal sphincter with the rectal tube *to stimulate contraction.* Then as the sphincter relaxes, tell the patient to breathe deeply through his mouth as you gently advance the tube.
- Advance the tube 2" to 4" (5 to 10 cm), aiming it toward the umbilicus (as shown below). Avoid forcing the tube *to prevent rectal wall trauma.* If it doesn't advance easily, allow a little solution to flow in *to relax the inner sphincter enough to allow passage.*

PEDIATRIC ALERT *For a child, insert the tube only 2" to 3" (5 to 7.5 cm); for an infant, insert it only 1" to 1½" (2.5 to 4 cm).*

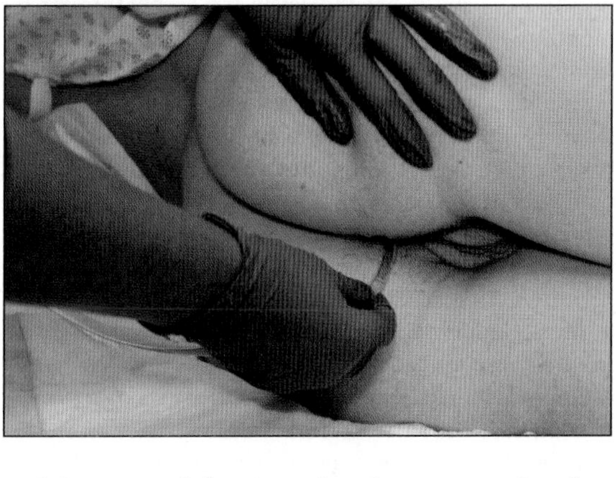

- If the patient feels pain or the tube meets continued resistance, notify the practitioner. *This may signal an unknown*

stricture or abscess. If the patient has poor sphincter control, use a plastic rectal tube guard.

- You can also use an indwelling urinary or rectal catheter as a rectal tube if your facility's policy permits. Insert the lubricated catheter as you would a rectal tube. Then gently inflate the catheter's balloon with 20 to 30 ml of water. Gently pull the catheter back against the patient's internal anal sphincter *to seal off the rectum.* If leakage still occurs with the balloon in place, add more water to the balloon in small amounts. When using either catheter, avoid inflating the balloon above 45 ml *because overinflation can compromise blood flow to the rectal tissues and may cause necrosis from pressure on the rectal mucosa.*
- If you're using a rectal tube, hold it in place throughout the procedure *because bowel contractions and the pressure of the tube against the anal sphincter can promote tube displacement.*
- Hold the solution container slightly above bed level, and release the tubing clamp. Then raise the container gradually to start the flow—usually at a rate of 75 to 100 ml/minute for a cleansing enema, but at the slowest possible rate for a retention enema *to avoid stimulating peristalsis and to promote retention.* Adjust the flow rate of an irrigating enema by raising or lowering the solution container according to the patient's retention ability and comfort. However, be sure not to raise it higher than 18″ (45.7 cm) for an adult, 12″ (30.5 cm) for a child, and 6″ to 8″ (15 to 20 cm) for an infant *because excessive pressure can force colon bacteria into the small intestine or rupture the colon.*
- Assess the patient's tolerance frequently during instillation. If he complains of discomfort, cramps, or the need to defecate, stop the flow by pinching or clamping the tubing. Then hold the patient's buttocks together, or firmly press toilet tissue against the anus. Instruct him to gently massage his abdomen and to breathe slowly and deeply through his mouth *to help relax his abdominal muscles and promote retention.* Resume administration at a slower flow rate after a few minutes when the discomfort passes, but interrupt the flow any time the patient complains of discomfort.
- If the flow slows or stops, the catheter tip may be clogged with feces or pressed against the rectal wall. Gently turn the catheter slightly *to free it without stimulating defecation.* If the catheter tip remains clogged, withdraw the catheter, flush it with solution, and reinsert it.
- After administering most of the prescribed amount of solution, clamp the tubing. Stop the flow before the container empties completely *to avoid introducing air into the bowel.*
- For a flush enema, stop the flow by lowering the solution container below bed level and allowing gravity to siphon the enema from the colon. Continue to raise and lower the container until gas bubbles cease or the patient feels more comfortable and abdominal distention subsides. Don't allow the solution container to empty completely before lowering it *because this may introduce air into the bowel.*
- For a cleansing enema, instruct the patient to retain the solution for 15 minutes, if possible.
- For a retention enema, instruct the patient to avoid defecation for the prescribed time or as follows: 30 minutes or longer for oil retention and milk and molasses; and 15 to 30 minutes for anthelmintic and emollient enemas. If you're using an indwelling catheter, leave the catheter in place *to promote retention.*
- If the patient is apprehensive, position him on the bedpan and allow him to hold toilet tissue or a rolled washcloth against his anus. Place the call signal within his reach. If he will be using the bathroom or the commode, instruct him to call for help before attempting to get out of bed *because the procedure may make the patient—particularly an elderly patient—feel weak or faint.* Also instruct him to call you if he feels weak at any time.
- When the solution has remained in the colon for the recommended time or for as long as the patient can tolerate it, assist the patient onto a bedpan or to the commode or bathroom as required.
- If an indwelling catheter is in place, deflate the balloon and remove the catheter if applicable.
- Provide privacy while the patient expels the solution. Instruct the patient not to flush the toilet.
- While the patient uses the bathroom, remove and discard any soiled linen and linen-saver pads.
- Assist the patient with cleaning, if necessary, and help him to bed. Make sure he feels clean and comfortable and can easily reach the call signal. Place a clean linen-saver pad under him *to absorb rectal drainage,* and tell him that he may need to expel additional stool or flatus later. Encourage him to rest *because the procedure may be tiring.*
- Cover the bedpan or commode and take it to the utility room for observation, or observe the contents of the toilet, as applicable. Carefully note fecal color, consistency, amount (minimal, moderate, or generous), and foreign matter, such as blood, rectal tissue, worms, pus, mucus, or other unusual matter.
- Send specimens to the laboratory, if ordered.
- Rinse the bedpan or commode with cold water, and then wash it in hot soapy water. Return it to the patient's bedside.
- Properly dispose of the enema equipment. If additional enemas are scheduled, store clean, reusable equipment in a closed plastic bag in the patient's bathroom. Discard your gloves and wash your hands.
- Ventilate the room or use an air freshener, if necessary.

Special considerations

- *Because patients with salt-retention disorders, such as heart failure, may absorb sodium from the saline enema solution,* administer the solution to such patients cautiously and monitor electrolyte status.
- Schedule a retention enema before meals because a full stomach may stimulate peristalsis and make retention difficult. Follow an oil-retention enema with a soap and water enema 1 hour later *to help expel the softened feces completely.*
- Administer less solution when giving a hypertonic enema *because osmotic pull moves fluid into the colon from body tissues, increasing the volume of colon contents.* Alternative means of instilling the solution include using a bulb syringe or a funnel with the rectal tube.
- For the patient who can't tolerate a flat position (for example, a patient with shortness of breath), administer the enema with the head of the bed in the lowest position he can safely and comfortably maintain. For a bedridden patient who needs to expel the enema into a bedpan, raise the head of the bed to approximate a sitting or squatting position. Don't give an enema to a patient who's in a sitting position, unless absolutely necessary, *because the solution won't flow high enough into the colon and will only distend the rectum and trigger rapid expulsion.*
- If the patient has hemorrhoids, instruct him to bear down gently during tube insertion. *This causes the anus to open and facilitates insertion.*
- If the patient fails to expel the solution within 1 hour because of diminished neuromuscular response, you may need to remove the enema solution. First, review your facility's policy *because you may need a practitioner's order.* Inform the practitioner when a patient can't expel an enema spontaneously *because of possible bowel perforation or electrolyte imbalance.* To siphon the enema solution from the patient's rectum, assist him to a side-lying position on the bed. Place a bedpan on a bedside chair so that it rests below mattress level. Disconnect the tubing from the solution container, place the distal end in the bedpan, and reinsert the rectal end into the patient's anus. If gravity fails to drain the solution into the bedpan, instill 30 to 50 ml of warm water (105° F [40.6° C] for an adult; 100° F [37.8° C] for a child or infant) through the tube. Then quickly direct the distal end of the tube into the bedpan. In both cases, measure the return *to make sure all of the solution has drained.*
- In patients with fluid and electrolyte disturbances, measure the amount of expelled solution *to assess for retention of enema fluid.*
- Double-bag all enema equipment, and label it as isolation equipment if the patient is on enteric precautions.
- If the practitioner orders enemas until returns are clear, give no more than three *to avoid excessive irritation of the rectal mucosa.* Notify the practitioner if the returned fluid isn't clear after three administrations.
- To administer a commercially prepared, small-volume enema, first remove the cap from the rectal tube. Insert the rectal tube into the rectum and squeeze the bottle *to deposit the contents in the rectum.* Remove the rectal tube, replace the used enema unit in its original container, and discard.

Home care

Describe the procedure to the patient and his family. Emphasize that administering an enema to a person in a sitting position or on the toilet could injure the rectal wall. Tell the patient how to prepare and care for the equipment.

Discuss relaxation techniques, and review measures for preventing constipation, including regular exercise, dietary modifications, and adequate fluid intake.

Complications

Enemas may produce dizziness or faintness; excessive irritation of the colonic mucosa resulting from repeated administration or from sensitivity to the enema's ingredients; hyponatremia or hypokalemia from repeated administration of hypotonic solutions; and cardiac arrhythmias resulting from vasovagal reflex stimulation after insertion of the rectal catheter. Colonic water absorption may result from prolonged retention of hypotonic solutions, which may, in turn, cause hypervolemia or water intoxication.

Documentation

Record the date and time of enema administration; special equipment used; type and amount of solution; retention time; approximate amount returned; color, consistency, and amount of the return; abnormalities within the return; any complications that occurred; and the patient's tolerance of the treatment.

Selected references

Fihn, J.G. "Pain and Cramping with Enema Administration," *Gastroenterology Nursing* 28(3):262, May-June 2005.

Higgins, D. "How to Administer an Enema," *Nursing Times* 102(20):24-25, May 2006.

Schmelzer, M., et al. "Safety and Effectiveness of Large-Volume Enema Solutions," *Applied Nursing Research* 17(4):265-74, November 2004.

Taylor, C., et al. *Fundamentals of Nursing: The Art and Science of Nursing,* 6th ed. Philadelphia: Lippincott Williams & Wilkins, 2008.

TRANSABDOMINAL ACCESS

TRANSABDOMINAL TUBE FEEDING AND CARE

To access the stomach, duodenum, or jejunum, the physician may place a tube through the patient's abdominal wall. This procedure may be done surgically or percutaneously.

A gastrostomy or jejunostomy tube is usually inserted during intra-abdominal surgery. The tube may be used for feeding during the immediate postoperative period, or it may provide long-term enteral access, depending on the type of surgery. Typically, the physician will suture the tube in place to prevent gastric contents from leaking.

In contrast, a percutaneous endoscopic gastrostomy (PEG) or jejunostomy (PEJ) tube can be inserted endoscopically without the need for laparotomy or general anesthesia. Typically, the insertion is done in the endoscopy suite or at the patient's bedside. A PEG or PEJ tube may be used for nutrition, drainage, and decompression. Contraindications to endoscopic placement include obstruction (such as an esophageal stricture or duodenal blockage), previous gastric surgery, morbid obesity, and ascites. These conditions would necessitate surgical placement.

With either type of tube placement, feedings may begin after 24 hours (or when peristalsis resumes).

After a time, the tube may need replacement, and the physician may recommend a similar tube, such as an indwelling urinary catheter or a mushroom catheter, or a gastrostomy button—a skin-level feeding tube. (See "Gastrostomy feeding button care," page 693.)

Nursing care includes providing skin care at the tube site, maintaining the feeding tube, administering feeding, monitoring the patient's response to feeding, adjusting the feeding schedule, and preparing the patient for self-care after discharge.

Equipment

For feeding: Feeding formula ▪ large-bulb or catheter-tip syringe ▪ 120 ml of water ▪ 4″ × 4″ gauze pads ▪ prescribed skin cleaning solution ▪ soap ▪ skin protectant ▪ hypoallergenic tape ▪ gravity-drip administration bags ▪ mouthwash, toothpaste, or mild salt solution ▪ stethoscope ▪ gloves ▪ optional: enteral infusion pump.

For decompression: Suction apparatus with tubing and straight drainage collection set.

Preparation of equipment

Always check the expiration date on commercially prepared feeding formulas. If the formula has been prepared by the dietitian or pharmacist, check the preparation date and time. Discard any opened formula that is more than 1 day old.

Commercially prepared administration sets and enteral pumps allow continuous formula administration. Place the desired amount of formula into the gavage container and purge air from the tubing. *To avoid contamination,* hang only a 4- to 6-hour supply of formula at a time.

Implementation

- Confirm the patient's identity using two patient identifiers according to your facility's policy.
- Provide privacy and wash your hands.
- Explain the procedure to the patient. Tell him, for example, that feedings usually start at a slow rate and increase as tolerated. After he tolerates continuous feedings, he may progress to intermittent feedings as ordered.
- Assess for bowel sounds with a stethoscope before feeding, and monitor for abdominal distention.
- Ask the patient to sit, or assist him into semi-Fowler's position, for the entire feeding. *This helps to prevent esophageal reflux and pulmonary aspiration of the formula.* For an intermittent feeding, have him maintain this position throughout the feeding and for 1 hour afterward.
- Put on gloves. Before starting the feeding, measure residual gastric contents. Attach the syringe to the feeding tube and aspirate. If the contents measure more than twice the amount infused, hold the feeding and recheck in 1 hour. If residual contents still remain too high, notify the practitioner. *Chances are the formula isn't being absorbed properly.* Keep in mind that residual contents will be minimal with PEJ tube feedings.
- Allow 30 ml of water to flow into the feeding tube *to establish patency.*
- Be sure to administer formula at room temperature. *Cold formula may cause cramping.*

Intermittent feedings

- Allow gravity to help the formula flow over 30 to 45 minutes. *Faster infusions may cause bloating, cramps, or diarrhea.*
- Begin intermittent feeding with a low volume (200 ml) daily. According to the patient's tolerance, increase the volume per feeding as needed *to reach the desired calorie intake.*
- When the feeding finishes, flush the feeding tube with 30 to 60 ml of water. *This maintains patency and provides hydration.*
- Cap the tube *to prevent leakage.*

- Rinse the feeding administration set thoroughly with hot water *to avoid contaminating subsequent feedings.* Allow it to dry between feedings.

Continuous feedings

- Measure residual gastric contents every 4 hours.
- To administer the feeding with a pump, set up the equipment according to the manufacturer's guidelines, and fill the feeding bag. To administer the feeding by gravity, fill the container with formula and purge air from the tubing.
- Monitor the gravity drip rate or pump infusion rate frequently *to ensure accurate delivery of formula.*
- Flush the feeding tube with 30 to 60 ml of water every 4 hours *to maintain patency and to provide hydration.*
- Monitor intake and output *to anticipate and detect fluid or electrolyte imbalances.*

Decompression

- To decompress the stomach, connect the PEG port to the suction device with tubing or straight gravity drainage tubing. Jejunostomy feeding may be given simultaneously via the PEJ port of the dual-lumen tube.

Tube exit site care

- Provide daily skin care.
- Gently remove the dressing by hand. Never cut away the dressing over the catheter *because you might cut the tube or the sutures holding the tube in place.*
- At least daily and as needed, clean the skin around the tube's exit site using a 4″ × 4″ gauze pad soaked in the prescribed cleaning solution. When healed, wash the skin around the exit site daily with soap. Rinse the area with water and pat dry. Apply skin protectant, if necessary.
- Anchor a gastrostomy or jejunostomy tube to the skin with hypoallergenic tape *to prevent peristaltic migration of the tube. This also prevents tension on the suture anchoring the tube in place.*
- Coil the tube, if necessary, and tape it to the abdomen *to prevent pulling and contamination of the tube.* PEG and PEJ tubes have toggle-bolt-like internal and external bumpers that make tape anchors unnecessary. (See *Caring for a PEG or PEJ site,* page 692.)

Special considerations

- If the patient vomits or complains of nausea, complains of feeling too full, or regurgitates, stop the feeding immediately and assess his condition. Flush the feeding tube and attempt to restart the feeding in 1 hour (measure residual gastric contents first). You may have to decrease the volume or rate of feedings. If the patient develops dumping syndrome, which includes nausea, vomiting, cramps, pallor, and diarrhea, the feedings may have been given too quickly.
- Provide oral hygiene frequently. Brush all surfaces of the teeth, gums, and tongue at least twice daily using mouthwash, toothpaste, or a mild salt solution.
- You can administer most tablets and pills through the tube by crushing them and diluting as necessary. (However, don't crush enteric-coated or sustained-release drugs, *which lose their effectiveness when crushed.*) Medications should be in liquid form for administration.
- Control diarrhea resulting from dumping syndrome by using continuous pump or gravity-drip infusions, diluting the feeding formula, or adding antidiarrheal medications.

Home care

Instruct the patient and his family members or other caregivers in all aspects of enteral feedings, including tube maintenance and site care. Specify signs and symptoms to report to the practitioner, define emergency situations, and review actions to take.

When the tube needs replacement, advise the patient that the physician may insert a replacement gastrostomy button or a latex, indwelling, or mushroom catheter after removing the initial feeding tube. The procedure may be done in the physician's office or your facility's endoscopy suite.

As the patient's tolerance of tube feeding improves, he may wish to try syringe feedings rather than intermittent feedings. If appropriate, teach him how to feed himself by the syringe method. (See *Teaching the patient about syringe feeding,* page 693.)

Complications

Common complications related to transabdominal tubes include GI or other systemic problems, mechanical malfunction, and metabolic disturbances. Cramping, nausea, vomiting, bloating, and diarrhea may be related to medication; rapid infusion rate; formula contamination, osmolarity, or temperature (too cold or too warm); fat malabsorption; or intestinal atrophy from malnutrition. Constipation may result from inadequate hydration or insufficient exercise.

Systemic problems may be caused by pulmonary aspiration, infection at the tube exit site, or contaminated formula. Proper positioning during feeding, verification of tube placement, meticulous skin care, and sterile formula preparation are ways to prevent these complications. Monitor for signs of infection, such as drainage, redness, tenderness, and warmth.

Typical mechanical problems include tube dislodgment, obstruction, or impairment. For example, a PEG or PEJ tube may migrate if the external bumper loosens. Occlusion may result from incompletely crushed and liquefied med-

Caring for a PEG or PEJ site

The exit site of a percutaneous endoscopic gastrostomy (PEG) or percutaneous endoscopic jejunostomy (PEJ) tube requires routine observation and care. Follow these care guidelines:

- Change the dressing daily while the tube is in place.
- After removing the dressing, carefully slide the tube's outer bumper away from the skin (as shown below) about ½" (1 cm).
- Examine the skin around the tube. Look for redness and other signs of infection or erosion.

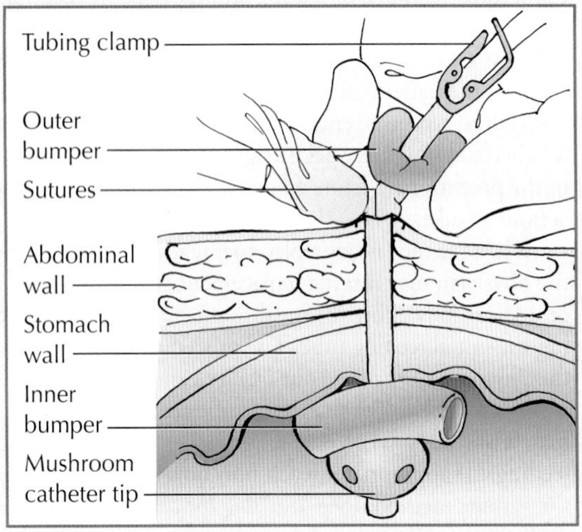

- Gently depress the skin surrounding the tube and inspect for drainage (as shown above right). Expect minimal wound drainage initially after implantation. This should subside in about 1 week.

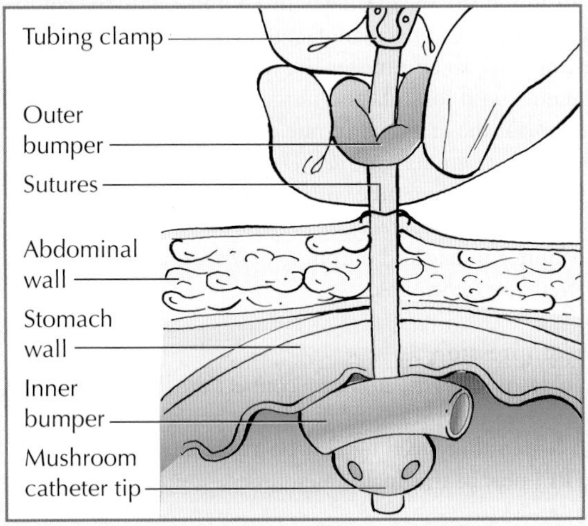

- Inspect the tube for wear and tear. (A tube that wears out will need replacement.)
- Clean the site with the prescribed cleaning solution.
- Rotate the outer bumper 90 degrees *(to avoid repeating the same tension on the same skin area)*, and slide the outer bumper back over the exit site.
- If leakage appears at the PEG site, or if the patient risks dislodging the tube, apply a sterile gauze dressing over the site. Don't put sterile gauze underneath the outer bumper. *Loosening the anchor this way allows the feeding tube free play, which could lead to wound abscess.*
- Write the date and time of the dressing change on the tape.

ication particles or inadequate tube flushing. Further, the tube may rupture or crack from age, drying, or frequent manipulation.

Monitor the patient for vitamin and mineral deficiencies, glucose tolerance, and fluid and electrolyte imbalances, which may follow bouts of diarrhea or constipation.

Documentation

On the intake and output record, note the date, time, and amount of each feeding and the water volume instilled. Maintain total volumes for nutrients and water separately to allow calculation of nutrient intake. In your notes, document the type of formula, the infusion method and rate, the patient's tolerance of the procedure and formula, and the amount of residual gastric contents. Also record complications and abdominal assessment findings. Note patient-teaching topics covered and the patient's progress in self-care.

Selected references

Reising, D.L., and Neal, R.S. "Enteral Tube Flushing: What You Think Are the Best Practices May Not Be," *AJN* 105(3):58-63, March 2005.

Teaching the patient about syringe feeding

If the patient plans to feed himself by syringe when he returns home, you'll need to teach him how to do this before he's discharged. Here are some points to emphasize.

Initial instructions

First, show the patient how to clamp the feeding tube, remove the syringe's bulb or plunger, and place the tip of the syringe into the feeding tube (as shown below). Then tell him to instill between 30 and 60 ml of water

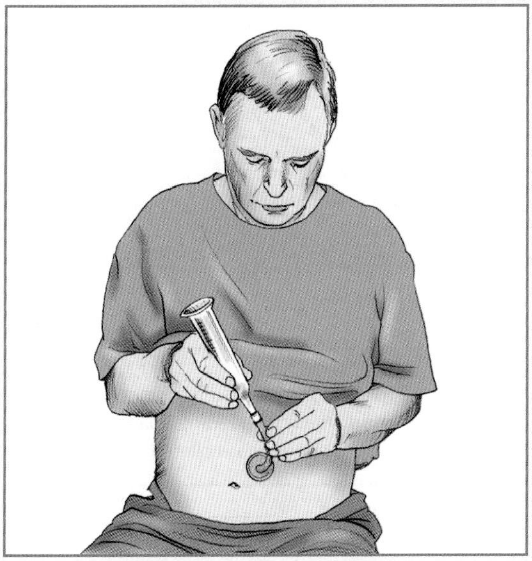

into the feeding tube *to make sure it stays open and patent.*

Next, tell him to pour the feeding solution into the syringe and begin the feeding (as shown above right). As the solution flows into the stomach, show him how to tilt the syringe *to allow air bubbles to escape*. Describe the discomfort that air bubbles may cause.

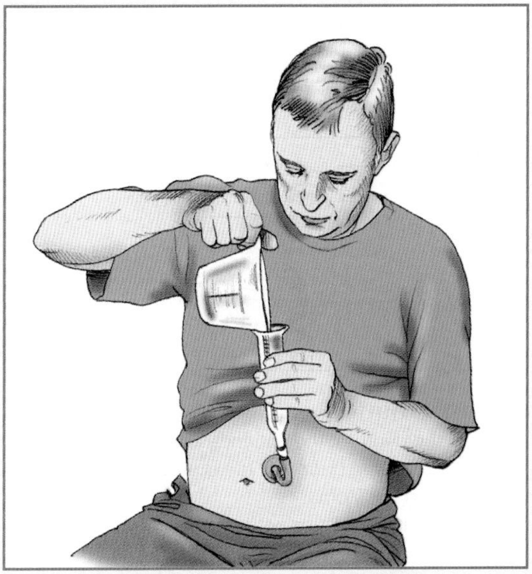

Tips for free flow

When about one-quarter of the feeding solution remains, direct the patient to refill the syringe. Caution him to avoid letting the syringe empty completely. *Doing so may result in abdominal cramping and gas.*

Show the patient how to increase and decrease the solution's flow rate by raising or lowering the syringe. Explain that he may need to dilute a thick solution *to promote free flow.*

Finishing up

Inform the patient that the feeding infusion process should take at least 15 minutes. If the process takes less than 15 minutes, dumping syndrome may result.

Show the patient the steps needed to finish the feeding, including how to flush the tube with water, clamp the tube, and clean the equipment for later use. If he's using disposable gear, urge him to discard it properly. Review instructions for storing unused feeding solution as appropriate.

Scolapio, J.S. "A Review of the Trends in the Use of Enteral and Parenteral Nutrition Support," *Journal of Clinical Gastroenterology* 38(5):403-407, May-June 2004.

Taylor, C., et al. *Fundamentals of Nursing: The Art and Science of Nursing,* 6th ed. Philadelphia: Lippincott Williams & Wilkins, 2008.

GASTROSTOMY FEEDING BUTTON CARE

A gastrostomy feeding button serves as an alternative feeding device for an ambulatory patient who's receiving long-term enteral feedings. Approved by the Food and Drug Ad-

How to reinsert a gastrostomy feeding button

If your patient's gastrostomy feeding button pops out (with coughing, for instance), you or he will need to reinsert the device. Here are some steps to follow.

Prepare the equipment

Collect the feeding button, an obturator, and water-soluble lubricant. If the button will be reinserted, wash it with soap and water and rinse it thoroughly.

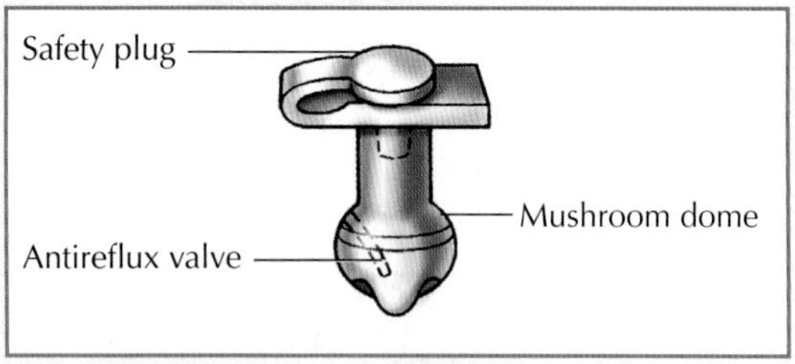

Insert the button

- Check the depth of the patient's stoma *to make sure you have a feeding button of the correct size.* Then clean around the stoma.
- Lubricate the obturator with a water-soluble lubricant, and distend the button several times *to ensure the patency of the antireflux valve within the button.*
- Lubricate the mushroom dome and the stoma. Gently push the button through the stoma into the stomach.

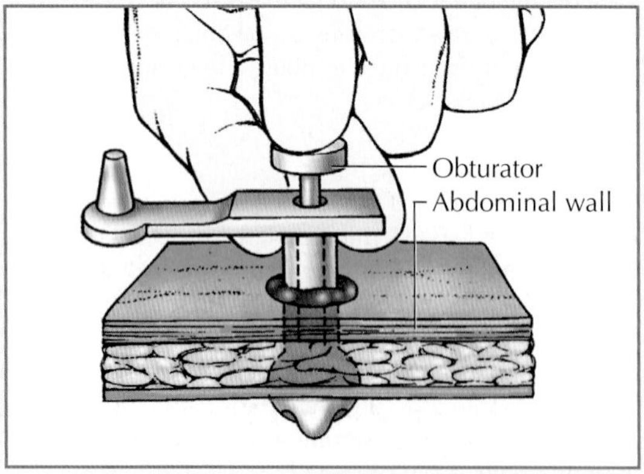

- Remove the obturator by gently rotating it as you withdraw it *to keep the antireflux valve from adhering to it.* If the valve sticks nonetheless, gently push the obturator back into the button until the valve closes.
- After removing the obturator, make sure the valve is closed. Then close the flexible safety plug, which should be relatively flush with the skin surface.

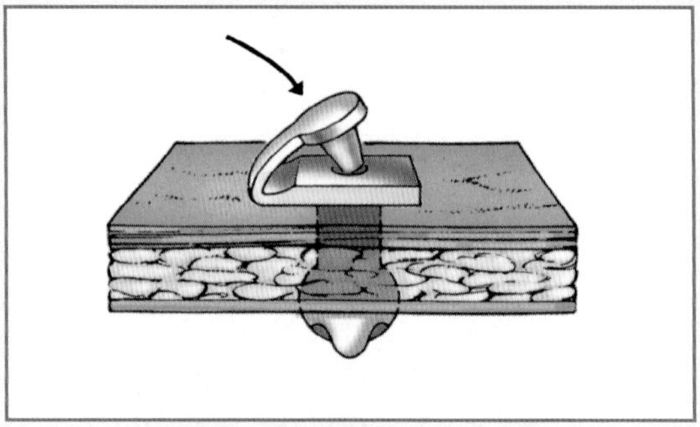

- If you need to administer a feeding right away, open the safety plug and attach the feeding adapter and feeding tube. Deliver the feeding, as ordered.

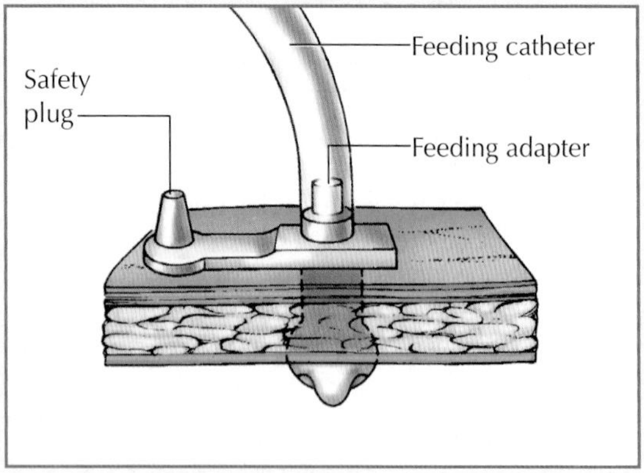

ministration for 6-month implantation, feeding buttons can be used to replace gastrostomy tubes if necessary.

The feeding button has a mushroom dome at one end and two wing tabs and a flexible safety plug at the other. When inserted into an established stoma, the button lies almost flush with the skin, with only the top of the safety plug visible.

The button usually can be inserted into a stoma in less than 15 minutes. Besides its cosmetic appeal, the device is easily maintained, reduces skin irritation and breakdown, and is less likely to become dislodged or to migrate than an ordinary feeding tube. A one-way, antireflux valve mounted just inside the mushroom dome prevents accidental leakage of gastric contents. The device usually requires replacement after 3 to 4 months, typically because the antireflux valve wears out.

Equipment

Gloves ■ feeding accessories, including adapter, feeding catheter, food syringe or bag, and formula ■ catheter clamp ■ cleaning equipment, including water, a syringe, cotton-tipped applicator, pipe cleaner, and mild soap or antiseptic solution ■ optional: pump.

Implementation

- Confirm the patient's identity using two patient identifiers according to your facility's policy.
- Explain the insertion, reinsertion, and feeding procedure to the patient. Tell him the physician will perform the initial insertion.
- Wash your hands and put on gloves.
- Elevate the head of the bed 30 to 45 degrees.
- Check for residual with the syringe. If greater than 50 to 100 ml, report to the practitioner and hold the feeding until reassessment.
- Attach the adapter and feeding catheter to the syringe or feeding bag. Clamp the catheter and fill the syringe or bag and catheter with formula. Refill the syringe before it's empty. *These steps prevent air from entering the stomach and distending the abdomen.*
- Open the safety plug, and attach the adapter and feeding catheter to the button. Elevate the syringe or feeding bag above stomach level, and gravity-feed the formula for 15 to 30 minutes, varying the height as needed *to alter the flow rate.* Use a pump for continuous infusion or for feedings lasting several hours.
- After the feeding, flush the button with 10 ml of water and clean the inside of the feeding catheter with a cotton-tipped applicator and water *to preserve patency and to dislodge formula or food particles.* Then lower the syringe or bag below stomach level *to allow burping.* Remove the adapter and feeding catheter. The antireflux valve should prevent gastric reflux. Then snap the safety plug in place *to keep the lumen clean and prevent leakage if the antireflux valve fails.* If the patient feels nauseated or vomits after the feeding, vent the button with the adapter and feeding catheter *to control emesis.*
- Maintain head of bed elevation of 30 to 45 degrees for at least 1 hour after feeding.
- Wash the catheter and syringe or feeding bag in warm soapy water and rinse thoroughly. Clean the catheter and adapter with a pipe cleaner. Rinse well before using for the next feeding. Soak the equipment once a week according to manufacturer's recommendations.

Special considerations

- If the button pops out while feeding, reinsert it, estimate the formula already delivered, and resume feeding. (See *How to reinsert a gastrostomy feeding button.*)
- Once daily, clean the peristomal skin with mild soap and water or antiseptic solution, and let the skin air-dry for 20 minutes *to avoid skin irritation.* Also clean the site whenever spillage from the feeding bag occurs.
- As the patient's weight or body mass index increases, monitor the site for embedded bumper (external). Report skin irritation and increased tension between the exit site and the bumper to the practitioner.

Home care

Before discharge, make sure the patient can insert and care for the gastrostomy feeding button. If necessary, teach him or a family member how to reinsert the button by first practicing on a model. Offer written instructions and answer his questions on obtaining replacement supplies.

Documentation

Record feeding time and duration, amount and type of feeding formula used, and patient tolerance. Maintain intake and output records as necessary. Note the appearance of the stoma and surrounding skin.

SELECTED REFERENCES

American Society for Parenteral and Enteral Nutrition. "Standards for Nutrition Support: Hospitalized Patients," *Nutrition in Clinical Practice* 10:208-19, December 1995.

Goldberg, E., et al. "Gastrostomy Tubes: Facts, Fallacies, Fistulas, and False Tracts," *Gastroenterology Nursing* 28(6):485-93, November-December 2005.

Guenter, P., and Silkroski, M. *Tube Feeding: Practical Guidelines and Nursing Protocols.* Gaithersburg, Md.: Aspen Pubs., Inc., 2001.

Holman, C., et al. "Promoting Adequate Nutrition: Using Artificial Feeding," *Nursing Older People* 17(10):31-32, January 2006.

Smeltzer, S.C., et al. *Brunner & Suddarth's Textbook of Medical-Surgical Nursing,* 11th ed. Philadelphia: Lippincott Williams & Wilkins, 2008.

COLOSTOMY AND ILEOSTOMY CARE

A patient with an ascending or transverse colostomy or an ileostomy must wear an external pouch to collect emerging fecal matter, which will be watery or pasty. Besides collect-

EQUIPMENT

Comparing ostomy pouching systems

Manufactured in many shapes and sizes, ostomy pouches are fashioned for comfort, safety, and easy application. For example, a disposable closed-end pouch may meet the needs of a patient who irrigates, who wants added security, or who wants to discard the pouch after each bowel movement. Another patient may prefer a reusable, drainable pouch. Some commonly available pouches are described below.

Disposable pouches

The patient who must empty his pouch often (because of diarrhea or a new colostomy or ileostomy) may prefer a one-piece, drainable, disposable pouch with a closure clamp attached to a skin barrier (shown below).

These transparent or opaque, odor-proof, plastic pouches come with attached adhesive or karaya seals. Some pouches have microporous adhesive. The bottom opening allows for easy draining. This pouch may be used permanently or temporarily, until stoma size stabilizes.

Also disposable and made of transparent or opaque odor-proof plastic, a one-piece disposable closed-end pouch may come in a kit with adhesive seal, belt tabs, skin barrier, or carbon filter for gas release. A patient with a regular bowel elimination pattern may choose this style for additional security and confidence.

A two-piece disposable drainable pouch with separate skin barrier (shown at right) permits frequent changes and also minimizes skin breakdown. Also made of transparent or opaque odor-proof plastic, this style comes with belt tabs and usually snaps to the skin barrier with a flange mechanism.

One-piece pouch

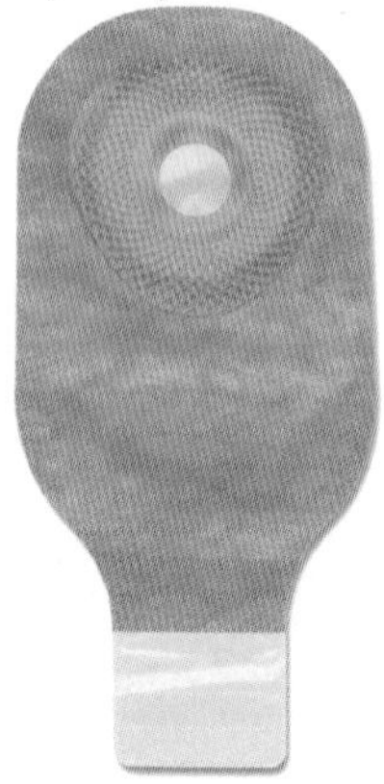

Skin barrier

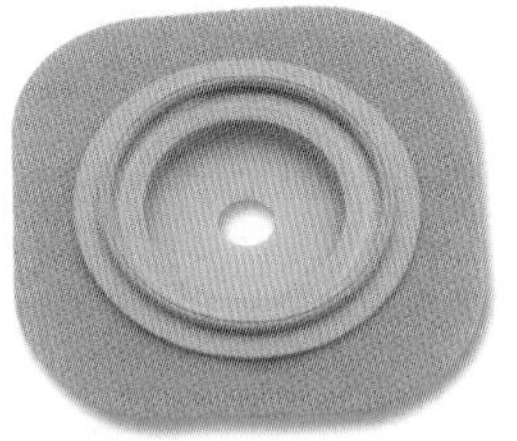

Disposable pouch

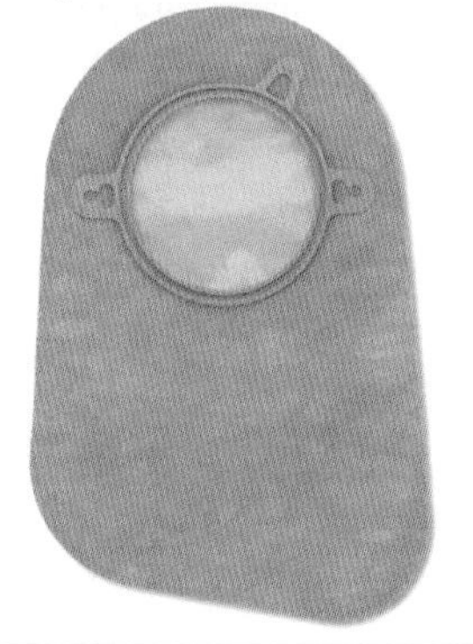

Photographs courtesy of Hollister, Incorporated, Libertyville, Ill.

ing waste matter, the pouch helps to control odor and protect the stoma and peristomal skin. Most disposable pouching systems can be used for 2 to 7 days; some models last even longer.

All pouching systems need to be changed immediately if a leak develops, and every pouch must be emptied when it's one-third to one-half full. The patient with an ileostomy may need to empty his pouch four or five times daily.

Naturally, the best time to change the pouching system is when the bowel is least active, usually between 2 to 4 hours after meals. After a few months, most patients can predict the best changing time.

The selection of a pouching system should take into consideration which system provides the best adhesive seal and skin protection for the individual patient. The type of pouch selected also depends on the stoma's location and structure, availability of supplies, wear time, consistency of effluent, personal preference, and finances.

Equipment

Pouching system ▪ stoma measuring guide ▪ stoma paste (if drainage is watery to pasty or stoma secretes excess mucus) ▪ scissors ▪ clippers ▪ washcloth and towel ▪ closure clamp ▪ toilet or bedpan ▪ water or pouch cleaning solution ▪ gloves ▪ facial tissues ▪ optional: paper tape, mild nonmoisturizing soap, liquid skin sealant, pouch deodorant.

Pouching systems may be drainable or closed-bottomed, disposable or reusable, adhesive-backed, and one-piece or two-piece. (See *Comparing ostomy pouching systems.*)

Implementation

■ Provide privacy and emotional support.

Fitting the pouch and skin barrier

■ For a pouch with an attached skin barrier, measure the stoma with the stoma measuring guide. Select the opening size that matches the stoma.

■ For an adhesive-backed pouch with a separate skin barrier, measure the stoma with the measuring guide and select the opening that matches the stoma. Trace the selected size opening onto the paper back of the skin barrier's adhesive side. Cut out the opening. (If the pouch has precut openings, which can be handy for a round stoma, select an opening that is ⅛″ larger than the stoma. If the pouch comes without an opening, cut the hole ⅛″ wider than the measured tracing.) The cut-to-fit system works best for an irregularly shaped stoma.

■ For a two-piece pouching system with flanges, see *Applying a skin barrier and pouch,* page 698.

■ Avoid fitting the pouch too tightly *because the stoma has no pain receptors. A constrictive opening could injure the stoma or skin tissue without the patient feeling warning discomfort.* Also avoid cutting the opening too big *because this may expose the skin to fecal matter and moisture.*

■ The patient with a descending or sigmoid colostomy who has formed stools and whose ostomy doesn't secrete much mucus may choose to wear only a pouch. In this case, make sure the pouch opening closely matches the stoma size.

■ Between 6 weeks and 1 year after surgery, the stoma will shrink to its permanent size. At that point, pattern-making preparations will be unnecessary unless the patient gains weight, has additional surgery, or injures the stoma.

Applying or changing the pouch

■ Collect all equipment.

■ Wash your hands and provide privacy.

■ Explain the procedure to the patient. As you perform each step, explain what you are doing and why *because the patient will eventually perform the procedure himself.*

■ Put on gloves.

■ Remove and discard the old pouch (as shown below).

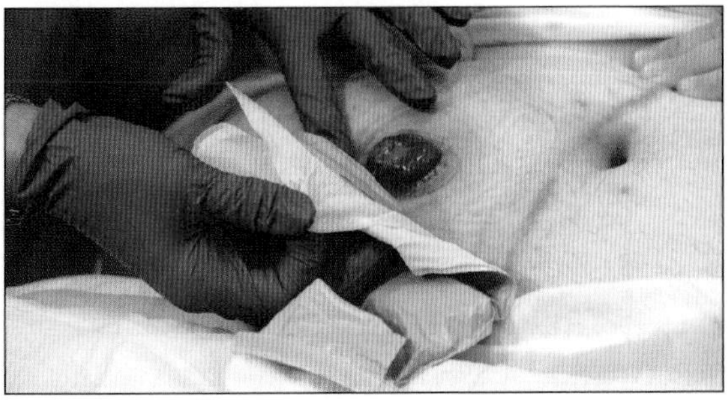

■ Wipe the stoma and peristomal skin gently with a facial tissue (as shown below).

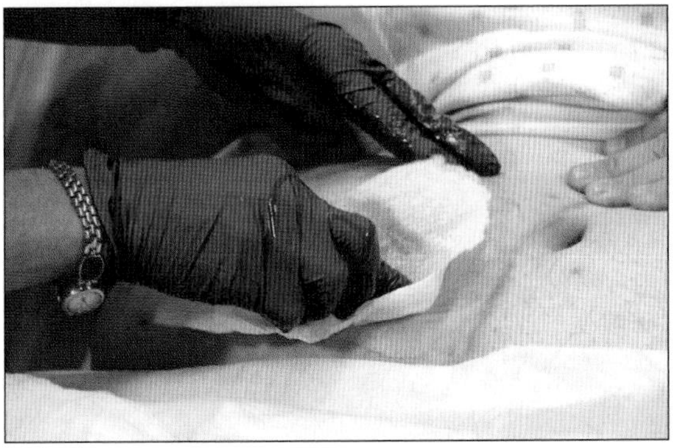

■ Carefully wash with mild soap and water and dry the peristomal skin by patting gently. Allow the skin to dry thoroughly. Inspect the peristomal skin and stoma (as shown below). If necessary, clip surrounding hair (in a direction away from the stoma) *to promote a better seal and avoid skin irritation from hair pulling against the adhesive.*

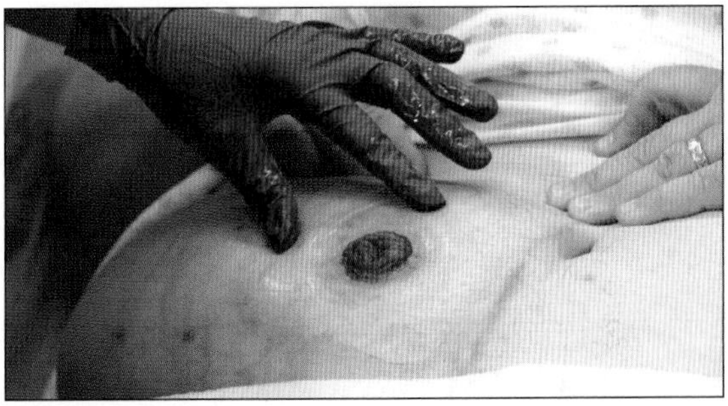

■ If applying a separate skin barrier, peel off the paper backing of the prepared skin barrier, center the barrier over the stoma, and press gently to ensure adhesion.

■ You may want to outline the stoma on the back of the skin barrier (depending on the product) with a thin ring of stoma paste *to provide extra skin protection.* (Skip this step if the patient has a sigmoid or descending colostomy, formed stools, and little mucus.)

■ Remove the paper backing from the adhesive side of the pouching system and center the pouch opening over the stoma. Press gently to secure.

■ For a pouching system with flanges, align the lip of the pouch flange with the bottom edge of the skin barrier flange. Gently press around the circumference of the pouch flange, beginning at the bottom, until the pouch securely adheres to the barrier flange. (The pouch will click into its secured position.) Holding the barrier against the skin, gently pull on the pouch *to confirm the seal between flanges.*

Applying a skin barrier and pouch

Fitting a skin barrier and ostomy pouch properly can be done in a few steps. Shown here is a two-piece pouching system with flanges, which is in common use.

Measure the stoma using a measuring guide.

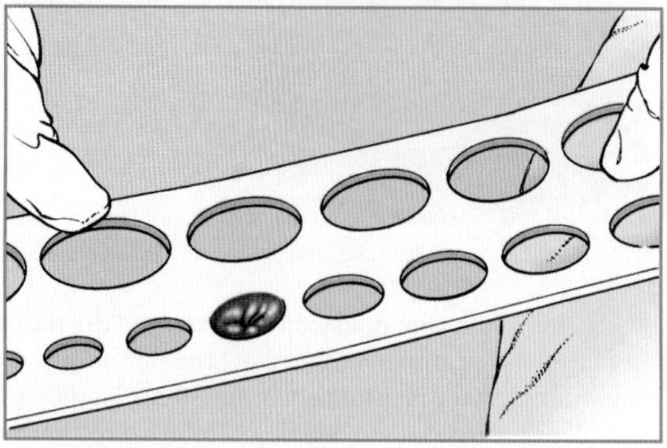

Trace the appropriate circle carefully on the back of the skin barrier.

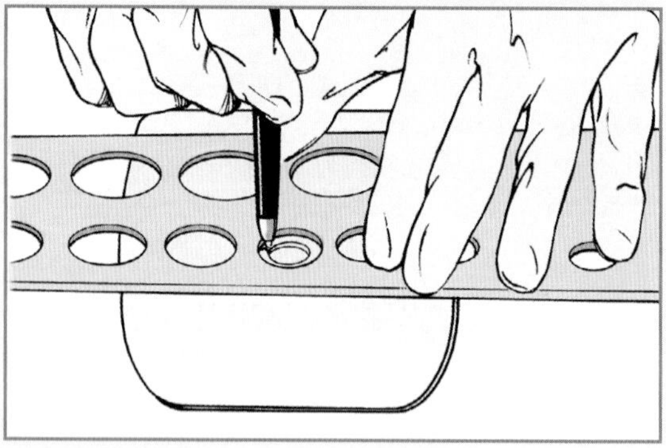

Cut the circular opening in the skin barrier. Bevel the edges *to keep them from irritating the patient.*

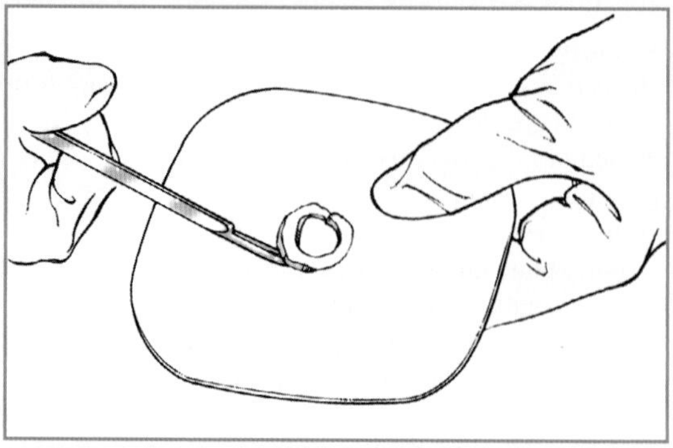

Remove the backing from the skin barrier and moisten it or apply barrier paste, as needed, along the edge of the circular opening.

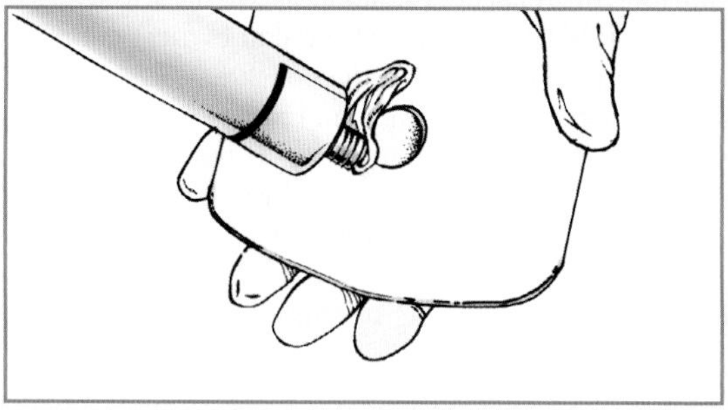

Center the skin barrier over the stoma, adhesive side down, and gently press it to the skin.

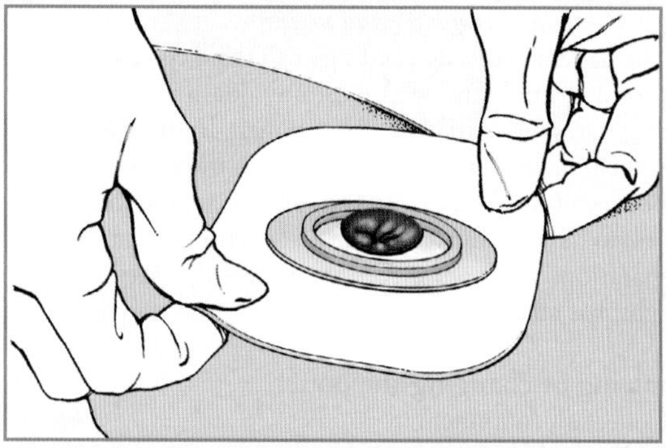

Gently press the pouch opening onto the ring until it snaps into place.

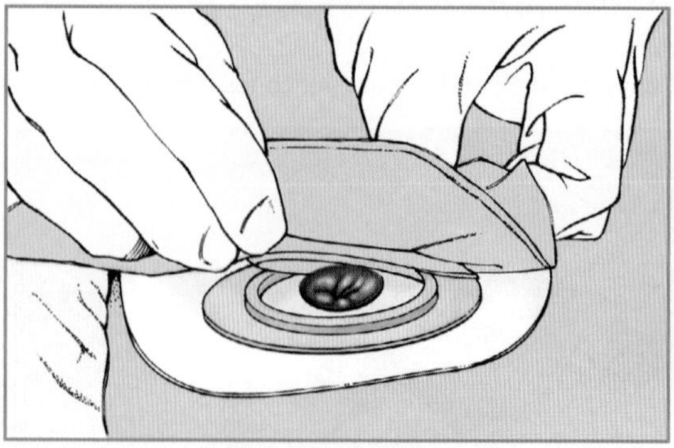

- Encourage the patient to stay quietly in position for about 5 minutes *to improve adherence. The patient's body warmth also helps to improve adherence and soften a rigid skin barrier.*
- Leave a bit of air in the pouch *to allow drainage to fall to the bottom.*
- Apply the closure clamp if necessary.
- If desired, apply paper tape in a picture-frame fashion to the pouch edges *for additional security.*

Emptying the pouch

- Put on gloves.
- Tilt the bottom of the pouch upward and remove the closure clamp (as shown below).

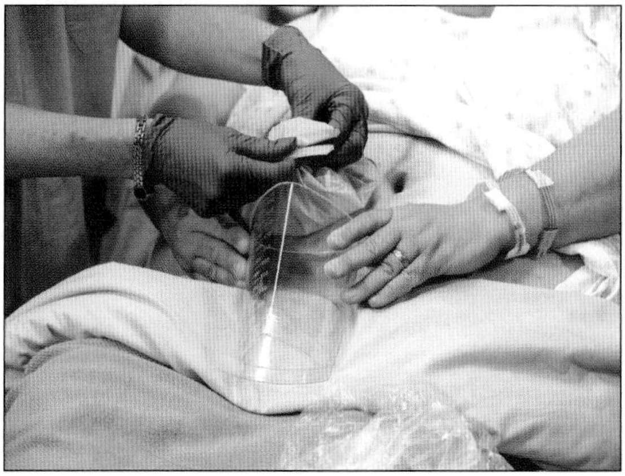

- Turn up a cuff on the lower end of the pouch and allow it to drain into the toilet or bedpan (as shown below).

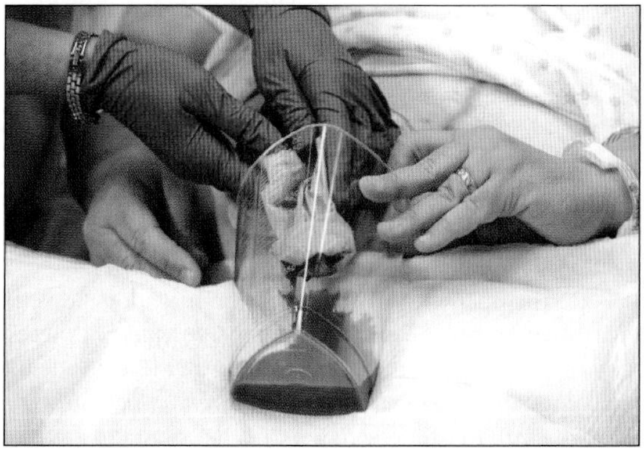

- Wipe the bottom of the pouch and reapply the closure clamp (as shown top of next column.

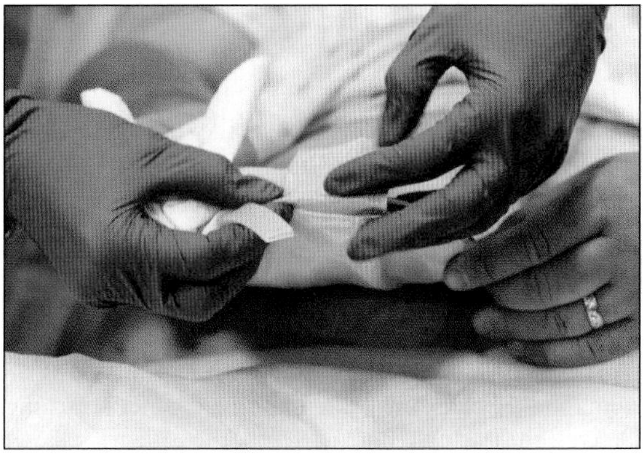

- If desired, the bottom portion of the pouch can be rinsed with cool tap water. Don't aim water up near the top of the pouch *because this may loosen the seal on the skin.*
- A two-piece flanged system can also be emptied by unsnapping the pouch. Let the drainage flow into the toilet.
- Release flatus through the gas release valve if the pouch has one. Otherwise, release flatus by tilting the pouch bottom upward, releasing the clamp, and expelling the flatus. To release flatus from a flanged system, loosen the seal between the flanges. (Some pouches have gas release valves.)
- Never make a pinhole in a pouch to release gas. *This destroys the odor-proof seal.*
- Remove and discard gloves.

Special considerations

- After performing and explaining the procedure to the patient, encourage the patient's increasing involvement in self-care.
- Use adhesive solvents and removers only after patch-testing the patient's skin *because some products may irritate the skin or produce hypersensitivity reactions.* Consider using a liquid skin sealant, if available, *to give skin tissue additional protection from drainage and adhesive irritants.*
- Remove the pouching system if the patient reports burning or itching beneath it or purulent drainage around the stoma. Notify the practitioner of any skin irritation, breakdown, rash, or unusual appearance of the stoma or peristomal area.
- Use commercial pouch deodorants, if desired. However, most pouches are odor-free, and odor should only be evident when you empty the pouch or if it leaks. Before discharge, suggest that the patient avoid odor-causing foods, such as fish, eggs, onions, and garlic.
- If the patient wears a reusable pouching system, suggest that he obtain two or more systems *so that he can wear one*

while the other dries after cleaning with soap and water or a commercially prepared cleaning solution.

Complications

Failure to fit the pouch properly over the stoma or improper use of a belt can injure the stoma. Be alert for a possible allergic reaction to adhesives and other ostomy products.

Documentation

Record the date and time of the pouching system change; note the character of drainage, including color, amount, type, and consistency. Also describe the appearance of the stoma and the peristomal skin. Document patient teaching. Describe the teaching content. Record the patient's response to self-care, and evaluate his learning progress.

SELECTED REFERENCES

Colwell, J.C., and Fichera, A. "Care of the Obese Patient with an Ostomy," *Journal of Wound, Ostomy, and Continence Nursing* 32(6):378-83, November-December 2005.

Pontierei-Lewis, V. "Basics of Ostomy Care," *Medsurg Nursing* 15(4):199-202, August 2006.

Taylor, C., et al. *Fundamentals of Nursing: The Art and Science of Nursing Care,* 6th ed. Philadelphia: Lippincott Williams & Wilkins, 2008.

Turnbull, G.B. "Using Education to Increase Self-Care for the Person with an Ostomy," *Ostomy/Wound Management* 52(9):16, 18, September 2006.

COLOSTOMY IRRIGATION

Irrigation of a colostomy can serve two purposes: It allows a patient with a descending or sigmoid colostomy to regulate bowel function, and it cleans the large bowel before and after tests, surgery, or other procedures.

Colostomy irrigation may begin as soon as bowel function resumes after surgery. However, most clinicians recommend waiting until bowel movements are more predictable. Initially, the nurse or the patient irrigates the colostomy at the same time every day, recording the amount of output and any spillage between irrigations. Between 4 and 6 weeks may pass before colostomy irrigation establishes a predictable elimination pattern.

Equipment

Colostomy irrigation set (contains an irrigation drain or sleeve, an ostomy belt [if needed] to secure the drain or sleeve, water-soluble lubricant, drainage pouch clamp, and irrigation bag with clamp, tubing, and cone tip) ▪ 1,000 ml (1 qt) of tap water irrigant warmed to about 105° F (37.8° C) ▪ normal saline solution (for cleansing enemas) ▪ I.V. pole or wall hook ▪ washcloth and towel ▪ water ▪ ostomy pouching system ▪ linen-saver pad ▪ gown, goggles, and gloves ▪ optional: bedpan or chair, mild nonmoisturizing soap, rubber band or clip, small dressing or bandage, stoma cap.

Preparation of equipment

Depending on the patient's condition, colostomy irrigation may be performed in bed using a bedpan or in the bathroom using the chair and the toilet.

Set up the irrigation bag with tubing and cone tip. If irrigation will take place with the patient in bed, place the bedpan beside the bed and elevate the head of the bed between 45 and 90 degrees, if allowed. If irrigation will take place in the bathroom, have the patient sit on the toilet or on a chair facing the toilet, whichever he finds more comfortable.

Fill the irrigation bag with warmed tap water (or normal saline solution, if the irrigation is for bowel cleansing). Hang the bag on the I.V. pole or wall hook. The bottom of the bag should be at the patient's shoulder level *to prevent the fluid from entering the bowel too quickly.* Most irrigation sets also have a clamp that regulates the flow rate.

Prime the tubing with irrigant *to prevent air from entering the colon and possibly causing cramps and gas pains.*

Implementation

- Confirm the patient's identity using two patient identifiers according to your facility's policy.
- Explain every step of the procedure to the patient *because he'll probably be irrigating the colostomy himself.*
- Provide privacy and wash your hands.
- If the patient is in bed, place a linen-saver pad under him *to protect the sheets from soiling.*
- Put on gloves and personal protective equipment.
- Remove the ostomy pouch if the patient uses one.
- Place the irrigation sleeve over the stoma. If the sleeve doesn't have an adhesive backing, secure the sleeve with an ostomy belt. If the patient has a two-piece pouching system with flanges, snap off the pouch and save it. Snap on the irrigation sleeve.
- Place the open-ended bottom of the irrigation sleeve in the bedpan or toilet *to promote drainage by gravity.* If necessary, cut the sleeve so that it meets the water level inside the bedpan or toilet. *Effluent may splash from a short sleeve or may not drain from a long sleeve.*
- Lubricate your gloved small finger with water-soluble lubricant and insert the finger into the stoma. If you're teaching the patient, have him do this *to determine the bowel angle at which to insert the cone safely.* Expect the stoma to tighten when the finger enters the bowel and then to relax in a few seconds.

- Lubricate the cone with water-soluble lubricant *to prevent it from irritating the mucosa.*
- Insert the cone into the top opening of the irrigation sleeve and then into the stoma. Angle the cone *to match the bowel angle.* Insert it gently but snugly.
- Unclamp the irrigation tubing and allow the water to flow slowly. If you don't have a clamp to control the irrigant's flow rate, pinch the tubing *to control the flow.* The water should enter the colon over 5 to 10 minutes. (If the patient reports cramping, slow or stop the flow, keep the cone in place, and have the patient take a few deep breaths until the cramping stops.) *Cramping during irrigation may result from a bowel that is ready to empty, water that is too cold, a rapid flow rate, or air in the tubing.*
- Have the patient remain stationary for 15 or 20 minutes *so that the initial effluent can drain.*
- If the patient is ambulatory, he can stay in the bathroom until all effluent empties, or he can clamp the bottom of the drainage sleeve with a rubber band or clip and return to bed. Explain that *ambulation and activity stimulate elimination.* Suggest that the nonambulatory patient lean forward or massage his abdomen *to stimulate elimination.*
- Wait about 45 minutes for the bowel to finish eliminating the irrigant and effluent. Then remove the irrigation sleeve.
- If the irrigation was intended to clean the bowel, repeat the procedure with warmed normal saline solution until the return solution appears clear.
- Using a washcloth, mild soap, and water, gently clean the area around the stoma. Rinse and dry the area thoroughly with a clean towel.
- Inspect the skin and stoma for changes in appearance. Usually dark pink to red, stoma color may change with the patient's status. Notify the practitioner of marked stoma color changes *because a pale hue may result from anemia, and substantial darkening suggests a change in blood flow to the stoma.*
- Apply a clean pouch. If the patient has a regular bowel elimination pattern, he may prefer a small dressing, bandage, or commercial stoma cap.
- Discard a disposable irrigation sleeve. Rinse a reusable irrigation sleeve and hang it to dry along with the irrigation bag, tubing, and cone.

Special considerations

- Irrigating a colostomy to establish a regular bowel elimination pattern doesn't work for all patients. If the bowel continues to move between irrigations, try decreasing the volume of irrigant. *Increasing the irrigant won't help because it serves only to stimulate peristalsis.* Keep a record of results. Also consider irrigating every other day.
- Irrigation may help to regulate bowel function in patients with a descending or sigmoid colostomy *because this is the bowel's stool storage area.* However, a patient with an ascending or transverse colostomy won't benefit from irrigation. Also, a patient with a descending or sigmoid colostomy who's missing part of the ascending or transverse colon may not be able to irrigate successfully *because his ostomy may function like an ascending or transverse colostomy.*
- If diarrhea develops, discontinue irrigations until stools form again. Keep in mind that irrigation alone won't achieve regularity for the patient. He must also observe a complementary diet and exercise regimen.
- If the patient has a strictured stoma that prohibits cone insertion, remove the cone from the irrigation tubing and replace it with a soft silicone catheter. Angle the catheter gently 2" to 4" (5 to 10 cm) into the bowel to instill the irrigant. Don't force the catheter into the stoma, and don't insert it farther than the recommended length *because you may perforate the bowel.*

Complications

Bowel perforation may result if a catheter is incorrectly inserted into the stoma. Fluid and electrolyte imbalances may result from using too much irrigant.

Documentation

Record the date and time of irrigation and the type and amount of irrigant. Note the stoma's color and the character of drainage, including the drainage color, consistency, and amount. Record any patient teaching. Describe teaching content and patient response to self-care instruction. Evaluate the patient's learning progress.

SELECTED REFERENCES

Craven, R.F., and Hirnle, C.J. *Fundamentals of Nursing: Human Health and Function,* 5th ed. Philadelphia: Lippincott Williams & Wilkins, 2006.

Karadag, A., et al. "Colostomy Irrigation: Results of 25 Cases with Particular Reference to Quality of Life," *Journal of Clinical Nursing* 14(4):479-85, April 2005.

Pullen, R.L., Jr. "Teaching Your Patient to Irrigate a Colostomy," *Nursing* 36(4):22, April 2006.

Taylor, C., et al. *Fundamentals of Nursing: The Art and Science of Nursing,* 6th ed. Philadelphia: Lippincott Williams & Wilkins, 2008.

CONTINENT ILEOSTOMY CARE

An alternative to a conventional ileostomy, a continent, or pouch, ileostomy (also called a *Koch ileostomy* or an *ileal pouch*) features an internal reservoir fashioned from the ter-

Understanding pouch construction

Depending on the patient and related factors during intestinal surgery, the surgeon may construct a pouch to collect fecal matter internally. To make such a pouch, the surgeon loops about 12″ (30.5 cm) of ileum and sutures the inner sides together.

He opens the loop with a U-shaped cut and seams the inside to create a smooth lining. Then he fashions a nipple or valve between what is becoming the pouch and what will be the stoma. He folds the open ileum over, sews the pouch closed, and fixes the pouch to the abdominal wall.

Because the pouch holds fecal matter in reserve, the patient benefits from not having to change and empty ostomy equipment. Instead, he empties and irrigates the pouch, as needed, by inserting a catheter though the stoma and into the pouch.

Initially after surgery, the nurse performs this procedure until the patient can do it himself.

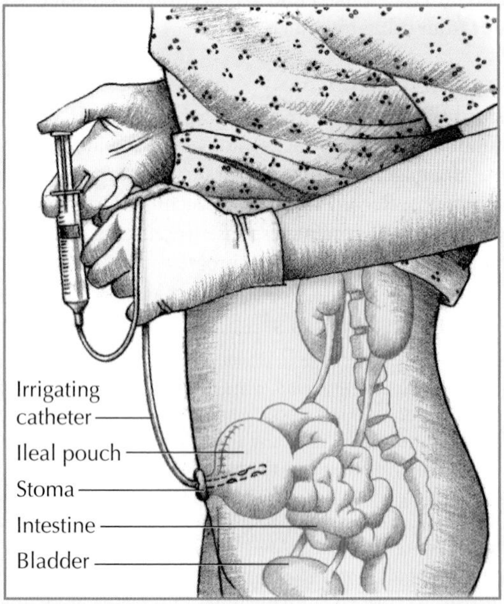

minal ileum. This procedure may be used for a patient who requires proctocolectomy for chronic ulcerative colitis or multiple polyposis. Other patients may have a traditional ileostomy converted to a continent ileostomy. This procedure is contraindicated in Crohn's disease or gross obesity. Patients who need emergency surgery and those who can't care for the pouch are also unlikely to have this procedure.

The length of preoperative hospitalization varies with the patient's condition. Nursing responsibilities include providing bowel preparation, antibiotic therapy, and emotional support. After surgery, nursing responsibilities include ensuring patency of the drainage catheter, assessing GI function, caring for the stoma and peristomal skin, managing pain resulting from surgery and, if necessary, perineal skin care.

Daily patient teaching on pouch intubation and drainage usually begins soon after surgery. Continuous drainage is maintained for about 2 to 6 weeks to allow the suture lines to heal. During this period, a drainage catheter is attached to low intermittent suction. After the suture line heals, the patient learns how to drain the pouch himself.

Equipment

For postoperative care: Bedside drainage bag ▪ normal saline solution ▪ 50 ml catheter-tipped syringe ▪ gloves ▪ water ▪ washcloth and towel ▪ skin sealant ▪ precut drain dressing ▪ 4″ × 4″ × 1″ foam ▪ Montgomery straps ▪ optional: catheter securement device.

Draining the pouch: Gloves ▪ drainage catheter ▪ water-soluble lubricant ▪ normal saline solution or water ▪ 50 ml catheter-tipped syringe ▪ dressing supplies (drain dressing, foam, Montgomery straps).

Implementation

Nursing interventions for a patient undergoing a continent ileostomy range from standard preoperative and postoperative care to pouch care and patient teaching.

Preoperative care

- Reinforce and, if necessary, supplement the physician's explanation of a continent ileostomy and its implications for the patient. (See *Understanding pouch construction.*)
- Make sure that the patient or a responsible family member has signed an appropriate consent form.
- Assess patient and family attitudes related to the operation and to the forthcoming changes in the patient's body image.
- Provide encouragement and support.

Postoperative care

- When the patient returns to his room, attach the drainage catheter emerging from the ileostomy to a bedside drainage bag.
- Irrigate the catheter with 30 ml of normal saline solution, as ordered and needed, *to prevent catheter obstruction and allow fluid return by gravity.* During the early postoperative

period, keep the pouch empty; drainage will be serosanguineous.
- Monitor fluid intake and output.
- Check the catheter frequently once the patient begins eating solid food *to ensure that neither mucus nor undigested food particles block it.*
- If the patient complains of abdominal cramps, distention, and nausea—symptoms of bowel obstruction—the catheter may be clogged. Gently irrigate with 20 to 30 ml of water or normal saline solution until the catheter drains freely. Then move the catheter slightly or rotate it gently *to help clear the obstruction.* Finally, try milking the catheter. If these measures fail, notify the physician.
- Check the stoma frequently for color, edema, and bleeding. Normally pink to red, a stoma that turns dark red or blue-red may have a compromised blood supply.
- To care for the stoma and peristomal skin, put on gloves. Remove the dressing, gently clean the peristomal area with water, and pat it dry. Use a skin sealant around the stoma *to prevent skin irritation.*
- One way to apply a stoma dressing is to slip a precut drain dressing around the catheter to cover the stoma. Cut a hole slightly larger than the lumen of the catheter in the center of a 4″ × 4″ × 1″ piece of foam. Disconnect the catheter from the drainage bag and insert the distal end of the catheter through the hole in the foam. Slide the foam pad onto the dressing. Secure the foam in place with Montgomery straps. Secure the catheter by wrapping the strap ties around it or by using a commercial catheter securing device. Then reconnect the catheter to the drainage bag. (The drainage catheter will be removed by the surgeon when he determines that the suture line has healed.)
- Assess the peristomal skin for irritation from moisture.
- *To reduce discomfort from gas pains,* encourage the patient to ambulate. Also recommend that he avoid swallowing air (*to minimize gas pains)* by chewing food well, limiting conversation while eating, and not drinking from a straw.

Draining the pouch

- Provide privacy, explain the procedure to the patient, and wash your hands.
- Put on gloves.
- Have the patient with a pouch conversion sit on the toilet *to help him feel more at ease during the procedure.*
- Remove the stoma dressing.
- Encourage the patient to relax his abdominal muscles *to allow the catheter to slide easily into the pouch.*
- Lubricate the tip of the drainage catheter tip with the water-soluble lubricant and insert it into the stoma. Gently push the catheter downward. (The direction of insertion may vary depending on the patient.)
- When the catheter reaches the nipple valve of the internal pouch or reservoir (after about 2″ or 2½″ [5 or 6.5 cm]), you'll feel resistance. Instruct the patient to take a deep breath as you exert gentle pressure on the catheter to insert it through the valve. If this fails, have the patient lie supine and rest for a few minutes. Then, with the patient still supine, try to insert the catheter again.
- Gently advance the catheter to the suture marking made by the surgeon.
- Let the pouch drain completely. This usually takes 5 to 10 minutes. With thick drainage or a clogged catheter, the process may take 30 minutes.
- If the tube clogs, irrigate with 30 ml of water or normal saline using the 50-ml catheter-tip syringe. Also, rotate and milk the tube. If these steps fail, remove, rinse, and reinsert the catheter.
- Remove the catheter after completing drainage.
- Measure output, subtracting the amount of irrigant used.
- Rinse the catheter thoroughly with warm water.
- Clean the peristomal area and apply a fresh stoma dressing.

Predischarge teaching

- Make sure the patient can properly intubate and drain the pouch himself.
- Provide the patient with appropriate equipment. If the postoperative drainage catheter is still in place, teach the patient how to care for it properly.
- Make sure the patient has a pouch-draining schedule, and give him appropriate pamphlets or video instructions on pouch care.
- Make sure he feels comfortable calling the practitioner, nurse, or appropriate other caregivers with questions or problems.
- Tell the patient where to obtain supplies.
- Refer the patient to a local ostomy group.
- Provide dietary counseling.

Special considerations

- Never aspirate fluid from the catheter *because the resulting negative pressure may damage inflamed tissue.*
- The first few times you intubate the pouch, the patient may be tense, making insertion difficult. Encourage relaxation. *To shorten drainage time,* have the patient cough, press gently on his abdomen over the pouch, or suddenly tighten his abdominal muscles and then relax them.
- Keep an accurate record of intake and output *to ensure fluid and electrolyte balance.* The average daily output should be 1,000 ml. Report inadequate or excessive output (more than 1,400 ml daily).

Understanding T-tube placement

The T tube is placed in the common bile duct, anchored to the abdominal wall, and connected to a closed drainage system.

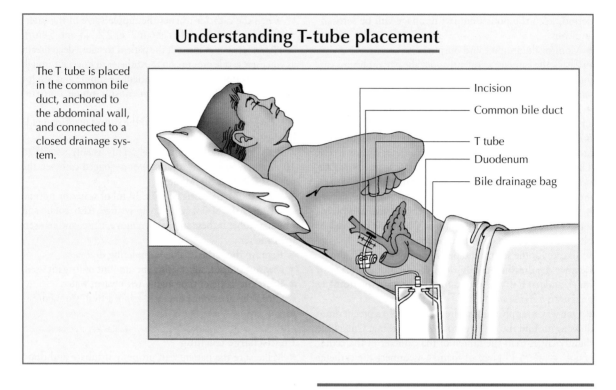

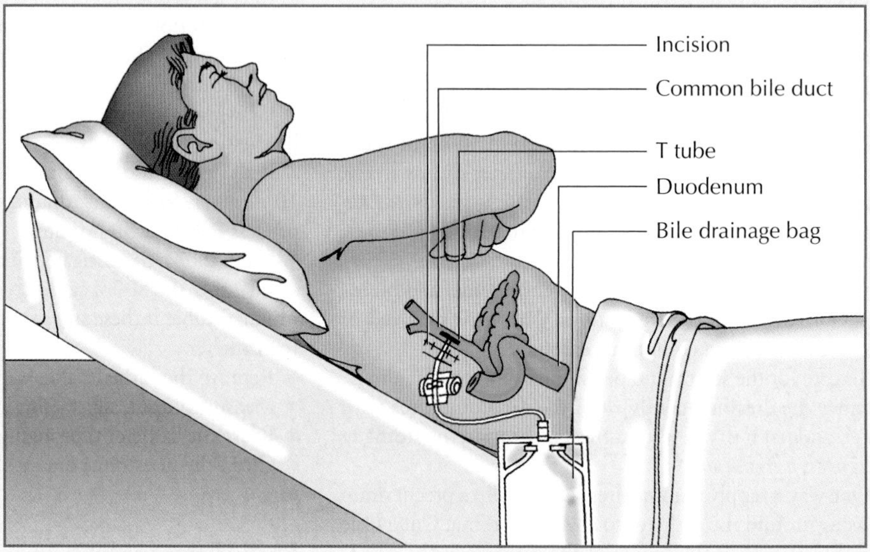

■ A leg drainage bag may be attached to the patient's thigh during ambulation.

Complications

Common postoperative complications include obstruction, fistula, pouch perforation, nipple valve dysfunction, abscesses, and bacterial overgrowth in the pouch.

Documentation

Record the date, time, and all aspects of preoperative and postoperative care: condition of the stoma and peristomal skin, diet, medications, intubations, patient teaching, and discharge planning.

SELECTED REFERENCES

Burch, J. "The Pre- and Postoperative Nursing Care for Patients with a Stoma," *British Journal of Nursing* 14(6):310-18, March-April 2005.

Herlufson, P., et al. "Study of Peristomal Skin Disorders in Patients with Permanent Stomas," *British Journal of Nursing* 15(16):854-62, September 2006.

Taylor, C., et al. *Fundamentals of Nursing: The Art and Science of Nursing,* 6th ed. Philadelphia: Lippincott Williams & Wilkins, 2008.

T-TUBE CARE

The T tube (or biliary drainage tube) may be placed in the common bile duct after cholecystectomy or choledochostomy. This tube facilitates biliary drainage during healing. The surgeon inserts the short end (crossbar) of the T tube in the common bile duct and draws the long end through the incision. The tube then connects to a closed gravity drainage system. (See *Understanding T-tube placement.*) Postoperatively, the tube remains in place between 7 and 14 days.

Equipment

Graduated collection container ■ small plastic bag ■ sterile gloves ■ clean gloves ■ clamp ■ sterile 4″ × 4″ gauze pads ■ transparent dressings ■ rubber band ■ normal saline solution ■ sterile cleaning solution ■ two sterile basins ■ antimicrobial swab ■ sterile precut drain dressings ■ hypoallergenic paper tape ■ skin protectant, such as petroleum jelly, zinc oxide, or aluminum-based gel ■ optional: Montgomery straps.

Preparation of equipment

Assemble equipment at the bedside. Open all sterile equipment. Place one sterile 4″ × 4″ gauze pad in each sterile basin. Using sterile technique, pour 50 ml of cleaning solution into one basin and 50 ml of normal saline solution into the other basin. Tape a small plastic bag on the table *to use for refuse.*

Implementation

■ Confirm the patient's identity using two patient identifiers according to your facility's policy.
■ Provide privacy and explain the procedure to the patient.
■ Wash your hands thoroughly.

Emptying drainage

■ Put on clean gloves.
■ Place the graduated collection container under the outlet valve of the drainage bag. Without contaminating the clamp, valve, or outlet valve, empty the bag's contents completely into the container and reseal the outlet valve. Carefully measure and record the character, color, and amount of drainage.
■ Discard your gloves.

Re-dressing the T tube

■ Wash your hands thoroughly *to prevent bacterial contamination of the incision.* Put on clean gloves.
■ Without dislodging the T tube, remove old dressings, and dispose of them in the small plastic bag. Remove the clean gloves.
■ Wash your hands again and put on sterile gloves. From this point on, follow sterile technique *to prevent bacterial contamination of the incision.*
■ Inspect the incision and tube site for signs of infection, including redness, edema, warmth, tenderness, induration, skin excoriation, or drainage. Assess for wound dehiscence or evisceration.
■ Use sterile cleaning solution, as prescribed, to clean and remove dried matter or drainage from around the tube. Always start at the tube site and gently wipe outward in a continuous motion *to prevent recontamination of the incision.*
■ Use normal saline solution to rinse off the prescribed cleaning solution. Dry the area with a sterile 4″ × 4″ gauze pad, and discard all used materials.
■ Using an antimicrobial swab, wipe the incision site in a circular motion. Allow the area to dry thoroughly.
■ Lightly apply a skin protectant, such as petroleum jelly, zinc oxide, or aluminum-based gel, *to protect the skin from injury caused by draining bile.*
■ Apply a sterile precut drain dressing on each side of the T tube *to absorb drainage.*
■ Apply a sterile 4″ × 4″ gauze pad or transparent dressing over the T tube and the drain dressings. Be careful not to kink the tubing, *which might block the drainage.* Also avoid putting the dressing over the open end of the T tube *because this end connects to the closed drainage system.*

TROUBLESHOOTING

Managing T-tube obstruction

If your patient's T tube blocks after cholecystectomy, notify the practitioner and take these steps while you wait for him to arrive:

■ Unclamp the T tube (if it was clamped before and after a meal) and connect the tube to a closed gravity-drainage system.
■ Inspect the tube carefully *to detect any kinks or obstructions.*
■ Prepare the patient for possible T-tube irrigation or direct X-ray of the common bile duct (cholangiography). Briefly describe these measures *to reduce the patient's apprehension and promote cooperation.*
■ Provide encouragement and support.

■ Secure the dressings with the hypoallergenic paper tape or Montgomery straps, if necessary.

Clamping the T tube

■ As ordered, occlude the tube lightly with a clamp or wrap a rubber band around the end. *Clamping the tube 1 hour before and after meals diverts bile back to the duodenum to aid digestion.*
■ Monitor the patient's response to clamping.
■ *To ensure patient comfort and safety,* check bile drainage amounts regularly. Be alert for such signs of obstructed bile flow as chills, fever, tachycardia, nausea, right-upper-quadrant fullness and pain, jaundice, dark foamy urine, and clay-colored stools. Report them immediately. (See *Managing T-tube obstruction.*)

Special considerations

■ Normal daily bile drainage ranges from 500 to 1,000 ml of viscous, green-brown liquid. The T tube usually drains 300 to 500 ml of blood-tinged bile in the first 24 hours after surgery. Report drainage that exceeds 500 ml in the first 24 hours after surgery. This amount typically declines to 200 ml or less after 4 days. Monitor fluid, electrolyte, and acid-base status carefully.
■ To prevent excessive bile loss (over 500 ml in first 24 hours) or backflow contamination, secure the T-tube drainage system at abdominal level. Bile will flow into the bag only when biliary pressure increases. As ordered, return excessive bile drainage (between 1,000 and 1,500 ml daily) to the patient

mixed with chilled fruit juice or, if possible, through a nasogastric tube.

- Provide meticulous skin care and frequent dressing changes. Observe for bile leakage, *which may indicate obstruction*. Assess tube patency and site condition hourly for the first 8 hours and then every 4 hours until the practitioner removes the tube. Protect the skin edges and avoid excessive taping *to prevent shearing the skin.*
- Monitor all urine and stools for color changes. Assess for icteric skin and sclera, *which may signal jaundice.*

Home care

Loose bowels occur commonly in the first few weeks after surgery. Teach the patient about signs and symptoms of T-tube and biliary obstruction, which he should report to the practitioner. Teach him how to care for the tube at home. In addition, caution him that bile stains clothing.

Complications

Obstructed bile flow, skin excoriation or breakdown, tube dislodgment, drainage reflux, and infection are the most common complications related to a biliary T tube.

Documentation

Record the date and time of each dressing change. Note the appearance of the wound and surrounding skin. Write down the color, character, and volume of bile collected. Also record the color of skin and mucous membranes around the T tube. Keep a precise record of temperature trends and the amount and frequency of urination and bowel movements.

SELECTED REFERENCES

Craven, R.F., and Hirnle, C.J. *Fundamentals of Nursing: Human Health and Function,* 5th ed. Philadelphia: Lippincott Williams & Wilkins, 2006.

Taylor, C., et al. *Fundamentals of Nursing: The Art and Science of Nursing,* 6th ed. Philadelphia: Lippincott Williams & Wilkins, 2008.

ABDOMINAL PARACENTESIS

A bedside procedure, abdominal paracentesis involves the aspiration of fluid from the peritoneal space through a needle, trocar, or cannula inserted into the abdominal wall. Used to diagnose and treat massive ascites resistant to other therapy, the procedure helps determine the cause of ascites while relieving the pressure created by ascites. It may also precede other procedures, including radiography, peritoneal dialysis, and surgery. With abdominal paracentesis, the health care team can also detect intra-abdominal bleeding after traumatic injury and obtain a peritoneal fluid specimen for laboratory analysis. The procedure must be performed cautiously in pregnant patients and in patients with bleeding tendencies, severely distended bowel, and in patients with an infection at the intended insertion site.

Nursing responsibilities during abdominal paracentesis include preparing the patient, monitoring his condition and providing emotional support during the procedure, assisting the physician, and obtaining specimens for laboratory analysis.

Equipment

Tape measure ▪ sterile gloves ▪ clean gloves ▪ mask ▪ gown ▪ goggles ▪ linen-saver pads ▪ four Vacutainer laboratory tubes ▪ two large glass Vacutainer bottles (1,000 ml or larger) ▪ dry, sterile dressing ▪ laboratory request forms ▪ antiseptic cleaning solution ▪ local anesthetic (multidose vial of 1% or 2% lidocaine with epinephrine) ▪ 4″ × 4″ sterile gauze pads ▪ sterile paracentesis tray ▪ sterile drapes ▪ marking pen ▪ 5-ml syringe with 21G or 25G needle ▪ sterile marker ▪ sterile labels ▪ optional: alcohol pad, 50-ml syringe, suture materials, salt-poor albumin.

A sterile paracentesis tray may be available. If a preassembled tray isn't available, you'll need to gather the following sterile supplies: trocar with stylet ▪ 16G to 20G needle ▪ 25G or 27G 1½″ needle ▪ 20G or 22G spinal needle ▪ scalpel ▪ No. 11 knife blade ▪ three-way stopcock.

Implementation

- Confirm the patient's identity using two patient identifiers according to your facility's policy.
- Explain the procedure to the patient *to ease his anxiety and promote cooperation.* Reassure him that he should feel no pain, but that he may feel a stinging sensation from the local anesthetic injection and pressure from the needle or trocar and cannula insertion. He may also sense pressure when the physician aspirates abdominal fluid.
- Be sure to obtain the patient's signed consent form.
- Instruct the patient to void before the procedure. Or, insert an indwelling urinary catheter, if ordered, *to minimize the risk of accidental bladder injury from the needle or trocar and cannula insertion.*
- Identify and record baseline values: vital signs, weight, and abdominal girth. (Use the tape measure to gauge the patient's abdominal girth at the umbilical level.) Indicate the abdominal area measured with a felt-tipped marking pen. *Baseline data will be used to monitor the patient's status.*
- Position the patient supine or on his side *to allow the fluid to accumulate in dependent areas.*
- Expose the patient's abdomen from diaphragm to pubis. Keep the rest of the patient covered *to avoid chilling him.*

■ Make the patient as comfortable as possible, and place a linen-saver pad under him *for protection from drainage.*
■ Remind the patient to stay as still as possible during the procedure *to prevent injury from the needle or trocar and cannula.*
■ Wash your hands. Open the paracentesis tray using sterile technique *to ensure a sterile field.* Next, put on gloves before assisting the physician as he prepares the patient's abdomen with antiseptic cleaning solution, drapes the operative site with sterile drapes, and administers the local anesthetic.
■ Label all medications, medication containers, and other solutions on and off the sterile field.
■ If the paracentesis tray doesn't contain a sterile ampule of anesthetic, wipe the top of a multidose vial of anesthetic solution with an alcohol pad, and invert the vial at a 45-degree angle. *This will allow the physician to insert the sterile 5-ml syringe with the 21G or 25G needle and withdraw the anesthetic without touching the nonsterile vial.*
■ Using the scalpel, the physician may make a small incision before inserting the needle or trocar and cannula (usually 1″ to 2″ [2.5 to 5 cm] below the umbilicus). Listen for a popping sound. *This signifies that the needle or trocar has pierced the peritoneum.*
■ Assist the physician with specimen collection in the appropriate containers. Wear clean gloves, gown, and goggles *to protect you from possible body fluid contamination.* If the physician orders substantial drainage, connect the three-way stopcock and tubing to the cannula. Run the other end of the tubing to a large sterile Vacutainer. Or aspirate the fluid with a three-way stopcock and 50-ml syringe.
■ Gently turn the patient from side to side *to enhance drainage* if necessary.
■ As the fluid drains, monitor the patient's vital signs every 15 minutes. Observe him closely for vertigo, faintness, diaphoresis, pallor, heightened anxiety, tachycardia, dyspnea, and hypotension—especially if more than 1,500 ml of peritoneal fluid was aspirated at one time. *This loss may induce a fluid shift and hypovolemic shock.*
■ Immediately report signs of shock to the physician; he may order you to administer salt-poor albumin I.V. *to prevent hypovolemia and a decline in renal function.*
■ When the procedure ends and the physician removes the needle or trocar and cannula, he may suture the incision. Wearing sterile gloves, apply the dry, sterile pressure dressing to the site. Help the patient assume a comfortable position.
■ Monitor the patient's vital signs and check the dressing for drainage every 15 minutes for 1 hour, every 30 minutes for 2 hours, every hour for 4 hours, and then every 4 hours for 24 hours *to detect delayed reactions to the procedure.* Be sure to note drainage color, amount, and character.
■ Label the Vacutainer specimen tubes, and send them to the laboratory with the appropriate laboratory request forms. If the patient is receiving antibiotics, note this on the request form. *This information will be considered during the fluid analysis.*
■ Make sure you remove and dispose of all equipment properly.

Special considerations

■ Throughout this procedure, try to help the patient remain still *to prevent accidental perforation of abdominal organs.*
■ If the patient shows any signs of hypovolemic shock, reduce the vertical distance between the needle or the trocar and cannula and the drainage collection container *to slow the drainage rate.* If necessary, stop the drainage.
■ *To prevent fluid shifts and hypovolemia,* limit aspirated fluid to between 1,500 and 2,000 ml. If peritoneal fluid doesn't flow easily, try repositioning the patient *to facilitate drainage.* Also verify suction in the Vacutainer collection bottle when you connect it to the drainage tubing, and be sure to use macrodrip tubing without a backflow device.
■ After the procedure, observe for peritoneal fluid leakage. If this develops, notify the physician. Always maintain daily patient weight and abdominal girth records. Compare these values with the baseline figures *to detect recurrent ascites.*

Complications

Removing large amounts of fluid may cause hypotension, oliguria, and hyponatremia. If an excessive amount of fluid (more than 2 L) is removed, ascitic fluid tends to form again, drawing fluid from extracellular tissue throughout the body. Other possible complications include perforation of abdominal organs by the needle or the trocar and cannula, wound infection, bleeding, and peritonitis.

Documentation

Record the date and time of the procedure, the puncture site location, and whether the wound was sutured. Document the amount, color, viscosity, and odor of aspirated fluid in your notes and in the fluid intake and output record. Note the number of specimens sent to the laboratory.

Record the patient's vital signs, weight, and abdominal girth measurements before and after the procedure. Also note his tolerance of the procedure, vital signs, and any signs and symptoms of complications during the procedure.

Tapping the peritoneal cavity

After administering a local anesthetic to numb the area near the patient's navel, the surgeon will make a smaller incision (about 3/4″ [2 cm]) through the skin and subcutaneous tissues of the abdominal wall in order to tap the peritoneal cavity. He'll retract the tissue, ligate several blood vessels, and use 4″ × 4″ gauze pads to absorb and keep incisional blood from entering the wound and producing a false-positive test result. Next, he'll direct the trocar through the incision into the pelvic midline until the instrument enters the peritoneum. Then, he'll advance the peritoneal catheter (via the trocar) 6″ to 8″ (15 to 20 cm) into the pelvis.

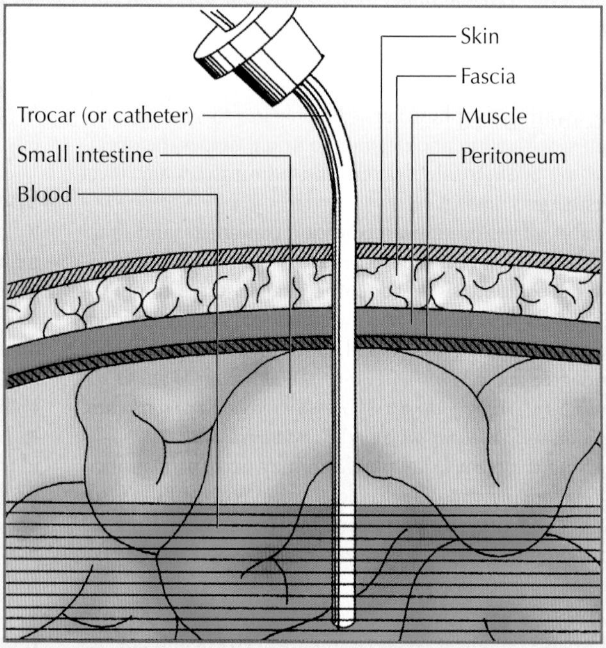

Selected references

Lynn-McHale Wiegand, D.J., and Carlson, K.K., eds. *AACN Procedure Manual for Critical Care,* 5th ed. Philadelphia: W.B. Saunders Co., 2005.

Stephenson, J., and Gilbert, J. "The Development of Clinical Guidelines on Paracentesis for Ascites Related to Malignancy," *Palliative Medicine* 16(3):213-18, May 2002.

Peritoneal lavage

Used mainly as a diagnostic procedure in a patient with blunt abdominal trauma, peritoneal lavage helps detect bleeding in the peritoneal cavity. Peritoneal lavage may also be used to warm the abdominal cavity in a patient with hypothermia, obtain a cytology specimen in a patient with cancer, and for irrigation in a patient with peritonitis or an intra-abdominal abscess. The test may proceed through several steps. Initially, the physician inserts a catheter through the abdominal wall into the peritoneal cavity and aspirates the peritoneal fluid with a syringe. If he can't see blood in the aspirated fluid, he then infuses a balanced saline solution and siphons the fluid from the cavity. He inspects the siphoned fluid for blood and also sends fluid samples to the laboratory for microscopic examination.

The medical team maintains strict sterile technique throughout this procedure to avoid introducing microorganisms into the peritoneum and causing peritonitis. (See *Tapping the peritoneal cavity.*)

Peritoneal lavage is contraindicated in a patient who has had multiple abdominal operations (adhesions), who has an abdominal wall hematoma, who's unstable and needs immediate surgery, who has coagulopathies, or who can't be catheterized before the procedure. The procedure requires great caution and a different technique if the patient is pregnant.

Equipment

Indwelling urinary catheter, catheter insertion kit, and drainage bag ▪ nasogastric (NG) tube ▪ gastric suction machine ▪ clippers ▪ I.V. pole ▪ macrodrip I.V. tubing ▪ I.V. solutions (1 L of warmed, balanced saline solution, usually lactated Ringer's solution or normal saline solution) ▪ peritoneal dialysis tray ▪ sterile gloves ▪ gown ▪ goggles ▪ antiseptic solution ▪ 3-ml syringe with 25G 1″ needle ▪ bottle of 1% lidocaine with epinephrine, if needed ▪ 8″ (20.3 cm) #14 intracatheter extension tubing and a small sterile hemostat (to clamp tubing) ▪ 30-ml syringe ▪ one 20G 1½″ needle ▪ sterile towels ▪ three containers for specimen collection, including one sterile tube for a culture and sensitivity specimen ▪ labels ▪ 4″ × 4″ gauze pads ▪ alcohol pads ▪ 2-0 and 3-0 sutures.

If using a commercially prepared peritoneal dialysis kit (containing a #15 peritoneal dialysis catheter, trocar, and extension tubing with roller clamp), make sure the macrodrip I.V. tubing doesn't have a reverse flow (or back-check) valve that prevents infused fluid from draining out of the peritoneal cavity.

Implementation

- Confirm the patient's identity using two patient identifiers according to your facility's policy.
- Make sure an informed consent is signed for the procedure.
- Provide privacy and wash your hands. Reinforce the physician's explanation of the procedure.
- Put on the gown and goggles.
- Before the procedure, advise the patient to expect a sensation of abdominal fullness. Also inform him that he may experience a chill if the lavage solution isn't warmed or doesn't reach his body temperature.
- Then catheterize the patient with the indwelling urinary catheter, and connect this catheter to the drainage bag. *This decreases the risk of the physician accidentally perforating the bladder during the procedure.*
- Insert the NG tube. Attach this tube to the gastric suction machine (set for low intermittent suction) *to drain the patient's stomach contents. Decompressing the stomach prevents vomiting and subsequent aspiration and minimizes the possibility of bowel perforation during trocar or catheter insertion.*
- Clip the hair, as ordered, from the area between the patient's umbilicus and pubis.
- Set up the I.V. pole. Attach the macrodrip tubing to the lavage solution container, and clear air from the tubing *to avoid introducing air into the peritoneal cavity during the lavage.*
- Using sterile technique, open the peritoneal dialysis tray.
- The physician will wipe the patient's abdomen from the costal margin to the pubic area and from flank to flank with the antiseptic solution. Then he'll drape the area with sterile towels from the dialysis tray *to create a sterile field.*
- Using sterile technique, hand the physician the 3-ml syringe and the 25G 1″ needle. If the peritoneal dialysis tray doesn't contain a sterile ampule of anesthetic, wipe the top of a multidose vial of 1% lidocaine with epinephrine with an alcohol pad, and invert the vial at a 45-degree angle. *This allows the physician to insert the needle and withdraw the anesthetic without touching the nonsterile vial.*

Interpreting peritoneal lavage results

If test findings in peritoneal lavage are abnormal, your patient may need laparotomy and further treatment. The most common abnormal findings include:

- unclotted blood, bile, or intestinal contents in aspirated peritoneal fluid (20 ml in an adult or 10 ml in a child)
- bloody or pinkish-red fluid returned from lavage—dark enough to obscure reading newsprint through it (if you can read newsprint through the fluid, test results are considered negative, although the physician may order more tests)
- green, cloudy, turbid, or milky peritoneal fluid return (normally appears clear to pale yellow)
- red blood cell count over 100,000/µl
- white blood cell count exceeding 500/µl
- bacteria in fluid (identified by culture and sensitivity testing or Gram stain).

If the patient's condition is stable, borderline positive results may suggest the need for additional tests, such as echography and arteriography. If test results are questionable or inconclusive, the physician may leave the catheter in place to repeat the procedure.

- The physician will inject the anesthetic directly below the umbilicus (or at an adjacent site if the patient has a surgical scar). When the area is numb, he'll make an incision, insert the catheter or trocar, withdraw fluid, and check the findings. If the findings are positive, the procedure ends, and you'll prepare the patient for laparotomy and further measures. Even if retrieved fluid looks normal, lavage will continue. (See *Interpreting peritoneal lavage results.*)
- Wearing gloves, connect the catheter extension tubing to the I.V. tubing, if ordered, and instill 700 to 1,000 ml (10 ml/kg body weight) of the warmed I.V. solution into the peritoneal cavity over 5 to 10 minutes. Then clamp the tubing with the hemostat.
- Unless contraindicated by the patient's injuries (such as a spinal cord injury, fractured ribs, or an unstable pelvic fracture), gently tilt the patient from side to side *to distribute the fluid throughout the peritoneal cavity.* (If the patient's condition contraindicates tilting, the physician may gently palpate the sides of the abdomen *to distribute the fluid.*)

■ After 5 to 10 minutes, place the I.V. container below the level of the patient's body, and open the clamp on the I.V. tubing. *Lowering the container helps excess fluid to drain.* Gently drain as much of the fluid as possible from the peritoneal cavity to the container. Be careful not to disconnect the tubing from the catheter. The peritoneal cavity may take 20 to 30 minutes to drain completely.

■ To obtain a fluid specimen, put on gloves and use a 30ml syringe and 20G 1½" needle to withdraw between 25 and 30 ml of fluid from a port in the I.V. tubing. Clean the top of each specimen container with an alcohol pad. Deposit fluid specimens in the containers, and send the specimens to the laboratory for culture and sensitivity analysis, Gram stain, red and white blood cell counts, amylase and bile level determinations, and spun-down sediment evaluation. *Note:* If you didn't obtain the culture and sensitivity specimen first, change the needle before drawing this fluid sample *to avoid contaminating the specimen.*

■ Label the specimens, and send them to the laboratory immediately. With positive test results, the physician will usually perform a laparotomy. If test results are normal, the physician will close the incision.

■ Wearing sterile gloves, dress the incision with a 4" × 4" gauze pad secured with 1" hypoallergenic tape.

■ Discard disposable equipment. Return reusable equipment to the appropriate department for cleaning and sterilization.

Special considerations

■ After lavage, monitor the patient's vital signs every 15 minutes until stable, or per your facility's policy. Report signs of shock (tachycardia, decreased blood pressure, diaphoresis, dyspnea or shortness of breath, and vertigo) at once. Assess the incisional site frequently for bleeding.

■ If the physician orders abdominal X-rays, they will probably precede peritoneal lavage. *X-ray films made after lavage may be unreliable because of air introduced into the peritoneal cavity.*

Complications

Bleeding from lacerated blood vessels may occur at the incisional site or intra-abdominally. A visceral perforation causes peritonitis and requires laparotomy for repair. If the patient has respiratory distress, infusion of a balanced saline solution may cause additional stress and trigger respiratory arrest.

The bladder may be lacerated or punctured if it isn't emptied completely before peritoneal lavage. Infection may develop at the incision site if strict sterile technique hasn't been used.

Documentation

Record the type and size of the peritoneal dialysis catheter used, the type and amount of solution instilled and withdrawn from the peritoneal cavity, and the amount and color of fluid returned. Document whether the fluid flowed freely into and out of the abdomen. Note which specimens were obtained and sent to the laboratory. Also note any complications encountered, and the nursing actions taken to handle them.

SELECTED REFERENCES

Hupuczi, P., and Papp, Z. "Postoperative Ascites Associated with Intraperitoneal Antiseptic Lavage," *Obstetrics and Gynecology* 105(5 Pt 2):1267-68, May 2005.

Lynn-McHale Wiegand, D.J., and Carlson, K.K., eds. *AACN Procedure Manual for Critical Care,* 5th ed. Philadelphia: W.B. Saunders Co., 2005.

McCullough, L., and Arora, S. "Diagnosis and Treatment of Hypothermia," *American Family Physician* 70(12):2325-332, December 2004.

INTRA-ABDOMINAL PRESSURE MONITORING

Intra-abdominal pressure monitoring measures the pressure in the abdominal compartment. It can be assessed indirectly in the patient with an indwelling urinary catheter by measuring the pressure in the bladder with a needle that connects a pressure transducer to the urinary catheter or by inserting an I.V. catheter into the sampling port. Pressure in the abdomen may rise from conditions such as intraperitoneal bleeding, third space fluid resuscitation, peritonitis, ascites, gaseous bowel distention, abdominal surgery, and trauma. If pressure in the abdominal cavity becomes greater than the pressure in the capillaries that perfuse the abdominal organs, ischemia and infarction may result. Increased intra-abdominal pressure can also lead to reduced cardiac output, increased systemic vascular resistance, increased vascular resistance, and reduced venous return. By measuring intra-abdominal pressure, the nurse can detect a rise in pressure and initiate lifesaving measures.

Equipment

Indwelling single- or multi-lumen urinary catheter with drainage bag ■ clean gloves ■ cardiac monitor ■ pressure cable for monitor interface ■ 500-ml bag of normal saline solution ■ appropriately sized pressure bag for size of saline bag ■ I.V. tubing ■ pressure tubing, pressure transducer with flush device, and stopcock ■ 60-ml luer-lock syringe ■ clamp ■ aseptic cleansing solution ■ 16 or 18 G needle or I.V. catheter or needleless adapter (when using a three-way indwelling urinary catheter, a sterile feeding "Y" connector is used in place of the I.V. catheter or needleless adapter) ▪ tape ▪ I.V. pole.

Several commercially prepared kits are available.

Preparation of equipment

Before setting up the monitoring system, wash your hands thoroughly. Maintain asepsis throughout preparation and wear the appropriate personal protective equipment. Assemble the equipment, taking care not to contaminate dead end caps, stopcocks, and syringes. Connect the I.V. tubing to the transducer, the transducer to a stopcock, then the stopcock to the pressure tubing and monitor cable. Attach a 60-ml syringe to the side port of the stopcock. Place the transducer in the transducer holder attached to the I.V. pole. Hang the 500-ml I.V. normal saline bag from an I.V. pole, attach the I.V. tubing, and flush the entire line system of air. Use the pressure bag to pressurize the system to 300 mm Hg. Attach the cable from the transducer to the monitor and select a 30 mm Hg scale for monitoring pressure.

Implementation

- Confirm the patient's identity using two patient identifiers according to your facility's policy.
- Explain the procedure to the patient, including the purpose of intra-abdominal pressure monitoring and anticipated duration of catheter placement, *to reduce anxiety and enhance cooperation.*
- Wash your hands thoroughly and put on clean gloves.
- Insert an indwelling urinary catheter, if the patient does not have one in place.
- Place the I.V. pole with the monitoring system next to the patient.
- With the patient supine, level and zero the transducer to the symphysis pubis to cancel out the effect of atmospheric pressure. *The supine position prevents the abdominal organs from exerting pressure down onto the bladder, falsely elevating the readings.*
- Cleanse the indwelling urinary catheter sampling port with antiseptic solution according to your facility's policy, and insert the needle, needleless adapter, or I.V. catheter into the port.
- Remove the stylet, if an I.V. catheter is used, and connect the I.V. catheter to the pressure tubing. Secure the connection with tape.
- When a three-way indwelling urinary catheter is used, cleanse the hub of the irrigation port and attach the pressure monitoring line directly into the irrigation hub using a sterile feeding tube "Y" connector. Secure the connection with tape.
- Clamp the urinary catheter just distal to the connection of the catheter and drainage bag *to keep saline from draining out of the bladder while filling the bladder.*
- Open the stopcock from the flush line to the syringe and fill the syringe from the I.V. normal saline solution bag.
- Close the stopcock to the transducer and open it to the pressure tubing and urinary catheter and instill 50 ml of normal saline solution into the bladder. *This volume will not overdistend the bladder and produce a falsely high reading.*
- Close the stopcock to the syringe and open it to the pressure tubing and the transducer.
- Obtain the intra-abdominal pressure with the patient in the supine position and the point of leveling at the symphysis pubis.
- Obtain a pressure reading at the end of expiration *to minimize the effects of respiration.* Fluctuation should be evident in the waveform with the heartbeat or respiratory pattern.
- After the reading is obtained, turn the stopcock off to the pressure tubing and catheter, release the clamp, and allow the instilled normal saline solution to drain.
- Measure the urinary output after subtracting the 50 ml of instilled normal saline solution *to maintain accurate intake and output.*
- Remove the needle or needleless adapter from the sampling port.
- If an I.V. catheter is being left in place, tape the connection securely.

Special considerations

- Report an increasing intra-abdominal pressure to the practitioner. While intra-abdominal pressures greater than 12 to 15 mm Hg are a concern, a pressure greater than 20 mm Hg is considered intra-abdominal hypertension, and decompression surgery may be indicated.
- Patients at risk for intra-abdominal hypertension should be assessed for signs of reduced organ perfusion, such as reduced or absent urinary output; increasing serum creatinine levels; hypotension; reduced cardiac output; increased central venous and pulmonary artery pressures; increased intracerebral pressure; increased serum lactate levels; increased peak airway pressure; decreased tidal volume; hypoxemia; hypercarbia; GI bleeding; and impaired peripheral circulation.
- If a patient can't lie supine to obtain a reading, take the reading with the head of the bed elevated. Document the position the patient was in for the reading, and obtain all further readings from this position.

Complications

Intra-abdominal pressures that exceed 20 mm Hg are usually associated with irreversible organ damage, leading to abdominal compartment syndrome and multiple organ dysfunction. With increased pressure readings and signs of reduced organ perfusion, surgical intervention may be required to preserve organ function and decrease morbidity and mortality associated with intra-abdominal hypertension and abdominal compartment syndrome. The presence of an indwelling urinary catheter and introduction of a needle or I.V. catheter into the closed drainage system increases the risk of infection.

Documentation

Describe any patient teaching performed. Record the date and time of the reading. Document if the system was leveled and zeroed and the patient's position during the reading. Note the amount of normal saline instilled. Record the intra-abdominal pressure reading. Frequent intra-abdominal pressure readings may be recorded on a frequent parameter assessment sheet. Note if anyone was notified of an abnormal reading, whether orders were given, treatments performed, and the patient's response. Record any vital signs and assessments done at the time of the reading. Record the urinary output after subtracting the instilled normal saline solution. Urinary output may also be documented on the frequent parameter assessment sheet. Chart any urinary catheter care performed. Note the patient's tolerance of the procedure. If a strip of the waveform is available, place it in the medical record, noting the date, time, and patient's name on the strip.

SELECTED REFERENCES

Balogh, Z., et al. "Continuous Intra-abdominal Pressure Measurement Technique," *American Journal of Surgery* 188(6):679-84, December 2004.

Lynn-McHale Wiegand, D.J., and Carlson, K.K., eds. *AACN Procedure Manual for Critical Care*, 5th ed. Philadelphia: W.B. Saunders Co., 2005.

Sugrue, M. "Abdominal Compartment Syndrome," *Current Opinion in Critical Care* 11(4):333-38, August 2005.

Walker, J., and Criddle, L.M. "Pathophysiology and Management of Abdominal Compartment Syndrome," *American Journal of Critical Care* 12(4):367-71, July 2003.

Wittman, D.H., and Iskander, G.A. "The Compartment Syndrome of the Abdominal Cavity: A State-of-the-Art Review," *Journal of Intensive Care Medicine* 15(4):201-20, July-August 2000.

Wolfe, T., et al. "Intra-abdominal Pressure Monitoring: The Key to Avoiding Abdominal Compartment Syndrome," *AACN News* 21(9), September 2004.

World Society of Abdominal Compartment Syndrome. Consensus Definitions. Available at *www.wsacs.org*.

11 ■ Renal and urologic care

Introduction

Because the renal and urologic systems produce, transport, collect, and excrete urine, their dysfunction will impair fluid, electrolyte, and acid-base balance as well as the elimination of waste. To restore or facilitate effective function of these systems, treatment of renal and urologic disorders usually involves temporary or permanent insertion of a urinary, peritoneal, or vascular catheter or tube. Catheterization also allows monitoring of renal and urologic systems and aids diagnosis of dysfunction.

Helping the patient cope

One goal in caring for a patient with a renal or urologic disorder is helping him accept an invasive procedure or adjust to a new body image. Begin to meet this goal by assessing the amount and kind of information he needs and can absorb about the procedure. Then present or reinforce this information and tell him what to expect.

For example, before insertion of an indwelling urinary catheter, tell the patient that he'll feel pressure during insertion that the catheter will cause a sense of fullness or the urge to void, that he must avoid dislodging the catheter, and that the collection bag must be lower than bladder level.

In a patient with a severe and chronic disorder, treatment usually requires permanent changes, such as urinary diversion, which may seriously affect his body image. To manage care effectively, you must help him cope with any distressing changes by helping him recognize the health benefits of the treatment. For example, a stoma may be initially unappealing, but you can help the patient see that living with the stoma is easier than living with the disease or symptoms that caused him to seek treatment in the first place.

Managing the procedure

Performing procedures skillfully is only one aspect of successfully managing renal and urologic disorders. You must also understand the purpose of each step of the procedure, the physiologic and scientific principles that support the procedure, and the associated indications, contraindications, and clinical ramifications. Additionally, you must accurately assess the patient's status, plan the appropriate approach to the procedure, implement the procedure, and evaluate its overall effect on the patient.

Based on the results of continued patient assessment, you can make valid clinical decisions and establish priorities that will contribute to a positive outcome. Your ability to assess a situation, analyze it critically, and establish priorities probably has the greatest impact on the success of the nursing process.

URINARY CATHETERS

Indwelling catheter insertion

Also known as a *Foley* catheter, an indwelling urinary catheter remains in the bladder to provide continuous urine drainage. A balloon inflated at the catheter's distal end prevents it from slipping out of the bladder after insertion.

Indwelling catheters are used most commonly to relieve bladder distention caused by urine retention and to allow continuous urine drainage when the urinary meatus is swollen from childbirth, surgery, or local trauma. Other indications for an indwelling catheter include urinary tract obstruction (by a tumor or enlarged prostate), urine retention or infection from neurogenic bladder paralysis caused by spinal cord injury or disease, and any illness in which the patient's urine output must be monitored closely.

An indwelling catheter is inserted using sterile technique and only when absolutely necessary. Insertion should be performed with extreme care to prevent injury and infection. To avoid trauma to the urethra and decrease the risk of infection, always use the smallest-sized catheter with the smallest balloon.

Equipment

Sterile indwelling catheter (latex or silicone #10 to #22 French [average adult sizes are #14 to #16 French]) ▪ syringe filled with 10 ml of sterile water (normal saline solution is sometimes used) ▪ washcloth ▪ towel ▪ soap and water ▪ two linen-saver pads ▪ clean gloves ▪ sterile gloves ▪ sterile drape ▪ sterile fenestrated drape ▪ sterile cotton-tipped applicators (or cotton balls and plastic forceps) ▪ antiseptic cleaning agent ▪ urine receptacle ▪ sterile water-soluble lubricant ▪ sterile drainage collection bag ▪ adhesive tape ▪ optional: urine specimen container and laboratory request form, leg band with Velcro closure, gooseneck lamp or flashlight, pillows or rolled blankets.

Prepackaged sterile disposable kits that usually contain all the necessary equipment are available. The syringes in these kits are prefilled with 10 ml of normal saline solution.

Preparation of equipment

Check the order on the patient's chart *to determine if a catheter size or type has been specified.* Then wash your hands, select the appropriate equipment, and assemble it at the patient's bedside.

Implementation

- Confirm the patient's identity using two patient identifiers according to your facility's policy.

■ Explain the procedure to the patient and provide privacy. Check his chart and ask when he voided last. Percuss and palpate the bladder *to establish baseline data.* Ask if he feels the urge to void.
■ Have a coworker hold a flashlight or place a gooseneck lamp next to the patient's bed *so that you can see the urinary meatus clearly in poor lighting.*
■ Place the female patient in the supine position, with her knees flexed and separated and her feet flat on the bed, about 2′ (61 cm) apart. If she finds this position uncomfortable, have her flex one knee and keep the other leg flat on the bed.
ELDER ALERT *The elderly patient may need pillows or blankets* **to provide support with positioning.**
■ You may need an assistant *to help the patient stay in position or to direct the light.*
■ Place the male patient in the supine position with his legs extended and flat on the bed. Ask the patient to hold the position *to give you a clear view of the urinary meatus and to prevent contamination of the sterile field.*
■ Put on clean gloves.
■ Use the washcloth to clean the patient's genital area and perineum thoroughly with soap and water. Dry the area with the towel. Then wash your hands.
■ Place the linen-saver pads on the bed between the patient's legs and under the hips. *To create the sterile field,* open the prepackaged kit or equipment tray and place it between the female patient's legs or next to the male patient's hip. If the sterile gloves are the first item on the top of the tray, put them on. Place the sterile drape under the patient's hips. Then drape the patient's lower abdomen with the sterile fenestrated drape so that only the genital area remains exposed. Take care not to contaminate your gloves (as shown below).

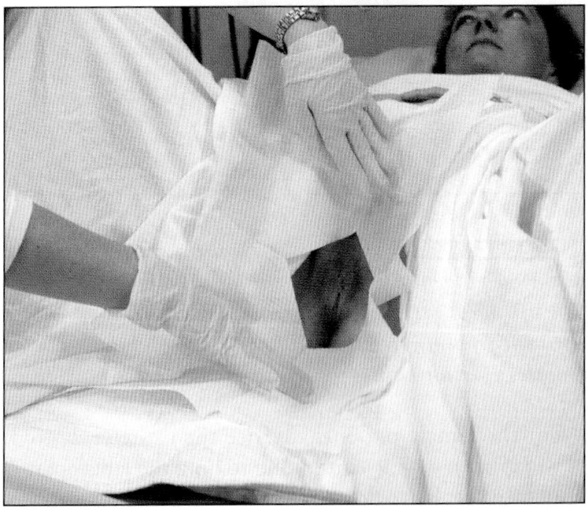

■ Open the rest of the kit or tray. Put on the sterile gloves if you haven't already done so.
■ Make sure the patient isn't allergic to iodine solution; if he is allergic, another antiseptic cleaning agent must be used.
■ Tear open the packet of antiseptic cleaning agent, and use it to saturate the sterile cotton balls or applicators. Be careful not to spill the solution on the equipment.
■ Open the packet of water-soluble lubricant and apply it to the catheter tip; attach the drainage bag to the other end of the catheter. (If you're using a commercial kit, the drainage bag may be attached.) Make sure all tubing ends remain sterile, and be sure the clamp at the emptying port of the drainage bag is closed *to prevent urine leakage from the bag.* Some drainage systems have an air-lock chamber *to prevent bacteria from traveling to the bladder from urine in the drainage bag.*

Note: Some urologists and nurses use a syringe prefilled with water-soluble lubricant and instill the lubricant directly into the male urethra, instead of on the catheter tip. *This method helps prevent trauma to the urethral lining as well as possible urinary tract infection.* Check your facility's policy.
■ Before inserting the catheter, inflate the balloon with normal saline solution *to inspect it for leaks.* To do this, attach the saline-filled syringe to the luer-lock, then push the plunger and check for seepage as the balloon expands. Aspirate the saline *to deflate the balloon.* Also inspect the catheter for resiliency. *Rough, cracked catheters can injure the urethral mucosa during insertion, which can predispose the patient to infection* (as shown below).

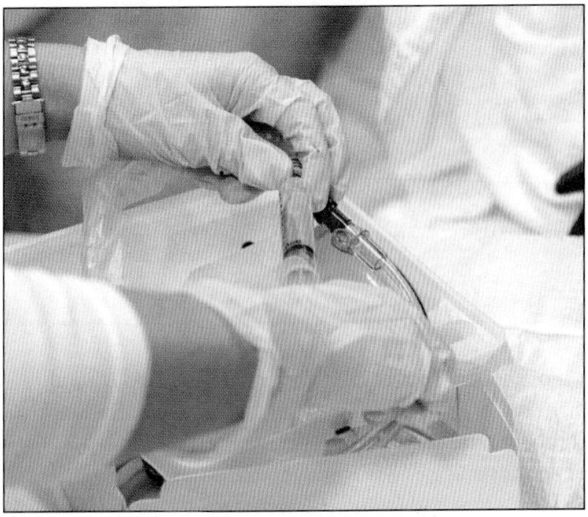

■ For the female patient, separate the labia majora and labia minora as widely as possible with the thumb, middle, and index fingers of your nondominant hand *so you have a full view of the urinary meatus.* Keep the labia well separated throughout the procedure (as shown below), *so they don't obscure the urinary meatus or contaminate the area when it's cleaned.*

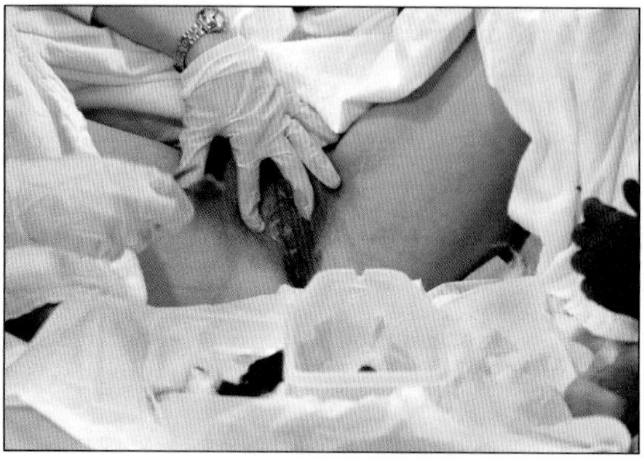

- With your dominant hand, use a sterile, cotton-tipped applicator (or pick up a sterile cotton ball with the plastic forceps) and wipe one side of the urinary meatus with a single downward motion (as shown below). Wipe the other side with another sterile applicator or cotton ball in the same way. Then wipe directly over the meatus with still another sterile applicator or cotton ball. Take care not to contaminate your sterile glove .

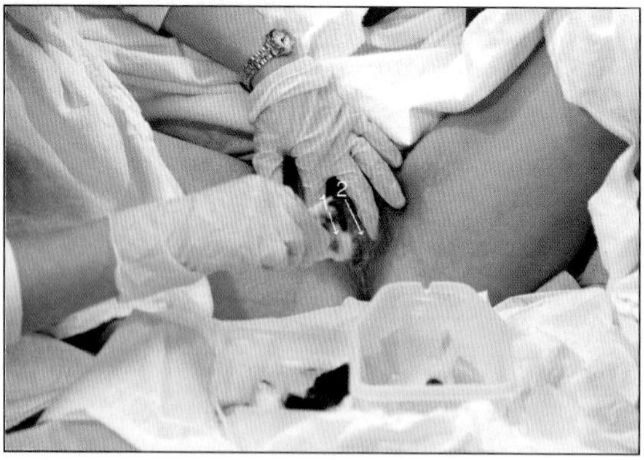

- For the male patient, hold the penis with your nondominant hand. If he's uncircumcised, retract the foreskin. Then gently lift and stretch the penis to a 60- to 90-degree angle. Hold the penis this way throughout the procedure *to straighten the urethra and maintain a sterile field.*
- Use your dominant hand to clean the glans with a sterile cotton-tipped applicator or a sterile cotton ball held in the forceps. Clean in a circular motion, starting at the urinary meatus and working outward (as shown top of next column).

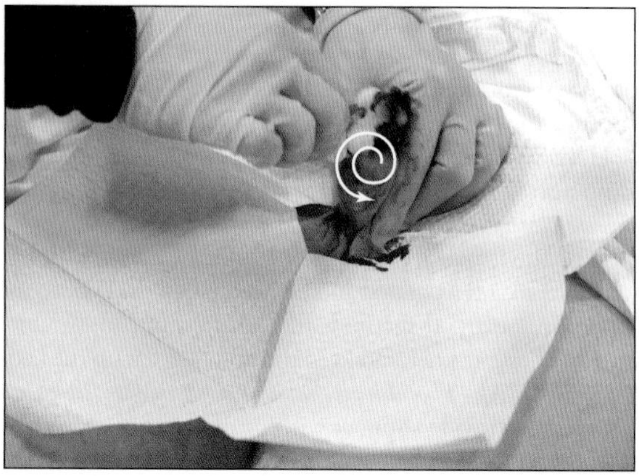

- Repeat the procedure, using another sterile applicator or cotton ball and taking care not to contaminate your sterile glove.
- Pick up the catheter with your dominant hand and prepare to insert the lubricated tip into the urinary meatus. *To facilitate insertion by relaxing the sphincter,* ask the patient to cough as you insert the catheter. Tell him to breathe deeply and slowly *to further relax the sphincter and spasms.* Hold the catheter close to its tip *to ease insertion and control its direction* (as shown below).

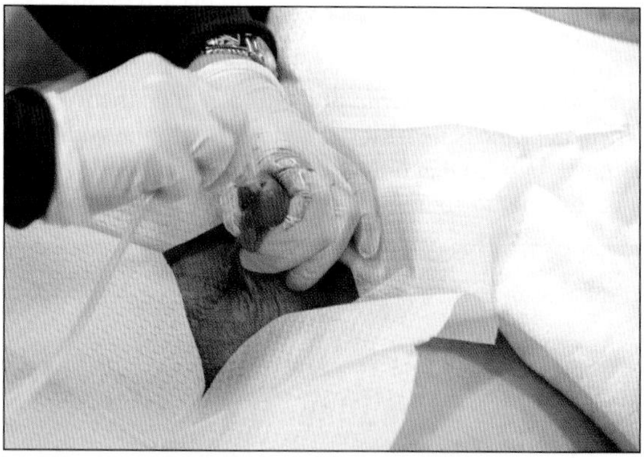

NURSING ALERT *Never force a catheter during insertion. Maneuver it gently as the patient bears down or coughs. If you still meet resistance, stop and notify the practitioner. Sphincter spasms, strictures, misplacement in the vagina (in females), or an enlarged prostate (in males) may cause resistance.*

- For the female patient, advance the catheter 2″ to 3″ (5 to 7.5 cm)—while continuing to hold the labia apart—until urine begins to flow. If the catheter is inadvertently inserted into the vagina, leave it there as a landmark. Then begin the procedure over again using new supplies.

■ For the male patient, advance the catheter to the bifurcation and check for urine flow. If the foreskin was retracted, replace it *to prevent compromised circulation and painful swelling.*
■ When urine stops flowing, attach the water-filled syringe to the luer-lock.
■ Push the plunger and inflate the balloon (as shown below) *to keep the catheter in place in the bladder.*

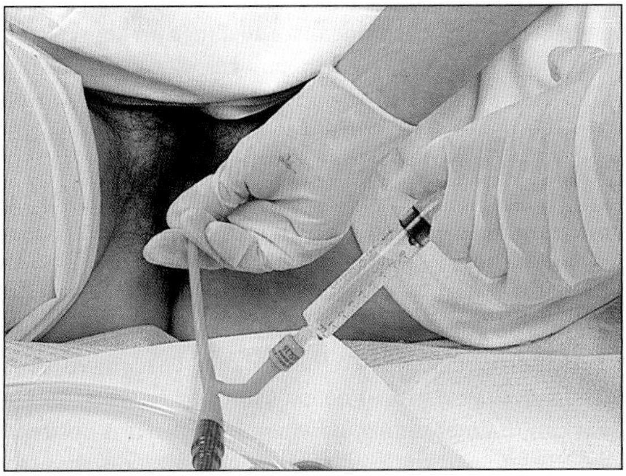

NURSING ALERT *Never inflate a balloon without first establishing urine flow,* which assures you that the catheter is in the bladder.
■ Hang the collection bag below bladder level *to prevent urine reflux into the bladder,* which can cause infection, and *to facilitate gravity drainage of the bladder.* Make sure the tubing doesn't get tangled in the bed's side rails.
■ Tape the catheter to the female patient's thigh *to prevent possible tension on the urogenital trigone.*
■ Tape the catheter to the male patient's abdomen or thigh *to prevent pressure on the urethra at the penoscrotal junction, which can lead to formation of urethrocutaneous fistulas. Taping this way also prevents traction on the bladder and alteration in the normal direction of urine flow in males.*
■ As an alternative, secure the catheter to the patient's thigh using a leg band with a Velcro closure. *This decreases skin irritation, especially in patients with long-term indwelling catheters.*
■ Dispose of all used supplies properly.

Special considerations

■ The balloon size determines the amount of solution or air needed for inflation, and the exact amount is usually printed on the distal extension of the catheter used for inflating the balloon. *Note:* Injecting a catheter with air makes identifying leaks difficult and doesn't guarantee deflation of the balloon for removal.

■ If necessary, ask the female patient to lie on her side with her knees drawn up to her chest during the catheterization procedure (as shown below). *This position may be especially helpful for elderly or disabled patients, such as those with severe contractures.*

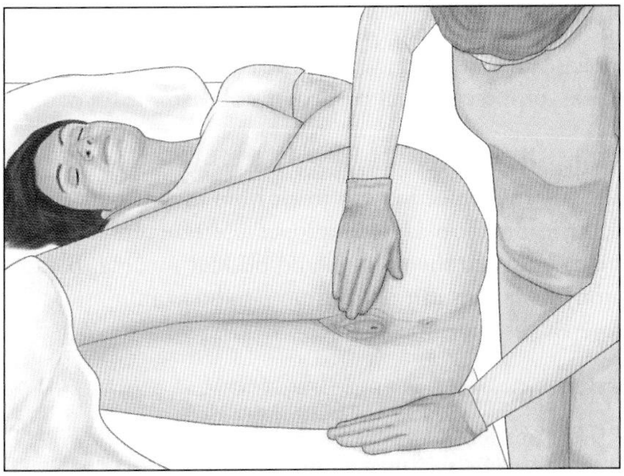

■ If the practitioner orders a urine specimen for laboratory analysis, obtain it from the urine receptacle with a specimen collection container at the time of catheterization, and send it to the laboratory with the appropriate laboratory request form. Connect the drainage bag when urine stops flowing.
■ Inspect the catheter and tubing periodically while they're in place *to detect compression or kinking that could obstruct urine flow.* Explain the basic principles of gravity drainage *so that the patient realizes the importance of keeping the drainage tubing and collection bag lower than his bladder at all times.* If necessary, provide the patient with detailed instructions for performing clean intermittent self-catheterization. (See "Self-catheterization," page 724.)
■ For monitoring purposes, empty the collection bag at least every 8 hours. Excessive fluid volume may require more frequent emptying *to prevent traction on the catheter,* which would cause the patient discomfort, and *to prevent injury to the urethra and bladder wall.* Some facilities encourage changing catheters at regular intervals, such as every 30 days, if the patient will have long-term continuous drainage.
NURSING ALERT *Observe the patient carefully for adverse reactions caused by removing excessive volumes of residual urine, such as hypovolemic shock. Check your facility's policy beforehand to determine the maximum amount of urine that may be drained at one time (some facilities limit the amount to 700 to 1,000 ml). Whether to limit the amount of urine drained is currently controversial. Clamp the catheter at the first sign of an adverse reaction, and notify the practitioner.*

Home care

If the patient will be discharged with a long-term indwelling catheter, teach him and his family all aspects of daily catheter maintenance, including care of the skin and urinary meatus, signs and symptoms of urinary tract infection or obstruction, how to irrigate the catheter (if appropriate), and the importance of adequate fluid intake *to maintain patency.* Explain that a home care nurse should visit every 4 to 6 weeks, or more often if needed, *to change the catheter.*

Complications

Urinary tract infection can result from the introduction of bacteria into the bladder. Improper insertion can cause traumatic injury to the urethral and bladder mucosa. Bladder atony or spasms can result from rapid decompression of a severely distended bladder.

Documentation

Record the date, time, and size and type of indwelling catheter used. Also describe the amount, color, and other characteristics of urine emptied from the bladder. Your facility may require only the intake and output sheet for fluid-balance data. If large volumes of urine have been emptied, describe the patient's tolerance for the procedure. Note whether a urine specimen was sent for laboratory analysis.

SELECTED REFERENCES

Clinical Practice Guidelines Task Force; Society of Urologic Nurses and Associates. "Female Urethral Catheterization," *Urologic Nursing* 26(4):314, August 2006.

Clinical Practice Guidelines Task Force; Society of Urologic Nurses and Associates. "Male Urethral Catheterization," *Urologic Nursing* 26(4):315, August 2006.

Doherty, W. "Urinary Catheterization in Male Patients," *Nursing Standards* 20(35):57-63, May 2006.

Garcia, M.M., et al. "Traditional Foley Drainage Systems—Do They Drain the Bladder?" *Journal of Urology* 177(1):203-207, January 2007.

Taylor, C., et al. *Fundamentals of Nursing: The Art and Science of Nursing Care*, 6th ed. Philadelphia: Lippincott Williams & Wilkins, 2008.

Woodward, S. "Use of Lubricant in Female Urethral Catheterization," *British Journal of Nursing* 14(19):1022-1023, October-November 2005.

INDWELLING CATHETER CARE AND REMOVAL

Intended to prevent infection and other complications by keeping the catheter insertion site clean, routine catheter care typically is performed daily after the patient's morning bath and immediately after perineal care. (Bedtime catheter care may have to be performed before perineal care.)

Studies suggest that catheter care should include daily cleaning of the meatal-catheter area. The use of topical antibiotics is discouraged because it hasn't been proven to be effective in decreasing infection. The equipment and the patient's genitalia require inspection twice daily.

Catheter surfaces and balloons that are exposed to urine will develop encrustations, and patients whose catheters develop a blockage have urine that's alkaline and high in concentrations of mucin, protein, and calcium salts. For this reason, it's recommended that catheterized patients drink lots of fluids to ensure increased urine output so that microorganisms are flushed out of the bladder.

Be sure to assess the catheter every day for crystals or encrustations by palpating it between your fingers and assessing for sandy or granular materials. Be careful not to break off any crystals. If encrustations are present on the catheter, it should be removed and replaced.

An indwelling urinary catheter should be removed when bladder decompression is no longer necessary, when the patient can resume voiding, or when the catheter is obstructed. Depending on the length of the catheterization, the practitioner may order bladder retraining before catheter removal.

Equipment

For catheter care: Soap and water ▪ sterile gloves ▪ sterile 4″ × 4″ gauze pads ▪ basin ▪ washcloth ▪ leg bag or adhesive tape ▪ collection bag ▪ waste receptacle ▪ optional: safety pin, rubber band, gooseneck lamp or flashlight, adhesive remover, specimen container.

For catheter removal: Gloves ▪ 10-ml syringe with a luer-lock ▪ bedpan ▪ linen-saver pad ▪ optional: clamp for bladder retraining.

Implementation

- Confirm the patient's identity using two patient identifiers according to your facility's policy.
- Explain the procedure and its purpose to the patient.
- Provide the patient with the necessary equipment for self-cleaning, if possible.
- Provide privacy.

Catheter care

- Make sure the lighting is adequate *so that you can see the perineum and catheter tubing clearly.* Place a gooseneck lamp at the bedside, if needed.
- Inspect the catheter for any problems, and check the urine drainage for mucus, blood clots, sediment, and turbidity. Then pinch the catheter between two fingers *to determine*

if the lumen contains any material. If you notice any of these conditions (or if your facility's policy requires it), obtain a urine specimen from the specimen collection port. Collect at least 3 ml of urine. Notify the practitioner about your findings.

- Inspect the outside of the catheter where it enters the urinary meatus for encrusted material and suppurative drainage. Also inspect the tissue around the meatus for irritation or swelling.
- Remove the leg band, or if adhesive tape was used to secure the catheter, remove the adhesive tape. Inspect the area for signs of adhesive burns—redness, tenderness, or blisters.
- Put on the sterile gloves. Clean the outside of the catheter and the tissue around the meatus using soap and water. *To avoid contaminating the urinary tract,* always clean by wiping away from—never toward—the urinary meatus using soap and water. Use a dry gauze pad to remove encrusted material.

NURSING ALERT *Don't pull on the catheter while you're cleaning it.* This can injure the urethra and the bladder wall. It can also expose a section of the catheter that was inside the urethra, so that when you release the catheter, the newly contaminated section will reenter the urethra, introducing potentially infectious organisms.

- Remove your gloves, reapply the leg band, and reattach the catheter to the leg band. If a leg band isn't available, tear a piece of adhesive tape from the roll.
- *To prevent skin hypersensitivity or irritation,* retape the catheter on the opposite side.

NURSING ALERT *Provide enough slack before securing the catheter* to prevent tension on the tubing, which could injure the urethral lumen or bladder wall.

- Most drainage bags have a plastic clamp on the tubing *to attach them to the sheet.* If this isn't available, wrap a rubber band around the drainage tubing, insert the safety pin through a loop of the rubber band, and pin the tubing to the sheet below bladder level. Then attach the collection bag, below bladder level, to the bed frame.
- If necessary, clean residue from the previous tape site with adhesive remover. Then dispose of all used supplies in a waste receptacle.

Catheter removal

- Wash your hands.
- Assemble the equipment at the patient's bedside. Explain the procedure and tell him that he may feel slight discomfort. Tell him that you'll check him periodically during the first 6 to 24 hours after catheter removal *to make sure he resumes voiding.*
- Put on gloves. Place a linen-saver pad under the patient's buttocks. Attach the syringe to the luer-lock mechanism on the catheter.
- Pull back on the plunger of the syringe. *This deflates the balloon by aspirating the injected fluid.* The amount of fluid injected is usually indicated on the tip of the catheter's balloon lumen and in the patient's chart.
- Grasp the catheter and pinch it firmly with your thumb and index finger *to prevent urine from flowing back into the urethra.* Before doing so, offer the patient a bedpan. Gently pull the catheter from the urethra. If you meet resistance, don't apply force; instead, notify the practitioner.
- Measure and record the amount of urine in the collection bag before discarding it. Remove and discard gloves, and wash your hands. For the first 24 hours after catheter removal, note the time and amount of each voiding.

Special considerations

- Some facilities require the use of specific cleaning agents for catheter care, so check your facility's policy manual before beginning this procedure.
- Use a closed drainage system, whenever possible, *to decrease the patient's chance of getting a urinary tract infection.*
- Avoid raising the drainage bag above bladder level. *This prevents reflux of urine, which may contain bacteria. To avoid damaging the urethral lumen or bladder wall,* always disconnect the drainage bag and tubing from the bed linen and bed frame before helping the patient out of bed.
- When possible, attach a leg bag *to allow the patient greater mobility.* If the patient will be discharged with an indwelling catheter, teach him how to use a leg bag. (See *Teaching about leg bags,* page 720.)
- Encourage patients with unrestricted fluid intake to increase intake to at least 3,000 ml per day. *This helps flush the urinary system and reduces sediment formation.*
- After catheter removal, assess the patient for incontinence (or dribbling), urgency, persistent dysuria or bladder spasms, fever, chills, or palpable bladder distention. The patient should void within 6 to 8 hours after catheter removal.
- When changing catheters after long-term use (usually 30 days), you may need a larger size catheter *because the meatus enlarges, causing urine to leak around the catheter.*

Home care

Instruct patients discharged with indwelling catheters to wash the urinary meatus and perineal area with soap and water twice daily and the anal area after each bowel movement.

Teaching about leg bags

A urine drainage bag attached to the leg provides the catheterized patient with greater mobility. *Because the bag is hidden under clothing,* it may also help him feel more comfortable about catheterization. Leg bags are usually worn during the day and are replaced at night with a standard collection device.

If your patient will be discharged with an indwelling catheter, teach him how to attach and remove a leg bag. To demonstrate, you'll need a bag with a short drainage tube, two straps, an alcohol pad, adhesive tape, and a screw clamp or hemostat.

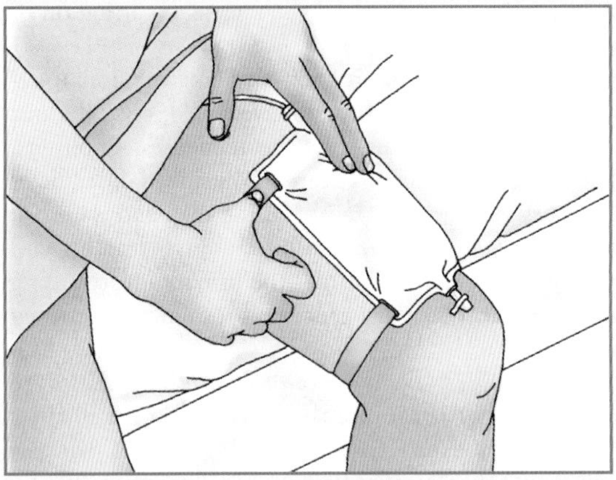

Attaching the leg bag

- Provide privacy and explain the procedure. Describe the advantages of a leg bag, but caution the patient that a leg bag is smaller than a standard collection device and may have to be emptied more frequently.
- Remove the protective covering from the tip of the drainage tube. Then show the patient how to clean the tip with an alcohol sponge, wiping away from the opening *to avoid contaminating the tube.* Show him how to attach the tube to the catheter.
- Place the drainage bag on the patient's calf or thigh. Have him fasten the straps securely (as shown), and show him how to tape the catheter to his leg. Emphasize that he must leave slack in the catheter to minimize pressure on the bladder, urethra, and related structures. *Excessive pressure or tension can lead to tissue breakdown.*
- Also tell him not to fasten the straps too tightly *to avoid interfering with his circulation.*

Avoiding complications

- Although most leg bags have a valve in the drainage tube that prevents urine reflux into the bladder, urge the patient to keep the drainage bag lower than his bladder at all times *because urine in the bag is a perfect growth medium for bacteria.* Caution him not to go to bed or take long naps while wearing the drainage bag.
- *To prevent a full leg bag from damaging the bladder wall and urethra,* encourage the patient to empty the bag when it's only one-half full. He should also inspect the catheter and drainage tube periodically for compression or kinking, *which could obstruct urine flow and result in bladder distention.*
- Tell the patient to wash the leg bag with soap and water or a bacteriostatic solution before each use *to prevent infection.*

Complications

Sediment buildup can occur anywhere in a catheterization system, especially in bedridden and dehydrated patients. To prevent this, keep the patient well hydrated if he isn't on fluid restriction. Change the indwelling catheter, as ordered, or when malfunction, obstruction, or contamination occurs.

Acute renal failure may result from a catheter obstructed by sediment. Be alert for sharply reduced urine flow from the catheter. Assess for bladder discomfort or distention.

Urinary tract infection can result from catheter insertion or from intraluminal or extraluminal migration of bacteria up the catheter. Signs and symptoms may include cloudy urine, foul-smelling urine, hematuria, fever, malaise, tenderness over the bladder, and flank pain.

Major complications in removing an indwelling catheter are failure of the balloon to deflate and rupture of the balloon. If the balloon ruptures, cystoscopy is usually performed *to ensure removal of any balloon fragments.*

Documentation

Record the care you performed, any modifications, patient complaints, and the condition of the perineum and urinary meatus. Note the character of the urine in the drainage bag, any sediment buildup, and whether a specimen was sent for laboratory analysis. Also record fluid intake and output. An hourly record is usually necessary for critically ill patients and those with renal insufficiency who are hemodynamically unstable.

SELECTED REFERENCES

Godfrey, H., and Fraczyk, L. "Preventing and Managing Catheter-associated Urinary Tract Infections," *British Journal of Community Nursing* 10(5):205-206, 208-12, May 2005.

Huang, W.C., et al. "Catheter-associated Urinary Tract Infections in Intensive Care Units Can Be Reduced by Prompting Physicians to Remove Unnecessary Catheters," *Infection Control and Hospital Epidemiology* 25(11):974-78, November 2004.

The Joanna Briggs Institute for Evidence Based Nursing and Midwifery. "Best Practice: Management of Short-Term Indwelling Urethral Catheters to Prevent Urinary Tract Infections," 4(1), 2000. Available at *www.joannabriggs.edu.au/best_practice/BPISIUC.php.*

Reilly, L., et al. "Reducing Foley Catheter Device Days in an Intensive Care Unit: Using the Evidence to Change Practice," *AACN Advances in Critical Care* 17(3):272-83, July-September 2006.

Ribby, K.J. "Decreasing Urinary Tract Infections through Staff Development, Outcomes, and Nursing Process," *Journal of Nursing Care Quality* 21(3):272-76 July-September 2006.

Robinson, J. "Removing Indwelling Urinary Catheters: Trial without Catheter in the Community," *British Journal of Community Nursing* 10(12):553-54, 556-57, December 2005.

Taylor, C., et al. *Fundamentals of Nursing: The Art and Science of Nursing Care,* 6th ed. Philadelphia: Lippincott Williams & Wilkins, 2008.

CATHETER IRRIGATION

To avoid introducing microorganisms into the bladder, the nurse irrigates an indwelling catheter to remove an obstruction, such as a blood clot that develops after bladder, kidney, or prostate surgery.

In some cases, the nurse may instill a medication that works directly on the bladder wall. Whenever possible, the catheter should be irrigated through a closed system to decrease the risk of infection.

Equipment

Ordered irrigating solution (such as normal saline solution) ▪ sterile basin ▪ two alcohol pads ▪ gloves ▪ linen-saver pad ▪ intake and output sheet ▪ 30- to 60-ml syringe ▪ 18G blunt-end needle (if system not needleless) ▪ clamp.

Commercially packaged kits containing sterile irrigating solution, a graduated receptacle, and a 50-ml catheter tip syringe may be available.

Preparation of equipment

Check the expiration date on the irrigating solution. *To prevent vesical spasms during instillation of solution,* warm it to room temperature. Never heat the solution on a burner or in a microwave oven. *Hot irrigating solution can injure the patient's bladder.*

Implementation

- Confirm the patient's identity using two patient identifiers according to your facility's policy.
- Wash your hands, and assemble the equipment at the bedside. Explain the procedure to the patient, and provide privacy.
- Expose the catheter's aspiration or needleless port and place the linen-saver pad under it *to protect the bed linens.*
- Create a sterile field at the patient's bedside. Using sterile technique, pour the prescribed amount of solution into the basin.
- Place the tip of the syringe into the solution, and fill the syringe with the appropriate amount of solution (as shown below).

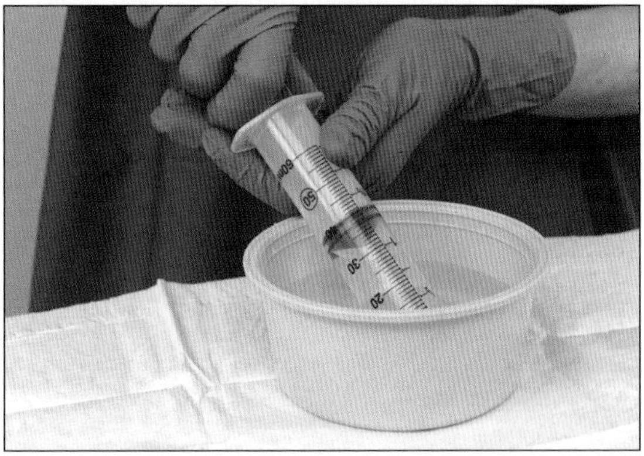

- Clean the aspiration or needleless port with an alcohol pad *to remove as many bacterial contaminants as possible* (as shown below).

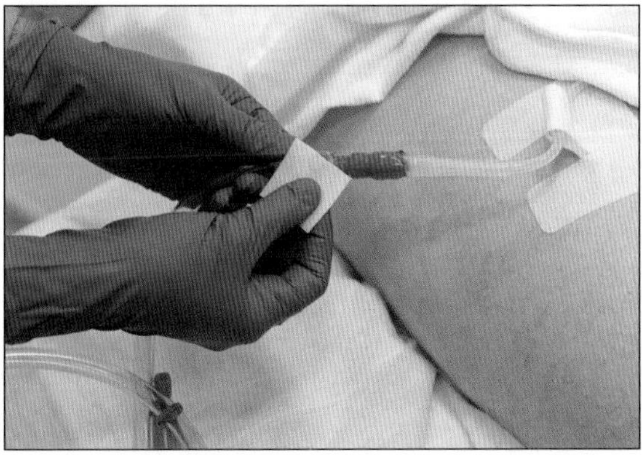

■ Clamp the catheter tubing below the port (as shown below).

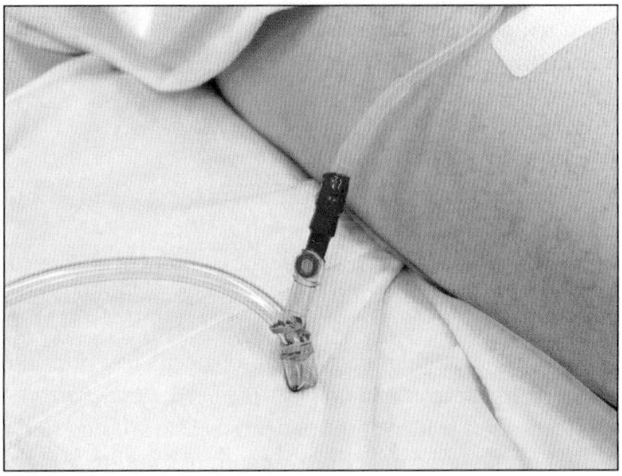

■ Attach the syringe to the needleless port, or insert the blunt-tip needle into the aspiration port if a needleless system isn't in place.
■ Instill the irrigating solution into the catheter. If necessary, refill the syringe and repeat this step until you've instilled the prescribed amount of irrigating solution.
■ Remove the syringe and unclamp the drainage tube *to allow the irrigant and urine to flow into the drainage bag* (as shown below).

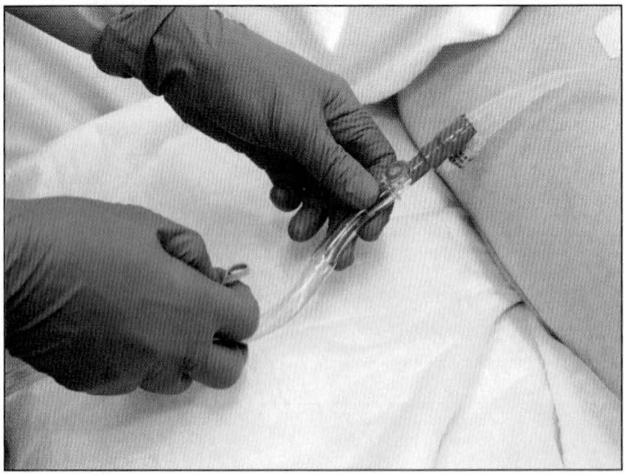

■ Make sure the catheter tubing is secured to the patient's leg and that the drainage bag is below the level of the bladder.
■ Dispose of all used supplies properly.

Special considerations

■ If you encounter any resistance during instillation of the irrigating solution, don't try to force the solution into the bladder. Instead, stop the procedure and notify the practitioner. If an indwelling catheter becomes totally obstructed, obtain an order to remove it and replace it with a new one *to prevent bladder distention, acute renal failure, urinary stasis, and subsequent infection.*
■ The practitioner may order a continuous irrigation system. *This decreases the risk of infection by eliminating the need to disconnect the catheter and drainage tube repeatedly.* (See "Continuous bladder irrigation" below.)
■ Encourage catheterized patients not on restricted fluid intake to increase intake to 3,000 ml per day *to help flush the urinary system and reduce sediment formation.*

Documentation

Note the amount, color, and consistency of return urine flow, and document the patient's tolerance for the procedure. Also note any resistance during instillation of the solution. If the return flow volume is less than the amount of solution instilled, note this on the intake and output balance sheets and in your notes.

SELECTED REFERENCES

Rew, M. "Caring for Catheterized Patients: Urinary Catheter Maintenance," *British Journal of Nursing* 14(2):87-92, January-February 2005.

Taylor, C., et al. *Fundamentals of Nursing: The Art and Science of Nursing Care*, 6th ed. Philadelphia: Lippincott Williams & Wilkins, 2008.

CONTINUOUS BLADDER IRRIGATION

Continuous bladder irrigation can help prevent urinary tract obstruction by flushing out small blood clots that form after prostate or bladder surgery. It may also be used to treat an irritated, inflamed, or infected bladder lining.

This procedure requires placement of a triple-lumen catheter. One lumen controls balloon inflation, one allows irrigant inflow, and one allows irrigant outflow. The continuous flow of irrigating solution through the bladder also creates a mild tamponade that may help prevent venous hemorrhage. (See *Setup for continuous bladder irrigation.*) Although the patient typically receives the catheter while he's in the operating room after prostate or bladder surgery, he may have it inserted at bedside if he isn't a surgical patient.

Equipment

Sterile irrigating solution ■ sterile tubing for use with bladder irrigating system ■ alcohol or antiseptic pad ■ drainage bag and tubing ■ I.V. pole.

Normal saline solution is usually prescribed for bladder irrigation after prostate or bladder surgery. Large volumes of irrigating solution are usually required during the first 24 to 48 hours after surgery.

Preparation of equipment
Before starting continuous bladder irrigation, double-check the irrigating solution against the practitioner's order. If the solution contains an antibiotic, check the patient's chart *to make sure he isn't allergic to the drug.*

Implementation
- Confirm the patient's identity using two patient identifiers according to your facility's policy.
- Wash your hands. Assemble all equipment at the patient's bedside. Explain the procedure and provide privacy.
- Insert the spike of the tubing into the container of irrigating solution.
- Squeeze the drip chamber on the spike of the tubing.
- Open the flow clamp and flush the tubing *to remove air, which could cause bladder distention.* Then close the clamp.
- To begin, hang the bag of irrigating solution on the I.V. pole.
- Clean the opening to the inflow lumen of the catheter with the alcohol or antiseptic pad.
- Insert the distal end of the tubing securely into the inflow lumen (third port) of the catheter.
- Make sure the catheter's outflow lumen is securely attached to the drainage bag tubing.
- Open the flow clamp under the container of irrigating solution, and set the drip rate as ordered.
- *To prevent air from entering the system,* don't let the primary container empty completely before replacing it.
- Empty the drainage bag about every 4 hours, or as often as needed. Use sterile technique *to avoid the risk of contamination.*
- Monitor vital signs at least every 4 hours during irrigation; increase the frequency if the patient becomes unstable.
- Monitor urine output at least hourly for the first 4 hours. Check for bladder distention or abdominal pain.

Special considerations
- Check the inflow and outflow lines periodically for kinks *to make sure the solution is running freely.* If the solution flows rapidly, check the lines frequently.
- As an alternative to flow clamp administration, an administration pump may be used, requiring the pump tubing to be primed. Set the flow rate as ordered by the practitioner. *The volume infused is used to help calculate the urine output.*

EQUIPMENT

Setup for continuous bladder irrigation

In continuous bladder irrigation, a triple-lumen catheter allows irrigating solution to flow into the bladder through one lumen and flow out through another, as shown in the inset. The third lumen is used to inflate the balloon that holds the catheter in place.

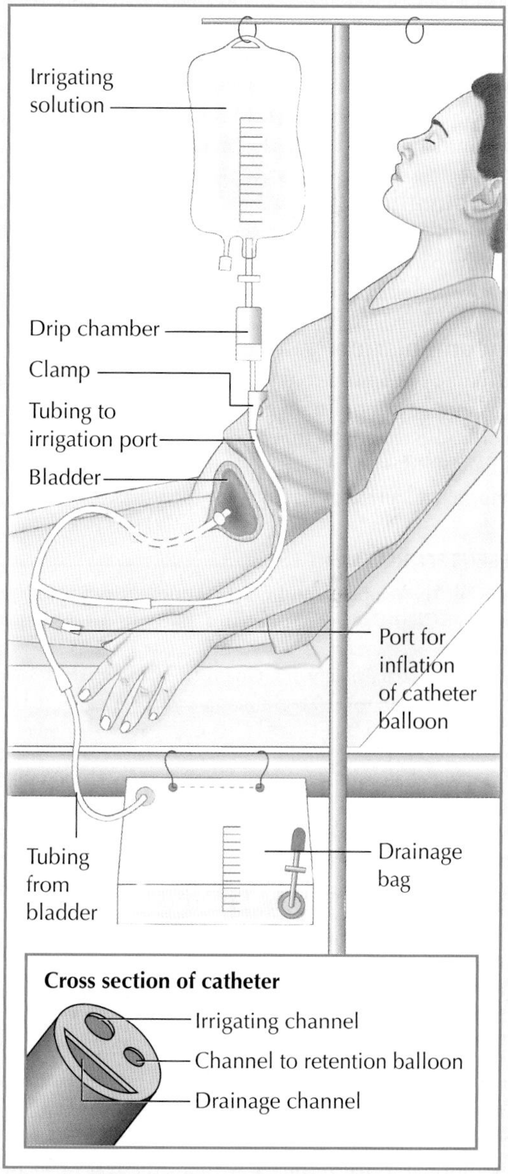

- Measure the outflow volume accurately. It should equal or, allowing for urine production, slightly exceed inflow volume. If inflow volume exceeds outflow volume postoperatively, suspect bladder rupture at the suture lines or renal damage, and notify the practitioner immediately.
- Also assess outflow for changes in appearance and for blood clots, especially if irrigation is being performed postoperatively to control bleeding. If drainage is bright red, irrigating solution should usually be infused rapidly with the clamp wide open until drainage clears. Notify the practitioner at once if you suspect hemorrhage. If drainage is clear, the solution is usually given at a rate of 40 to 60 drops/minute. The practitioner typically specifies the rate for antibiotic solutions.
- Encourage oral fluid intake of 2 to 3 qt (2 to 3 L)/day unless contraindicated by another medical condition.

Complications

Interruptions in a continuous irrigation system can predispose the patient to infection. Obstruction in the catheter's outflow lumen can cause bladder distention.

Documentation

Each time you finish a container of solution, record the date, time, and amount of fluid given on the intake and output record. Also record the time and amount of fluid each time you empty the drainage bag. Note the appearance of the drainage and any complaints the patient has.

Selected references

Cutts, B. "Developing and Implementing a New Bladder Irrigation Chart," *Nursing Standard* 20(8):48-52, November 2005.

Defoor, W., et al. "Safety of Gentamicin Bladder Irrigations in Complex Urological Cases," *Journal of Urology* 175(5):1861-864, May 2006.

Smeltzer, S.C., et al. *Brunner & Suddarth's Textbook of Medical-Surgical Nursing*, 11th ed. Philadelphia: Lippincott Williams & Wilkins, 2008.

Self-catheterization

A patient with impaired or absent bladder function may catheterize himself for routine bladder drainage. Because clean intermittent catheterization is safer than an indwelling catheter to prevent urinary tract infections (UTIs), it's a recommended alternative by the Centers for Disease Control and Prevention. The two major advantages of self-catheterization are that patient independence is maintained and bladder control is regained. In addition, self-catheterization allows normal sexual intimacy without the fear of incontinence, decreases the chance of urinary reflux, reduces the use of aids and appliances and, in many cases, allows the patient to return to work.

Self-catheterization requires thorough and careful teaching by the nurse. The patient will probably use clean technique for self-catheterization at home, but he must use sterile technique in the hospital because of the increased risk of infection.

Equipment

Rubber catheter ▪ washcloth ▪ soap and water ▪ small packet of water-soluble lubricant ▪ plastic storage bag ▪ optional: drainage container, paper towels, rubber or plastic sheets, gooseneck lamp, catheterization record, mirror.

Preparation of equipment

Instruct the patient to keep a supply of catheters at home and to use each catheter only once before cleaning it. Advise him to wash the used catheter in warm, soapy water, rinse it inside and out, and then dry it with a clean towel and store it in a plastic bag until the next time it's needed. *Because catheters become brittle with repeated use,* tell the patient to check them often and to order a new supply well in advance.

Implementation

- Tell the patient to begin by trying to urinate into the toilet or, if a toilet isn't available or he needs to measure urine quantity, to urinate into a drainage container. Then he should wash his hands thoroughly with soap and water and dry them.
- Demonstrate how the patient should perform the catheterization, explaining each step clearly and carefully. Position a gooseneck lamp nearby if room lighting is inadequate *to make the urinary meatus clearly visible.* Arrange the patient's clothing so that it's out of the way.

Teaching the female patient

- Demonstrate and explain to the female patient that she should separate the vaginal folds as widely as possible with the fingers of her nondominant hand *to obtain a full view of the urinary meatus.* She may need to use a mirror *to visualize the meatus.* Ask if she's right- or left-handed, and then tell her which is her nondominant hand. While holding her labia open with the nondominant hand, she should use the dominant hand to wash the perineal area thoroughly with a soapy washcloth, using downward strokes. Tell her to rinse the area with the washcloth, using downward strokes as well.
- Show her how to squeeze some lubricant onto the first 3″ (7.6 cm) of the catheter and then how to insert the catheter. (See *Teaching self-catheterization.*)

■ When the urine stops draining, tell her to remove the catheter slowly, get dressed, and wash the catheter with warm, soapy water. Then she should rinse it inside and out and dry it with a paper towel.

Teaching the male patient

■ Tell a male patient to wash and rinse the end of his penis thoroughly with soap and water, pulling back the foreskin, if appropriate. He should keep the foreskin pulled back during the procedure.
■ Show him how to squeeze lubricant onto a paper towel and have him roll the first 7″ to 10″ (17.5 to 25 cm) of the catheter in the lubricant. Tell him that copious lubricant will make the procedure more comfortable for him. Then show him how to insert the catheter.
■ When the urine stops draining, tell him to remove the catheter slowly and, if necessary, pull the foreskin forward again. Have him get dressed and wash and dry the catheter as described above.

Special considerations

■ Impress upon the patient that the timing of catheterization is critical *to prevent overdistention of the bladder, which can lead to infection.* Self-catheterization is usually performed every 4 to 6 hours around the clock (or more often at first).
■ Female patients should be able to identify the body parts involved in self-catheterization: labia majora, labia minora, vagina, and urinary meatus.
■ Keep in mind the difference between boiling and sterilization. Boiling kills bacteria, viruses, and fungi, but does not kill spores, whereas sterilization does. However, for catheter cleaning done in the patient's home, boiling is a sufficient safeguard against spreading infections.
■ Advise the patient to store cleaned catheters only after they're completely dry *to prevent growth of gram-negative organisms.*
■ Stress the importance of regulating fluid intake, as ordered, *to prevent incontinence while maintaining adequate hydration.* However, explain that incontinent episodes may occur occasionally. For managing incontinence, the practitioner or a home health care nurse can help develop a plan such as more frequent catheterizations. After an incontinent episode, tell the patient to wash with soap and water, pat himself dry with a towel, and expose the skin to the air for as long as possible. Bedding and furniture can be protected by covering them with rubber or plastic sheets and then covering the rubber or plastic with fabric.
■ Also stress the importance of taking medications, as ordered, *to increase urine retention and help prevent incontinence.* Advise the patient to avoid calcium-rich and phos-

Teaching self-catheterization

Teach a woman to hold the catheter in her dominant hand as if it were a pencil or a dart, about ½″ (1.3 cm) from its tip. Keeping the vaginal folds separated, she should slowly insert the lubricated catheter about 3″ (7.6 cm) into the urethra. Tell her to press down with her abdominal muscles to empty the bladder, allowing all urine to drain through the catheter and into the toilet or drainage container.

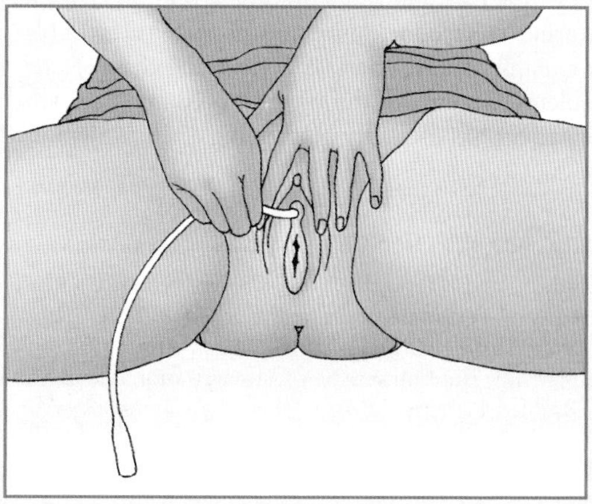

Teach a man to hold his penis in his nondominant hand, at a right angle to his body. He should hold the catheter in his dominant hand as if it were a pencil or a dart and slowly insert it 7″ to 10″ (17.5 to 25 cm) into the urethra until urine begins flowing. Then he should gently advance the catheter about 1″ (2.5 cm) farther, allowing all urine to drain into the toilet or drainage container.

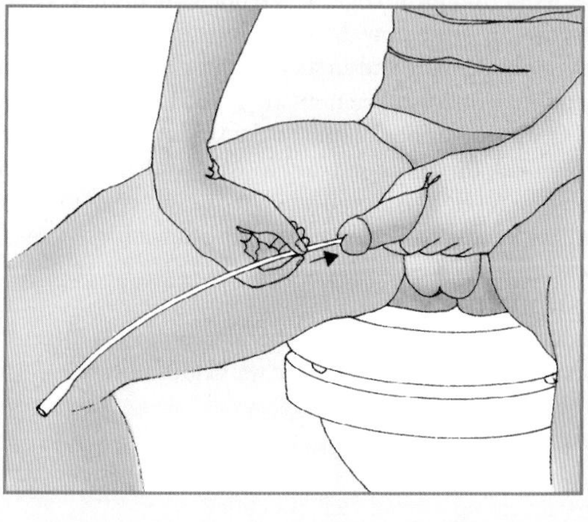

phorus-rich foods, as ordered, *to reduce the chance of renal calculus formation.*

Complications

Overdistention of the bladder can lead to urinary tract infection and urine leakage. Improper hand washing or equipment cleaning can also cause urinary tract infection. Incorrect catheter insertion can injure the urethral or bladder mucosa.

Documentation

Record the date and times of catheterization, character of the urine (color, odor, clarity, presence of particles or blood), the amount of urine (increase, decrease, no change), and any problems encountered during the procedure. Note whether the patient has difficulty performing a return demonstration.

SELECTED REFERENCES

Heard, L., and Buhrer, R. "How Do We Prevent UTI in People Who Perform Intermittent Catheterization?" *Rehabilitation Nursing* 30(2):44-45, 61, March-April 2005.

Robinson, J. "Intermittent Self-Catheterization Appliances for Disabled Patients," *British Journal of Community Nursing* 11(12):520-23, December 2006.

Robinson, J. "Intermittent Self-Catheterization: Principles and Practice," *British Journal of Community Nursing* 11(4):144, 146, 148 passim, April 2006.

Taylor, C., et al. *Fundamentals of Nursing: The Art and Science of Nursing Care*, 6th ed. Philadelphia: Lippincott Williams & Wilkins, 2008.

BLADDER ULTRASONOGRAPHY

Urine retention, a potentially life-threatening condition, may result from neurologic or psychological disorders or obstruction of urine flow. Medications such as anticholinergics, antihistamines, and antidepressants may also cause urine retention. Urinary catheterization, while a traditional method for measuring urine volume in the bladder, places the patient at risk for infection. Noninvasive bladder ultrasonography, however, provides an accurate assessment of urine volume with reduced risk of urinary tract infection.

Equipment

BladderScan (ultrasound) unit with scanhead ▪ ultrasonic transmission gel ▪ alcohol pad ▪ washcloth ▪ gloves.

Implementation

- Confirm the patient's identity using two patient identifiers according to your facility's policy.
- Bring the ultrasound unit to the bedside. Explain the procedure *to the patient to help reduce his anxiety.* Wash your hands.
- Provide privacy. If this is a postvoiding scan, ask the patient to void and assist him with this, if necessary. Position the patient in a supine position.
- Put on gloves and clean the rounded end of the scanhead with an alcohol pad.
- Expose the patient's suprapubic area.
- Turn on the ultrasound by pressing the button (designated by a dot within a circle) on the far left and press SCAN.
- Place ultrasonic gel on the scanhead *to promote an airtight seal for optimal sound-wave transmission.*
- Tell the patient that the gel will feel cold when placed on the abdomen. Locate the symphysis pubis, and place the scanhead about 1″ (2.5 cm) superior to the symphysis pubis.
- Locate the icon (a rough figure of a patient) on the probe, and make sure the head of the icon points toward the head of the patient.
- Press the scanhead button marked with a soundwave pattern to activate the scan. Hold the scanhead steady until you hear the beep.
- Look at the aiming icon and screen, which displays the bladder position and volume.
- Reposition the probe, and scan until the bladder is centered in the aiming screen. The largest measurement will be saved.
- Press DONE when finished.
- The ultrasound will display the measured urine volume and the longitudinal and horizontal axis scans.
- Press PRINT to obtain a hard copy of your results.
- Turn off the ultrasound. Use an alcohol pad to clean the gel off the scanhead.
- Using a washcloth, remove the gel from the patient's skin.
- Remove your gloves and wash your hands.

Special considerations

- Some scanners require you to choose a sex for the patient. If the patient has had a hysterectomy, choose male.

Documentation

Write the patient's name, the date, and the time on the printout, and attach it to the patient's medical record. Document the procedure and urine volume, as well as any treatment, in the patient's medical record.

SELECTED REFERENCES

Addison, R. "Assessing Continence with Bladder Ultrasound," *Nursing Times* 103(19):44-45, May 2007.

Graf, J. "Efficient Bladder Ultrasonography," *Pediatrics* 116(3):797, September 2005.

Oh-Oka, H., and Fujisawa, M. "Study of Low Bladder Volume Measurement Using 3-Dimensional Ultrasound Scanning Device: Improvement in Measurement Accuracy through Training when Bladder Volume Is 150 ml or Less," *Journal of Urology* 177(2):595-99, February 2007.

Taylor, C., et al. *Fundamentals of Nursing: The Art and Science of Nursing Care*, 6th ed. Philadelphia: Lippincott Williams & Wilkins, 2008.

SURGICAL URINARY DIVERSION

NEPHROSTOMY AND CYSTOSTOMY TUBE CARE

Two urinary diversion techniques—nephrostomy and cystostomy—ensure adequate drainage from the kidneys or bladder and help prevent urinary tract infection or kidney failure. (See *Urinary diversion techniques.*)

A nephrostomy tube drains urine directly from a kidney when a disorder inhibits the normal flow of urine. The tube is usually placed percutaneously, though sometimes it is surgically inserted through the renal cortex and medulla into the renal pelvis from a lateral incision in the flank. The usual indication is obstructive disease, such as calculi in the ureter or ureteropelvic junction, or an obstructing tumor. Draining urine with a nephrostomy tube also allows kidney tissue damaged by obstructive disease to heal.

A cystostomy tube drains urine from the bladder, diverting it from the urethra. This type of tube is used after certain gynecologic procedures, bladder surgery, prostatectomy, and for severe urethral strictures or traumatic injury. Inserted about 2″ (5 cm) above the symphysis pubis, a cystostomy tube may be used alone or with an indwelling urethral catheter.

Equipment

For dressing changes: Antiseptic swabs ▪ paper bag ▪ linen-saver pad ▪ clean gloves (for dressing removal) ▪ sterile gloves (for new dressing) ▪ precut 4″ × 4″ drain dressings or transparent semipermeable dressings ▪ adhesive tape (preferably hypoallergenic).

For nephrostomy-tube irrigation: 3-ml syringe ▪ antiseptic swab ▪ normal saline solution ▪ gloves ▪ optional: hemostat.

Commercially prepared sterile dressing kits may be available.

Urinary diversion techniques

A cystostomy or a nephrostomy can be used to create a permanent diversion, to relieve obstruction from an inoperable tumor, or to provide an outlet for urine after cystectomy. A temporary diversion can relieve obstruction from a calculus or ureteral edema.

In a *cystostomy,* a catheter is inserted percutaneously through the suprapubic area into the bladder. In a *nephrostomy,* a catheter is inserted percutaneously through the flank into the renal pelvis.

Cytostomy

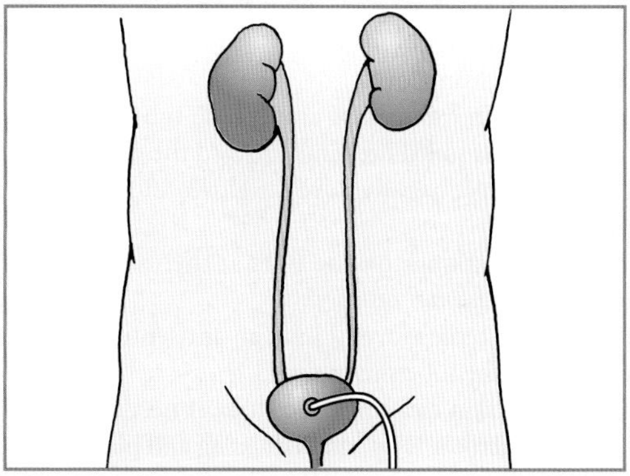

Nephrostomy

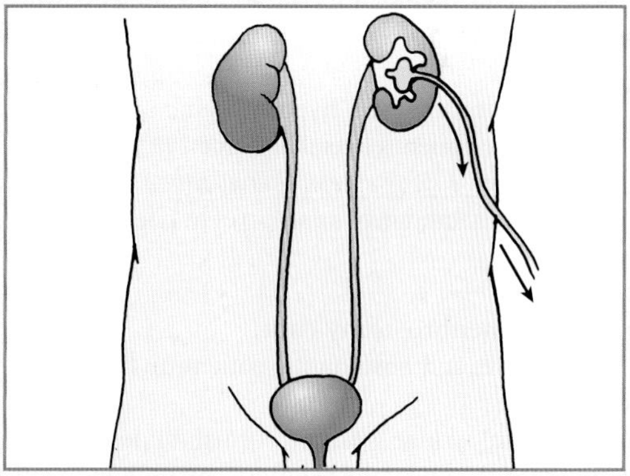

Preparation of equipment

Wash your hands, and assemble all equipment at the patient's bedside. Open the antiseptic swabs, the drain dressings, and sterile gloves. If you're using a commercially packaged dressing kit, open it using sterile technique.

Open the paper bag and place it away from the other equipment *to avoid contaminating the sterile field.*

Implementation

- Confirm the patient's identity using two patient identifiers according to your facility's policy.
- Provide privacy and explain the procedure.
- Wash your hands.

Changing a dressing

- Help the patient to lie on his back (for a cystostomy tube) or on the side opposite the tube (for a nephrostomy tube) *so that you can see the tube clearly and change the dressing more easily.*
- Place the linen-saver pad under the patient *to absorb excess drainage and keep him dry.*
- Put on the clean gloves.
- Carefully remove the tape around the tube, and then remove the wet or soiled dressing. Discard the tape and dressing into the paper bag. Remove the gloves and discard them into the bag.
- Note the markings on the tube at the insertion site *to check for its accidental dislodging.*
- Put on the sterile gloves. Using an antiseptic swab, clean the site from the tube site outward.
- Repeat the skin cleaning procedure, if needed.
- Pick up a sterile 4″ × 4″ drain dressing and place it around the tube. If necessary, overlap two drain dressings *to provide maximum absorption.* Or, depending on your facility's policy, apply a transparent semipermeable dressing over the site and tubing *to allow observation of the site without removing the dressing.*
- Secure the dressing with hypoallergenic tape. Then tape the tube to the patient's lateral abdomen *to prevent tension on the tube.* (See *Taping a nephrostomy tube.*)
- Dispose of all equipment appropriately. Clean the patient, as necessary.

Irrigating a nephrostomy tube

- Put on gloves and position the patient on his side opposite the tube.
- Fill the 3-ml syringe with the normal saline solution.
- Clean the junction of the nephrostomy tube and drainage tube with the antiseptic swab, and disconnect the tubes.
- Insert the syringe into the nephrostomy tube opening, and instill 2 to 3 ml of saline solution into the tube.
- Slowly aspirate the solution back into the syringe. *To avoid damaging the renal pelvis tissue,* never pull back forcefully on the plunger.
- If the solution doesn't return, remove the syringe from the tube and reattach it to the drainage tubing *to allow the solution to drain by gravity.*
- Dispose of all equipment appropriately.

Special considerations

- Change dressings once per day or more often if needed.

NURSING ALERT *Never irrigate a nephrostomy tube with more than 5 ml of solution because the capacity of the renal pelvis is usually between 4 and 8 ml.* **(Remember: The purpose of irrigation is to keep the tube patent, not to lavage the renal pelvis.)**

- When necessary, irrigate a cystostomy tube as you would an indwelling urinary catheter. Be sure to perform the irrigation gently *to avoid damaging any suture lines.*
- Check a nephrostomy tube frequently for kinks or obstructions. Kinks are likely to occur if the patient lies on the insertion site. Suspect an obstruction when the amount of urine in the drainage bag decreases or the amount of urine around the insertion site increases. Pressure created by urine backing up in the tube can damage nephrons. Gently curve a cystostomy tube *to prevent kinks.*
- If a blood clot or mucus plug obstructs a nephrostomy or cystostomy tube, try milking the tube *to restore its patency.* With your nondominant hand, hold the tube securely above the obstruction *to avoid pulling the tube out of the incision.* Then place the flat side of a closed hemostat under the tube, just above the obstruction, pinch the tube against the hemostat, and slide both your finger and the hemostat toward you, away from the patient.
- Typically, cystostomy tubes for postoperative urologic patients should be checked hourly for 24 hours *to ensure adequate drainage and tube patency.* To check tube patency, note the amount of urine in the drainage bag, and check the patient's bladder for distention.
- Keep the drainage bag below the level of the kidney at all times *to prevent urine reflux.*
- If the tube becomes dislodged, cover the site with a sterile dressing and notify the practitioner immediately.

Home care

Tell the home care patient to clean the insertion site with soap and water, check for skin breakdown, and change the dressing daily; then show him how to take these steps. Also teach him how to change the leg bag or drainage bag. He can use a leg bag during the day and a larger drainage bag at night. Whether he uses a drainage bag or larger container, tell him to wash it daily with a 1:3 vinegar and water solution, rinse it with plain water, and dry it thoroughly. *This prevents crystalline buildup.* Encourage patients with unrestricted fluid intake to increase intake to at least 3 qt (3 L)

Taping a nephrostomy tube

To tape a nephrostomy tube directly to the skin, cut a wide piece of hypoallergenic adhesive tape twice lengthwise to its midpoint.

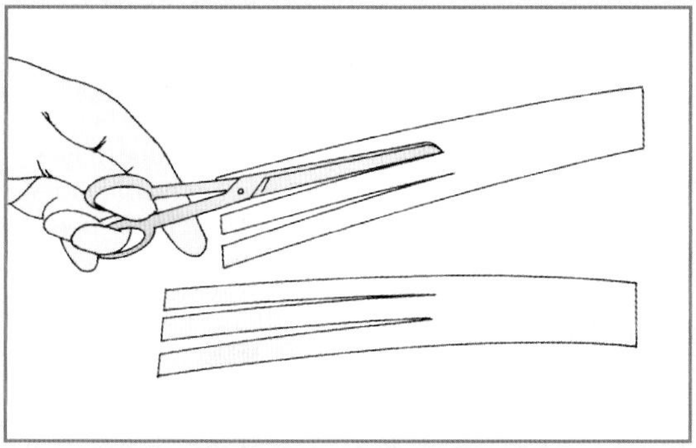

Apply the uncut end of the tape to the skin so that the midpoint meets the tube. Wrap the middle strip around the tube in spiral fashion. Tape the other two strips to the patient's skin on both sides of the tube.

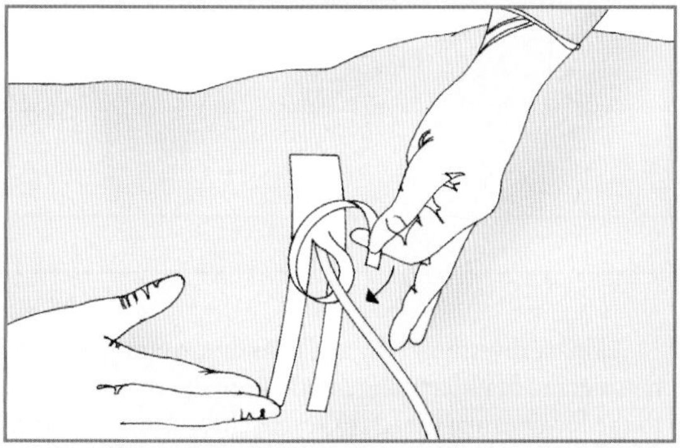

For greater security, repeat this step with a second piece of tape, applying it in the reverse direction. You may also apply two more strips of tape perpendicular to and over the first two pieces.

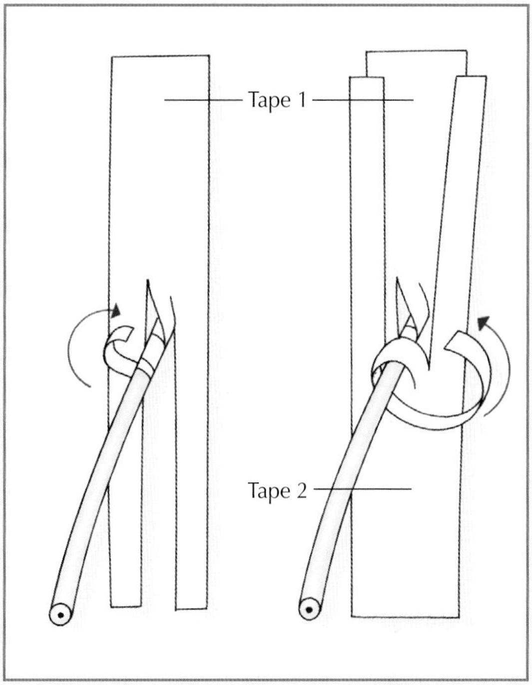

Always apply another strip of tape lower down on the tube in the direction of the drainage tube *to further anchor the tube.* Don't put tension on any sutures that prevent tube distention.

per day *to help flush the urinary system and reduce sediment formation.*

Stress the importance of reporting to the practitioner signs of infection (red skin or white, yellow, or green drainage at the insertion site) or tube displacement (drainage that smells like urine).

Complications

The patient has an increased risk of infection *because nephrostomy and cystostomy tubes provide a direct opening to the kidneys and bladder.*

Documentation

Describe the color and amount of drainage from the nephrostomy or cystostomy tube, and record any color changes as they occur. Similarly, if the patient has more than one tube, describe the drainage (color, amount, and character) from each tube separately. If irrigation is necessary, record the amount and type of irrigant used and whether or not you obtained a complete return.

Types of permanent urinary diversion

Two types of urinary diversions—the ileal conduit and the continent urinary diversion—are described here. Another recently developed type of continent urinary diversion (not pictured here) is "hooked" back to the urethra, obviating the need for a stoma.

Ileal conduit

A segment of the ileum is excised, and the two ends of the ileum that result from excision of the segment are sutured closed. Then the ureters are dissected from the bladder and anastomosed to the ileal segment. One end of the ileal segment is closed with sutures; the opposite end is brought through the abdominal wall, thereby forming a stoma.

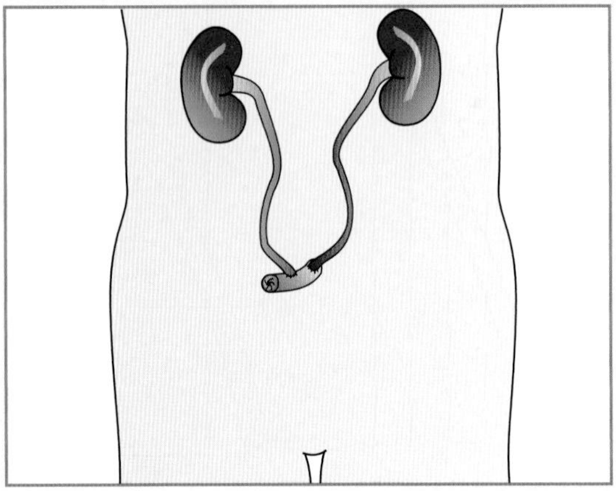

Continent urinary diversion

A tube is formed from part of the ascending colon and ileum. One end of the tube is brought to the skin to form the stoma. At the internal end of this tube, a nipple valve is constructed *so urine won't drain out unless a catheter is inserted through the stoma into the newly formed bladder pouch*. The urethral neck is sutured closed.

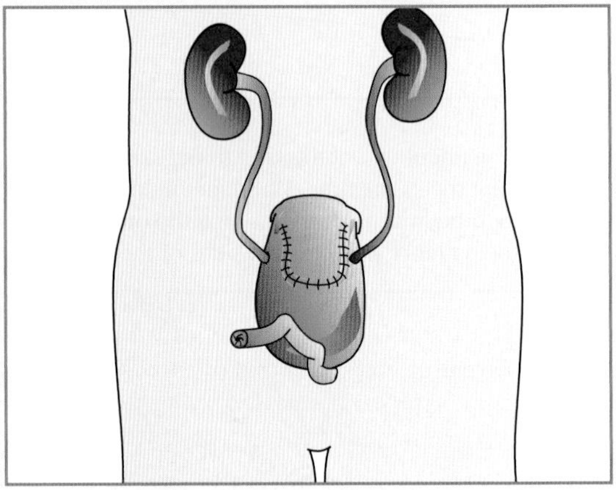

Selected references

Hautman, R. "Urinary Diversion," *Urology* 29(1Suppl):17-19, January 2007.

Taylor, C., et al. *Fundamentals of Nursing: The Art and Science of Nursing Care*, 6th ed. Philadelphia: Lippincott Williams & Wilkins, 2008.

Urinary diversion stoma care

Urinary diversions provide an alternative route for urine flow when a disorder, such as an invasive bladder tumor, impedes normal drainage. A permanent urinary diversion is indicated in any condition that requires a total cystectomy. In conditions requiring temporary urinary drainage or diversion, a suprapubic or urethral catheter is usually inserted to divert the flow of urine temporarily. The catheter remains in place until the incision heals.

Urinary diversions may also be indicated for patients with neurogenic bladder, congenital anomaly, traumatic injury to the lower urinary tract, or severe chronic urinary tract infection. Ileal conduit and continent urinary diversion are the two types of permanent urinary diversions with stomas. (See *Types of permanent urinary diversion*.) These procedures usually require the patient to wear a urine-collection appliance and to care for the stoma created during surgery. Evaluation by the wound ostomy continence nurse will facilitate site selection and postoperative stoma care.

Equipment

Soap and warm water ▪ waste receptacle (such as an impervious or wax-coated bag) ▪ linen-saver pad ▪ hypoallergenic paper tape ▪ antiseptic swab ▪ ruler ▪ scissors ▪ urine-collection appliance (with or without antireflux valve) ▪ graduated cylinder ▪ cottonless gauze pads (some rolled, some flat) ▪ washcloth ▪ skin barrier in liquid, paste, wafer, or sheet form ■ two pairs of gloves ■ optional: adhesive solvent, irrigating syringe, hair dryer, clippers, regular gauze pads, vinegar, deodorant tablets.

Commercially packaged stoma care kits are available. In place of soap and water, you can use adhesive remover pads, if available, or cotton gauze saturated with adhesive solvent.

Some appliances come with a semipermeable skin barrier (impermeable to liquid but permeable to vapor and oxygen, which is essential for maintaining skin integrity). Wafer-type barriers may offer more protection against irritation than adhesive appliances. For example, a carbon-zinc barrier is economical and easy to apply. Its puttylike consistency allows it to be rolled between the palms to form a "washer" that can encircle the base of the stoma. This barrier can withstand enzymes, acids, and other damaging discharge material. All semipermeable barriers are easily removed along with the adhesive, causing less damage to the skin.

Preparation of equipment

Assemble all the equipment on the patient's overbed table. Tape the waste receptacle to the table *for ready access.* Provide privacy for the patient, and wash your hands. Measure the diameter of the stoma with a ruler. Cut the opening of the appliance with the scissors—it shouldn't be more than ⅛" to ⅙" (0.3 to 0.4 cm) larger than the diameter of the stoma. Moisten the faceplate of the appliance with a small amount of solvent or water *to prepare it for adhesion. Performing these preliminary steps at the bedside allows you to demonstrate the procedure and show the patient that it isn't difficult, which will help him relax.*

Implementation

■ Wash your hands again. Explain the procedure to the patient as you go along, and offer constant reinforcement and reassurance *to counteract negative reactions that may be elicited by stoma care.*

■ Place the bed in low Fowler's position so the patient's abdomen is flat. *This position eliminates skin folds that could cause the appliance to slip or irritate the skin and allows the patient to observe or participate.*

■ Put on the gloves and place the linen-saver pad under the patient's side, near the stoma. Open the drain valve of the appliance being replaced *to empty the urine into the graduated cylinder.* Then, *to remove the appliance,* apply soap and water or adhesive solvent as you gently push the skin back from the pouch. If the appliance is disposable, discard it into the waste receptacle. If it's reusable, clean it with soap and lukewarm water and let it air-dry.

NURSING ALERT To avoid irritating the patient's stoma, *avoid touching it with adhesive solvent. If adhesive remains on the skin, gently rub it off with a dry gauze pad. Discard used gauze pads in the waste receptacle.*

■ *To prevent a constant flow of urine onto the skin while you're changing the appliance,* wick the urine with an absorbent, lint-free material. (See *Wicking urine from a stoma.*)

■ Use water to carefully wash off any crystal deposits that may have formed around the stoma. If urine has stagnated and has a strong odor, use soap to wash it off. Be sure to rinse thoroughly *to remove any oily residue that could cause the appliance to slip.*

■ Follow your facility's skin care policy to treat any minor skin problems.

■ Dry the peristomal area thoroughly with a gauze pad *because moisture will keep the appliance from sticking.* Use a hair dryer if you wish. Remove any hair from the area with clippers *to prevent hair follicles from becoming irritated when the pouch is removed, which can cause folliculitis.*

Wicking urine from a stoma

Use a piece of rolled, cottonless gauze to wick urine from a stoma. Working by capillary action, wicking absorbs urine while you prepare the patient's skin to hold a urine-collection appliance.

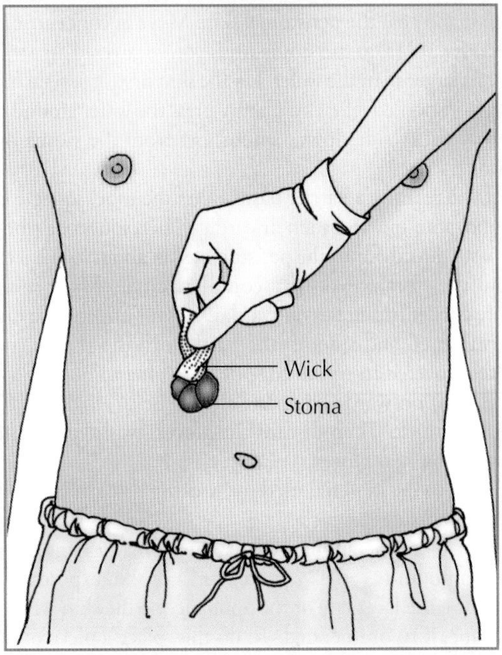

- Inspect the stoma *to see if it's healing properly and to detect complications.* Check the color and the appearance of the suture line, and examine any moisture or effluent. Inspect the peristomal skin for redness, irritation, and intactness.
- Apply the skin barrier. If you apply a wafer or sheet, cut it to fit over the stoma. Remove any protective backing and set the barrier aside with the adhesive side up. If you apply a liquid barrier (such as Skin-Prep), saturate a gauze pad with it and coat the peristomal skin. Move in concentric circles outward from the stoma until you've covered an area 2″ (5 cm) larger than the wafer. Let the skin dry for several minutes—it should feel tacky. Gently press the wafer around the stoma, sticky side down, smoothing from the stoma outward.
- If you're using a barrier paste, open the tube, squeeze out a small amount, and then discard it. Then squeeze a ribbon of paste directly onto the peristomal skin about ½″ (1.3 cm) from the stoma, making a complete circle. Make several more concentric circles outward. Dip your fingers into lukewarm water, and smooth the paste until the skin is completely covered from the edge of the stoma to 3″ to 4″ (7.5 to 10 cm) outward. The paste should be ¼″ to ½″ (0.6 to 1.3 cm) thick. Then discard the gloves, wash your hands, and put on new gloves.
- Remove the material used for wicking urine, and place it into the waste receptacle.
- Now place the appliance over the stoma, leaving only a small amount (⅜″ to ¾″ [1 to 2 cm]) of skin exposed.
- Secure the faceplate of the appliance to the skin with paper tape, if recommended. To do this, place a piece of tape lengthwise on each edge of the faceplate so that the tape overlaps onto the skin.
- The pouch has a ridge that fits over the rim of barrier adhesive and snaps securely into place.
- Dispose of the used materials appropriately.

Special considerations

- The patient's attitude toward his urinary diversion stoma plays a big part in determining how well he'll adjust to it. *To encourage a positive attitude,* help him get used to the idea of caring for his stoma and the appliance as though they are natural extensions of himself. When teaching him to perform the procedure, give him written instructions and provide positive reinforcement after he completes each step. Suggest that he perform the procedure in the morning when urine flows most slowly.
- Help the patient choose between disposable and reusable appliances by telling him the advantages and disadvantages of each. Emphasize the importance of correct placement and of a well-fitted appliance *to prevent seepage of urine onto the skin.* When positioned correctly, most appliances remain in place for at least 3 days and for as long as 5 days if no leakage occurs. After 5 days, the appliance should be changed.
- Because urine flows constantly, it accumulates quickly, becoming even heavier than stools. *To prevent the weight of the urine from loosening the seal around the stoma and separating the appliance from the skin,* tell the patient to empty the appliance through the drain valve when it is one-third to one-half full.
- Instruct the patient to connect his appliance to a urine-collection container before he goes to sleep. *The continuous flow of urine into the container during the night prevents the urine from accumulating and stagnating in the appliance.*
- Teach the patient sanitary and dietary measures that can protect the peristomal skin and control the odor that commonly results from alkaline urine, infection, or poor hygiene. Reusable appliances should be washed with soap and lukewarm water, then air-dried thoroughly *to prevent brittleness.* Soaking the appliance in vinegar and water or placing deodorant tablets in it can further dissipate stubborn odors. Generous fluid intake also helps to reduce odors by diluting the urine.
- If the patient has a continent urinary diversion, make sure you know how to meet his special needs. (See *Caring for the patient with a continent urinary diversion.*)
- Inform the patient about support services provided by ostomy clubs and the American Cancer Society. Members of these organizations routinely visit hospitals and other health care facilities to explain ostomy care and the types of appliances available and to help patients learn to function normally with a stoma.

Home care

The patient or a family member can learn to care for a urinary diversion stoma at home. However, the patient's emotional adjustment to the stoma must be given special consideration before he can be expected to maintain it properly. Arrange for a visiting nurse or an enterostomal therapist to assist the patient at home.

Complications

Because intestinal mucosa is delicate, an ill-fitting appliance can cause bleeding. This is especially likely to occur with an ileal conduit, the most common type of urinary diversion stoma, *because a segment of the intestine forms the conduit.* Peristomal skin may become reddened or excoriated from too-frequent changing or improper placement of the appliance, poor skin care, or allergic reaction to the appliance or adhesive. Constant leakage around the appliance can result from improper placement of the appliance or from poor skin turgor.

Caring for the patient with a continent urinary diversion

In this procedure, an alternative to the traditional ileal conduit, a pouch created from the ascending colon and terminal ileum serves as a new bladder, which empties through a stoma. To drain urine continuously, several drains are inserted into this reconstructed bladder and left in place for 3 to 6 weeks until the new stoma heals. The patient will be discharged from the hospital with the drains in place. He'll return to have them removed and to learn to catheterize his stoma.

First hospitalization

- Immediately after surgery, monitor intake and output from each drain. Be alert for decreased output, *which may indicate that urine flow is obstructed.*
- Watch for common postoperative complications, such as infection or bleeding. Also watch for signs of urinary leakage, which include increased abdominal distention, and urine appearing around the drains or midline incision.
- Irrigate the drains, as ordered.
- Clean the area around the drains daily—first with antiseptic solution and then with sterile water. Apply a dry, sterile dressing to the area. Use precut 4″ × 4″ drain dressings around the drain *to absorb leakage.*
- *To increase the patient's mobility and comfort,* connect the drains to a leg bag.

Second hospitalization or outpatient

- After the patient's drains are removed, teach him how to catheterize the stoma. Begin by gathering the following equipment on a clean towel: rubber catheter (usually #14 or #16 French), water-soluble lubricant, washcloth, stoma covering (nonadherent gauze pad or panty liner), hypoallergenic adhesive tape, and an irrigating solution (optional).
- Apply water-soluble lubricant to the catheter tip *to facilitate insertion.*
- Remove and discard the stoma cover. Using the washcloth, clean the stoma and the area around it, starting at the stoma and working outward in a circular motion.
- Hold the urine-collection container under the catheter; then slowly insert the catheter into the stoma. Urine should then begin to flow into the container. If it doesn't, gently rotate the catheter or redirect its angle. If the catheter drains slowly, it may be plugged with mucus. Irrigate it with sterile saline solution or sterile water to clear it. When the flow stops, pinch the catheter closed and remove it.

Home care

- Teach the patient how to care for the drains and their insertion sites during the 3 to 6 weeks he'll be at home before their removal, and teach him how to attach them to a leg bag. Also teach him how to recognize the signs of infection and obstruction.
- After the drains are removed, teach the patient how to empty the pouch, and establish a schedule. Initially, he should catheterize the stoma and empty the pouch every 2 to 3 hours. Later, he should catheterize every 4 hours while awake and also irrigate the pouch each morning and evening, if ordered. Instruct him to empty the pouch whenever he feels a sensation of fullness.
- Tell the patient that the catheters are reusable, but only after they've been cleaned. He should clean the catheter thoroughly with warm, soapy water, rinse it thoroughly, and hang it to dry over a clean towel. He should store cleaned and dried catheters in plastic bags. Tell him he can reuse catheters for up to 1 month before discarding them. However, he should immediately discard any catheter that becomes discolored or cracked.

Documentation

Record the appearance and color of the stoma and whether it's inverted, flush with the skin, or protruding. If it protrudes, note by how much it protrudes above the skin. (The normal range is ½″ to ¾″ [1.5 to 2 cm].) Record the appearance and condition of the peristomal skin, noting any redness or irritation or complaints by the patient of itching or burning.

SELECTED REFERENCES

Pahernik, S., et al. "Conversion from Colonic or Ileal Conduit to Continent Cutaneous Urinary Diversion," *Journal of Urology* 171(6 Pt 1):2293-297, June 2004.

Richbourne, L. "Difficulties Experienced by the Ostomate after Hospital Discharge," *Journal of Wound Ostomy Continence* 34(1):70-79, January-February 2007.

Smeltzer, S., et al. *Textbook of Medical-Surgical Nursing,* 11th ed. Philadelphia: Lippincott Williams & Wilkins, 2008.

How peritoneal dialysis works

Peritoneal dialysis works through a combination of diffusion and osmosis.

Diffusion

In diffusion, particles move through a semipermeable membrane from an area of high-solute concentration to an area of low-solute concentration.

In peritoneal dialysis, the water-based dialysate being infused contains glucose, sodium chloride, calcium, magnesium, acetate or lactate, and no waste products. Therefore, the waste products and excess electrolytes in the blood cross through the semipermeable peritoneal membrane into the dialysate. Removing the waste-filled dialysate and replacing it with fresh solution keeps the waste concentration low and encourages further diffusion.

Osmosis

In osmosis, fluids move through a semipermeable membrane from an area of low-solute concentration to an area of high-solute concentration. In peritoneal dialysis, dextrose is added to the dialysate to give it a higher solute concentration than the blood, creating a high osmotic gradient. Water migrates from the blood through the membrane at the beginning of each infusion, when the osmotic gradient is highest.

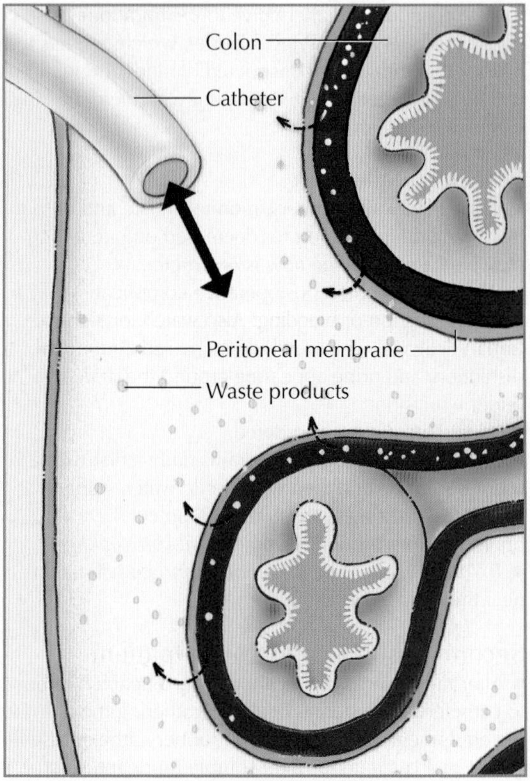

DIALYSIS

PERITONEAL DIALYSIS

Peritoneal dialysis is indicated for patients with chronic renal failure who have cardiovascular instability, vascular access problems that prevent hemodialysis, fluid overload, or electrolyte imbalances. In this procedure, dialysate—the solution instilled into the peritoneal cavity by a catheter—draws waste products, excess fluid, and electrolytes from the blood across the semipermeable peritoneal membrane. (See *How peritoneal dialysis works.*) After a prescribed period, the dialysate is drained from the peritoneal cavity, removing impurities with it. The dialysis procedure is then repeated, using a new dialysate each time, until waste removal is complete, and fluid, electrolyte, and acid-base balance has been restored.

The catheter is inserted in the operating room in an acute situation or at the patient's bedside with a nurse assisting. With special preparation, the nurse may perform dialysis, either manually or using an automatic or semiautomatic cycle machine.

Equipment

For catheter placement and dialysis: Prescribed dialysate (in 1- or 2-L bottles or bags, as ordered) ▪ warmer, heating pad, or water bath ▪ at least three face masks ▪ medication, such as heparin, if ordered ▪ dialysis administration set with drainage bag ▪ two pairs of sterile gloves ▪ I.V. pole ▪ fenestrated sterile drape ▪ vial of 1% or 2% lidocaine ▪ antiseptic pads ▪ 3-ml syringe with 25G 1″ needle ▪ ordered type of multi-eyed, nylon, peritoneal catheter (see *Comparing peritoneal dialysis catheters*) ▪ scalpel (with #11 blade) ▪ peritoneal stylet ▪ sutures or hypoallergenic tape ▪ antiseptic solution ▪ precut drain dressings ▪ protective cap for catheter ▪ 4″ × 4″

EQUIPMENT

Comparing peritoneal dialysis catheters

The first step in any type of peritoneal dialysis is insertion of a catheter to allow instillation of dialyzing solution. The surgeon may insert one of the three catheters described here.

Tenckhoff catheter

To implant a Tenckhoff catheter, the surgeon inserts the first 6¾″ (17 cm) of the catheter into the patient's abdomen. The next 2¾″ (7-cm) segment, which may have a Dacron cuff at one or both ends, is imbedded subcutaneously. Within a few days after insertion, the patient's tissues grow around the cuffs, forming a tight barrier against bacterial infiltration. The remaining 3⅞″ (10 cm) of the catheter extends outside of the abdomen and is equipped with a metal adapter at the tip that connects to dialyzer tubing.

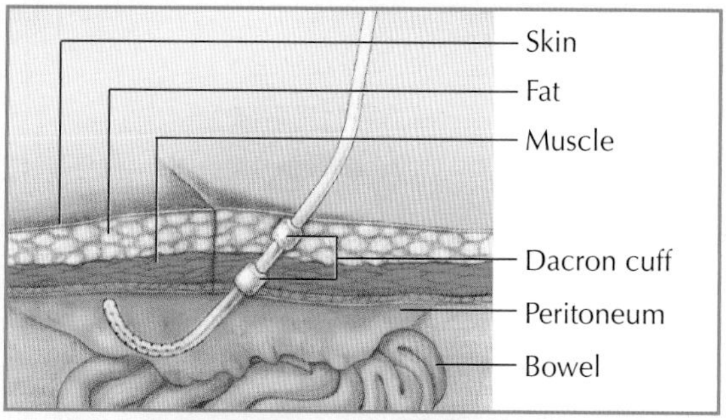

Flanged-collar catheter

To insert this kind of catheter, the surgeon positions its flanged collar just below the dermis so that the device extends through the abdominal wall. He keeps the distal end of the cuff from extending into the peritoneum, where it could cause adhesions.

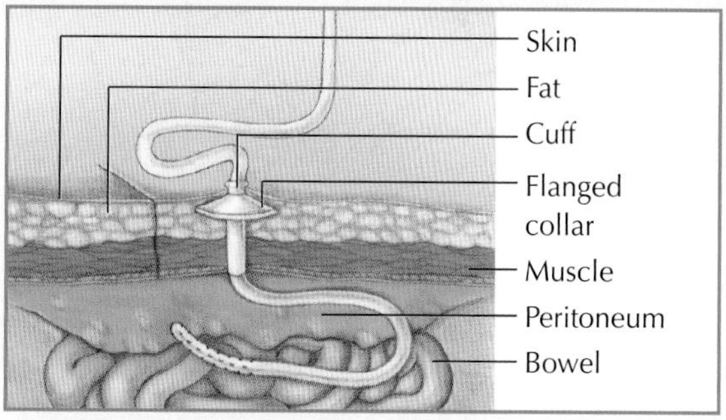

Column-disk peritoneal catheter

To insert a column-disk peritoneal catheter (CDPC), the surgeon rolls up the flexible disk section of the implant, inserts it into the peritoneal cavity, and retracts it against the abdominal wall. The implant's first cuff rests just outside the peritoneal membrane, and its second cuff rests just underneath the skin.

Because the CDPC doesn't float freely in the peritoneal cavity, it keeps inflowing dialyzing solution from being directed at the sensitive organs, which increases patient comfort during dialysis.

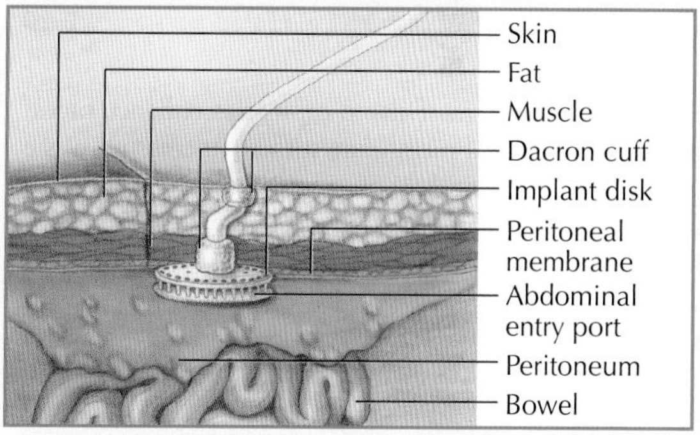

gauze pads ▪ small, sterile plastic clamp ▪ sterile labels ▪ sterile marker ▪ optional: 10-ml syringe with 22G ½″ needle, specimen container, label, laboratory request form.

For dressing changes: One pair of sterile gloves ▪ sterile cotton-tipped applicators or sterile 2″ × 2″ gauze pads ▪ two precut drain dressings ▪ adhesive tape ▪ antiseptic solution or normal saline solution ▪ two sterile 4″ × 4″ gauze pads.

All equipment must be sterile. Commercially packaged dialysis kits or trays are available.

Preparation of equipment

Bring all equipment to the patient's bedside. Make sure the dialysate is at body temperature. *This decreases patient discomfort during the procedure and reduces vasoconstriction of*

Setup for peritoneal dialysis

This illustration shows the proper setup for peritoneal dialysis.

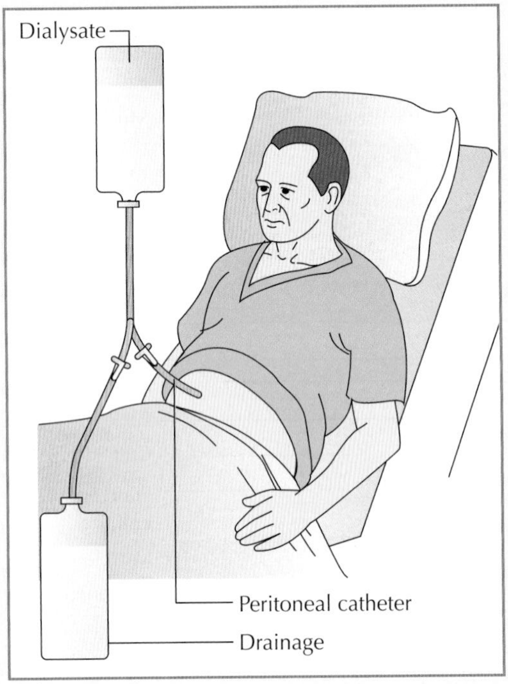

the peritoneal capillaries. Dilated capillaries enhance blood flow to the peritoneal membrane surface, increasing waste clearance into the peritoneal cavity. Place the container in a warmer or a water bath, or wrap it in a heating pad set at 98.6° F (37° C) for 30 to 60 minutes *to warm the solution.*

Implementation

- Confirm the patient's identity using two patient identifiers according to your facility's policy.
- Explain the procedure to the patient. Assess and record vital signs, weight, and abdominal girth *to establish baseline levels.*
- Review recent laboratory values (blood urea nitrogen, serum creatinine, sodium, potassium, and complete blood count).

Catheter placement and dialysis

- Have the patient try to urinate. *This reduces the risk of bladder perforation during insertion of the peritoneal catheter.* If he can't urinate, and you suspect that his bladder isn't empty, obtain an order for straight catheterization *to empty his bladder.*
- Place the patient in the supine position, and have him put on one of the sterile face masks.
- Wash your hands.
- Inspect the warmed dialysate, which should appear clear and colorless.
- Put on a sterile face mask. Prepare to add any prescribed medication to the dialysate, using strict sterile technique *to avoid contaminating the solution.* Label all medications, medication containers, and other solutions on and off the sterile field. Medications should be added immediately before the solution will be hung and used. Disinfect multiple-dose vials by soaking them in antiseptic solution for 5 minutes. Heparin is typically added to the dialysate *to prevent accumulation of fibrin in the catheter.*
- Prepare the dialysis administration set. (See *Setup for peritoneal dialysis.*)
- Close the clamps on all lines. Place the drainage bag below the patient *to facilitate gravity drainage,* and connect the drainage line to it. Connect the dialysate infusion lines to the bottles or bags of dialysate using sterile technique. Hang the bottles or bags on the I.V. pole at the patient's bedside. *To prime the tubing,* open the infusion lines, and allow the solution to flow until all lines are primed. Then close all clamps.
- At this point, the physician puts on a mask and a pair of sterile gloves. He cleans the patient's abdomen with antiseptic solution and drapes it with a sterile drape.
- Wipe the stopper of the lidocaine vial with antiseptic solution and allow it to dry. Invert the vial and hand it to the physician so he can withdraw the lidocaine, using the 3-ml syringe with the 25G 1″ needle.
- The physician anesthetizes a small area of the patient's abdomen below the umbilicus. He then makes a small incision with the scalpel, inserts the catheter into the peritoneal cavity—using the stylet to guide the catheter—and sutures or tapes the catheter in place.
- If the catheter is already in place, clean the site with antiseptic solution in a circular outward motion, according to your facility's policy, before each dialysis treatment.
- Connect the catheter to the administration set, using strict sterile technique *to prevent contamination of the catheter and the solution, which could cause peritonitis.*
- Open the drain dressing and the 4″ × 4″ gauze pad packages. Put on the other pair of sterile gloves. Apply the precut drain dressings around the catheter. Cover them with the gauze pads and tape them securely.
- Unclamp the lines to the patient. Rapidly instill 500 ml of dialysate into the peritoneal cavity *to test the catheter's patency.*

- Clamp the lines to the patient. Immediately unclamp the lines to the drainage bag *to allow fluid to drain into the bag.* Outflow should be brisk.
- Having established the catheter's patency, clamp the lines to the drainage bag and unclamp the lines to the patient *to infuse the prescribed volume of solution over a period of 5 to 10 minutes.* As soon as the dialysate container empties, clamp the lines to the patient immediately *to prevent air from entering the tubing.*
- Allow the solution to dwell in the peritoneal cavity for the prescribed time (10 minutes to 4 hours). *This lets excess fluid, electrolytes, and accumulated wastes move from the blood through the peritoneal membrane and into the dialysate.*
- Warm the solution for the next infusion.
- At the end of the prescribed dwell time, unclamp the line to the drainage bag and allow the solution to drain from the peritoneal cavity into the drainage bag (normally 30 to 40 minutes).
- Repeat the infusion-dwell-drain cycle immediately after outflow until the prescribed number of fluid exchanges have been completed.
- If the physician (or your facility's policy) requires a dialysate specimen, you'll usually collect one after every 10 infusion-dwell-drain cycles (*always* during the drain phase), after every 24-hour period, or as ordered. To do this, attach the 10-ml syringe to the 22G 1½" needle, and insert it into the injection port on the drainage line, using strict sterile technique, and aspirate the drainage sample. Transfer the sample to the specimen container, label it appropriately, and send it to the laboratory with a laboratory request form.
- After completing the prescribed number of exchanges, clamp the catheter and put on sterile gloves. Disconnect the administration set from the peritoneal catheter. Place the sterile protective cap over the catheter's distal end.
- Dispose of all used equipment appropriately.

Dressing changes

- Explain the procedure to the patient and wash your hands.
- If necessary, carefully remove the old dressings *to avoid putting tension on the catheter and accidentally dislodging it and to avoid introducing bacteria into the tract through movement of the catheter.*
- Put on the sterile gloves.
- Saturate the sterile applicators or the 2" × 2" gauze pads with antiseptic solution, and clean the skin around the catheter, moving in concentric circles from the catheter site outward. Remove any crusted material carefully.
- Inspect the catheter site for drainage and the tissue around the site for redness and swelling.
- Place two precut drain dressings around the catheter site. Tape the 4" × 4" gauze pads over them *to secure the dressings.*

Special considerations

- During and after dialysis, monitor the patient and his response to treatment. Peritoneal dialysis is usually contraindicated in patients who have had extensive abdominal or bowel surgery or extensive abdominal trauma.
- Monitor the patient's vital signs every 10 to 15 minutes for the first 1 to 2 hours of exchanges, then every 2 to 4 hours, or more frequently if necessary. Notify the practitioner of any abrupt changes in the patient's condition.
- *To reduce the risk of peritonitis,* use strict sterile technique during catheter insertion, dialysis, and dressing changes. Masks should be worn by all personnel in the room whenever the dialysis system is opened or entered. Change the dressing at least every 24 hours or whenever it becomes wet or soiled. Frequent dressing changes will also help prevent skin excoriation from any leakage.
- *To prevent respiratory distress,* position the patient for maximal lung expansion. Promote lung expansion through turning and deep-breathing exercises. In some patients, decreasing volumes may be necessary.

NURSING ALERT *If the patient suffers severe respiratory distress during the dwell phase of dialysis, drain the peritoneal cavity and notify the practitioner. Monitor any patient on peritoneal dialysis who is being weaned from a ventilator.*

- *To prevent protein depletion,* the practitioner may order a high-protein diet or a protein supplement. He will also monitor serum albumin levels.
- Dialysate is available in three concentrations—4.25% dextrose, 2.5% dextrose, and 1.5% dextrose. The 4.25% solution usually removes the largest amount of fluid from the blood because its glucose concentration is highest. If your patient receives this concentrated solution, monitor him carefully *to prevent excess fluid loss.* Also, some of the glucose in the 4.25% solution may enter the patient's bloodstream, causing hyperglycemia severe enough to require an insulin injection or an insulin addition to the dialysate.
- Patients with low serum potassium levels may require the addition of potassium to the dialysate solution *to prevent further losses.*
- Monitor fluid volume balance, blood pressure, and pulse *to help prevent fluid imbalance.* Assess fluid balance at the end of each infusion-dwell-drain cycle. Fluid balance is positive if less than the amount infused was recovered; it's negative if more than the amount infused was recovered. Notify the practitioner if the patient retains 500 ml or more of fluid for three consecutive cycles or if he loses at least 1 liter of fluid for three consecutive cycles.

- Weigh the patient daily *to help determine how much fluid is being removed during dialysis treatment.* Note the time and any variations in the weighing technique next to his weight on his chart.
- If inflow and outflow are slow or absent, check the tubing for kinks. You can also try raising the I.V. pole or repositioning the patient *to increase the inflow rate.* Repositioning the patient or applying manual pressure to the lateral aspects of the patient's abdomen may also help increase drainage. If these maneuvers fail, notify the practitioner. *Improper positioning of the catheter or an accumulation of fibrin may obstruct the catheter.*
- Always examine outflow fluid (effluent) for color and clarity. Normally it's clear or pale yellow, but pink-tinged effluent may appear during the first three or four cycles. If the effluent remains pink-tinged, or if it's grossly bloody, suspect bleeding into the peritoneal cavity and notify the practitioner. Also notify the practitioner if the outflow contains feces, *which suggests bowel perforation*, or if it's cloudy, *which suggests peritonitis.* Obtain a sample for culture and Gram stain. Send the sample in a labeled specimen container to the laboratory with a laboratory request form.
- Patient discomfort at the start of the procedure is normal. If the patient experiences pain during the procedure, determine when it occurs, its quality and duration, and whether it radiates to other body parts. Then notify the practitioner. Pain during infusion usually results from a dialysate that's too cool or acidic. Pain may also result from rapid inflow; slowing the inflow rate may reduce the pain. Severe, diffuse pain with rebound tenderness and cloudy effluent may indicate peritoneal infection. Pain that radiates to the shoulder often results from air accumulation under the diaphragm. Severe, persistent perineal or rectal pain can result from improper catheter placement.
- The patient undergoing peritoneal dialysis will require a great deal of assistance in his daily care. *To minimize his discomfort,* perform daily care during a drain phase in the cycle, *when the patient's abdomen is less distended.*

Home care

Teach the patient and his family how to use sterile technique throughout the procedure, especially for cleaning and dressing changes, *to prevent complications such as peritonitis.* Also teach them the signs and symptoms of peritonitis (cloudy fluid, fever, and abdominal pain and tenderness) and infection (redness and drainage). Stress the importance of notifying the practitioner immediately if such signs or symptoms arise.

Inform the patient about the advantages of an automated continuous cycler for home use. Instruct the patient to record his weight and blood pressure daily and to check regularly for swelling of the extremities. Teach him to keep an accurate record of intake and output.

Complications

Peritonitis, the most common complication, usually follows contamination of the dialysate, but it may develop if solution leaks from the catheter exit site and flows back into the catheter tract. Respiratory distress may result when dialysate in the peritoneal cavity increases pressure on the diaphragm, which decreases lung expansion.

Protein depletion may result from the diffusion of protein in the blood into the dialysate solution through the peritoneal membrane. As much as 14 g of protein may be lost daily—more in patients with peritonitis.

Constipation is a major cause of inflow-outflow problems; therefore, *to ensure regular bowel movements,* give a laxative or stool softener, as needed.

Excessive fluid loss from the use of 4.25% solution may cause hypovolemia, hypotension, and shock. Excessive fluid retention may lead to blood volume expansion, hypertension, peripheral edema, and even pulmonary edema and congestive heart failure.

Other possible complications include electrolyte imbalance and hyperglycemia, which can be identified by frequent blood tests.

Documentation

Record the amount of dialysate infused and drained, any medications added to the solution, and the color and character of effluent. Also record the patient's daily weight and fluid balance. Use a peritoneal dialysis flowchart to compute total fluid balance after each exchange. Note the patient's vital signs and tolerance of the treatment as well as other pertinent observations.

Selected references

Finkelstein, F.O., et al. "The Role of Chronic Peritoneal Dialysis in the Management of the Patient with Chronic Kidney Disease," *Contributions in Nephrology* 150:235-39, 2006.

Lynn-McHale Wiegand, D.J., and Carlson, K.K., eds. *AACN Procedure Manual for Critical Care*, 5th ed. Philadelphia: W.B. Saunders Co., 2005.

Saxena, R. et al. "Peritoneal Dialysis: A Viable Renal Replacement Therapy," *The American Journal of the Medical Sciences* 330(1):36-47, July 2005.

Smeltzer, S.C., et al. *Brunner & Suddarth's Textbook of Medical-Surgical Nursing*, 11th ed. Philadelphia: Lippincott Williams & Wilkins, 2008.

Three major steps of continuous ambulatory peritoneal dialysis

A bag of dialysate is attached to the tube entering the patient's abdominal area so that the fluid flows into the peritoneal cavity.

While the dialysate remains in the peritoneal cavity, the patient can roll up the bag, place it under his shirt, and go about his normal activities.

Unroll the bag and suspend it below the pelvis *to allow the dialysate to drain from the peritoneal cavity back into the bag*

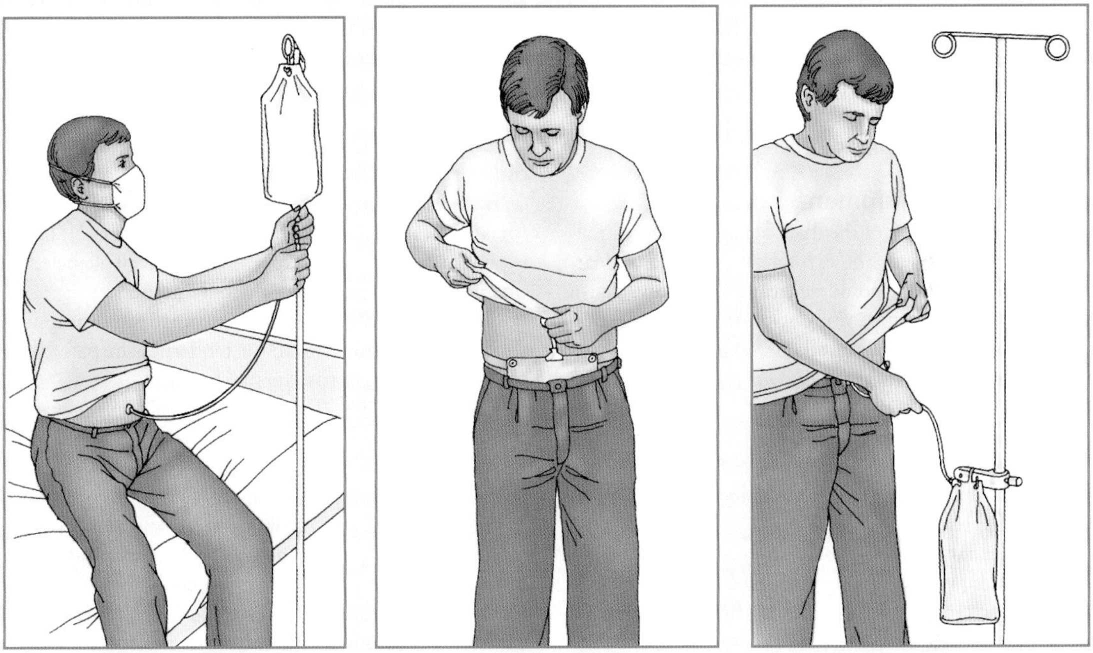

CONTINUOUS AMBULATORY PERITONEAL DIALYSIS

Continuous ambulatory peritoneal dialysis (CAPD) requires insertion of a permanent peritoneal catheter (such as a Tenckhoff catheter) to circulate dialysate in the peritoneal cavity constantly. Inserted under local anesthetic, the catheter is sutured in place and its distal portion tunneled subcutaneously to the skin surface. There it serves as a port for the dialysate, which flows in and out of the peritoneal cavity by gravity. (See *Three major steps of continuous ambulatory peritoneal dialysis.*)

CAPD is used most commonly for patients with end-stage renal disease. CAPD can be a welcome alternative to hemodialysis, because it gives the patient more independence and requires less travel for treatments. It also provides more stable fluid and electrolyte levels than conventional hemodialysis.

Patients or family members can usually learn to perform CAPD after only 2 weeks of training. In addition, because the patient can resume normal daily activities between solution changes, CAPD helps promote independence and a return to a near-normal lifestyle. It also costs less than hemodialysis.

Conditions that may prohibit CAPD include recent abdominal surgery, abdominal adhesions, an infected abdominal wall, diaphragmatic tears, ileus, and respiratory insufficiency.

Equipment

To infuse dialysate: Prescribed amount of dialysate (usually in 2-L bags) ■ heating pad or commercial warmer ■ three face masks ■ 42″ (106.7-cm) connective tubing with drain clamp ▪ six to eight packages of sterile 4″ × 4″ gauze pads ▪ medication, if ordered ▪ antiseptic pads ▪ hypoallergenic tape ▪ plastic snap-top container ▪ antiseptic solution ▪ sterile basin ▪ container of alcohol ▪ sterile gloves ▪ belt or fabric pouch ▪ two sterile waterproof paper drapes (one fenestrated) ▪ optional: syringes, labeled specimen container.

To discontinue dialysis temporarily: Three sterile waterproof paper barriers (two fenestrated) ▪ 4″ × 4″ gauze pads (for cleaning and dressing the catheter) ▪ two face masks ▪ sterile basin ▪ hypoallergenic tape ▪ antiseptic solution ▪ sterile gloves ▪ sterile rubber catheter cap.

All equipment for infusing the dialysate and discontinuing the procedure must be sterile. Commercially prepared sterile CAPD kits are available.

Preparation of equipment

Check the concentration of the dialysate against the practitioner's order. Also check the expiration date and appearance of the solution—it should be clear, not cloudy. Warm the solution to body temperature with a heating pad or a commercial warmer if one is available. Don't warm the solution in a microwave oven *because the temperature is unpredictable.*

To minimize the risk of contaminating the bag's port, leave the dialysate container's wrapper in place. *This also keeps the bag dry, which makes examining it for leakage easier after you remove the wrapper.*

Wash your hands and put on a surgical mask. Remove the dialysate container from the warming setup, and remove its protective wrapper. Squeeze the bag firmly *to check for leaks.*

If ordered, use a syringe to add any prescribed medication to the dialysate, using sterile technique *to avoid contamination.* (The ideal approach is to add medication under a laminar flow hood.) Disinfect multiple-dose vials in a 5-minute antiseptic soak. Insert the connective tubing into the dialysate container. Open the drain clamp to prime the tube. Then close the clamp.

Place an antiseptic pad on the dialysate container's port. Cover the port with a dry gauze pad, and secure the pad with tape. Remove and discard the surgical mask. Tear the tape *so it will be ready to secure the new dressing.* Commercial devices with antiseptic pads are available for covering the dialysate container and tubing connection.

Implementation

- Confirm the patient's identity using two patient identifiers according to your facility's policy.
- Weigh the patient *to establish a baseline level.* Weigh him at the same time every day *to help monitor fluid balance.*

Infusing dialysate

- Assemble all equipment at the patient's bedside, and explain the procedure to him. Prepare the sterile field by placing a waterproof, sterile paper drape on a dry surface near the patient. Take care to maintain the drape's sterility.
- Fill the snap-top container with antiseptic solution, and place it on the sterile field. Place the basin on the sterile field. Then place four pairs of sterile gauze pads in the sterile basin, and saturate them with the antiseptic solution. Drop the remaining gauze pads on the sterile field. Loosen the cap on the alcohol container, and place it next to the sterile field.
- Put on a clean surgical mask and provide one for the patient.
- Carefully remove the dressing covering the peritoneal catheter and discard it. Be careful not to touch the catheter or skin. Check skin integrity at the catheter site, and look for signs of infection such as purulent drainage. If drainage is present, obtain a swab specimen, put it in a labeled specimen container, and notify the practitioner.
- Put on the sterile gloves and palpate the insertion site and subcutaneous tunnel route for tenderness or pain. If these symptoms occur, notify the practitioner.

NURSING ALERT ***If the patient experiences drainage, tenderness, or pain, don't proceed with the infusion without specific orders.***

- Wrap one gauze pad saturated with antiseptic solution around the distal end of the catheter, and leave it in place for 5 minutes. Clean the catheter and insertion site with the rest of the gauze pads, moving in concentric circles away from the insertion site. Use straight strokes to clean the catheter, beginning at the insertion site and moving outward. Use a clean area of the pad for each stroke. Loosen the catheter cap one notch and clean the exposed area. Place each used pad at the base of the catheter *to help support it.* After using the third pair of pads, place the fenestrated paper drape around the base of the catheter. Continue cleaning the catheter for another minute with one of the remaining pads soaked with antiseptic solution.
- Remove the antiseptic pad on the catheter cap, remove the cap, and use the remaining antiseptic pad to clean the end of the catheter hub. Attach the connective tubing from the dialysate container to the catheter. Be sure to secure the luer-lock connector tightly.
- Open the drain clamp on the dialysate container *to allow solution to enter the peritoneal cavity by gravity* over a period of 5 to 10 minutes. Leave a small amount of fluid in the bag *to make folding it easier.* Close the drain clamp.
- Fold the bag and secure it with a belt, or tuck it in the patient's clothing or a small fabric pouch.

■ After the prescribed dwell time (usually 4 to 6 hours), unfold the bag, open the clamp, and allow peritoneal fluid to drain back into the bag by gravity.
■ When drainage is complete, attach a new bag of dialysate and repeat the infusion.
■ Discard used supplies appropriately.

Discontinuing dialysis temporarily
■ Wash your hands, put on a surgical mask, and provide one for the patient. Explain the procedure to him.
■ Using sterile gloves, remove and discard the dressing over the peritoneal catheter.
■ Set up a sterile field next to the patient by covering a clean, dry surface with a waterproof drape. Be sure to maintain the drape's sterility. Place all equipment on the sterile field, and place the 4″ × 4″ gauze pads in the basin. Saturate them with the antiseptic solution. Open the 4″ × 4″ gauze pads to be used as the dressing, and drop them onto the sterile field. Tear pieces of tape, as needed.
■ Tape the dialysate tubing to the side rail of the bed *to keep the catheter and tubing off the patient's abdomen.*
■ Change to another pair of sterile gloves. Then place one of the fenestrated drapes around the base of the catheter.
■ Use a pair of antiseptic pads to clean about 6″ (15 cm) of the dialysis tubing. Clean for 1 minute, moving in one direction only, away from the catheter. Then clean the catheter, moving from the insertion site to the junction of the catheter and dialysis tubing. Place used pads at the base of the catheter *to prop it up.* Use two more pairs of pads to clean the junction for a total of 3 minutes.
■ Place the second fenestrated paper drape over the first at the base of the catheter. With the fourth pair of pads, clean the junction of the catheter and 6″ of the dialysate tubing for another minute.
■ Disconnect the dialysate tubing from the catheter. Pick up the catheter cap and fasten it to the catheter, making sure it fits securely over both notches of the hard plastic catheter tip.
■ Clean the insertion site and a 2″ (5-cm) radius around it with antiseptic pads, working from the insertion site outward. Let the skin air-dry before applying the dressing.
■ Remove the tape and discard used supplies appropriately.

Special considerations
■ Absolute contraindications for CAPD include:
– documented loss of peritoneal function or extensive abdominal adhesions that limit dialysate flow
– physical or mental incapacity to perform peritoneal dialysis and no assistance available at home
– mechanical defects that prevent effective dialysis, which can't be corrected, or increase the risk of infection (such as surgically irreparable hernia, omphalocele, gastroschisis, diaphragmatic hernia, and bladder extrophy).
■ Relative contraindications for CAPD include:
– fresh intra-abdominal foreign bodies (for example, 4-month wait after abdominal vascular prostheses, recent ventricular-peritoneal shunt)
– peritoneal leaks or infection, or infection of the abdominal wall or skin
– body size limitations—either a patient who's too small to tolerate adequate dialysate, or a patient who's too large to be effectively dialyzed
–inability to tolerate the necessary volumes of dialysate for peritoneal dialysis to be successful
– inflammatory or ischemic bowel disease, or recurrent episodes of diverticulitis
– morbid obesity in short individuals, or patients suffering from severe malnutrition.
■ If inflow and outflow are slow or absent, check the tubing for kinks. You can also try raising the solution or repositioning the patient *to increase the inflow rate.* Repositioning the patient or applying manual pressure to the lateral aspects of the patient's abdomen may also help increase drainage.

Home care
Teach the patient and family how to use sterile technique throughout the procedure, especially for cleaning and dressing changes, *to prevent complications such as peritonitis.* Also teach them the signs and symptoms of peritonitis—cloudy fluid, fever, abdominal pain, and tenderness—and stress the importance of notifying the practitioner immediately if such symptoms arise. Also encourage them to call the practitioner immediately if redness and drainage occur because these are also signs of infection.

Inform the patient about the advantages of an automated continuous cycler system for home use. (See *Continuous-cycle peritoneal dialysis,* page 742.)

Instruct the patient to record his weight and blood pressure daily and to check regularly for swelling of the extremities. Teach him to keep an accurate record of intake and output.

Complications
Peritonitis is the most frequent complication of CAPD. Although treatable, it can permanently scar the peritoneal membrane, decreasing its permeability and reducing the efficiency of dialysis. Untreated peritonitis can cause septicemia and death.

Excessive fluid loss may result from a concentrated (4.25%) dialysate solution, improper or inaccurate moni-

Continuous-cycle peritoneal dialysis

Continuous ambulatory peritoneal dialysis is easier for the patient who uses an automated continuous cycler system. When set up, this system runs the dialysis treatment automatically until all the dialysate is infused. The system remains closed throughout the treatment, *which cuts the risk of contamination.* Continuous-cycle peritoneal dialysis (CCPD) can be performed while the patient is awake or asleep. The system's alarms warn about general system, dialysate, and patient problems.

The cycler can be set to an intermittent or continuous dialysate schedule at home or in a health care facility. The patient typically initiates CCPD at bedtime and undergoes three to seven exchanges, depending on his prescription. Upon awakening, the patient infuses the prescribed dialysis volume, disconnects himself from the unit, and carries the dialysate in his peritoneal cavity during the day.

The continuous cycler follows the same sterile care and maintenance procedures as the manual method.

toring of inflow and outflow, or inadequate oral fluid intake. Excessive fluid retention may result from improper or inaccurate monitoring of inflow and outflow, or excessive salt or oral fluid intake.

Documentation

Record the type and amount of fluid instilled and returned for each exchange, the time and duration of the exchange, and any medications added to the dialysate. Note the color and clarity of the returned exchange fluid and check it for mucus, pus, and blood. Also note any discrepancy in the balance of fluid intake and output, as well as any signs or symptoms of fluid imbalance, such as weight changes, decreased breath sounds, peripheral edema, ascites, and changes in skin turgor. Record the patient's weight, blood pressure, and pulse rate after his last fluid exchange for the day.

Selected references

Finkelstein, F.O., et al. "The Role of Chronic Peritoneal Dialysis in the Management of the Patient with Chronic Kidney Disease," *Contributions in Nephrology* 150:235-39, 2006.

National Kidney and Urologic Diseases Information Clearinghouse. "Peritoneal Dialysis Dose and Adequacy," *NIH Publications* No. 04-4587, May 2004. Available at *www.kidney.niddk.nih.gov/Kudiseases/pubs/peritonealdose/.*

National Kidney Foundation. "Clinical Practice Guidelines for Peritoneal Dialysis Adequacy Update 2000," *American Journal of Kidney Diseases* 37(1 Supp 1):S65-S136, January 2001.

Selby, N.M., et al. "Automated Peritoneal Dialysis Has Significant Effects on Systemic Hemodynamics," *Peritoneal Dialysis International* 26(3):306-308, May-June 2006.

Hemodialysis

Hemodialysis is performed to remove toxic wastes from the blood of patients in renal failure. This potentially lifesaving procedure removes blood from the body, circulates it through a purifying dialyzer, and then returns the blood to the body. Various access sites can be used for this procedure. (See *Hemodialysis access sites.*) The access can be temporary or long term, depending on the patient's need. Catheters are usually used when temporary access is warranted and arteriovenous (AV) fistulas are preferred for long-term access.

The underlying mechanism in hemodialysis is differential diffusion across a semipermeable membrane, which extracts by-products of protein metabolism, such as urea and uric acid, as well as creatinine and excess body water. This process restores or maintains the balance of the body's buffer system and electrolyte level. Hemodialysis thus promotes a rapid return to normal serum values and helps prevent complications associated with uremia. (See *How hemodialysis works,* page 744.)

Hemodialysis provides temporary support for patients with acute reversible renal failure. It's also used for regular long-term treatment of patients with chronic end-stage renal disease. Hemodialysis may also be necessary to remove toxic substances from the blood in patients suffering from various acute poisoning or barbiturate or analgesic overdose. The patient's condition (rate of creatinine generation, weight gain) determines the number and duration of hemodialysis treatments.

There are several types of double-lumen catheters that can be used for dialysis access depending on the patient's condition, the physician's preference, and the anticipated length of time the catheter will be needed. The internal diameter of each lumen is approximately 12G to allow for high flow rates. The catheters have two ports—one colored red and one colored blue. The red port is used for withdrawing the patient's blood and sending it to the dialyzer, and the blue port is used for returning the dialyzed blood to the patient.

Hemodialysis access sites

Hemodialysis requires vascular access. The site and type of access may vary, depending on the expected duration of dialysis, the surgeon's preference, and the patient's condition.

Subclavian vein catheterization

Using the Seldinger technique, the physician or surgeon inserts an introducer needle into the subclavian vein. He then inserts a guide wire through the introducer needle and removes the needle. Using the guide wire, he then threads a 5″ to 12″ (12- to 30-cm) plastic or Teflon catheter (with a Y hub) into the patient's vein.

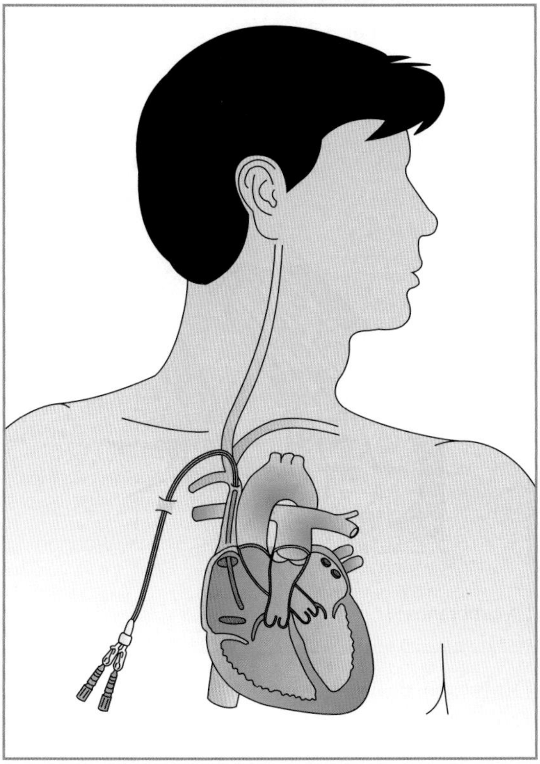

Arteriovenous fistula

To create a fistula, the surgeon makes an incision into the patient's wrist or lower forearm, then a small incision in the side of an artery and another in the side of a vein. He sutures the edges of the incisions together to make a common opening 3 to 7 mm long.

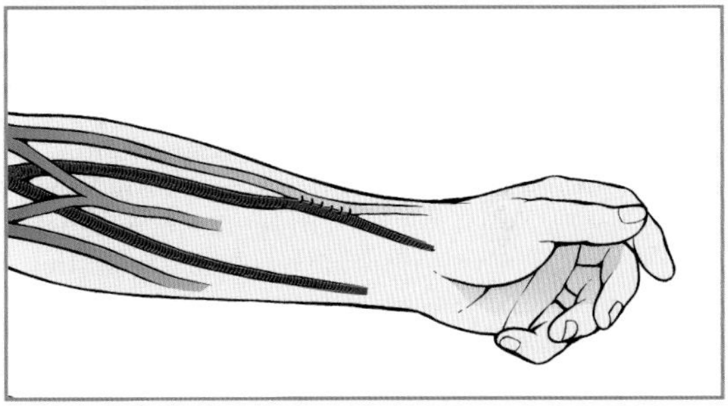

Arteriovenous graft

To create a graft, the surgeon makes an incision in the patient's forearm, upper arm, or thigh. He then tunnels a natural or synthetic graft under the skin and sutures the distal end to an artery and the proximal end to a vein.

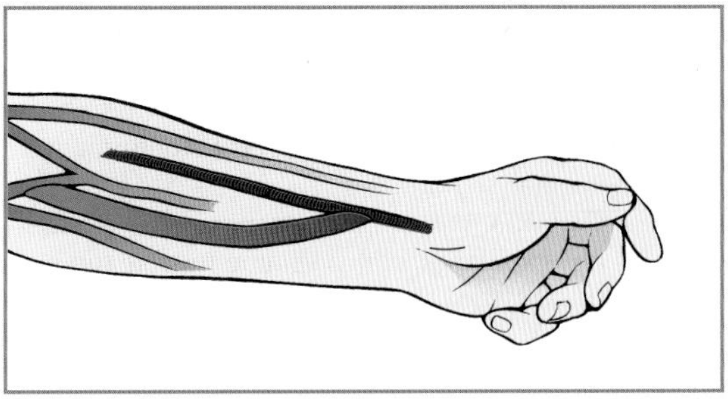

Typically, double-lumen catheters are placed in the internal jugular, subclavian, or common femoral veins. The internal jugular site is preferable to the subclavian site in patients who do, or will, have permanent dialysis accesses placed in their arms. Most double-lumen catheters are considered temporary dialysis accesses. However, a double-lumen, tunneled catheter with a Dacron cuff may be used for months. This catheter is tunneled from the skin insertion site to the selected vein, and the Dacron cuff on the catheter under the skin acts as a barrier to infection.

A primary AV fistula dialysis access is created by the surgical anastomosis of an artery and a vein and is typically used for long-term hemodialysis. Careful preoperative evaluation of the veins and arteries of the arm is necessary to ensure adequate maturation and functioning of the fistula. Indeed, a

How hemodialysis works

In hemodialysis, blood flows from the patient to an external dialyzer (or artificial kidney) through an arterial access site. Inside the dialyzer, blood and dialysate flow countercurrently, divided by a semipermeable membrane. The composition of the dialysate resembles normal extracellular fluid. The blood contains an excess of specific solutes (metabolic waste products and some electrolytes), and the dialysate contains electrolytes that may be at abnormal levels in the patient's bloodstream. The dialysate's electrolyte composition can be modified to raise or lower electrolyte levels, depending on need.

Excretory function and electrolyte homeostasis are achieved by *diffusion*, the movement of a molecule across the dialyzer's semipermeable membrane from an area of higher solute concentration to an area of lower concentration. Water (solvent) crosses the membrane from the blood into the dialysate by *ultrafiltration*. This process removes excess water, waste products, and other metabolites through *osmotic pressure* and *hydrostatic pressure*. Osmotic pressure is the movement of water across the semipermeable membrane from an area of lesser solute concentration to one of greater solute concentration. Hydrostatic pressure forces water from the blood compartment into the dialysate compartment. Cleaned of impurities and excess water, the blood returns to the body through a venous site.

Types of dialyzers

There are two types of dialyzers: the hollow-fiber and the flat-plate or parallel flow-plate. The flat-plate and hollow-fiber dialyzers may be used several times on each patient. Heparin is used to prevent clot formation during hemodialysis.

The *hollow-fiber dialyzer*, the most common type, contains fine capillaries, with a semipermeable membrane enclosed in a plastic cylinder. Blood flows through these capillaries as the system pumps diasylate in the opposite direction on the outside of the capillaries.

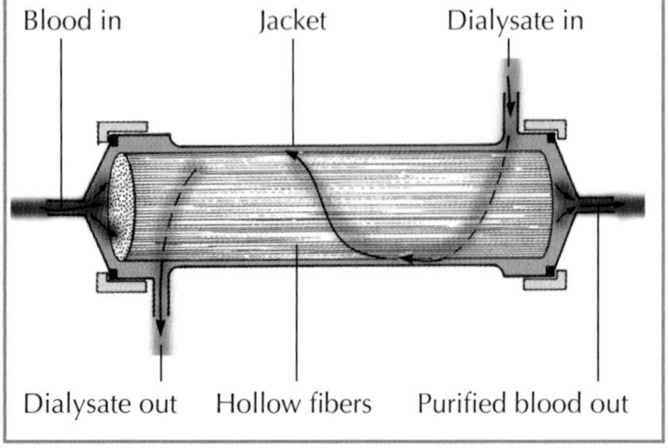

The *flat-plate* or *parallel flow-plate dialyzer* has two or more layers of semipermeable membrane, bound by a semirigid or rigid structure. Blood ports are located at both ends, between the membranes. Blood flows between the membranes, and dialysate flows in the opposite direction along the outside of the membranes.

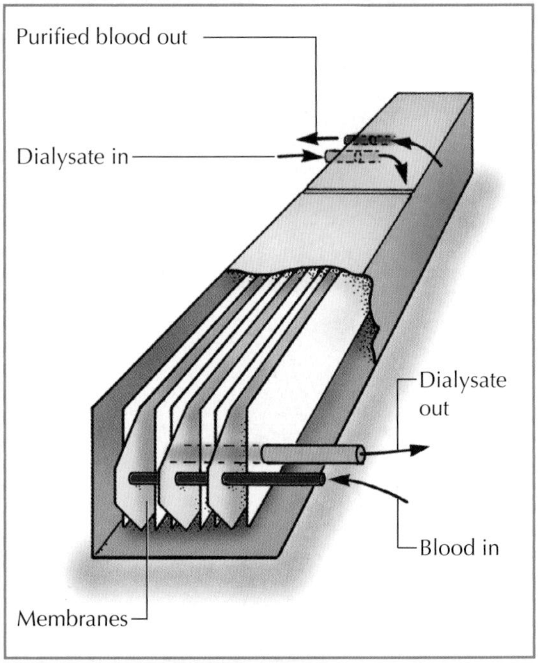

Dialysate delivery systems

Three system types can be used to deliver dialysate. The *batch system* uses a reservoir for recirculating dialysate. The *regenerative system* uses sorbents to purify and regenerate recirculating dialysate. The *proportioning system* (the most common) mixes concentrate with water to form dialysate, which then circulates through the dialyzer and goes down a drain after a single pass, followed by fresh dialysate.

fistula may require weeks or months to mature and be usable for hemodialysis.

A bridge graft may be necessary in a patient whose vessels are inadequate for fistula construction. A synthetic graft is surgically anastomosed to the selected artery and vein to form a bridge between them. Arm vessels are most commonly used and are preferable to the legs. The graft material itself is cannulated during dialysis. Although some grafts may be used within days of their creation, most require several weeks of maturation before they can be used for dialysis. The incidence of thrombosis and infection are higher with AV bridge grafts than with AV fistulas.

Specially prepared personnel usually perform this procedure in a hemodialysis unit. However, if the patient is acutely ill and unstable, hemodialysis can be done at bedside in the intensive care unit. Special hemodialysis units are available for use at home.

Equipment

For preparing the hemodialysis machine: Hemodialysis machine with appropriate dialyzer ▪ I.V. solution, administration sets, lines, and related equipment ▪ dialysate ▪ optional: heparin, 3-ml syringe with needle, medication label, hemostats.

For hemodialysis with a double-lumen catheter: Sterile gloves ▪ clean gloves ▪ gown ▪ sterile drape ▪ sterile 4″ × 4″ gauze pads ▪ antiseptic swabs ▪ stethoscope ▪ sphygmomanometer ▪ two 3-ml syringes ▪ two 5-ml syringes with prescribed anticoagulant flush.

For hemodialysis with an AV access: Two 19G winged fistula needles ▪ two 10-ml syringes ▪ prescribed anticoagulant flush solution ▪ linen-saver pad ▪ antiseptic swabs ▪ sterile 4″ × 4″ gauze pads ▪ sterile drape ▪ tourniquet ▪ sterile gloves ▪ clean gloves ▪ gown ▪ stethoscope ▪ two pair of hemostats ▪ adhesive tape.

Discontinuing dialysis with a double-lumen catheter: Two 10-ml syringes with normal saline solution ▪ two 5-ml syringes with prescribed anticoagulant flush solution ▪ two sterile Luer-Loc caps ▪ antiseptic swabs ▪ stethoscope ▪ sphygmomanometer ▪ supplies for catheter site care ▪ antiseptic solution ▪ sterile drape ▪ sterile 4″ × 4″ gauze pads ▪ optional: supplies for drainage culture.

Discontinuing dialysis with an AV access: Clean gloves ▪ two pairs of hemostats ▪ 4″ × 4″ gauze pads ▪ dry, sterile dressing ▪ stethoscope ▪ sphygmomanometer.

Preparation of equipment

Prepare the hemodialysis equipment following the manufacturer's instructions and your facility's policy. Maintain strict sterile technique *to prevent introducing pathogens into the patient's bloodstream during dialysis.* Be sure to test the dialyzer and dialysis machine for residual disinfectant after rinsing, and test all the alarms.

Implementation

- Gather the appropriate equipment.
- Confirm the patient's identity using two patient identifiers according to your facility's policy.
- Explain the procedure to the patient.
- Weigh the patient. *To determine ultrafiltration requirements,* compare his present weight to his weight after the last dialysis and his target weight. Record his baseline vital signs, taking his blood pressure while he's sitting and standing. Auscultate his heart for rate, rhythm, and abnormalities. Observe respiratory rate, rhythm, and quality. Auscultate the lungs for crackles, which may indicate fluid overload. Assess for edema. Check his mental status and note any problems occurring since the last dialysis; evaluate previous laboratory data.
- Help the patient into a comfortable position (supine or sitting in recliner chair with feet elevated). Make sure the access site is well supported and resting on a clean drape.
- Use standard precautions in all cases *to prevent transmission of infection.* Wash your hands before beginning.

Beginning hemodialysis with a double-lumen catheter

- Clamp the catheter tubing *to prevent air from entering either lumen of the catheter.*
- Prepare a sterile field with the sterile drapes and place the sterile 4″ × 4″ gauze pads on it.
- Identify the red and the blue ports and place them near the sterile field. Place the dialyzer arterial and venous blood lines near the field.
- Put on sterile gloves and clean each catheter extension tube, clamp, and luer-lock injection cap with antiseptic according to your facility's policy. Place a sterile drape beneath the catheter tubing.
- Remove and discard the luer-lock cap on the red port and replace it with a 3-ml syringe. Unclamp the red port, aspirate 1.5 to 3 ml of blood, and re-clamp the port. Remove the syringe.
- Connect one 5-ml syringe with anticoagulant flush to the red port, aspirate 1.5 to 3 ml of blood, and gently instill the flush. Re-clamp the red port.
- Remove and discard the luer-lock cap on the blue port and replace it with a 3-ml syringe. Gently aspirate 1.5 to 3 ml of blood and re-clamp the port. Remove the syringe.
- Connect the other 5-ml syringe with anticoagulant flush to the blue port, aspirate 1.5 to 3 ml of blood, and gently instill the flush. Re-clamp the blue port.

- Remove the syringe from the red port, and attach the red port to the line leading to the arterial port of the dialyzer.
- Remove the syringe from the blue port, and attach the blue port to the line leading to the venous port of the dialyzer.
- Administer the prescribed anticoagulant into the dialyzer. *This prevents clotting in the extracorporeal circuit.*
- Secure the tubing to the patient *to reduce tension on the connections and prevent trauma to the catheter insertion site.* Open the clamps to the arterial and venous dialyzer tubing.
- Begin the hemodialysis treatment according to your facility's policy.
- Monitor the patient's condition and vital signs according to your facility's policy.
- Administer medications and obtain clotting times during hemodialysis, as ordered.

Beginning hemodialysis with an AV access

- Assess the AV access site for patency. Check for the quality of the thrill and auscultate the bruit. Check for the presence of swelling, edema, erythema, or drainage.
- Prepare the two fistula needles by attaching a 10-ml syringe to each. Draw up the prescribed flush solution into each syringe, and prime and clamp the tubing.
- Place the patient's access limb on a sterile drape.
- Put on sterile gloves.
- Using aseptic technique, clean a 3″ × 10″ area of the skin over the AV access with antiseptic swabs. Begin at the proposed needle insertion site, and swab outward in concentric circles for 1 full minute. Discard the swab.
- Using a second antiseptic swab, repeat the previous skin cleaning procedure for a second full minute. Discard the swab.
- If the access is an AV fistula, apply a tourniquet above the fistula *to distend the veins and facilitate the puncture.* Avoid occluding the fistula.
- Put on clean gloves.
- Remove the needle guard on the first fistula needle (arterial), and squeeze the wings together. Insert the arterial needle into the fistula or graft at least 1″ from the arterial-venous anastomotic site. Be careful not to puncture the posterior wall of the access.
- Release the tourniquet, and flush the needle with anticoagulant solution to prevent clotting. Clamp the arterial needle tubing with a hemostat and secure the wing tips of the needle to the skin with adhesive tape *to prevent accidental dislodging of the needle.*
- Perform the second access (venous) puncture with the other fistula needle, a few inches proximal to the arterial needle. Be careful not to puncture the posterior wall of the access.
- Flush the needle with anticoagulant solution. Clamp the venous needle tubing with the second hemostat, and secure the wing tips of the venous needle to the patient's skin with adhesive tape.
- Remove the syringe from the end of the arterial needle tubing, uncap the arterial dialyzer tubing, and connect the two lines. Tape the connection securely *to prevent accidental separation of the tubing.*
- Remove the syringe from the end of the venous needle tubing, uncap the venous dialyzer tubing, and connect the two lines. Tape the connection securely *to prevent accidental separation of the tubing.*
- Remove the hemostats from the tubing and begin the hemodialysis treatment.
- Monitor the patient's condition and vital signs according to your facility's policy.
- Administer medications and obtain clotting times, as ordered.

Discontinuing hemodialysis with a double-lumen catheter

- Wash your hands, and put on appropriate personal protective equipment.
- Open the syringes, the luer-lock caps, and gauze pads and place on a sterile field.
- Fill the two 5-ml syringes with the prescribed amount of anticoagulant flush.
- Fill the two 10-ml syringes with normal saline solution.
- Clamp the tubing to the red and the blue catheter ports and the blood lines to the dialyzer.
- Place a sterile drape beneath the ports.
- Clean the connection points on the catheter, the clamps, and the blood lines with antiseptic solution.
- Place a clean drape under the catheter and place two sterile 4″ × 4″ gauze pads beneath the catheter ports.
- Soak the other 4″ × 4″ gauze pads with antiseptic.
- Put on sterile gloves.
- Grasp the red port connection with the gauze pad, and disconnect it from the arterial dialyzer tubing.
- Attach the 10-ml syringe (with normal saline) to the red port on the catheter and slowly flush the tubing.
- Replace the 10-ml syringe on the red port with the 5-ml syringe filled with the prescribed anticoagulant flush and instill it. Remove the syringe, and cap the port with a sterile luer-lock cap.
- Grasp the blue port connection with the gauze pad and disconnect it from the venous dialyzer tubing.
- Attach the 10-ml syringe (with normal saline) to the blue catheter port and slowly flush the tubing.
- Replace the 10-ml syringe on the blue port with the 5-ml syringe filled with the prescribed anticoagulant flush and

instill it. Remove the syringe, and cap the port with a sterile luer-lock cap. Clamp both ports.

- When catheter care is complete, redress the insertion site and obtain a drainage sample for culture, if necessary.
- Obtain the patient's post-dialysis weight, vital signs, and neurologic, respiratory, and hemodynamic parameters and compare them to his predialysis baseline.
- Rinse and disinfect the delivery system according to the manufacturer's instructions.

Discontinuing hemodialysis utilizing an AV access

- Wash your hands.
- Turn the blood pump on the hemodialysis machine to 50 to 100 ml/minute.
- Put on clean gloves.
- Remove the tape from the connection site of the arterial lines. Clamp the needle tubing with the hemostat and disconnect the lines. The blood in the arterial line will continue to flow toward the dialyzer, followed by a column of air. Clamp the blood line with another hemostat just before the blood reaches the point where the saline enters the line.
- Unclamp the saline solution to allow a small amount of saline to flow through the line. Unclamp the hemostat on the dialyzer line. *This allows all blood to flow into the dialyzer where it passes through the filter and back to the patient through the venous line.*
- After the blood is re-transfused, clamp the venous needle tubing and the dialyzer's venous line with hemostats and turn off the blood pump.
- Remove the tape from the connection site of the venous lines and disconnect the lines.
- Remove the venipuncture needle completely, and then apply pressure to the site with a folded 4″ × 4″ gauze pad using two fingers. If inadequate pressure is used, a hematoma may develop. If excessive pressure is used, the access may thrombose. You should be able to continue to feel a thrill both above and below the compression site while holding pressure. Bleeding usually stops within 10 minutes.
- Apply a dry, sterile dressing to the site. Avoid circumferential taping of the dressing.
- Repeat the procedure on the arterial needle and site.
- When dialysis is complete, weigh the patient, obtain vital signs (including blood pressure sitting and standing, and assess his mental status. Compare these to the pre-dialysis assessment data.
- Rinse and disinfect the delivery system according to the manufacturer's instructions.

Special considerations

- Obtain blood samples from the patient, as ordered. Samples are usually drawn before beginning hemodialysis.

NURSING ALERT *Use strict sterile technique during preparation of the machine* to avoid pyrogenic reactions and bacteremia with septicemia resulting from contamination. *Discard equipment that has fallen on the floor or that has been disconnected and exposed to the air.*

- Immediately report any machine malfunction or equipment defect.

NURSING ALERT *Make sure you complete each step correctly.* Overlooking a single step or performing it incorrectly can cause unnecessary blood loss or inefficient treatment from poor clearances or inadequate fluid removal. *For example, never allow a saline solution bag to run dry while priming and soaking the dialyzer* because this can cause air to enter the patient portion of the dialysate system. *Ultimately, failure to perform hemodialysis accurately can lead to patient injury and even death.*

- Continue necessary drug administration during dialysis unless the drug would be removed in the dialysate; if so, administer the drug after dialysis.
- Don't inject I.V. fluids or medications into either port of the double-lumen catheter.
- If, while instilling the anticoagulant flush into either port, you meet resistance, stop flushing immediately. Clamp the port, replace the sterile luer-lock cap, and notify the practitioner. Place "do not use" message on the port until its patency is verified.
- If the patient receives meals during dialysis, make sure they're light.

Home care

Before the patient leaves the hospital, teach him how to care for his vascular access site. Instruct him to keep the incision clean and dry *to prevent infection,* and to clean it daily until it heals completely and the sutures are removed (usually 10 to 14 days after surgery). He should notify the physician of pain, swelling, redness, or drainage in the accessed arm. Teach him how to use a stethoscope to auscultate for bruits and how to palpate a thrill.

Explain that once the access site heals, he may use the arm freely. In fact, exercise is beneficial *because it helps stimulate vein enlargement.* Remind him not to allow any treatments or procedures on the accessed arm, including blood pressure monitoring or needle punctures. Also tell him to avoid putting excessive pressure on the arm. He shouldn't sleep on it, wear constrictive clothing on it, or lift heavy objects. He also should avoid getting wet for several hours after dialysis.

Teach the patient exercises for the affected arm *to promote vascular dilation and enhance blood flow.* He may start by squeezing a small rubber ball or other soft object for 15 minutes, when advised by the physician.

If the patient will be performing hemodialysis at home, thoroughly review all aspects of the procedure with the patient and his family. Give them the phone number of the dialysis center. Emphasize that training for home hemodialysis is a complex process requiring 2 to 3 months *to ensure that the patient or family member performs it safely and competently.* Keep in mind that this procedure is stressful.

Complications

Bacterial endotoxins in the dialysate may cause fever. Rapid fluid removal and electrolyte changes during hemodialysis can cause early dialysis disequilibrium syndrome. Signs and symptoms include headache, nausea, vomiting, restlessness, hypertension, muscle cramps, backache, and seizures.

Excessive removal of fluid during ultrafiltration can cause hypovolemia and hypotension. Diffusion of the sugar and sodium content of the dialysate solution into the blood can cause hyperglycemia and hypernatremia and subsequent hyperosmolarity.

Cardiac arrhythmias can occur due to electrolyte and pH changes in the blood. They may also develop if the patient is taking antiarrhythmics because the dialysate removes these drugs during the treatment. Angina may develop in patients with anemia or who have preexisting arteriosclerotic cardiovascular disease because of the physiologic stress on the blood during purification and ultrafiltration. Patients with reduced oxygen levels resulting from extracorporeal blood flow or membrane sensitivity may require oxygen administration during hemodialysis.

Some complications of hemodialysis can be fatal. For example, an air embolism can result if the dialyzer retains air, if tubing connections become loose, or if the saline solution container empties. Symptoms include chest pain, dyspnea, coughing, and cyanosis.

Hemolysis can result from obstructed flow of the dialysate concentrate or from incorrect setting of the conductivity alarm limits. Symptoms include chest pain, dyspnea, cherry red blood, arrhythmias, acute decrease in hematocrit, or hyperkalemia.

Hyperthermia can result from overheating of the dialysate and is potentially fatal. Exsanguination can result from separations of the blood lines or from rupture of the blood lines or dialyzer membrane.

Improper access site cannulation or needle site care may cause hematoma, pseudoaneurysm formation, or even rupture of the graft and excessive bleeding.

Documentation

Record the time treatment began and any problems with it. Note the patient's vital signs and weight before and during treatment. Note the time blood samples were taken for testing, the test results, and treatment for any complications that arose. Record the time the treatment was completed and the patient's response to it.

Selected references

Hadaway, L. "Technology of Flushing Vascular Access Devices," *Journal of Infusion Nursing* 29(3):129-45, May-June 2006.

Kaveh, K., et al. "The New Arteriovenous Fistula: The Need for Earlier Intervention," *Seminars in Dialysis* 18:1, 3-7, 2005.

Konner, K. "History of Vascular Access for Haemodyalisis," *Nephrology, Dialysis, Transplantation* 20(12):2629-35, December 2005.

Lynn-McHale Wiegand, D.J., and Carlson, K.K., eds. *AACN Procedure Manual for Critical Care,* 5th ed. Philadelphia: W.B. Saunders Co., 2005.

Nation Kidney Foundation NKF/KDOQI Guidelines. Clinical Practice Guidelines and Clinical Practice Recommendation for Hemodialysis Adequacy, 2006 update. *www.kidney.org/professionals/kdoqi/guideline_upHD_PD_VA/index.htm*

Safdar, N., et al. "The Pathogenesis of Catheter-related Bloodstream Infection with Non-cuffed Short-Term Central Venous Catheters," *Intensive Care Medicine* 30(1):62-67, 2004.

Continuous renal replacement therapy

Continuous renal replacement therapy (CRRT) is used to treat patients who suffer from acute renal failure. Unlike the more traditional intermittent hemodialysis (IHD), CRRT is administered round the clock, providing patients with continuous therapy and sparing them the destabilizing hemodynamic and electrolytic changes characteristic of IHD. CRRT is used for patients who are unable to tolerate traditional hemodialysis, such as those who have hypotension. For such patients, CRRT is typically the only choice of treatment; however, it can also be used on many patients who can tolerate IHD. CRRT methods vary in complexity. The techniques include the following:

- Slow continuous ultrafiltration (SCUF) uses arteriovenous access and the patient's blood pressure to circulate blood through a hemofilter. Because the goal with this therapy is the removal of fluids, the patient doesn't receive any replacement fluids.
- Continuous arteriovenous hemofiltration (CAVH) uses the patient's blood pressure and arteriovenous access to circulate blood through a flow resistance hemofilter. Howev-

er, to maintain the patency of the filter and the systemic blood pressure, the patient receives replacement fluids.

- Continuous venovenous hemofiltration (CVVH) fuses SCUF and CAVH. A double-lumen catheter is used to provide access to a vein, and a pump moves blood through the hemofilter.
- Continuous arteriovenous hemodialysis (CAVH-D) combines hemodialysis with hemofiltration. In this technique, the infusion pump moves dialysate solution concurrent to blood flow, adding the ability to continuously remove solute while removing fluid. Like CAVH, it can also be performed in patients with hypotension and fluid overload.
- Continuous venovenous hemodialysis (CVVH-D) is similar to CAVH-D, except that a vein provides the access while a pump is used to move dialysate solution concurrent with blood flow.

NURSING ALERT *CVVH or CVVH-D is being used instead of CAVH or CAVH-D in many facilities to treat critically ill patients. CVVH has several advantages over CAVH: It doesn't require arterial access, CVVH can be performed in patients with low mean arterial pressures and CVVH has a better solute clearance than CAVH.*

Equipment

CRRT equipment ▪ heparin flush solution ▪ occlusive dressings for catheter insertion sites ▪ sterile and clean gloves ▪ mask and gown, as needed ▪ antiseptic solution ▪ sterile gauze pads ▪ tape ▪ filtration replacement fluid (FRF), as ordered ▪ infusion pump.

Preparation of equipment

Prime the hemofilter and tubing according to the manufacturer's instructions.

Implementation

- Confirm the patient's identity using two patient identifiers according to your facility's policy.
- Wash your hands. Assemble your equipment at the patient's bedside according to manufacturer's recommendations and your facility's policy, and explain the procedure. (See *Setup for CAVH and CVVH,* pages 750 and 751.)
- If necessary, assist with inserting the catheters into the femoral artery and vein, using strict sterile technique. (In some cases, an arteriovenous fistula or double-lumen catheter may be used instead of the femoral route.) If ordered, flush both catheters with the heparin flush solution to prevent clotting.
- Apply occlusive dressings to the insertion sites, and mark the dressings with the date and time. Secure the tubing and connections with tape *to prevent accidental dislodging.*
- Weigh the patient, take baseline vital signs, and make sure all necessary laboratory studies have been done (usually, electrolyte levels, coagulation factors, complete blood count, blood urea nitrogen, and creatinine studies). Monitor the patient's condition and vital signs hourly.
- Put on sterile gloves and mask. Prepare the connection sites by cleaning them with gauze pads soaked in antiseptic solution, then connect them to the exit port of each catheter.
- Using sterile technique, connect the arterial and venous lines to the hemofilter.
- Turn on the hemofilter and monitor the blood-flow rate through the circuit. The flow rate is typically between 500 and 900 ml/hour.
- Inspect the ultrafiltrate during the procedure. It should remain clear yellow, with no gross blood. Pink-tinged or bloody ultrafiltrate may signal a membrane leak in the hemofilter, which permits bacterial contamination. If a leak occurs, notify the practitioner and discontinue the treatment immediately.
- Assess all pulses—dorsalis pedis, posterior tibial, popliteal, and femoral—in the affected leg every hour for the first 4 hours, then every 2 hours thereafter.
- Assess the affected leg for signs of obstructed blood flow, such as pain, coolness, pallor, and weak pulse. Check the groin area on the affected side for signs of hematoma. Ask the patient whether he has pain at the insertion sites.
- Calculate the amount of FRF every hour, as ordered, or according to your facility's policy. Infuse the prescribed amount and type of FRF through the infusion pump into the arterial side of the circuit.
- Assess hemodynamic parameters, including pulmonary artery pressure (PAP), central venous pressure (CVP), pulmonary artery wedge pressure (PAWP), and blood pressure hourly, or more frequently if indicated. Be alert for indications of hypovolemia (such as dropping blood pressure and decrease in PAP, CVP, and PAWP) *from too-rapid removal of ultrafiltrate,* or hypervolemia *due to excessive fluid replacement with a decrease in ultrafiltrate.*
- Institute continuous cardiac monitoring *to detect arrhythmias indicative of electrolyte imbalances.*

Special considerations

- *Because blood flows through an extracorporeal circuit during CAVH and CVVH,* the blood in the hemofilter may need to be anticoagulated. To do this, infuse heparin in low doses (usually starting at 500 units/hour) into an infusion port on the arterial side of the setup. Measure thrombin clotting time or the activated clotting time (ACT). *This ensures that the circuit, not the patient, is anticoagulated.* A normal ACT is 100 seconds; during CRRT, keep it between 100 and 300 seconds, depending on the patient's clotting times. If the

EQUIPMENT

Setup for CAVH and CVVH

Continuous renal replacement therapy is frequently performed using one of the two systems described here.

Continuous arteriovenous hemofiltration

In continuous arteriovenous hemofiltration (CAVH), the physician inserts two large-bore, single-lumen catheters (as shown below). One catheter is inserted into an artery—most commonly, the femoral artery. The other catheter is inserted into a vein, usually the femoral, subclavian, or internal jugular vein. During CAVH, the patient's arterial blood pressure serves as a natural pump, driving blood through the arterial line. A hemofilter removes water and toxic solutes (ultrafiltrate) from the blood. Replacement fluid is infused into a port on the arterial side. The same port can be used to infuse heparin. The venous line carries the replacement fluid and purified blood to the patient.

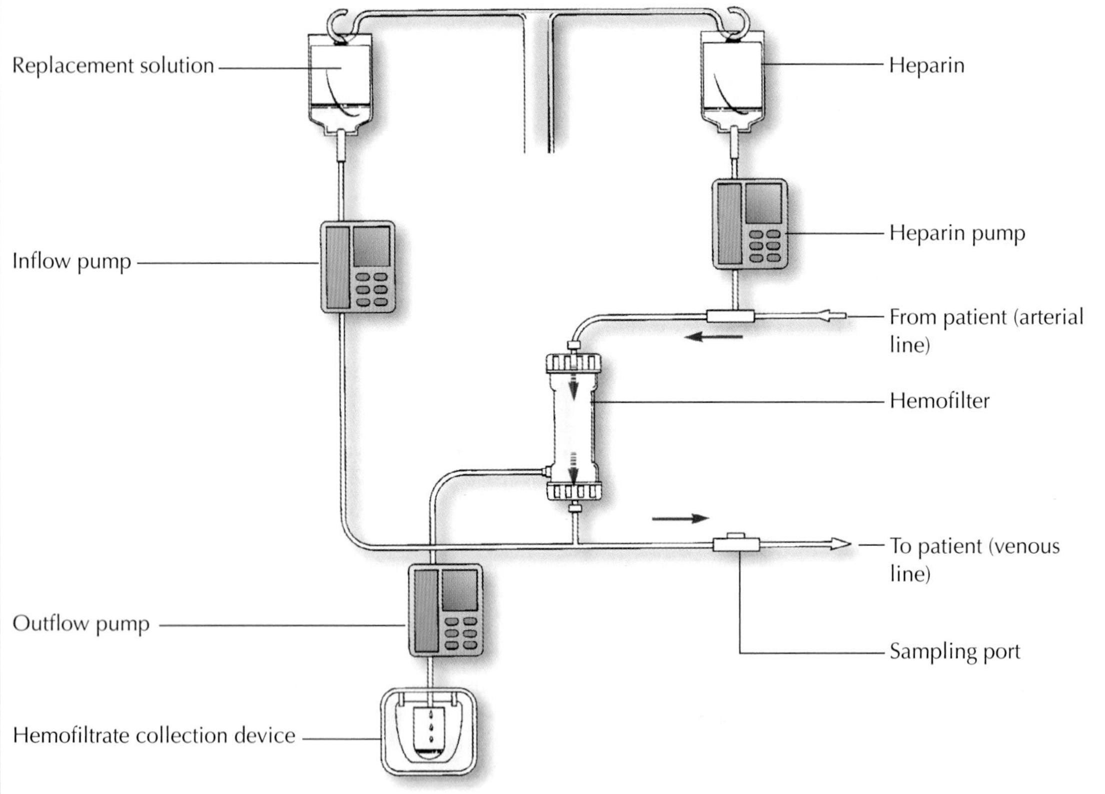

ACT is too high or too low, the practitioner will adjust the heparin dose accordingly.

- Another way to prevent clotting in the hemofilter is to infuse medications or blood through another venous access device rather than the venous line, if possible.
- A third way to help prevent clots in the hemofilter, and also to prevent kinks in the catheter, is to make sure the patient doesn't bend the affected leg more than 30 degrees at the hip.

Continuous venovenous hemofiltration

In continuous venovenous hemofiltration (CVVH), the physician inserts a special double-lumen catheter into a large vein—commonly the subclavian, femoral, or internal jugular vein (as shown below). Because the catheter is in a vein, an external pump is used to move blood through the system. The patient's venous blood moves through the "arterial" lumen to the pump, which then pushes the blood through the catheter to the hemofilter. Here, water and toxic solutes (ultrafiltrate) are removed from the patient's blood and drain into a collection device. Blood cells aren't removed because they are too large to pass through the filter. As the blood exits the hemofilter, it's then pumped through the "venous" lumen back to the patient.

Several components of the pump provide safety mechanisms. Pressure monitors on the pump maintain the flow of blood through the circuit at a constant rate. An air detector traps air bubbles before the blood returns to the patient. A venous trap collects any blood clots that may be in the blood. A blood-leak detector signals when blood is found in the ultrafiltrate; a venous clamp operates if air is detected in the circuit or if there is any disconnection in the blood line.

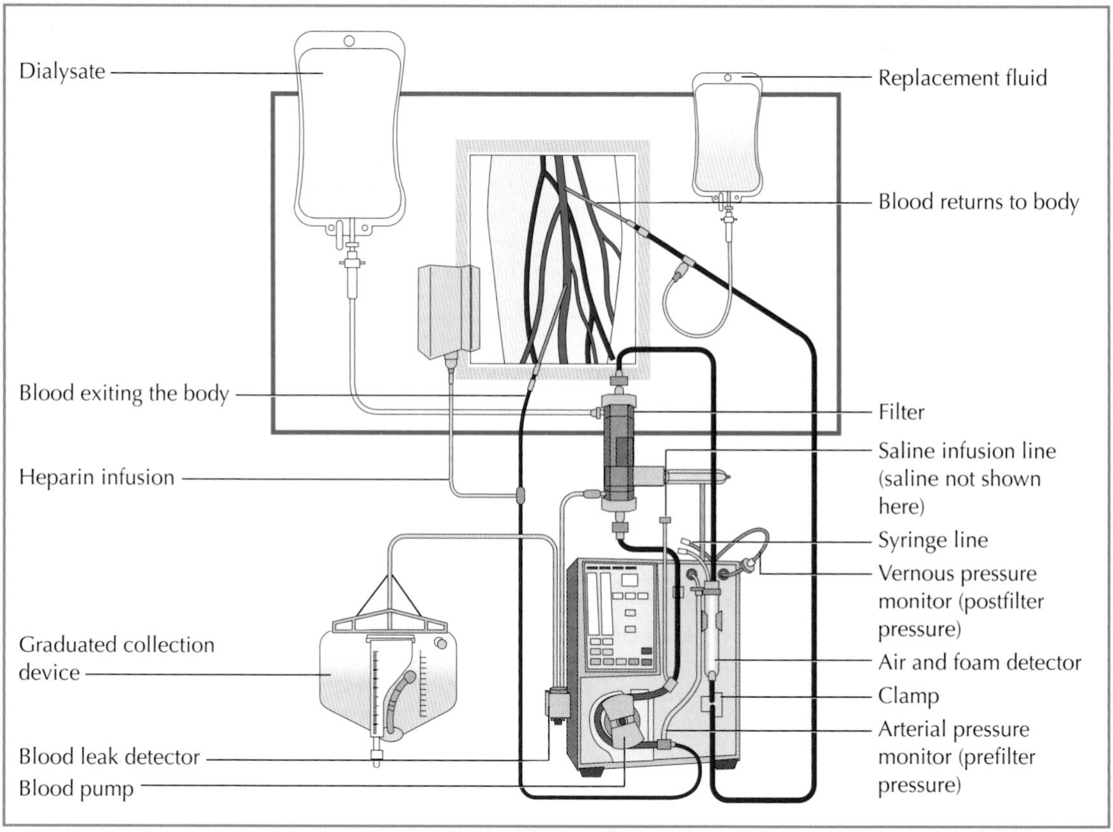

■ If the ultrafiltrate flow rate decreases, raise the bed *to increase the distance between the collection device and the hemofilter.* Lower the bed *to decrease the flow rate.*

NURSING ALERT *Clamping the ultrafiltrate line is contraindicated with some types of hemofilters* because pressure may build up in the filter, clotting it and collapsing the blood compartment.

■ Obtain serum electrolyte levels every 4 to 6 hours, or as ordered; anticipate adjustments in replacement fluid or dialysate based on the results.

Preventing complications of CRRT

Measures to avoid complications of CRRT are listed below.

COMPLICATION	NURSING INTERVENTIONS
Hypotension	▪ Monitor blood pressure. ▪ Temporarily decrease the blood pump's speed for transient hypotension. ▪ Increase the vasopressor support.
Hypothermia	▪ Use an inline fluid warmer placed on the blood return line to the patient or an external warming blanket.
Fluid and electrolyte imbalances	▪ Monitor the patient's fluid levels every 4 to 6 hours. ▪ Monitor the patient's sodium, lactate, potassium, and calcium levels and replace as necessary.
Acid-base imbalances	▪ Monitor the patient's bicarbonate and arterial blood gas levels.
Air embolism	▪ Observe for air in the system. ▪ Use luer-lock devices on catheter openings.
Hemorrhage	▪ Check all connections and keep the dialysis lines visible.
Infection	▪ Perform sterile dressing changes.

▪ If the patient is receiving CVVH and the pressure alarm sounds, check the catheter for kinks, disconnections, or other problems. Determine which alarm sounded—the arterial or the venous pressure alarm. If the arterial pressure alarm sounds, check the arterial lumen; if the venous pressure alarm sounds, check the venous lumen. *A sudden rise in pressure indicates some blockage in the catheter or tubing. A dramatic and significant drop in pressure suggests a disconnection or opening of a port.*

▪ Inspect the site dressing every 4 to 8 hours for infection and bleeding. *To prevent infection,* perform skin care at the catheter insertion sites every 48 hours, using sterile technique. Cover the sites with an occlusive dressing.

Complications

Possible complications of CRRT include bleeding, hemorrhage, hemofilter occlusion, infection, and thrombosis. (See *Preventing complications of CRRT.*)

Documentation

Record the time the treatment began and ended, fluid balance information, vital signs, times of dressing changes, complications, medications given, and the patient's tolerance of the procedure.

SELECTED REFERENCES

Lynn-McHale Wiegand, D.J., and Carlson, K.K., eds. *AACN Procedure Manual for Critical Care*, 5th ed. Philadelphia: W.B. Saunders Co., 2005.

Rickard, C.M., et al. "Preventing Hypothermia During Continuous Veno-Venous Haemofiltration: A Randomized Controlled Trial," *Journal of Advanced Nursing* 47(4):393-400, August 2004.

Waldrop, J., et al. "A Comparison of Continuous Renal Replacement Therapy to Intermittent Dialysis in the Management of Renal Insufficiency in the Acutely Ill Surgical Patient," *The American Surgeon* 71(1):36-39, January 2005.

12 ■ Orthopedic care

Introduction

Orthopedics began as a specialty for the prevention and treatment of children's musculoskeletal deformities. However, this branch of medicine has expanded dramatically to include the prevention, treatment, and care of musculoskeletal conditions affecting patients of all ages.

The American Nurses Association defines orthopedic nursing as the diagnosis and treatment of human responses to actual and potential health problems related to musculoskeletal function. More specifically, orthopedic nursing focuses on promoting wellness and self-care and on preventing further injury and illness in patients with degenerative, traumatic, inflammatory, neuromuscular, congenital, metabolic, and oncologic disorders.

Traditionally, orthopedic nurses have needed to operate special mechanical and traction equipment. Today, they need to understand principles of internal and external fixation, prosthetics, orthotics, immobilization, and implantation.

Despite the evolution of complex surgical procedures and mechanical devices that characterize modern orthopedic care, some things remain the same. A patient hospitalized for any orthopedic procedure—whether it's cast application, traction, or arthroplasty—is vulnerable to similar complications, such as:

- joint stiffness and skin breakdown from impaired physical mobility
- fractures from mishandling of osteoporotic extremities
- neurovascular compromise from pressure on major blood vessels and nerves caused by immobilization devices or compartmental edema
- infection of surgical wounds or skeletal pin tracts
- prolonged healing time from failure to observe sound principles of immobilization.

In addition, the patient's level of understanding and the effectiveness of his coping skills must be assessed.

Consistent care

Without exception, orthopedic complications can be prevented or minimized by appropriate and consistent assessment, monitoring, and therapy. For example, the orthopedic patient's neurovascular status must be assessed at regular intervals; otherwise, signs and symptoms of neurovascular compromise may go undetected until irreversible damage occurs. Consistent orthopedic care remains the surest way to promote rapid healing and successful rehabilitation.

Ready for an emergency

Orthopedic nursing care is characterized by the high incidence of emergency procedures that you're likely to perform. The first step—always—in administering emergency care at the scene of an accident is immediate assessment for a life-threatening condition. Don't move the patient unless danger is imminent because this might worsen the injury and increase pain. If the patient must be moved, assess him for possible spinal injury so that appropriate transfer techniques can be used. After determining that no life-threatening injury exists, conduct an initial head-to-toe assessment, comparing bilaterally where applicable.

Always evaluate neurovascular status. (Check the five Ps: pain, pallor, pulse, paresthesia, and paralysis.) Assess the injury thoroughly, and use strict sterile technique when caring for all open wounds to prevent infection. If you suspect a bone injury, apply a splint to reduce injury and immobilize the bone.

In nonemergencies, performing orthopedic procedures correctly can ease pain, prevent further injury, and encourage proper healing.

Support procedures

Clavicle strap application

Also called a *figure-eight strap*, a clavicle strap reduces and immobilizes fractures of the clavicle. It does this by elevating, extending, and supporting the shoulders in position for healing, known as the position of attention. A commercially available figure-eight strap or a 4″ elastic bandage may serve as a clavicle strap. This strap is contraindicated for an uncooperative patient.

Equipment

Powder or cornstarch ▪ figure-eight clavicle strap or 4″ elastic bandage ▪ safety pins, if necessary ▪ tape ▪ cotton batting or padding ▪ marking pen ▪ analgesics, as ordered ▪ optional: scissors.

Implementation

- Gather the equipment.
- Confirm the patient's identity using two patient identifiers according to your facility's policy.
- Explain the procedure to the patient and provide privacy.
- Help the patient take off his shirt, or cut off the shirt if movement is too painful.
- Assess neurovascular integrity by palpating skin temperature; noting the color of the hand and fingers; palpating the radial, ulnar, and brachial pulses bilaterally; and then comparing the affected with the unaffected side. Ask the pa-

tient about any numbness or tingling distal to the injury, and assess his motor function.

- Determine the patient's degree of comfort, and administer analgesics, as ordered.
- Demonstrate how to assume the position of attention. Instruct the patient to sit upright and assume this position gradually *to minimize pain.*
- Gently apply powder, as appropriate, to the axillae and shoulder area *to reduce friction from the clavicle strap.* You can use cornstarch if the patient is allergic to powder.

Applying a figure-eight strap

- Place the apex of the triangle between the scapulae, and drape the straps over the shoulders. Bring the strap with the Velcro or buckle end under one axilla and through the loop; then pull the other strap under the other axilla and through the loop. (See *Types of clavicle straps.*)
- Gently adjust the straps so they support the shoulders in the position of attention.
- Bring the straps back under the axillae toward the anterior chest, making sure that they maintain the position of attention.

Applying a 4″ elastic bandage

- Roll both ends of the elastic bandage toward the middle, leaving between 12″ and 18″ (30.5 to 45.5 cm) unrolled.
- Place the unrolled portion diagonally across the patient's back, from right shoulder to left axilla.
- Bring the lower end of the bandage under the left axilla and back over the left shoulder; loop the upper end over the right shoulder and under the axilla.
- Pull the two ends together at the center of the back *so that the bandage supports the position of attention.*

Completing a figure-eight strap or elastic bandage

- Secure the ends using safety pins, Velcro pads, or a buckle, depending on the equipment. Make sure a buckle or any sharp edges face away from the skin. Tape the secured ends to the underlying strap or bandage.
- Place cotton batting or padding under the straps, as well as under the buckle or pins, *to avoid skin irritation.*
- Use a pen to mark the strap at the site of the loop of the figure-eight strap or the site where the elastic bandage crosses on the patient's back. *If the strap loosens, this mark helps you tighten it to the original position.*
- Assess neurovascular integrity, *which may be impaired by a strap that is too tight.* If neurovascular integrity is compromised when the strap is correctly applied, notify the practitioner. *He may want to change the treatment.*

EQUIPMENT

Types of clavicle straps

Clavicle straps provide support to the shoulder to help heal a fractured clavicle. These straps are available ready-made, or they can be made from a wide bandage.

Commercially made clavicle straps have a short back panel and long straps that extend around the patient's shoulders and axillae. They have Velcro pads or buckles on the ends for easy fastening.

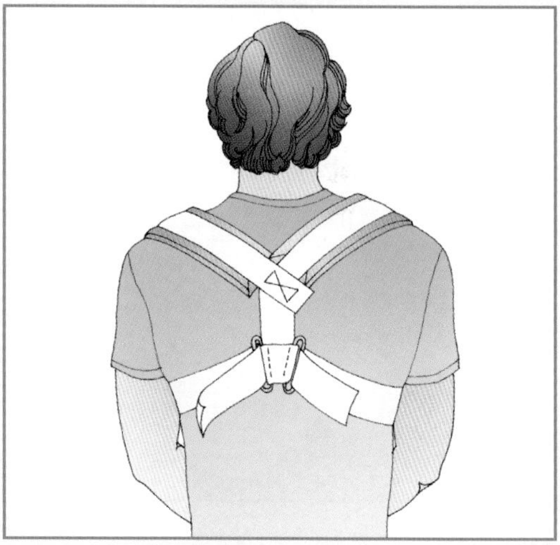

When making a clavicle strap with a wide elastic bandage, start in the middle of the patient's back. After wrapping the bandage around the shoulders, fasten the ends with safety pins.

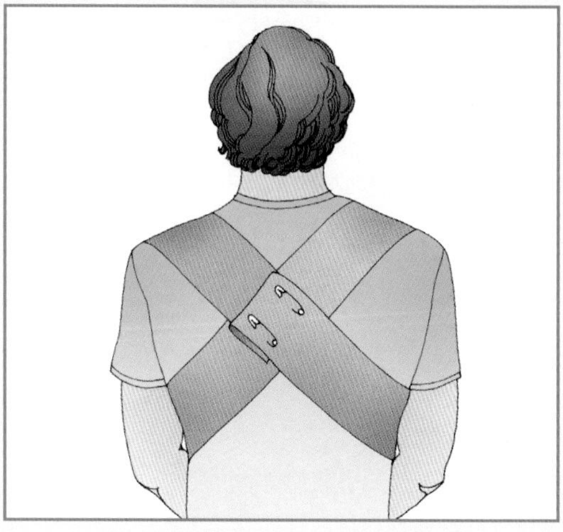

EQUIPMENT

Types of cervical collars

Cervical collars are used to support an injured or weakened cervical spine and to maintain alignment during healing.

Made of rigid plastic, the molded cervical collar holds the patient's neck firmly, keeping it straight, with the chin slightly elevated and tucked in.

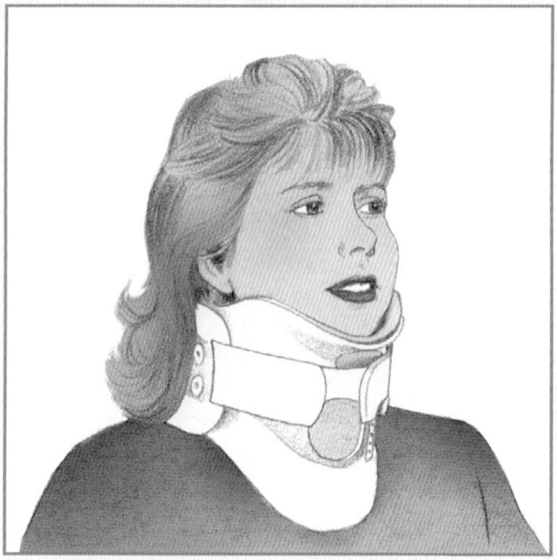

The soft cervical collar, made of spongy foam, provides gentler support and reminds the patient to avoid cervical spine motion.

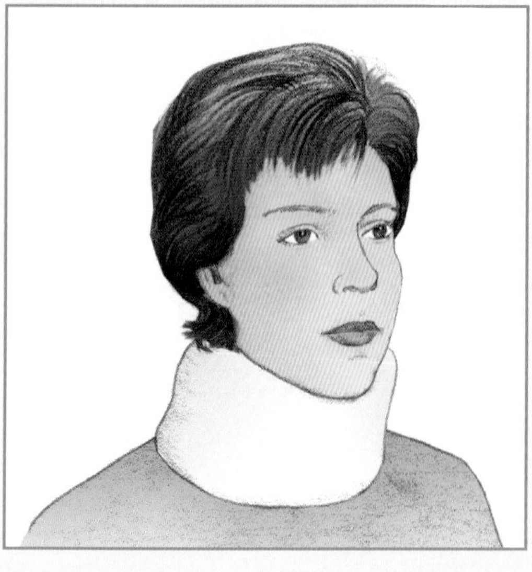

Special considerations

- If possible, perform the procedure with the patient standing. However, this may not be feasible *because the pain from the fracture can cause syncope.*
- An adult with a clavicle strap made from an elastic bandage may require a sling *to help support the weight of the arm, enhance immobilization, and reduce pain. Inadequate immobilization can cause improper healing.*
- Instruct the patient not to remove the clavicle strap until instructed to do so by his practitioner. Explain that, with help, he can maintain proper hygiene by lifting segments of the strap to remove the cotton and by washing and powdering the skin daily. Explain that fresh cotton should be applied after cleaning.
- For a hospitalized patient, check the pen markings every 8 hours *to monitor the position of the strap.* Assess neurovascular integrity. Teach the outpatient how to assess his own neurovascular integrity and to recognize symptoms to report promptly to the practitioner.

Documentation

In the appropriate section of the emergency department sheet or in your notes, record the date and time of strap application, type of clavicle strap, use of powder and padding, bilateral neurovascular integrity before and after the procedure, and instructions to the patient.

Selected references

Canadian Orthopedic Trauma Society. "Nonoperative Treatment Compared with Plate Fixation of Displaced Midshaft Clavicular Fractures: A Multicenter Randomized Clinical Trial," *Journal of Bone and Joint Surgery* 89(1):1-10, January 2007.

Duke University Medical Center Division of Orthopaedic Surgery. *Wheeless' Textbook of Orthopaedics.* Durham, N.C.: Data Trace Internet Publishing, LLC. Available at *www.wheelessonline.com.*

CERVICAL COLLAR APPLICATION

A cervical collar may be used for an acute injury (such as strained cervical muscles) or a chronic condition (such as arthritis or cervical metastasis). Or, it may augment such splinting devices as a spine board to prevent potential cervical spine fracture or spinal cord damage.

Designed to hold the neck straight with the chin slightly elevated and tucked in, the collar immobilizes the cervical spine, decreases muscle spasms, and relieves some pain; it also prevents further injury and promotes healing. As symptoms of an acute injury subside, the patient may gradually discontinue wearing the collar, alternating periods of wear with increasing periods of removal, until he no longer needs the collar.

Equipment

Cervical collar in the appropriate size ▪ optional: cotton (for padding). (See *Types of cervical collars.*)

Implementation

▪ Confirm the patient's identity using two patient identifiers according to your facility's policy.
▪ Check the patient's neurovascular status before application.
▪ Instruct the patient to position his head slowly to face directly forward.
▪ Place the cervical collar in front of the patient's neck *to ensure that the size is correct.*
▪ Fit the collar snugly around the neck and attach the Velcro fasteners or buckles at the back of the neck.
▪ Check the patient's airway and his neurovascular status *to ensure that the collar isn't too tight.*

Special considerations

▪ For a sprain or a potential cervical spine fracture, make sure the collar isn't too high in front *because this may hyperextend the neck.* In a neck sprain, such hyperextension may cause ligaments to heal in a shortened position. In a potential cervical spine fracture, hyperextension may cause serious neurologic damage.
▪ If the patient complains of pressure, the collar may be too tight. Remove and reapply it. If the patient complains of skin irritation or friction, the collar itself may be irritating him. Apply protective cotton padding between the irritated skin and the collar.

Home care

Teach the patient how to apply the collar and how to do a neurovascular check. Have the patient demonstrate how to apply the collar after you have instructed him. Some collars are complex and the patient (or caregiver) may need to practice if he will be responsible for application. If indicated, advise sleeping without a pillow.

Documentation

Note the type and size of the cervical collar and the time and date of application in your notes. Record the results of neurovascular checks. Document patient comfort, the collar's snugness, and all patient instructions.

Selected references

Powers, J., et al. "The Incidence of Skin Breakdown Associated with Use of Cervical Collars," *Journal of Trauma Nursing* 13(4):198-200, October-December 2006.

Smeltzer, S.C., et al. *Brunner & Suddarth's Textbook of Medical-Surgical Nursing*, 11th ed. Philadelphia: Lippincott Williams & Wilkins, 2008.

SPLINT APPLICATION

By immobilizing the site of an injury, a splint alleviates pain and allows the injury to heal in proper alignment. It also minimizes possible complications, such as excessive bleeding into tissues, restricted blood flow caused by bone pressing against vessels, and possible paralysis from an unstable spinal cord injury. In cases of multiple serious injuries, a splint or spine board allows caretakers to move the patient without risking further damage to bones, muscles, nerves, blood vessels, and skin.

A splint can be applied to immobilize a simple or compound fracture, a dislocation, or a subluxation. (See *Types of splints,* page 758.) During an emergency, any injury suspected of being a fracture, dislocation, or subluxation should be splinted. No contraindications exist for rigid splints; don't use traction splints for upper extremity injuries and open fractures.

Equipment

Rigid splint, Velcro support splint, spine board, or traction splint ▪ bindings ▪ padding ▪ sandbags or rolled towels or clothing ▪ optional: roller gauze, cloth strips, sterile or clean compress, ice bag, scissors.

Several commercial splints are widely available. In an emergency, any long, sturdy object, such as a tree limb, mop handle, or broom—even a magazine—can be used to make a rigid splint for an extremity; a door can be used as a spine board.

An inflatable semirigid splint, called an air splint, sometimes can be used to secure an injured extremity. (See *Using an air splint,* page 759.) Velcro straps, 2″ roller gauze, or 2″ cloth strips can be used as bindings. When improvising, avoid using twine or rope, if possible, *because they can restrict circulation.*

Implementation

▪ Confirm the patient's identity using two patient identifiers according to your facility's policy.
▪ Obtain a complete history of the injury, if possible, and begin a thorough head-to-toe assessment, inspecting for obvious deformities, swelling, or bleeding.
▪ Ask the patient if he can move the injured area (typically an extremity). Compare it bilaterally with the uninjured extremity, where applicable. Gently palpate the injured area; inspect for swelling, obvious deformities, bleeding, discoloration, and evidence of fracture or dislocation.

EQUIPMENT

Types of splints

Three kinds of splints are commonly used to help provide support for injured or weakened limbs or to help correct deformities.

A *rigid splint* can be used to immobilize a fracture or dislocation in an extremity, as shown at right. Ideally, two people should apply a rigid splint to an extremity.

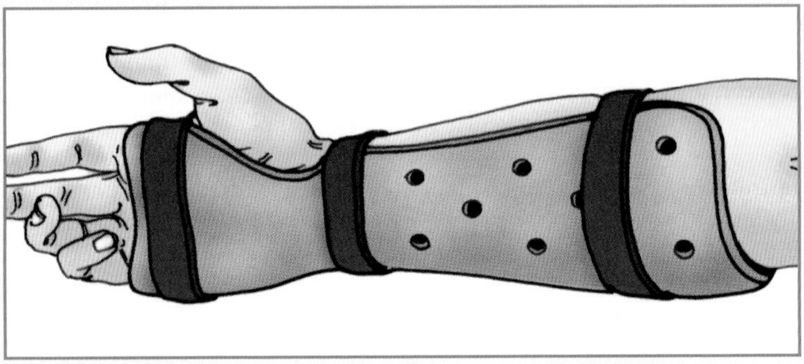

A *traction splint* immobilizes a fracture and exerts a longitudinal pull that reduces muscle spasms, pain, and arterial and neural damage. Used primarily for femoral fractures, a traction splint may also be applied for a fractured hip or tibia. Two trained people should apply a traction splint.

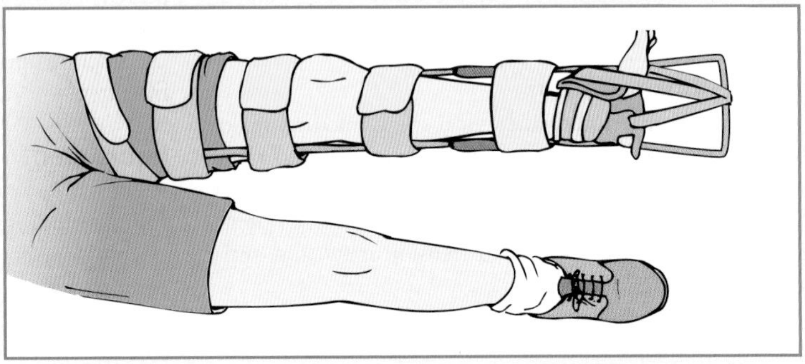

A *spine board,* applied for a suspected spinal fracture, is a rigid splint that supports the injured person's entire body. Three people should apply a spine board.

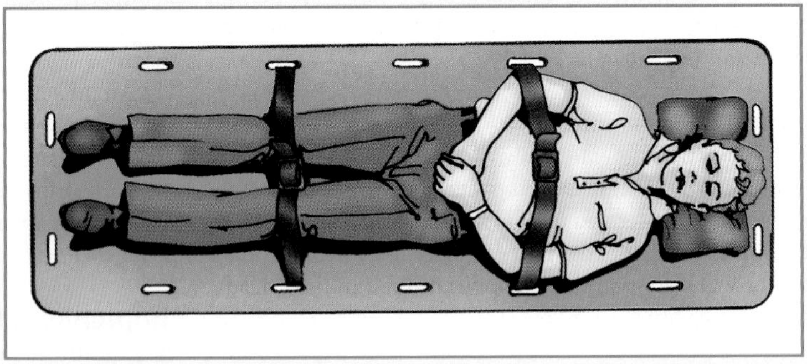

■ Remove or cut away clothing from the injury site, if necessary. Check neurovascular integrity distal to the site. Explain the procedure to the patient *to allay his fears.*

■ If an obvious bone misalignment causes the patient acute distress or severe neurovascular problems, align the extremity in its normal anatomic position, if possible. Stop, however, if this causes further neurovascular deterioration. Don't try to straighten a dislocation *to avoid damaging displaced vessels and nerves.* Also, don't attempt reduction of a contaminated bone end *because this may cause additional laceration of soft tissues, vessels, and nerves as well as gross contamination of deep tissues.*

■ Choose a splint that will immobilize the joints above and below the fracture; pad the splint as necessary *to protect bony prominences.*

Applying a rigid splint

■ Support the injured extremity and apply firm, gentle traction.
■ Have an assistant place the splint under, beside, or on top of the extremity, as ordered.
■ Tell the assistant to apply the bindings *to secure the splint.* Don't let them obstruct circulation.

Applying a spine board

■ Pad the spine board carefully, especially the areas that will support the lumbar region and knees, *to prevent uneven pressure and discomfort.*
■ If the patient is lying on his back, place one hand on each side of his head and apply gentle traction to the head and neck, keeping the head aligned with the body. Have one assistant logroll the patient onto his side while another slides the spine board under the patient. Then instruct the assistants to roll the patient onto the board while you maintain traction and alignment.
■ If the patient is prone, logroll him onto the board so he ends up in a supine position.
■ *To maintain body alignment,* use strips of cloth to secure the patient on the spine board; *to keep head and neck aligned,* place sandbags or rolled towels or clothing on both sides of his head.

Applying a traction splint

■ Place the splint beside the injured leg. (Never use a traction splint on an arm *because the major axillary plexus of nerves and blood vessels can't tolerate countertraction.*) Adjust the splint to the correct length, and then open and adjust the Velcro straps.
■ Have an assistant keep the leg motionless while you pad the ankle and foot and fasten the ankle hitch around them. (You may leave the shoe on.)
■ Tell the assistant to lift and support the leg at the injury site as you apply firm, gentle traction.
■ While you maintain traction, tell the assistant to slide the splint under the leg, pad the groin *to avoid excessive pressure on external genitalia,* and gently apply the ischial strap.
■ Have the assistant connect the loops of the ankle hitch to the end of the splint.
■ Adjust the splint to apply enough traction to secure the leg comfortably in the corrected position.
■ After applying traction, fasten the Velcro support splints *to secure the leg closely to the splint.*

Using an air splint

In an emergency, an air splint can be applied to immobilize a fracture or control bleeding, especially from a forearm or lower leg. This compact, comfortable splint is made of double-walled plastic and provides gentle, diffuse pressure over an injured area. The appropriate splint is chosen, wrapped around the affected extremity, secured with Velcro or other strips, and then inflated. The fit should be snug enough to immobilize the extremity without impairing circulation.

An air splint (shown below) may actually control bleeding better than a local pressure bandage. Its clear plastic construction simplifies inspection of the affected site for bleeding, pallor, or cyanosis. An air splint also allows the patient to be moved without further damage to the injured limb.

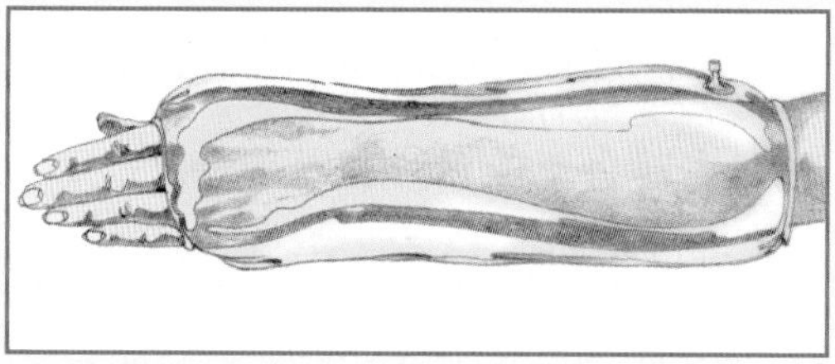

NURSING ALERT *Don't use a traction splint for a severely angulated femur or knee fracture.*

Special considerations

■ At the scene of an accident, always examine the patient completely for other injuries. Avoid unnecessary movement or manipulation, *which might cause additional pain or injury.*
■ Always consider the possibility of cervical injury in an unconscious patient. If possible, apply the splint before repositioning the patient.
■ If the patient requires a rigid splint but one isn't available, use another body part as a splint. To splint a leg in this manner, pad its inner aspect and secure it to the other leg with roller gauze or cloth strips.
■ After applying any type of splint, monitor vital signs frequently *because bleeding in fractured bones and surrounding tissues may cause shock.* Also monitor the neurovascular status of the fractured limb by assessing skin color and checking for numbness in the fingers or toes. *Numbness or paral-*

Assessing neurovascular status

When assessing an injured extremity, include the following steps, and compare your findings bilaterally:

- Inspect the color of fingers or toes.
- *To detect edema,* note the size of the digits.
- Simultaneously touch the digits of the affected and unaffected extremities and compare temperature.
- Check capillary refill by pressing on the distal tip of one digit until it's white. Then release the pressure and note how soon the normal color returns. It should return quickly in both the affected and unaffected extremities.
- Check sensation by touching the fingers or toes and asking the patient how they feel. Note reports of any numbness or tingling.
- *To check proprioception,* tell the patient to close his eyes; then move one digit and ask him which position it's in.
- *To test movement,* tell the patient to wiggle his toes or move his fingers.
- Palpate the distal pulses *to assess vascular patency.*

Record your findings for the affected and the unaffected extremities, using standard terminology to avoid ambiguity. Warmth, free movement, rapid capillary refill, and normal color, sensation, and proprioception indicate sound neurovascular status.

ysis distal to the injury indicates pressure on nerves. (See *Assessing neurovascular status.*)

- Transport the patient to a hospital as soon as possible. Apply ice to the injury. Regardless of the apparent extent of the injury, don't allow the patient to eat or drink anything until the practitioner evaluates him.
- Indications for removing a splint include evidence of improper application or vascular impairment. Apply gentle traction, and remove the splint carefully under a practitioner's direct supervision.

Complications

Multiple transfers and repeated manipulation of a fracture may result in fat embolism, indicated by shortness of breath, agitation, and irrational behavior. This complication usually occurs 24 to 72 hours after injury or manipulation.

Documentation

Record the circumstances and cause of the injury. Document the patient's complaints, noting whether symptoms are localized. Record neurovascular status before and after applying the splint. Note the type of wound and the amount and type of drainage, if any. Document the time of splint application. If the bone end should slip into surrounding tissue or if transportation causes any change in the degree of dislocation, be sure to note it.

Selected references

Bong, M., et al. "A Comparison of Immediate Post-Reduction Splinting Constructs for Controlling Initial Displacement of Fractures of the Distal Radius: A Prospective Randomized Study of Long Arm Versus Short Arm Splinting," *Journal of Hand Surgery* 31(5):766-70, May-June 2006.

Borschneck, A. "Traction Splint: Proper Splint Design and Application Are the Keys," *Journal of Emergency Medical Services* 29(8):70, 72-75, August 2004.

Burton, J., et al. "A Statewide Prehospital Emergency Medical Service Selective Patient Spine Immobilization Protocol," *Journal of Trauma-Injury Infection and Critical Care* 61(1):161-67, July 2006.

Del Rossi, G., et al. "Spine Board Transfer Techniques and the Unstable Cervical Spine," *Spine* 29(7):E134-E138, April 2004.

Lee, C., et al. "Prehospital Management of Lower Limb Fracture," *Emergency Medicine Journal* 22(9):660-63, September 2005.

Russ, S., et al. "Patterns and Risks in Spinal Trauma: The Emergency Transport Perspective," *Archives of Disease in Childhood* 90(9):985, September 2005.

Smeltzer, S.C., et al. *Brunner & Suddarth's Textbook of Medical-Surgical Nursing,* 11th ed. Philadelphia: Lippincott Williams & Wilkins, 2008.

CAST PREPARATION

A cast is a hard mold that encases a body part, usually an extremity, to provide immobilization without discomfort. It can be used to treat injuries (including fractures), correct orthopedic conditions (such as deformities), or promote healing after general or plastic surgery, amputation, or nerve and vascular repair.

Casts may be constructed of plaster, fiberglass, or other synthetic materials. Plaster, a commonly used material, is inexpensive, nontoxic, nonflammable, easy to mold, and rarely causes allergic reactions or skin irritation. However, fiberglass is lighter, stronger, and more resilient than plaster. Because fiberglass dries rapidly, it's more difficult to mold, but it can bear body weight immediately if needed. (See *Types of cylindrical casts.*)

EQUIPMENT

Types of cylindrical casts

Made of plaster, fiberglass, or synthetic material, casts may be applied almost anywhere on the body—to support a single finger or the entire body. Common casts are shown below.

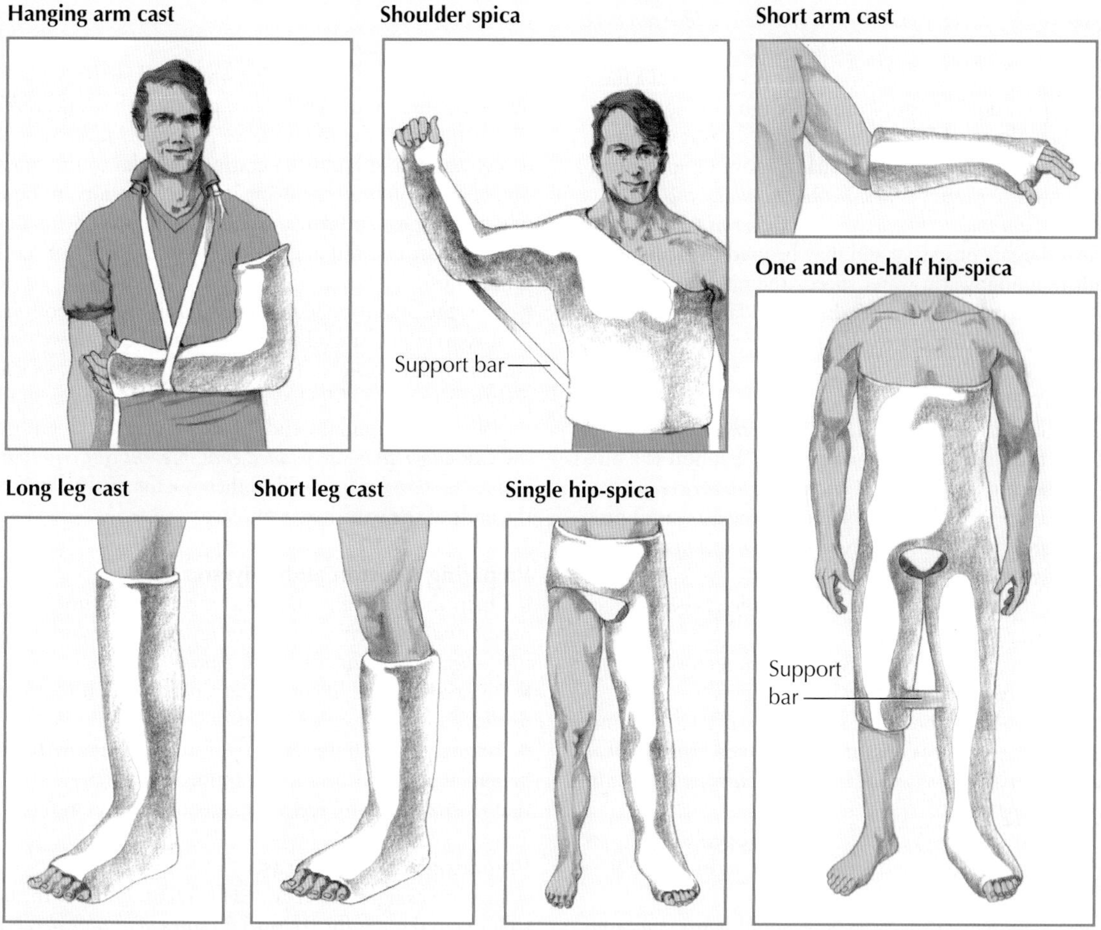

Typically, a practitioner applies a cast, and a nurse prepares the patient and the equipment and assists during the procedure. With special preparation, a nurse may apply or change a standard cast, but an orthopedist must reduce and set the fracture.

Contraindications for casting may include skin diseases, peripheral vascular disease, diabetes mellitus, open or draining wounds, and susceptibility to skin irritations. However, these aren't strict contraindications; the practitioner must weigh the potential risks and benefits for each patient.

Equipment

Tubular stockinette ▪ casting material ▪ plaster rolls ▪ plaster splints (if necessary) ▪ bucket of water ▪ sink equipped with plaster trap ▪ linen-saver pad ▪ sheet wadding ▪ sponge or felt padding (if necessary) ▪ local anesthetic (if necessary) ▪ pillows or bath blankets ▪ optional: rubber gloves, cast stand.

Gather the tubular stockinette, cast material, and plaster splints in the appropriate sizes. Tubular stockinettes range from 2″ to 12″ (5 to 30.5 cm) wide; plaster rolls, from 2″ to

6″ (5 to 15 cm) wide; and plaster splints, from 3″ to 6″ (7.5 to 15 cm) wide. Wear rubber gloves, especially if applying a fiberglass cast.

Preparation of equipment

Gently squeeze the packaged casting material to make sure the envelopes don't have any air leaks. *Humid air penetrating such leaks can cause plaster to become stale, which can make it set too quickly, form lumps, fail to bond with lower layers, or set as a soft, friable mass.* (Baking a stale plaster roll at a medium temperature for 1 hour can make it usable again.)

Follow the manufacturer's directions for water temperature when preparing plaster. Usually, room temperature or slightly warmer water is best *because it allows the cast to set in about 7 minutes without excessive exothermia.* (Cold water retards the rate of setting and may be used to facilitate difficult molding; warm water speeds the rate of setting and raises skin temperature under the cast.) Place all equipment within the practitioner's reach.

Implementation

- Explain the procedure *to allay the patient's fears.* If plaster is being used, make sure he understands that heat will build under the cast *because of a chemical reaction between the water and plaster.* Also begin explaining some aspects of proper cast care *to prepare him for patient teaching and to assess his knowledge level.*
- Cover the appropriate parts of the patient's bedding and gown with a linen-saver pad.
- If the cast is applied to the wrist or arm, remove rings that may interfere with circulation in the fingers.
- Assess the condition of the skin in the affected area, noting any redness, contusions, or open wounds. *This will make it easier to evaluate any complaints the patient may have after the cast is applied.*
- If the patient has severe contusions or open wounds, prepare him for a local anesthetic if the practitioner will administer one.
- Assess neurovascular status *to establish baseline measurements.* Palpate the distal pulses; assess the color, temperature, and capillary refill of the appropriate fingers or toes; and check neurologic function, including sensation and motion in the affected and unaffected extremities.
- Help the practitioner position the limb, as ordered. (Commonly, the limb is immobilized in the neutral position.)
- Support the limb in the prescribed position while the practitioner applies the tubular stockinette and sheet wadding. The stockinette should extend beyond the ends of the cast *to pad the edges.* (If the patient has an open wound or a severe contusion, the practitioner may not use the stockinette.) He then wraps the limb in sheet wadding, starting at the distal end, and applies extra wadding to the distal and proximal ends of the cast area as well as any points of prominence. As he applies the sheet wadding, check for wrinkles.
- If needed, help the practitioner place an extra layer of sponge or felt padding over the area where the cast scissors will be used.
- Prepare the various cast materials, as ordered.

Preparing a plaster cast

- Place a roll of plaster casting on its end in the bucket of water. Be sure to immerse it completely. When air bubbles stop rising from the roll, remove it, gently squeeze out the excess water, and hand the casting material to the practitioner, who will begin applying it to the extremity. As he applies the first roll, prepare a second roll in the same manner. (Stay at least one roll ahead of the practitioner during the procedure.)
- After the practitioner applies each roll, he'll smooth it to remove wrinkles, spread the plaster into the cloth webbing, and empty air pockets. If he's using plaster splints, he'll apply them in the middle layers of the cast. Before wrapping the last roll, he'll pull the ends of the tubular stockinette over the cast edges *to create padded ends, prevent cast crumbling, and reduce skin irritation.* He'll then use the final roll to keep the ends of the stockinette in place.

Preparing a cotton and polyester cast

- Open these casting materials one roll at a time *because cotton and polyester casting must be applied within 3 minutes—before humidity in the air hardens the tape.*
- Immerse the roll in cold water, and squeeze it four times *to ensure uniform wetness.*
- Remove the dripping material from the bucket. Tell the patient that it will be applied immediately. Forewarn him that the material will feel warm, giving off heat as it sets.

Preparing a fiberglass cast

- If you're using water-activated fiberglass, immerse the tape rolls in tepid water for 10 to 15 minutes *to initiate the chemical reaction that causes the cast to harden.* Open one roll at a time. Avoid squeezing out excess water before application.
- If you're using light-cured fiberglass, you can unroll the material more slowly. This casting remains soft and malleable until it's exposed to ultraviolet light, which sets it.

Completing the cast

- As necessary, "petal" the cast's edges *to reduce roughness and to cushion pressure points.* (See *How to petal a cast.*)
- Use a cast stand or your palm to support the cast in the therapeutic position until it becomes firm to the touch (usually 6 to 8 minutes).

■ *To check circulation in the casted limb,* palpate the distal pulse and assess the color, temperature, and capillary refill of the fingers or toes. Determine neurologic status by asking the patient if he's experiencing paresthesia in the extremity or decreased motion of the extremity's uncovered joints. Assess the unaffected extremity in the same manner and compare findings.

■ Elevate the limb above heart level with pillows or bath blankets, as ordered, *to facilitate venous return and reduce edema.* Make sure pressure is evenly distributed under the cast *to prevent molding.*

■ The practitioner will then order X-rays *to ensure proper positioning.*

■ Instruct the patient to notify the practitioner of any pain, foul odor, drainage, or burning sensation under the cast. (After the cast hardens, the practitioner may cut a window in it to inspect the painful or burning area.)

■ Pour water from the plaster bucket into a sink containing a plaster trap. Don't use a regular sink *because plaster will block the plumbing.*

Special considerations

■ A fiberglass cast dries immediately after application. A plaster extremity cast dries in approximately 24 to 48 hours; a plaster spica or body cast, in 48 to 72 hours. During this drying period, the cast must be properly positioned *to prevent a surface depression that could cause pressure areas or dependent edema.* Neurovascular status must be assessed, drainage monitored, and the condition of the cast checked periodically.

■ After the cast dries completely, it looks white and shiny and no longer feels damp or soft. Care consists of monitoring for changes in the drainage pattern, preventing skin breakdown near the cast, and averting the complications of immobility.

■ Patient teaching must begin immediately after the cast is applied and should continue until the patient or a family member can care for the cast.

■ Never use the bed or a table to support the cast as it sets *because molding can result, causing pressure necrosis of underlying tissue.* Also, don't use rubber- or plastic-covered pillows before the cast hardens *because they can trap heat under the cast.*

■ If a cast is applied after surgery or traumatic injury, remember that the most accurate way to assess for bleeding is to monitor vital signs. A visible blood spot on the cast can be misleading: One drop of blood can produce a circle 3″ (7.6 cm) in diameter.

■ Casts may need to be opened to assess underlying skin and pulses, or to relieve pressure in a specific area. In a windowed cast, a specific area is cut out to allow inspection of underlying skin or relieve pressure. A bivalved cast is split medially and laterally, creating anterior and posterior sections. One of the sections may be removed to relieve pressure while the remaining section maintains immobilization.

■ The practitioner usually removes the cast at the appropriate time, with a nurse assisting. (See *Removing a plaster*

EQUIPMENT

How to petal a cast

Rough cast edges can be cushioned by petaling them with adhesive tape or moleskin. To do this, first cut several 4″× 4″ (10 × 5 cm) strips. Round off one end of each strip to keep it from curling. Then, making sure the rounded end of the strip is on the outside of the cast, tuck the straight end just inside the cast edge.

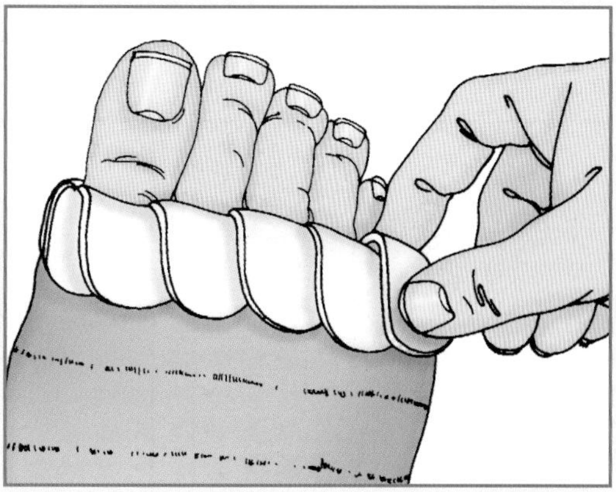

Smooth the moleskin with your finger until you're sure it's secured inside and out. Repeat the procedure, overlapping the moleskin pieces until you've gone all the way around the cast edge.

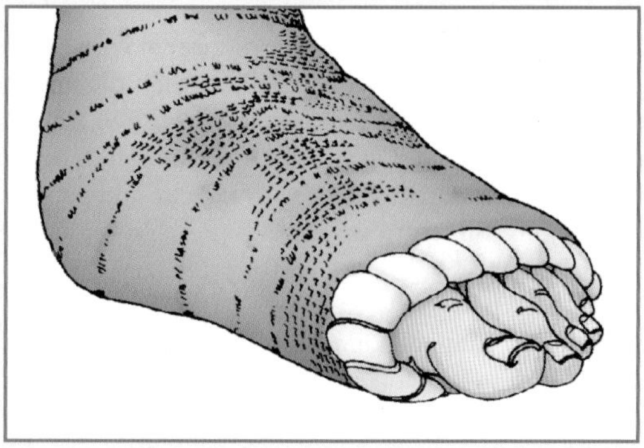

Removing a plaster cast

Typically, a cast is removed when a fracture heals or requires further manipulation. Less common indications include cast damage, a pressure ulcer under the cast, excessive drainage or bleeding, and a constrictive cast.

Explain the procedure to the patient. Tell him he'll feel some heat and vibration as the cast is split with the cast saw. If the patient is a child, tell him that the saw is very noisy but won't cut the skin beneath. Warn the patient that when the padding is cut, he'll see discolored skin and signs of poor muscle tone. Reassure him that you'll stay with him. The illustrations below show how a plaster cast is removed.

The practitioner cuts one side of the cast, then the other. As he does so, closely monitor the patient's anxiety level.

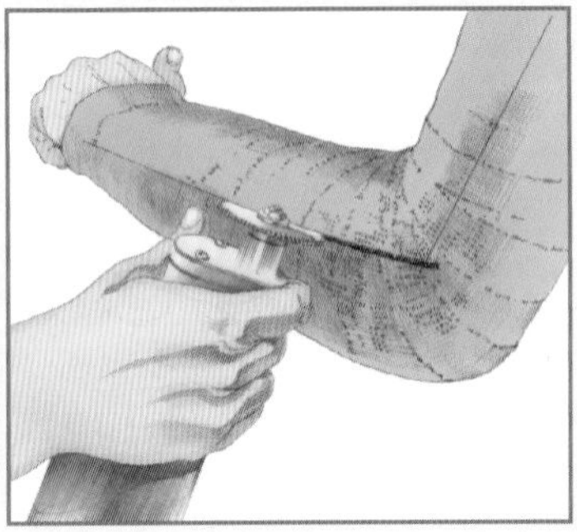

Next, the practitioner opens the cast pieces with a spreader.

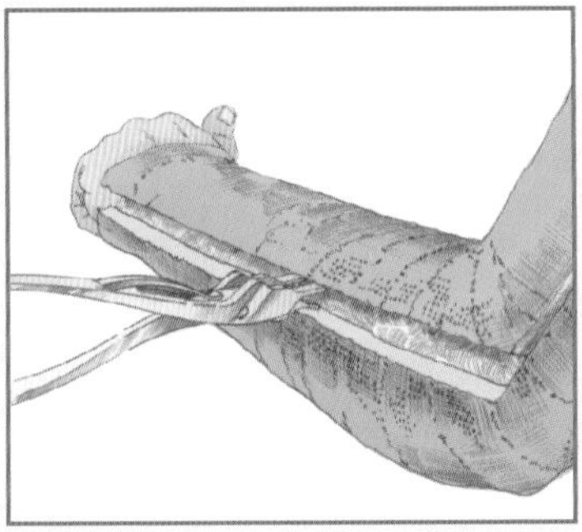

Finally, using cast scissors, the practitioner cuts through the cast padding.

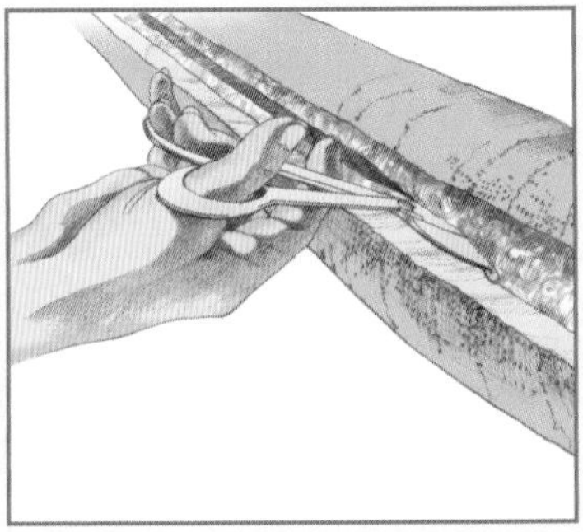

When the cast is removed, provide skin care to remove accumulated dead skin and to begin restoring the extremity's normal appearance.

cast.) Tell the patient that when the cast is removed, his casted limb will appear thinner and flabbier than the uncasted limb. In addition, his skin will appear yellowish or gray from the accumulated dead skin and oils from the glands near the skin surface. Reassure him that with exercise and good skin care, his limb will return to normal.

Home care

Before the patient goes home, teach him how to care for his cast. Tell him to keep the casted limb elevated above heart level to minimize swelling. Raise a casted leg by having the patient lie in a supine position with his leg on top of pillows. Prop a casted arm so that the hand and elbow are higher than the shoulder.

Instruct the patient to call the practitioner if he can't move his fingers or toes, if he has numbness or tingling in the affected limb, or if he has symptoms of infection such as fever, unusual pain, or a foul odor from the cast. Advise him to maintain muscle strength by continuing any recommended exercises.

If the cast needs repair (if it loosens and slips) or if the patient has any questions about cast care, advise him to notify his practitioner. Warn him not to get the cast wet. *Moisture will weaken or destroy it.* If the practitioner approves, tell the patient he may cover the cast with a plastic bag or cast cover for showering or bathing.

Urge the patient not to insert anything (such as a back scratcher or powder) into the cast to relieve itching. *Foreign matter can damage the skin and cause an infection.* Tell him, though, that he can apply alcohol on the skin at the cast edges. Warn the patient not to chip, crush, cut, or otherwise break any area of the cast and not to bear weight on the cast unless instructed to do so by the practitioner.

If the patient must use crutches, instruct him to remove throw rugs from the floor and to rearrange furniture to reduce the risk of tripping and falling. If the patient has a cast on his dominant arm, he may need help with bathing, toileting, eating, and dressing.

Complications

Complications of improper cast application include compartment syndrome, palsy, paresthesia, ischemia, ischemic myositis, pressure necrosis and, eventually, misalignment or nonunion of fractured bones.

Documentation

Record the date and time of cast application and skin condition of the extremity before the cast was applied. Note any contusions, redness, or open wounds; results of neurovascular checks, before and after application, for the affected and unaffected extremities; location of any special devices, such as felt pads or plaster splints; and any patient teaching provided.

Selected references

Smeltzer, S.C., et al. *Brunner & Suddarth's Textbook of Medical-Surgical Nursing,* 11th ed. Philadelphia: Lippincott Williams & Wilkins, 2008.

Smith, G., et al. "Fiberglass Cast Application," *American Journal of Emergency Medicine* 23(3): 347-50, May 2005.

TRACTION AND FIXATION

MECHANICAL TRACTION

Mechanical traction exerts a pulling force on a part of the body—usually the spine, pelvis, or long bones of the arms and legs. It can be used to reduce fractures, treat dislocations, correct or prevent deformities, improve or correct contractures, or decrease muscle spasms. Depending on the injury or condition, an orthopedist may order either skin or skeletal traction.

Applied directly to the skin and thus indirectly to the bone, skin traction is ordered when a light, temporary, or noncontinuous pulling force is required. Contraindications for skin traction include a severe injury with open wounds, an allergy to tape or other skin traction equipment, circulatory disturbances, dermatitis, and varicose veins.

In skeletal traction, an orthopedist inserts a pin or wire through the bone and attaches the traction equipment to the pin or wire to exert a direct, constant, longitudinal pulling force. Indications for skeletal traction include fractures of the tibia, femur, and humerus. Infections such as osteomyelitis contraindicate skeletal traction.

Nursing responsibilities for this procedure include setting up the traction frame. (See *Traction frames,* page 766.) The design of the patient's bed usually dictates whether to use a claw clamp or I.V.-post-type frame. (The claw-type Balkan frame is rarely used.) Setup of the specific traction can be done by a nurse with special skills, an orthopedic technician, or the practitioner. Instructions for setting up these traction units usually accompany the equipment.

After the patient is placed in the specific type of traction ordered by the orthopedist, the nurse is responsible for preventing complications from immobility; for routinely inspecting the equipment; for adding traction weights, as ordered; and, in patients with skeletal traction, for monitoring the pin insertion sites for signs of infection. (See *Comparing types of traction,* page 767.)

Equipment

For a claw-type basic frame: 102" (260-cm) plain bar ▪ two 66" (170-cm) swivel-clamp bars ▪ two upper-panel clamps ▪ two lower-panel clamps.

For an I.V.-type basic frame: 102" plain bar ▪ 27" (70-cm) double-clamp bar ▪ 48" (122-cm) swivel-clamp bar ▪ two 36" (92-cm) plain bars ▪ four 4" (10-cm) I.V. posts with clamps ▪ cross clamp.

For an I.V.-type Balkan frame: Two 102" plain bars ▪ two 27" double-clamp bars ▪ two 48" swivel-clamp bars ▪ five 36" plain bars ▪ four 4" I.V. posts with clamps ▪ eight cross clamps.

For all frame types: Trapeze with clamp ▪ wall bumper or roller.

For skeletal traction care: Sterile cotton-tipped applicators ▪ prescribed antiseptic solution ▪ sterile gauze pads ▪ antimicrobial solution ▪ optional: antimicrobial ointment.

Preparation of equipment

Arrange with central supply or the appropriate department to have the traction equipment transported to the patient's room on a traction cart. If appropriate, gather the equipment for pin-site care at the patient's bedside. Pin-site care protocols may vary with each hospital or practitioner.

Implementation

- Confirm the patient's identity using two patient identifiers according to your facility's policy.
- Explain the purpose of traction to the patient. Emphasize the importance of maintaining proper body alignment after the traction equipment is set up.

Setting up a claw-type basic frame

- Attach one lower-panel and one upper-panel clamp to each 66" swivel-clamp bar.
- Fasten one bar to the footboard and one to the headboard by turning the clamp knobs clockwise until they're tight and

EQUIPMENT

Traction frames

You may encounter three types of traction frames, as described here.

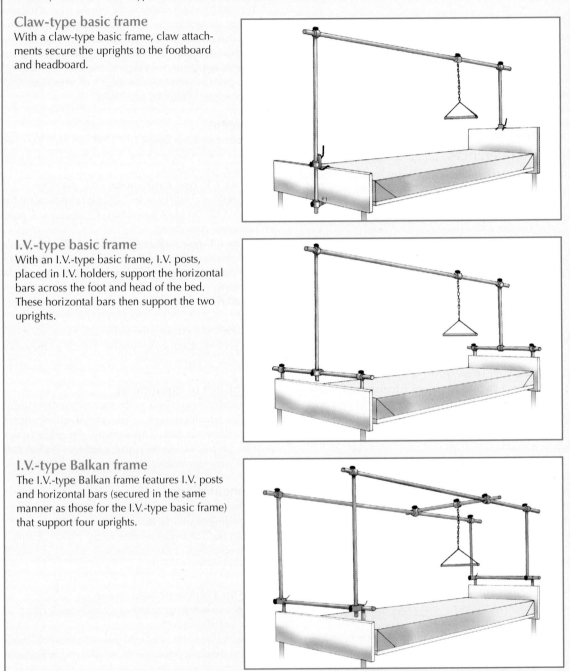

Claw-type basic frame

With a claw-type basic frame, claw attachments secure the uprights to the footboard and headboard.

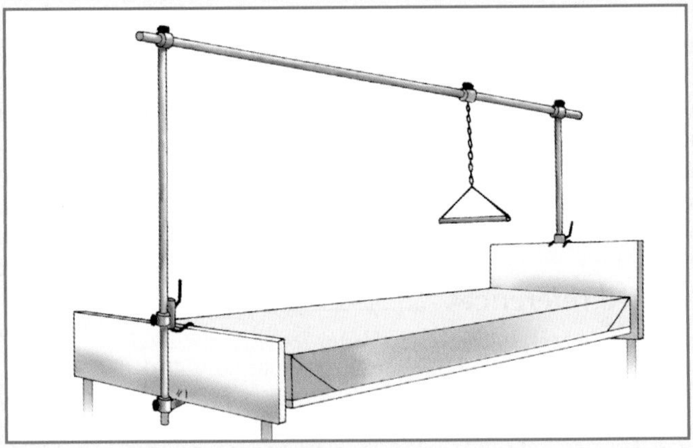

I.V.-type basic frame

With an I.V.-type basic frame, I.V. posts, placed in I.V. holders, support the horizontal bars across the foot and head of the bed. These horizontal bars then support the two uprights.

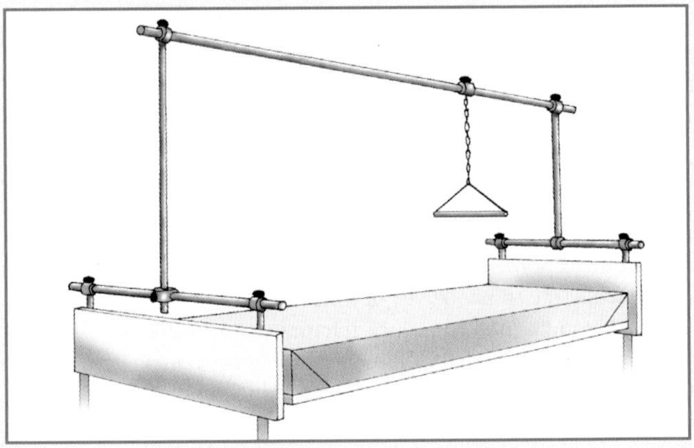

I.V.-type Balkan frame

The I.V.-type Balkan frame features I.V. posts and horizontal bars (secured in the same manner as those for the I.V.-type basic frame) that support four uprights.

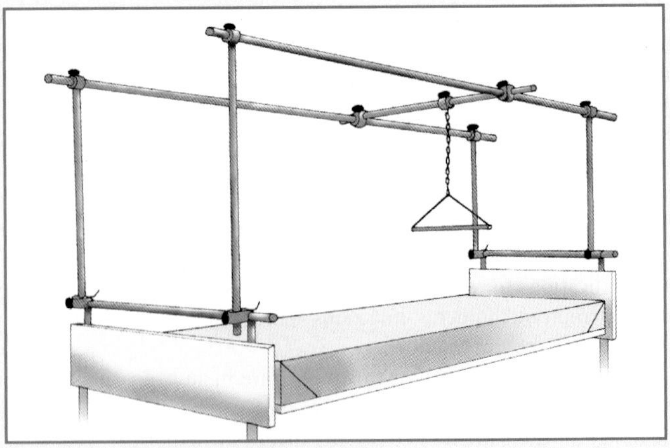

EQUIPMENT

Comparing types of traction

Traction restricts movement of a patient's affected limb or body part and may confine the patient to bed rest for an extended period. The limb is immobilized by pulling with equal force on each end of the injured area—an equal mix of traction and countertraction. Weights provide the pulling force. Countertraction is produced by using other weights or by positioning the patient's body weight against the traction pull.

Skin traction

Skin traction immobilizes a body part intermittently over an extended period through direct application of a pulling force on the skin. The force may be applied using adhesive or nonadhesive traction tape or other skin traction devices, such as a boot, belt, or halter.

Adhesive attachment allows more continuous traction, whereas nonadhesive attachment allows easier removal for daily skin care.

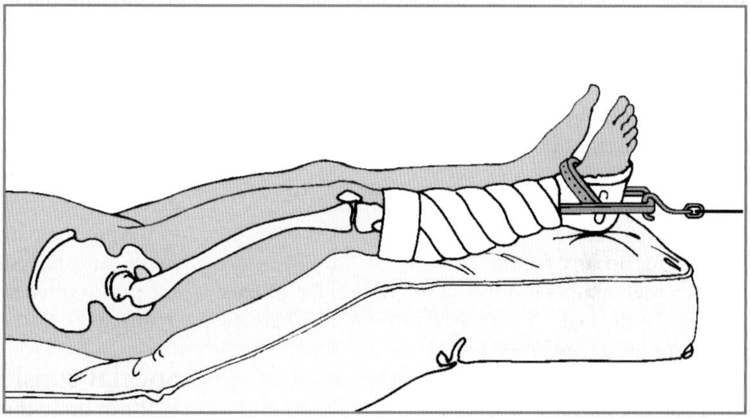

Skeletal traction

Skeletal traction immobilizes a body part for prolonged periods by attaching weighted equipment directly to the patient's bones. This may be accomplished with pins, screws, wires, or tongs. The amount of weight applied is determined by body size and the extent of the injury.

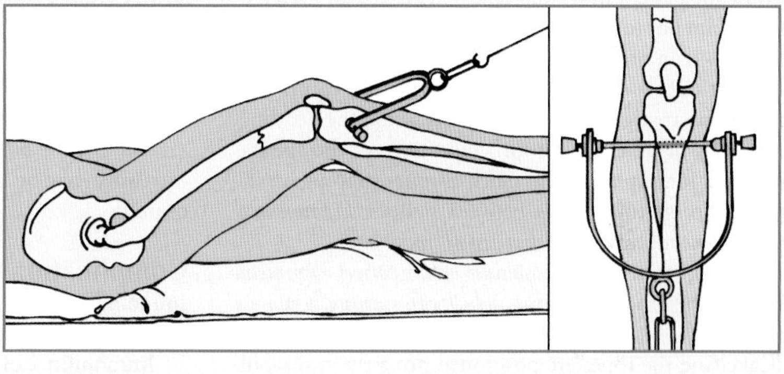

then pulling back on the upper clamp's rubberized bar until it's tight.

- Secure the 102″ horizontal plain bar atop the two vertical bars, making sure that the clamp knobs point up.
- Using the appropriate clamp, attach the trapeze to the horizontal bar about 2′ (60 cm) from the head of the bed.

Setting up an I.V.-type basic frame

- Attach one 4″ I.V. post with clamp to each end of both 36″ horizontal plain bars.
- Secure an I.V. post in each I.V. holder at the bed corners. Using a cross clamp, fasten the 48″ vertical swivel-clamp bar to the middle of the horizontal plain bar at the foot of the bed.
- Fasten the 27″ vertical double-clamp bar to the middle of the horizontal plain bar at the head of the bed.
- Attach the 102″ horizontal plain bar to the tops of the two vertical bars, making sure the clamp knobs point up.
- Using the appropriate clamp, attach the trapeze to the horizontal bar about 2′ from the head of the bed.

Setting up an I.V.-type Balkan frame

- Attach one 4″ I.V. post with clamp to each end of two 36″ horizontal plain bars.
- Secure an I.V. post in each I.V. holder at the bed corners.

■ Attach a 48″ vertical swivel-clamp bar, using a cross clamp, to each I.V. post clamp on the horizontal plain bar at the foot of the bed.
■ Fasten one 36″ horizontal plain bar across the midpoints of the two 48″ swivel-clamp bars, using two cross clamps.
■ Attach a 27″ vertical double-clamp bar to each I.V. post clamp on the horizontal bar at the head of the bed.
■ Using two cross clamps, fasten a 36″ horizontal plain bar across the midpoints of two 27″ double-clamp bars.
■ Clamp a 102″ horizontal plain bar onto the vertical bars on each side of the bed; make sure the clamp knobs point up.
■ Use two cross clamps to attach a 36″ horizontal plain bar across the two overhead bars, about 2′ from the head of the bed.
■ Attach the trapeze to this 36″ horizontal bar.

After setting up any frame

■ Attach a wall bumper or roller to the vertical bar or bars at the head of the bed. *This protects the walls from damage caused by the bed or equipment.*

Caring for the patient in traction

■ Show the patient how much movement he's allowed and instruct him not to readjust the equipment. Also tell him to report any pain or pressure from the traction equipment.
■ At least once a shift, make sure the traction equipment connections are tight and that no parts touch the bedding, the patient, or other inappropriate portions of the apparatus. Check for impingements, such as ropes rubbing on the footboard or getting caught between pulleys. *Friction and impingement reduce the effectiveness of traction.*
■ Inspect the traction equipment *to ensure correct alignment.*
■ Inspect the ropes for fraying, *which can eventually cause a rope to break.*
■ Make sure the ropes are positioned properly in the pulley track. *An improperly positioned rope changes the degree of traction.*
■ *To prevent tampering and aid stability and security*, make sure all rope ends are taped above the knot.
■ Inspect the equipment regularly to make sure the traction weights hang freely. *Weights that touch the floor, bed, or each other reduce the amount of traction.*
■ About every 2 hours, check the patient for proper body alignment and reposition the patient as necessary. *Misalignment causes ineffective traction and may keep the fracture from healing properly.*
■ *To prevent complications from immobility,* assess neurovascular integrity routinely. The patient's condition, the hospital routine, and the practitioner's orders determine the frequency of neurovascular assessments.
■ Provide skin care, encourage coughing and deep-breathing exercises, and assist with ordered range-of-motion exercises for unaffected extremities. Typically, an order for elastic support stockings is written. Check elimination patterns and provide laxatives, as ordered.
■ For the patient with skeletal traction, make sure the protruding pin or wire ends are covered with cork *to prevent them from tearing the bedding or injuring the patient and staff.*
■ Check the pin site and surrounding skin regularly for signs of infection.
■ If ordered, clean the pin site and surrounding skin. Pin-site care varies, but you'll usually follow guidelines like these: Use sterile technique; avoid digging at pin sites with the cotton-tipped applicator; if ordered, clean the pin site and surrounding skin with a cotton-tipped applicator dipped in ordered antiseptic; if ordered, apply antimicrobial ointment to the pin sites; apply a loose sterile dressing, or dress with sterile gauze pads soaked in antiseptic solution. Perform pin-site care as often as necessary, depending on the amount of drainage.

Special considerations

■ When using skin traction, apply ordered weights slowly and carefully *to avoid jerking the affected extremity.* Arrange the weights so they don't hang over the patient, *to avoid injury in case the ropes break.*
■ When applying Buck's traction, make sure the line of pull is always parallel to the bed and not angled downward *to prevent pressure on the heel.* Placing a flat pillow under the extremity may be helpful as long as it doesn't alter the line of pull.

Complications

Immobility during traction may result in pressure ulcers, osteoporosis, and muscle atrophy, weakness, or contractures.

Immobility can also cause:

■ GI disturbances such as constipation
■ urinary problems, including stasis and calculi
■ respiratory problems, such as stasis of secretions and hypostatic pneumonia
■ circulatory disturbances, including stasis and thrombophlebitis.

Prolonged immobility, especially after traumatic injury, may promote depression or other emotional disturbances. Skeletal traction may cause osteomyelitis originating at the pin or wire sites.

Documentation

In the patient record, document the amount of traction weight used daily, noting the application of additional weights and the patient's tolerance. Document equipment inspec-

EQUIPMENT

Types of external fixation

The physician's selection of an external fixation device depends on the severity of the patient's fracture and on the type of bone alignment needed.

Universal day frame

A universal day frame is used to manage tibial fractures. This frame allows the physician to readjust the position of bony fragments by angulation and rotation. The compression-distraction device allows compression and distraction of bony fragments.

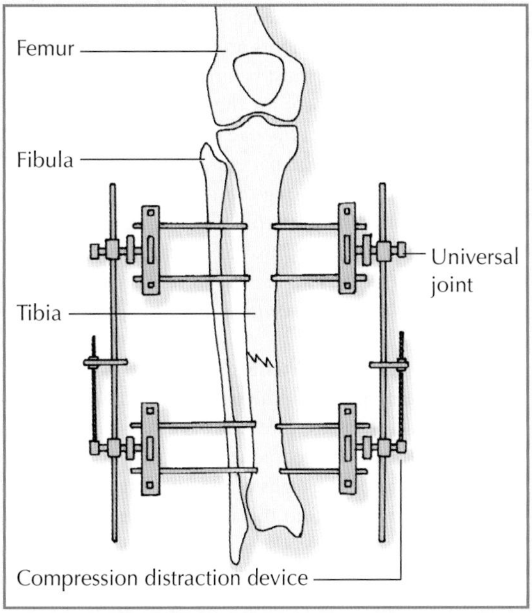

Portsmouth external fixation bar

A Portsmouth external fixation bar is used to manage complicated tibial fractures. The locking nut adjustment on the mobile carriage only allows bone compression, so the physician must accurately reduce bony fragments before applying the device.

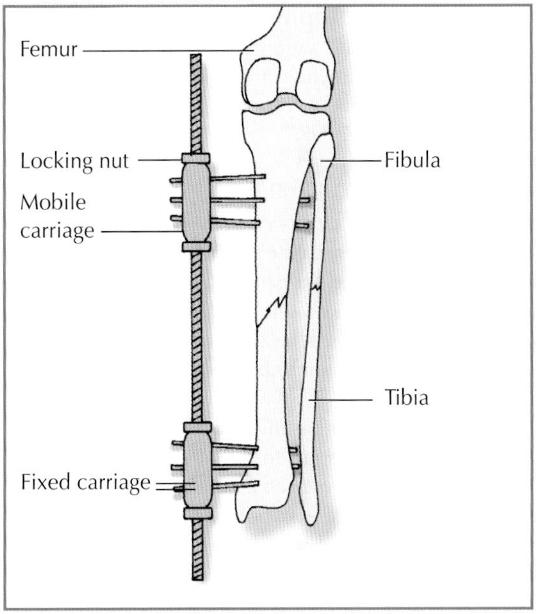

tions and patient care, including routine checks of neurovascular integrity, skin condition, respiratory status, and elimination patterns. If applicable, note the condition of the pin site and any care given.

Selected references

Maher, A.B., et al. *Orthopaedic Nursing,* 3rd ed. Philadelphia: W.B. Saunders Co., 2002.

EXTERNAL FIXATION

In external fixation, a practitioner inserts metal pins and wires through skin and muscle layers into the broken bones and affixes them to an adjustable external frame that maintains their proper alignment during healing. (See *Types of external fixation.*) This procedure is used most commonly to treat open, unstable fractures with extensive soft tissue damage, comminuted closed fractures, and septic, nonunion fractures and to facilitate surgical immobilization of a joint. Specialized types of external fixators may be used to lengthen leg bones or immobilize the cervical spine.

An advantage of external fixation over other immobilization techniques is that it stabilizes the fracture while allowing full visualization and access to open wounds. It also facilitates early ambulation, thus reducing the risk of complications from immobilization.

The Ilizarov fixator is a special type of external fixation device. This device is a combination of rings and tensioned transosseous wires used primarily in limb lengthening, bone transport, and limb salvage. Highly complex, it provides gradual distraction resulting in good-quality bone formation with a minimum of complications.

Equipment

Sterile cotton-tipped applicators ▪ prescribed antiseptic cleaning solution ▪ sterile gauze pads ▪ ice bag ▪ analgesic or opioid ▪ optional: antimicrobial ointment.

Equipment varies with the type of fixator and the type and location of the fracture. Typically, sets of pins, stabilizing rods, and clips are available from manufacturers. Don't reuse pins.

Preparation of equipment

Make sure the external fixation set includes all the equipment it's supposed to include and that the equipment has been sterilized according to your facility's procedure.

Implementation

- Confirm the patient's identity using two patient identifiers according to your facility's policy.
- Explain the procedure to the patient *to reduce his anxiety.* Assure him that he'll feel little pain after the fixation device is in place and that he'll be able to adjust to the apparatus.
- Tell the patient that he'll be able to move about with the apparatus in place, which may help him resume normal activities more quickly.
- After the fixation device is in place, perform neurovascular checks every 2 to 4 hours for 24 hours, then every 4 to 8 hours, as appropriate, *to assess for possible neurologic damage.* Assess color, motion, sensation, digital movement, edema, capillary refill, and pulses of the affected extremity. Compare with the unaffected side.
- Apply an ice bag to the surgical site, as ordered, *to reduce swelling, relieve pain, and lessen bleeding.*
- Administer analgesics or opioids, as ordered, before exercising or mobilizing the affected extremity *to promote comfort.*
- Monitor the patient for pain not relieved by analgesics or opioids and for burning, tingling, or numbness, *which may indicate nerve damage or circulatory impairment.*
- Elevate the affected extremity, if appropriate, *to minimize edema.*
- Perform pin-site care, as ordered, *to prevent infection.* Pin-site care varies, but you'll usually follow guidelines such as these: Use sterile technique; avoid digging at pin sites with the cotton-tipped applicator; if ordered, clean the pin site and surrounding skin with a cotton-tipped applicator dipped in ordered antiseptic solution; if ordered, apply an antimicrobial ointment to the pin sites; apply a loose sterile dressing, or dress with sterile gauze pads soaked in antimicrobial solution. Perform pin-site care as often as necessary, depending on the amount of drainage.
- Also check for redness, tenting of the skin, prolonged or purulent drainage from the pin site, swelling, elevated body or pin-site temperature, and any bowing or bending of pins, which may stress the skin.

For the patient with an Ilizarov fixator

- When the device has been placed and preliminary calluses have begun to form at the insertion sites (in 5 to 7 days), gentle distraction is initiated by turning the appropriate screws one-quarter turn (1 mm) every 4 to 6 hours, as ordered.
- Teach the patient that he must be consistent in turning the screws every 4 to 6 hours around the clock. Make sure he understands that he must be strongly committed to compliance with the protocol for the procedure to be successful. *Because the treatment period may be prolonged (4 to 10 months),* discuss with the patient and family members the psychological effects of long-term care.
- Don't administer nonsteroidal anti-inflammatory drugs (NSAIDs) to patients who are being treated with the Ilizarov Fixator. *NSAIDs may decrease the necessary inflammation caused by the distraction, resulting in delayed bone formation.*

Special considerations

- Before discharge, teach the patient and family members how to provide pin-site care. This is a sterile procedure in the hospital, but clean technique can be used at home. Teach them how to recognize signs of pin-site infection.
- Tell the patient to keep the affected limb elevated when sitting or lying down.
- Encourage the patient to stop smoking and provide smoking cessation materials *because smoking delays bone healing.*

Complications

Complications of external fixation include:

- loosening of pins and loss of fracture stabilization
- infection of the pin tract or wound
- skin breakdown
- nerve damage
- muscle impingement.

Ilizarov fixator pin sites are more prone to infection *because of the extended treatment period and because of the pins' movement to accomplish distraction.* The pins are also more likely to break *because of their small diameter.* Also, the large number of pins used increases the patient's risk of neurovascular compromise.

EQUIPMENT

Types of internal fixation devices

Choice of a specific internal fixation device depends on the location, type, and configuration of the fracture.

In trochanteric or subtrochanteric fractures, the surgeon may use a hip pin or nail, with or without a screw plate. A pin or plate with extra nails stabilizes the fracture by impacting the bone ends at the fracture site.

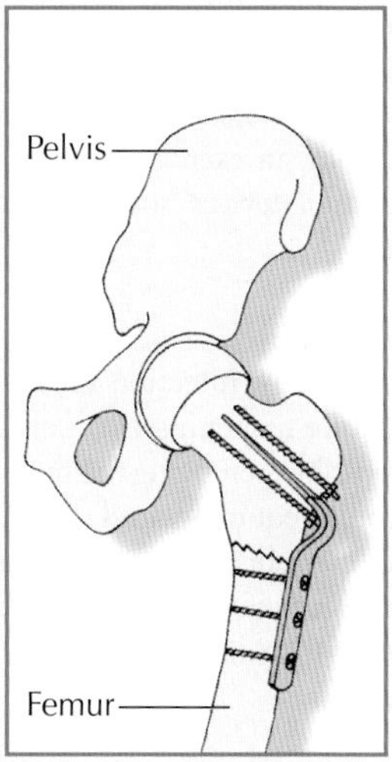

In an uncomplicated fracture of the femoral shaft, the surgeon may use an intramedullary rod. This device permits early ambulation with partial weight bearing.

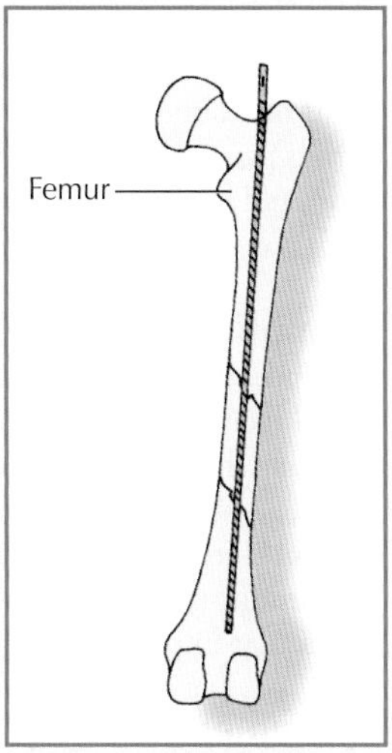

Another choice for fixation of a long-bone fracture is a screw plate, shown here on the tibia.

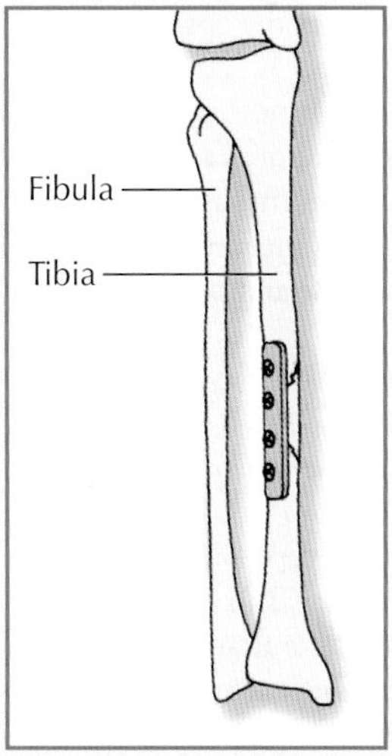

In an arm fracture, the surgeon may fix the involved bones with a plate, rod, or nail. Most radial and ulnar fractures may be fixed with plates, whereas humeral fractures are commonly fixed with rods.

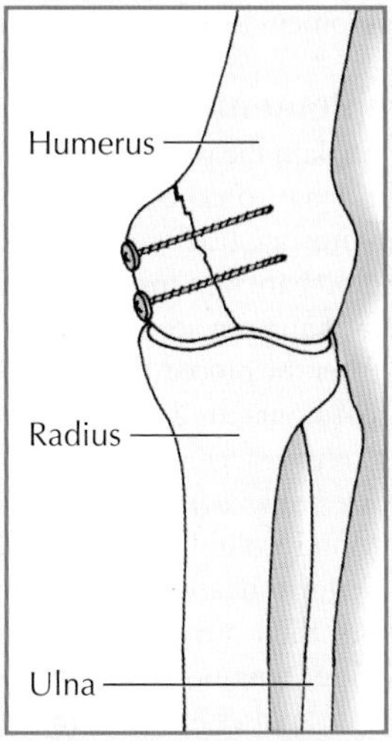

Documentation

Assess and document the condition of the pin sites and skin. Document the patient's reaction to the apparatus and to ambulation as well as his understanding of teaching instructions.

Selected references

Holmes, S.B., et al. "Skeletal Pin Site Care: National Association of Orthopaedic Nurses Guidelines for Orthopaedic Nursing," *Orthopaedic Nursing* 24(2):99-102, March-April 2005.

Maher, A.B., et al. *Orthopaedic Nursing,* 3rd ed. Philadelphia: W.B. Saunders Co., 2002.

Patterson, H. "Impact of External Fixation on Adolescents: An Integrative Research Review," *Orthopaedic Nursing* 25(5):300-308, September-October 2006.

U.S. National Library of Medicine and National Institute of Health. "External Fixation Device," Medline Plus-Medical Encyclopedia. Last updated June 10, 2005. Available at *http://medlineplus.gov/*.

INTERNAL FIXATION

In internal fixation, also known as surgical reduction or open reduction–internal fixation, the physician implants fixation devices—using no external framework—to stabilize the fracture. Internal fixation devices include nails, screws, pins, wires, and rods, all of which may be used in combination with metal plates. These devices remain in the body indefinitely unless the patient experiences adverse reactions after the healing process is complete. (See *Types of internal fixation devices.*)

Internal fixation is typically used to treat fractures of the face and jaw, spine, arm or leg bones, and fractures involving a joint (most commonly, the hip). Internal fixation permits earlier mobilization and can shorten hospitalization, particularly in elderly patients with hip fractures.

Equipment

Ice bag ▪ pain medication (analgesic or opioid) ▪ incentive spirometer ▪ compression stockings.

Patients with leg fractures may also need the following: overhead frame with trapeze ▪ pressure-relief mattress ▪ crutches or walker ▪ pillow (hip fractures may require abductor pillows).

Preparation of equipment

Equipment is collected and prepared in the operating room.

Implementation

- Explain the procedure to the patient *to allay his fears.* Tell him what to expect during postoperative assessment and monitoring, teach him how to use an incentive spirometer, and prepare him for proposed exercise and progressive ambulation regimens if necessary.
- After the procedure, monitor the patient's vital signs every 2 to 4 hours for 24 hours, then every 4 to 8 hours, according to your facility's protocol. *Changes in vital signs may indicate hemorrhage or infection.*
- Monitor fluid intake and output every 4 to 8 hours.
- Perform neurovascular checks every 2 to 4 hours for 24 hours, then every 4 to 8 hours as appropriate. Assess color, motion, sensation, digital movement, edema, capillary refill, and pulses of the affected area. Compare findings with the unaffected side.
- Apply an ice bag to the operative site, as ordered, *to reduce swelling, relieve pain, and lessen bleeding.*
- Administer opioids, as ordered, before exercising or mobilizing the affected area *to promote comfort.* If the patient is using patient-controlled analgesia, instruct him to administer a dose before exercising or mobilizing.
- Monitor the patient for pain unrelieved by opioids and for burning, tingling, or numbness, *which may indicate infection or impaired circulation.*
- Elevate the affected limb on a pillow, if appropriate, *to minimize edema.*
- Check surgical dressings for excessive drainage or bleeding. Also check the incision site for signs of infection, such as erythema, drainage, edema, and unusual pain.
- Assist and encourage the patient to perform range-of-motion and other muscle strengthening exercises, as ordered, *to promote circulation, improve muscle tone, and maintain joint function.*
- Teach the patient to perform progressive ambulation and mobilization using an overhead frame with trapeze, or crutches or a walker, as appropriate.
- Continue anticoagulant therapy, as ordered by the practitioner.
- Teach the patient signs and symptoms of venous thromboembolism.

Special considerations

- *To avoid the complications of immobility after surgery,* have the patient use an incentive spirometer. Apply compression stockings, as appropriate. The patient may also require a pressure-relief mattress.

Home care

Before discharge, teach the patient and family members how to care for the incision site and recognize signs and symptoms of wound infection. Also teach them about administering pain medication, practicing an exercise regimen (if any), and using assistive ambulation devices (such as crutches or a walker), if appropriate.

Complications

Wound infection and, more critically, infection involving metal fixation devices may require reopening the incision, draining the suture line and, possibly, removing the fixation device. Any such infection would require wound dressings and antibiotic therapy. Other complications may include malunion, nonunion, fat or pulmonary embolism, neurovascular impairment, and chronic pain.

Documentation

In the patient record, document perioperative findings on cardiovascular, respiratory, and neurovascular status. Note which pain management techniques were used. Describe wound appearance and alignment of the affected bone. Note the patient's response to teaching about appropriate exercise, care of the infection site, use of assistive devices (if appropriate), and symptoms that should be reported to the practitioner.

Selected references

Geerts, W.H., et al. "Seventh AACP Conference on Antithrombotic and Thrombolytic Therapy: Prevention of Venous Thromboembolism," *Chest* 126(3Suppl):338S-400S, September 2004.

Maher, A.B., et al. *Orthopaedic Nursing,* 3rd ed. Philadelphia: W.B. Saunders Co., 2002.

OTHER ORTHOPEDIC PROCEDURES

STUMP AND PROSTHESIS CARE

Patient care directly after limb amputation includes wound healing, pain control, reducing edema, and stump shaping and conditioning. Postoperative care of the stump will vary slightly, depending on the amputation site (arm or leg) and the type of dressing applied to the stump (elastic bandage or plaster cast).

After the stump heals, it requires only routine daily care, such as proper hygiene and continued muscle-strengthening exercises. The prosthesis—when in use—also requires daily care. Typically, a plastic prosthesis, the most common type, must be cleaned and lubricated and checked for proper fit. As the patient recovers from the physical and psychological trauma of amputation, he will need to learn correct procedures for routine daily care of the stump and the prosthesis.

Equipment

For postoperative stump care: Pressure dressing ▪ abdominal (ABD) pad ▪ suction equipment, if ordered ▪ overhead trapeze ▪ 1″ adhesive tape, bandage clips, or safety pins ▪ sandbags or trochanter roll (for a leg) ▪ elastic stump shrinker or 4″ elastic bandage ▪ optional: tourniquet (as a last resort to control bleeding).

For stump and prosthesis care: Mild soap or alcohol pads ▪ stump socks or athletic tube socks ▪ two washcloths ▪ two towels ▪ appropriate lubricating oil.

Implementation

- Confirm the patient's identity using two patient identifiers according to your facility's policy.
- Perform routine postoperative care. Frequently assess respiratory status and level of consciousness, monitor vital signs and I.V. infusions, check tube patency, and provide for the patient's comfort, pain management, and safety.

Monitoring stump drainage

- *Because gravity causes fluid to accumulate at the stump,* frequently check the amount of blood and drainage on the dressing. Notify the practitioner if accumulations of drainage or blood increase rapidly. If excessive bleeding occurs, notify the practitioner immediately, and apply a pressure dressing or compress the appropriate pressure points. If this doesn't control bleeding, use a tourniquet only as a last resort. Keep a tourniquet available.
- Tape the ABD pad over the moist part of the dressing, as needed. *Providing a dry area helps prevent bacterial infection.*
- Monitor the suction drainage equipment, and note the amount and type of drainage.

Positioning the extremity

- Evaluate the extremity for the first 24 hours *to reduce swelling and promote venous return.*
- *To prevent contractures,* position an arm with the elbow extended and the shoulder abducted.
- *To correctly position a leg,* elevate the foot of the bed slightly and place sandbags or a trochanter roll against the hip *to prevent external rotation.*

NURSING ALERT ***Don't place a pillow under the thigh to flex the hip*** **because this can cause hip flexion contracture.** ***For the same reason, tell the patient to avoid prolonged sitting.***

- After a below-the-knee amputation, maintain knee extension *to prevent hamstring muscle contractures.*
- After any leg amputation, place the patient on a firm surface in the prone position for at least 2 hours per day, with his legs close together and without pillows under his stomach, hips, knees, or stump, unless this position is contraindicated. *This position helps prevent hip flexion, contractures, and abduction; it also stretches the flexor muscles.*

Assisting with prescribed exercises

- After arm amputation, encourage the patient to exercise the remaining arm *to prevent muscle contractures.* Help the patient perform isometric and range-of-motion (ROM) exercises for both shoulders, as prescribed by the physical therapist, *because use of the prosthesis requires both shoulders.*
- After leg amputation, stand behind the patient and, if necessary, support him with your hands at his waist during balancing exercises.
- Instruct the patient to exercise the affected and unaffected limbs *to maintain muscle tone and increase muscle strength.* A patient with a leg amputation may perform push-ups, as ordered (in the sitting position, arms at his sides), or pull-ups on the overhead trapeze *to strengthen his arms, shoulders, and back in preparation for using crutches.*

Wrapping and conditioning the stump

- If the patient doesn't have a rigid cast, apply an elastic stump shrinker *to prevent edema and shape the limb in preparation for the prosthesis.* Wrap the stump so that it narrows toward the distal end. *This helps to ensure comfort when the patient wears the prosthesis.*
- Instead of using an elastic stump shrinker, you can wrap the stump in a 4″ elastic bandage. To do this, stretch the bandage to about two-thirds its maximum length as you

Wrapping a stump

Proper stump care helps protect the limb, reduces swelling, and prepares the limb for a prosthesis. As you perform the procedure, teach it to the patient.

Start by obtaining two 4″ elastic bandages. Center the end of the first 4″ bandage at the top of the patient's thigh. Unroll the bandage downward over the stump and to the back of the leg.

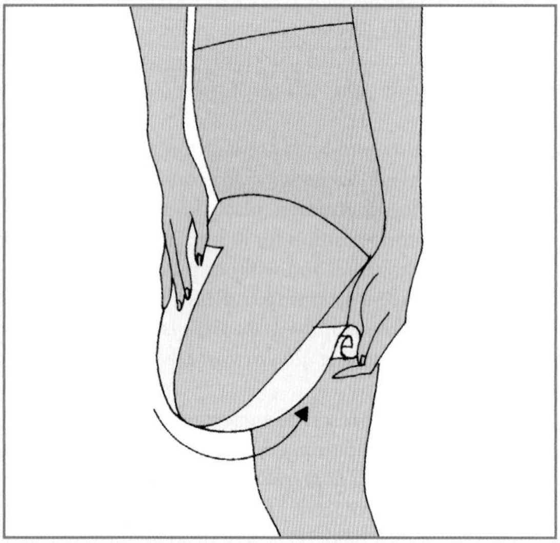

Make three figure-eight turns to adequately cover the ends of the stump. As you wrap, be sure to include the roll of flesh in the groin area. Use enough pressure to ensure that the stump narrows toward the end *so that it fits comfortably into the prosthesis*.

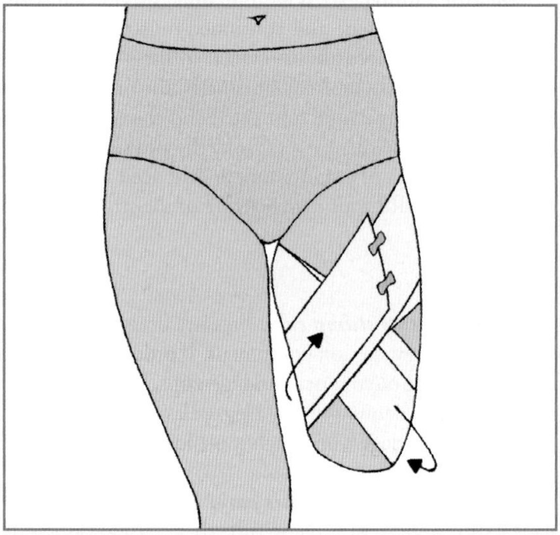

wrap it diagonally around the stump, with the greatest pressure distally. (Depending on the size of the leg, you may need to use two 4″ bandages.) Secure the bandage with clips, safety pins, or adhesive tape. Make sure the bandage covers all portions of the stump smoothly *because wrinkles or exposed areas encourage skin breakdown.* (See *Wrapping a stump.*)

- The use of an immediate postoperative prosthesis has proved effective in decreasing the time until final prosthetic fitting.
- If the patient experiences throbbing after the stump is wrapped, remove the bandage immediately and reapply it less tightly. *Throbbing indicates impaired circulation.*
- Check the bandage regularly. Rewrap it when it begins to bunch up at the end (usually about every 12 hours for a moderately active patient) or as necessary.
- After removing the bandage to rewrap it, massage the stump gently, always pushing toward the suture line rather than away from it. *This stimulates circulation and prevents scar tissue from adhering to the bone.*
- When healing begins, instruct the patient to push the stump against a pillow. Then have him progress gradually to pushing against harder surfaces, such as a padded chair, then a hard chair. *These conditioning exercises will help the patient adjust to experiencing pressure and sensation in the stump.*

Caring for the healed stump

- Bathe the stump but never shave it *to prevent a rash.* If possible, bathe the stump at the end of the day *because the warm water may cause swelling, making reapplication of the prosthesis difficult.*
- Rub the stump with alcohol daily *to toughen the skin, reducing the risk of skin breakdown.* (Avoid using powders or lotions *because they can soften or irritate the skin.*) *Because al-*

Use the second 4″ bandage to anchor the first bandage around the waist. For a below-the-knee amputation, use the knee to anchor the bandage in place. Secure the bandage with clips, safety pins, or adhesive tape. Check the stump bandage regularly, and rewrap it if it bunches at the end.

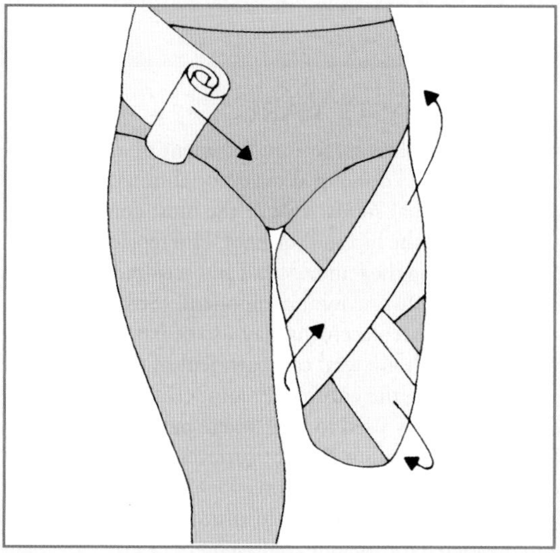

cohol may cause severe irritation in some patients, instruct the patient to watch for and report this sign.

- Inspect the stump for redness, swelling, irritation, and calluses. Report any of these to the practitioner. Following the first cast change, many surgeons will have the patient begin partial weight-bearing, if the wound appears stable.
- Continue muscle-strengthening exercises *so the patient can build the strength he'll need to control the prosthesis.*
- Change and wash the patient's elastic bandages every day *to avoid exposing the skin to excessive perspiration, which can be irritating.* Wash them in warm water and gentle nondetergent soap; lay them flat on a towel to dry. *Machine washing or drying may shrink the elastic bandages. To shape the stump,* have the patient wear an elastic bandage 24 hours per day except while bathing.

Caring for the plastic prosthesis

- Wipe the plastic socket of the prosthesis with a damp cloth and mild soap or alcohol *to prevent bacterial accumulation.*
- Wipe the insert (if the prosthesis has one) with a dry cloth.
- Dry the prosthesis thoroughly; if possible, allow it to dry overnight.
- Maintain and lubricate the prosthesis, as instructed by the manufacturer.
- Check for malfunctions and adjust or repair the prosthesis, as necessary, *to prevent further damage.*
- Check the condition of the shoe on a foot prosthesis frequently, and change it as necessary.

Applying the prosthesis

- Apply a stump sock. Keep the seams away from bony prominences.
- If the prosthesis has an insert, remove it from the socket, place it over the stump, and insert the stump into the prosthesis.
- If it has no insert, merely slide the prosthesis over the stump. Secure the prosthesis onto the stump according to the manufacturer's directions.

Special considerations

- If a patient arrives at the hospital with a traumatic amputation, the amputated part may be saved for possible reimplantation. (See *Caring for a severed body part,* page 262.)
- Teach the patient how to care for his stump and prosthesis properly. Make sure he knows signs and symptoms that indicate problems in the stump. Explain that a 10-lb (4.5-kg) change in body weight will alter his stump size and require a new prosthesis socket *to ensure a correct fit.*
- Exercise of the remaining muscles in an amputated limb must begin the day after surgery. A physical therapist will direct these exercises. For example, arm exercises progress from isometrics to assisted ROM to active ROM. Leg exercises include rising from a chair, balancing on one leg, and ROM exercises of the knees and hips.
- For a below-the-knee amputation, you may substitute an athletic tube sock for a stump sock by cutting off the elastic band. If the patient has a rigid plaster of Paris dressing, perform normal cast care. Check the cast frequently to make sure it doesn't slip off. If it does, apply an elastic bandage immediately and notify the practitioner *because edema will develop rapidly.*

Home care

Emphasize to the patient that proper care of his stump can speed healing. Tell him to inspect his stump carefully every day, using a mirror, and to continue proper daily stump care. Instruct him to call the practitioner if the incision appears to be opening, looks red or swollen, feels warm, is painful to touch, or is seeping drainage.

Tell the patient to massage the stump toward the suture line *to mobilize the scar and prevent its adherence to bone.* Advise him to avoid exposing the skin around the stump to excessive perspiration, *which can be irritating.* Tell him to change his elastic bandages or stump socks during the day to avoid this.

Tell the patient that he may experience twitching, spasms, phantom limb pain, or phantom limb sensations such as warmth, cold, or itching, as his stump muscles adjust to amputation. Such measures as imagery, biofeedback, or distraction may be helpful in relieving phantom limb pain or other sensations. Advise him that he can decrease these symptoms with heat, massage, or gentle pressure. If his stump is sensitive to touch, tell him to rub it with a dry washcloth for 4 minutes three times per day.

Stress the importance of performing prescribed exercises to help minimize complications, maintain muscle strength and tone, prevent contractures, and promote independence. Also stress the importance of positioning to prevent contractures and edema.

Complications

The most common postoperative complications include hemorrhage, stump infection, contractures, and a swollen or flabby stump.

Complications that may develop at any time after an amputation include:

- skin breakdown or irritation from lack of ventilation
- friction from an irritant in the prosthesis
- a sebaceous cyst or boil from tight socks
- psychological problems, such as denial, depression, or withdrawal
- phantom limb pain caused by stimulation of nerves that once carried sensations from the distal part of the extremity.

Documentation

Record the date, time, and specific procedures of all postoperative care, including amount and type of drainage, condition of the dressing, need for dressing reinforcement, and appearance of the suture line and surrounding tissue. Document pain assessment. Note any signs of skin irritation or infection, any complications and the nursing action taken, the patient's tolerance of exercises, and his psychological reaction to the amputation.

During routine daily care, document the date, time, type of care given, and condition of the skin and suture line, noting any signs of irritation, such as redness or tenderness. Note the patient's progress in caring for the stump or prosthesis.

Selected references

Bryant, G. "Stump Care," *AJN* 101(2):67-71, February 2001.

Goldberg, T., et al. "Postoperative Management of Lower Extremity Amputation," *Physical Medicine and Rehabilitation Clinics of North America* 11(3):559-68, August 2000.

Harker, J. "Wound Healing Complications Associated with Lower Limb Amputation." Available at: *http://www.worldwidewounds.com/2006/september/Harker/Wound-Healing-Complications-Limb-Amputation.html.* September 2006.

Maher, A.B., et al. *Orthopaedic Nursing,* 3rd ed. Philadelphia: W.B. Saunders Co., 2002.

Arthroplasty care

Arthroplasty involves surgical replacement of all or part of the joint, which is done to decrease or eliminate pain and improve functional status. Two of the most commonly replaced joints are the hip and the knee. Hip replacement may be total, replacing the femoral head and acetabulum, or partial, replacing only one joint component. (See *Total hip replacement.*) Knee replacement may also be partial, replacing either the medial or lateral compartment of the knee joint, or total, replacing the entire knee joint. Total knee replacement is commonly used to treat severe pain, joint contractures, and deterioration of joint surfaces—conditions that prohibit full extension or flexion.

According to the National Institutes of Health (NIH), to be considered for total hip replacement (THR), a patient should have some radiographic evidence of joint damage and moderate to severe pain or disability (or both) that isn't relieved by nonsurgical measures. The measures should include use of assistive devices (walkers), nonsteroidal anti-inflammatory drugs, physical therapy, and a reduction in physical activity. NIH statistics show that THR is most commonly used for patients with osteoarthritis. Other indications include:

- rheumatoid arthritis
- avascular necrosis
- traumatic arthritis
- certain hip fractures
- benign and malignant bone tumors
- arthritis associated with Paget's disease
- ankylosing spondylitis
- juvenile rheumatoid arthritis.

Arthroplasty care includes maintaining alignment of the affected joint, assisting with exercises, and providing routine postoperative care.

Nursing responsibilities include teaching the patient safe mobility while performing activities of daily living, home care, and exercises that may continue for several years, depending on the type of arthroplasty performed and the patient's conditioning.

Equipment

Traction frame with trapeze ▪ comfort device (such as static air mattress overlay, low-air-loss bed, or sheepskin) ▪ bed sheets ▪ incentive spirometer ▪ continuous passive motion (CPM) machine ▪ compression stocking ▪ sterile dressings ▪ hypoallergenic tape ▪ ice bag ▪ skin lotion ▪ warm water ▪ crutches or walker ▪ pain medications ▪ closed-wound drainage system ▪ I.V. antibiotics ▪ pillow ▪ abduction splint ▪ anticoagulants ▪ optional: slings.

After total knee replacement, a knee immobilizer may be applied in the operating room, or the leg may be placed in CPM.

Preparation of equipment

After the patient goes to the operating room, make a Balkan frame with a trapeze on his bed frame. *This will allow him some mobility after the operation.* Then make the bed, using a comfort device and clean sheets. Have the bed taken to the operating room. *This enables immediate placement of the patient on his hospital bed after surgery and eliminates the need for an additional move from his recovery room bed.*

Implementation

- Check vital signs every 15 minutes twice, every 30 minutes until they stabilize, and then every 2 to 4 hours and routinely thereafter, according to hospital protocol. Report any changes in vital signs *because they may indicate infection and hemorrhage.*
- Encourage the patient to perform deep-breathing and coughing exercises. Assist with incentive spirometry, as ordered, *to prevent respiratory complications.*
- Perform bilateral neurovascular assessment every 2 hours for the first 48 hours and then every 4 hours *for signs of complications.* Check the affected leg for color, temperature, toe movement, sensation, edema, capillary filling, and pedal pulse, and compare to unaffected extremity. Investigate any complaints of pain, burning, numbness, or tingling.
- Apply the compression stockings to the unaffected leg, as ordered, *to promote venous return and prevent phlebitis and pulmonary emboli.* Once every 8 hours, remove the stockings, inspect the legs for pressure ulcers, and reapply.
- Administer pain medications, as ordered.
- Administer I.V. antibiotics, as ordered, for at least 24 hours after surgery *to minimize the risk of wound infection.*

Total hip replacement

To form a totally artificial hip, the surgeon cements a femoral head prosthesis in place to articulate with a cup, which he then cements into the deepened acetabulum. He may avoid using cement by implanting a prosthesis with a porous coating that promotes bony ingrowth.

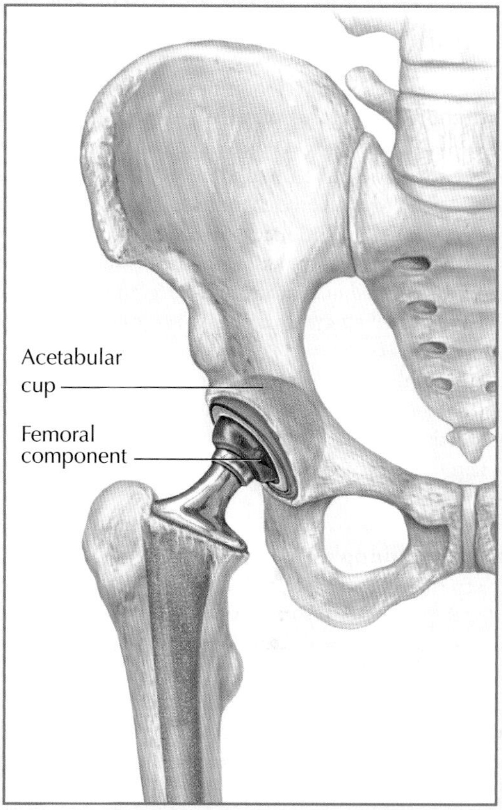

- Administer anticoagulant therapy, as ordered, *to minimize the risk of thrombophlebitis and embolus formation.* Observe for bleeding and for symptoms of phlebitis, such as warmth, swelling, tenderness, redness, and a positive Homans' sign. Monitor lab results such as complete blood count, prothrombin time, or partial thromboplastin time.
- Check dressings for excessive bleeding. Circle any drainage on the dressing and mark it with your initials, the date, and the time. As needed, apply more sterile dressings, using hypoallergenic tape. Report excessive bleeding to the practitioner.

- Observe the closed-wound drainage system for discharge color. *Proper drainage prevents hematoma. Purulent discharge and fever may indicate infection.* Empty and measure drainage, as ordered, using sterile technique *to prevent infection.* (For more information, see "Closed-wound drain management," page xxx.)
- Monitor fluid intake and output daily; include wound drainage in the output measurement.
- Apply an ice bag, as ordered, to the affected site for the first 48 hours *to reduce swelling, relieve pain, and control bleeding.*
- Every 2 hours, turn the patient no more than 45 degrees toward each side and keep him in this position as long as he's comfortable. *These position changes enhance comfort, prevent pressure ulcers, and help prevent respiratory complications.*
- Help the patient use the trapeze to lift himself every 2 hours. Then provide skin care for the back and buttocks, using warm water and lotion, as indicated.
- Instruct the patient to perform muscle-strengthening exercises for affected and unaffected extremities, as ordered, *to help maintain muscle strength and range of motion and to help prevent phlebitis.*
- Before ambulation, give a mild analgesic, as ordered, *because movement is very painful.* Encourage the patient during exercise.
- Help the patient with progressive ambulation, using adjustable crutches or a walker when needed.

After hip arthroplasty

- Keep the affected leg in abduction and in the neutral position *to stabilize the hip and keep the cup and femur head in the acetabulum.* Place a pillow between the patient's legs *to maintain hip abduction.*
- If the patient desires, elevate the head of the bed 45 degrees for comfort. (Some physicians permit 60-degree elevation.) Keep it elevated no more than 30 minutes at a time *to prevent excessive hip flexion.*

NURSING ALERT ***Don't let the hip flex more than 90 degrees* because the prosthesis might dislocate.**

- On the day after surgery, have the patient begin plantar flexion and dorsiflexion exercises of the foot on the affected leg. When ordered, instruct him to begin quadriceps exercises. Progressive ambulation protocols vary. Most patients are permitted to begin transfer and progressive ambulation with assistive devices on the first day.

After total knee replacement

- Elevate the affected leg, as ordered, *to reduce swelling.*
- Instruct the patient to begin quadriceps exercises and straight leg-raising when ordered (usually on the second postoperative day). Encourage flexion-extension exercises when ordered (usually after the first dressing change).
- If the practitioner orders use of the CPM machine, he will adjust the machine daily *to gradually increase the degree of flexion of the affected leg.* Typically, patients can dangle their feet on the first day after surgery and begin ambulation with partial weight-bearing as tolerated (cemented knee) or toe-touch ambulation only (uncemented knee) by the second day. The patient may need to wear a knee immobilizer for support when walking; otherwise, he should be in CPM for most of the day and night or during waking hours only. Check your hospital's protocol.
- The degree of flexion, extension, and weight-bearing status will depend on the practitioner's specific orders, surgical approach used, and preference.

Special considerations

- Before surgery, explain the procedure to the patient. Emphasize that frequent assessment—including the monitoring of vital signs, neurovascular integrity, and wound drainage—is normal after the operation.
- Inform the patient that he'll receive I.V. antibiotics for about 2 days. Make sure he understands that pharmacologic and nonpharmacologic methods will be available to help pain control. Explain the need for immobilizing the affected leg and exercising the unaffected one, as appropriate.
- Before discharge, instruct the patient regarding home care and exercises.

Complications

Immobility after arthroplasty may result in such complications as shock, pulmonary embolism, pneumonia, phlebitis, paralytic ileus, urine retention, and bowel impaction. A deep wound or infection at the prosthesis site is a serious complication that may force removal of the prosthesis. Dislocation of a total hip prosthesis may occur after violent hip flexion or adduction or during internal rotation. Signs of dislocation include inability to rotate the hip or bear weight, shortening of the leg, and increased pain.

Fat embolism, a potentially fatal complication resulting from release of fat molecules in response to increased intermedullary canal pressure from the prosthesis, may develop within 72 hours after surgery. Watch for such signs and symptoms as apprehension, diaphoresis, fever, dyspnea, pulmonary effusion, tachycardia, cyanosis, seizures, decreased level of consciousness, and a petechial rash on the chest and shoulders.

Documentation

Record the patient's neurovascular status, maintenance of traction (for cup arthroplasty and hip replacement), or knee immobilization (for knee replacement). Describe the patient's position (especially the position of the affected leg), skin care and condition, respiratory care and condition, and the use of elastic stockings. Document all exercises performed and their effect; also record ambulatory efforts, the type of support used, and the amount of traction weight.

On the appropriate flowchart, record vital signs and fluid intake and output. Note the turning and skin care schedule and the current exercise and ambulation program. Also include the physician's orders for the amount of traction and the degree of flexion permitted. Record discharge instructions and how well the patient seems to understand them.

Selected references

Ennis, R. "Postoperative Deep Vein Thrombosis Prophylaxis: A Retrospective Analysis in 1,000 Consecutive Hip Fracture Patients Treated in a Community Hospital Setting," *Journal of the Southern Orthopaedic Association* 12(1):10-17, Spring 2003.

Geerts, W.H., et al. Seventh ACCP Conference on Antithrombotic and Thrombolytic Therapy. "Prevention of Venous Thromboembolism," *Chest* 126(3 Suppl):338S-400S, September 2004.

Institute for Clinical Systems Improvement (ICSI). "Venous Thromboembolism Prophylaxis," Bloomington, Minn.: Institute for Clinical Systems Improvement, June 2006. *www.icsi.org/venous_thromboembolism_prophylaxis_4.html*

Maher, A.B., et al. *Orthopaedic Nursing,* 3rd ed. Philadelphia: W.B. Saunders Co., 2002.

ELECTRICAL BONE GROWTH STIMULATION

By imitating the body's natural electrical forces, this procedure initiates or accelerates the healing process in a fractured bone that fails to heal. About 1 in 20 fractures may fail to heal properly, possibly as a result of infection, insufficient reduction or fixation, pseudarthrosis, or severe tissue trauma around the fracture. Electrical bone growth stimulation is also used to help bones grow together after such procedures as spinal fusion.

Three basic electrical bone stimulation techniques are available: fully implantable direct current stimulation; semi-invasive percutaneous stimulation; and noninvasive electromagnetic coil stimulation. (See *Methods of electrical bone growth stimulation,* page 780.) Choice of technique depends on the fracture type and location, the physician's preference, and the patient's ability and willingness to comply. The invasive device requires little or no patient involvement. With the other two methods, however, the patient must manage his own treatment schedule and maintain the equipment. Treatment time averages 3 to 6 months.

Equipment

For direct current stimulation: The equipment set consists of a small generator and leadwires that connect to a titanium cathode wire that is surgically implanted into the nonunited bone site.

For percutaneous stimulation: The set consists of an external anode skin pad with a leadwire, lithium battery pack, and one to four Teflon-coated stainless steel cathode wires that are surgically implanted.

For electromagnetic stimulation: The set consists of a generator that plugs into a standard 110-volt outlet and two strong electromagnetic coils placed on either side of the injured area. The coils can be incorporated into a cast, cuff, or orthotic device.

Preparation of equipment

All equipment comes in sets with instructions provided by the manufacturer. Follow the instructions carefully. Make sure all parts are included and are sterilized according to hospital policy and procedure.

Implementation

- Confirm the patient's identity using two patient identifiers according to your facility's policy.
- Tell the patient whether he'll have an anesthetic and, if possible, which kind.

Direct current stimulation

- Implantation is performed with the patient under general anesthesia. Afterward, the physician may apply a cast or external fixator to immobilize the limb. The patient is usually hospitalized for 2 to 3 days after implantation. Weight bearing may be ordered as tolerated.
- After the bone fragments join, the generator and leadwire can be removed under local anesthesia. The titanium cathode remains implanted.

Percutaneous stimulation

- Remove excessive body hair from the injured site before applying the anode pad. Avoid stressing or pulling on the anode wire. Instruct the patient to change the anode pad every 48 hours. Tell him to report any local pain to his physician and not to bear weight for the duration of treatment.

Electromagnetic stimulation

- Show the patient where to place the coils, and tell him to apply them for 3 to 10 hours each day, as ordered by his physician. Many patients find it most convenient to perform the procedure at night.
- Urge the patient not to interrupt the treatments for more than 10 minutes at a time.
- Teach the patient how to use and care for the generator.

Methods of electrical bone growth stimulation

Electrical bone growth stimulation may be invasive or noninvasive.

Invasive system

An invasive system involves placing a spiral cathode inside the bone at the fracture site. A wire leads from the cathode to a battery-powered generator, also implanted in local tissues. The patient's body completes the circuit.

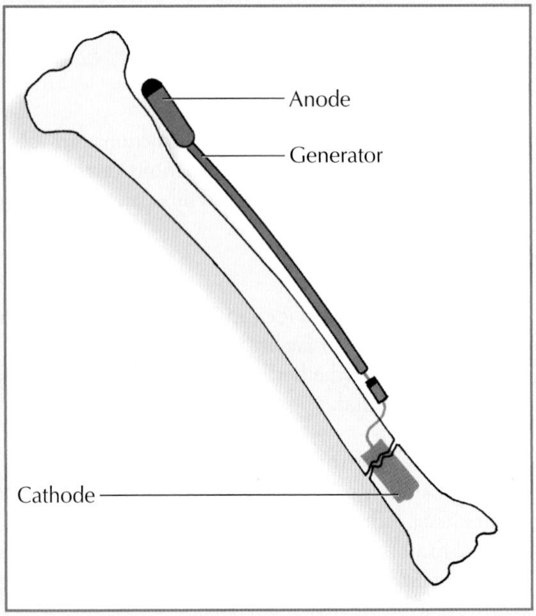

Noninvasive system

A noninvasive system may include a cuff-like transducer or fitted ring that wraps around the patient's limb at the level of the injury. Electric current penetrates the limb.

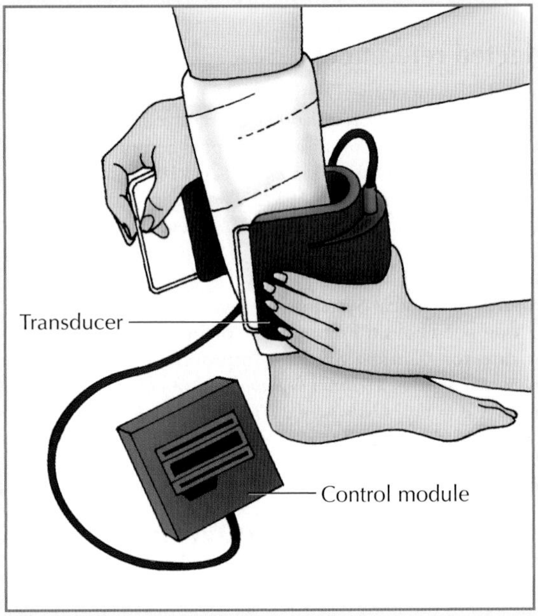

- Relay the physician's instructions for weight bearing. Usually, the physician will advise against bearing weight until evidence of healing appears on X-rays.

Special considerations

- A patient with direct current electrical bone stimulation shouldn't undergo electrocauterization, diathermy, or magnetic resonance imaging (MRI). *Electrocautery may "short" the system; diathermy may potentiate the electrical current, possibly causing tissue damage; and MRI will interfere with or stop the current.*
- Percutaneous electrical bone stimulation is contraindicated in patients with any kind of inflammatory process. Ask the patient if he's sensitive to nickel or chromium; *both are present in the electrical bone stimulation system.*
- Electromagnetic coils are contraindicated for a pregnant patient, a patient with a tumor, or a patient with an arm fracture and a pacemaker.

Home care

Teach the patient how to care for his cast or external fixation devices and for the electrical generator. Urge him to follow treatment instructions faithfully.

Complications

Complications associated with any surgical procedure, including increased risk of infection, may occur with direct current electrical bone stimulation equipment. Local irritation or skin ulceration may occur around cathode pin sites with percutaneous devices. No complications are associated with use of electromagnetic coils.

Documentation

Record the type of electrical bone stimulation equipment provided, including date, time, and location, as appropriate. Note the patient's skin condition and tolerance of the procedure. Also record instructions given to the patient and his family as well as their ability to understand and act on those instructions.

Selected references

Mackenzie, D., and Veninga, F.D. "Reversal of Delayed Union of Anterior Cervical Fusion Treated with Pulsed Electromagnetic Field Stimulation: A Case Report," *Southern Medical Journal* 97(5):519-24, May 2004.

Maher, A.B., et al. *Orthopedic Nursing*, 3rd ed. Philadelphia: W.B. Saunders Co., 2002.

CONTINUOUS PASSIVE MOTION DEVICE

A continuous passive motion (CPM) device is frequently used after joint surgery—particularly after total knee arthroplasty. The device increases range of motion in the joint as the flexion and extension settings are adjusted during therapy. In addition, the negative effects of immobility are minimized due to increased circulation from the passive movement of the limb. There's also stimulation of healing within the articular cartilage and reduction in adhesions and swelling.

The practitioner determines the amount of flexion and extension of the joint and the cycle rate (the number of revolutions per minute) as well as the length of time it's to be used.

Although the CPM device is usually used on the knee, it may be appropriate for other joints as well.

Equipment

CPM device ▪ single patient use soft-goods kit ▪ tape measure ▪ goniometer ▪ nonsterile gloves, if indicated.

Implementation

- Check the practitioner's order for the CPM settings, frequency, and duration.
- Gather the appropriate equipment.
- Apply the soft goods padding to the CPM device.
- Confirm the patient's identity using two patient identifiers according to your facility's policy.
- Explain the procedure to the patient *to reduce anxiety and encourage compliance.*
- Assess the patient's pain level and administer prescribed analgesic, if needed. Allow time for the full effect of the analgesic to occur before starting the machine.
- Wash your hands and put on gloves, if indicated, *to prevent possible contact with blood or body fluids.*
- Provide privacy. Place the bed at a comfortable working height.
- Determine the distance between the gluteal crease and the popliteal space using the measuring tape.
- Also measure the length of the lower leg from the knee to ¼″ beyond the bottom of the foot.
- Adjust the thigh length and foot plate position on the CPM machine based on your measurements.
- Position the patient in the middle of the bed.
- Support the affected extremity, elevating it to allow placement of the padded CPM device on the bed. Gently lower the leg onto the device (as shown below).

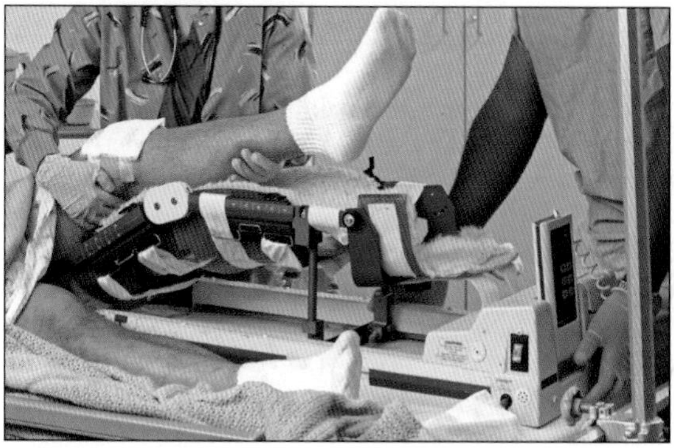

- Make sure the knee is resting at the hinged joint of the CPM machine and that the leg is slightly abducted.
- Adjust the footplate to maintain a neutral position for the patient's foot. Assess the patient's position to make sure the leg is not internally or externally rotated *to prevent injury* (as shown below).

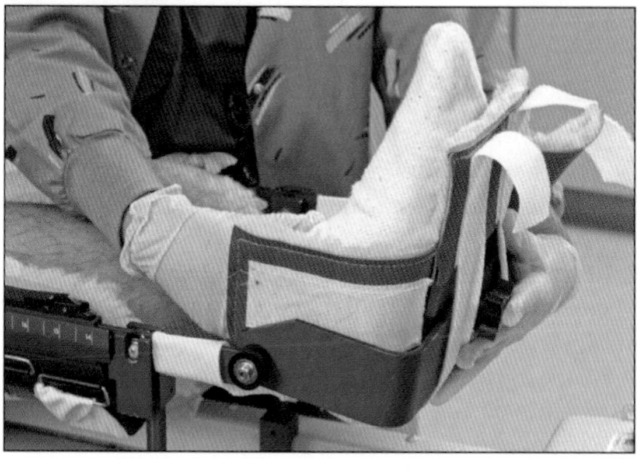

- Secure the restraining straps under the CPM device and around the leg *to hold the leg in position.* Check that two fingers fit between the strap and the leg *to prevent injury from excessive pressure from the strap* (as shown below).

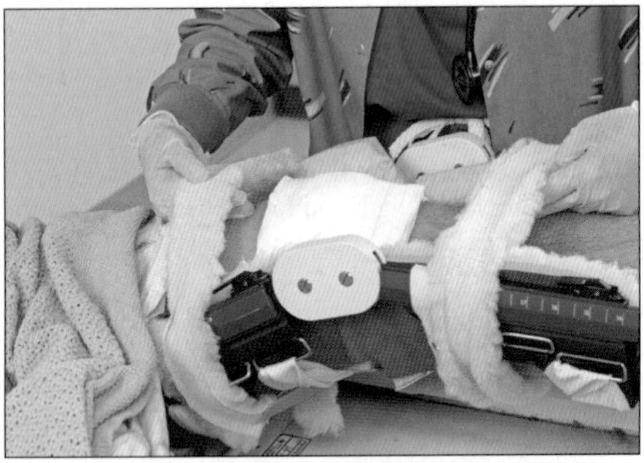

- Turn the unit on at the main power switch and set the controls to the level prescribed by the practitioner.
- Instruct the patient in the use of the STOP/GO button.
- Set the device to ON and start the therapy by pressing the GO button. Monitor the patient and the device through the first few cycles. Verify the angel of flexion when the device reaches its greatest height by measuring with a goniometer *to ensure the device is set to the prescribed parameters* (as shown below).

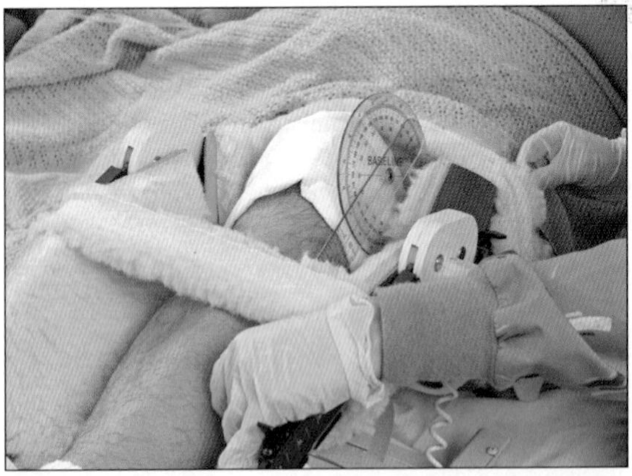

- Return the bed to the lowest position *for patient safety.* Make sure the call bell and other necessary items are within easy reach.
- Check the patient's level of comfort frequently, and perform skin and neurovascular assessment at least every 8 hours or according to your facility's policy.
- Remove gloves and wash your hands.

Special considerations

- The use of the CPM device is in addition to physical therapy during the rehabilitation process.
- Encourage the patient to use the CPM machine, as prescribed, *to promote healing and function of the joint. Effective and timely pain control is important to ensuring the patient's cooperation.*
- Instruct the patient in use of the device and patient controls. Make the patient aware of setting changes and goals of CPM therapy.
- Teach the patient to report signs and symptoms of neurovascular impairmen, such as numbness or tingling, sudden pain, or coolness of the affected limb.

Documentation

Record settings and the patient's tolerance of the CPM device. Note skin and incision condition and neurovascular assessment. Document pain assessment, nursing actions taken, and outcomes. Also record any patient teaching provided.

Selected references

Altizer, L. "Patient Education for Total Hip or Knee Replacement," *Orthopaedic Nursing* 23(4):283-88, July-August 2004.

Denis, M., et al. "Effectiveness of Continuous Passive Motion and Conventional Physical Therapy after Total Knee Arthroplasty: A Randomized Clinical Trial," *Physical Therapy* 86(2):174-85, February 2006.

Milne, S., et al. "Continuous Passive Motion Following Total Knee Arthroplasty," *Cochrane Database of Systematic Reviews* (2):CD004260, 2003.

Taylor, C., et al. *Fundamentals of Nursing: The Art and Science of Nursing Care*, 6th ed. Philadelphia: Lippincott Williams & Wilkins, 2008.

13 ■ Skin care

Introduction

Besides helping to shape a patient's self-image, the skin performs many physiologic functions. For example, it protects internal body structures from the environment and from potential pathogens. It also regulates body temperature and homeostasis and serves as an organ of sensation and excretion. As a result, meticulous skin care is essential to overall health. When skin integrity is compromised by pressure ulcers, burns, or other lesions, you'll need to take steps to prevent or control infection, promote new skin growth, control pain, and provide emotional support.

Controlling infection

Because the skin is the body's first line of defense against infection, any damage to its integrity increases the risk of infection, which could delay healing, worsen pain, and even threaten the patient's life. Most burn deaths, for example, result from complications of infection rather than from the burns themselves.

Infection control requires sterile technique to avoid introducing new pathogens into an already contaminated wound. This is achieved by thorough hand washing with an antiseptic agent and by the use of sterile equipment during wound care.

Promoting new skin growth

To enhance natural healing, skin wounds need regular dressing changes (extra changes for soiled dressings), thorough cleaning and, if necessary, debridement to remove debris, reduce bacterial growth, and encourage tissue repair. Using warm solutions for wound cleaning increases circulation to the site, which promotes delivery of oxygen and the nutrients required to support tissue repair.

Controlling pain

To control pain effectively, you need to evaluate each patient's response to pain and adapt your techniques accordingly. If the patient has minor skin discomfort such as pruritus, an analgesic or topical medication, reassurance, or distraction techniques may provide him with adequate relief. If he has moderate pain, he may benefit from comfortable positioning and ample rest. However, if he has severe pain, only strong opioid analgesics may provide relief.

Providing emotional support

A patient with a painful and disfiguring skin disorder may have to deal with depression, frustration, and anger. Along with physical support, such a patient needs continuing emotional support as he develops coping mechanisms to accommodate an altered self-image. Severe disfigurement, which is common in a burn patient, may require emotional support and psychological counseling throughout a slow and painful recovery period. The expectation and reality of scars (or other evidence of skin injury or disease) influence the patient's self-acceptance as well as his acceptance by others. Sensitivity to the patient's needs and respect for his manner of coping are among your most important challenges.

PRESSURE ULCERS

Pressure ulcer care

A pressure ulcer is a lesion caused by unrelieved pressure that results in damage to underlying tissues. Most pressure ulcers develop over bony prominences, where friction and shearing force combine with pressure to break down skin and underlying tissues. Approximately 95% of pressure ulcers occur in the lower part of the body, with the sacrum or the heel being the two most frequent sites that experience skin breakdown.

Successful pressure ulcer treatment involves relieving pressure, restoring circulation and, if possible, resolving or managing related disorders. Typically, the effectiveness and duration of treatment depend on the pressure ulcer's characteristics. Ideally, prevention is the key to avoiding extensive therapy. Preventive strategies include recognizing the risk, decreasing the effects of pressure, assessing nutritional status, avoiding excessive bed rest, and preserving skin integrity. Although many systems have been developed for the classification or "staging" of wounds, the system currently recommended by the Agency for Healthcare Research and Quality and the Wound, Ostomy, and Continence Nurses Society is a four-stage system based on the tissue layers involved. (See *Assessing pressure ulcers.*)

The Braden scale, on the other hand, is the assessment tool of choice for determining the risk of developing pressure sores; it's also used to direct implementation of preventive strategies. (See *Braden scale: Predicting pressure sore risk,* pages 788 and 789.)

Treatment includes methods to decrease pressure, such as frequent repositioning to shorten pressure duration, and the use of special equipment to reduce pressure intensity. Treatment may involve special pressure-reducing devices, such as beds, mattresses, mattress overlays, and chair cushions. Other therapeutic measures include decreasing risk factors and use of topical treatments, wound cleansing, debridement, and the use of dressings to support moist wound healing. (See *Guide to topical agents for pressure ulcers,* page 787.)

Assessing pressure ulcers

To select the most effective treatment for a pressure ulcer, you first need to assess its characteristics. The pressure ulcer staging system described here, used by the National Pressure Ulcer Advisory Panel and the Agency for Health Care Policy and Research, reflects the anatomic depth of exposed tissue. Keep in mind that if the wound contains necrotic tissue, you won't be able to determine the stage until you can see the wound base.

Suspected deep tissue injury

Deep tissue injury is characterized by a purple or maroon localized area of intact skin or a blood-filled blister caused by damage of underlying soft tissue from pressure or shear. The injury may be preceded by tissue that's painful, firm, mushy, boggy, or warm or cool compared to adjacent tissue. Further, it may be difficult to detect in individuals with dark skin tones.

Stage I

A stage I pressure ulcer is characterized by intact skin with nonblanchable redness of a localized area, usually over a bony prominence. Darkly pigmented skin may not have visible blanching, but its color may differ from the surrounding area.

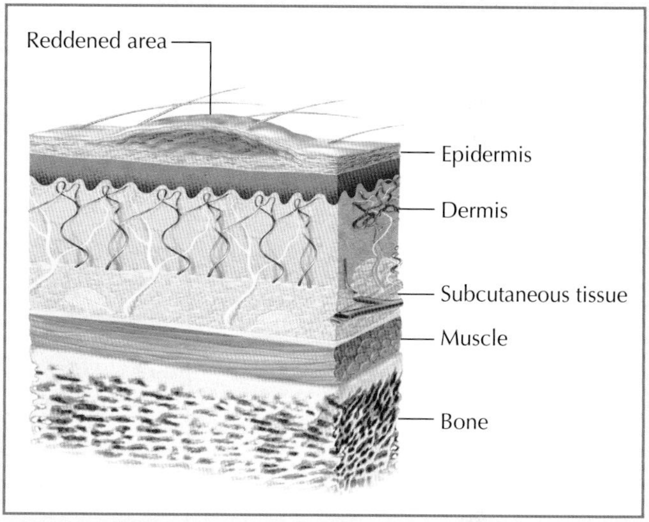

Stage II

A stage II pressure ulcer is characterized by partial-thickness loss of the dermis, presenting as a shallow, open ulcer with a red-pink wound bed without slough. It may also present as an intact or open serum-filled blister.

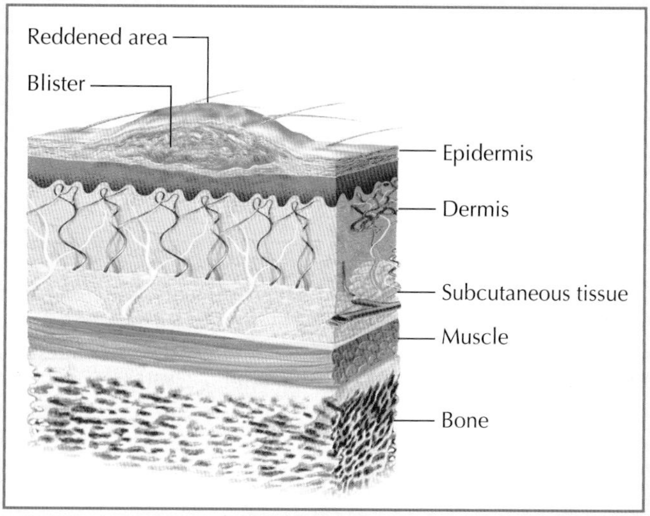

(continued)

Assessing pressure ulcers *(continued)*

Stage III

A stage III pressure ulcer is characterized by full-thickness tissue loss. Subcutaneous fat may be visible, but bone, tendon, and muscle aren't exposed. Slough may be present but doesn't obscure the depth of tissue loss. Undermining and tunneling may be present. The depth of a stage III ulcer varies by anatomical location.

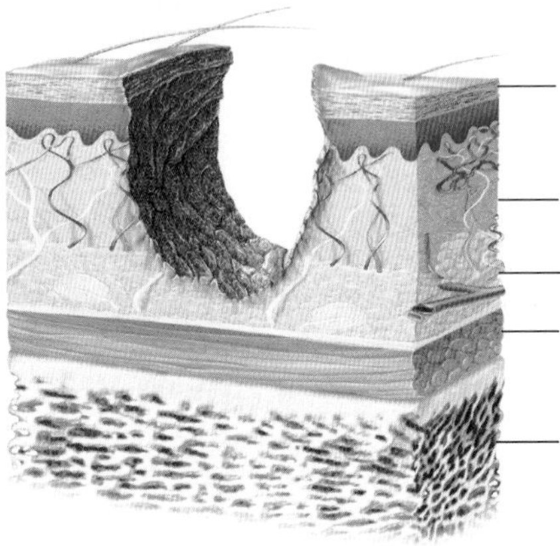

Stage IV

A stage IV pressure ulcer involves full-thickness tissue loss with exposed bone, tendon, or muscle. Slough or eschar may be present on some parts of the wound bed. Undermining and tunneling are also common. The depth of a stage IV ulcer varies by anatomical location.

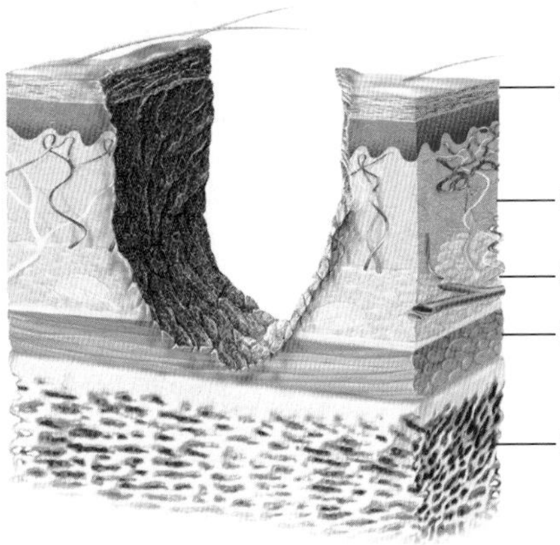

Unstageable

An unstageable ulcer is characterized by full-thickness tissue loss in which the base of the ulcer in the wound bed is covered by slough, eschar, or both. Until enough slough or eschar is removed to expose the base of the wound, the true depth, and therefore stage, can't be determined.

Nurses usually perform or coordinate treatments according to your facility's policy. The procedures detailed below address cleaning and dressing the pressure ulcer. Always follow the standard precautions guidelines of the Centers for Disease Control and Prevention.

Equipment

Hypoallergenic tape or elastic netting ▪ overbed table ▪ piston-type irrigating system ▪ two pairs of gloves ▪ normal saline solution, as ordered ▪ sterile 4″ × 4″ gauze pads ▪ sterile cotton swab ▪ selected topical dressing ▪ linen-saver pads ▪ impervious plastic trash bag ▪ disposable wound-measuring device ▪ optional: skin sealant.

Preparation of equipment

Assemble equipment at the patient's bedside. Cut tape into strips for securing dressings. Loosen lids on cleaning solutions and medications *for easy removal.* Loosen existing dressing edges and tapes before putting on gloves. Attach an im-

Guide to topical agents for pressure ulcers

Several agents are available for topical treatment of pressure ulcers. Nursing considerations and care vary for each type, so be sure to follow the manufacturer's recommendations.

TOPICAL AGENTS	NURSING CONSIDERATIONS
Antibiotics silver sulfadiazine, triple antibiotics	■ Consider a 2-week trial of topical antibiotics for clean or exudated pressure ulcers that aren't responding to moist-wound healing therapy.
Circulatory stimulants (Granulex, Proderm)	■ Use these agents to promote blood flow. Both contain balsam of Peru and castor oil, but Granulex also contains trypsin, an enzyme that facilitates debridement.
Enzymes collagenase (Santyl)	■ Apply collagenase in thin layers after cleaning the wound with normal saline solution. ■ Avoid concurrent use of collagenase with agents that decrease enzymatic activity, including detergents, hexachlorophene, antiseptics with heavy-metal ions, iodine, and such acid solutions as Burow's solution. ■ Use collagenase cautiously near the patient's eyes. If contact occurs, flush the eyes repeatedly with normal saline solution or sterile water.
Exudate absorbers dextranomer beads (Debrisan)	■ Use dextranomer beads on secreting ulcers. Discontinue use when secretions stop. ■ Clean—but don't dry—the ulcer before applying dextranomer beads. Don't use in tunneling ulcers. ■ Remove gray-yellow beads (which indicate saturation) by irrigating with sterile water or normal saline solution. ■ Use cautiously near the eyes. If contact occurs, flush the eyes repeatedly with normal saline solution or sterile water.
Isotonic solutions normal saline solution	■ This agent moisturizes tissue without injuring cells.

pervious plastic trash bag to the overbed table *to hold used dressings and refuse.*

Implementation

■ Confirm the patient's identity using two patient identifiers according to your facility's policy.
■ Premedicate the patient, if necessary.
■ Before any dressing change, wash your hands and review the principles of standard precautions. (See chapter 2, Infection control.)

Cleaning the pressure ulcer

■ Provide privacy, and explain the procedure to the patient *to allay his fears and promote cooperation.*
■ Position the patient in a way that maximizes his comfort while allowing easy access to the pressure ulcer site.
■ Cover bed linens with a linen-saver pad *to prevent soiling.*
■ Open the normal saline solution container and the piston syringe. Carefully pour normal saline solution into an irrigation container *to avoid splashing.* (The container may be clean or sterile, depending on your facility's policy.) Put the piston syringe into the opening provided in the irrigation container.
■ Open the packages of supplies.
■ Put on gloves and remove the old dressing, exposing the pressure ulcer. Discard the soiled dressing in the impervious plastic trash bag *to avoid contaminating the sterile field and spreading infection.*

(Text continues on page 790.)

Braden scale: Predicting pressure sore risk

The Braden scale, shown below, is the most reliable of several instruments used to assess the risk of developing pressure sores. The numbers to the left of each description are the points to be tallied; the lower the score, the greater the risk.

Patient's name ______________________ **Evaluator's name** ______________________

Sensory perception Ability to respond meaningfully to pressure-related discomfort	**1. Completely limited** Patient is unresponsive (doesn't moan, flinch, or grasp in response) to painful stimuli because of diminished level of consciousness or sedation. OR Patient has a limited ability to feel pain over most of body surface.	**2. Very limited** Patient responds only to painful stimuli; can't communicate discomfort except through moaning or restlessness. OR Patient has a sensory impairment that limits ability to feel pain or discomfort over half of body.
Moisture Degree to which skin is exposed to moisture	**1. Constantly moist** Patient's skin is kept moist almost constantly by perspiration or urine; dampness is detected every time he's moved or turned.	**2. Very moist** Patient's skin is usually but not always moist; linen must be changed at least once per shift.
Activity Degree of physical activity	**1. Bedfast** Patient is confined to bed.	**2. Chairfast** Patient's ability to walk severely limited or nonexistent; can't bear own weight and must be assisted into a chair or wheelchair.
Mobility Ability to change and control body position	**1. Completely immobile** Patient doesn't make even slight changes in body or extremity position without assistance.	**2. Very limited** Patient makes occasional slight changes in body or extremity position but can't make frequent or significant changes independently.
Nutrition Usual food intake pattern	**1. Very poor** Patient never eats a complete meal; rarely eats more than one-third of any food offered; eats two servings or less of protein (meat or dairy products) per day; takes fluids poorly; doesn't take a liquid dietary supplement. OR Patient is NPO or maintained on clear liquids or I.V. fluids for more than 5 days.	**2. Probably inadequate** Patient rarely eats a complete meal and generally eats only about one-half of any food offered; protein intake includes only three servings of meat or dairy products per day; occasionally will take a dietary supplement. OR Patient receives less than optimum amount of liquid diet or tube feeding.
Friction and shear	**1. Problem** Patient requires moderate to maximum assistance in moving; complete lifting without sliding against sheets is impossible; frequently slides down in bed or chair, requiring frequent repositioning with maximum assistance; spasticity, contractures, or agitation leads to almost constant friction.	**2. Potential problem** Patient moves feebly or requires minimum assistance during a move; skin probably slides to some extent against sheets, chair restraints, or other devices; maintains relatively good position in chair or bed most of the time but occasionally slides down.

		Date of Assessment			
3. Slightly limited Patient responds to verbal commands but can't always communicate discomfort or the need to be turned. OR Patient has some sensory impairment that limits ability to feel pain or discomfort in one or two extremities.	**4. No impairment** Patient responds to verbal commands; has no sensory deficit that would limit ability to feel or voice pain or discomfort.				
3. Occasionally moist Patient's skin is occasionally moist; linen requires an extra change approximately once per day.	**4. Rarely moist** Patient's skin is usually dry; linen requires changing only at routine intervals.				
3. Walks occasionally Patient walks occasionally during the day, but for very short distances, with or without assistance; spends majority of each shift in a bed or chair.	**4. Walks frequently** Patient walks outside room at least twice per day and inside room at least once every 2 hours during waking hours.				
3. Slightly limited Patient makes frequent (although slight) changes in body or extremity position independently.	**4. No limitations** Patient makes major and frequent changes in body or extremity position without assistance.				
3. Adequate Patient eats more than one-half of most meals; eats four servings of protein (meat and dairy products) per day; occasionally refuses a meal but will usually take a supplement if offered. OR Patient is on a tube feeding or total parenteral nutrition regimen that probably meets most nutritional needs.	**4. Excellent** Patient eats most of every meal and never refuses a meal; usually eats four or more servings of meat and dairy products per day; occasionally eats between meals; doesn't require supplementation.				
3. No apparent problem Patient moves in bed and in chair independently and has sufficient muscle strength to lift up completely during move; maintains good position in bed or chair at all times.					
	Total Score				

Understanding pressure ulcer debridement

Because moist necrotic tissue promotes the growth of pathologic organisms, removing such tissue aids pressure ulcer healing. A pressure ulcer can be debrided using various methods. The patient's condition and the goals of care determine which method to use. Sharp debridement is indicated for patients with an urgent need for debridement, such as those with sepsis or cellulitis. Otherwise, another method, such as mechanical, enzymatic, or autolytic debridement, may be used. Sometimes, several methods are used in combination. Debridement isn't indicated for ulcers that exhibit adequate granulation tissue.

Sharp debridement

The most rapid method, sharp debridement removes thick, adherent eschar and devitalized tissue through the use of a scalpel; curved, blunt-tipped scissors; or another sharp instrument. Small amounts of necrotic tissue can be debrided at the bedside; extensive amounts must be debrided in the operating room.

Mechanical debridement

Typically, mechanical debridement involves the use of wet-to-dry dressings. Gauze moistened with normal saline solution is applied to the wound and then removed after it dries and adheres to the wound bed. The goal is to debride the wound as the dressing is removed. Mechanical debridement has certain disadvantages; for example, it's often painful, and it may take a long time to completely debride the ulcer.

Enzymatic debridement

Enzymatic debridement removes necrotic tissue by breaking down tissue elements. Topical enzymatic debriding agents are placed on the necrotic tissue. If eschar is present, it must be crosshatched to allow the enzyme to penetrate the tissue.

Autolytic debridement

Autolytic debridement involves the use of moisture-retentive dressings to cover the wound bed. Necrotic tissue is then removed through self-digestion of enzymes in the wound fluid. Although autolytic debridement takes longer than other debridement methods, it's appropriate for patients who can't tolerate any other method. If the ulcer is infected, autolytic debridement isn't the treatment of choice.

- Inspect the wound. Note the color, amount, and odor of drainage and necrotic debris. Measure the wound perimeter with the disposable wound-measuring device.
- Using the piston syringe, apply full force to irrigate the pressure ulcer *to remove necrotic debris and help decrease bacteria in the wound.* For nonnecrotic wounds, use gentle pressure *to prevent damage to new tissue.*
- Remove and discard your soiled gloves, and put on a fresh pair.
- Insert a sterile cotton swab into the wound to assess wound tunneling or undermining. *Tunneling usually signals wound extension along fascial planes.*
- Next, reassess the condition of the skin and the ulcer. Note the character of the clean wound bed and the surrounding skin.
- If you observe adherent necrotic material, notify a wound care specialist or a practitioner *to ensure appropriate debridement.* (See *Understanding pressure ulcer debridement.*)
- Prepare to apply the appropriate topical dressing. Directions for applying topical moist saline gauze, hydrocolloid, transparent, alginate, foam, and hydrogel dressings follow. For other dressings or topical agents, follow your facility's policy or the manufacturer's instructions.

Applying a moist saline gauze dressing

- Irrigate the pressure ulcer with normal saline solution. Blot the surrounding skin dry with a sterile 4″ × 4″ gauze pad.
- Moisten the gauze dressing with normal saline solution.
- Gently place the dressing over the surface of the ulcer. *To separate surfaces within the wound,* gently place a dressing between opposing wound surfaces. *To avoid damage to tissues,* don't pack the gauze tightly.
- Change the dressing often enough to keep the wound moist. (See *Choosing a pressure ulcer dressing.*)

Applying a hydrocolloid dressing

- Irrigate the pressure ulcer with normal saline solution. Blot the surrounding skin dry with a sterile 4″ × 4″ gauze pad.
- Choose a clean, dry, presized dressing, or cut one to overlap the pressure ulcer by about 1″ (2.5 cm). Remove the dressing from its package, pull the release paper from the

Choosing a pressure ulcer dressing

Choosing the proper dressing for a wound should be guided by four questions:

- What does the wound need (does it need to be drained, protected, kept moist?)
- What does the dressing do?
- How well does the product do it?
- What is available and practical?

Gauze dressings

Made of absorptive cotton or synthetic fabric, gauze dressings are permeable to water, water vapor, and oxygen and may be impregnated with petroleum jelly or another agent. When uncertain about which dressing to use, you may apply a gauze dressing moistened in saline solution until a wound specialist recommends definitive treatment. *To prevent skin maceration and future breakdown,* avoid placing the moist dressing on the skin surrounding the wound.

Hydrocolloid dressings

Hydrocolloid dressings are adhesive, moldable wafers that are made of a carbohydrate-based material and usually have waterproof backings. They're impermeable to oxygen, water, and water vapor and most have some absorptive properties.

Transparent film dressings

Transparent film dressings are clear, adherent, nonabsorptive, polymer-based dressings that are permeable to oxygen and water vapor but not to water. Their transparency allows visual inspection. Because they can't absorb drainage, these dressings are used on partial-thickness wounds with minimal exudate.

Alginate dressings

Made from seaweed, alginate dressings are nonwoven, absorptive dressings that are available as soft, white sterile pads or ropes. They absorb excessive exudate and may be used on infected wounds. As these dressings absorb exudate, they turn into a gel that keeps the wound bed moist and promotes healing. When exudate is no longer excessive, switch to another type of dressing.

Foam dressings

Foam dressings are spongelike polymer dressings that may be impregnated or coated with other materials. Somewhat absorptive, they may be adherent. These dressings promote moist wound healing and are useful when a nonadherent surface is desired.

Hydrogel dressings

Hydrogel dressings are water-based, nonadherent, polymer-based dressings that have some absorptive properties. They're available as a gel in a tube, as flexible sheets, and as saturated gauze packing strips. They may have a cooling effect, which eases pain.

adherent side of the dressing, and apply the dressing to the wound. *To minimize irritation,* carefully smooth out wrinkles as you apply the dressing.

- If the dressing's edges need to be secured with tape, apply a skin sealant to the intact skin around the ulcer. After the area dries, tape the dressing to the skin. *The sealant protects the skin and promotes tape adherence.* Avoid using tension or pressure when applying the tape.
- Remove your gloves and discard them in the impervious plastic trash bag. Dispose of refuse according to your facility's policy, and wash your hands.
- Change a hydrocolloid dressing every 2 to 7 days as necessary—for example, if the patient complains of pain, the dressing no longer adheres, or leakage occurs. Discontinue if signs of infection are present.

Applying a transparent dressing

- Irrigate the pressure ulcer with normal saline solution. Blot the surrounding skin dry with a sterile 4″ × 4″ gauze pad.
- Select a dressing to overlap the ulcer by 2″ (5 cm).
- Gently lay the dressing over the ulcer. *To prevent shearing force,* don't stretch the dressing. Press firmly on the edges of the dressing *to promote adherence.* Although this type of dressing is self-adhesive, you may have to tape the edges *to prevent them from curling.*
- If necessary, aspirate accumulated fluid with a 21G needle and syringe. After aspirating the pocket of fluid, clean the aspiration site with an alcohol pad and cover it with another strip of transparent dressing.
- Change the dressing every 3 to 7 days, depending on the amount of drainage.

Applying an alginate dressing

- Irrigate the pressure ulcer with normal saline solution. Blot the surrounding skin dry with a sterile 4″ × 4″ gauze pad.
- Apply the alginate dressing to the ulcer surface. Cover the area with a secondary dressing (such as gauze pads), as ordered. Secure the dressing with tape or elastic netting.
- If the wound is draining heavily, change the dressing once or twice daily for the first 3 to 5 days. As drainage decreases, change the dressing less frequently—every 2 to 4 days or as ordered. When the drainage stops or the wound bed looks dry, stop using alginate dressing.

Applying a foam dressing

- Irrigate the pressure ulcer with normal saline solution. Blot the surrounding skin dry with a sterile 4″ × 4″ gauze pad.
- Gently lay the foam dressing over the ulcer.
- Use tape, elastic netting, or gauze to hold the dressing in place.
- Change the dressing when the foam no longer absorbs the exudate.

Applying a hydrogel dressing

- Irrigate the pressure ulcer with normal saline solution. Blot the surrounding skin dry with a sterile 4″ × 4″ gauze pad.
- Apply gel to the wound bed.
- Cover the area with a secondary dressing.
- Change the dressing daily, or as needed, *to keep the wound bed moist.*
- If the dressing you select comes in sheet form, cut the dressing to match the wound base; *otherwise, the intact surrounding skin can become macerated.*
- Hydrogel dressings also come in a prepackaged, saturated gauze for wounds that require "dead space" to be filled. Follow the manufacturer's directions for usage.

Preventing pressure ulcers

- Turn and reposition the patient every 1 to 2 hours unless contraindicated. For a patient who can't turn himself or who is turned on a schedule, use a pressure-reducing device, such as air, gel, or a 4″ (10.2-cm) foam mattress overlay. Low- or high-air-loss bed therapy may be indicated *to reduce excessive pressure and promote evaporation of excess moisture.* As appropriate, implement active or passive range-of-motion exercises *to relieve pressure and promote circulation. To save time,* combine these exercises with bathing if applicable.
- When turning the patient, lift him rather than slide him *because sliding increases friction and shear.* Use a turning sheet and get help from coworkers, if necessary.
- Use pillows *to position the patient and increase his comfort.* Be sure to eliminate sheet wrinkles that could increase pressure and cause discomfort.
- Post a turning schedule at the patient's bedside. Adapt position changes to his situation. Emphasize the importance of regular position changes to the patient and his family, and encourage their participation in the treatment and prevention of pressure ulcers by having them perform a position change correctly, after you have demonstrated how.
- Avoid placing the patient directly on his trochanter. Instead, place him on his side, at about a 30-degree angle.
- Except for brief periods, avoid raising the head of the bed more than 30 degrees *to prevent shearing pressure.*
- Direct the patient confined to a chair or wheelchair to shift his weight every 15 minutes *to promote blood flow to compressed tissues.* Show a paraplegic patient how to shift his weight by doing push-ups in the wheelchair. If the patient needs your help, sit next to him and help him shift his weight to one buttock for 60 seconds; then repeat the procedure on the other side. Provide him with pressure-relieving cushions, as appropriate. However, avoid seating the patient on a rubber or plastic doughnut, *which can increase localized pressure at vulnerable points.*
- Adjust or pad appliances, casts, or splints, as needed, *to ensure proper fit and avoid increased pressure and impaired circulation.*
- Tell the patient to avoid heat lamps and harsh soaps *because they dry the skin.* Applying lotion after bathing will help keep his skin moist. Also tell him to avoid vigorous massage *because it can damage capillaries.*
- If the patient's condition permits, recommend a diet that includes adequate calories, protein, and vitamins. Dietary therapy may involve nutritional consultation, food supplements, enteral feeding, or total parenteral nutrition.
- If diarrhea develops or if the patient is incontinent, clean and dry soiled skin. Then apply a protective moisture barrier *to prevent skin maceration.*
- Make sure the patient, family members, and caregivers learn pressure ulcer prevention and treatment strategies *so that they understand the importance of care, the choices that are available, the rationales for treatments, and their own role in selecting goals and shaping the care plan.*

Special considerations

- Avoid using elbow and heel protectors that fasten with a single narrow strap. *The strap may impair neurovascular function in the involved hand or foot.*
- Avoid using artificial sheepskin. *It doesn't reduce pressure, and it may create a false sense of security.*
- Repair of stage III and stage IV ulcers may require surgical intervention—such as direct closure, skin grafting, and

flaps—depending on the patient's needs. They may also be treated with growth factors, electrical stimulation, heat therapy, or vacuum-assisted wound closure.

Complications

Infection may cause foul-smelling drainage, persistent pain, severe erythema, induration, and elevated skin and body temperatures. Advancing infection or cellulitis can lead to septicemia. Severe erythema may signal worsening cellulitis, which indicates that the offending organisms have invaded the tissue and are no longer localized.

Documentation

Record the date and time of initial and subsequent treatments. Note the specific treatment given. Detail preventive strategies performed. Document the pressure ulcer's location and size (length, width, and depth); color and appearance of the wound bed; amount, odor, color, and consistency of drainage; and condition of the surrounding skin. Reassess pressure ulcers at least weekly.

Update the care plan, as required. On the clinical record, note changes in the condition or size of the pressure ulcer and elevations of skin temperature. Document when the practitioner was notified of pertinent abnormal observations. Record the patient's temperature daily on the graphic sheet *to allow easy assessment of body temperature patterns.*

SELECTED REFERENCES

Ayello, E.A., and Baronoski, S. "Examining the Problem of Pressure Ulcers," *Advances in Skin & Wound Care* 18(4):192, May 2005.

Benbow, M. "Guidelines for the Prevention and Treatment of Pressure Ulcers," *Nursing Standard* 20(52):42-44, September 2006.

Bouza, C., et al. "Efficacy of Advanced Dressings in the Treatment of Pressure Ulcers: A Systematic Review," *Journal of Wound Care* 14(5):193-99, May 2005.

Clance, H.F., et al. "Pressure Ulcers: Implementation of Evidence-Based Nursing Practice," *Journal of Advanced Nursing* 49(6):578-90, March 2005.

Fletcher, J. "Understanding Wound Dressings: Foam Dressings," *Nursing Times* 101(24):50-51, June 2005.

Kaya, A.Z., et al. "The Effectiveness of a Hydrogel Dressing Compared with Standard Management of Pressure Ulcers," *Journal of Wound Care* 14(1):42-44, January 2005.

Keast, D.H., et al. "Best Practice Recommendations for the Prevention and Treatment of Pressure Ulcers: Update 2006," *Advances in Skin & Wound Care* 20(8):447-60, August 2007.

Lyder, C., and van Rijswijk, L. "Pressure Ulcer Prevention and Care: Preventing and Managing Pressure Ulcers in Long-term Care: An Overview of the Revised Federal Regulation," *Ostomy/Wound Management* Suppl:2-6, April 2005.

Parnell, L.K., et al. "Preliminary Use of a Hydrogel Containing Enzymes in the Treatment of Stage II and Stage III Pressure Ulcers," *Ostomy/Wound Management* 51(8):50-60, August 2005.

Wound, Ostomy, and Continence Nurses Society (WOCN). *Position Statement: Clean vs Sterile: Management of Chronic Wounds.* Glenview Ill.: WOCN, 2005.

Wound, Ostomy, and Continence Nurses Society (WOCN). *Guidelines for Prevention and Management of Pressure Ulcers.* Glenview Ill.: WOCN, 2003. *www.guideline.gov/summary/summary.aspx?doc_id=3860*

UNNA'S BOOT

Named for dermatologist Paul Gerson Unna, this boot can be used to treat uninfected, nonnecrotic leg and foot ulcers that result from such conditions as venous insufficiency and stasis dermatitis. A commercially prepared, medicated gauze compression dressing, Unna's boot wraps around the affected foot and leg. Alternatively, a preparation known as *Unna's paste* (gelatin, zinc oxide, calamine lotion, and glycerin) may be applied to the ulcer and covered with lightweight gauze. The boot's effectiveness results from compression applied by the bandage combined with moisture supplied by the paste.

Unna's boot is contraindicated in patients allergic to any ingredient used in the paste and in patients with arterial ulcers, weeping eczema, or cellulitis.

Equipment

Scrub sponge with ordered cleaning agent ■ normal saline solution ■ commercially prepared gauze bandage saturated with Unna's paste (or Unna's paste and lightweight gauze) ■ bandage scissors ■ gloves ■ elastic bandage to cover Unna's boot ■ optional: extra gauze for excessive drainage.

Implementation

- Confirm the patient's identity using two patient identifiers according to your facility's policy.
- Explain the procedure to the patient and provide privacy.
- Wash your hands, and put on gloves.
- Assess the ulcer and the surrounding skin. Evaluate ulcer size, drainage, and appearance. Perform a neurovascular assessment of the affected foot *to ensure adequate circulation.* If you don't detect a pulse in the foot, check with the ordering practitioner before applying Unna's boot.
- Clean the affected area gently with the sponge and cleaning agent *to retard bacterial growth and to remove dirt and wound debris, which may create pressure points after you apply the bandage.* Rinse with normal saline solution.

How to wrap Unna's boot

After cleaning the patient's skin thoroughly, flex his knee. Then, starting with the foot positioned at a right angle to the leg, wrap the medicated gauze bandage firmly—not tightly—around the patient's foot. Make sure the dressing covers the heel. Continue wrapping upward, overlapping the dressing slightly with each turn. Smooth the boot with your free hand as you go (as shown below).

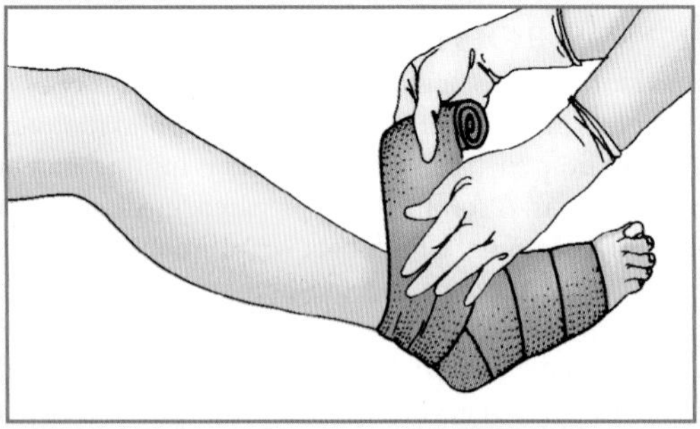

Stop wrapping about 1″ (2.5 cm) below the knee. If necessary, make a 2″ (5-cm) slit in the boot just below the knee *to relieve constriction that may develop as the dressing hardens.*

If drainage is excessive, you may wrap a roller gauze dressing over the boot. As the final layer, wrap an elastic bandage in a figure-eight pattern.

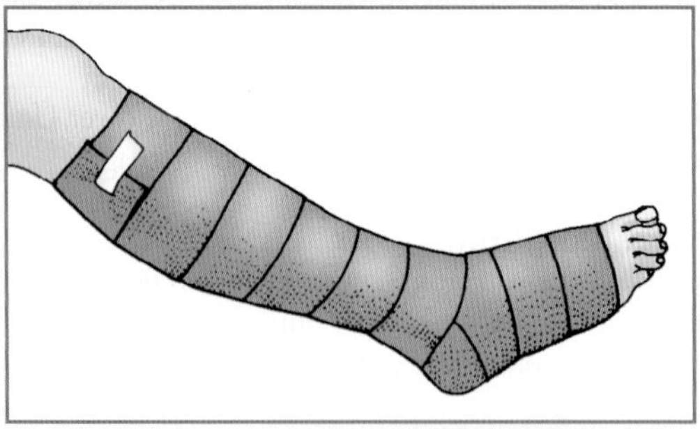

- If a commercially prepared gauze bandage isn't ordered, spread Unna's paste evenly on the leg and foot. Then cover the leg and foot with the lightweight gauze. Apply three to four layers of paste interspersed with layers of gauze. Commercially prepared bandages are impregnated with the paste.
- Apply gauze or the prepared bandage in a spiral motion, from just above the toes to the knee. Be sure to cover the heel. The wrap should be snug but not tight. *To cover the area completely,* make sure that each turn overlaps the previous one by half the bandage width. (See *How to wrap Unna's boot.*)
- Continue wrapping the patient's leg up to the knee, using firm, even pressure. Stop the dressing 1″ (2.5 cm) below the popliteal fossa *to prevent irritation when the knee is bent.* Mold the boot with your free hand as you apply the bandage *to make it smooth and even.*
- Cover the boot with an elastic bandage *to provide external compression.*
- Instruct the patient to remain in bed with his leg outstretched and elevated on a pillow until the paste dries (approximately 30 minutes). Observe the patient's foot for signs of impairment, such as cyanosis, loss of feeling, and swelling. *These signs indicate that the bandage is too tight and must be removed.*
- Leave the boot on for 5 to 7 days, or as ordered. Instruct the patient to walk on and handle the boot carefully *to avoid damaging it.* Tell him the boot will stiffen but won't be as hard as a cast.
- Change the boot weekly, or as ordered, *to assess the underlying skin and ulcer healing.* Remove the boot by unwrapping the bandage from the knee back to the foot.

Special considerations

- If the boot is applied over a swollen leg, it must be changed as the edema subsides—if necessary, more frequently than every 5 days.
- Don't make reverse turns while wrapping the bandage. *This could create excessive pressure areas that may cause discomfort as the bandage hardens.*
- For bathing, instruct the patient to cover the boot with a plastic kitchen trash bag sealed at the knee with an elastic bandage *to avoid wetting the boot. A wet boot softens and loses its effectiveness.* If the patient's safety is a concern, instruct him to take a sponge bath.

Complications

Contact dermatitis may result from hypersensitivity to Unna's paste.

Documentation

Record the date and time of application and the presence of a pulse in the affected foot. Specify which leg you bandaged. Describe the appearance of the patient's skin before and after boot application. List the equipment used (a commercially prepared bandage or Unna's paste and lightweight gauze). Describe any allergic reaction that the patient had.

Burn care at the scene

By acting promptly when a burn injury occurs, you can improve a patient's chance of uncomplicated recovery. Emergency care at the scene should include steps to stop the burn from worsening; assessment of the patient's airway, breathing, and circulation (ABCs); a call for help from an emergency medical team; and emotional and physiologic support for the patient.

Stop the burning process

- If the victim is on fire, tell him to fall to the ground and roll to put out the flames. *(If he panics and runs, air will fuel the flames, worsening the burn and increasing the risk of inhalation injury.)* Or, if you can, wrap the victim in a blanket or other large covering *to smother the flames and protect the burned area from dirt.* Keep his head outside the blanket *so that he doesn't breathe toxic fumes.* As soon as the flames are out, unwrap the patient *so that the heat can dissipate.*
- Cool the burned area with any nonflammable liquid. *This decreases pain and stops the burn from growing deeper or larger.*
- If possible, remove any potential sources of heat, such as jewelry, belt buckles, and some types of clothing. *Besides adding to the burning process, these items may cause constriction as edema develops.* If the patient's clothing adheres to his skin, don't try to remove it. Rather, cut around it.
- Cover the wound with a tablecloth, sheet, or other smooth, nonfuzzy material.

Assess the damage

- Call for help as quickly as possible. Send someone to contact the emergency medical service (EMS).
- Assess the patient's ABCs, and perform cardiopulmonary resuscitation, if necessary. Then check for other serious injuries, such as fractures, spinal cord injury, lacerations, blunt trauma, and head contusions.
- Estimate the extent and depth of the burns. If flames caused the burns and the injury occurred in a closed space, assess for signs of inhalation injury: singed nasal hairs, burns on the face or mouth, soot-stained sputum, coughing or hoarseness, wheezing, or respiratory distress.
- If the patient is conscious and alert, try to get a brief medical history as soon as possible.
- Reassure the patient that help is on the way. Provide emotional support by staying with him, answering questions, and explaining what's being done for him.
- When help arrives, give the EMS a report on the patient's status.

SELECTED REFERENCES

Adelman, A. "Compression Treatment for Venous Leg Ulcers," *Journal of Family Practice* 45(6):471, December 1997.

Barr, D.M. "The Unna's Boot as a Treatment for Venous Ulcers," *Nurse Practitioner* 21(7):55-56, 61-64, 71-72, July 1996.

Davis, J., and Gray, M. "Is the Unna's Boot Bandage as Effective as a Four-Layer Wrap for Managing Venous Leg Ulcers?" *Journal of Wound, Ostomy and Continence Nursing* 32(3):152-56, May-June 2005.

Fletcher, A., et al. "A Systematic Review of Compression Treatment for Venous Leg Ulcers," *British Medical Journal* 315(7108):576-80, September 1997.

BURNS

BURN CARE

The goals of burn care are to maintain the patient's physiologic stability, repair skin integrity, prevent infection, and promote maximal functioning and psychosocial health. Competent care immediately after a burn occurs can dramatically improve the success of overall treatment. (See *Burn care at the scene.*)

All burn victims should be evaluated initially as a trauma patient following the systematic approach developed by the American College of Surgeons Committee. The primary survey focuses mainly on maintaining the patient's airway, breathing, and circulation. When the burn is caused by a chemical agent, the priority is to remove the offending agent and institute water lavage to the affected area. The secondary survey focuses on a head-to-toe assessment, followed by efforts to stop the burn and extension of the injury. Specific elements of the survey should include burn severity, which is determined by the depth and extent of the burn, determination of a possible inhalation injury, and other factors, such as age, complications, coexisting illnesses, and the possibility of abuse. (See *Estimating burn surfaces in adults and children,* page 796. See also *Evaluating burn severity,* page 797.)

Estimating burn surfaces in adults and children

You need to use different formulas to compute burned body surface area (BSA) in adults and children because the proportion of BSA varies with growth.

Rule of Nines

You can quickly estimate the extent of an adult patient's burn by using the "Rule of Nines." This method quantifies BSA in percentages either in fractions of nine or in multiples of nine. To use this method, mentally assess your patient's burns by the body chart shown below. Add the corresponding percentages for each body section burned. Use the total—a rough estimate of burn extent—to calculate initial fluid replacement needs.

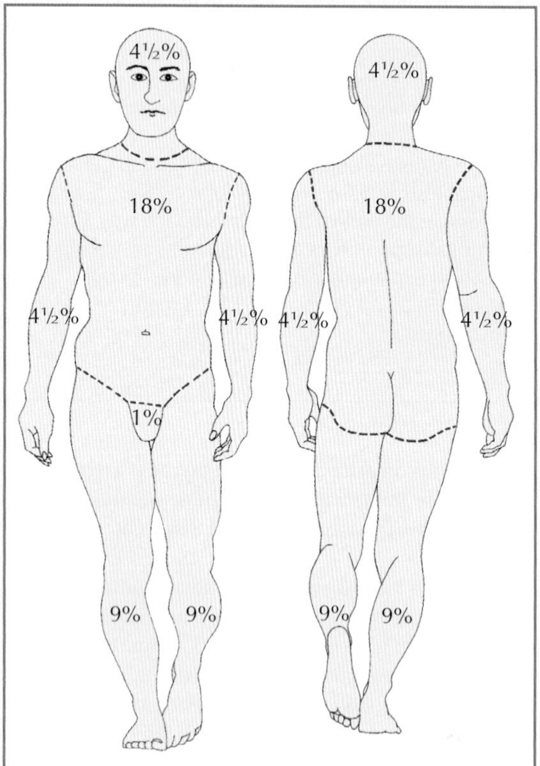

Lund-Browder chart

The Rule of Nines isn't accurate for infants and children because their body shapes differ from those of adults. An infant's head, for example, accounts for about 17% of his total BSA, compared with 7% for an adult. Instead, use the Lund-Browder chart shown here.

Percentage of burned body surface by age

At birth	0 to 1 year	1 to 4 years	5 to 9 years	10 to 15 years	Adult
A: Half of head					
9½%	8½%	6½%	5½%	4½%	3½%
B: Half of one thigh					
2¾%	3¼%	4%	4¼%	4½%	4¾%
C: Half of one leg					
2½%	2½%	2¾%	3%	3¼%	3½%

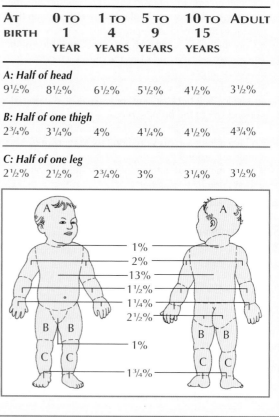

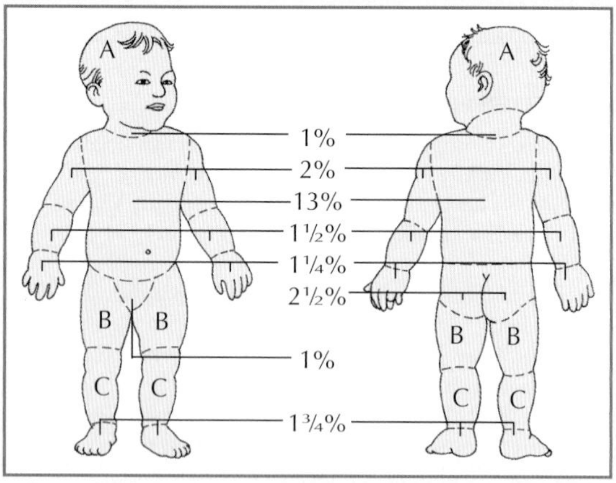

According to the American Burn Association, you'll need to carefully monitor your patient's respiratory status, especially if he has suffered smoke inhalation. Be aware that a patient with burns involving more than 20% of his total body surface area usually needs fluid resuscitation, which aims to support the body's compensatory mechanisms without overwhelming them. Expect to give fluids (such as lactated Ringer's solution) to keep the patient's urine output at 30 to 50 ml/hour, and expect to monitor blood pressure and heart rate. You'll also need to control body temperature because skin loss interferes with temperature regulation. Use warm fluids, heat lamps, and hyperthermia blankets, as ap-

Evaluating burn severity

To judge a burn's severity, assess its depth and extent as well as the presence of other factors.

Superficial partial-thickness burn

Does the burned area appear pink or red with minimal edema? Is the area sensitive to touch and temperature changes? If so, your patient most likely has a superficial partial-thickness, or first-degree, burn affecting only the epidermal skin layer.

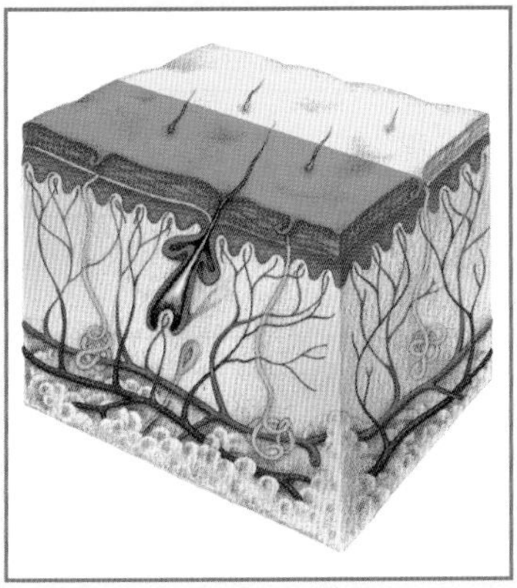

Deep partial-thickness burn

Does the burned area appear pink or red, with a mottled appearance? Do red areas blanch when you touch them? Does the skin have large, thick-walled blisters with subcutaneous edema? Does touching the burn cause severe pain? Is the hair still present? If so, the person most likely has a deep partial-thickness, or second-degree, burn, affecting the epidermal and dermal layers.

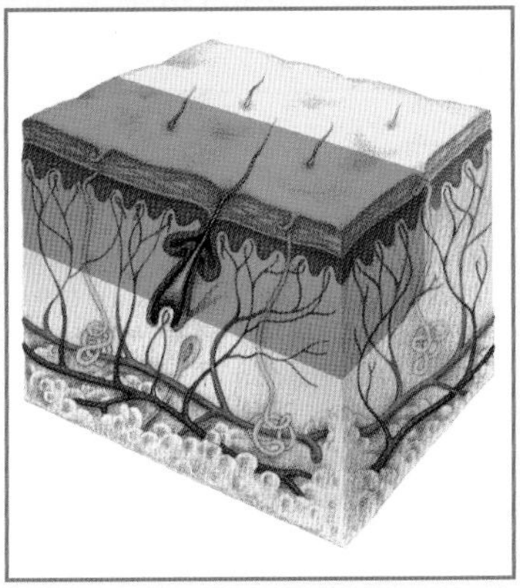

Full-thickness burn

Does the burned area appear red, waxy white, brown, or black? Does red skin remain red with no blanching when you touch it? Is the skin leathery with extensive subcutaneous edema? Is the skin insensitive to touch? Does the hair fall out easily? If so, your patient most likely has a full-thickness, or third-degree, burn, affecting all skin layers.

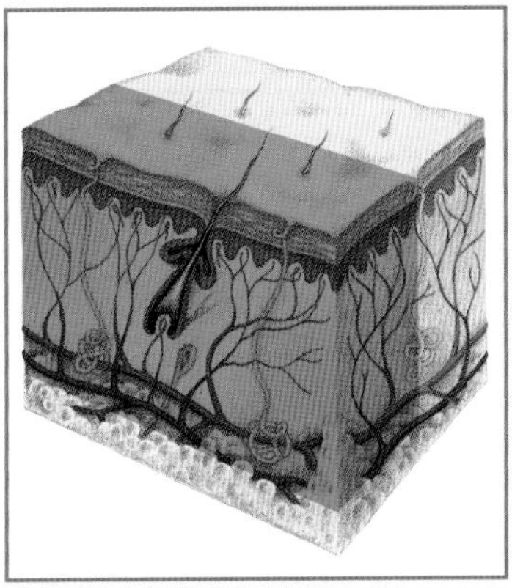

propriate, to keep the patient's temperature above 97° F (36.1° C), if possible. Additionally, you'll frequently review laboratory values, such as serum electrolyte levels, to detect early changes in the patient's condition.

Infection can increase wound depth, cause rejection of skin grafts, slow healing, worsen pain, prolong hospitalization, and even lead to death. To help prevent infection, use strict aseptic technique during care, dress the burn site as ordered, monitor and rotate I.V. lines regularly, and carefully assess the burn extent, body system function, and the patient's emotional status.

Early post-burn positioning is extremely important to prevent contractures. Careful positioning and regular exercise for burned extremities help maintain joint function and minimize deformity. When the extremities aren't being exercised, they should be maintained in maximal extension, using splints, if necessary. Pay particular attention to the hands and neck because they're the most prone to rapid contracture. (See *Positioning the burn patient to prevent deformity,* page 798.)

Skin integrity is repaired through aggressive wound debridement, followed by maintenance of a clean wound bed until the wound heals or is covered with a skin graft.

Early excision and debridement of the wound in the first 48 hours has been shown to decrease blood loss and reduce hospital stay; however, this procedure should only be used on wounds that are clearly full-thickness burns. Surgery takes place as soon as possible after fluid resuscitation. Most wounds are managed with twice-daily dressing changes using topical antibiotics. Burn dressings encourage healing by barring

Positioning the burn patient to prevent deformity

For each of the potential deformities listed below, you can use the corresponding positioning and interventions to help prevent the deformity.

BURNED AREA	POTENTIAL DEFORMITY	PREVENTIVE POSITIONING	NURSING INTERVENTIONS
Neck	■ Flexion contraction of neck ■ Extensor contraction of neck	■ Extension ■ Prone with head slightly raised	■ Remove pillow from bed. ■ Place pillow or rolled towel under upper chest to flex cervical spine, or apply cervical collar.
Axilla	■ Adduction and internal rotation	■ Shoulder joint in external rotation and 100- to 130-degree abduction	■ Use an I.V. pole, bedside table, or sling to suspend arm.
	■ Adduction and external rotation	■ Shoulder in forward flexion and 100- to 130-degree abduction	■ Use an I.V. pole, bedside table, or sling to suspend arm.
Pectoral region	■ Shoulder protraction	■ Shoulders abducted and externally rotated	■ Remove pillow from bed.
Chest or abdomen	■ Kyphosis	■ Same as for pectoral region, with hips neutral (not flexed)	■ Use no pillow under head or legs.
Lateral trunk	■ Scoliosis	■ Supine; affected arm abducted	■ Put pillows or blanket rolls at sides.
Elbow	■ Flexion and pronation	■ Arm extended and supinated	■ Use an elbow splint, arm board, or bedside table.
Wrist	■ Flexion ■ Extension	■ Splint in 15-degree extension ■ Splint in 15-degree flexion	■ Apply a hand splint. ■ Apply a hand splint.
Fingers	■ Adhesions of the extensor tendons; loss of palmar grip	■ Metacarpophalangeal joints in maximum flexion; interphalangeal joints in slight flexion; thumb in maximum abduction	■ Apply a hand splint; wrap fingers separately.
Hip	■ Internal rotation, flexion, and adduction; possibly joint subluxation if contracture is severe	■ Neutral rotation and abduction; maintain extension by prone position	■ Put a pillow under buttocks (if supine) or use trochanter rolls or knee or long leg splints.
Knee	■ Flexion	■ Maintain extension	■ Use a knee splint with no pillows under legs.
Ankle	■ Plantar flexion if foot muscles are weak or their tendons are divided	■ 90-degree dorsiflexion	■ Use a footboard or ankle splint.

germ entry and by removing exudate, eschar, and other debris that host infection. After thorough wound cleaning, topical antibacterial agents are applied, and the wound is covered with absorptive, coarse mesh gauze. Roller gauze typically tops the dressing and is secured with elastic netting or tape.

Equipment

Normal saline solution ▪ bowl ▪ scissors ▪ tissue forceps ▪ ordered topical medication ▪ burn gauze ▪ roller gauze ▪ elastic netting or tape ▪ fine mesh gauze ▪ cotton-tipped applicators ▪ ordered pain medication ▪ three pairs of gloves ▪ cotton bath blanket ▪ 4″ × 4″ gauze pads ▪ gown ▪ mask ▪ surgical cap ▪ heat lamps ▪ impervious plastic trash bag.

A sterile field is required; so, all equipment and supplies used to clean and dress the wound should be sterile.

Preparation of equipment

Warm normal saline solution by immersing unopened bottles in warm water. Assemble equipment on the dressing table. Make sure the treatment area has adequate light *to allow accurate wound assessment.* Open equipment packages using sterile technique. Arrange supplies on a sterile field in order of use.

To prevent cross-contamination, plan to dress the cleanest areas first and the dirtiest or most contaminated areas last. *To help prevent excessive pain or cross-contamination,* you may need to perform the dressing in stages to avoid exposing all wounds at the same time.

Implementation

- Confirm the patient's identity using two patient identifiers according to your facility's policy.
- Administer the ordered pain medication about 20 minutes before beginning wound care *to maximize patient comfort and cooperation.*
- Explain the procedure to the patient and provide privacy.
- Turn on overhead heat lamps *to keep the patient warm.* Make sure they don't overheat the patient.
- Pour warmed normal saline solution into the sterile bowl in the sterile field.
- Wash your hands.

Removing a dressing without hydrotherapy

- Put on a gown, mask, and sterile gloves.
- Remove dressing layers down to the innermost layer by cutting the outer dressings with sterile blunt scissors. Lay open the dressings.
- If the inner layer appears dry, soak it with warm normal saline solution *to ease removal.*
- Remove the inner dressing with sterile tissue forceps or your gloved hand.
- *Because soiled dressings harbor infectious microorganisms,* dispose of the dressings carefully in the impervious plastic trash bag according to your facility's policy. Dispose of your gloves, and wash your hands.
- Put on a new pair of sterile gloves. Using gauze pads moistened with normal saline solution, gently remove any exudate and old topical medication.
- Carefully remove all loose eschar with sterile forceps and scissors, if ordered. (See "Mechanical debridement," page 805.)
- Assess wound condition. The wound should appear clean, with no debris, loose tissue, purulence, inflammation, or darkened margins.
- Before applying a new dressing, remove your gown, gloves, and mask. Discard them properly, and put on a clean mask, surgical cap, gown, and sterile gloves.

Applying a wet dressing

- Soak fine-mesh gauze and the elastic gauze dressing in a large sterile basin containing the ordered solution (for example, silver nitrate).
- Wring out the fine-mesh gauze until it's moist but not dripping, and apply it to the wound. Warn the patient that he may feel transient pain when you apply the dressing.
- Wring out the elastic gauze dressing, and position it to hold the fine-mesh gauze in place.
- Roll an elastic gauze dressing over these two dressings *to keep them intact.*
- Cover the patient with a cotton bath blanket *to prevent chills.* Change the blanket if it becomes damp. Use an overhead heat lamp, if necessary.
- Change the dressings frequently, as ordered, *to keep the wound moist,* especially if you're using silver nitrate. *Silver nitrate becomes ineffective, and the silver ions may damage tissue if the dressings become dry.* (*To maintain moisture,* some protocols call for irrigating the dressing with solution at least every 4 hours through small slits cut into the outer dressing.)

Applying a dry dressing with a topical medication

- Remove old dressings, and clean the wound (as described previously).
- Apply the ordered medication to the wound in a thin layer (about 2 to 4 mm thick) with your sterile gloved hand. Then apply several layers of burn gauze over the wound *to contain the medication but allow exudate to escape.*
- Remember to cut the dry dressing to fit only the wound areas; don't cover unburned areas.

■ Cover the entire dressing with roller gauze, and secure it with elastic netting or tape.

Providing arm and leg care

■ Apply the dressings from the distal to the proximal area *to stimulate circulation and prevent constriction.* Wrap the burn gauze once around the arm or leg so the edges overlap slightly. Continue wrapping in this way until the gauze covers the wound.

■ Apply a dry roller gauze dressing *to hold the bottom layers in place.* Secure with elastic netting or tape.

Providing hand and foot care

■ Wrap each finger separately with a single layer of a 4″ × 4″ sterile gauze pad *to allow the patient to use his hands and to prevent webbing contractures.*

■ Place the hand in a functional position, and secure this position using a dressing. Apply splints, if ordered.

■ Put gauze between each toe, as appropriate, *to prevent webbing contractures.*

Providing chest, abdomen, and back care

■ Apply the ordered medication to the wound in a thin layer. Then cover the entire burned area with sheets of burn gauze.

■ Wrap the area with roller gauze or apply a specialty vest dressing *to hold the burn gauze in place.*

■ Secure the dressing with elastic netting or tape. Make sure the dressing doesn't restrict respiratory motion, especially in very young or elderly patients or in those with circumferential injuries.

Providing facial care

■ If the patient has scalp burns, clip the hair around the burn, as ordered. Clip other hair until it's about 2″ (5 cm) long *to prevent contamination of burned scalp areas.*

■ Shave facial hair if it comes in contact with burned areas.

■ Typically, facial burns are managed with milder topical agents (such as triple antibiotic ointment) and are left open to air. If dressings are required, make sure they don't cover the eyes, nostrils, or mouth.

Providing ear care

■ Clip the hair around the affected ear.

■ Remove exudate and crusts with cotton-tipped applicators dipped in normal saline solution.

■ Place a 4″ × 4″ layer of gauze behind the auricle *to prevent webbing.*

■ Apply the ordered medication to 4″ × 4″ gauze pads, and place the pads over the burned area. Before securing the dressing with a roller bandage, position the patient's ears normally *to avoid damaging the auricular cartilage.*

■ Assess the patient's hearing ability.

Providing eye care

■ Clean the area around the eyes and eyelids with a cotton-tipped applicator and normal saline solution every 4 to 6 hours, or as needed, *to remove crusts and drainage.*

■ Administer ordered eye ointments or drops.

■ If the eyes can't be closed, apply lubricating ointments or drops, as ordered.

■ Be sure to close the patient's eyes before applying eye pads *to prevent corneal abrasion.* Don't apply any topical ointments near the eyes without a practitioner's order.

Providing nasal care

■ Check the nostrils for inhalation injury: inflamed mucosa, singed vibrissae, and soot.

■ Clean the nostrils with cotton-tipped applicators dipped in normal saline solution. Remove crusts.

■ Apply the ordered ointments.

■ If the patient has a nasogastric tube, use tracheostomy ties to secure the tube. Be sure to check the ties frequently for tightness resulting from swelling of facial tissue. Clean the area around the tube every 4 to 6 hours.

Special considerations

■ Thorough assessment and documentation of the wound's appearance are essential *to detect infection and other complications.* A purulent wound or green-gray exudate indicates infection, an overly dry wound suggests dehydration, and a wound with a swollen, red edge suggests cellulitis. Suspect a fungal infection if the wound is white and powdery. Healthy granulation tissue appears clean, pinkish, faintly shiny, and free of exudate.

■ *Because blisters protect underlying tissue,* leave them intact unless they impede joint motion, become infected, or cause patient discomfort.

■ Keep in mind that the patient with healing burns has increased nutritional needs. He'll require extra protein and carbohydrates *to accommodate an almost doubled basal metabolism.*

■ If you must manage a burn with topical medications, exposure to air, and no dressing, watch for such problems as wound adherence to bed linens, poor drainage control, and partial loss of topical medications.

Home care

Begin discharge planning as soon as the patient enters the facility to help him (and his family) make a smooth transition from facility to home. To encourage therapeutic com-

HOME CARE

Successful burn care after discharge

You can help the patient make a successful transition from hospital to home by encouraging him to follow the wound care and self-care guidelines below.

Wound care

- Instruct the patient or a family member to follow this procedure when changing dressings:
- Clean the bathtub, shower, or washbasin thoroughly, and then assemble the required equipment (topical medication, if ordered, and dressing supplies). Open the supplies aseptically on a clean surface.
- Wash your hands. Remove the old dressing and discard it.
- Using a clean washcloth and mild soap and water, wash the wound to remove all the old medication. Try to remove any loose skin, too. Then pat the skin dry with a clean towel.
- Check the burned area for signs of infection: redness, heat, foul odor, increased pain, and difficulty moving the area. If any of these signs is present, notify the practitioner after completing the dressing change.
- Wash your hands. If ordered, apply a thin layer of topical medication to the burned area.
- Cover the burned area with thin layers of gauze, and wrap it with a roller bandage. Finally, secure the dressing with tape or elastic netting.

Self-care

To enhance healing, instruct the patient to eat well-balanced meals with adequate carbohydrates and proteins, to eat between-meal snacks, and to include at least one protein source in each meal and snack. Tell him to avoid tobacco, alcohol, and caffeine *because they constrict peripheral blood flow.*

Advise the patient to wash new skin with mild soap and water. *To prevent excessive skin dryness,* instruct him to use a lubricating lotion and to avoid lotions containing alcohol or perfume. Caution the patient to avoid bumping or scratching regenerated skin tissue.

Recommend nonrestrictive, nonabrasive clothing, which should be laundered in a mild detergent. Advise the patient to wear protective clothing during cold weather *to prevent frostbite.* Warn the patient not to expose new skin to strong sunlight and to always use a sunscreen with a sun protection factor of 20 or higher. Also, tell him not to expose new skin to irritants, such as paint, solvents, strong detergents, and antiperspirants. Recommend cool baths or ice packs *to relieve itching.*

To minimize scar formation, the patient may need to wear a pressure garment—usually for 23 hours per day for 6 months to 1 year. Instruct him to remove it only during daily hygiene. Suspect that the garment is too tight if it causes cold, numbness, or discoloration in the fingers or toes or if its seams and zippers leave deep, red impressions for more than 10 minutes after the garment is removed.

pliance, prepare him to expect scarring, teach him wound management and pain control, and urge him to follow the prescribed exercise regimen. Provide encouragement and emotional support, and urge the patient to join a burn survivor support group. Teach the family or caregivers how to encourage, support, and provide care for the patient. (See *Successful burn care after discharge.*)

Complications

Infection is the most common burn complication.

Documentation

Record the date and time of all care provided. Describe wound condition, special dressing-change techniques, topical medications administered, positioning of the burned area, and the patient's tolerance of the procedure.

SELECTED REFERENCES

ABA. "Practice Guidelines for Burn Care," *Journal of Burn Care and Rehabilitation* 22(3Suppl): May-June 2001.

Hemington-Gorse, S.J. "Colloid or Crystalloid for Resuscitation of Major Burns," *Journal of Wound Care* 14(6):256-58, June 2005.

Lipley, N. "New Guidelines for Managing Patients with Burns," *Emergency Nurse* 14(10):3, March 2007.

Mendez-Eastman, S. "Burn Injuries," *Plastic Surgical Nursing* 25(3):133-39, July-September 2005.

Tenqvall, O.M., et al. "Differences in Pain Patterns for Infected and Non-infected Patients with Burn Injuries," *Pain Management Nursing* 7(4):176-82, December 2006.

Biological burn dressings

Biological dressings provide a temporary protective covering for burn wounds and clean granulation tissue. They also temporarily secure fresh skin grafts and protect graft donor sites. Three organic materials (pigskin, cadaver skin, and amniotic membrane) and one synthetic material (Biobrane) are commonly used. (See *Comparing biological dressings.*) Besides stimulating new skin growth, these dressings act like normal skin; they reduce heat loss, block infection, and minimize fluid, electrolyte, and protein losses.

Amniotic membrane or fresh cadaver skin is usually applied to the patient in the operating room, although it may be applied in a treatment room. Pigskin or Biobrane may be applied in either the operating room or a treatment room. Before applying a biological dressing, the caregiver must clean and debride the wound. The frequency of dressing changes depends on the type of wound and the dressing's specific function.

Equipment

Ordered analgesic ▪ cap ▪ mask ▪ two pairs of sterile gloves ▪ sterile or clean gown ▪ shoe covers ▪ biological dressing ▪ sterile normal saline solution ▪ sterile basin ▪ Xeroflo gauze ▪ sterile forceps ▪ sterile scissors ▪ sterile hemostat ▪ elastic netting.

Preparation of equipment

Place the biological dressing in the sterile basin containing sterile normal saline solution (or open the Biobrane package). Using sterile technique, open the sterile dressing packages. Arrange the equipment on the dressing cart, and keep the cart readily accessible. Make sure the treatment area has adequate light *to allow accurate wound assessment and dressing placement.*

Implementation

- Confirm the patient's identity using two patient identifiers according to your facility's policy.
- If this is the patient's first treatment, explain the procedure *to allay his fears and promote cooperation.* Provide privacy.
- If ordered, administer an analgesic to the patient 20 minutes before beginning the procedure or give an analgesic I.V. immediately before the procedure *to increase the patient's comfort and tolerance levels.*
- Wash your hands and put on cap, mask, gown, shoe covers, and sterile gloves.
- Clean and debride the wound *to reduce bacteria.* Remove and dispose of gloves. Wash your hands and put on a fresh pair of sterile gloves.
- Place the dressing directly on the wound surface. Apply pigskin dermal with the shiny side down; apply Biobrane nylon-backed with the dull side down. Roll the dressing directly onto the skin if applicable. Place the dressing strips so that the edges touch but don't overlap. Use sterile forceps if necessary. Smooth the dressing. Eliminate folds and wrinkles by rolling out the dressing with the hemostat handle, the forceps handle, or your sterile-gloved hand *to cover the wound completely and ensure adherence.*
- Use the scissors to trim the dressing around the wound so that the dressing fits the wound without overlapping adjacent areas.
- Place Xeroflo gauze directly over an allograft, pigskin graft, or amniotic membrane. Place a few layers of gauze on top *to absorb exudate,* and wrap with a roller gauze dressing. Secure the dressing with tape or elastic netting. During daily dressing changes, the dressing will be removed down to the Xeroflo gauze, and the gauze will be replaced after the Xeroflo is inspected for drainage, adherence, and signs of infection.
- Place a nonadhesive dressing (such as Exu-dry) over the Biobrane *to absorb drainage and provide stability.* Wrap the dressing with a roller gauze dressing, and secure it with tape or elastic netting. During daily dressing changes, the dressing will be removed down to the Biobrane and the site inspected for signs of infection. After the Biobrane adheres (usually in 2 to 3 days), it doesn't need to be covered with a dressing.
- Position the patient comfortably, elevating the area if possible. *This reduces edema, which may prevent the biological dressing from adhering.*

Special considerations

- Handle the biological dressing as little as possible.

Home care

Instruct the patient or caregiver to assess the site daily for signs of infection, swelling, blisters, drainage, and separation. Make sure the patient knows whom to contact if these complications develop.

Complications

Infection may develop under a biological dressing. Observe the wound carefully during dressing changes for signs of infection. If wound drainage appears purulent, remove the dressing, clean the area with normal saline solution or another prescribed cleaning solution, as ordered, and apply a fresh biological dressing.

Comparing biological dressings

Different types of biological dressings are available and are used as appropriate for the type of graft required. Nursing considerations for each type are listed below.

TYPE	DESCRIPTION AND USES	NURSING CONSIDERATIONS
Cadaver (homograft)	▪ Obtained at autopsy up to 24 hours after death ▪ Applied in the operating room or at the bedside to debrided, untidy wounds ▪ Available as fresh cryopreserved homografts in tissue banks nationwide ▪ Provides protection, especially to granulation tissue after escharotomy ▪ May be used in some patients as a test graft for autografting ▪ Covers excised wounds immediately	▪ Observe for exudate. ▪ Watch for signs of rejection. ▪ Keep in mind that the gauze dressing may be removed every 8 hours to observe the graft.
Pigskin (heterograft or xenograft)	▪ Applied in the operating room or at the bedside ▪ Comes fresh or frozen in rolls or sheets ▪ Can cover and protect debrided, untidy wounds, mesh autografts, clean (eschar-free) partial-thickness burns, and exposed tendons	▪ Reconstitute frozen form with normal saline solution 30 minutes before use. ▪ Watch for signs of rejection. ▪ Cover with gauze dressing or leave exposed to air, as ordered.
Amniotic membrane (homograft)	▪ Available from the obstetric department ▪ Must be sterile and come from an uncomplicated birth; serologic tests must be done ▪ Bacteriostatic condition doesn't require antimicrobials ▪ May be used to protect partial-thickness burns or (temporarily) granulation tissue before autografting ▪ Applied by the physician to clean wounds only	▪ Change the membrane every 48 hours. ▪ Cover the membrane with a gauze dressing or leave it exposed, as ordered. ▪ If you apply a gauze dressing, change it every 48 hours.
Biobrane (biosynthetic membrane)	▪ Comes in sterile, prepackaged sheets in various sizes and in glove form for hand burns ▪ Used to cover donor graft sites, superficial partial-thickness burns, debrided wounds awaiting autograft, and meshed autografts ▪ Provides significant pain relief ▪ Applied by the nurse	▪ Apply taut against the skin. ▪ Leave the membrane in place for 3 to 14 days, possibly longer. ▪ Don't use this dressing for preparing a granulation bed for subsequent autografting.

Documentation

Record the time and date of dressing changes. Note areas of application, quality of adherence, and purulent drainage or other signs of infection. Describe the patient's tolerance of the procedure.

SELECTED REFERENCES

Chiu, T., and Burd, A. "'Xenograft' Dressing in the Treatment of Burns," *Clinical Dermatology* 23(4):419-23, July-August 2005.

Demling, R.H., et al. "Clinical Use of Biobrane." Available at *www.burnsurgery.org/Modules/BurnWound%201/sect_viii.htm.*

Mendez-Eastman, S. "Burn Injuries," *Plastic Surgical Nursing* 25(3):133-39, July-September 2005.

HYDROTHERAPY

Treating diseases or injuries by immersing part or all of the patient's body in water is known as hydrotherapy. Sometimes used to debride serious burns and to hasten healing, hydrotherapy also promotes circulation and comfort in patients with peripheral vascular disease and musculoskeletal disorders such as arthritis. Although hydrotherapy usually involves immersing the patient in a tub of water ("tubbing"), showers or other water-spray techniques may replace tubbing in some health care facilities and burn centers.

The nurse or physical therapist usually assists the patient into the tub or shower area if he's ambulatory. If he isn't ambulatory, he can enter the water using a stretcher or hoist device. Hydrotherapy is usually limited to 30 minutes or fewer to prevent chilling.

Hydrotherapy is contraindicated in the presence of sudden changes: fever, electrolyte or fluid imbalance, or unstable vital signs. Always follow the standard precautions guidelines. (See chapter 2, Infection control.)

Equipment

Water tank or tub or shower table ▪ stretcher ▪ headrest ▪ hydraulic hoist ▪ gown ▪ surgical cap ▪ mask ▪ gloves ▪ debridement instruments ▪ razor, shaving cream, mild soap, shampoo, and washcloth (for general cleaning) ▪ fluffed gauze pads ▪ cotton-tipped applicators ▪ sterile sheets ▪ warm, sterile bath blankets ▪ optional: analgesic.

Barriers, sheets, and bath blankets may be sterile or clean, depending on the patient's condition and your facility's infection-control policies.

Preparation of equipment

Thoroughly clean and disinfect the tub or shower, its equipment, and the tub or shower room before each treatment *to prevent cross-contamination.* After cleaning, fill the tub with warm water (98° to 104° F [36.6° to 40° C]).

Attach the headrest to the sides of the tub. Warm the bath blankets and ensure that the room is warm enough *to avoid chilling the patient.*

Implementation

- Confirm the patient's identity using two patient identifiers according to your facility's policy.
- If this is the patient's first treatment, explain the procedure to him *to allay his fears and promote cooperation.*
- As necessary (before debridement, for example), administer an analgesic about 20 minutes before the procedure.
- Check the patient's vital signs.
- If the patient is receiving an I.V. infusion, make sure he has enough I.V. solution to last through the procedure.
- Transfer the patient to a stretcher, and transport him to the therapy room. If he's ambulatory, he may walk unassisted, provided that the therapy room is nearby.
- Wash your hands, and put on your gown, gloves, mask, and surgical cap.
- Remove the outer dressings and dispose of them properly before immersing the patient. Leave the inner gauze layer on the wound unless it can be easily removed.
- Assist the patient into the tub. Position him so that the headrest supports his head. Allow him to soak for 3 to 5 minutes.
- Remove remaining gauze dressings, if any, from the patient's wounds.
- If ordered, place the tub's agitator into the water and turn it on. *The motor may burn out if it's turned on out of the water.* Some tubs have aerators to agitate the water.
- Clean all unburned areas first (encourage the patient to do this if he can). Wash unburned skin, and clip or shave hair near the wound. Shave facial hair, shampoo the scalp, and give mouth care, as appropriate. Provide perineal care, and clean inside the patient's nose and the folds of the ears and eyes with cotton-tipped applicators.
- Gently scrub burned areas with fluffed gauze pads *to remove topical agents, exudates, necrotic tissue, and other debris.* Debride the wound after turning off the agitator.
- Exercise the patient's extremities with active or passive range of motion, depending on his condition and exercise tolerance. Alternatively, you may have the physical therapist exercise the patient.
- After you've completed the treatment, use the hoist to raise the patient above the water.
- With the patient still suspended over the water, spray-rinse his body *to remove debris from shaving, cleaning, and debridement.*
- Transfer the patient to a stretcher covered with a clean sheet and bath blanket, and cover him with a warm sterile sheet (a blanket may be added for warmth). Pat unburned areas dry *to prevent chilling.*
- Remove the wet or damp linens, and cover the patient with dry linens. Remove your gown, gloves, and mask before transporting the patient back to his room.
- Have the tub drained, cleaned, and disinfected according to your facility's policy.

Special considerations

- Remain with the patient at all times *to prevent accidents in the tub.* Limit hydrotherapy to 20 to 30 minutes. Watch the patient closely for adverse reactions.
- If necessary, weigh the patient during hydrotherapy *to assess nutritional status and fluid shift.* Use a hoist that has a table scale.

■ Whirlpool treatments should be discontinued when the wounds are assessed as clean *because the whirlpool's agitating water may result in trauma to the regenerating tissue.*

Complications

Incomplete disinfection of tub, drains, and faucets, or cross-contamination from members of the tubbing team, may cause infection. The patient may chill easily from decreased resistance to temperature changes. A fluid or electrolyte imbalance (or both) may result from a chemical imbalance between the patient and the tub solution.

Documentation

Record the date, time, and patient's reaction. Note the patient's condition (vital signs and wound appearance). Document any wound infection or bleeding. Note treatments given, such as debridement, and dressing changes. Record any special treatments in the nursing care plan.

SELECTED REFERENCES

Gwynne, B., and Newton, M. "An Overview of the Common Methods of Wound Debridement," *British Journal of Nursing* 15(19):S4-S10, October-November 2006.

MECHANICAL DEBRIDEMENT

Debridement involves removing necrotic tissue by mechanical, chemical, or surgical means to allow underlying healthy tissue to regenerate. Mechanical debridement procedures include irrigation, hydrotherapy, and excision of dead tissue with forceps and scissors. The procedure may be done at the bedside or in a specially prepared room.

Depending on the type of burn, a combination of debridement techniques may be used. Other debridement techniques include chemical debridement (with wound-cleaning beads or topical agents that absorb exudate and debris) or surgical excision and skin grafting (usually reserved for deep burns or ulcers). Typically, the patient receives a local or general anesthetic.

Burn wound debridement removes eschar (hardened, dead tissue). This prevents or controls infection, promotes healing, and prepares the wound surface to receive a graft. Ideally, the wound should be debrided daily during the dressing change. Frequent, regular debridement guards against possible hemorrhage resulting from more extensive and forceful debridement. It also reduces the need to conduct extensive debridement under anesthesia.

Closed blisters over partial-thickness burns shouldn't be debrided. (For additional information, see "Hydrotherapy.")

Equipment

Ordered pain medication ■ two pairs of sterile gloves ■ two gowns or aprons ■ mask ■ cap ■ sterile scissors ■ sterile forceps ■ 4″ × 4″ sterile gauze pads ■ sterile solutions and medications, as ordered ■ hemostatic agent, as ordered ■ tweezers ■ #15 blade (for fine debriding) ■ #10 or 20 blade (for thin slices of tissue).

Be sure to have the following equipment immediately available to control hemorrhage: needle holder ■ gut suture with needle ■ silver nitrate sticks.

Implementation

■ Confirm the patient's identity using two patient identifiers according to your facility's policy.
■ Explain the procedure to the patient *to allay his fears and promote cooperation.* Teach him distraction and relaxation techniques, if possible, *to minimize his discomfort.*
■ Provide privacy. Administer an analgesic 20 minutes before debridement begins, or give an I.V. analgesic immediately before the procedure.
■ Keep the patient warm. Expose only the area to be debrided *to prevent chilling and fluid and electrolyte loss.*
■ Wash your hands, and put on a cap, mask, gown or apron, and sterile gloves.
■ Remove the burn dressings and clean the wound. (For detailed directions, see "Burn care," page 795.)
■ Remove your gown or apron and dirty gloves, and change to another gown or apron and sterile gloves.
■ Lift loosened edges of eschar with forceps. Use the blunt edge of scissors or forceps to probe the eschar. Cut the dead tissue from the wound with the scissors. Leave a ¼″ (0.6 cm) edge on remaining eschar *to avoid cutting into viable tissue.*
■ *Because debridement removes only dead tissue,* bleeding should be minimal. If bleeding occurs, apply gentle pressure on the wound with sterile 4″ × 4″ gauze pads. Then apply the hemostatic agent or silver nitrate sticks. If bleeding persists, notify the practitioner, and maintain pressure on the wound until he arrives. Excessive bleeding or spurting vessels may require ligation.
■ Perform additional procedures, such as application of topical medications and dressing replacements, as ordered.

Special considerations

■ Work quickly, with an assistant if possible, to complete this painful procedure as soon as possible. Try to limit the procedure time to 20 minutes.
■ Acknowledge the patient's discomfort, and provide emotional support.
■ Debride no more than a 4″ (10.2-cm) square area at one time.

Understanding types of grafts

A burn patient may receive one or more of the graft types described below.

Split-thickness

The type used most commonly for covering open burns, a split-thickness graft includes the epidermis and part of the dermis. It may be applied as a sheet (usually on the face or neck *to preserve the cosmetic result*) or as a mesh. A mesh graft has tiny slits cut in it, which allow the graft to expand up to nine times its original size. Mesh grafts prevent fluids from collecting under the graft and typically are used over extensive full-thickness burns.

Full-thickness

This graft type includes the epidermis and the entire dermis. Consequently, the graft contains hair follicles, sweat glands, and sebaceous glands, which typically aren't included in split-thickness grafts. Full-thickness grafts are usually used for small deep burns.

Pedicle-flap

This full-thickness graft includes not only skin and subcutaneous tissue, but also subcutaneous blood vessels *to ensure a continued blood supply to the graft.* Pedicle-flap grafts may be used during reconstructive surgery *to cover previous defects.*

Complications

Infection may develop despite the use of sterile technique and equipment. In addition, some blood loss may occur if debridement exposes an eroded blood vessel or if you inadvertently cut a vessel. Fluid and electrolyte imbalances may result from exudate lost during the procedure.

Documentation

Record the date and time of wound debridement, the area debrided, and solutions and medications used. Describe wound condition, noting signs of infection or skin breakdown. Record the patient's tolerance of and reaction to the procedure. Note indications for additional therapy.

Selected references

Anderson, I. "Debridement Methods in Wound Care," *Nursing Standards* 20(24):65-66, 68, February 2006.

Brem, H., and Lyder, C. "Protocol for the Successful Treatment of Pressure Ulcers," *American Journal of Surgery* 188(1ASuppl):9-17, July 2004.

Steed, D.L. "Debridement," *American Journal of Surgery* 187(5A):71S-74S, May 2004.

Skin graft care

A skin graft consists of healthy skin taken from either the patient (autograft) or a donor (allograft) and applied to a part of the patient's body, where the graft resurfaces an area damaged by burns, traumatic injury, or surgery. Care procedures for an autograft or an allograft are essentially the same. However, an autograft requires care for two sites: the graft site and the donor site.

Skin grafts are indicated where skin loss has occurred due to burns or for reconstructive purposes following trauma, infection (such as necrotizing fasciitis), malformation, deformity, congenitally deformed tissue, removal of malignant lesions, and plastic surgery in which direct closure by suturing isn't possible.

The graft itself may be one of several types: split-thickness, full-thickness, or pedicle-flap. (See *Understanding types of grafts.*) Successful grafting depends on various factors, including clean wound granulation with adequate vascularization, complete contact of the graft with the wound bed, sterile technique to prevent infection, adequate graft immobilization, and skilled care.

The size and depth of the patient's burns determine whether the burns will require grafting. Grafting usually occurs at the completion of wound debridement. The goal is to cover all wounds with an autograft or allograft within 2 weeks. With enzymatic debridement, grafting may be performed 5 to 7 days after debridement is complete; with surgical debridement, grafting can occur the same day as the surgery.

Depending on your facility's policy, a practitioner or a specially trained nurse may change graft dressings. The dressings usually stay in place for 5 to 7 days after surgery to avoid disturbing the graft site. Meanwhile, the donor graft site needs diligent care. (See *How to care for a donor graft site.*)

Equipment

Ordered analgesic ▪ clean and sterile gloves ▪ sterile gown ▪ cap ▪ mask ▪ sterile forceps ▪ sterile scissors ▪ sterile scalpel ▪ sterile 4″ × 4″ gauze pads ▪ Xeroflo gauze ▪ elastic gauze dressing ▪ warm normal saline solution ▪ moisturizing cream ▪ topical medication ▪ optional: sterile cotton-tipped applicators.

Implementation

- Confirm the patient's identity using two patient identifiers according to your facility's policy.
- Explain the procedure to the patient and provide privacy.
- Administer an analgesic, as ordered, 20 to 30 minutes before beginning the procedure. Alternatively, give an I.V. analgesic immediately before the procedure.
- Wash your hands.
- Put on the sterile gown and the clean mask, cap, and gloves.
- Gently lift off all outer dressings. Soak the middle dressings with warm saline solution. Remove these carefully and slowly *to avoid disturbing the graft site.* Leave the Xeroflo intact *to avoid dislodging the graft.*
- Remove and discard the clean gloves, wash your hands, and put on the sterile gloves.
- Assess the condition of the graft. If you see purulent drainage, notify the practitioner.
- Remove the Xeroflo with sterile forceps, and clean the area gently. If necessary, soak the Xeroflo with warm saline solution *to facilitate removal.*
- Inspect an allograft for signs of rejection, such as infection and delayed healing. Inspect a sheet graft frequently for blebs. If ordered, evacuate them carefully with a sterile scalpel. (See *Evacuating fluid from a sheet graft,* page 808.)
- Place fresh Xeroflo over the site *to promote wound healing and prevent infection.* Cover this with elastic gauze and a roller bandage.
- Clean any completely healed areas, and apply a moisturizing cream to them *to keep the skin pliable and to retard scarring.*

Special considerations

- *To avoid dislodging the graft,* hydrotherapy is usually discontinued, as ordered, for 3 to 4 days after grafting. Avoid using a blood pressure cuff over the graft. Don't tug or pull dressings during dressing changes. Keep the patient from lying on the graft.
- If the graft dislodges, apply sterile skin compresses *to keep the area moist until the surgeon reapplies the graft.* If the graft affects an arm or a leg, elevate the affected extremity *to reduce postoperative edema.* Check for bleeding and signs of neurovascular impairment: increasing pain, numbness or tingling, coolness, and pallor.

Home care

Teach the patient how to apply moisturizing cream. Stress the importance of using a sunscreen with a sun protection factor of 20 or higher on all grafted areas *to avoid sunburn and discoloration.*

How to care for a donor graft site

Autografts are usually taken from another area of the patient's body with a dermatome, an instrument that cuts a uniform, split-thickness skin portion—typically about 0.013 to 0.05 cm thick. Autografting makes the donor site a partial-thickness wound, which may bleed, drain, and cause pain.

This site needs scrupulous care to prevent infection, which could convert the site to a full-thickness wound. Depending on the graft's thickness, tissue may be obtained from the donor site again in as few as 10 days.

Usually, Xeroflo gauze is applied postoperatively. The outer gauze dressing can be taken off on the first postoperative day; the Xeroflo will protect the new epithelial proliferation.

Dressing the wound

Care for the donor site as you care for the autograft, using dressing changes at the initial stages to prevent infection and promote healing. Follow these guidelines:

- Wash your hands, and put on sterile gloves.
- Remove the outer gauze dressings within 24 hours. Inspect the Xeroflo for signs of infection; then leave it open to the air *to speed drying and healing.*
- Leave small amounts of fluid accumulation alone. Using sterile technique, aspirate larger amounts through the dressing with a small-gauge needle and syringe.
- Apply a lanolin-based cream daily to completely healed donor sites *to keep skin tissue pliable and to remove crusts.*

Complications

Graft failure may result from traumatic injury, hematoma or seroma formation, infection, an inadequate graft bed, rejection, or compromised nutritional status.

Documentation

Record the time and date of all dressing changes. Document all medications used, and note the patient's response to the medications. Describe the condition of the graft, and note any signs of infection or rejection. Record any additional treatment, and note the patient's reaction to the graft.

Evacuating fluid from a sheet graft

When small pockets of fluid (called *blebs*) accumulate beneath a sheet graft, you'll need to evacuate the fluid using a sterile scalpel and sterile cotton-tipped applicators. First, carefully perforate the center of the bleb with the scalpel.

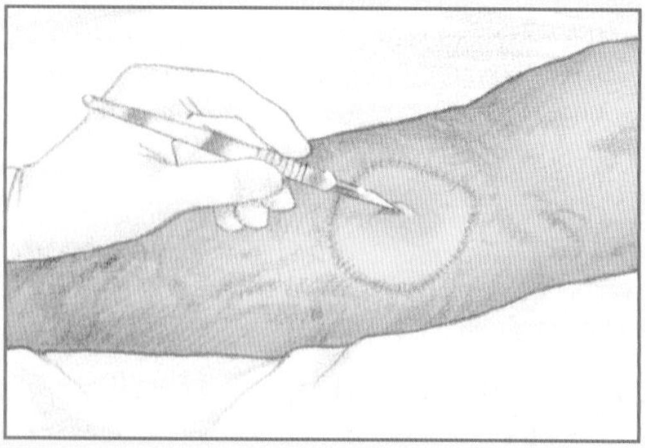

Gently express the fluid with the cotton-tipped applicators.

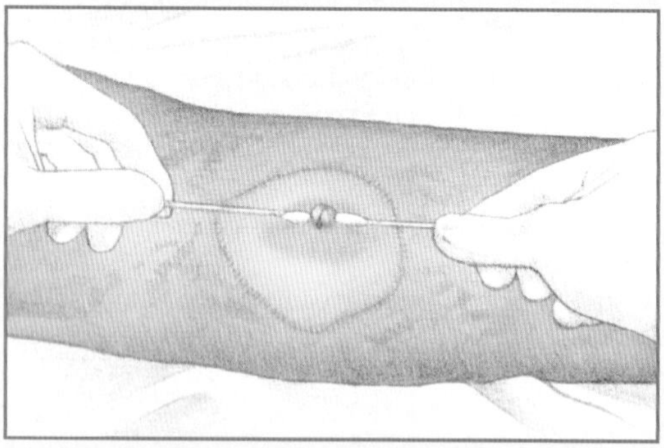

Never express fluid by rolling the bleb to the edge of the graft. *This disturbs healing in other areas.*

Selected references

Hall, B. "Wound Care for Burn Patients in Acute Rehabilitation Settings," *Rehabilitation Nursing* 30(3):114-19, May-June 2005.

Mendez-Eastman, S. "Full-Thickness Skin Grafting: A Procedural Review," *Plastic Surgical Nursing* 24(2):41-45, April 2004.

Siegel, J.D., et al. "Guideline for Isolation Precautions: Preventing Transmission of Infectious Agents in Healthcare Settings 2007." Available at *www.cdc.gov/ncidod/dhqp/pdf/guidelines/Isolation2007.pdf.*

OTHER THERAPIES

Ultraviolet light therapy

Ultraviolet (UV) light causes profound biological changes, including temporary suppression of epidermal basal cell division followed by a later increase in cell turnover, and UV light–induced immune suppression. As a result, such skin conditions as psoriasis, mycosis fungoides, atopic dermatitis, and uremic pruritus may respond to therapy that uses timed exposure to UV light rays.

Emitted by the sun, the UV spectrum is subdivided into three bands—A, B, and C—each of which affects the skin differently. Ultraviolet A (UVA) radiation (with a relatively long wavelength of 320 to 400 nm) rapidly darkens preformed melanin pigment, may augment ultraviolet B (UVB) in causing sunburn and skin aging, and may induce phototoxicity in the presence of some drugs. UVB radiation (with a wavelength of 280 to 320 nm) causes sunburn and erythema. Ultraviolet C (UVC) radiation (with a wavelength of 200 to 280 nm) is normally absorbed by the earth's ozone layer and doesn't reach the ground. However, UVC kills bacteria and is used in operating-room germicidal lamps.

The drug methoxsalen, a psoralens agent, creates artificial sensitivity to UVA by binding with the deoxyribonucleic acid in epidermal basal cells. Treating skin with a photosensitizing agent such as methoxsalen and UVA is called psoralen plus UVA (PUVA) therapy (or photochemotherapy). Administered before a UV light treatment, methoxsalen photosensitizes the skin to enhance therapeutic effect.

Other drugs used in photochemotherapy in combination with PUVA include acitretin (Soriatane), an oral vitamin A derivative, and methotrexate.

Contraindications to PUVA and UVB therapy include a history of photosensitivity diseases, skin cancer, arsenic ingestion, or cataracts or cataract surgery; current use of photosensitivity-inducing drugs; and previous skin irradiation (which can induce skin cancer). Ultraviolet light therapy is also contraindicated in pregnant women, patients who have undergone previous ionizing chemotherapy, and patients who are using photosensitizing or immunosuppressant drugs.

Equipment

For UVA radiation: Fluorescent black-light lamp ▪ high-intensity UVA fluorescent bulbs.

For UVB radiation: Fluorescent sunlamp or hot quartz lamp ▪ sunlamp bulbs.

For all UV treatments: Oral or topical phototherapeutic medications, if necessary ■ body-size light chamber or smaller light box ■ dark, polarized goggles ■ sunscreen, if necessary ■ hospital gown ■ towels.

Preparation of equipment

The patient can undergo UV light therapy in the hospital, in a physician's office, or at home. Typically set into a reflective cabinet, the light source consists of a bank of high-intensity fluorescent bulbs. (At home, the patient may use a small fluorescent sunlamp.)

Check the practitioner's orders to confirm the light treatment type and dose. For PUVA, the initial dose is based on the patient's skin type and is increased according to the treatment protocol and the patient's tolerance. (See *Comparing skin types.*) The practitioner calculates the UVB dose based on skin type estimation or by determining a minimal erythema dose—the smallest amount of UV light needed to produce mild erythema.

Implementation

■ Confirm the patient's identity using two patient identifiers according to your facility's policy.
■ Inform the patient that UV light treatments produce a mild sunburn that will help reduce or resolve skin lesions.
■ Review the patient's health history for contraindications to UV light therapy. Also ask whether he's currently taking photosensitizing drugs, such as anticonvulsants, certain antihypertensives, phenothiazines, salicylates, sulfonamides, tetracyclines, tretinoin, and various cancer drugs.
■ If the patient will have PUVA therapy, make sure he took methoxsalen (with food) 1½ hours before treatment.
■ To begin therapy, instruct the patient to disrobe and put on a hospital gown. Have him remove the gown or expose just the treatment area after he's in the phototherapy unit. Make sure he wears goggles *to protect his eyes* and a sunscreen, towels, or the hospital gown *to protect vulnerable skin areas.* All male patients receiving PUVA must wear protection over the groin area.
■ If the patient is having local UVB treatment, position him at the correct distance from the light source. For instance, for facial treatment with a sunlamp, position the patient's face about 12″ (30.5 cm) from the lamp. For body treatment, position the patient's body about 30″ (76 cm) from either the sunlamp or the hot quartz lamp.
■ During therapy, make sure the patient wears goggles at all times. You should also wear goggles if you're observing him through light-chamber windows. If the patient must stand for the treatment, ask him to report any dizziness *to ensure his safety.*

Comparing skin types

A person's skin type influences his sensitivity to ultraviolet radiation.

SKIN TYPE	SUNBURN AND TANNING HISTORY
I	Always burns; never tans; sensitive ("Celtic" skin)
II	Burns easily; tans minimally
III	Burns moderately; tans gradually to light brown (average Caucasian skin)
IV	Burns minimally; always tans well to moderately brown (olive skin)
V	Rarely burns; tans profusely to dark (brown skin)
VI	Never burns; deeply pigmented; not sensitive (black skin)

■ After delivering the prescribed UV dose, help the patient out of the unit and instruct him to shield exposed areas of skin from sunlight for 8 hours after therapy.

Special considerations

■ Overexposure to UV light (sunburn) can result from prolonged treatment and an inadequate distance between the patient and light sources. It can also result from the use of photosensitizing drugs or from overly sensitive skin.
■ Prevent eye damage by using gray or green polarized lenses during UVB therapy or UV-opaque sunglasses during PUVA therapy. The patient undergoing PUVA therapy should wear these glasses for 24 hours after treatment *because methoxsalen can cause photosensitivity.*
■ Tell the patient to look for marked erythema, blistering, peeling, or other signs of overexposure 4 to 6 hours after UVB therapy and 24 to 48 hours after UVA therapy. In either case, the erythema should disappear within another 24 hours. Inform him that mild dryness and desquamation will occur in 1 or 2 days. Teach him appropriate skin care measures. (See *Skin care guidelines,* page 810.) Advise him to notify the practitioner if overexposure occurs. Typically, the practitioner recommends stopping treatment for a few days and then starting over at a lower exposure level.

HOME CARE

Skin care guidelines

A patient who is receiving ultraviolet light treatments must know how to protect his skin from injury. Provide your patient with the following skin care tips:

- Encourage the patient to use emollients and drink plenty of fluids *to combat dry skin and maintain adequate hydration.* Warn him to avoid hot baths or showers and to use soap sparingly *because heat and soap promote dry skin.*
- Instruct the patient to notify his physician before taking any medication, including aspirin, *to prevent heightened photosensitivity.*
- If the patient is receiving PUVA therapy, review his methoxsalen dosage schedule. Explain that deviating from it could result in burns or ineffective treatment. Urge him to wear appropriate sunglasses outdoors for at least 24 hours after taking methoxsalen. Recommend yearly eye examinations *to detect cataract formation.*
- If the patient uses a sunlamp at home, advise him to let the lamp warm for 5 minutes before treatment. Stress the importance of exposing his skin to the light for the exact amount of time prescribed by the physician. Instruct the patient to protect his eyes with goggles and to use a dependable timer or have someone else time his therapy. Above all, urge him never to use the sunlamp when he's tired *to avoid falling asleep under the lamp and sustaining a burn.*
- Teach the patient first aid for localized burning: Tell him to apply cool water soaks for 20 minutes or until skin temperature cools. For more extensive burns, recommend tepid tap water baths after notifying the physician about the burn. After the patient bathes, suggest using an oil-in-water moisturizing lotion (not a petroleum-jelly-based product, which can trap radiant heat).
- Tell the patient to limit natural-light exposure, to use a sunscreen when he's outdoors, and to notify his physician immediately if he discovers any unusual skin lesions.
- Advise the patient to avoid harsh soaps and chemicals, such as paints and solvents, and to discuss ways to manage physical and psychological stress, which may exacerbate skin disorders.

- Before giving methoxsalen or etretinate, check to ensure that baseline liver function studies have been done. Keep in mind that both drugs are hepatotoxic agents and are never given together. Liver function and blood lipid studies are required before treatment with acitretin and at regular intervals during treatment. Liver function studies and a complete blood count are required before and during methotrexate treatment.

Complications

Erythema is the major adverse effect of UVB therapy. Minimal erythema without discomfort is acceptable, but treatments are suspended if marked edema, swelling, or blistering occurs.

Erythema, nausea, and pruritus are the three major short-term adverse effects of PUVA. Long-term adverse effects are similar to those caused by excessive exposure to sun—premature aging (xerosis, wrinkles, and mottled skin), lentigines, telangiectasia, increased risk of skin cancer, and ocular damage if eye protection isn't used. The patient can minimize effects by using emollients, sunscreens, and cover-ups.

Documentation

Record the date and time of initial and subsequent treatments, the UV wavelength used, and the name and dose of any oral or topical medications given. Record the exact duration of therapy, the distance between the light source and the skin, and the patient's tolerance. Note safety measures used such as eye protection. Also describe the patient's skin condition before and after treatment. Note improvements and adverse reactions, such as increased pruritus, oozing, and scaling.

SELECTED REFERENCES

Lagan, K.M., et al. "Low Intensity Laser Therapy/Combined Phototherapy in the Management of Chronic Venous Ulceration: A Placebo-Controlled Study," *Journal of Clinical Laser Medical Surgery* 20(3):109-16, June 2002.

LASER THERAPY

Using the highly focused and intense energy of a laser beam, the surgeon can treat various skin lesions. Laser surgery has several advantages. As a surgical instrument, the laser offers precise control. It spares normal tissue, speeds healing, and deters infection by sterilizing the operative site. In addition, by sealing tiny blood vessels as it vaporizes tissue, the laser beam leaves a nearly bloodless operative field. In addition, the procedure can be performed on an outpatient basis.

The lasers used most commonly to treat skin lesions are vascular, pigment, and carbon dioxide (CO_2) lasers. (See *Understanding types of laser therapy.*)

In general, laser surgery is safe, although bleeding and scarring can result. One pronounced hazard—to the patient and treatment staff alike—is eye damage or other injury caused by unintended laser beam reflection. For this reason, everyone in the surgical suite, including the patient, must wear special goggles to filter laser light. The surgeon must use special nonreflective instruments. Access to the room must be strictly controlled, and all windows must be covered.

Equipment
Laser ▪ filtration face masks ▪ protective eyewear ▪ laser vacuum ▪ extra vacuum filters ▪ surgical drape ▪ sterile gauze ▪ prescribed cleaning solution ▪ nonadherent dressings ▪ surgical tape ▪ cotton-tipped applicators ▪ nonreflective surgical instruments ▪ sterile gloves.

Preparation of equipment
Before the procedure begins, prepare the tray. It should include a local anesthetic, as ordered, and dry and wet gauze. The gauze will be used *to control bleeding, protect healthy tissue, and abrade and remove any eschar,* which would otherwise inhibit laser absorption. Prepare surgical instruments as needed.

Implementation
- Confirm the patient's identity using two patient identifiers according to your facility's policy.
- Put on gown, filtration face mask, and protective eyewear.
- Tell the patient how the laser works and name its benefits. Point out the equipment and outline the procedure *to help allay the patient's concerns.*
- Just before the surgeon begins, position the patient comfortably, drape him, and place sterile gauze, if needed, around the operative site. Confirm that everyone in the room—including the patient—has safety goggles on *to filter the laser light.*
- Lock the door to the surgical suite *to keep unprotected persons from inadvertently entering the room.*
- After the surgeon administers the anesthetic and it takes effect, activate the laser vacuum. The CO_2 laser has a vacuum hose attached to a separate apparatus. Use this apparatus *to clear the surgical site.* The vacuum has a filter that traps and collects most of the vaporized tissue. Change the filter whenever suction decreases, and follow your facility's guidelines for filter disposal.
- When the surgeon finishes the procedure, apply direct pressure with sterile gauze to any bleeding wound for 20 minutes. (Wear sterile gloves.) If the wound continues to bleed, notify the surgeon.
- After the bleeding is controlled, use sterile technique to clean the area with a cotton-tipped applicator dipped in the prescribed cleaning solution. Then size and cut a nonadherent dressing. Spread a thin layer of antibiotic ointment on one side of the dressing. Place the ointment side over the wound and secure the dressing with surgical tape.
- Vascular and pigment lasers won't result in a wound; only superficial skin changes will occur.

Understanding types of laser therapy

Laser therapy has become an essential tool for treating many types of skin lesions. The number of lasers used in dermatology is ever growing, and each type is used for specific conditions. The term *laser* is an acronym for light amplification by the stimulated emission of radiation. When directed toward the skin, most of this light energy is absorbed by chromophores, substances that absorb specific wavelengths of light. This is the basis of selective photothermolysis, which has revolutionized cutaneous laser surgery. Melanin is the target chromophore in pigmented lesions, and oxyhemoglobin in microvessels is the target chromophore in vascular lesions.

It's important to be familiar with the various types of lasers and the indications for each.

Lasers for vascular lesions
The laser most frequently used for vascular lesions is the pulsed dye laser (PDL). Other types include copper vapor, argon, KTP, krypton, neodymium: yttrium-aluminum-garnet (Nd:YAG), and argon-pumped tunable dye laser. The type of laser used depends on the type of vascular lesion. Port-wine stains, hemangiomas, venous lake, rosacea, teleangiectasia, and Kaposi's sarcoma are examples of vascular lesions that may be treated with laser therapy.

Lasers for pigmented lesions
Lasers that are effective in treating tattoos and dermal and epidermal pigmented lesions include Q-switched ruby, Q-switched Nd:YAG, and Q-switched alexandrite PDL. Among the pigmented lesions appropriate for laser treatment are nevi of Ota, melasma, solar lentigo, café-au-lait spots, Becker's nevi, and epidermal nevi.

Special considerations

- The surgeon uses the laser beam much as he would a scalpel to excise the lesion. Explain that the laser causes a burnlike wound that can be deep. Inform the patient that the wound will appear charred. Tell the patient that some of the eschar will be removed during the initial postoperative cleaning and that more will gradually dislodge at home.
- Warn the patient to expect a burning odor and smoke during the procedure. A machine called a smoke evacuator, which sounds like a vacuum cleaner, will clear it away. Advise the patient that he may sense heat from the laser. Urge him to tell the surgeon at once if pain develops.
- The nurse must have thorough knowledge of how each laser operates and of laser safety considerations for both the patient and the health care providers.

Home care

Teach the patient how to dress his wound or care for his skin daily as ordered by the surgeon. Tell him that he can take showers but shouldn't immerse the wound site in water *to promote wound healing and prevent infection.*

- If the wound bleeds at home, demonstrate how to apply direct pressure on the site with clean gauze or a washcloth for 20 minutes. If pressure doesn't control the bleeding, tell the patient to call his practitioner.
- If the patient's foot or leg was operated on, urge him to keep the extremity elevated and to use it as little as possible *because pressure can inhibit healing.*
- Warn the patient to protect the treated area from exposure to the sun *to avoid changes in pigmentation.* Tell him to call the practitioner if a fever of 100° F (37.8° C) or higher persists longer than 1 day.

Complications

Pain, bruising, redness, and blistering may occur after laser surgery. Scarring, pigment changes, and infection are rare complications of laser surgery.

Documentation

Most patients who have laser surgery for skin lesions are treated as outpatients. Note the patient's skin condition before and after the procedure. Also document any bleeding, record the type of dressing applied, and list the patient's complaints of pain. Note whether the patient understands home care instructions.

Selected references

Huikeshoven, M., et al. "Redarkening of Port-Wine Stains 10 Years after Pulsed-Dye Laser Treatment," *New England Journal of Medicine* 356(12):1235-40, March 2007.

Wiper, A., et al. "Amiodarone-Induced Skin Pigmentation: Q-switched Laser Therapy, an Effective Treatment Option," *Heart* 93(1):15, January 2007.

14 ■ Eye, ear, and nose care

INTRODUCTION

Because the eyes transmit about 70% of the sensory information reaching the brain, visual impairment can severely limit a person's ability to function independently and to perceive and react to his surroundings. Similarly, untreated hearing loss can drastically impair communication and social interaction. Inner-ear disorders may disrupt equilibrium and the ability to move freely. Likewise, nasal disorders can interfere with respiration, reduce vitality, and cause marked discomfort.

When caring for a patient with a sensory loss, remember that he's actually experiencing multiple impairments because sensory impairment also impairs perception. The combined loss significantly alters a person's daily activities and threatens his security and self-image.

Because eye, ear, and nose disorders are as common as they are troublesome, you're likely to perform the procedures presented in this chapter whether you practice in a hospital, clinic, extended-care facility, or other setting. You may be called on to assist with or perform eye, ear, or nose procedures in situations ranging from emergencies to routine checkups. These procedures call for the utmost care and precision to prevent infection and injury and to preserve function.

Overcoming perceptual barriers

Performing procedures that diagnose, treat, or even briefly cause sensory impairment requires you to give clear, simple instructions and explanations. You'll also need to provide ample reassurance to a patient who's certain to feel apprehensive about his ability to care for himself and function independently. In an emergency, effective communication becomes even more important because you'll be dealing with a patient suddenly disoriented by sensory and perceptual impairments.

Providing clear patient teaching

You can make an important contribution to the patient's understanding of eye, ear, and nasal disorders. As you implement various procedures, inform your patient about preventive care measures. Teach him to recognize signs and symptoms of sensory disorders. Urge him to schedule regular examinations to detect problems early. Remind him to use safety equipment at work and, as appropriate, at home.

Always provide thorough explanations. A simple fact or tip that to you seems almost too obvious to mention may actually offer valuable insight to the patient. When the patient leaves you, he should be better able to prevent, cope with, and manage the sensory disorder he has as well as any that could arise in the future.

EYE CARE

HOT AND COLD EYE COMPRESSES

Whether applied hot or cold, eye compresses are soothing and therapeutic. Hot compresses may be used to relieve discomfort. Because heat increases circulation (which enhances absorption and decreases inflammation), hot compresses may promote drainage of superficial infections. On the other hand, cold compresses can reduce swelling or bleeding and relieve itching. Because cold numbs sensory fibers, cold compresses may be ordered to ease periorbital discomfort between prescribed doses of pain medication. Typically, a hot or cold compress should be applied for 20-minute periods, four to six times per day. Ocular infection calls for the use of sterile technique.

Equipment

For hot compresses: Gloves ▪ prescribed solution, usually sterile water or normal saline solution ▪ sterile bowl ▪ sterile 4″ × 4″ gauze pads ▪ towel.

For cold compresses: Small plastic bag (such as a sandwich bag) or glove ▪ ice chips ▪ ½″ hypoallergenic tape ▪ towel ▪ sterile 4″ × 4″ gauze pads ▪ sterile water, normal saline solution, or prescribed ophthalmic irrigant ▪ gloves.

Preparation of equipment

For hot compresses: Place a capped bottle of sterile water or normal saline solution in a bowl of hot water or under a stream of hot tap water. Allow the solution to become warm, not hot (no higher than 120° F [48.9° C]). Pour the warm water or saline solution into a sterile bowl, filling the bowl about halfway. Place some sterile gauze pads in the bowl.

For cold compresses: Place ice chips in a plastic bag (or a glove if necessary) to make an ice pack. Keep the ice pack small *to avoid excessive pressure on the eye.* Remove excess air from the bag or glove, and knot the open end. Cut a piece of hypoallergenic tape to secure the ice pack. Place all equipment on the bedside stand near the patient.

Implementation

- Confirm the patient's identity using two patient identifiers according to your facility's policy.
- Explain the procedure to the patient, make him comfortable, and provide privacy.
- When applying hot compresses, have the patient sit if possible. When applying cold compresses, have the patient lie supine. Support his head with a pillow, and turn his head slightly to the unaffected side. *This position will help hold the compress in place.*

Applying an eye patch

With a practitioner's order, you may apply an eye patch for various reasons: to protect the eye after injury or surgery, to prevent accidental damage to an anesthetized eye, to promote healing, to absorb secretions, or to prevent the patient from touching or rubbing his eye.

A thicker patch, called a pressure patch, may be used to help corneal abrasions heal, compress postoperative edema, or control hemorrhage from traumatic injury. Application requires an ophthalmologist's prescription and supervision.

To apply a patch, choose a gauze pad of appropriate size for the patient's face, place it gently over the closed eye (as shown), and secure it with two or three strips of tape. Extend the tape from midforehead across the eye to below the earlobe.

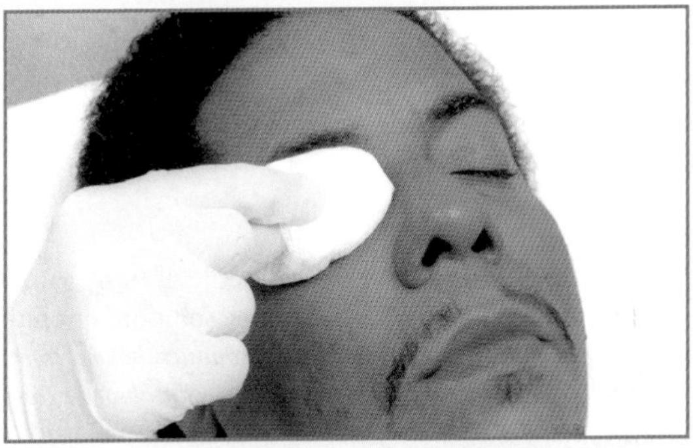

A pressure patch, which is markedly thicker than a single-thickness gauze patch, exerts extra tension against the closed eye. After placing the initial gauze pad, build it up with additional gauze pieces. Tape it firmly so that the patch exerts even pressure against the closed eye (as shown).

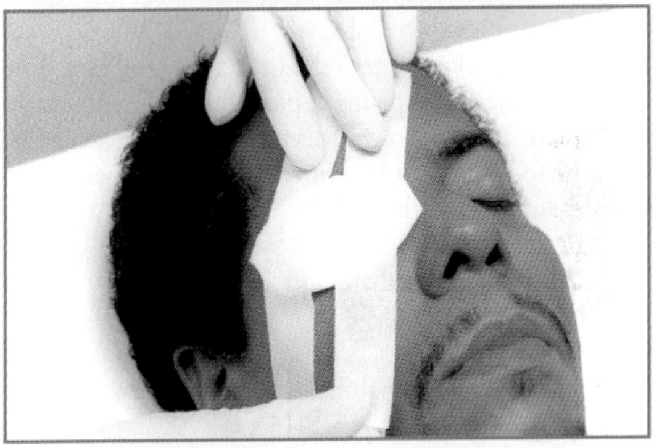

For increased protection of an injured eye, place a plastic or metal shield (as shown) on top of the gauze pads and apply tape over the shield.

Occasionally, you may use a head dressing to secure a pressure patch. *The dressing applies additional pressure or, in burn patients, holds the patch in place without tape.*

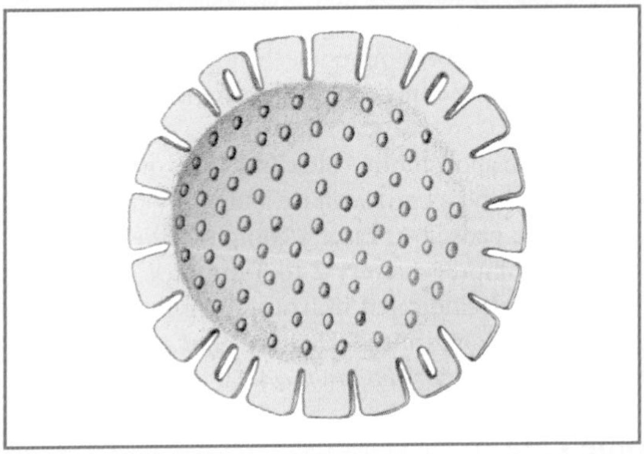

- Drape a towel around the patient's shoulders *to catch any spills.* Wash your hands and put on gloves.
- If the patient has an eye patch, remove it.

Applying hot compresses

- Take two 4″ × 4″ gauze pads from the basin. Squeeze out the excess solution.
- Instruct the patient to close his eyes. Gently apply the pads—one on top of the other—to the affected eye. (If the patient complains that the compress feels too hot, remove it immediately.)
- Change the compress every few minutes, as necessary, for the prescribed length of time. After removing each compress, check the patient's skin for signs that the compress solution is too hot.

Applying cold compresses

- Moisten the middle of one of the sterile 4″ × 4″ gauze pads with the sterile water, normal saline solution, or ophthalmic irrigating solution. *This helps to conduct the cold from the ice pack. Keep the edges dry so that they can absorb excess moisture.*
- Tell the patient to close his eyes; then place the moist gauze pad over the affected eye.
- Place the ice pack on top of the gauze pad, and tape it in place. If the patient complains of pain, remove the ice pack. Some patients may have an adverse reaction to cold.
- After 15 to 20 minutes, remove the tape, ice pack, and gauze pad and discard them.

Concluding the procedure

- Use the remaining sterile 4″ × 4″ gauze pads to clean and dry the patient's face.
- If ordered, apply ophthalmic ointment or an eye patch. (See *Applying an eye patch,* page 815.)

Special considerations

- When applying hot compresses, change the prescribed solution as frequently as necessary *to maintain a constant temperature.*
- If ordered to apply moist, cold compresses directly to the patient's eyelid, fill a bowl with ice and water and soak the 4″ × 4″ gauze pads in it. Place a compress directly on the lid; change compresses every 2 to 3 minutes. Cold compresses are contraindicated in treating eye inflammation, such as keratitis and iritis, *because the capillary constriction inhibits delivery of nutrients to the cornea.*

Home care

When teaching a patient to apply warm compresses at home, explain that he can substitute a clean bowl and washcloth for the sterile equipment. If both eyes are infected, emphasize the importance of using separate equipment for each eye. *Inform the patient that this will keep him from passing infection back and forth between the eyes.* Direct him to wash his hands thoroughly before and after treating each eye.

Documentation

Record the time and duration of the procedure. Describe the eye's appearance before and after treatment. Note any ointments (and amounts) or dressings applied to the eye. Record the patient's tolerance of the procedure.

SELECTED REFERENCES

Gardner, J.S. "Hospital Infection Control Practices Advisory Committee Guidelines for Isolation Precautions in Hospitals," *Infection Control and Hospital Epidemiology* 17:53-80, January 1996.

Taylor, C., et al. *Fundamentals of Nursing,* 6th ed. Philadelphia: Lippincott Williams & Wilkins, 2008.

EYE IRRIGATION

Used mainly to flush secretions, chemicals, and foreign objects from the eye, eye irrigation also provides a way to administer medications for corneal and conjunctival disorders. In an emergency, tap water may serve as an irrigant.

The amount of solution needed to irrigate an eye depends on the contaminant. Secretions require a moderate volume; major chemical burns require a copious amount. Usually, an I.V. bottle or bag of normal saline solution (with I.V. tubing attached) supplies enough solution for continuous irrigation of a chemical burn. (See *Three devices for eye irrigation.*)

Equipment

Gloves ▪ towels ▪ eyelid retractor ▪ 60-ml sterile syringe ▪ sterile basin ▪ emesis basin ▪ optional: proparacaine topical anesthetic.

For moderate-volume irrigation: Prescribed sterile ophthalmic irrigant ▪ sterile cotton-tipped applicators.

For copious irrigation: One or more 1,000-ml bottles or bags of normal saline solution ▪ standard I.V. infusion set without needle ▪ I.V. pole.

Commercially prepared bottles of sterile ophthalmic irrigant are available. All solutions should be at body temperature: 98.6° F (37° C).

Preparation of equipment

Read the label on the sterile ophthalmic irrigant. Double-check its sterility, strength, and expiration date.

EQUIPMENT

Three devices for eye irrigation

Depending on the type and extent of injury, the patient's eye may need to be irrigated using different devices.

Squeeze bottle

For moderate-volume irrigation — to remove eye secretions, for example — apply sterile ophthalmic irrigant to the eye directly from the squeeze bottle container. Direct the stream at the inner canthus, and position the patient so that the stream washes across the cornea and exits at the outer canthus (as shown at right).

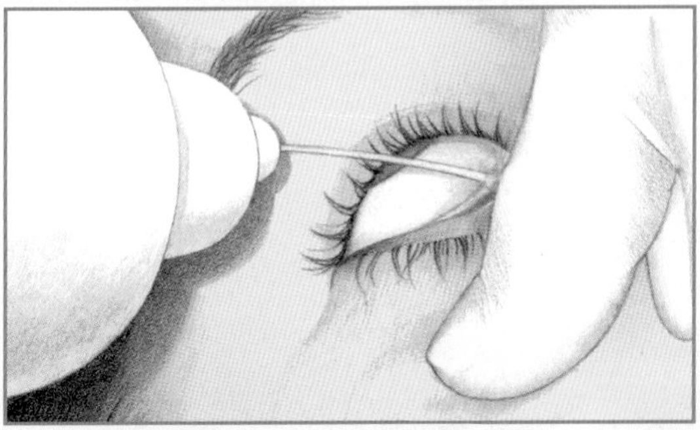

I.V. tube

For copious irrigation — to treat chemical burns, for example — set up an I.V. bag and tubing without a needle. Use the procedure described for moderate irrigation to flush the eye for at least 15 minutes (as shown at right).

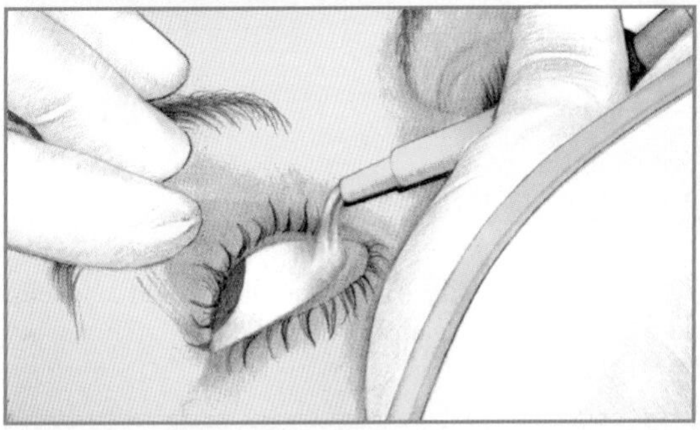

Morgan lens

Connected to irrigation tubing, a Morgan lens permits continuous lavage and also delivers medication to the eye. Use an adapter to connect the lens to the I.V. tubing and the solution container. Begin the irrigation at the prescribed flow rate. To insert the device, ask the patient to look down as you insert the lens under the upper eyelid. Then have him look up as you retract and release the lower eyelid over the lens (as shown at right).

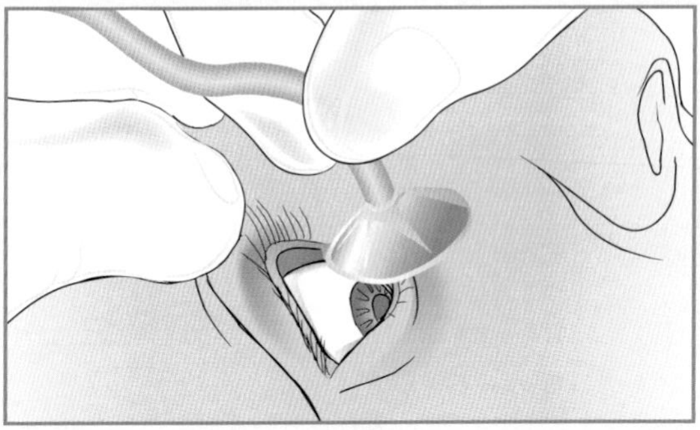

For moderate-volume irrigation: Pour the sterile irrigant into the sterile basin. Fill the syringe with 30 to 60 ml of irrigant. If you're using a commercially prepared bottle of sterile irrigant, remove the cap from the irrigant container and place the container within easy reach. (Be sure to keep the tip of the container sterile.)

For copious irrigation: Use sterile technique to set up the I.V. tubing and the bag or bottle of normal saline solution. Hang the container on an I.V. pole, fill the I.V. tubing with the solution, and adjust the drip regulator valve *to ensure an adequate but not forceful flow.* Place all other equipment within easy reach.

Implementation

■ Confirm the patient's identity using two patient identifiers according to your facility's policy.

■ Wash your hands, put on gloves, and explain the procedure to the patient. If the patient has a chemical burn, ease his anxiety by explaining that irrigation prevents further damage.

■ Assist the patient in lying supine. Turn his head slightly toward the affected side, as shown below, *to prevent solution flowing over his nose and into the other eye.*

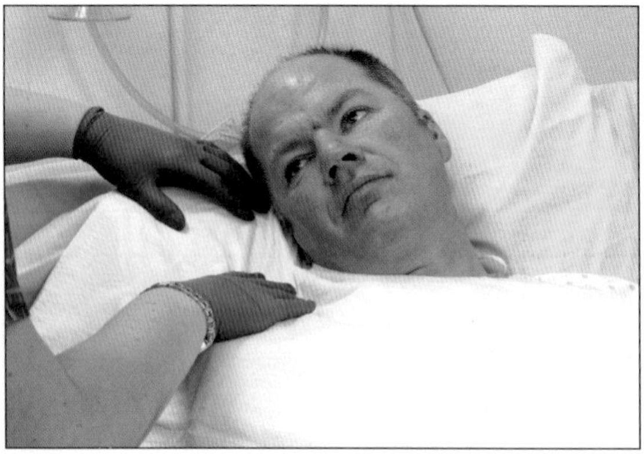

■ Place a towel under the patient's head, and hold or let him hold the emesis basin against his affected side, as shown below, *to catch excess solution.*

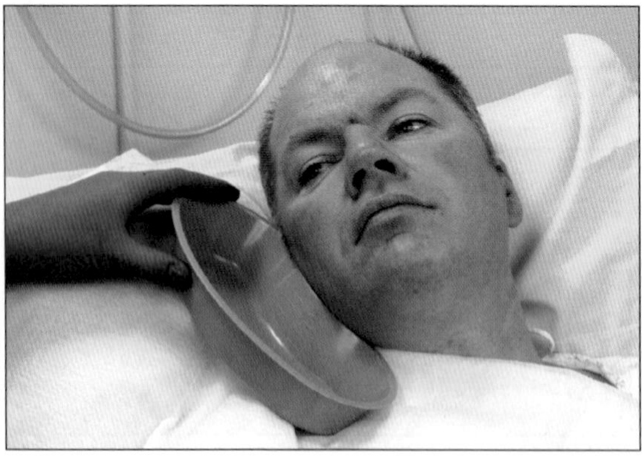

■ Using the thumb and index finger of your nondominant hand, separate the patient's eyelids, as shown top of next column.

■ If ordered, instill proparacaine eyedrops *as a comfort measure.* Use them only once *because repeated use retards healing.*

■ To irrigate the conjunctival cul-de-sac, continue holding the eyelids apart with your thumb and index finger.

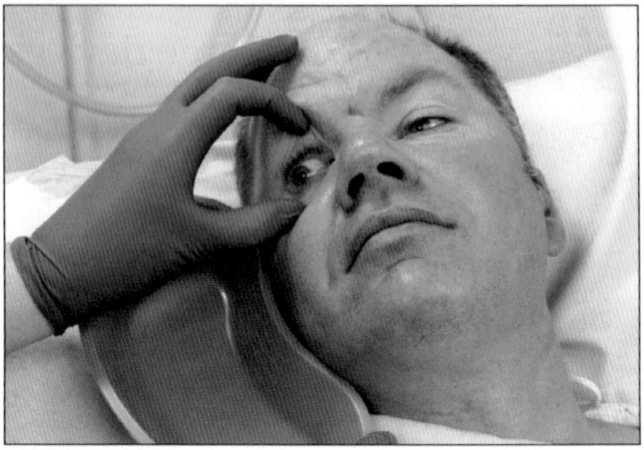

■ To irrigate the upper eyelid (the superior fornix), use an eyelid retractor. Steady the hand holding the retractor by resting it on the patient's forehead. *The retractor prevents the eyelid from closing involuntarily when solution touches the cornea and conjunctiva.*

For moderate irrigation

■ Holding the syringe about 1″ (2.5 cm) from the eye, direct a constant, gentle stream at the inner canthus, as shown below, *so that the solution flows across the cornea to the outer canthus.*

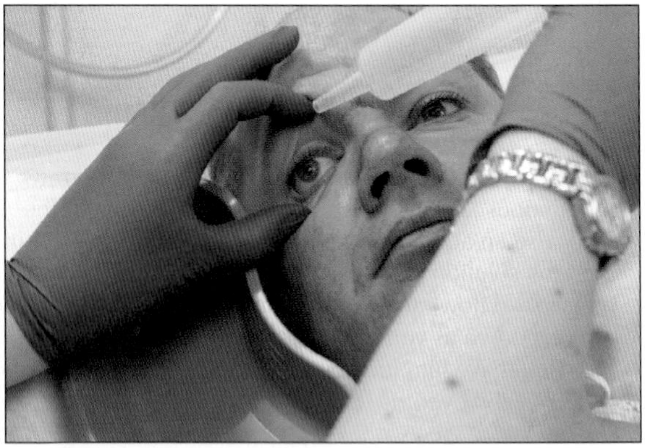

■ Evert the lower eyelid and then the upper eyelid *to inspect for retained foreign particles.*

■ Remove any foreign particles by gently touching the conjunctiva with sterile, wet cotton-tipped applicators. Don't touch the cornea.

■ Resume irrigating the eye until it's clean of all visible foreign particles.

For copious irrigation

■ Hold the control valve on the I.V. tubing about 1″ above the eye, and direct a constant, gentle stream of normal saline solution at the inner canthus *so that the solution flows across the cornea to the outer canthus.*

- Ask the patient to rotate his eye periodically while you continue the irrigation. *This action may dislodge foreign particles.*
- Evert the lower eyelid and then the upper eyelid *to inspect for retained foreign particles. (This inspection is especially important when the patient has caustic lime in his eye.)*

Concluding the procedure

- After eye irrigation, gently dry the eyelid with cotton balls or facial tissues, wiping from the inner to the outer canthus. Use a new cotton ball or tissue for each wipe. *This reduces the patient's need to rub his eye.*
- Remove and discard your gloves and goggles.
- When indicated, arrange for follow-up care.
- Wash your hands *to avoid burning from residual chemical contaminants.*

Special considerations

- When irrigating both eyes, have the patient tilt his head toward the side being irrigated *to avoid cross-contamination.*
- For chemical burns, irrigate each eye for at least 15 minutes with normal saline solution *to dilute and wash the harsh chemical.* (After irrigating for a chemical burn, note the time, date, and chemical for your own reference *in case you develop contact dermatitis.*)

Documentation

Note the duration of irrigation, the type and amount of solution, and characteristics of the drainage. Record your assessment of the patient's eye before and after irrigation. Note his response to the procedure.

Selected references

Taylor, C., et al. *Fundamentals of Nursing,* 6th ed. Philadelphia: Lippincott Williams & Wilkins, 2008.

EAR CARE

Ear irrigation

Irrigating the ear involves washing the external auditory canal with a stream of solution to clean the canal of discharges, to soften and remove impacted cerumen, or to dislodge a foreign body. Irrigation may also be used to relieve localized inflammation and discomfort. The procedure must be performed carefully to avoid causing patient discomfort or vertigo and to avoid increasing the risk of otitis externa. Because irrigation may contaminate the middle ear if the tympanic membrane is ruptured, an otoscopic examination always precedes ear irrigation.

This procedure is contraindicated when a foreign body (such as a pea) obstructs the auditory canal because a foreign body attracts and absorbs moisture. In contact with an irrigant or other solution, it swells, causing intense pain and complicating removal of the object by irrigation. Ear irrigation is also contraindicated if the patient has a cold, a fever, an ear infection, or an injured or ruptured tympanic membrane. The presence of a hearing aid battery in the ear also contraindicates irrigation because battery acid could leak, and irrigation would spread caustic material throughout the canal.

Equipment

Ear irrigation syringe (rubber bulb) ■ gloves ■ otoscope with aural speculum ■ prescribed irrigant ■ large basin ■ linen-saver pad and bath towel ■ emesis basin ■ cotton balls or cotton-tipped applicators ■ 4" × 4" gauze pad ■ optional: adjustable light (such as a gooseneck lamp).

Preparation of equipment

Select the appropriate syringe, and obtain the prescribed irrigant. Put the container of irrigant into the large basin filled with hot water *to warm the solution to body temperature (98.6° F [37° C]).* Avoid extreme temperature changes *because they can affect inner ear fluids, causing nausea and dizziness.*

Test the temperature of the solution by sprinkling a few drops on your inner wrist. Inspect equipment for breaks or cracks.

Implementation

- Confirm the patient's identity using two patient identifiers according to your facility's policy.
- Explain the procedure to the patient, provide privacy, wash your hands, and put on gloves, if necessary.
- If you haven't already done so, use the otoscope to inspect the auditory canal that will be irrigated.
- Help the patient to a sitting position. *To prevent the solution from running down his neck,* tilt his head slightly forward and toward the affected side. If he can't sit, have him lie on his back and tilt his head slightly forward and toward the affected ear.
- Make sure you have adequate lighting.
- If the patient is sitting, place the linen-saver pad (covered with the bath towel) on his shoulder and upper arm, under the affected ear. If he's lying down, cover his pillow and the area under the affected ear.
- Have the patient hold the emesis basin close to his head under the affected ear as shown top of next page.

How to irrigate the ear canal

Follow these guidelines for irrigating the ear canal:

■ Gently pull the auricle up and back *to straighten the ear canal* (as shown below). (For a child, pull the ear down and back.)

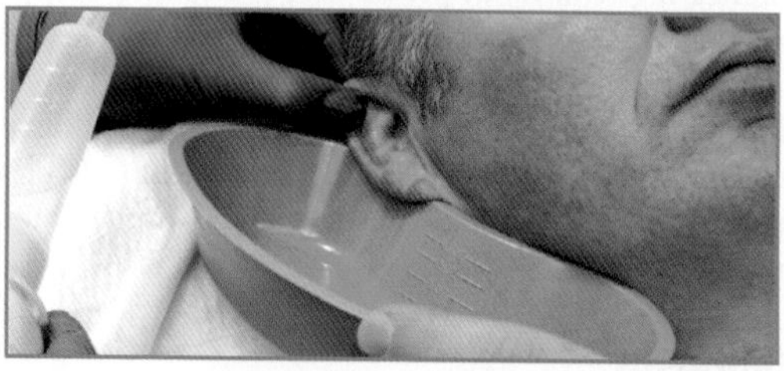

■ Have the patient hold an emesis basin beneath the ear *to catch returning irrigant.* Position the tip of the irrigating syringe at the meatus of the auditory canal (as shown below). Don't block the meatus *because you'll impede backflow and raise pressure in the canal.*

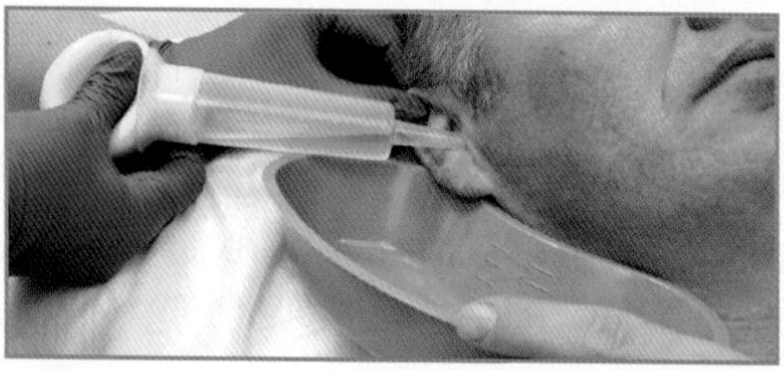

■ Tilt the patient's head toward you, and point the syringe tip upward and toward the posterior ear canal (as shown below). *This angle prevents damage to the tympanic membrane and guards against pushing debris farther into the canal.*

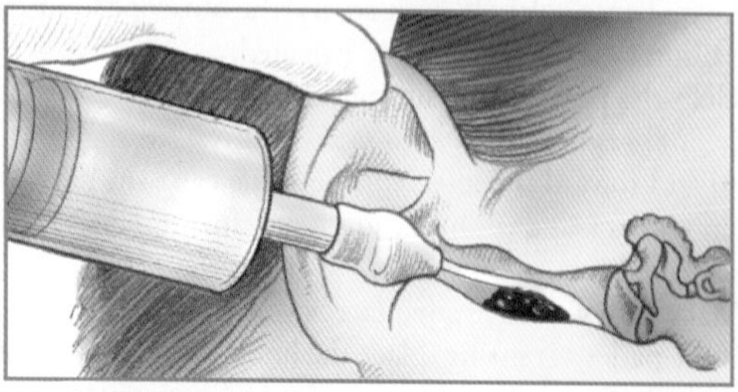

■ Direct a steady stream of irrigant against the upper wall of the ear canal, and inspect return fluid for cloudiness, cerumen, blood, or foreign matter.

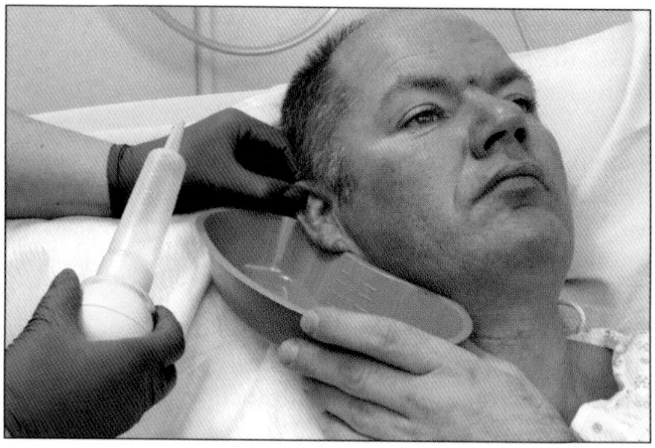

■ *To avoid getting foreign matter into the ear canal,* clean the auricle and the meatus of the auditory canal with a cotton ball or cotton-tipped applicator moistened with normal saline solution or the prescribed irrigating solution.

■ Draw the irrigant into the syringe and expel any air.

■ Straighten the auditory canal; then insert the syringe tip and start the flow. (See *How to irrigate the ear canal.*)

■ During irrigation, observe the patient for signs of pain or dizziness. If he reports either, stop the procedure, recheck the temperature of the irrigant, inspect the patient's ear with the otoscope, and resume irrigation, as indicated.

■ When the syringe is empty, remove it and inspect the return flow. Then, refill the syringe, and continue the irrigation until the return flow is clear. Never use more than 500 ml of irrigant during this procedure.

■ Remove the syringe, and inspect the ear canal for cleanliness with the otoscope.

■ Dry the patient's auricle and neck.

■ Remove the bath towel and place a 4″ × 4″ gauze pad under his ear *to promote drainage of residual debris and solution.*

Special considerations

■ Avoid dropping or squirting irrigant on the tympanic membrane. *This may startle the patient and cause discomfort.*

■ If the practitioner directs you to place a cotton pledget in the ear canal to retain some of the solution, pack the cotton loosely. Instruct the patient not to remove it.

■ If irrigation doesn't dislodge impacted cerumen, the practitioner may order you to instill several drops of glycerin, carbamide peroxide (Debrox), or a similar preparation two to three times daily for 2 to 3 days, and then to irrigate the ear again.

Complications

Possible complications include vertigo, nausea, otitis externa, and otitis media (if the patient has a perforated or ruptured tympanic membrane). Forceful instillation of irrigant can rupture the tympanic membrane.

Documentation

Record the date and time of irrigation. Note which ear you irrigated. Also note the volume and the solution used, the appearance of the canal before and after irrigation, the appearance of the return flow, the patient's tolerance of the procedure, and any comments he made about his condition, especially related to his hearing acuity.

SELECTED REFERENCES

Keegan, D.A., and Bannister, S.L. "A Novel Method for the Removal of Ear Cerumen," *Canadian Medical Association Journal* 173(12):1496-97, December 2005.

Taylor, C., et al. *Fundamentals of Nursing,* 6th ed. Philadelphia: Lippincott, Williams & Wilkins, 2008.

NOSE CARE

NASAL IRRIGATION

Irrigation of the nasal passages soothes irritated mucous membranes and washes away crusted mucus, secretions, and foreign matter. Left unattended, these deposits may impede sinus drainage and nasal airflow and cause headaches, infections, and unpleasant odors. Irrigation may be done with a bulb syringe or an electronic oral irrigating device.

Nasal irrigation benefits patients with either acute or chronic nasal conditions, including sinusitis, rhinitis, Wegener's granulomatosis, and Sjögren's syndrome. In addition, the procedure may help people who regularly inhale toxins or allergens—paint fumes, sawdust, pesticides, or coal dust, for example. Nasal irrigation is routinely recommended after some nasal surgeries to enhance healing by removal of postoperative eschar and to aid remucosolization of the sinus cavities and ostia.

Contraindications for nasal irrigation may include advanced destruction of the sinuses, frequent nosebleeds, and foreign bodies in the nasal passages (which could be driven farther into the passages by the irrigant). However, some patients with these conditions may benefit from irrigation.

Equipment

Bulb syringe or an oral irrigating device (such as a Water Pik) ■ rigid or flexible disposable irrigation tips (for one-patient use) ■ hypertonic saline solution ■ plastic sheet ■ towels ■ facial tissue ■ bath basin ■ gloves.

Preparation of equipment

Warm the saline solution to about 105° F (40.6° C). If you'll be irrigating with a bulb syringe, draw some irrigant into the bulb and then expel it. *This will rinse any residual solution from the previous irrigation and warm the bulb.*

If you're using an oral irrigating device, plug the instrument into an electrical outlet in an area near the patient. Then run about 1 cup (236.6 ml) of saline solution through the tubing *to rinse residual solution from the lines and warm the tubing.* Next, fill the reservoir of the device with warm saline solution.

Implementation

- Confirm the patient's identity using two patient identifiers according to your facility's policy.
- Wash your hands, and put on gloves.
- Explain the procedure to the patient, and place a towel on his upper body *to protect his clothing from getting wet.* Place a plastic sheet on the bed, if indicated.
- Have the patient sit comfortably near the equipment in a position that allows the bulb or catheter tip to enter his nose and the returning irrigant to flow into the bath basin or sink. (See *Positioning the patient for nasal irrigation,* page 822.)
- Remind the patient to keep his mouth open and to breathe rhythmically during irrigation. *This causes the soft palate to seal the throat, thus allowing the irrigant to stream out the opposite nostril and carry discharge with it.*
- Instruct the patient not to speak or swallow during the irrigation *to avoid forcing infectious material into the sinuses or eustachian tubes.*
- *To avoid injuring the nasal mucosa,* remove the irrigating tip from the patient's nostril if he reports the need to sneeze or cough.

Using a bulb syringe

- Fill the bulb syringe with saline solution, and insert the tip about ½" (1.3 cm) into the patient's nostril.
- Squeeze the bulb until a gentle stream of warm irrigant washes through the nose. Avoid forceful squeezing, *which may drive debris from the nasal passages into the sinuses or eustachian tubes and introduce infection.* Alternate the nostrils until the return irrigant runs clear.

Using an oral irrigating device

- Insert the irrigation tip into the nostril about ½" to 1" (1.5 to 2.5 cm) and turn on the irrigating device. Begin with a low pressure setting (increasing the pressure as needed) *to obtain a gentle stream of irrigant.* Again, be careful not to drive material from the nose into the sinuses or eustachian tubes. Irrigate both nostrils.

Positioning the patient for nasal irrigation

Whether you're teaching a patient to perform nasal irrigation with a bulb syringe or an oral irrigating device, the irrigation will progress more easily when the patient learns how to hold her head for optimal safety, comfort, and effectiveness.

Help the patient to sit upright with her head bent forward over the basin or sink and flexed on her chest, as shown below. Her nose and ear should be on the same vertical plane.

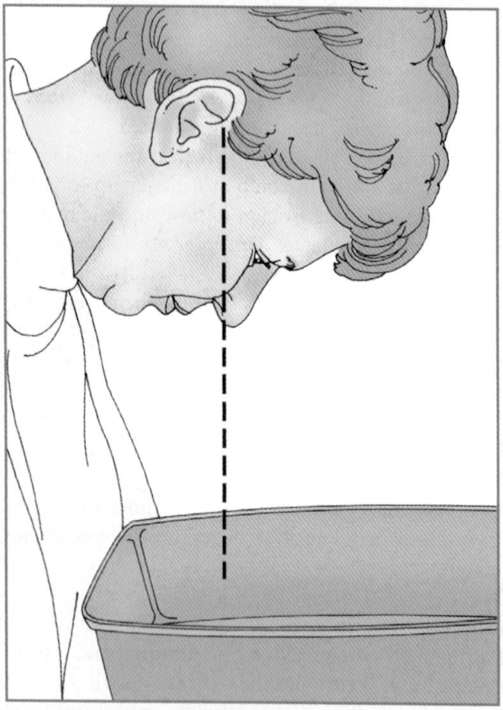

Explain that she's less likely to breathe in the irrigant when holding her head in this position. *This position should also keep the irrigant from entering the eustachian tubes, which will now lie above the level of the irrigation stream.*

- Inspect returning irrigant. Changes in color, viscosity, or volume may signal an infection and should be reported to the practitioner. Also report blood or necrotic material.

Concluding the procedure

- After irrigation, have the patient wait a few minutes before blowing excess fluid from both nostrils at once. *Gentle blowing through both nostrils prevents fluid or pressure buildup in the sinuses. This action also helps to loosen and expel crusted secretions and mucus.*
- Clean the bulb syringe or irrigating device with soap and water, and then disinfect, as recommended. Rinse and dry.

Special considerations

- Expect fluid to drain from the patient's nose for a brief time after the irrigation and before he blows his nose.
- Be sure to insert the irrigation tip far enough *to ensure that the irrigant cleans the nasal membranes before draining out.* A typical amount of irrigant is 500 to 1,000 ml.

Home care

To continue nasal irrigations at home, teach the patient how to prepare saline solution. Tell him to fill a clean 1-L plastic bottle with bottled or distilled water, add 1 tsp of canning salt, and shake the solution until the salt dissolves. Teach him how to disinfect used irrigating devices.

Documentation

Note the time and duration of the procedure and the amount of irrigant used. Describe the appearance of the returned solution. Record your assessment of the patient's comfort level and breathing ease before and after the procedure. Document any patient teaching provided.

Selected references

Taylor, C., et al. *Fundamentals of Nursing,* 6th ed. Philadelphia: Lippincott Williams & Wilkins, 2008.

Nasal packing

In the highly vascular nasal mucosa, even seemingly minor injuries can cause major bleeding and blood loss. When routine therapeutic measures, such as direct pressure, cautery, and vasoconstrictive drugs, fail to control epistaxis (nosebleed), the patient's nose may have to be packed to stop anterior bleeding (which runs out of the nose) or posterior bleeding (which runs down the throat). If blood drains into the nasopharyngeal area or lacrimal ducts, the patient may also appear to bleed from the mouth and eyes.

Most nasal bleeding originates at a plexus of arterioles and venules in the anteroinferior septum. Only about 1 in 10 nosebleeds occurs in the posterior nose, which usually bleeds more heavily than the anterior location.

A nurse typically assists a physician with anterior or posterior nasal packing. (See *Types of nasal packing.*) She may

EQUIPMENT

Types of nasal packing

Nosebleeds may be controlled with anterior or posterior nasal packing.

Anterior nasal packing

The physician may treat an anterior nosebleed by packing the anterior nasal cavity with a 3′ to 4′ (0.9- to 1.2-m) strip of antibiotic-impregnated petroleum gauze (shown below) or with a nasal tampon.

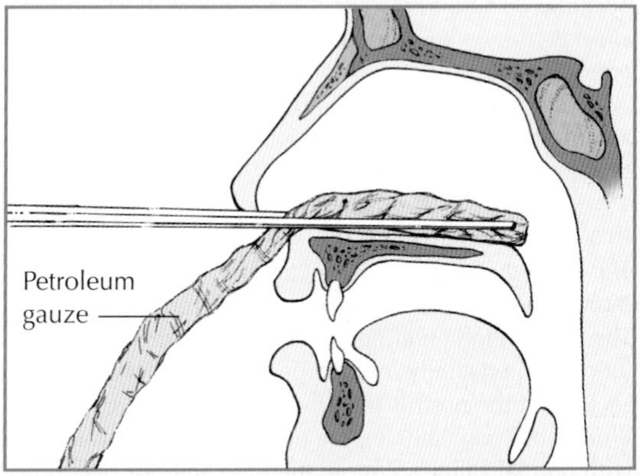

A nasal tampon is made of tightly compressed absorbent material with or without a central breathing tube. The physician inserts a lubricated tampon along the floor of the nose and, with the patient's head tilted backward, instills 5 to 10 ml of antibiotic or normal saline solution. *This causes the tampon to expand, stopping the bleeding.* The tampon should be moistened periodically, and the central breathing tube should be suctioned regularly.

In a child or a patient with blood dyscrasias, the physician may fashion an absorbable pack by moistening a gauzelike, regenerated cellulose material with a vasoconstrictor. Applied to a visible bleeding point, this substance will swell to form a clot. The packing is absorbable and doesn't need removal.

Posterior nasal packing

Posterior packing consists of a gauze roll shaped and secured by three sutures (one suture at each end and one in the middle) or a balloon-type catheter. To insert the packing, the physician advances one or two soft catheters into the patient's nostrils (shown at top of next column). When the catheter tips appear in the nasopharynx, the physician grasps them with a Kelly clamp or bayonet forceps and pulls them forward through the mouth. He secures the two end sutures to the catheter tip and draws the catheter back through the nostrils.

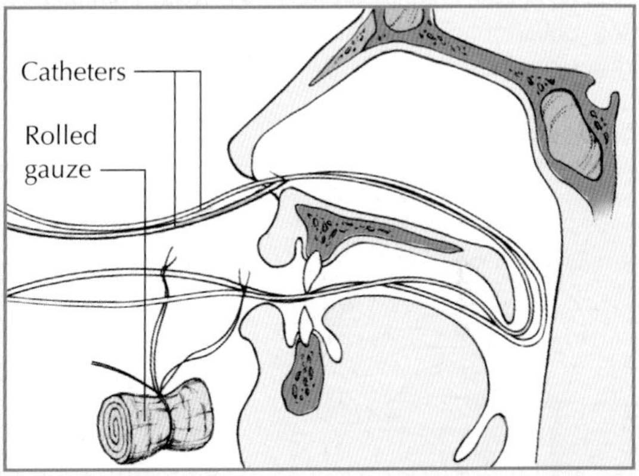

This step brings the packing into place with the end sutures hanging from the patient's nostril. (The middle suture emerges from the patient's mouth to free the packing, when needed.)

The physician may weight the nose sutures with a clamp. Then he will pull the packing securely into place behind the soft palate and against the posterior end of the septum (nasal choana).

After he examines the patient's throat (*to ensure that the uvula hasn't been forced under the packing*), he inserts anterior packing and secures the whole apparatus by tying the posterior pack strings around rolled gauze or a dental roll at the nostrils (shown below).

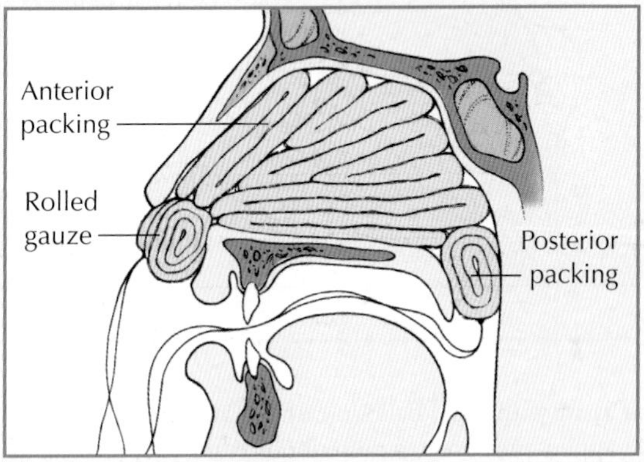

EQUIPMENT

Nasal balloon catheters

To control epistaxis, the physician may use a balloon catheter instead of nasal packing. Self-retaining and disposable, the catheter may have a single or double balloon to apply pressure to bleeding nasal tissues. If bleeding is still uncontrolled, the physician may choose to use arterial ligation, cryotherapy, or arterial embolization.

When inserted and inflated, the single-balloon catheter (shown below) compresses the blood vessels while a soft, collapsible external bulb prevents the catheter from dislodging posteriorly.

Single-balloon catheter

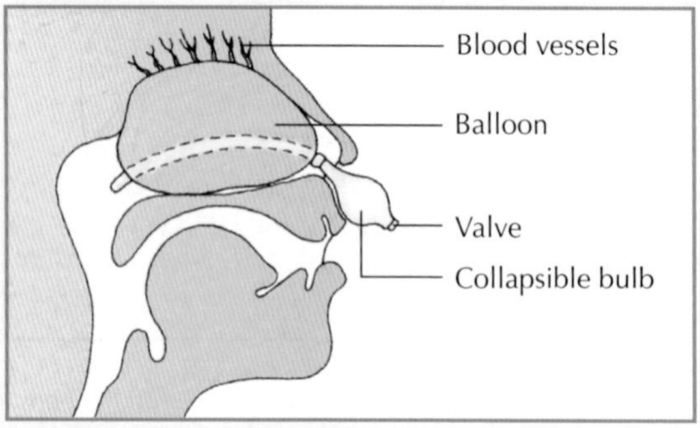

The double-balloon catheter (shown below) is used for simultaneous anterior and posterior nasal packing. The posterior balloon compresses the posterior vessels serving the nose, including the bleeding vessels; the anterior balloon compresses bleeding intranasal vessels. This catheter contains a central airway for breathing comfort.

Double-balloon catheter

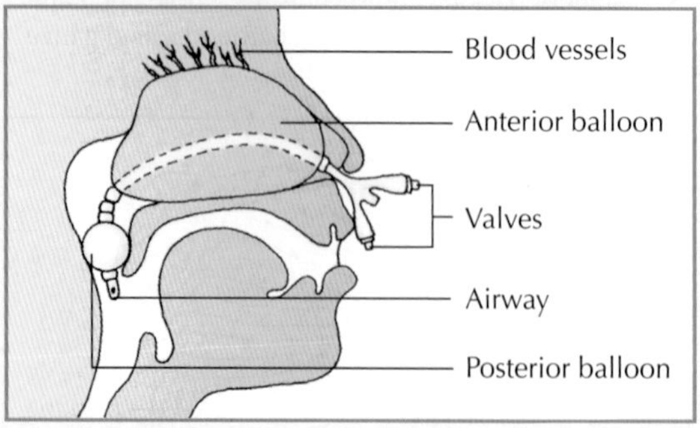

Assisting with insertion

To assist with inserting a single- or double-balloon catheter, prepare the patient as you would for nasal packing. Be sure to discuss the procedure thoroughly *to alleviate the patient's anxiety and promote his cooperation.*

Explain that the catheter tip will be lubricated with an antibiotic or a water-soluble lubricant *to ease passage and prevent infection.*

Providing routine care

The tip of the single-balloon catheter will be inserted into the nostrils until it reaches the posterior pharynx. Then the balloon will be inflated with normal saline solution, pulled gently into the posterior nasopharynx, and secured at the nostrils with the collapsible bulb. With a double-balloon catheter, the posterior balloon is inflated with normal saline solution; then the anterior balloon is inflated.

To check catheter placement, mark the catheter at the nasal vestibule during insertion; then inspect for that mark during catheter care, and observe the oropharynx for the posteriorly placed balloon. Assess the nostrils for irritation or erosion. Remove secretions by gently suctioning the airway of a double-balloon catheter or by dabbing away crusted external secretions if the patient has a catheter with no airway.

To prevent damage to nasal tissue, the physician may order the balloon deflated for 10 minutes every 24 hours. If bleeding recurs or remains uncontrolled, reinflate the balloon and contact the physician, who may add packing.

Recognizing complications

The patient may report difficulty breathing, swallowing, or eating, and the nasal mucosa may sustain damage from pressure. Balloon deflation may dislodge clots and nasal debris into the oropharynx, which could prompt coughing, gagging, or vomiting.

also assist with nasal balloon catheterization, a procedure that applies pressure to a posterior bleeding site. (See *Nasal balloon catheters.*)

Whichever procedure the patient undergoes, you should provide ongoing encouragement and support to reduce his discomfort and anxiety. You should also perform ongoing assessment to determine the procedure's success and to detect possible complications.

Equipment

For anterior and posterior packing: Gowns ▪ goggles ▪ masks ▪ sterile gloves ▪ nasal speculum and tongue blades (may be in preassembled head and neck examination kit) ▪ directed illumination source (such as headlamp or strong flashlight) or fiber-optic nasal endoscope, light cables, and light source ▪ suction apparatus with sterile suction-connecting tubing and sterile nasal aspirator tip ▪ sterile cotton-tipped applicators ▪ local anesthetic spray (topical 4% lidocaine) or vial of local anesthetic solution (such as 2% lidocaine or 1% to 2% lidocaine with epinephrine 1:100,000) ▪ 10-ml syringe with 22G 1½" needle ▪ silver nitrate sticks ▪ electrocautery device with grounding plate and small tip ▪ topical nasal decongestant (such as 0.5% phenylephrine) ▪ antibiotic ointment ▪ absorbable hemostatic (such as Gelfoam, Avitene, Surgicel, or thrombin) ▪ petroleum jelly ▪ water-soluble lubricant ▪ equipment for measuring vital signs.

For assessment and bedside use: Tongue blades ▪ flashlight ▪ long hemostats or sponge forceps ▪ 60-ml syringe for deflating balloons (if applicable) ▪ if nasal tampons are in place: saline bullets for applying moisture, and small flexible catheters for suctioning central breathing tube ▪ drip pad or moustache dressing supplies ▪ mouth care supplies ▪ water or artificial saliva ▪ external humidification ▪ equipment for drawing blood.

Preparation of equipment

Wash your hands. Assemble all equipment at the patient's bedside. Make sure the headlamp works. Plug in the suction apparatus, and connect the tubing from the collection bottle to the suction source. Test the suction equipment to make sure it works properly. At the bedside, create a sterile field. (Use the sterile towels or the sterile tray.) Using sterile technique, place all sterile equipment on the sterile field.

If the physician will inject a local anesthetic rather than spray it into the nose, place the 22G 1½" needle attached to the 10-ml syringe on the sterile field. When the physician readies the syringe, clean the stopper on the anesthetic vial, and hold the vial so he can withdraw the anesthetic. *This practice allows the physician to avoid touching his sterile gloves to the nonsterile vial.*

Open the packages containing the sterile suction-connecting tubing and aspirating tip, and place them on the sterile field. Fill the sterile bowl with normal saline solution *so that the suction tubing can be flushed as necessary.* Thoroughly lubricate the anterior or posterior packing with antibiotic ointment.

If the patient needs a nasal balloon catheter, test the balloon for leaks by inflating the catheter with normal saline solution. Remove the solution before insertion.

Implementation

- Ensure that all people caring for the patient wear gowns, gloves, and goggles during insertion of packing *to prevent possible contamination from splattered blood.*
- Check the patient's vital signs, and observe for hypotension with postural changes. Hypotension suggests significant blood loss. Also monitor airway patency *because the patient will be at risk for aspirating or vomiting swallowed blood.*
- Explain the procedure to the patient, and offer reassurance *to reduce his anxiety and promote cooperation.*
- If ordered, administer a sedative or tranquilizer *to reduce the patient's anxiety and decrease sympathetic stimulation, which can exacerbate a nosebleed.*
- Help the patient sit with his head tilted forward *to minimize blood drainage into the throat and prevent aspiration.*
- Turn on the suction apparatus and attach the connecting tubing *so the physician can aspirate the nasal cavity to remove clots before locating the bleeding source.*
- To inspect the nasal cavity, the physician will use a nasal speculum and an external light source or a fiber-optic nasal endoscope. To remove collected blood and help visualize the bleeding vessel, he will use suction or cotton-tipped applicators. The nose may be treated early with a topical vasoconstrictor, such as phenylephrine, *to slow bleeding and aid visualization.*

For anterior nasal packing

- Help the physician apply topical vasoconstricting agents *to control bleeding* or to use chemical cautery with silver nitrate sticks.
- *To enhance the vasoconstrictor's action,* apply manual pressure to the nose for about 10 minutes.
- If bleeding persists, you may help insert an absorbable nasal pack directly on the bleeding site. The pack swells to form an artificial clot.
- If these methods fail, prepare to assist with electrocautery or insertion of anterior nasal packing. (Even if only one side is bleeding, both sides may require packing to control bleeding.)
- While the anterior pack is in place, use the cotton-tipped applicators to apply petroleum jelly to the patient's lips and nostrils *to prevent drying and cracking.*

For posterior nasal packing

- Wash your hands, and put on sterile gloves.

HOME CARE

Preventing recurrent nosebleeds

Review these self-care guidelines with your patient to reduce his risk of developing recurrent nosebleeds:

- *Because nosebleeds can result from dry mucous membranes,* suggest that the patient use a cool mist vaporizer or humidifier, as needed, especially in dry environments.
- Teach the patient how to minimize pressure on nasal passages. Advise him, for instance, to avoid constipation and consequent straining during defecation. Recommend a fiber-rich diet and adequate fluid intake, and warn him to avoid extreme physical exertion for 24 hours after the nosebleed stops. Caution him to avoid aspirin (*which has anticoagulant properties*), alcoholic beverages, and tobacco for at least 5 days.
- If the patient gets a nosebleed despite these precautions, tell him to keep his head higher than his heart and, using his thumb and forefinger, to press the soft portion of the nostrils together and against the facial bones. (Recommend against direct pressure if he has a facial injury or nasal fracture.) Tell him to maintain pressure for up to 10 minutes and then to reassess bleeding. If it's uncontrolled, he should reapply pressure for another 10 minutes with ice between the thumb and forefinger.
- After a nosebleed or after nasal packing is removed, caution the patient to avoid rubbing or picking his nose, putting a handkerchief or tissue in his nose, or blowing his nose forcefully for at least 48 hours. After this time, he may blow his nose gently and use salt-water nasal spray to clear nasal clots.

- If the physician identifies the bleeding source in the posterior nasal cavity, lubricate the soft catheters *to ease insertion.*
- Instruct the patient to open his mouth and to breathe normally through his mouth during catheter insertion *to minimize gagging as the catheters pass through the nostril.*
- Help the physician insert the packing, as directed.
- Help the patient assume a comfortable position with his head elevated 45 to 90 degrees. Assess him for airway obstruction or any respiratory changes.
- Monitor the patient's vital signs regularly *to detect changes that may indicate hypovolemia or hypoxemia.*

Special considerations

- Patients with posterior packing usually are hospitalized for monitoring. If mucosal oozing persists, apply a moustache dressing by securing a folded gauze pad over the nasal vestibules with tape or a commercial nasal dressing holder. Change the pad when soiled.
- Test the patient's call bell *to make sure he can summon help, if needed.* Also keep emergency equipment (flashlight, tongue blade, syringe, and hemostats) at the patient's bedside *to speed packing removal if it becomes displaced and occludes the airway.*
- Once the packing is in place, compile assessment data carefully to help detect the underlying cause of nosebleeds. Mechanical factors include a deviated septum, injury, and a foreign body. Environmental factors include drying and erosion of the nasal mucosa. Other possible causes are upper respiratory tract infection, anticoagulant or salicylate therapy, blood dyscrasias, cardiovascular or hepatic disorders, tumors of the nasal cavity or paranasal sinuses, chronic nephritis, and familial hemorrhagic telangiectasia.
- If significant blood loss occurs or if the underlying cause remains unknown, expect the physician to order a complete blood count and coagulation profile as soon as possible. Blood transfusion may be necessary. After the procedure, the physician may order arterial blood gas analysis *to detect any pulmonary complications* and arterial oxygen saturation monitoring *to assess for hypoxemia.* If necessary, prepare to administer supplemental humidified oxygen with a face mask and to give antibiotics and decongestants, as ordered.
- *Because a patient with nasal packing must breathe through his mouth,* provide thorough mouth care often. Artificial saliva, room humidification, and ample fluid intake also relieve dryness caused by mouth breathing.
- Until the pack is removed, the patient should be on modified bed rest. As ordered, administer moderate doses of nonaspirin analgesics, decongestants, and sedatives along with prophylactic antibiotics *to prevent sinusitis or related infections.*
- Nasal packing is usually removed in 2 to 5 days. After an anterior pack is removed, instruct the patient to avoid rubbing or picking his nose, inserting any object into his nose, and blowing his nose forcefully for 48 hours, or as ordered.

Home care

Tell the patient to expect reduced ability to detect smell and taste. Make sure he has a working smoke detector at home. Advise him to eat soft foods *because his eating and swallowing abilities will be impaired.* Instruct him to drink fluids often or to use artificial saliva to cope with dry mouth. Teach him measures to prevent nosebleeds, and instruct him to seek medical help if these measures fail to stop bleeding. (See *Preventing recurrent nosebleeds.*)

Complications

The pressure of a posterior pack on the soft palate may lead to hypoxemia. Patients with posterior packing are at special risk for aspiration of blood. Patients with underlying pulmonary conditions, such as chronic obstructive pulmonary disease and asthma, are at special risk for exacerbation of the condition or for hypoxemia while nasal packing is in place. Hypoxemia can be detected with pulse oximetry. Signs and symptoms include tachycardia, confusion, cyanosis, and restlessness.

Airway obstruction may occur if a posterior or anterior nasal pack slips backward. The patient may complain of difficulty swallowing, pain, or discomfort. In patients with posterior packs, otitis media may develop. Other possible complications include hematotympanum and pressure necrosis of nasal structures, especially the septum.

Sedation may cause hypotension in a patient with significant blood loss and may also increase the patient's risk of aspiration and hypoxemia.

Documentation

Record the type of pack used *to ensure its removal at the appropriate time.* On the intake and output record, document the estimated blood loss and all fluid administered. Note the patient's vital signs, his response to sedation or position changes, the results of any laboratory tests, and any drugs administered, including topical agents. Record any complications. Document discharge instructions and clinical follow-up plans.

SELECTED REFERENCES

Beer, H.L., et al. "Blood Loss Estimation in Epistaxis Scenarios," *The Journal of Laryngology and Otology* 119(1):16-18, January 2005.

Hudson, J.W. "Epistaxis: Diagnosis and Treatment," *Journal of Oral Maxillofacial Surgery* 64(6):995, June 2006.

Kucik, C.J., and Clenney, T. "Management of Epistaxis," *American Family Physician* 71(2): 305-11, January 2005.

Thomas, L., et al. "Avoiding Alar Necrosis with Post-nasal Packs," *The Journal of Laryngology and Otology* 119(9):727-28, September 2005.

15 ■ Psychiatric care

INTRODUCTION

In today's society, more people than ever before experience mental health problems. Mental health disorders are behavioral or psychological syndromes or patterns that are characterized by the presence of current distress (a painful symptom), a disability in functioning, or significantly increased risk of suffering, pain, disability, loss of freedom, or even death. Whatever the original cause, mental disorders are considered a sign of a behavioral, psychological, or biological dysfunction in the individual.

Psychiatric nursing is a specialized area of nursing practice that is recognized by the National Institute of Mental Health as an essential field of study. As a psychiatric nurse, you have a distinct role in providing psychiatric care for the patient diagnosed with a mental disorder. Your patients may include individuals, families, groups, and even communities. You may practice in diverse settings, including psychiatric hospitals, community mental health centers, general hospitals, community health agencies, outpatient clinics, homes, schools, prisons, health maintenance organizations, primary care practices, private practices, crisis units, and industrial centers. You will face situations that will require you to assume many roles, such as staff nurse, administrator, consultant, in-service educator, clinical practitioner, researcher, program evaluator, primary care provider, and liaison between the patient and other members of the health care team, and family members.

Considering the psychiatric patient

To effectively care for your patients, you must consider not only the psychological aspects but the physiologic aspects of your patient's health. For example, a patient who seeks medical help for chest pain may also need to be assessed for anxiety and depression. Providing care for these patients requires the development of a practical, orderly method for dealing with problems that can be diverse and complex. Your responsibilities include planning, implementing, and evaluating care, and also establishing a meaningful therapeutic relationship with the patient. Furthermore, you'll need to develop a keen awareness of your own attitudes and feelings to prevent frustration from getting in the way of your efforts when confronted with difficult situations.

Implementing change

It's important to keep abreast of the rapid changes taking place in psychiatric nursing. There have been developments in neurobiology that have revolutionized diagnosis and treatment. A newer system of classifying mental disorders has been established, which emphasizes observable data and deemphasizes subjective and theoretical impressions. Advancements in drug therapy for acute psychiatric disorders, as well as a new emphasis on the holistic approach to promote a closer relationship between psychiatry and other branches of medicine, are all changes that you can implement in your nursing care to impact the well-being of your psychiatric patients.

Providing psychiatric care

As a nurse providing psychiatric care, you may be involved in functions that involve direct and indirect care, including:

- maintaining a therapeutic setting
- working to solve the patient's current problem
- fulfilling a surrogate parent role
- using somatic therapies to alleviate the patient's health problems
- educating consumers about factors that influence mental health
- promoting change to improve socioeconomic conditions
- providing leadership and clinical supervision to colleagues
- conducting psychotherapy
- engaging in social and community mental health efforts
- participating in continuing education, in-service, and nursing administration
- performing consultations and research.

Your primary care functions may include providing health education, improving socioeconomic conditions, offering consumer education about normal growth and development, giving referrals before symptoms develop, supporting family members, and engaging in community and political activities.

Your secondary nursing functions may include screening and evaluating patients promptly; providing emergency treatment, crisis intervention, and a therapeutic milieu; supervising medication administration; preventing suicide; counseling on a time-limited basis; conducting psychotherapy; and initiating community and organization interventions such as helping to set up shelters for the homeless.

Finally, your tertiary functions may include establishing vocational training, psychosocial rehabilitation, and aftercare programs.

Treating psychiatric disorders

The psychological treatment of mental and emotional disorders involves a range of approaches from in-depth psychoanalysis to 1-day crisis counseling. Regardless of the approach, most types of psychotherapy aim to change a patient's attitudes, feelings, or behavior. The therapist may act as a neutral observer or an active participant. The success of therapy depends largely on the compatibility between patient and therapist, the treatment goals selected, and the patient's commitment.

As a psychiatric nurse, you may be directly or indirectly involved in the therapeutic treatments described here.

Individual therapy

Individual therapy requires a series of counseling sessions that may be short- or long-term. It involves mutually agreed-upon goals, with the therapist mediating the patient's disturbed patterns of behavior to promote personality growth and development.

Cognitive therapy

Cognitive therapy aims to reduce the patient's depression or distress by identifying and changing his negative generalizations, personalizations, and expectations. Cognitive theory states that depression stems from the patient's lack of self-worth and belief that the future is bleak and hopeless. Cognitive therapists assign homework that includes making lists of pleasurable activities and reducing automatic negative thoughts and conclusions.

Group therapy

Guided by a psychotherapist, a group of people (ideally 4 to 10) experiencing similar emotional problems meet to discuss their concerns with one another. Duration varies from a few weeks for acute conditions requiring hospitalization, to several years. Group therapy is especially useful in treating addictions.

Family therapy

The goal of family therapy is to alter relationships within the family and to change the problematic behavior of one or more family members. Family therapy is useful in treating adjustment disorders of childhood or adolescence, marital discord, and abuse situations. It may be short-term or long-term.

Crisis intervention

Crisis intervention seeks to help the patient develop adequate coping skills to resolve an immediate, pressing problem. The crisis can be a developmental one (such as a marriage or death of a family member) or a situational one (such as a natural disaster or an illness). This type of therapy seeks to enable the patient to return to the level of functioning that existed before the crisis. It usually involves the patient and therapist only, but may include family members. Therapy may consist of one session, or multiple sessions that take place over a course of several months.

Milieu therapy

Whether used in the hospital or in a community setting, milieu therapy refers to the use of the patient's environment as a tool for overcoming mental and emotional disorders. Specifically, the patient's surroundings become a therapeutic community, with the patient himself involved in planning, implementing, and evaluating his treatment as well as in sharing with staff and other patients the responsibility for establishing group rules and policies. This helps the patient learn to interact appropriately with staff and other patients. Staff members usually wear street clothes instead of uniforms, keep units unlocked, and run activities in a community room, which is the center for meetings, recreation, and meals. Staff members also provide individual, group, and occupational therapy.

Responding to psychiatric needs

Caring for the needs of the psychiatric patient is an important contribution to nursing and to society as a whole. With an increased number of dysfunctional families, single parents, troubled children, and homeless, as a result of altered traditional family structure and the loss of the extended family, psychiatric nurses have an increased workload, not only in the health care setting but in society as well. In addition, alcohol and substance abuse cases continue to rise in the younger population, as the elderly population faces problems of increasing isolation, fear of violent crime, and loneliness. Combat veterans, rape victims, and child abuse victims struggle to cope with the trauma they have experienced. The loss of effective support systems strains a person's ability to cope and often, people need help coping, even with minor problems. You'll be required to provide care that involves monitoring, safety, and treatment methods to alleviate the problems that psychiatric patients face. Clearly, the need for psychiatric care expands as the problems of society continue to increase.

MONITORING

DEPRESSION OR HOSTILITY OBSERVATION AND PRECAUTIONS

Caring for a patient diagnosed with depression or hostility requires safety precautions and close observation to prevent him from harming himself or others. In addition to close observation and assessment, frequent interaction with the patient is required.

Implementation

- Explain your actions to the patient before and during your observation.
- Remove all potentially harmful objects from the patient and his surroundings. The patient should be dressed in pajamas unless otherwise ordered by the practitioner.

- Observe and interact with the patient every 15 minutes around the clock. Be especially attentive when the patient is in the rest room.
- Restrict the patient to the unit at all times except in an emergency or when otherwise ordered by the practitioner.
- Observe the patient closely during meals, and ensure that all tableware and eating utensils used by the patient are returned. The patient shouldn't leave the unit for meals.
- Allow visitors as the patient's condition permits and per the practitioner's orders. Keep the patient on the unit and continue to monitor him every 15 minutes.
- Encourage the patient to express his feelings and thoughts about homicide, suicide, agitation, destructive behavior, depression, and hope for the future.

Documentation

Document your observations in the patient's progress notes every shift. Note the patient's sleeping and eating patterns, changes in energy level, and interactions with others as well as his expressions about his feelings of self-worth and anger.

Selected references

Holcomb, S.S. "Identification and Treatment of Depression," *The Nurse Practitioner* 31(12):42-44, December 2006.

Jacobs. D.G., et al. *Practice Guideline for the Treatment of Patients with Suicidal Behaviors.* November 2003. Available at *http://www.psych.org/psych_pract/treatg/pg/SuicidalBehavior_05-15-06.pdf*

Karasu, T., et al. *Practice Guideline for the Treatment of Patients with Major Depressive Disorder,* 2nd ed. April 2000. Available at *http://www.psych.org/psych_pract/treatg/pg/MDD2e_05-15-06.pdf*

Elopement monitoring

Elopement monitoring is necessary to prevent patients at risk from leaving the unit without authorization. A patient at risk for elopement must be placed on risk status by the practitioner to prevent him from leaving the unit. The following procedure should be implemented when a patient is restricted to the unit.

Implementation

- Explain the reasons for the patient's restriction to the unit *to help relieve his fear and anxiety.*
- Observe the patient closely, especially when exit doors are open, and check on his whereabouts every 15 minutes.
- Encourage the patient to express his thoughts and feelings about elopement and involve him in unit activities *to expend energy.*

NURSING ALERT *If the patient needs to leave the unit, escort him with another staff member.*

- Have the patient dress in pajamas and a robe or scrubs *to discourage elopement.*
- If the patient manages to elope, make all reasonable efforts to apprehend and return him to the unit. If a search is needed, follow your facility's policy for notifying security or the local police department.
- When the patient is found and returned, assess his status, examine him for injuries, and check to make sure he has nothing with which he could harm himself or others. Reassure the patient that he continues to need hospital care.

Documentation

Document the patient's elopement risk and any unusual occurrences. Document the verbal expressions of his feelings, desire to elope, aggressive thoughts and actions, hallucinations, and tolerance of restriction to the unit.

Selected references

APA Task Force on Psychiatric Emergency Services. Report and Recommendations Regarding Psychiatric Emergency and Crisis Services. Available at *http://www.psych.org/downloads/EmergencyServicesFinal.pdf*

Shives, L.R. *Basic Concepts of Psychiatric-Mental Health Nursing,* 7th ed. Philadelphia: Lippincott Williams & Wilkins, 2007.

Special nursing observation

Psychiatric patients who are critically ill and require intensive care, are at risk for suicide, or who may intentionally or unintentionally harm themselves need special nursing observation. The seriousness of the patient's condition must never be underestimated. Constant, vigilant, high-quality observation, intervention, and documentation are required.

Implementation

- Fully explain the special nursing observation status to the patient before and during the entire procedure.
- Keep the patient under constant visual observation throughout the duration of this procedure. Position yourself close enough to the patient so you can intervene immediately, if necessary, *to prevent harm.* Constant observation and proper positioning should be maintained 24 hours per day, including times the patient spends bathing, toileting, sleeping, pacing, and conducting other activities.
- Remove all contraband or potentially harmful articles and possessions from the patient and his surroundings. Search the patient and his surroundings at least once every 24 hours. Search especially dangerous patients frequently *to maintain safety.* Look for potentially dangerous articles, such as dis-

posable razors, nail files, combs, and sharp objects. Document the findings of your search.

■ Be sure to provide relief for the assigned nurse for meals and other tasks *because observation must be continuous.* Communicate the patient's status during the relief change.

■ Restrict the patient to a closed section of the unit at all times. Visitors may be permitted with a specific order from the practitioner. If visitors are allowed, the nurse must stay and observe the patient during contact with visitors. Observe the patient closely during mealtimes, and make sure all tableware and eating utensils used by the patient are removed from the area after meals.

■ Don't allow your patient to leave the unit except for emergency appointments and essential tests that can't be performed on the unit. Obtain a practitioner's order if the patient must leave the restricted area, and accompany him off the unit with another staff member.

Special considerations

■ A practitioner's order is necessary before placing a patient on special status. The nurse must assess the patient immediately after receiving the practitioner's order and then place the patient on special nursing observation.

■ When a patient requires special nursing observation for homicidal risk, the practitioner must write an order stating, "Place on special nursing observation for homicidal observation."

■ A practitioner's order is required before discontinuing special nursing observation.

Documentation

Document your observations and assessment each shift, or more often, as indicated. Note the patient's level of depression, the presence or absence of suicidal thoughts, specific interventions, and the patient's behavior, mental status, sleep pattern, appetite, and energy level. Describe progress or lack thereof in resolving problems identified in the treatment and nursing care plan. Document each search of the patient's environment and possessions. After removing the patient from special nursing observation, document his progress every 7 days.

SELECTED REFERENCES

Bisconer, S.W., et al. "Managing Aggression in a Psychiatric Hospital Using a Behavior Plan: A Case Study," *Journal of Psychiatric and Mental Health Nursing* 13(5):515-21, October 2006.

Jacobs. D.G., et al. *Practice Guideline for the Treatment of Patients with Suicidal Behaviors.* November 2003. Available at *http://www.psych.org/psych_pract/treatg/pg/SuicidalBehavior_05-15-06.pdf.*

Karasu, T., et al. *Practice Guideline for the Treatment of Patients with Major Depressive Disorder,* 2nd ed. April 2000. Available at *http://www.psych.org/psych_pract/treatg/pg/MDD2e_05-15-06.pdf.*

MacKay, I., et al. "Constant or Special Observations of Inpatients Presenting a Risk of Aggression or Violence: Nurses' Perceptions of the Rules of Engagement," *Journal of Psychiatric and Mental Health Nursing* 12(4):464-71, August 2005.

SAFETY

MANAGING VIOLENT AND ASSAULTIVE PATIENTS

To manage violent and assaultive behavior in patients, the nursing staff must use the least amount of force possible to bring the situation under control. The key to managing this type of situation is encouraging the patient to talk about his feelings rather than acting them out. It's important to treat the patient with respect and dignity during this stressful situation.

Implementation

■ Talk with the patient to ascertain what's upsetting him. Assess his behavioral controls and ability to cooperate. Speak in a calm, reassuring — but firm — manner.

■ Encourage the patient to vent his hostility verbally. Divert his attention or help him to redirect his energy to appropriate activities or exercise.

■ Provide a private, nonstimulating environment in which the patient can relax or talk.

■ Be honest with the patient, answer his questions truthfully, and don't provide false promises.

■ Define limits in a firm but nonthreatening manner.

■ Allow the patient to lie down in a quiet room. You may remain with the patient or observe him frequently. (See "Seclusion for assaultive or violent behavior," page 834.)

■ Assess the need for medication or chemical restraint and notify the practitioner. The practitioner is responsible for ensuring that an acutely disturbed patient receives appropriate medication and amounts *to prevent as much violent behavior as possible.*

■ Give the medication, as needed, before using seclusion or physical restraints. Oral liquid medication is preferred over tablets, capsules, or the I.M. route.

■ If all efforts fail to assist the patient in regaining or maintaining self-control, use seclusion or physical restraints. (See "Seclusion for assaultive or violent behavior," page 834, and "Restraint use for assaultive or violent behavior," page 836.)

■ Obtain a practitioner's order for seclusion or restraints, and plan the strategy for approach and application away from the patient. *It's challenging to the patient, not reassuring, if he perceives that there will be a struggle to control his behavior.*

- Make sure you have enough available help but have them remain on the periphery and assist, as directed, in a show of force. Tell the patient quietly and calmly what you're going to do and keep repeating it as you approach him.
- Use firm but humane physical holds to place the patient in seclusion or restraints.
- If the patient responds inappropriately to seclusion by becoming harmful to himself, remove him from seclusion and place him in restraints and a private room. When a patient is in physical restraints, give a chemical restraint *to reduce the amount of time spent in physical restraints.*
- Obtain a practitioner's order within 1 hour of initiation of restraint or seclusion. Verbal orders must be cosigned within 8 hours of initiation. Each order must state a time limit and can't exceed 4 hours for an adult. A registered nurse may continue this order for two 4-hour periods, according to the practitioner's order, if reassessment by the registered nurse indicates continued need. After a maximum of 12 hours, the practitioner must conduct a face-to-face assessment of the patient and write a new order and progress note.
- Review the incident with the patient after control is achieved.
- If the problem can't be solved using the actions described, contact your local police department.

Special considerations

Make every effort to calm the patient using the following techniques before the use of restraint or seclusion:

- Treat the patient with dignity and respect.
- Convey a willingness to understand the patient and show concern for his welfare.
- Keep communications simple, concise, and clear.
- Strive to establish trust. Don't threaten the patient.
- Avoid power struggles. Don't argue with the patient.
- Convey the expectation that if he doesn't maintain self-control, you'll take measures to prevent him from harming himself or others.
- Allow the patient time to express his feelings and deal with his frustrations.
- Quietly clear the area of other patients and any objects that could be used to inflict harm.
- Define clear limits with the patient.
- Continue to assess the patient's level of behavioral controls and his ability to cooperate.

Documentation

Document the patient's behavior as soon as possible and be specific. Document all interventions and the patient's response to these interventions.

Selected references

APA Task Force on Psychiatric Emergency Services. *Report and Recommendations Regarding Psychiatric Emergency and Crisis Services.* August 2002. Available at *http://www.psych.org/downloads/EmergencyServicesFinal.pdf.*

Bisconer, S.W., et al. "Managing Aggression in a Psychiatric Hospital Using a Behavior Plan: A Case Study," *Journal of Psychiatric and Mental Health Nursing* 13(5):515-21, October 2006.

The Joint Commission. *Comprehensive Accreditation Manual for Hospitals: The Official Handbook.* Standard PC.12.10 to PC.12.190, 2007.

MacKay, I., et al. "Constant or Special Observations of Inpatients Presenting a Risk of Aggression or Violence: Nurses' Perceptions of the Rules of Engagement," *Journal of Psychiatric and Mental Health Nursing* 12(4):464-71, August 2005.

Nelstrop, L., et al. "A Systematic Review of the Safety and Effectiveness of Restraint and Seclusion as Interventions for the Short-term Management of Violence in Adult Psychiatric Inpatient Settings and Emergency Departments," *Worldwide Views on Evidence-based Nursing* 3(1):8-18, 2006.

Vergare, M.J., et al. *Practice Guideline for the Psychiatric Evaluation of Adults,* 2nd ed. June 2006. Available at *http://www.psych.org/psych_pract/treatg/pg/PsychEval2ePG_04-28-06.pdf.*

Seclusion for assaultive or violent behavior

Seclusion is a temporary, therapeutic safety measure used for the management of severely disturbed behavior that's harmful to the patient or others or disrupts the therapeutic environment. Seclusion is used only after less-restrictive measures are ineffective in containing or redirecting the behavior. Seclusion shouldn't be used as a punishment or to control behavior for the convenience of the nursing staff. Don't use seclusion for patients who are acutely suicidal or intoxicated, physically ill, or have uncontrolled seizure disorders.

Clinical rationales for seclusion include:

- unpredictable or assaultive behavior
- behavior that's dangerous to the patient or others
- verbally or physically threatening behavior with poor control or a confirmed history of violence
- intoxication by alcohol or drugs with poor, tenuous, or absent behavioral controls
- manic behavior with poor controls and a history of violence
- poor, tenuous, or absent behavior controls that haven't responded to less-restrictive measures, such as medication or quiet room use
- the patient's request.

Whenever possible, seclusion should be used before restraints. Nursing measures that may be used as alternatives to seclusion include:

- verbal interventions
- listening to and monitoring the patient
- social engagement (such as conversation)
- administering medications as needed
- initiating noncompetitive tasks, such as puzzles, cards, and art
- removing stimuli or moving the patient to a quiet area
- implementing physical outlets, such as treadmill use, walking, or involvement in recreational activities.

Equipment

Seclusion room and bed ▪ optional: standard precautions supplies, including gloves, gowns, masks, and eye protectors if contact with blood or body fluids is possible.

Implementation

- Explain to the patient what you're going to do and why. Use a firm, yet kind approach *to alleviate anxiety.* For example, you may say, "You'll remain in seclusion until you can regain control."
- Approach the patient with two or more staff members simultaneously from the side. Convey an attitude that prevents increased anxiety and panic.

NURSING ALERT *Never approach a patient alone to escort him to the seclusion room.*

- If necessary, pass one hand under the patient's arm and grasp the arm just below the elbow. The palm of your hand should be on the anterior part of the patient's arm. Grasp the lower arm at the wrist with your other hand and walk the patient to the seclusion room. Avoid holding the soft parts of the arm *because these bruise easily.* Don't position yourself where the patient can bite, kick, or hold on to you.
- Assess your patient for injuries and document descriptively. Continually assess for injuries, especially if the patient complains of injury.
- Remove all potentially harmful items from the patient's pockets and possession and store these in a safe place until the patient regains self-control. Such items may include nail clippers, jewelry, keys, and a prosthesis that could be used to inflict self-injury or be damaged or lost. Remove cash and other loose valuables as well as the patient's shoes, belt, and bra, if applicable. Document and inventory the items removed.
- Dress the patient in comfortable, safe clothing appropriate for seclusion, such as a shirt, pants, and underwear (no bra) or pajamas and socks.
- Keep the door to the seclusion room locked at all times.
- Observe the patient every 15 minutes through the window of the locked door or by a remote camera and monitor system. When using a remote camera and monitor system, the patient should be visible and the monitor turned *to prevent other patients or visitors from viewing the patient.* If the patient isn't visible or is in distress, do a one-to-one observation. When doing this, ensure your safety by using a security emergency call system before entering the room. Make sure other staff members are available to assist you immediately. While in the seclusion room, make sure the viewing window on the seclusion room door can't be occluded from the inside.
- Offer the patient fluids frequently *to prevent dehydration.* Monitor intake and output.
- Patients in seclusion are given a break for 15 minutes every 2 hours. Assess the patient before and after the break *to determine whether seclusion should be continued.*
- If the patient's condition permits, he may be allowed to leave the seclusion room to take his meals. Give assistance during meals and observe the patient closely. Count all tableware and eating utensils before and after the meal *to assure safety.* Assess for the need to use a spoon only. Meals in the seclusion room should only be served with plastic tableware and tray.
- Always have adequate help when removing the patient from the seclusion room for breaks and meals.
- The patient should be released from seclusion as soon as his condition permits.

Special considerations

- A practitioner's order is required to place a patient in seclusion. If a verbal order is obtained, include the exact date and time of seclusion. All orders for seclusion must be time limited and shouldn't exceed 4 hours for adults. Follow your facility's policy regarding time limits and procedures for seclusion orders.

NURSING ALERT *In an emergency or crisis situation, a nurse may place a patient in seclusion. In such a case, a written or verbal order must be obtained within 1 hour. (Follow your facility's policy regarding the cosigning time limit for verbal orders.)*

- A registered nurse is responsible for the total care of the patient who requires seclusion. This includes assessment, assignment, planning, implementation, communication, evaluation, documentation, and supervision.
- Patients in seclusion have a right to respectful care that maintains dignity. An attitude of kindness, acceptance, and sincere interest in the patient as an individual should be shown at all times.
- Don't place a patient in restraints while he's in seclusion.

Documentation

Use a flow sheet or checklist to document your care and assessments. Documentation should include the patient's name, date, rationale for seclusion, time placed in seclusion, and time removed. Record the patient's condition, his behavior before and during seclusion, and his behavior while in break periods. Document any alternatives to seclusion used, evidence of break periods every 2 hours, preventive nursing measures used, and safety measures.

Document your observations every 15 minutes. Also document intake and output, unusual physical conditions or injuries, and removal of possessions for safety. For the first 24 hours after removal from seclusion, document changes in mental status, level of behavioral controls, effectiveness of medication, response to the nursing care plan, appropriate patient education, and other pertinent observations every shift.

SELECTED REFERENCES

APA Task Force on Psychiatric Emergency Services. *Report and Recommendations Regarding Psychiatric Emergency and Crisis Services.* August 2002. Available at *http://www.psych.org/downloads/EmergencyServicesFinal.pdf.*

Bisconer, S.W., et al. "Managing Aggression in a Psychiatric Hospital Using a Behavior Plan: A Case Study," *Journal of Psychiatric and Mental Health Nursing* 13(5):515-21, October 2006.

Huckshorn, K.A. "Reducing Seclusion Restraint in Mental Health Settings: Core Strategies for Prevention," *Journal of Psychosocial Nursing and Mental Health Services* 42(9):22-33, Spetember 2004.

The Joint Commission. *Comprehensive Accreditation Manual for Hospitals: The Official Handbook.* Standard PC.12.10 to PC.12.190, 2007.

MacKay, I., et al. "Constant or Special Observations of Inpatients Presenting a Risk of Aggression or Violence: Nurses' Perceptions of the Rules of Engagement," *Journal of Psychiatric and Mental Health Nursing* 12(4):464-71, August 2005.

Vergare, M.J., et al. *Practice Guideline for the Psychiatric Evaluation of Adults,* 2nd ed. June 2006. Available at *http://www.psych.org/psych_pract/treatg/pg/PsychEval2ePG_04-28-06.pdf.*

RESTRAINT USE FOR ASSAULTIVE OR VIOLENT BEHAVIOR

Using restraints on an assaultive or violent patient is a temporary, therapeutic safety measure used for the management of severely disturbed behavior that's harmful to the patient or others or disrupts the therapeutic environment. Restraints should be used only after less-restrictive measures have proven ineffective in containing or redirecting the behavior.

NURSING ALERT *Restraints shouldn't be used as a punishment or to control a patient's behavior for the convenience of the nursing staff.*

Clinical rationales for restraint use include:

- unpredictable or assaultive behavior
- behavior that's dangerous to the patient or others
- self-destructive behavior
- verbally or physically threatening behavior with poor control or confirmed history of violence
- intoxication by alcohol or drugs with poor, tenuous, or absent behavioral controls
- manic behavior with poor controls and a history of violence
- suicidal behavior with poor impulse control, serious verbal threat, intact plan, or history of attempts
- poor, tenuous, or absent behavior controls that haven't responded to less-restrictive measures, such as medication or quiet room use
- the patient's request.

Restraints should be viewed as a last resort — nursing measures should be implemented to modify the patient's behavior before using restraints. Nursing measures that may be used as alternatives to restraints include:

- verbal interventions
- listening to and monitoring the patient
- social engagement (such as conversation)
- administering medications
- initiating noncompetitive tasks such as puzzles, cards, or art
- removing stimuli or moving the patient to a quiet area
- implementing physical outlets, such as treadmill use, walking, and involvement in recreational activities.

Equipment

Leather anklets, belts, and wristlets ▪ restraint key ▪ body lotion ▪ optional: standard precaution supplies, including gloves, gowns, masks, eye protectors.

Preparation of equipment

Assemble restraints, as needed, check lock, and place in order for application. Lower the bed to the lowest position.

Implementation

- Secure sufficient help to apply restraints depending on the situation at hand. Never approach the patient alone.
- Explain to the patient what you are doing and why. Use a firm yet kind approach. You may say, "You'll remain in restraints until you can regain control."
- Approach the patient from the side and convey an attitude that will prevent increased anxiety and possible panic.
- When possible, pass one hand under the patient's arm and grasp the arm just below the elbow (the palm of your hand should be on the anterior part of his arm). Grasp the lower arm at the wrist with your other hand. Walk the pa-

tient to his room and place him in bed. Avoid holding the soft parts of the arm *because these bruise easily.* Don't place yourself where the patient can bite, kick, or hold on to you.

- If the patient is out of control and combative, use appropriate holds or takedowns, as necessary, according to your facility's policy.
- After selecting a length that fits the arm, apply the wristlets with the metal loop on the inside of the wrist. Make certain these aren't tight enough to impair circulation or loose enough that the patient can slip his hand out.
- If you're using two-point restraints to move the patient to the bed, pass the belt loop through the metal loop on one wristlet, loop the belt over, follow the waistline with the belt, and then pass the belt through the other wristlet loop; again make a loop in the belt and fasten the buckle by locking it. Check to make sure the belt isn't too tight and is smooth against the body. The buckle of the belt should be at either side of patient.
- After placing the patient in bed, pass the belt through the wristlets and fasten the belt around the bed frame on each side of the bed. Lock the buckle. Use the same procedure to secure the anklets to the bed.
- Assess the patient for injuries and document a description if an injury is discovered. Report complaints of injury or actual injury to the practitioner. Complete an events report or incident report as per your facility's policy and procedure.
- Remove all potentially harmful items from the patient's pockets and possession and store them in a safe place until the patient regains self-control. Such items may include nail clippers, jewelry, keys, a prosthesis that could be used to inflict self-injury or be damaged or lost, cash, and other loose valuables. Remove the patient's shoes, belt, and bra, if applicable. Document and inventory items that are removed.
- Observe closely for signs of circulatory impairment, brush burns, redness, irritation, and edema. As indicated, provide skin care using massage or lotion while the patient is restrained and also when restraints are removed.
- Offer fluids frequently *to prevent dehydration.* Record the patient's intake and output.
- Loosen or remove restraints at mealtimes. Give assistance during meals and count all tableware and eating utensils before and after each meal *to assure safety.* Assess for the need to use a spoon only.
- Assist the patient with toileting and personal needs such as bathing. Use rest periods to provide for these needs as much as possible.
- Provide rest periods by removing restraints every hour *to allow the patient to move about.* Examine the patient before the rest period *to decide how the break will occur and afterward to determine if restraints need to be continued.* If the patient is sleeping, quietly unlock the buckles with the key so the patient can turn in bed. If the patient hasn't regained sufficient control to remove all the restraints at one time, release one limb at a time *to ensure all four limbs have a period of movement.*
- To walk your patient while in restraints, remove his feet from the restraints, secure his hands to the belt around the waist, and assist the patient with ambulation.
- Observe the patient constantly either by direct one-to-one supervision or by a remote camera and monitor system. When using a remote camera and monitor system, make sure the patient is visible at all times and the monitor is turned *so that other patients or visitors can't view the patient.* If the patient is in distress, a direct observation check must be done. When the patient is restrained, all defenses have been removed; therefore, you must continually provide for the patient's safety. When using a remote camera and monitor system, lock the room door *to provide for patient safety.*
- The patient should be released from restraints as soon as his condition permits, according to the practitioner's order.

Special considerations

- A practitioner's order is required to place a patient in restraints. If a verbal order is obtained, include the exact date and time of restraint. All orders for restraints must be time limited and shouldn't exceed 4 hours for adults, 2 hours for children and adolescents ages 9 to 17, and 1 hour for children under age 9. Follow your facility's time limits and procedures for restraint orders.

NURSING ALERT *A patient may be placed in restraints by a registered nurse in an emergent or crisis situation. In such a case, a written or verbal order must be obtained within 1 hour. (Follow your facility's policy for the co-signing time limit for verbal orders.) If a verbal order is obtained, include the exact date and time of restraint.*

- A registered nurse is responsible for the total care of the patient who requires restraints, including assessment, assignment, planning, implementation, communication, evaluation, documentation, and supervision.
- Patients who are restrained in bed using a soft body tie should be placed in a bed with a full side rail. If using a split side rail, use padded covers *to prevent injury or entrapment between the rails.*

Documentation

Document using progress notes and a restraint flow sheet or checklist. Include the patient's name, date, type of restraint, time placed in restraints, time removed, rationale for restraints, and alternative nursing measures used in an effort to avoid restraint use. Note acute psychotic behavior or assaultive behavior toward himself or others before and during placement and the patient's behavior while in restraints and during rest periods. Document assessments before and after rest periods and evidence that restraints were removed or loosened every hour. Include documentation of examinations for injuries and outcomes.

Document nursing care and safety measures, intake and output, and unusual conditions. After restraints are removed, document every shift, including your assessment of the patient's mental status, level of behavioral controls, effectiveness of medication, other pertinent observations, patient education, and responses to the nursing care plan.

SELECTED REFERENCES

APA Task Force on Psychiatric Emergency Services. *Report and Recommendations Regarding Psychiatric Emergency and Crisis Services.* August 2002. Available at *http://www.psych.org/downloads/EmergencyServicesFinal.pdf.*

Bisconer, S.W., et al. "Managing Aggression in a Psychiatric Hospital Using a Behavior Plan: A Case Study," *Journal of Psychiatric and Mental Health Nursing* 13(5):515-21, October 2006.

The Joint Commission. *Comprehensive Accreditation Manual for Hospitals: The Official Handbook.* Standard PC.12.10 to PC.12.190, 2007.

Nelstrop, L., et al. "A Systematic Review of the Safety and Effectiveness of Restraint and Seclusion as Interventions for the Short-term Management of Violence in Adult Psychiatric Inpatient Settings and Emergency Departments," *Worldwide Views on Evidence-based Nursing* 3(1):8-18, 2006.

Vergare, M.J., et al. *Practice Guideline for the Psychiatric Evaluation of Adults,* 2nd ed. June 2006. Available at *http://www.psych.org/psych_pract/treatg/pg/PsychEval2ePG_04-28-06.pdf.*

SHAVING RESTRICTED-AREA PSYCHIATRIC PATIENTS

Shaving improves a patient's cleanliness and morale but presents a special challenge when you're caring for a patient in a restricted area. Supervision is needed to ensure safety for the patient and you. Always use standard precautions; wearing gloves, gowns, masks, and eye protectors as needed if contact with blood or body fluids is possible.

Equipment

Brush ▪ 70% isopropyl alcohol ▪ cart containing razors ▪ razors (disposable safety or electric) ▪ bath towels ▪ washcloths ▪ shaving cream ▪ disposable gloves ▪ optional: preshave and aftershave lotions.

Preparation of equipment

Assemble all equipment. Label equipment with the patient's name and identification number and keep in a locked cart.

Keep electric razor heads clean by using a brush and 70% isopropyl alcohol. Soak in alcohol for 10 minutes and let air-dry. Discard disposable razors in a puncture-resistant sharps container when dull.

Implementation

- Explain to the patient that the razor is to be used in the area provided and returned to the person issuing the razor. Don't allow the patient to keep a razor in his room or with his possessions.
- Issue the patient's individually owned razor from a locked cart.
- Supply the patient with shaving cream, towels, washcloths, shaving lotion, and other needed supplies.
- Apply gloves and assist the patient, as necessary. If the patient doesn't need assistance, supervise him carefully the entire time he has the razor.
- Return the razor to the locked cart and return the locked cart to the designated area.

Documentation

Keep a safety data sheet and document by signing your name when the razor is returned to the locked cart.

SELECTED REFERENCES

Pridding, A., et al. "Mental Health Nursing Roles and Functions in Acute Inpatient Units: Caring for People with Intellectual Disability and Mental Health Problems-A Literature Review," *The International Journal of Psychiatric Nursing Research* 12(2):1459-71, January 2007.

TREATMENTS

ELECTROCONVULSIVE THERAPY

In electroconvulsive therapy (ECT), an electric shock is delivered to the patient's brain by way of electrodes placed on his temples. Electrodes may be placed bilaterally or unilaterally. ECT is an effective way to treat patients with affective disorders and selected schizophrenias or related psychoses.

A physician is primarily responsible for administering ECT, but safe and effective therapy requires an interdisciplinary approach and cooperation. The nurse's role is to provide care during the assessment, preparation, treatment, and recovery. The treatment team also includes a certified registered nurse-anesthetist (CRNA) and, possibly, a nurse practitioner (NP).

The physician's role is to obtain appropriate consent, order pretreatment and posttreatment regimens, titrate drug doses, administer treatment, and determine when the patient may be released from the post-ECT recovery unit. The CRNA is responsible for ensuring a patent airway, administering positive pressure oxygen during the treatment and until the patient is breathing well on his own, and administering specific drugs during the procedure. If an NP is part of the team, she's responsible for making sure all equipment, drugs, and emergency equipment are available, preparing the patient by attaching electrocardiograph (ECG) and EEG monitors, explaining the procedure to the patient, and completing a preprocedure assessment.

Equipment

EEG/ECG machine ▪ five connection wires (three ECG and two EEG) ▪ rubber headband ▪ two stimulus electrodes ▪ conduction gel ▪ ECG monitor and disposable ECG electrodes ▪ crash cart with emergency drug kit and defibrillator ▪ suction machine with sterile pharyngeal catheters ▪ endotracheal intubation tray ▪ rubber mouthpiece ▪ electronic blood pressure monitor ▪ oxygen source and tubing with positive pressure equipment ▪ two pairs of gloves ▪ alcohol pads ▪ 21G needles ▪ butterfly infusion set ▪ sterile 3-cc, 5-cc, and 10-cc syringes ▪ methohexital ▪ succinylcholine (Anectine) ▪ glycopyrrolate (Robinul) ▪ dantrolene (Dantrium) ▪ tape ▪ sterile water or normal saline solution for injection ▪ tourniquet ▪ patient's medical record ▪ documentation records ▪ stretcher ▪ optional: protective equipment, such as gloves, gowns, masks, and eye protectors.

Preparation of equipment

Plug the EEG/ECG machine into a 120-volt wall socket. Plug the stimulus output electrode leads into the machine's outlet — marked stimulus output. Plug the stimulus monitor electrode leads into the machine's receptacle — labeled patient monitor input — which monitors the EEG and ECG. Check the dual channel chart recorder to ensure that it's properly loaded with heat sensitive graph paper. The paper will show a red warning line when a new roll of paper is needed. Press the master power switch to activate the display panels and chart recorder. *The panel switches light up when the power switch is pressed.* Briefly turn on the chart recorder using the manual switch to advance the paper *to ensure that the machine is working properly.*

Set the treatment parameters, as ordered, for pulse width (ms), frequency (Hz), duration (sec), and current (amp). These parameters represent the total volume of electrical stimulus applied, which differs depending on the patient's age, medication use, seizure threshold, and other factors. Plug in the electronic blood pressure monitor. Make sure the crash cart, with emergency drug kit, defibrillator, suction equipment, endotracheal intubation tray, and oxygen is readily available and that needed medications are properly prepared. (See *Preparing medications for ECT*, page 840.)

Implementation

- Check the order.
- Gather the appropriate equipment.
- After arrival in the ECT room, confirm the patient's identity and check his nothing-by-mouth status.
- Explain the procedure to the patient *to allay his anxiety.*
- Make sure the physician has obtained a signed informed consent form.
- Make sure the patient's history (including allergies to medications or latex), physical examination, and dental evaluation are documented in his chart.
- Make sure the following diagnostic tests have been completed and assessed: complete blood count, thyroid profile, urinalysis, ECG, pseudocholinesterase activity determination (especially in patients with severe liver disease, malnutrition, or a history of sensitivity to muscle relaxants or similar substances), chest X-ray, spine radiographs, EEG, and cranial computed tomography scan.
- Wash your hands and put on gloves. Help the patient remove dentures, partial plates, or other foreign objects from his mouth *to prevent choking.*
- Remove and dispose of gloves.
- Make sure the patient removes all jewelry, metal objects, and prosthetic devices before the procedure *to prevent injury.*
- Have the patient dress in a hospital gown and ask him to void *to prevent incontinence during the procedure.*
- Help the patient onto the stretcher.
- Put on gloves, attach the patient to an electronic blood pressure monitor, and check his baseline vital signs.
- Attach the patient to a pulse oximeter to monitor his respiratory status during the procedure *because the drugs used cause respiratory depression.*
- Insert an I.V. catheter using sterile technique.
- Attach the patient to the ECG monitor.
- Attach the EEG electrodes and stimulus electrodes to the rubber headband. Coat the electrodes with conduction gel and place the band around the patient's head. Place the large, silver-colored stimulus electrodes on each temple at about eye-level. Space the small, brown-colored EEG electrodes across the forehead.
- Connect the stimulus electrodes to the stimulus output receptacle on the machine.

Preparing medications for ECT

Even though the physician or certified registered nurse-anesthetist administers medications during electroconvulsive therapy (ECT), you should become familiar with the medications that can be used so you can assess the patient for adverse effects. Brief descriptions of the most commonly used drugs appear below.

DRUG	ACTIONS	ADVERSE EFFECTS
Dantrolene (Dantrium)	Direct-acting skeletal muscle relaxant that's effective against malignant hyperthermia	■ Seizures ■ Muscle weakness ■ Drowsiness ■ Fatigue ■ Headache ■ Hepatitis ■ Nervousness ■ Insomnia
Glycopyrrolate (Robinul)	Has desirable cholinergic blocking effects because it reduces secretions in the respiratory system as well as oral and gastric secretions; also prevents a drop in heart rate caused by vagal nerve stimulation during anesthesia	■ Dilated pupils ■ Tachycardia ■ Urine retention ■ Anaphylaxis ■ Confusion (in elderly patients) ■ Dry mouth
Methohexital	Rapid, ultra-short-acting barbiturate anesthetic agent	■ Hypotension ■ Tachycardia ■ Respiratory arrest ■ Bronchospasm ■ Anxiety ■ Hypersensitivity reaction ■ Emergence delirium
Succinylcholine (Anectine)	Ultra-short-acting depolarizing skeletal muscle relaxant; given I.V., causes rapid, flaccid paralysis	■ Bradycardia ■ Arrhythmias ■ Cardiac arrest ■ Prolonged respiratory depression ■ Malignant hyperthermia ■ Anaphylaxis

■ Run the EEG/ECG machine in the self-test mode. When the machine is ready, it displays the message "Self Test Passed" and prints the date, time, treatment parameters, a brief ECG strip, and EEG monitors.

■ The CRNA or physician will then administer glycopyrrolate, followed by methohexital. Methohexital acts very rapidly. Expect an abrupt loss of consciousness when the appropriate dose is infused.

■ After the patient is unconscious, succinylcholine is administered. *A tremor or fasciculation of various muscle groups occurs due to the depolarizing effect of this drug. Succinylcholine also causes complete flaccid paralysis,* so mechanical ventilation is started at this time. A rubber mouthpiece is inserted and positive pressure oxygen is given.

■ The physician initiates the stimulus, and mild seizurelike activity occurs for about 30 seconds. The patient's jaw and extremities must be supported while avoiding contact with metal.

- Monitor vital signs as well as ECG and EEG rhythm strips. Assess the patient's skin for burns.
- When spontaneous ventilation returns, usually in 3 to 5 minutes, discontinue the I.V. infusion. Continue to monitor vital signs.
- As the patient becomes more alert, speak quietly and explain what's happening. Remove the rubber mouthpiece.
- Place the patient on his side *to maintain a patent airway.* Measure and document his vital signs every 15 minutes until they stabilize.
- Discharge the patient from the recovery area when he's able to move all four extremities voluntarily, can breathe and cough adequately, is roused and oriented when called, has an Aldrete score of 7 or greater, has stable vital signs and temperature within 1° F (0.6° C) of the pretreatment value, and has a normal swallowing reflex. A physician's order is required to release the patient from the recovery area.
- One hour after treatment, obtain and record the patient's vital signs. Check the patient's temperature *to assess for malignant hyperthermia.* Then continue to check vital signs every hour as necessary, until stable.

Special considerations

- If the patient is taking benzodiazepines before the procedure, obtain an order to begin tapering, and discontinue the drug 3 to 4 days before the procedure. *Benzodiazepines and anticonvulsants (such as lorazepam and phenytoin) negatively affect the patient's response to treatment.*
- Contraindications to ECT include brain tumors, space-occupying lesions, and other brain diseases that cause increased intracranial pressure. The seriousness of any physical illness, such as heart, liver, or kidney disease as well as that of the psychiatric disorder, must be weighed against each other before ECT is initiated.

NURSING ALERT *Malignant hyperthermia is an uncommon but potentially life-threatening complication that can follow the administration of anesthetic agents or a depolarizing muscle relaxant such as succinylcholine. An oral temperature above 100° F (37.8° C) within 1 hour after treatment should be reported to the physician immediately. Malignant hyperthermia is a medical emergency that requires multiple personnel to care for the patient and administer dantrolene to treat the disorder. Follow your facility's policy and procedure for a malignant hyperthermia crisis.*

Documentation

Document using flow sheets or progress notes. Include the patient's vital signs and responses during the treatment sequence, recovery, and post-recovery. Assess and document the patient's physical and mental status and any behavioral changes or lack of such changes.

SELECTED REFERENCES

American Psychiatric Association. *A Task Force Report on the Practice of Electroconvulsive Therapy: Recommendations for Treatment, Training, and Privileging,* 2nd ed., 2001. Available at *http://www.psych.org/psych_pract/treatg/pg/ect.cfm.*

The Joint Commission. *Comprehensive Accreditation Manual for Hospitals: The Official Handbook.* Standard PC.13.50 to PC.13.60, 2007.

Karasu, T., et al. *Practice Guideline for the Treatment of Patients with Major Depressive Disorder,* 2nd ed. Available at *http://www.psych.org/psych_pract/treatg/pg/MDD2e_05-15-06.pdf.*

Ness, D.E. "ECT in Patients with Depression and Borderline Personality Disorder," *American Journal of Psychiatry* 162(9):1762, September 2005.

GROUP WORK TECHNIQUES

A small group setting helps to address the specific therapeutic needs of each of its members, who are experiencing similar emotional problems. Groups meet to discuss their concerns with one another and can work on resocialization, reality orientation, sensory retraining, life review, counseling, education, rehabilitation, or other topics as needed. The choice of group activities is determined by the health care provider based on the patients' interests, assessed needs, mental and physical capabilities, and care plan. (See *Group therapy activities,* pages 842 to 845.)

Equipment

Quiet space for up to 10 or more persons ▪ chairs and space for wheelchairs ▪ optional: props and audio visual aids, as needed.

Preparation of equipment

Plan the group activity and prepare needed materials.

Implementation

- Select patients who will benefit from and cooperate with the group.
- Arrange seating and check the environment for lighting and noise.
- Prepare audiovisual equipment.
- Inform patients about the group activity before the scheduled time.
- Encourage attendance by exploring the purpose of the group and the plans for the day.

Group therapy activities

The table below lists various types of group therapy activities and describes the purpose, patient-selection criteria, content, and desired patient outcomes.

GROUP THERAPY	PURPOSE	CRITERIA FOR PATIENT SELECTION
Classroom reality orientation	Classroom reality orientation provides a structured setting to help the patient recall or retain personal identity, improve awareness of time references, foster an interest in his surroundings, build self-esteem and personal dignity, encourage socialization, and increase independence in activities of daily living.	Patients who are confused or disoriented due to any cause, regardless of age or diagnosis, may be selected for participation in a classroom reality orientation group. Patients with significant memory loss may also be selected. The expectations and format of the group activity vary according to the patient's physical and mental limitations. Patients who need sensory stimuli and are able to sit in the group area may be included.
Exercise	An exercise group promotes physical and mental health by increasing the patient's activity tolerance and functional ability and promoting a feeling of well-being.	The selection of patients for an exercise group is based on the goals of the group, such as increasing heart rate and strengthening the heart muscle, improving or maintaining body flexibility, and increasing the social network (especially for a group with elderly patients).
Health-related self-help	A health-related self-help group provides health teaching through group discussion. The focus of the discussion is on a specific health-related topic or common condition, symptom, or experience. The group provides a means for mobilizing psychological resources to overcome personal health problems or concerns or to promote health promotion.	Patients with a common need rising from a health problem, condition, experience, or interest may be selected to join a health-related self-help group.
Reminiscence	Reminiscence provides a therapeutic means of exchanging ideas and discussing life experiences, which aids in the development of self-esteem and renewal of the patient's past identity. This group activity helps to decrease withdrawal and provides an opportunity to socialize and communicate; activates recall or relating of past experiences; and aids in conflict resolution in later life.	Patients selected for a reminiscence group are alert and oriented or have minimal confusion. These patients are able to hear or see, recall the past, and have been assessed to need "normal group experience." The group needs a mix of patients who are withdrawn, impaired, or verbally suppressive.

- Seek assistance from others, as needed, *to gain patient cooperation.*
- Welcome the patients and introduce yourself.
- Follow the selected format and discussion using resource information.
- Assess and evaluate the group on ongoing and individual bases.

CONTENT	DESIRED PATIENT OUTCOMES
The depth of information presented in classroom reality orientation depends on the patient's degree of disorientation. The activity provides intensive orientation to time, place, and person using verbal interaction and environmental props. The leader should follow the members' cues to keep the interest of the group and provide reorientation. Repetition is an effective tool. Include kind, human contact through touch with talking. Avoid mechanical repetition of information. Call patients by titles and correct names. Introduce yourself each day. Give praise and recognition for each positive response and avoid negative statements. Correct confused rambling speech with accurate information about time, place, and person.	Desired patient outcomes include verbal or nonverbal responses; identification of time-, place-, and person-related items; increased attention span; responses to touch and verbal praise; accurate responses following repetition of information by leader; and diminished confusion with less rambling speech.
A group leader directs and demonstrates all exercises. A simple warm-up followed by a consistent routine of exercises using music is usually successful. The group leader may introduce himself at the beginning to promote a positive atmosphere. Further reading and a specific plan by the leader is required to conduct this group.	Desired patient outcomes include expressing a feeling of accomplishment, increased activity tolerance, improved range of motion and mobility, improved mood, and a more positive attitude.
The content of a health-related self-help group depends on the group's needs. Discuss and share concerns with "like" group members, giving ideas for coping, suggesting alternatives, expressing feelings, and suggesting practical day-to-day ways of dealing with difficulties resulting from health-related issues.	Desired patient outcomes include demonstrating alternative lifestyles, expressing greater knowledge and understanding, exhibiting increased self-control, demonstrating improved health practices, and seeking mutual aid from others, as appropriate.
Reminiscence group discussion is informal and centers on past life experiences for the members' age group. The leader may use objects or events as stimuli to promote reminiscing and life review. Choose topics that are common to the group, such as a first date, learning to drive, favorite president, elementary school days, holidays, celebrations, namesakes, names or nicknames, and childhood experiences.	Desired patient outcomes include increased attention span, improved physical appearance, decreased withdrawal, increased social interaction, increased appetite, ability and willingness to communicate or share a feeling of accomplishment, and an enhanced positive self-concept when working through and mastering personal losses.

(continued)

Documentation

Document in the progress notes, under the heading of patient education or on a patient education flow sheet, information about the patient's response to other group members and his participation in the session.

Group therapy activities *(continued)*

GROUP THERAPY	PURPOSE	CRITERIA FOR PATIENT SELECTION
Remotivation	Remotivation is a group activity that helps the patient take a renewed interest in his surroundings by discussing simple, objective, everyday-life occurrences that aren't related to the patient's emotional difficulties. It provides an opportunity for verbal expression and socialization in a structured setting. Specific objectives to gain or retain mental activity, enhance self-esteem, and improve the patient's self-image may be achieved through a structured program of discussion.	Remotivation is appropriate for apathetic patients who are disinterested in the world around them. Patients should be willing to join the group; able to hear and speak; oriented to time, place, and person; and lack a preoccupation with hallucination. A mix of talkers and listeners is helpful.
Rehabilitation	Rehabilitation group activities are used to teach new coping skills or enhance previously learned basic skills. Activities may involve relearning basic tasks involving sensory motor skills or preparing a caregiver to provide care for a discharged patient. The focus is on self-help.	Patients who need new coping skills may be selected for a rehabilitation group.
Counseling	A counseling group provides the opportunity to examine and explore the behavior of group members with a view toward the permanent change of maladaptive behaviors. Insight occurs when the patient is able to see the connection between unconscious feelings, wishes, and conflicts and conscious behaviors and the consequences of those behaviors.	Patients selected for a counseling group exhibit maladaptive behavior.

SELECTED REFERENCES

Korran, L.M., et al. *Practice Guideline for the Treatment of Patients with Obsessive-Compulsive Disorder.* Available at *http://www.psych.org/psych_pract/treatg/pg/OCDPracticeGuidelineFinal05-04-07.pdf.*

McLeod, T., et al. "Cognitive Behavioural Therapy Group Work with Voice Hearers. Part 1," *British Journal of Nursing* 16(4): 248-52, February-March 2007.

McLeod, T., et al. "Cognitive Behavioural Therapy Group Work with Voice Hearers. Part 2," *British Journal of Nursing* 16(5): 292-95, March 2007.

QUIET ROOM USE

A quiet room provides an area of decreased external stimuli for a patient who's experiencing external or internal stimulus overload. The quiet room is used in the first stages of escalating behavior, when verbal intervention is effective and the patient is in control of his behavior. Chemical intervention may also be used to control escalating behavior while the patient is in the quiet room. The major difference between the use of the quiet room and the use of a seclusion room is that the doors of the quiet room are never locked.

Equipment

Quiet room with a clean observation mirror that gives the nurse an unobstructed view of the patient.

Preparation of equipment

The quiet room must be free from auditory and visual stimuli and have doors that are never locked.

CONTENT	DESIRED PATIENT OUTCOMES
Remotivation is usually done in five specific steps that produce a climate of acceptance: 1. Read aloud to bridge reality. 2. Discuss the world in which we live. 3. Consider the work world. 4. Express appreciation and pleasure. 5. Avoid topics that focus on individual problems and family relationships but include such general topics as vacations, gardens, sports, rocks, pets, the sea, transportation, weather, and animals.	Desired patient outcomes include increased attention span, participation in discussion, appropriate responses to props, increased expression of pleasure, discussion of reality, and appropriate communication.
Rehabilitation group activities may include structured educational content, demonstrations of self-help skills, and verbal support from the group. Each member can share ideas or demonstrations for coping with practical, everyday living with the group.	Desired patient outcomes include decreased verbalization or complaints of pain, improved compliance with the treatment regimen, and improved self-control.
The content of a counseling group includes verbal examination and exploration of the behavior of group members. Group members may share and discuss concerns with peers and give ideas for coping, expressing feelings appropriately, and practicing day-to-day ways of dealing with difficulties.	Desired patient outcomes include the appropriate verbalization of feelings and improved self-control of behaviors.

Implementation

- Make sure adequate help is available to place your patient in the quiet room, especially if he hasn't requested this placement. *A patient displaying escalating behavior can be unpredictable and may strike out because of fear brought on by stimulus overload.*
- Explain to the patient what you're doing and why. Assure him that the door will be unlocked. Explain that you or another nurse will observe him and be available to assist him in regaining control. Instruct him to stay in the room until you say he can come out. *These steps will alleviate any further anxiety.*
- Escort the patient to the quiet room.
- Remove any potentially harmful objects from the patient's possession.
- Allow the patient to have time to himself in the quiet room. Assess the level of escalation the patient has reached.
- Observe the patient every 15 minutes until he's removed from the quiet room by his request or by your judgment. During observation, verbally interact with the patient *to assess his state of behavior.*

Special considerations

- The quiet room is never used as a form of punishment.
- The quiet room shouldn't be used when the patient requires one-to-one observation.
- Use proper judgment and assessment to prevent misuse of the quiet room by patients seeking bed rest or wishing to withdraw from a structured routine treatment.

Documentation

Document the initial behavior that necessitated the use of the quiet room, the patient's behavior while in the quiet room, and the effectiveness of the use of the quiet room.

Record 15-minute assessments, as needed, and any use of as-needed medication.

SELECTED REFERENCES

Champagne, T., and Stromberg, N. "Sensory Approaches in Inpatient Psychiatric Settings: Innovative Alternatives to Seclusion and Restraint," *Journal of Psychosocial Nursing and Mental Health Services* 42(9):34-44, September 2004.

REALITY ORIENTATION

Reality orientation is used to help a confused person retain or regain an awareness of his own identity, surroundings, and correct time reference. It also encourages socialization, reinforces socially acceptable behavior, encourages independence in activities of daily living, and helps to build confidence, dignity, and self-esteem.

Equipment

Reality orientation props such as clocks ■ directional signs ■ pictures ■ cards ■ mementos ■ bulletin boards ■ newspapers ■ magazines ■ televisions ■ radios ■ night lights ■ calendars ■ mirrors ■ paintings.

The above equipment should be used frequently in the patient's environment, such as in hallways, rooms, and dining rooms, *to aid in orientation as the patient moves about.*

NURSING ALERT ***Label orientation tools using large lettering for patients with vision deficits.***

Implementation

- Assess the patient's current orientation status by observing for specific behaviors, such as wandering, getting lost, using rambling speech, or withdrawing from social situations. Ask questions about time, place, and person as well as recent and remote memories.
- If the patient is confused, use reality orientation props and orient him through verbal interaction. For example, say, "Mr. George, look at the calendar; today is Monday. Your wife will come to visit you on Wednesday." Or "This is your bed, Mrs. Peters. See your name on the end of the bed?" Orient the patient frequently, in every interaction, 24 hours per day.
- Teach family members and visitors how to reorient the patient.

NURSING ALERT ***Ensure consistency in all interventions by establishing and maintaining a regular routine for daily activities and by avoiding changes of room, unit, or furniture.***

- Address the patient by his correct title and full name *to promote self-esteem, dignity, and orientation.*
- Always identify yourself and your role, and state what you expect the patient to do. Explain one step at a time, employing good eye contact, touch, and a positive attitude.
- Provide a calm environment, but recognize that it's also important to plan for and provide some stimulation *to prevent monotony.*
- Socialize and talk with the patient and relate time, place, and person to current activities.
- Give praise and recognition, such as a smile, warm handshake, pat on the back, or sincere verbal praise for each positive response. *Positive reinforcement helps to improve self-esteem and increases the likelihood that the positive response will be repeated.*
- Encourage the patient to take an interest in his personal appearance by using a mirror to maintain awareness of his body image. Encourage self-care within the patient's known limitations.
- Correct rambling speech or actions. Offer reminders in a nonthreatening and noncritical way.

Special considerations

Patients who need reality orientation are found in all age-groups, but primarily are elderly patients. Two categories of people may benefit from reality orientation. One category includes patients who are confused or disoriented from any cause, regardless of their age or diagnosis. The patient's confusion can result from such conditions as arteriosclerosis, sensory deprivation, overmedication, metabolic imbalance, nutritional deficiency, or emotional stress. The other category includes patients who are oriented but face a stressful situation, which could cause confusion. Examples are changes in living arrangements, surgery, loss of a spouse, or even visual or hearing problems. Both groups are encountered in all areas of nursing, including extended care, medical-surgical, and psychiatric units as well as urgent care and clinic settings.

Documentation

Document all interventions as well as the patient's response in progress notes. An interdisciplinary treatment care plan should also be written with attainable goals and interventions. Update this, as needed, according to your facility's policy.

SELECTED REFERENCES

O'Connell, B., et al. "Clinical Usefulness and Feasibility of Using Reality Orientation with Patients Who Have Dementia in Acute Care Settings," *International Journal of Nursing Practice* 13(3):182-92, June 2007.

Patton, D. "Reality Orientation: Its Use and Effectiveness within Older Person Mental Health Care," *Journal of Clinical Nursing* 15(11):1440-49, November 2006.

16 ■ Maternal-neonatal care

INTRODUCTION

Because of its profound emotional implications for mother and child, maternal-neonatal care requires expertise that goes beyond clinical skills. Such care must combine clinical competence, sensitivity, and good judgment. It must consider the patient's sexuality and self-image and recognize changing social attitudes and values — especially those concerning conventional and alternative methods of conception and childbirth.

Changing maternal care

More than 4 million infants are born in the United States each year. Many are born with considerably less medical intervention than was customary in previous decades, and many were conceived with considerably more intervention. As a result, nurses today must be prepared to implement or assist with a wide range of procedures.

If you're working with a pregnant patient, you'll need to use your teaching skills. For instance, you may be called on to organize and direct natural childbirth classes or to teach the mother-to-be how to breathe and control pain during childbirth. You may teach fathers and other support persons to participate in childbirth by providing comfort and direction.

You may also be asked to give information about childbirth options. Although most births still occur in a hospital, many parents inquire about delivery in a birth center. Usually located in the maternity unit of a hospital or sponsored by a childbirth association, a birth center combines the advantages of a homelike setting with the emergency medical and nursing interventions available in a hospital. Today's nurse may staff or direct the birth center.

Historically, the midwife has been a fixture in remote or poor communities. Today's professional nurse-midwife, however, brings advanced technical skills and certification to diverse communities — urban center to country town alike. She may work in collaboration with — or be supervised by — a physician or a group. In some areas, she may even practice independently. In fact, several states permit insurers to make direct payment to the nurse-midwife for her services.

Changing neonatal care

Accompanying the changes in maternity care are changes in neonatal care — thanks to advanced knowledge and techniques for improving fetal monitoring and promoting neonatal survival. New clinical evaluation methods, combined with new electronic and biochemical monitoring techniques, allow improved neonatal care. To make use of these advances, you must be familiar with neonatal physiology, procedures, and equipment.

FETAL ASSESSMENT

FETAL HEART RATE

Fetal heart rate (FHR) is the best way to determine fetal well-being during gestation and labor. It may be assessed by auscultating with a fetoscope or a Doppler ultrasound stethoscope placed on the maternal abdomen. The fetoscope utilizes bone conduction to assist in hearing the opening and closing of the fetal ventricular heart valves. The Doppler device uses ultrasound technology to detect heart motion, such as moving heart walls or valves. Both methods have been approved by the American College of Obstetricians and Gynecologists and the Association of Women's Health, Obstetric, and Neonatal Nurses.

Normal FHR ranges from 110 to 160 beats/minute. Auscultation easily can be used to detect fetal tachycardia (heart rate greater than 160 beats/minute) and bradycardia (heart rate less than 110 beats/minute), and it allows the examiner to determine whether the rhythm is regular or irregular.

Auscultation requires the ability to distinguish among the fetal heart sounds generated. FHR must also be distinguished from similar sounds created by the maternal pulse in the uterine vessels. The uterine bruit, or souffle sounds that are simultaneous with the maternal pulse, could be confused with the FHR. Practitioners should check maternal and fetal heart rates because false conclusions about fetal status could be reached if the maternal sounds are considered to be fetal heart sounds.

Baseline rhythm can also be assessed with auscultation. The presence of an irregularity in the baseline rate can be detected best when listening with an auscultation device that allows practitioners to hear the actual heart sounds.

Because auscultation can detect gross (but often late) fetal distress signs (tachycardia and bradycardia), the technique remains useful in an uncomplicated, low-risk pregnancy. In a high-risk pregnancy, indirect external or direct internal electronic fetal monitoring gives more accurate information on fetal status.

Equipment

Fetoscope or Doppler stethoscope ▪ water-soluble lubricant (for ultrasound instrument) ▪ watch with second hand. (See *Instruments for hearing fetal heart tones.*)

Implementation

- Confirm the patient's identity using two patient identifiers according to your facility's policy.
- Explain the procedure to the patient, wash your hands, and provide privacy. Reassure the patient that you may repo-

EQUIPMENT

Instruments for hearing fetal heart tones

The fetoscope and the Doppler stethoscope are basic instruments for auscultating fetal heart tones and assessing fetal heart rate.

Fetoscope

A fetoscope can detect fetal heartbeats as early as the 20th gestational week. As an assessment tool during labor, the fetoscope is helpful for hearing fetal heart tones when contractions are mild and infrequent.

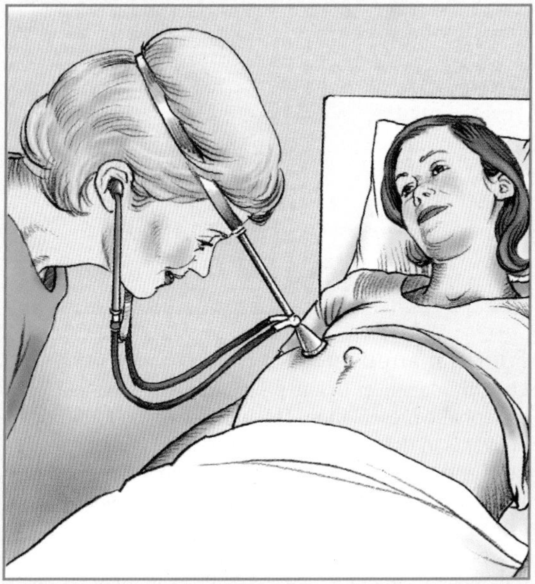

Doppler stethoscope

A Doppler stethoscope can detect fetal heartbeats as early as the 10th gestational week. Useful throughout labor, the Doppler stethoscope has greater sensitivity than the fetoscope.

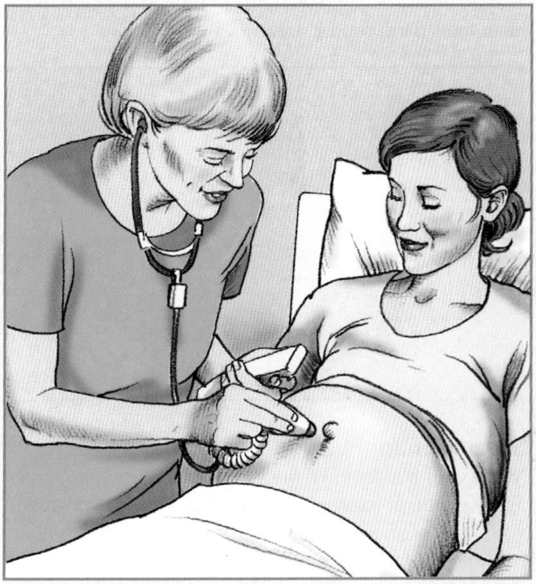

sition the listening instrument frequently *to hear the loudest fetal heart tones.*

■ Assist the patient to a supine position, placing a wedge under the right hip, and drape her in a way that minimizes exposure. If you're using a Doppler stethoscope, apply the water-soluble lubricant to the patient's abdomen. *This gel or paste creates an airtight seal between the skin and the instrument and promotes optimal ultrasound wave conduction and reception.*

Calculating FHR during gestation

■ To assess FHR in a fetus age 20 weeks or older, place the earpieces in your ears and position the bell of the fetoscope or Doppler stethoscope on the abdominal midline above the pubic hairline. After 20 weeks, when you can palpate fetal position, use Leopold's maneuvers *to locate the back of the fetal thorax.* Then position the listening instrument over the fetal back. (See *Performing Leopold's maneuvers,* page 850.)

■ *Because the presentation and position of the fetus may change,* most clinicians don't perform Leopold's maneuvers until 32 to 34 weeks' gestation.

■ Using a Doppler stethoscope, place the earpieces in your ears, and press the bell gently on the patient's abdomen. Start listening at the midline, midway between the umbilicus and the symphysis pubis. If you're using a fetoscope, place the earpieces in your ears with the fetoscope positioned centrally on your forehead. Gently press the bell about ½″ (1.3 cm) into the patient's abdomen. Remove your hands from the fetoscope *to avoid extraneous noise.*

■ Move the bell of either instrument slightly from side to side, as necessary, *to locate the loudest heart tones.* After locating these tones, palpate the maternal pulse.

Performing Leopold's maneuvers

You can determine fetal position, presentation, and attitude by performing Leopold's maneuvers. Ask the patient to empty her bladder, assist her to a supine position, and expose her abdomen. Then perform the four maneuvers in order.

First maneuver

Face the patient and warm your hands. Place them on her abdomen to determine fetal position in the uterine fundus. Curl your fingers around the fundus. With the fetus in vertex position, the buttocks feel irregularly shaped and firm. With the fetus in breech position, the head feels hard, round, and movable.

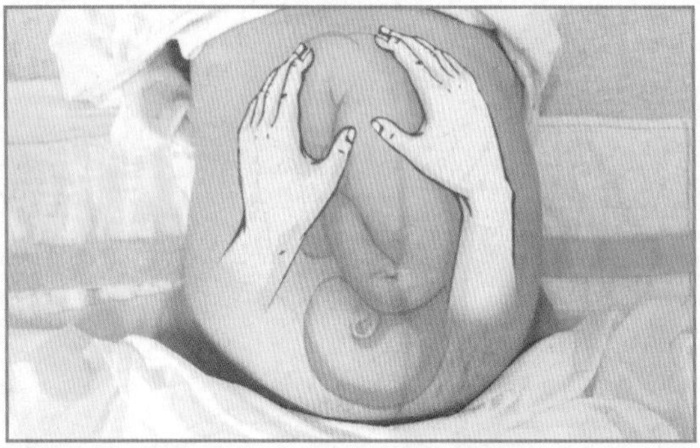

Second maneuver

Move your hands down the sides of the abdomen, and apply gentle pressure. If the fetus lies in vertex position, you'll feel a smooth, hard surface on one side — the fetal back. Opposite, you'll feel lumps and knobs — the knees, hands, feet, and elbows. If the fetus lies in breech position, you may not feel the back at all.

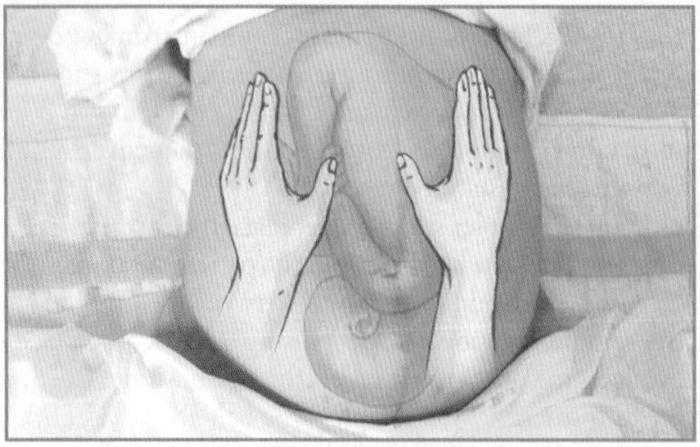

Third maneuver

Spread apart the thumb and fingers of one hand. Place them just above the patient's symphysis pubis. Bring your fingers together. If the fetus lies in vertex position and hasn't descended, you'll feel the head. If the fetus lies in vertex position and has descended, you'll feel a less distinct mass.

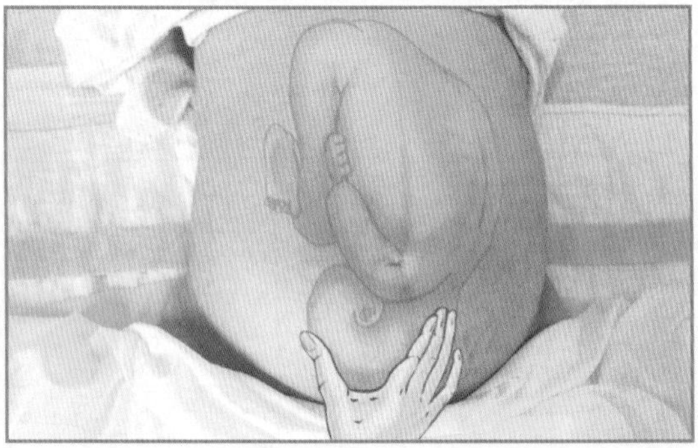

Fourth maneuver

Use this maneuver in late pregnancy when the fetus is in cephalic presentation. The purpose of the fourth maneuver is to determine flexion or extension of the fetal head and neck. Place your hands on both sides of the lower abdomen. Apply gentle pressure with your fingers as you slide your hands downward, toward the symphysis pubis. If the head and neck are flexed, your hands will meet obstruction—the cephalic prominence—on the side opposite the fetal back. If the head and neck are extended, the cephalic prominence will be palpated on the same side as the fetal back. Flexion of the fetal head and neck facilitates vaginal delivery.

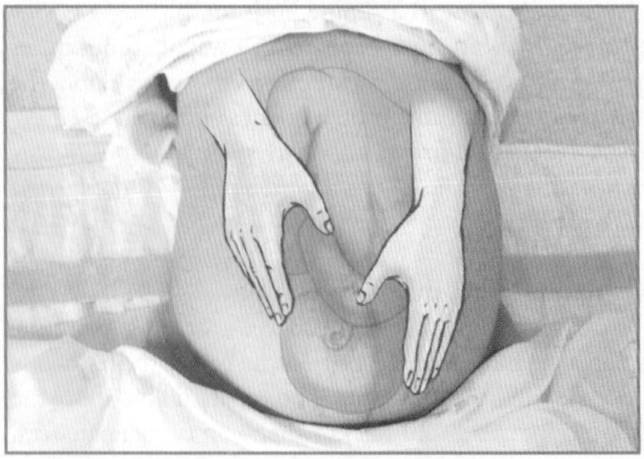

■ While monitoring the maternal pulse rate *(to avoid confusing maternal heart tones with fetal heart tones),* count the fetal heartbeats for at least 15 seconds. If the maternal radial pulse and FHR are the same, try to locate the fetal thorax by using Leopold's maneuvers; then reassess FHR. Usually, the fetal heart beats faster than the maternal heart does. Record FHR.

Counting FHR during labor

■ Allow the mother and her support person to listen to the fetal heart if they wish. *This helps to make the fetus a greater reality for them.* Record their participation.

■ Place the fetoscope or Doppler stethoscope on the abdomen — midway between the umbilicus and symphysis pubis *for cephalic presentation,* or at the umbilicus or above *for breech presentation.* Locate the loudest heartbeats, and simultaneously palpate the maternal pulse *to ensure that you're monitoring fetal rather than maternal pulse.*

■ Monitor maternal pulse rate, and count fetal heartbeats for 60 seconds during the relaxation period between contractions *to determine baseline FHR.* In a low-risk labor, assess FHR every 60 minutes during the latent phase, every 30 minutes during the active phase, and every 15 minutes during the second stage of labor. In a high-risk labor, assess FHR every 30 minutes during the latent phase, every 15 minutes during the active phase, and every 5 minutes during the second stage of labor.

■ Auscultate FHR during a contraction and for 30 seconds afterward *to identify the response to the contraction.*

■ Notify the practitioner immediately if you observe marked changes in FHR from baseline values (especially during or immediately after a contraction when signs of fetal distress typically occur). If fetal distress develops, begin indirect or direct electronic fetal monitoring.

■ Repeat the procedure, as ordered.

■ Also auscultate before administration of medications, before ambulation, and before artificial rupture of membranes.

■ Auscultate after rupture of membranes, after any changes in the characteristics of the contractions, after vaginal examinations, and after administration of medications.

Special considerations

■ If you're auscultating FHR with a Doppler stethoscope, be aware that obesity and hydramnios can interfere with sound-wave transmission, making accurate results more difficult to obtain. If the practitioner orders continuous FHR monitoring, apply the ultrasound transducer to the patient's abdomen. The monitor will provide a printed record of FHR.

■ The tocotransducer should be applied to monitor the contractile pattern at this time *to monitor fetal response to maternal contractions and assess fetal well-being.*

Documentation

Record FHR and maternal pulse rate on the flowchart. Record each auscultation, and note tolerance to activity or treatment.

SELECTED REFERENCES

ACOG Practice Bulletin. Clinical Management for Obstetrician-Gynecologists No. 70 "Intrapartum Fetal Heart Rate Monitoring," *Obstetrics and Gynecology* 105(5pt1):1161-69, December 2005.

DeVoe, L., et al. "United States Multicenter Clinical Usage Study of the STAW21 Electronic Fetal Monitoring System," *American Journal of Obstetrics and Gynecology* 195(3):729-34, September 2006.

Hofmeyr, G. "Evidence-Based Intrapartum Care," *Best Practice & Research. Clinical Obstetrics & Gynaecology* 19(1):103-15, February 2005.

Mattson, S., and Smith, J., eds. *Core Curriculum for Maternal-Newborn Nursing,* 3rd ed. Philadelphia: W.B. Saunders Co., 2004.

AMNIOCENTESIS

A needle aspiration of amniotic fluid for laboratory analysis, amniocentesis is usually performed between 14 and 20 weeks' gestation. This procedure can detect neural tube and chromosomal defects as well as certain metabolic and other disorders. The procedure can also identify the sex of the fetus and assist in assessing fetal health. When performed in the final trimester, amniocentesis helps to evaluate fetal lung maturity and detect Rh hemolytic disease.

Indications for amniocentesis include maternal age over 35 (associated with Down syndrome), a family history of neural tube or chromosomal defects, or inborn errors of metabolism. Another test, chorionic villi sampling, may also detect fetal disorders. (See *Understanding chorionic villi sampling,* page 852.) Either procedure may be performed in a labor and delivery suite, in the ultrasound department, or in a physician's office.

Contraindications for amniocentesis include an anterior uterine wall completely covered by the placenta and insufficient amniotic fluid. The risks of this procedure must be weighed against its expected benefits if the mother is infected with human immunodeficiency virus.

Equipment

Hospital gown ■ two sets of sterile gloves, sterile gowns, and masks ■ stethoscope ■ Doppler stethoscope and other appropriate ultrasound equipment ■ fetoscope or electronic fetal monitor ■ antiseptic solution with sterile container ■ local anesthetic ■ alcohol ■ 10-ml syringe ■ sterile 20G or 22G

Understanding chorionic villi sampling

Laboratory analysis of chorionic villi specimens can detect genetic, metabolic, and blood disorders—such as Down syndrome, Duchenne's muscular dystrophy, sickle cell anemia, alpha (and some beta) thalassemias, and phenylketonuria. Performed at 10 to 12 weeks' gestation, the procedure can yield results in just a few days.

To obtain the tissue specimens, the physician typically uses ultrasound or endoscopic imaging to guide a plastic catheter through the cervical canal into the uterus (as shown). He aspirates a small portion of chorionic tissue from the fetus, taking care not to contaminate the specimen with maternal tissue.

Before the test, make sure that the patient has given her written consent, provide emotional support, and answer any questions. Arrange for ordered blood studies. Instruct the patient to drink 1 qt (1 L) of water 30 minutes before the test *because a full bladder allows a better view of the uterus.* Also, Rh-negative women should receive RhoGAM beforehand to reduce the risk of isoimmunization.

Assess vital signs before, during, and after the procedure. Watch for vaginal bleeding.

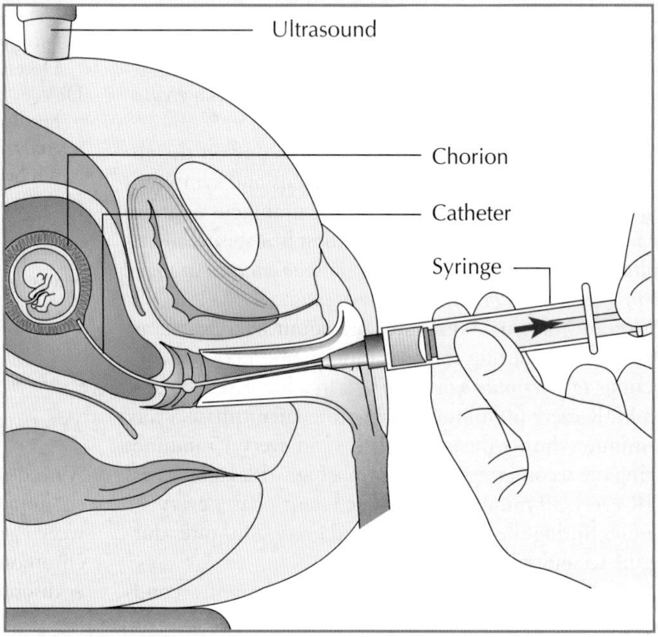

4″ spinal needle with stylet ▪ 22G or 25G needle ▪ sterile 20-ml syringe ▪ clean amber glass specimen container for Rh sensitization and lecithin/sphingomyelin (L/S) ratio tests ▪ three sterile glass specimen tubes (for genetic tests) ▪ laboratory request forms ▪ adhesive bandage ▪ towel.

Preassembled amniocentesis trays are available.

Preparation of equipment

If you don't have an amber specimen container, cover the outside of a clean test tube or glass container with adhesive tape or aluminum foil. *Protecting aspirated amniotic fluid from light prevents the breakdown of such pigments as bilirubin.* Properly label all specimen containers, tubes, and medications on and off the sterile field.

Implementation

- Confirm the patient's identity using two patient identifiers according to your facility's policy.
- Explain the procedure to the patient. Confirm that she understands the risk of complications. Emphasize that the physician may need to repeat the procedure and that amniotic fluid analysis can't detect all birth defects.
- Make sure you have the patient's signed informed consent form.
- *To reduce the risk of bladder puncture,* ensure that the patient voids before the procedure if the pregnancy exceeds 20 weeks (*before 20 weeks, a full bladder may help to hold the uterus steady*).
- Provide privacy and instruct the patient to put on a hospital gown. Assist her to a supine position and place a folded towel under her right hip. *This tips her slightly to the left and moves the uterus off the vena cava, preventing supine hypotension syndrome.*
- Obtain baseline maternal vital signs. Next, determine the baseline fetal heart rate (FHR) with the Doppler stethoscope or the fetoscope.

■ Instruct the patient to fold her hands on her chest or rest her hands behind her head. Tell her to remain still.
■ The physician will use ultrasonography to locate the fetus and placenta. After he identifies an amniotic fluid pocket, he can determine the appropriate needle-insertion depth. Next, he'll put on the sterile gown, sterile gloves, and mask and clean the skin with an antiseptic solution.
■ If the patient is receiving a local anesthetic, clean the diaphragm of the multidose vial of anesthetic solution with alcohol. Provide a 10-ml syringe and a 22G or 25G needle. Then invert the bottle *to allow the physician to withdraw the anesthetic.*
■ Scrub your hands and put on a sterile gown, sterile gloves, and mask *to assist the physician with amniocentesis, a sterile procedure.*
■ After the anesthetic takes effect, the physician, guided by ultrasonographic imaging, will advance the 20G needle with a stylet through the abdomen and uterine wall into the amniotic sac (as shown below). Then he'll remove the stylet. When a drop of amniotic fluid appears, he'll attach the 20-ml syringe to the needle and aspirate the fluid.

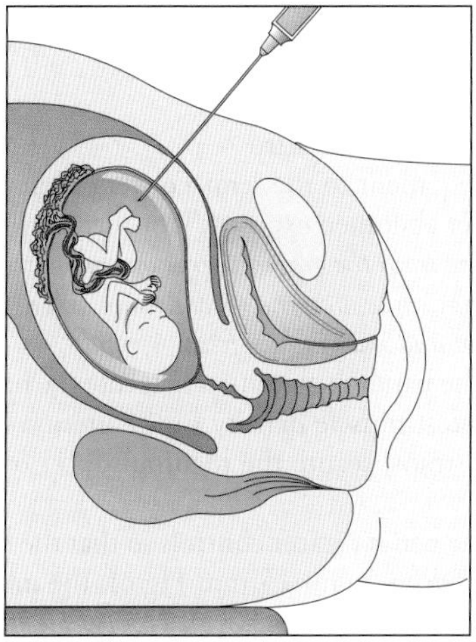

■ If the patient is having genetic studies, open the sterile specimen tubes. After the physician transfers amniotic fluid to the tubes, use sterile technique when closing the tubes *to avoid contamination, which can yield aberrant test results.*
■ If the patient is having Rh sensitization or L/S ratio tests, open the amber or covered specimen container so the physician can transfer the amniotic fluid. Close the container at once *to protect the fluid from light, which may cause pigments in the fluid, such as bilirubin, to break down and skew test results.*
■ When the physician withdraws the needle, place an adhesive bandage over the insertion site.
■ Complete the laboratory request forms, and send the specimens to the laboratory immediately. *Speedy transport is important because if the amniotic fluid contains blood or meconium, immediate centrifugation can preserve the specimen for analysis.*
■ Assess maternal vital signs and FHR every 15 minutes for 30 minutes *to detect changes from the baseline values.* FHR changes, such as tachycardia and bradycardia, signal distress. If these signs appear, notify the physician, and continue to monitor FHR.
■ Electronically monitor the patient for uterine irritability and the fetus for changes in heart rate pattern. Monitoring should continue for a few hours after the procedure *to allow early intervention if complications occur.* Normally, maternal vital signs should remain stable.
■ Instruct the patient to report signs and symptoms of complications: vaginal discharge (fluid or blood), decreased fetal movement, contractions, or fever and chills.
■ Help the patient dress in preparation for discharge.

Special considerations

■ Monitor the patient for signs and symptoms of supine hypotension, such as light-headedness, nausea, and diaphoresis.
■ If the patient will receive a dose of RhoGAM, explain that this passive immunizing agent may help prevent an Rh incompatibility between her and the fetus that would cause antibody formation in her blood. This condition is known as *erythroblastosis fetalis* (hydrops fetalis or hemolytic disease of the newborn).
■ Inform the patient, her family, and her support person, as appropriate, that test results should be available in 2 to 4 weeks. Provide emotional support, as needed.

Complications

Although amniocentesis is an invasive procedure, it rarely produces maternal or fetal complications. Maternal complications, which affect less than 1% of patients, include amniotic fluid embolism, hemorrhage, infection, premature labor, abruptio placentae, placenta or umbilical cord trauma, bladder or intestinal puncture, and Rh isoimmunization. Rare fetal complications include intrauterine fetal death, amnionitis, injury from needle puncture, amniotic fluid leakage, bleeding, spontaneous abortion, and premature birth.

Documentation

Record the physician's name and the date and time of the procedure. Document baseline maternal vital signs and FHR, and note any changes in baseline data. List the ordered laboratory tests. Note the amount and appearance of the specimen and when it was transported to the laboratory. Document discharge instructions to the patient and how she tolerated the procedure.

SELECTED REFERENCES

Eddelman, K.A., et al. "Pregnancy Loss Rates after Midtrimester Amniocentesis," *Obstetrics and Gynecology* 108(5):1067-72, November 2005.

Harris, A., et al. "Clinical Correlates of Pain with Amniocentesis," *American Journal of Obstetrics and Gynecology* 191(2):542-45, August 2004.

Kirkham, C., et al. "Evidence-Based Prenatal Care: Part 1. General Prenatal Care and Counseling Issues," *American Family Physician* 71(7):1307-16, April 2005.

EXTERNAL FETAL MONITORING

An indirect, noninvasive procedure, external fetal monitoring uses two devices strapped to the mother's abdomen to evaluate fetal well-being during labor. One device, an ultrasound transducer, transmits high-frequency sound waves through soft body tissues to the fetal heart. The waves rebound from the heart, and the transducer relays them to a monitor. The other, a pressure-sensitive tocotransducer, responds to the pressure exerted by uterine contractions and simultaneously records their duration and frequency. (See *Applying external fetal monitoring devices.*) The monitoring apparatus traces fetal heart rate (FHR) and uterine contraction data onto the same printout paper.

Indications for external fetal monitoring include high-risk pregnancy, oxytocin-induced labor, maternal medical illness, and antepartal nonstress, contraction stress tests, and psychological factors, such as tobacco, alcohol, drug use, and lack of prenatal care. Many labor and delivery units use external fetal monitoring for all patients. The procedure has no contraindications, but it may be difficult to perform on patients with hydramnios, on obese patients, or on hyperactive or premature fetuses.

Equipment

Electronic fetal monitor ■ ultrasound transducer ■ tocotransducer ■ conduction gel ■ transducer straps ■ damp cloth ■ printout paper.

Preparation of equipment

Because fetal monitor features and complexity vary, review the operator's manual before proceeding. If the monitor has two paper speeds, select the slower speed (typically 3 cm/minute) *to ensure an easy-to-read tracing.* At higher speeds (for example, 1 cm/minute), the printed tracings are difficult to decipher and interpret accurately.

Then plug the tocotransducer cable into the uterine activity jack and the ultrasound transducer cable into the phono-ultrasound jack. Attach the straps to the tocotransducer and the ultrasound transducer.

Label the printout paper with the patient's identification number or birth date and name, the date, maternal vital signs and position, the paper speed, and the number of the strip paper *to maintain accurate, consecutive monitoring records.*

If your facility has central monitoring capabilities, enter the patient data into the central computer *to ensure accurate labeling of monitor strips.*

Implementation

- Confirm the patient's identity using two patient identifiers according to your facility's policy.
- Explain the procedure to the patient, and provide emotional support. Inform her that the monitor may make noise if the pen set tracer moves above or below the printed paper. Reassure her that this doesn't indicate fetal distress. As appropriate, explain other aspects of the monitor *to help reduce maternal anxiety about fetal well-being.*
- Make sure the patient has signed a consent form, if required.
- Wash your hands and provide privacy.

Beginning the procedure

- Assist the patient to the semi-Fowler or left-lateral position with her abdomen exposed. Don't let her lie supine *because pressure from the gravid uterus on the maternal inferior vena cava may cause maternal hypotension and decreased uterine perfusion and may induce fetal hypoxia.*
- Palpate the patient's abdomen to locate the fundus — the area of greatest muscle density in the uterus. Then, using transducer straps, secure the tocotransducer over the fundus.
- Adjust the pen set tracer controls so that the baseline values read between 5 and 15 mm Hg on the monitor strip. *This prevents triggering the alarm that indicates the tracer has dropped below the paper's margins.* The proper setting varies among tocotransducers.
- Apply conduction gel to the ultrasound transducer crystals *to promote an airtight seal and optimal sound-wave transmission.*
- Use Leopold's maneuvers to palpate the fetal back, through which fetal heart sounds resound most audibly.
- Start the monitor. Then apply the ultrasound transducer directly over the site having the strongest heart tones.
- Activate the control that begins the printout. On the printout paper, note any coughing, position changes, drug administration, vaginal examinations, and blood pressure readings that may affect interpretation of the tracings.

EQUIPMENT

Applying external fetal monitoring devices

To ensure clear tracings that define fetal status and labor progress, be sure to precisely position external monitoring devices, such as an ultrasound transducer or a tocotransducer.

Fetal heart monitor

Palpate the uterus to locate the fetus's back. If possible, place the ultrasound transducer over this site where the fetal heartbeat sounds the loudest. Then tighten the belt. Use the fetal heart tracing on the monitor strip to confirm the transducer's position.

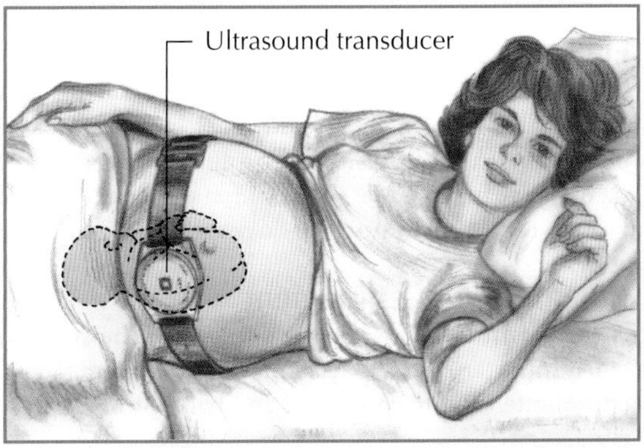

Labor monitor

A tocotransducer records uterine motion during contractions. Place the tocotransducer over the uterine fundus where it contracts, either midline or slightly to one side. Place your hand on the fundus, and palpate a contraction to verify proper placement. Secure the tocotransducer's belt; then adjust the pen set so that the baseline values read between 5 and 15 mm Hg on the monitor strip.

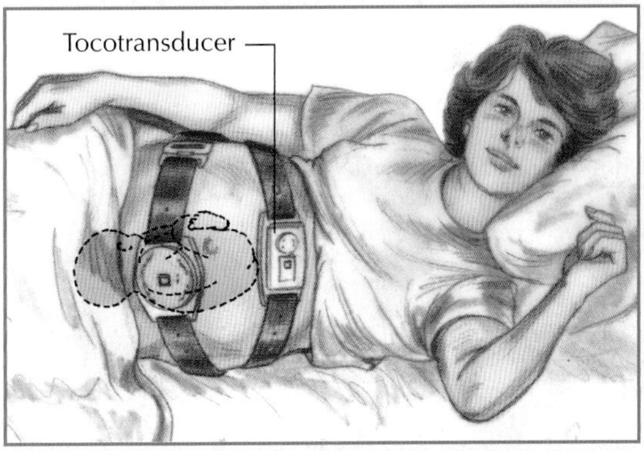

■ Explain to the patient and her support person how to time and anticipate contractions with the monitor. Inform them that the distance from one dark vertical line to the next on the printout grid represents 1 minute. The support person can use this information to prepare the patient for the onset of a contraction and to guide and slow her breathing as the contraction subsides.

Monitoring the patient

■ Observe the tracings to identify the frequency and duration of uterine contractions, but palpate the uterus to determine intensity of contractions.

■ Mentally note the baseline FHR — the rate between contractions — *to compare with suspicious-looking deviations.* FHR normally ranges from 110 to160 beats/minute.

■ Assess periodic accelerations or decelerations from the baseline FHR. Compare the FHR patterns with those of the uterine contractions. Note the time relationship between the onset of an FHR deceleration and the onset of a uterine contraction, the time relationship of the lowest level of an FHR deceleration to the peak of a uterine contraction, and the range of FHR deceleration. *These data help distinguish fetal distress from benign head compression.*

■ Move the tocotransducer and the ultrasound transducer *to accommodate changes in maternal or fetal position.* Readjust both transducers every hour, and assess the patient's skin for reddened areas caused by the strap pressure. Document skin condition.

■ Clean the ultrasound transducer periodically with a damp cloth *to remove dried conduction gel, which can interfere with ultrasound transmission.* Apply fresh gel as necessary. After using the ultrasound transducer, place the cover over it.

Special considerations

■ If the monitor fails to record uterine activity, palpate for contractions. Check for equipment problems as the manufacturer directs, and readjust the tocotransducer.

■ If the patient reports discomfort in the position that provides the clearest signal, try to obtain a satisfactory 5- or 10-minute tracing with the patient in this position before assisting her to a more comfortable position. As the patient progresses through labor and abdominal pressure increases, the pen set tracer may exceed the alarm boundaries. Reassure the patient that the pen set tracer doesn't accurately measure uterine contraction pressure.

Documentation

Make sure you number each monitor strip in sequence and label each printout sheet with the patient's identification number or birth date and name, the date, the time, and the paper speed. Record the time of any vaginal examinations, membrane rupture, drug administration, and maternal or fetal movements. Also record maternal vital signs and the intensity of uterine contractions. Document each time that you moved or readjusted the tocotransducer and ultrasound transducer, and summarize this information in your notes.

SELECTED REFERENCES

ACOG Practice Bulleting. Clinical Management for Obstetrician-Gynecologists. No. 70. "Intrapartum Fetal Heart Rate Monitoring," *Obstetrics and Gynecology* 105(5Pt1):1161-60, December 2005.

AWHONN Fetal Heart Monitoring—Principles and Practices, 3rd ed. Washington, D.C., 2003.

Mattson, S., and Smith, J., eds. *Core Curriculum for Maternal-Newborn Nursing,* 3rd ed. Philadelphia: W.B. Saunders Co., 2004.

Snelgrove-Clance, E., and Scott-Findlay, S. "Fetal Health Surveillance: The Use of Research Evidence in Practice," *AWHONN Lifelines* 9(5):400-403, October-November 2005.

INTERNAL FETAL MONITORING

Also called *direct fetal monitoring,* this sterile, invasive procedure uses a spiral electrode and an intrauterine catheter to evaluate fetal status during labor. By providing an electrocardiogram (ECG) of the fetal heart rate (FHR), internal electronic fetal monitoring assesses fetal response to uterine contractions more accurately than external fetal monitoring. It precisely measures intrauterine pressure, tracks labor progress, and allows evaluation of short- and long-term FHR variability.

Internal fetal monitoring is indicated whenever direct, beat-to-beat FHR monitoring is required. Specific indications include maternal diabetes or hypertension, fetal postmaturity, suspected intrauterine growth retardation, and meconium-stained fluid. However, internal monitoring is performed only if the amniotic sac has ruptured, the cervix is dilated at least 2 cm, and the presenting part of the fetus is at least at the −1 station.

Contraindications for internal fetal monitoring include maternal blood dyscrasias, suspected fetal immune deficiency, placenta previa, face presentation or uncertainty about the presenting part, maternal human immunodeficiency virus–positive status, and cervical or vaginal herpetic lesions.

A spiral electrode is the most commonly used device for internal fetal monitoring. Shaped like a corkscrew, the electrode is attached to the presenting fetal part (usually the scalp). It detects the fetal heartbeat and then transmits it to the monitor, which converts the signals to a fetal ECG waveform.

A pressure-sensitive intrauterine catheter, though not as widely used as the tocotransducer, is the most accurate method of determining the true intensity of contractions. It's especially helpful in dysfunctional labor and in preventing or rapidly determining the need for a cesarean delivery. However, the risk of infection or uterine perforation associated with this device is high.

Equipment

Electronic fetal monitor ▪ spiral electrode and a drive tube ▪ disposable leg plate pad or reusable leg plate with Velcro belt ▪ conduction gel ▪ antiseptic solution ▪ hypoallergenic tape ▪ two pairs of sterile gloves ▪ intrauterine catheter connection cable and pressure-sensitive catheter ▪ graph paper.

Preparation of equipment

If the monitor has two paper speeds, set the speed at 3 cm/minute *to ensure a readable tracing.* A tracing at 1 cm/minute is more condensed and harder to interpret accurately.

Connect the intrauterine cable to the uterine activity outlet on the monitor. Wash your hands and open the sterile equipment, maintaining sterile technique.

Implementation

- Confirm the patient's identity using two patient identifiers according to your facility's policy.
- Describe the procedure to the patient and her partner, if present, and explain how the equipment works. Tell the patient that a practitioner will perform a vaginal examination *to identify the position of the fetus.*
- Make sure the patient is fully informed about the procedure, and obtain a signed consent form.
- Label the printout paper with the patient's identification number or name and birth date, the date, the paper speed, and the number on the monitor strip.

Monitoring contractions

- Assist the patient into the lithotomy position for a vaginal examination. The practitioner puts on sterile gloves.
- Attach the connection cable to the appropriate outlet on the monitor marked UA (uterine activity). Connect the cable to the intrauterine catheter. Next, zero the catheter with

EQUIPMENT

Applying an internal electronic fetal monitor

During internal electronic fetal monitoring, a spiral electrode monitors the fetal heart rate and an intrauterine pressure catheter monitors uterine contractions.

Inserting the spiral electrode

The spiral electrode is inserted after a vaginal examination that determines the position of the fetus. As shown below, the electrode is attached to the presenting fetal part, usually the scalp or buttocks.

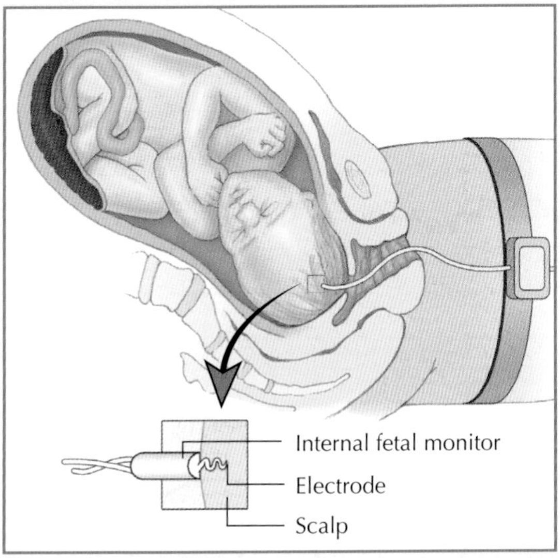

Inserting the intrauterine pressure catheter

The intrauterine pressure catheter is inserted up to a premarked level on the tubing and then connected to a monitor that interprets uterine contraction pressures (as shown below).

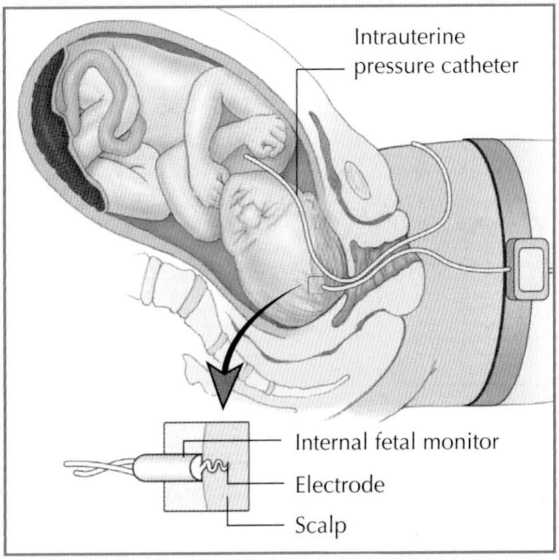

a gauge provided on the distal end of the catheter. *This will help determine the resting tone of the uterus, which is usually 5 to 15 mm Hg.*

- Cover the patient's perineum with a sterile drape if your facility's policy so dictates. Then clean the perineum with antiseptic solution, according to your facility's policy. Using sterile technique, the practitioner inserts the catheter into the uterine cavity while performing a vaginal examination. The catheter is advanced to the black line on the catheter and secured with hypoallergenic tape along the inner thigh.
- Observe the monitoring strip to verify proper placement of the catheter guide and to ensure a clear tracing. Periodically evaluate the monitoring strip to determine the exact amount of pressure exerted with each contraction. Note all such data on the monitoring strip and on the patient's medical record.
- The intrauterine catheter is usually removed during the second stage of labor or at the practitioner's discretion. Dispose of the catheter, and clean and store the cable according to your facility's policy. (See *Applying an internal electronic fetal monitor.*)

Monitoring FHR

- Apply conduction gel to the leg plate. Then secure the leg plate to the patient's inner thigh with Velcro straps or 2″ tape. Connect the leg plate cable to the ECG outlet on the monitor.
- Inform the patient that she'll undergo a vaginal examination *to identify the fetal presenting part* (which is usually the scalp or buttocks), *to determine the level of fetal descent,* and *to apply the electrode.* Explain that this examination is done to ensure that the electrode isn't attached to the suture lines, fontanels, face, or genitalia of the fetus. The spiral electrode will be placed in a drive tube and advanced through the vagina to the fetal presenting part. *To secure the electrode,*

Reading a fetal monitor strip

Presented in two parallel recordings, the fetal monitor strip records the fetal heart rate (FHR) in beats per minute in the top recording and uterine activity (UA) in millimeters of mercury (mm Hg) in the bottom recording. You can obtain information on fetal status and labor progress by reading the strips horizontally and vertically.

Reading horizontally on the FHR or the UA strip, each small block represents 10 seconds. Six consecutive small blocks, separated by a dark vertical line, represent 1 minute. Reading vertically on the FHR strip, each block represents an amplitude of 10 beats/minute. Reading vertically on the UA strip, each block represents 5 mm Hg of pressure.

Assess the baseline FHR (the "resting" heart rate) between uterine contractions when fetal movement diminishes. This baseline FHR (normal range: 120 to 160 beats/minute) pattern serves as a reference for subsequent FHR tracings produced during contractions.

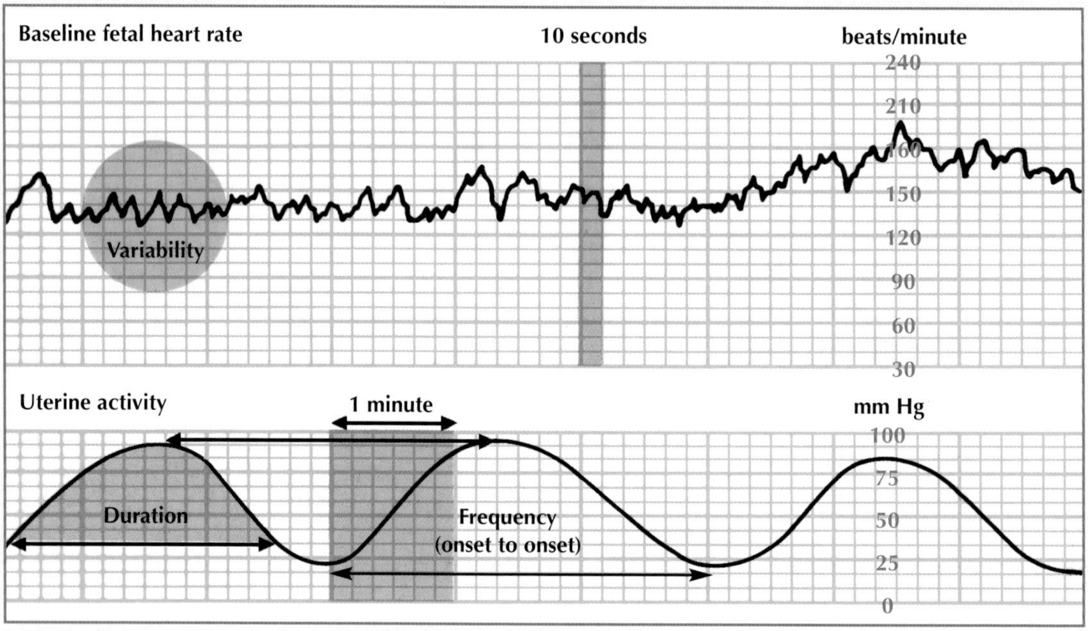

mild pressure will be applied and the drive tube will be turned clockwise 360 degrees.

- After the electrode is in place and the drive tube has been removed, connect the color-coded electrode wires to the corresponding color-coded leg plate posts.
- Turn on the recorder, and note the time on the printout paper.
- Help the patient to a comfortable position, and evaluate the strip *to verify proper placement and a clear FHR tracing.*

Monitoring the patient

- Begin by noting the frequency, duration, and intensity of uterine contractions. Normal intrauterine pressure ranges from 8 to 12 mm Hg. (See *Reading a fetal monitor strip.*)
- Next, check the baseline FHR. Assess periodic accelerations or decelerations from the baseline FHR.
- Compare the FHR pattern with the uterine contraction pattern. Note the interval between the onset of an FHR deceleration and the onset of a uterine contraction; the interval between the lowest level of an FHR deceleration and the peak of a uterine contraction; and the range of FHR deceleration.
- Check for FHR variability, which is a measure of fetal oxygen reserve and neurologic integrity and stability. (See *Identifying baseline FHR irregularities.*)
- When removing the spinal electrode, perform a vaginal examination and turn the electrode counterclockwise or until it releases from the fetal presenting part. Don't pull on

Identifying baseline FHR irregularities

IRREGULARITY	POSSIBLE CAUSES	CLINICAL SIGNIFICANCE	NURSING INTERVENTIONS
BASELINE TACHYCARDIA beats/minute 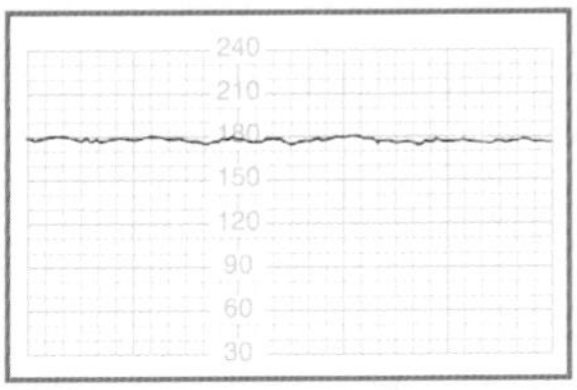 	■ Early fetal hypoxia ■ Maternal fever ■ Parasympathetic agents, such as atropine and scopolamine ■ Beta-adrenergics, such as terbutaline ■ Amnionitis (inflammation of inner layer of fetal membrane, or amnion) ■ Maternal hyperthyroidism ■ Fetal anemia ■ Fetal heart failure ■ Fetal arrhythmias	Persistent tachycardia without periodic changes doesn't usually adversely affect fetal well-being, especially when associated with maternal fever. However, tachycardia is an ominous sign when associated with late decelerations, severe variable decelerations, or lack of variability.	■ Intervene to alleviate the cause of fetal distress, and provide supplemental oxygen as ordered. Administer I.V. fluids as prescribed. ■ Discontinue oxytocin infusion *to reduce uterine activity.* ■ Turn the patient onto her left side and elevate her legs. ■ Continue to observe the fetal heart rate (FHR). ■ Document interventions and outcomes. ■ Notify the practitioner; further medical intervention may be necessary.
BASELINE BRADYCARDIA beats/minute 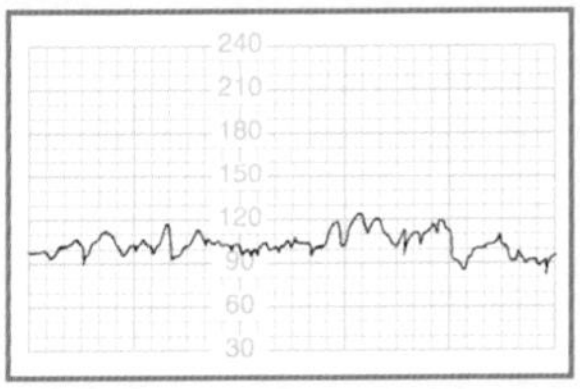 	■ Late fetal hypoxia ■ Beta-adrenergic blocking agents, such as propranolol, and anesthetics ■ Maternal hypotension ■ Prolonged umbilical cord compression ■ Fetal congenital heart block	Bradycardia with good variability and no periodic changes doesn't signal fetal distress if FHR remains higher than 80 beats/minute. However, bradycardia caused by hypoxia and acidosis is an ominous sign when associated with loss of variability and late decelerations.	■ Intervene to correct the cause of fetal distress. Administer supplemental oxygen, as ordered. Start an I.V. line and administer fluids, as prescribed. ■ Discontinue oxytocin infusion *to reduce uterine activity.* ■ Turn the patient onto her left side, and elevate her legs. ■ Continue observing the FHR. ■ Document interventions and outcomes. ■ Notify the practitioner; further medical intervention may be necessary.

(continued)

Identifying baseline FHR irregularities *(continued)*

IRREGULARITY	POSSIBLE CAUSES	CLINICAL SIGNIFICANCE	NURSING INTERVENTIONS
EARLY DECELERATIONS beats/minute 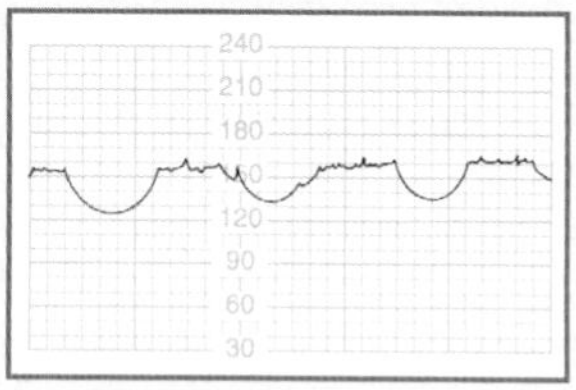 mm Hg 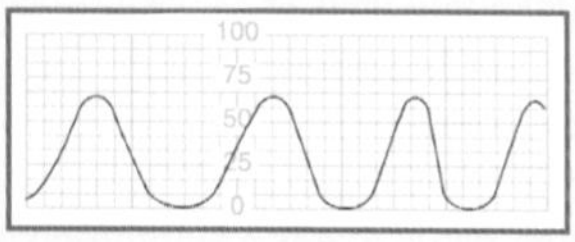	▪ Fetal head compression	Early decelerations are benign, indicating fetal head compression at dilation of 4 to 7 cm.	▪ Reassure the patient that the fetus isn't at risk. ▪ Observe the FHR. ▪ Document the frequency of decelerations.
LATE DECELERATIONS beats/minute 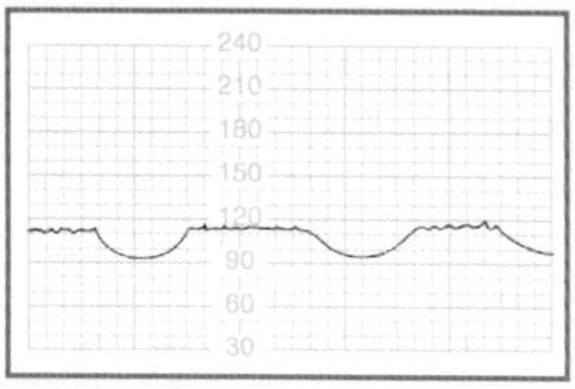 mm Hg 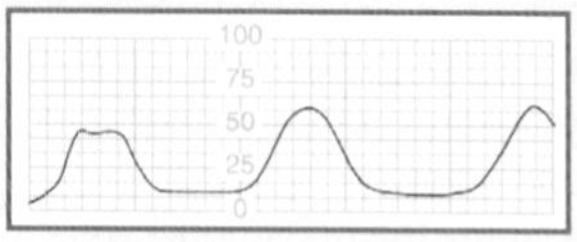	▪ Uteroplacental circulatory insufficiency (placental hypoperfusion) caused by decreased intervillous blood flow during contractions or a structural placental defect such as abruptio placentae ▪ Uterine hyperactivity caused by excessive oxytocin infusion ▪ Maternal hypotension ▪ Maternal supine hypotension	Late decelerations indicate uteroplacental circulatory insufficiency and may lead to fetal hypoxia and acidosis if the underlying cause isn't corrected.	▪ Turn the patient onto her left side *to increase placental perfusion and decrease contraction frequency.* ▪ Increase the I.V. fluid rate *to boost intravascular volume and placental perfusion, as prescribed.* ▪ Administer oxygen by mask *to increase fetal oxygenation, as ordered.* ▪ Assess for signs of the underlying cause, such as hypotension or uterine tachysystole. ▪ Take other appropriate measures such as discontinuing oxytocin, as prescribed. ▪ Document interventions and outcomes. ▪ Notify the practitioner; further medical intervention may be necessary. Prepare for possible prompt delivery of the neonate if late decelerations continue.

Identifying baseline FHR irregularities *(continued)*

IRREGULARITY	POSSIBLE CAUSES	CLINICAL SIGNIFICANCE	NURSING INTERVENTIONS
VARIABLE DECELERATIONS beats/minute 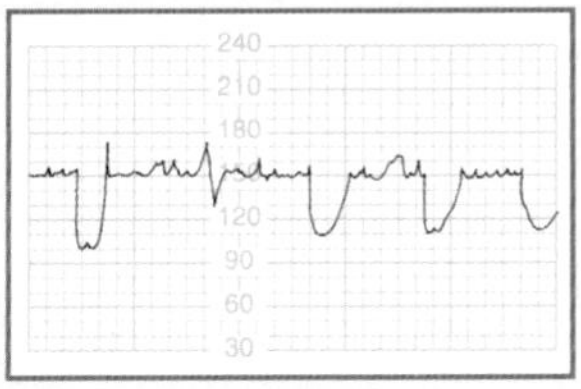 mm Hg 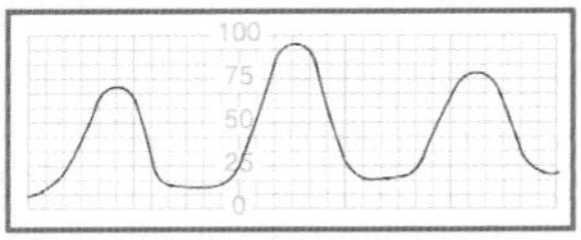	■ Umbilical cord compression causing decreased fetal oxygen perfusion	Variable decelerations are the most common deceleration pattern in labor because of contractions and fetal movement.	■ Help the patient change position. No other intervention is necessary unless you detect fetal distress. ■ Assure the patient that the fetus tolerates cord compression well. Explain that cord compression affects the fetus the same way that breath holding affects her. ■ Assess the deceleration pattern for reassuring signs: a baseline FHR that isn't increasing, short-term variability that isn't decreasing, abruptly beginning and ending decelerations, and decelerations lasting less than 50 seconds. If assessment doesn't reveal reassuring signs, notify the practitioner. ■ Start I.V. fluids and administer oxygen by mask at 10 to 12 L/minute, as prescribed. ■ Document interventions and outcomes. ■ Discontinue oxytocin infusion to decrease uterine activity.

the electrode. If it won't disconnect easily from the presenting part, it may be removed after delivery under direct visualization. The electrode should be removed just before a cesarean delivery. It should be brought through the uterine incision. If unable to detach, cut the wire at the perineum and notify the practitioner.

Special considerations

■ Interpret FHR and uterine contractions at regular intervals. Guidelines of the Association of Women's Health, Obstetric, and Neonatal Nurses specify that high-risk patients need continuous FHR monitoring, whereas low-risk patients should have FHR auscultated every 30 minutes after a contraction during the first stage and every 15 minutes after a contraction during the second stage.

■ First determine the baseline FHR within10 beats/minute; then assess the degree of baseline variability. Note the presence or absence of short-term or long-term variability. Identify periodic FHR changes such as decelerations (early, late, variable, or mixed) and nonperiodic changes such as a sinusoidal pattern.

■ Keep in mind that acute fetal distress can result from any change in the baseline FHR that causes fetal compromise. If necessary, take steps to counteract FHR changes.

■ If vaginal delivery isn't imminent (within 30 minutes) and fetal distress patterns don't improve, cesarean delivery will be necessary.

Complications

Maternal complications of internal fetal monitoring may include uterine perforation and intrauterine infection. Fetal complications may include abscess, hematoma, and infection.

Documentation

Document all activity related to monitoring. (A fetal monitoring strip becomes part of the patient's permanent record, so it's considered a legal document.) Be sure to record the type of monitoring your patient received as well as all interventions. Identify the monitoring strip with the patient's name, her practitioner's name, your name, and the date and time. Also document the paper speed and electrode placement.

Record the patient's vital signs at regular intervals. Note her pushing efforts, and record any change in her position. Document any I.V. line insertion and any changes in the I.V. solution or infusion rate. Note the use of oxytocin, regional anesthetics, or other medications.

After a vaginal examination, document cervical dilation and effacement as well as fetal station, presentation, and position. Also document membrane rupture, including the time it occurred and whether it was spontaneous or artificial. Note the amount, color, and odor of the fluid. If an internal electronic fetal monitor was used, document electrode placement.

SELECTED REFERENCES

ACOG Practice Bulleting. Clinical Management for Obstetrician-Gynecologists. No. 70. "Intrapartum Fetal Heart Rate Monitoring," *Obstetrics and Gynecology* 105(5 Pt 1):1161-69, December 2005.

AWHONN Fetal Heart Monitoring-Principles and Practices, 3rd ed. Washington, D.C., 2003.

Mattson, S., and Smith, J., eds. *Core Curriculum for Maternal-Newborn Nursing,* 3rd ed. Philadelphia: W.B. Saunders Co., 2004.

LABOR AND DELIVERY

UTERINE CONTRACTION PALPATION

Periodic, involuntary uterine contractions characterize normal labor and cause progressive cervical effacement and dilation, impelling the fetus to descend. Uterine palpation can tell you the frequency, duration, and intensity of contractions and the relaxation time between them. The character of contractions varies with the stage of labor and the body's response to labor-inducing drugs, if administered. As labor advances, contractions become more intense, occur more often, and last longer. (See *Quick guide to stages of labor.*)

Equipment

Watch with a second hand ■ sheet (for draping).

Implementation

■ Review the patient's admission history *to determine the onset, frequency, duration, and intensity of contractions.* Also, note where contractions feel strongest or exert the most pressure.

■ Wash your hands and provide privacy.

■ Describe the palpation procedure to the patient. *Because she may be ticklish or sensitive to touch,* forewarn her that you'll palpate her abdominal area over the uterus.

■ Assist the patient to a comfortable side-lying position *to relieve pressure on the inferior vena cava and promote uteroplacental circulation. This position also relieves direct pressure on the sacral area from the fetal head and eases backache.*

■ Drape the patient with a sheet.

■ Plant the palmar surface of your fingers on the uterine fundus, and palpate lightly *to assess contractions.* Note the uterine tightening and abdominal lifting that occur with contractions. Each contraction has three phases: increment (rising), acme (peak), and decrement (letting down or ebbing).

■ Palpate several contractions. Simultaneously use the second hand on your watch to assess and measure such contraction qualities as frequency, duration, and intensity.

■ *To assess frequency,* time the interval between the beginning of one contraction and the beginning of the next. In normal labor, contractions begin slowly and gradually occur more frequently with briefer relaxation intervals.

■ *To assess duration,* time the period from when the uterus begins tightening until it begins relaxing. As labor progresses, contractions usually last longer.

■ *To assess intensity,* press your fingertips into the uterine fundus when the uterus tightens. During mild contractions, the fundus indents easily and feels like a chin; during moderate contractions, the fundus indents less easily and feels like a nose; during strong contractions, the fundus resists indenting and feels like a forehead. At the conclusion of the contraction, check the fundus *to confirm that the uterus relaxes and becomes soft between contractions.*

■ Determine how the patient copes with discomfort by assessing her breathing and relaxation techniques, if any. *This*

Quick guide to stages of labor

Normal labor advances through the four stages summarized below. Offer your patient encouragement and progress reports throughout the stages.

First stage

Regular contractions, which repeat at 5- to 10-minute intervals and last between 10 and 30 seconds, signal the onset of labor's first stage. This stage has three phases: latent, active, and transitional. In primiparous patients, the first stage of labor ranges from 3.3 to 19.7 hours; in multiparous patients, it ranges from 0.1 to 14.3 hours.

In the *latent phase* (characterized by irregular, brief, and mild contractions), the cervix dilates to 3 or 4 cm. Other signs and symptoms include abdominal cramping and backache. The patient may expel the mucus plug during this phase. This phase averages 9 hours in primiparous patients and 6 hours in multiparous patients.

During the *active phase,* cervical dilation increases to about 7 cm. Contractions occur every 2 to 5 minutes, last 40 to 60 seconds, and become moderately intense. In primiparous patients, this phase averages 3 hours; in multiparous patients, 2 hours.

In the *transitional phase,* the cervix dilates completely (8 to 10 cm). Uterine contractions grow intense, last between 60 and 90 seconds, and repeat at least every 2 minutes. The patient may thrash about, lose control of breathing techniques, and experience nausea and vomiting. This phase typically lasts about 1 hour in primiparous patients and about 30 minutes in multiparous patients.

Second stage

In the second stage of labor, contractions occur every 1½ to 2 minutes and last up to 90 seconds. This stage commonly ends within 1 hour for all patients.

Signs and symptoms signaling onset of the second stage include increased bloody show, rupture of membranes (if they're still intact), severe rectal pressure and flaring, and reflexive bearing down with each contraction. The fetal head approaches the perineal floor and emerges at the vaginal opening. The second labor stage concludes with birth.

Third stage

Strong but less painful contractions expel the placenta, which normally emerges within 20 minutes after the neonate emerges. Signs indicating normal separation of the placenta from the uterine wall include lengthening of the umbilical cord, a sudden gush of dark blood from the vagina, and a palpable change in uterine shape from disklike to globular.

Fourth stage

The fourth stage begins with placental expulsion and extends through the next 4 hours, while the patient's body rests and begins adjusting to the postpartum state.

may help guide your intervention choices. Continue to provide ongoing emotional support in any event.

- Observe the patient's response to contractions to evaluate whether she needs an analgesic, anesthetic, or other appropriate measure, such as repositioning and back massage.
- Assess contractions at least hourly during the latent phase of first-stage labor and every 30 minutes throughout the active phase. During second-stage labor, assess contractions every 15 minutes.

Special considerations

- *Because the patient may become irritable or anxious during the transitional phase of first-stage labor—when the cervix dilates fully—and because abdominal palpation may aggravate her distress,* assess contractions only as necessary. If appropriate, teach her support person to palpate and record contractions.
- If any contraction lasts longer than 90 seconds and isn't followed by uterine muscle relaxation, notify the practitioner immediately *so that he can evaluate maternal and fetal well-being.* Also report a brief relaxation period between contractions *because inadequate relaxation intervals increase the risk of fetal hypoxia and exhaust the mother.*
- Be aware that false labor (or Braxton Hicks) contractions occur at irregular intervals and vary in intensity. They're felt over the abdomen and are typically relieved by walking. Membranes remain intact, and there's no show of blood or progressive cervical dilation or effacement.

Documentation

Record the frequency, duration, and intensity of contractions. Keep track of the relaxation time between contractions, and describe the patient's response to contractions.

SELECTED REFERENCES

Mattson, S., and Smith, J., eds. *Core Curriculum for Maternal-Newborn Nursing,* 3rd ed. Philadelphia: W.B. Saunders Co., 2004.

VAGINAL EXAMINATION

During first-stage labor, a practitioner or a nurse with special skills performs a vaginal examination to assess cervical dilation, effacement, membrane status, and fetal presentation, position, and engagement.

Important considerations during the examination include respecting the patient's privacy, providing simple explanations for her and her support person, maintaining eye contact when possible, and using sterile technique. With experience, the typical examiner develops a well-honed routine for collecting necessary information. This enables the examination to proceed precisely and efficiently. (See *Step-by-step vaginal examination.*)

Contraindications to a vaginal examination include excessive vaginal bleeding, which may signal placenta previa.

Equipment

Sterile gloves and clean disposable gloves ■ sterile water-soluble lubricant or sterile water ■ mild soap and water or cleaning solution ■ linen-saver pads ■ antiseptic solution ■ sterile gauze.

Implementation

- Confirm the patient's identity using two patient identifiers according to your facility's policy.
- Explain the procedure to the patient, and give her an opportunity to empty her bladder. *A distended bladder may interfere with accurate examination findings.*
- Wash your hands and provide privacy for the patient.
- Use Leopold's maneuvers to identify the fetal presenting part and position. Then help the patient into a lithotomy position for the vaginal examination.
- Place a linen-saver pad under the patient's buttocks, and put on sterile gloves.
- Inform the patient when you're about to touch her *to avoid startling her.*
- Clean the perineum with mild soap and water or cleaning solution using clean disposable gloves.
- Put on sterile gloves.
- Lubricate the index and middle fingers of your examining hand with sterile water or sterile water-soluble lubricant *to facilitate insertion.* If the membranes are ruptured, use an antiseptic solution.
- Spread the labia gently apart with your nondominant hand *to avoid contaminating your examining hand.*
- Ask the patient to relax by taking several deep breaths and slowly releasing the air. Then insert your lubricated fingers (palmar surface down) into the vagina. Keep your uninserted fingers flexed *to avoid the rectum.*
- Palpate the cervix, keeping in mind that it may assume a posterior position in early labor and be difficult to locate. When you find the cervix, note its consistency. The cervix gradually softens throughout pregnancy, reaching a buttery consistency before labor begins. (See *Cervical effacement and dilation,* page 866.)
- After identifying the presenting fetal part and position, evaluating dilation and effacement, assessing fetal engagement and station, and verifying membrane status, gently withdraw your fingers. Let the patient clean her perineum herself with sterile gauze if she can walk to the bathroom. If she's confined to bed, you can clean her perineum and change the linen-saver pad.
- *To encourage the patient and help reduce her anxiety,* describe how labor is progressing, and define the stage and phase, if appropriate.

Special considerations

- In early labor, perform the vaginal examination between contractions, focusing primarily on the extent of cervical dilation and effacement. At the end of first-stage labor, perform the examination during a contraction, when the uterine muscle pushes the fetus downward. This examination will focus on assessing fetal descent.
- If the amniotic membrane ruptures during the examination, record the fetal heart rate (FHR). Then note the time, and describe the color, odor, and approximate amount of fluid. If FHR becomes unstable, notify the practitioner, determine fetal station, and check for umbilical cord prolapse. After the membranes rupture, perform the vaginal examination only when labor changes significantly *to minimize the risk of introducing intrauterine infection.*

Complications

Placental tears and hemorrhage may occur if the procedure is performed during excessive vaginal bleeding.

Documentation

After each examination, record the percentage of effacement, dilation, the station of the presenting fetal part, amniotic membrane status, and the patient's tolerance of the procedure.

Step-by-step vaginal examination

Begin the vaginal examination — usually in early labor — by inserting your gloved index and middle fingers palm side down into the vagina (as shown below). Use your nondominant hand to gently but firmly press on the uterus to steady the fetal presenting part against the cervix for examination.

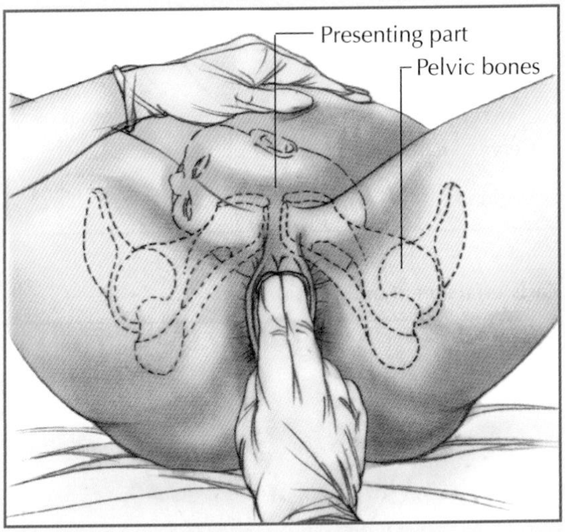

Confirm the presenting part and position

Rotate your fingers to palpate and confirm the fetal presenting part (a fetal head feels firm, the buttocks soft) and position (left, right, anterior, posterior, or transverse) identified by using Leopold's maneuvers (as shown below).

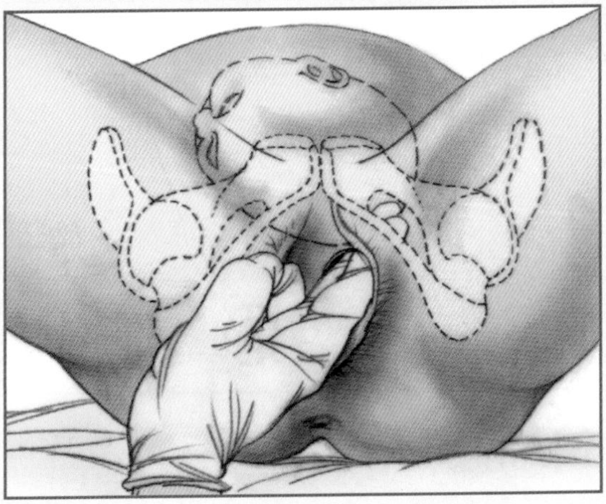

Assess cervical effacement and dilation

Estimate cervical dilation by palpating the internal os. Each fingerbreadth of dilation averages 1.5 to 2 cm, depending on the width of the examiner's finger.

Next, determine the percentage of effacement by palpating the ridge of tissue around the cervix. Assign a low percentage of effacement to defined and thick cervical tissue. Indistinct, wafer-thin cervical tissue scores 100%.

Assess fetal engagement and station

Estimate the extent of fetal engagement (descent of the fetal presenting part into the pelvis). Then palpate the presenting part, and grade the fetal station (where the presenting part lies in relation to the ischial spines of the maternal pelvis) (as shown below). A zero grade indicates that the presenting part lies level with the ischial spines.

Station grades range from –3 (3 cm above the maternal ischial spines) to +4 (4 cm below the maternal ischial spines, causing the perineum to bulge).

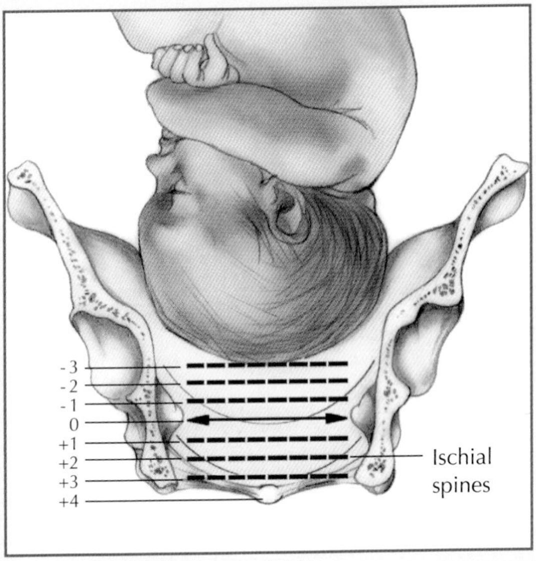

Evaluate membrane status

If appropriate, also check amniotic membrane status. If you feel a bulging, slick surface over the presenting fetal part, you know the membranes remain intact.

Cervical effacement and dilation

As labor advances, so do cervical effacement and dilation, thereby facilitating birth. During effacement, the cervix shortens and its walls become thin, progressing from 0% effacement (palpable and thick) (as shown top right) to 100% effacement (fully indistinct—or effaced—and paper thin) (as shown bottom right). Full effacement obliterates the constrictive uterine neck to create a smooth, unobstructed passage for the fetus.

At the same time, dilation occurs. This progressive widening of the cervical canal—from the upper internal cervical os to the lower external cervical os—advances from 0 to 10 cm. As the cervical canal opens, resistance decreases, which further eases fetal descent.

No effacement or dilation

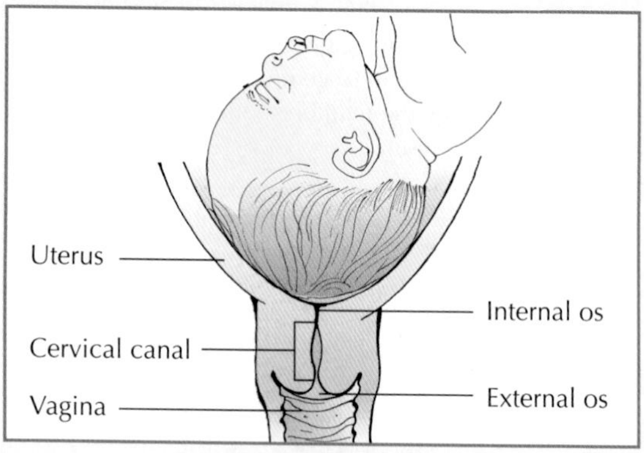

Early effacement and dilation

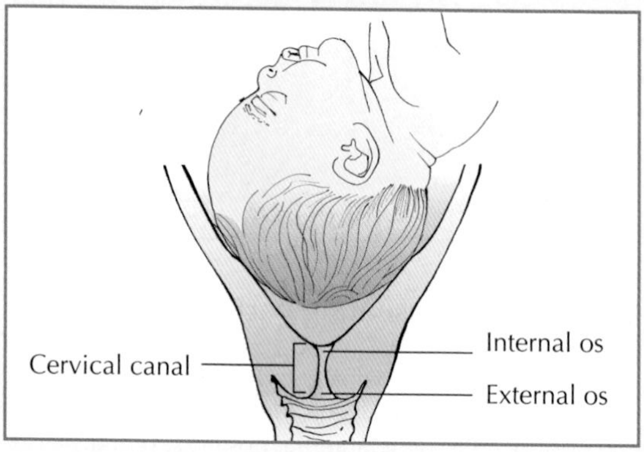

Full effacement and dilation

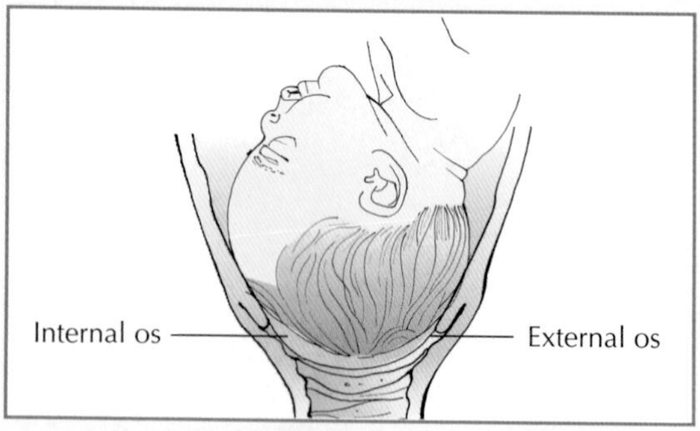

SELECTED REFERENCES

Mattson, S., and Smith, J., eds. *Core Curriculum for Maternal-Newborn Nursing,* 3rd ed. Philadelphia: W.B. Saunders Co., 2004.

Pillitteri, A. *Maternal & Child Health Nursing: Care of the Childbearing and Childrearing Family,* 5th ed. Philadelphia: Lippincott Williams & Wilkins, 2007.

TOCOLYTIC THERAPY

Tocolytic therapy involves the use of medications to suppress preterm uterine activity, thereby preventing preterm contractions and labor. Several drugs may be used, including magnesium sulfate, terbutaline, nifedipine, or indomethacin (See *Tocolytic drugs.*) Tocolytic therapy may prolong pregnancy for 2 to 7 days, thus allowing the patient to receive steroids to improve fetal lung maturity.

Tocolytic therapy is contraindicated if the gestation is less than 20 weeks, cervical dilation is greater than 4 cm, or cervical effacement is greater than 50%.

Equipment

I.V. line ■ medication, as ordered by practitioner ■ tubes for laboratory studies, as ordered.

Tocolytic drugs

This chart highlights the major drugs used to halt uterine contractions.

DRUG	INDICATIONS	EFFECTS ON THE MOTHER	EFFECTS ON THE FETUS	ANTIDOTE
Terbutaline	Beta2-receptor stimulator that causes smooth-muscle relaxation	Tachycardia, diarrhea, nervousness and tremors, nausea and vomiting, headache, hyperglycemia or hypoglycemia, hypokalemia, and pulmonary edema	Tachycardia, hypoxia, hypoglycemia, and hypocalcemia	Propranolol (Inderal)
Magnesium sulfate	Central nervous system (CNS) depressant that prevents reflux of calcium into the myometrial cells, thereby keeping the uterus relaxed Prostaglandin synthesis inhibitor; typically not used after 32 weeks' gestation to avoid premature closure of the ductus arteriosus	Drowsiness, flushing, warmth, nausea, headache, slurred speech, and blurred vision (toxicity is manifested by CNS depression, respirations less than 12 breaths/minute, hyporeflexia, oliguria, cardiac arrhythmias, and cardiac arrest)	Hypotonia and bradycardia	Calcium gluconate
Indomethacin	Nonsteroidal anti-inflammatory that decreases production of prostaglandins, which are lipid compounds associated with the initiation of labor	Nausea, vomiting, and dyspepsia; additive CNS effects if given with magnesium sulfate	Premature closure of ductus arteriosus	None; discontinuation of drug necessary
Nifedipine	Calcium channel blocker that decreases the production of calcium — a substance associated with the initiation of labor	Headache, flushing; additive CNS effects if given with magnesium sulfate	Minimal	None; discontinuation of drug necessary

Administering terbutaline

I.V. terbutaline may be ordered for a woman in premature labor. When administering this drug, follow these steps:

- Obtain baseline maternal vital signs, fetal heart rate (FHR), and laboratory studies, including serum glucose and electrolyte levels and hematocrit.
- Institute external monitoring of uterine contractions and FHR.
- Prepare the drug with lactated Ringer's solution instead of dextrose and water *to prevent additional glucose load and possible hyperglycemia.*
- Administer the drug as an I.V. piggyback infusion into a main I.V. solution *so that the drug can be discontinued immediately if the patient experiences adverse reactions.*
- Use microdrip tubing and infusion pump *to ensure an accurate flow rate.*
- Expect to adjust infusion flow rate every 10 minutes until contractions cease or adverse reactions become problematic.
- Monitor maternal vital signs every 15 minutes while infusion rate is being increased and then every 30 minutes thereafter until contractions cease; monitor FHR every 15 to 30 minutes.
- Auscultate breath sounds for evidence of crackles or changes; monitor the patient for complaints of dyspnea and chest pain.
- Be alert for maternal pulse rate greater than 120 beats/minute, blood pressure less than 90/60 mm Hg, or persistent tachycardia or tachypnea, chest pain, dyspnea, or abnormal breath sounds *because these could indicate developing pulmonary edema.* Notify the practitioner immediately.
- Watch for fetal tachycardia or late or variable decelerations in FHR pattern *because these could indicate uterine bleeding or fetal distress necessitating an emergency birth.*
- Monitor intake and output closely, every hour during the infusion, and then every 4 hours thereafter.
- Expect to continue the infusion for 12 to 24 hours after contractions have ceased and then switch to oral therapy.
- Administer the first dose of oral therapy 30 minutes before discontinuing the I.V. infusion.
- Instruct the patient on how to take the oral therapy, continuing therapy until 37 weeks' gestation or until fetal lung maturity has been confirmed by amniocentesis; alternatively, if the patient is prescribed subcutaneous terbutaline therapy via a continuous pump, teach the patient how to use the pump.
- Teach the patient how to measure her pulse rate before each dose of oral terbutaline, or at the recommended times with subcutaneous therapy; instruct the patient to call the practitioner if her pulse rate exceeds 120 beats/minute or she experiences palpitations or severe nervousness.

Implementation

- Confirm the patient's identity using two patient identifiers according to your facility's policy.
- Assess baseline uterine contractions and fetal heart rate (FHR) patterns.
- Explain the drug therapy ordered, including the route to be used and possible adverse effects.
- Insert an I.V. catheter for the patient who is to receive magnesium sulfate or terbutaline
- Obtain laboratory studies, such as complete blood count, hemoglobin and hematocrit, and serum electrolytes.
- Obtain a baseline electrocardiogram and cultures of urine, vaginal, and cervix, as ordered.
- Closely observe the patient in preterm labor for signs of fetal or maternal distress and provide comprehensive supportive care.
- Provide guidance about the hospital stay, potential for delivery of a preterm neonate, and the possible need for neonatal intensive care.
- Encourage the patient to assume the side-lying position *to maximize placental blood flow and relieve pressure on the cervix.*
- During attempts to suppress preterm labor, make sure the patient maintains bed rest; provide appropriate diversionary activities.
- Administer tocolytic agent, as ordered. Give nifedipine and indomethacin orally; administer magnesium sulfate I.V. piggybacked into a primary line; give terbutaline subcutaneously or I.V. piggybacked into a primary line.
- When administering terbutaline, monitor blood pressure, pulse rate, respirations, FHR, and uterine contraction pattern. (See *Administering terbutaline.*)

■ Monitor the status of contractions, notifying the practitioner if the patient experiences more than four contractions per hour. If the patient's pulse rises above 120 beats/minute or her systolic blood pressure drops below 90 mm Hg, or if the fetus's heart rate rises above 180 beats/minute or drops below 110 beats/minute, notify the practitioner.

Special considerations

■ Minimize adverse reactions by keeping the patient in a side-lying position as much as possible *to ensure adequate placental perfusion.*
■ Administer fluids, as ordered, *to ensure adequate hydration*; monitor intake and output *to prevent fluid overload.*
■ Frequently assess deep tendon reflexes when administering magnesium sulfate. (See *Safety with magnesium.*)
■ Prepare patient for possible delivery if therapy is unsuccessful; if preterm labor continues, expect to administer corticosteroids *to promote lung maturity in the fetus.*
■ If labor is not stopped and a preterm neonate is delivered, monitor the neonate for signs of magnesium toxicity, including neuromuscular and respiratory depression.

Home care

If labor is suppressed, begin discharge teaching with the woman and her support person about tocolytic therapy at home; anticipate referral for home care follow-up. Instruct the woman in drug dosage, frequency, route, and possible adverse effects. Teach the patient how to monitor contraction pattern, pulse rate, and fetal movement. Also teach about the signs and symptoms of true labor. Finally, review activity restrictions and danger signs to report to health care provider.

Documentation

Document the drug, dose, route, site, and date and time of drug administration, and document status of contractions, mother's vital signs and fetal heart rate according to institutional policy.

Safety with magnesium

Use caution when administering I.V. magnesium therapy by following these guidelines.
■ Always administer the drug as a piggyback infusion so that if the patient develops signs and symptoms of toxicity, the drug can be discontinued immediately.
■ Obtain a baseline serum magnesium level before initiating therapy, and monitor frequently thereafter.
■ Keep in mind that to be effective as an anticonvulsant, the serum magnesium level should be between 5 and 8 mg/dl. A level above 8 mg/dl indicates toxicity and places the patient at risk for respiratory depression, cardiac arrhythmias, and cardiac arrest.
■ Assess the patient's deep tendon reflexes. Ideally, this should be the patellar reflex. However, if the patient has received epidural anesthesia, test the biceps or triceps reflex. Diminished or hypoactive reflexes suggest magnesium toxicity.
■ Assess for ankle clonus by rapidly dorsiflexing the patient's ankle three times in succession and then remove your hand, observing foot movement. If no further motion is noted, ankle clonus is absent; if the foot continues to move voluntarily, clonus is present. Moderate (three to five) or severe (six or more) movements may suggest magnesium toxicity.
■ Have calcium gluconate readily available at the patient's bedside. Anticipate administering this antidote for magnesium toxicity.

SELECTED REFERENCES

American College of Obstetrics & Gynecology (ACOG). "Management of Preterm Labor," *ACOG Practice Bulletin No. 43,* Washington, D.C.: May 2003. Available at *www.guideline.gov/summary/summary.aspx?doc_id=3993.*

Berkman, N.D., et al. "Tocolytic Treatment for the Management of Preterm Labor: A Review of the Evidence," *American Journal of Obstetrics and Gynecology* 188(6):1648-59, June 2003.

How, H.Y., et al. "Tocolysis in Women with Preterm Labor between 32 0/7 and 34 6/7 Weeks of Gestation: A Randomized Controlled Pilot Study," *American Journal of Obstetrics and Gynecology* 194(4):976-81, April 2006.

Smith, G.N., et al. "Randomized Double-Blind Placebo-Controlled Trial of Transdermal Nitroglycerin for Preterm Labor," *American Journal of Obstetrics and Gynecology* 196(1):37.e1-8, January 2007.

OXYTOCIN ADMINISTRATION

The hormone oxytocin stimulates the uterus to contract, thereby facilitating cervical dilation. The practitioner may order synthetic oxytocin (Pitocin or Syntocinon) to induce or augment labor or to control bleeding and enhance uterine contraction after the placenta is delivered. Usually, the nurse administers oxytocin I.V. To regulate dosage and to help prevent uterine hyperstimulation, she always uses an infusion pump. Additional nursing responsibilities include managing the infusion and monitoring maternal and fetal responses.

Indications for oxytocin administration include the following maternal and fetal conditions:

- *Maternal conditions*—gestational hypertension, premature rupture of membranes, preeclampsia or eclampsia, and maternal medical problems, such as diabetes, renal disease, chronic hypertension, and chronic obstructive cardiopulmonary disease. Other maternal situations in which induction may be considered include risk of rapid labor and delivery and being far from the health care facility. If induction is scheduled in these conditions, confirmation of term gestation and fetal lung maturity should be done.
- *Fetal conditions*—postterm gestation, macrosomia, fetal demise, fetal anomaly, blood group sensitization, nonreassuring fetal testing, fetal hydrops, and intrauterine growth restriction.

Assessment of the pregnant patient scheduled for an induction should include a determination of labor readiness. One way to determine the woman's readiness for delivery is by using the Bishop scoring method. (See *Bishop Score.*) This assessment includes determination of the woman's cervical dilation, effacement, station, and consistency of the position of the cervix. A score of four or less indicates that the cervix isn't ready for labor and delivery.

Contraindications include placenta previa or vasa previa, diagnosed cephalopelvic disproportion, fetal distress, previous classic uterine incision or uterine surgery, transverse fetal lie, prolapsed umbilical cord, or active genital herpes. Oxytocin should be administered cautiously and requires special attention to a patient who has an overdistended uterus or a history of cervical surgery, uterine surgery, or grand multiparity, breech presentation, maternal heart disease, polyhydramnios, presenting part above the pelvic inlet, severe hypertension, or abnormal fetal heart rate (FHR) patterns not necessitating emergency delivery.

Equipment

Administration set for primary I.V. line ▪ infusion pump and tubing ▪ I.V. solution, as ordered ▪ external or internal fetal monitoring equipment ▪ oxytocin ▪ 20G 1″ needle ▪ label ▪ venipuncture equipment with an 18G through-the-needle catheter ▪ optional: autosyringe.

Preparation of equipment

Prepare the oxytocin solution, as ordered. Rotate the I.V. bag *to disperse the drug throughout the solution.* Label the I.V. container with the name of the medication. Then attach the infusion pump tubing to the I.V. container, and connect the tubing to the pump.

Because infusion pump features vary, review the operator's manual before proceeding. Attach the 20G 1″ needle to the tubing to piggyback it to the primary I.V. line, or use an autosyringe connected to the primary I.V. line. Then set up the equipment for internal or external fetal monitoring.

Implementation

- Confirm the patient's identity using two patient identifiers according to your facility's policy.
- Explain the procedure to the patient and provide privacy. Wash your hands. Describe the equipment, and forewarn the patient that she may feel a pinch from the venipuncture.

Administering oxytocin during labor and delivery

- Help the patient to a lateral-tilt position, and support her hip with a pillow. Don't let her lie in a supine position. *In the supine position, the gravid uterus presses on the maternal great vessels, producing maternal hypotension and reduced uterine perfusion.*
- Identify and record FHR, and assess uterine contractions occurring in a 20-minute span *to establish baseline fetal status and evaluate spontaneous maternal uterine activity.*
- Start the primary I.V. line using an 18G through-the-needle catheter. Use this line to deliver not only oxytocin but also fluids, blood, or other medications, as needed.
- Piggyback the oxytocin solution (metered by the infusion pump) to the primary I.V. line at the Y injection site closest to the patient. *Piggybacking maintains I.V. line patency (which you'll need to preserve if you discontinue the oxytocin infusion). Also, using the Y injection site nearest the venipuncture ensures that the primary line holds the lowest concentration of oxytocin if you must stop the infusion.*
- Begin the oxytocin infusion, as ordered (either high-dose or low-dose regimen). If starting the patient on a low-dose regimen, begin the infusion at 0.5 to 1.0 mU/minute with incremental increases (for the desired results) at 30- to 40-minute intervals in increments of 1 mU/minute; or, begin the oxytocin administration at 1 to 2 mU/minute and increase the dose by 2 mU/minute every 15 minutes.
- If starting the patient on high-dose oxytocin, begin the infusion at 6 mU/minute, increasing the dose by 6 mU every 15 minutes; or, begin the infusion at 6 mU/minute and increase the dose by 1, 3, or 6 mU every 20 to 40 minutes. The maximum dose is usually 20 mU/minute.
- *Because oxytocin begins acting immediately,* be prepared to start monitoring uterine contractions.
- Increase the oxytocin dosage as ordered and based on your assessment of the contraction pattern and fetal response. When induced labor simulates normal labor (contractions occurring every 2 to 3 minutes and lasting 40 to 60 seconds) and cervical dilation progresses at least 1 cm/hour in first-stage, active-phase labor, you can stop increasing the dosage.

Bishop Score

This scoring system was created to determine whether the cervix is "ripe"—that is, ready for cervical dilation. If a woman's total score is eight or more, the cervix is considered to be ready for birth and should respond to induction.

SCORING FACTOR	SCORE 0	1	2	3
Dilation (cm)	0	1 to 2	3 to 4	5 to 6
Effacement (%)	0 to 30	40 to 50	60 to 70	80
Station	–3	–2	–1 to 0	+1 to +2
Consistency	Firm	Medium	Soft	
Position	Posterior	Midposition	Anterior	

Adapted with permission from Searing, K.A. "Induction vs. Post-Date Pregnancies: Exploring the Controversy of Who's Really at Risk," *AWHONN Lifelines* 5(2):44-48, April-May 2001. Originally published by Bishop, E.H. "Pelvic Scoring for Elective Induction," *Obstetrics and Gynecology* 24:266, 1964.

However, continue the infusion at the dosage and rate that maintain the activity closest to normal labor.

- Before each increase, be sure to time the frequency and duration of contractions, palpate the uterus *to identify contraction intensity,* and assess maternal vital signs and fetal heart rhythm and rate *to ensure safety and to anticipate possible complications.* If you're using an external fetal monitor, the uterine activity strip or grid should show contractions occurring every 2 to 3 minutes. The contractions should last for about 60 seconds and be followed by uterine relaxation. If you're using an internal fetal monitor, look for an optimal baseline value ranging from 5 to 15 mm Hg. Your aim is to verify uterine relaxation between contractions.
- Assist with comfort measures, such as repositioning the patient on her other side, as needed.
- Continue assessing maternal and fetal responses to the oxytocin. For example, every 10 to 15 minutes, evaluate FHR, maternal response to increased contraction activity and subsequent discomfort, and maternal pulse rate and pattern, blood pressure, respiration rate and quality, and uterine contractions. Also, review the infusion rate *to prevent uterine hyperstimulation.* Signs of hyperstimulation include contractions less than 2 minutes apart and lasting 90 seconds or longer, uterine pressure that doesn't return to baseline between contractions, and intrauterine pressure that rises over 75 mm Hg.
- *To reduce uterine irritability,* try to increase uterine blood flow. Do this by changing the patient's position and increasing the infusion rate of the primary I.V. line. Avoid exceeding the maximum total infusion of 20 mU/minute.
- *To manage hyperstimulation,* discontinue the infusion, administer oxygen, and notify the practitioner.
- After hyperstimulation resolves, resume the oxytocin infusion. Depending on maternal and fetal conditions, select one of the following methods: Resume the infusion beginning with oxytocin 0.5 mU/minute, increase the dosage to 1 mU/minute every 15 minutes, and increase the rate as before; resume the infusion at one-half of the last dosage given and increase the rate as before; or resume the infusion at the dosage given before hyperstimulation signs occurred. Check your facility's policy for the appropriate method.
- Monitor and record intake and output. Output should be at least 30 ml/hour. Oxytocin has an antidiuretic effect at rates of 16 mU/minute and more, so you may need to administer an electrolyte-containing I.V. solution *to maintain electrolyte balance.*

Administering oxytocin after delivery

- As ordered after delivery, administer 10 to 40 units of oxytocin added to 1,000 ml of physiologic electrolyte solution. Infuse at a rate titrated to decrease postpartum bleeding or uterine atony after placental delivery. As an alternative, ad-

Conversion formulas for oxytocin administration

To ensure that all members of the health care team speak the same language when administering oxytocin, use the following formulas, as needed, to convert milliliters (ml) per minute or drops (gtt) per minute to milliunits (mU) per minute. Conversion to mU per minute gives the actual drug dosage instead of the fluid dosage.

The conversion formula you use may be dictated by the infusion pump you use. Synthetic oxytocin for I.V. administration comes in a concentration of 10 units/ml in 10-ml vials, in 0.5- and 1-ml ampules, and in 1-ml disposable syringes.

To calculate oxytocin dilution (in mU/ml):

$$\frac{\text{\# of units oxytocin}}{\text{ml of fluid}} \times 1{,}000 = \text{mU/ml}$$

To convert ml/minute to mU/minute:

$$\frac{\text{mU}}{\text{ml}} \times \frac{\text{ml}}{\text{minute}} = \frac{\text{mU}}{\text{minute}}$$

To convert gtt/minute to mU/minute:

$$\frac{\text{gtt}}{\text{minute}} \times \frac{\text{mU}}{\text{ml}} \times \frac{\text{ml}}{\text{gtt}} = \frac{\text{mU}}{\text{minute}}$$

minister 10 units of oxytocin I.M. until you can establish the I.V. line.

Special considerations

- Most health care facilities require the use of an infusion pump *to ensure accurate dosage and titration.* (See *Conversion formulas for oxytocin administration.*)
- Without an infusion pump, administer oxytocin through a minidrop system (60 drops/ml) or an autosyringe, and observe the patient closely. Without an electronic fetal monitor, frequently palpate and assess contractions. Auscultate FHR every 5 to 15 minutes. (See "Fetal heart rate," page 848.)

Complications

Oxytocin can cause uterine hyperstimulation that may progress to tetanic contractions, which last longer than 2 minutes. Other potential complications include fetal distress, abruptio placentae, and uterine rupture.

Watch for signs of oxytocin hypersensitivity such as elevated blood pressure. Rarely, oxytocin leads to maternal seizures or coma from water intoxication.

Documentation

Monitor uterine activity response to oxytocin infusion rate. Document the baseline FHR, variability, accelerations, decelerations, and changes in FHR response to uterine contraction pattern. Document interventions related to assessment of contractile pattern and fetal response, and record maternal response to contractions, blood pressure, pulse rate and pattern, and respiratory rate and quality on the labor progression chart. Record oxytocin infusion rate and intake and output amounts.

SELECTED REFERENCES

Briggs, G.G., and Wan, S.R. "Drug Therapy during Labor and Delivery, Part 1," *American Journal of Health System Pharmacists* 63(11):1038-47, June 2006.

Jackson, K.W., Jr., et al. "A Randomized Controlled Trial Comparing Oxytocin Administration before and after Placental Delivery in the Prevention of Postpartum Hemorrhage," *American Journal of Obstetric Gynecology* 185(4):873-77, October 2001.

Mattson, S., and Smith, J., eds. *Core Curriculum for Maternal-Newborn Nursing,* 3rd ed. Philadelphia: W.B. Saunders Co., 2004.

Maughan, K.L., et al. "Preventing Postpartum Hemorrhage: Managing the Third Stage of Labor," *American Family Doctor* 73(6):1025-28, March 2006.

Simpson, K.R. "The Context and Clinical Evidence for Common Nursing Practices During Labor," *The American Journal of Maternal Child Nursing* 30(6):356-63, November-December 2005.

Smith, J.G., and Merrill, D.C. "Oxytocin for Induction of Labor," *Clinical Obstetrics and Gynecology* 49(3):594-608, September 2006.

AMNIOTOMY

In amniotomy, the practitioner uses a sterile amniohook to rupture the amniotic membranes. This controversial but common procedure prompts amniotic fluid drainage, which enhances the intensity, frequency, and duration of uterine contractions by reducing uterine volume.

Amniotomy is performed to induce or augment labor when the membranes fail to rupture spontaneously. It helps to expedite labor after dilation begins, and it facilitates insertion of an intrauterine catheter and a spiral electrode for direct fetal monitoring.

Oxytocin infusion may precede amniotomy or follow it by 6 to 8 hours if labor fails to progress. If birth doesn't occur within 24 hours after amniotomy, the practitioner may decide to perform a cesarean delivery to reduce the risk of infection.

When deciding whether to perform amniotomy, the practitioner considers such factors as fetal presentation, position, and station; the degree of cervical dilation and effacement; contraction frequency and intensity; the fetus's gestational age; existing complications; and maternal and fetal vital signs.

Amniotomy is contraindicated in high-risk pregnancies, unless more accurate fetal assessment using internal fetal monitoring is necessary. It's also contraindicated when the presenting fetal part is unengaged because of the risk of transverse lie and umbilical cord prolapse.

Equipment

Antiseptic solution ▪ linen-saver pads ▪ bedpan ▪ soap and water ▪ 4″ × 4″ gauze pads ▪ external electronic fetal monitoring equipment or a fetoscope or Doppler stethoscope ▪ sterile gloves ▪ sterile amniohook.

Preparation of equipment

Assemble the equipment at the patient's bedside.

Implementation

- Reinforce the practitioner's explanation of the procedure, and answer the patient's questions. Wash your hands and put on sterile gloves.
- Clean the perineum with soap and water or 4″ × 4″ gauze pads moistened with antiseptic solution.
- Position the patient and the bedpan so that the bedpan receives the amniotic fluid. Then elevate the head of the bed about 25 degrees *to tilt the pelvis for easier vaginal access.* Alternatively, place linen-saver pads under the patient if the bedpan is too uncomfortable, and then permit the amniotic fluid to drain onto the linen-saver pads.
- Note the baseline fetal heart rate (FHR) *to evaluate fetal status before and after amniotomy.* Use external fetal monitoring throughout the procedure. Otherwise, use the fetoscope or Doppler stethoscope before and after the procedure.
- Using sterile technique, open the amniohook package. Then, wearing sterile gloves, the practitioner removes the amniohook from the package.
- If ordered, apply pressure to the uterine fundus as the practitioner inserts the amniohook vaginally to the cervical os. *This helps to keep the fetal presenting part engaged and reduces the risk of cord prolapse.* Then, carefully avoiding contact with the fetal presenting part, the practitioner ruptures the amniotic membrane at the internal os.
- Without external electronic fetal monitoring equipment, use a fetoscope or Doppler stethoscope to evaluate FHR for at least 60 seconds after the membrane ruptures *to detect bradycardia.* Otherwise, check the monitor tracing for large, variable decelerations in FHR that suggest cord compression. If these FHR changes occur, the practitioner will perform a vaginal examination *to check for cord prolapse.*
- Clean and dry the perineal area, and remove the bedpan. When necessary, replace the linen-saver pad under the patient's buttocks *to promote comfort and hygiene.*
- Inspect the amniotic fluid for meconium, blood, or foul odor. Note the color, and measure the amount of fluid.
- Take the patient's temperature every 2 hours *to detect infection.* If her temperature rises to 100° F (37.8° C), begin hourly checks. Continue to monitor uterine contractions and labor progress.

Special considerations

During a vaginal examination after amniotomy, maintain strict sterile technique *to prevent uterine infection.* For the same reason, minimize the number of examinations.

Complications

Umbilical cord prolapse—a life-threatening potential complication of amniotomy—is an emergency requiring immediate cesarean delivery *to prevent fetal death.* It occurs when amniotic fluid, gushing from the ruptured sac, sweeps the cord down through the cervix. The risk of prolapse is higher if the fetal head isn't engaged in the pelvis before the rupture occurs. Intrauterine infection can result from failure to use sterile technique for amniotomy or from prolonged labor after amniotomy.

Documentation

Record FHR before, and at frequent intervals immediately after, amniotomy (every 5 minutes for 20 minutes and then every 30 minutes). Note any meconium or blood in the amniotic fluid. Measure the amount of fluid, and note whether the fluid has an odor. Record maternal temperature every 2 hours and labor progress, as appropriate.

SELECTED REFERENCES

National Institute for Health and Clinical Excellence. "Inherited Clinical Guideline: Induction of Labor." 2004. Available at *www.nice.org.uk/page.aspx?o=17321.*

Vincent, M. "Amniotomy: To Do or Not to Do?" *RCM Midwives* 8(5):228-89, May 2005.

AMNIOINFUSION

Amnioinfusion is the replacement of amniotic fluid volume through an intrauterine infusion. It involves the infusion of an isotonic solution, such as normal saline or lactated Ringer's solution, via a pressure catheter into the amniotic cavity.

Amnioinfusion is indicated when umbilical cord compression is a factor or when repetitive variable decelerations aren't alleviated by maternal position changes and oxygen administration. It also helps to relieve umbilical cord compression in such conditions as oligohydramnios associated with postmaturity, intrauterine growth retardation, and premature rupture of membranes. Although this procedure can be done to dilute meconium before aspiration occurs, a recent study suggested that for women in labor who had thick meconium staining of their amniotic fluid, amnioinfusion *did not* decrease perinatal death, severe meconium aspiration syndrome, or other major neonatal or maternal disorders.

Equipment

Fetal heart rate monitor ▪ sterile intrauterine pressure catheter ▪ normal saline solution or Ringer's lactate at room temperature ▪ I.V. tubing.

Implementation

- Explain the procedure and rationale for its use.
- Prepare the patient for the procedure, and encourage her to lie in a lateral recumbent position.
- Inform the patient that she will feel fluid flowing out of her vagina during the procedure.
- Make sure that solution for infusion is warmed to the patient's body temperature *to avoid chilling.*
- Institute continuous fetal heart rate (FHR) monitoring if not already in place; obtain a baseline FHR tracing.
- The physician ruptures the membranes if they have not ruptured spontaneously and then inserts a sterile pressure catheter through the cervix into the uterus.
- The catheter is attached via I.V. tubing to a warmed isotonic solution.
- The fluid is administered rapidly, usually 500 ml initially, and then flow rate is titrated based on FHR patterns.
- Assist with infusion, and adjust flow rate, as ordered, to maintain an FHR pattern that shows no variable decelerations.

Special considerations

- Continuously monitor FHR and uterine contractions.
- Assess temperature at least every hour *to detect infection.*
- Monitor the patient for a continuous flow of fluid through the vagina.
- Provide comfort measures, including frequent bed linen changes.
- Notify the physician if the fluid suddenly stops — an indication that the fetal head is engaged and fluid is collecting in the uterus, which could lead to hydramnios and possible uterine rupture.

Complications

As with an invasive procedure, amnioinfusion may cause infection. Other possible complications include hydramnios and uterine rupture.

Documentation

Keep accurate intake and output records during the procedure. Document FHR along with the maternal vital signs and response to treatment.

SELECTED REFERENCES

Fraser, W.D., et al. "Amnioinfusion for the Prevention of Meconium Aspiration Syndrome," *New England Journal of Medicine* 353(9):909-17, September 2005.

Mattson, S., and Smith, J., eds. *Core Curriculum for Maternal-Newborn Nursing,* 3rd ed. Philadelphia: W.B. Saunders Co., 2004.

Weismiller, D.G. "Transcervical Amnioinfusion," *American Family Physician* 57(3):504-10, February 1998.

VACUUM EXTRACTION

Vacuum extraction, also called *vacuum-assisted birth,* is an alternative to forceps delivery. It's associated with a lower incidence of vaginal, cervical, and third-and fourth-degree lacerations; less maternal discomfort, because the cup doesn't occupy additional space in the birth canal; and less anesthesia than that required for forceps delivery. However, vacuum extraction is associated with a marked caput succedaneum of the neonate's head, lasting as long as 7 days after birth.

Tentorial tears are also possible due to the extreme pressure, and renewed bleeding from the scalp can occur if used for a fetus that has undergone fetal blood sampling. Further, its use in preterm neonates is problematic because of the extreme softness of their skulls.

Equipment

Vacuum extractor ▪ pressure regulator ▪ suction source.

Implementation

- Explain the procedure to the patient and her partner.
- Monitor uterine contractions and fetal heart rate frequently.
- Inform her that the pressure and traction will be applied during contractions; encourage the woman to push when directed.

■ Assess the patient for possible contraindications to the procedure, including true cephalopelvic disproportion, nonvertex presentations, maternal or suspected fetal coagulation problems, hydrocephalus (known or suspected), and trauma to the fetal scalp.
■ Inform the patient and her partner that the neonate may have a misshapen head *due to application of the suction.*
■ Encourage the woman to participate in the labor process as much as possible.
■ A plastic vacuum cup connected to a suction source via tubing is applied to the fetal head over the posterior fontanelle. (See *Understanding vacuum extraction.*)
■ Negative pressure of approximately 50 to 60 mm Hg is exerted, *causing air beneath the cup to be removed.*
■ The cup adheres tightly to the fetal head.
■ In conjunction with contractions, the physician applies traction until the head is delivered.
■ Once the head is delivered, the vacuum cup is removed.
■ After delivery of the neonate, provide postpartum care as usual.
■ Inspect the neonate's head for evidence of caput succedaneum, which is a common finding after vacuum extraction.

Special considerations
■ Assess the neonate for possible complications, such as cephalhematoma, and for signs of trauma and infection.
■ Monitor the neonate for signs of listlessness or poor sucking, *which may indicate cerebral irritation.*
■ Offer support to the parents regarding the neonate's misshapen head; reassure the parents that the swelling on the neonate's head will soon resolve.
■ Inform neonatal caregivers and personnel that vacuum extraction was used.

Complications
Cephalhematomas and subgleal hemorrhages (rare) may occur. Scalp bruising and lacerations and maternal perineal and vaginal lacerations may also occur.

Documentation
Document that the delivery was performed with vacuum extraction assistance. Document the amount of pressure used and the condition of the neonate at delivery.

Understanding vacuum extraction

With vacuum extraction, a suction cup is applied to the fetal head at the posterior fontanel. Negative pressure via suction is used, and traction is applied to achieve delivery.

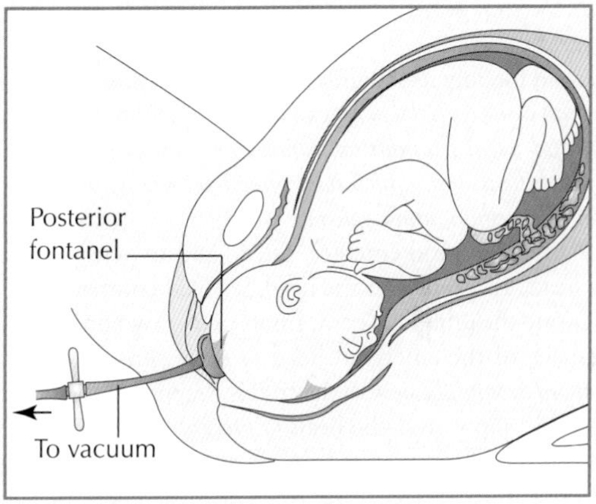

Selected references

Caughey, A.B., et al. "Forceps Compared with Vacuum: Rates of Neonatal and Maternal Morbidity," *Obstetrics and Gynecology* 106(5 Pt 1):908-12, November 2005.

Groom, K., et al. "A Prospective Randomised Controlled Trial of the Kiwi Omnicup Versus Conventional Ventouse Cups for Vacuum-Assisted Vaginal Delivery," *British Journal of Obstetrics and Gynecology* 113(2):183-89, February 2006.

Simonson, C., et al. "Neonatal Complications of Vacuum-Assisted Delivery," *Obstetrics and Gynecology* 109(3):626-33, March 2007.

EMERGENCY DELIVERY
Emergency delivery may occur when labor progresses very quickly and you must deliver the neonate. Your objectives include establishing a clean, safe, and private birth area; promoting a controlled delivery; and preventing injury, infection, and hemorrhage.

Equipment
Sterile gloves ■ sterile Kelly forceps ■ sterile scissors ■ bulb syringe ■ blankets ■ towel.

Implementation
■ Have another nurse call the practitioner while you stay with the patient at all times.
■ Offer support and reassurance *to help relieve the patient's anxiety.* Encourage the patient to pant during contractions *to promote a controlled delivery.* When possible, provide privacy, wash your hands, and put on gloves.

■ Position the patient comfortably on the bed.

NURSING ALERT *Don't collapse the foot section of the bed.*

■ Check for signs of imminent delivery—bulging perineum, increase in bloody show, urge to push, and crowning of the presenting part.

■ As the fetal head reaches and begins to pass the perineum, instruct the patient to pant or blow through the contractions *because forceful bearing down could cause extensive maternal lacerations.* Place one hand gently on the perineum *to cover the fetal head, control birth speed, and prevent sudden expulsion.*

■ Avoid forcibly restraining fetal descent *because undue pressure can cause cephalohematoma or scalp lacerations, head trauma, and vagal stimulation. Undue pressure can also occlude the umbilical cord, which may cause fetal bradycardia, circulatory depression, and hypoxia.*

■ As the fetal head emerges, use a hand to gently support the head. Try to deliver the head between contractions.

■ Locate the umbilical cord. Insert one or two fingers along the back of the emergent head *to make sure the cord isn't wrapped around the neck.* If the cord is wrapped loosely around the neck, slip it over the head *to prevent strangulation during delivery.* If it's wrapped tightly around the neck, clamp the cord in two paces using Kelly clamps. Then use sterile scissors to cut the cord between the clamps.

■ Carefully support the head with both hands as it rotates to one side (external rotation). Gently suction mucus and amniotic fluid from the nose and mouth with a bulb syringe *to prevent aspiration.*

■ Instruct the patient to bear down with the next contraction *to aid delivery of the shoulders.* Position your hands on either side of the neonate's head and support the neck. Exert gentle downward pressure *to deliver the anterior shoulder.* Then exert gentle upward pressure *to deliver the posterior shoulder.*

■ *Remember that amniotic fluid and vernix are slippery,* so take care to support the neonate's body securely after freeing the shoulders.

■ Keep the neonate in a slightly head-down position *to encourage mucus to drain from the respiratory tract.* Wipe excess mucus from his face. If the neonate doesn't breathe spontaneously, gently pat the soles of the feet or stroke the back. *Never suspend a neonate by his feet.*

■ Dry and cover the neonate quickly with a blanket. Ensure that his head is well covered *to minimize exposure and prevent heat loss.*

■ Cradle the neonate at the level of the maternal uterus until the umbilical cord stops pulsating. *This prevents the neonatal blood from flowing to or from the placenta, leading to hypovolemia or hypervolemia, respectively.* Hypovolemia can lead to circulatory collapse and neonatal death; hypervolemia can cause hyperbilirubinemia.

■ Place the neonate on the mother's abdomen in a slightly head-down position.

■ Clamp the umbilical cord at two points, 1″ to 2″ (2.5 to 5 cm) apart. Place the first clamp 4″ to 6″ (10 to 15 cm) from the neonate. *Clamping the cord prevents autotransfusion, which may cause hemolysis and hyperbilirubinemia.*

■ Cut the umbilical cord between the two clamps, using sterile scissors.

■ Watch for signs of placental separation, such as a slight gush of dark blood from the vagina, cord lengthening, and a firm uterine fundus rising within the abdominal area. Usually, the placenta separates from the uterus within 5 minutes after delivery (though it may take as long as 30 minutes). When you see these signs, encourage the patient to bear down *to expel the placenta.* As she does, apply gentle downward pressure on her abdomen *to aid placental delivery.* Never tug on the umbilical cord to initiate or aid placental delivery *because this may invert the uterus or sever the cord from the placenta.*

■ Examine the expelled placenta for intactness. *Retained placental fragments may cause hemorrhage or lead to intrauterine infection.*

■ Palpate the maternal uterus *to make sure it's firm.* Gently massage the atonic uterus *to encourage contraction and prevent hemorrhage.* Encourage breast-feeding, if appropriate, *to stimulate uterine contraction.*

■ Check the patient for excessive bleeding from perineal lacerations. Apply a perineal pad, if available, and instruct the patient to press her thighs together. Provide comfort and reassurance, and offer fluids if available.

Special considerations

■ Never introduce any object into the vagina to facilitate delivery. *Doing so increases the risk of intrauterine infection as well as injury to the cervix, uterus, fetus, umbilical cord, or placenta.*

■ If the patient begins to deliver and the neonate is in a breech position, carefully support the fetal buttocks with both hands. Gently lift the body *to deliver the posterior shoulder.* Then lower the neonate slightly *to deliver the anterior shoulder.* Flexion of the head usually follows. Never apply traction to the body *to avoid lodging the head in the cervix.* Allow the neonate to rotate and emerge spontaneously.

■ If the umbilical cord emerges first, elevate the presenting part throughout delivery *to prevent occluding the cord and causing fetal hypoxia. This obstetric emergency usually necessitates a cesarean delivery.* Continue to displace the presenting part of the cord until the practitioner arrives.

■ If the neonate fails to breathe spontaneously after birth, begin cardiopulmonary resuscitation. (See "Cardiopulmonary resuscitation, infant," page 924.)

Documentation

Give the medical care team the following information if possible: the time of delivery; the presentation and position of the fetus; any delivery complications, such as the cord wrapped around the neonate's neck; the color, character, and amount of amniotic fluid; and the mother's blood type and Rh factor if known. Note the time of placental expulsion, the placental appearance and intactness, the amount of postpartum bleeding, the status of uterine firmness (tone) and contractions, and the mother's response.

Document the sex of the neonate, his estimated Apgar score, and any resuscitative measures used. Record whether the mother began breast-feeding the neonate. Also identify and quantify any fluids given to the mother.

SELECTED REFERENCES

Klossner, N.J. *Introductory Maternity Nursing.* Philadelphia: Lippincott Williams & Wilkins, 2006.

Mattson, S., and Smith, J., eds. *Core Curriculum for Maternal-Newborn Nursing,* 3rd ed. Philadelphia: W.B. Saunders Co., 2004.

Simpson, K.R. "The Context and Clinical Evidence for Common Nursing Practices during Labor," *American Journal of Maternal and Child Nursing* 30(6):356-63, November-December 2005.

POSTPARTUM FUNDAL ASSESSMENT

After delivery, the uterus gradually shrinks and descends into its prepregnancy position in the pelvis — a process known as involution. The nurse evaluates normal involutional progress by palpating and massaging the uterus to identify uterine size, firmness, and descent.

Involution normally begins immediately after delivery, when the firmly contracted uterus lies midway between the umbilicus and the symphysis pubis. Soon the uterus rises to the umbilicus; after the first postpartum day, it begins returning to the pelvis. The average descent rate is 1 cm or fingerbreadth daily — slightly slower if the patient had a cesarean delivery. By the 10th postpartum day, the now unpalpable uterus lies deep in the pelvis, at or below the symphysis pubis.

When the uterus fails to contract or remain firm during involution, uterine bleeding or hemorrhage can result. That's because placental separation after delivery exposes large uterine blood vessels, which uterine contractions close off (like a tourniquet). Fundal massage, administration of synthetic oxytocin, or the release of natural oxytocic substances during breast-feeding help to maintain or stimulate contractions.

Typical nursing procedures that coincide with fundal palpation and massage include caring for the perineum and evaluating healing.

Equipment

Gloves ■ analgesics ■ perineal pad ■ optional: urinary catheter.

Implementation

■ Confirm the patient's identity using two patient identifiers according to your facility's policy.

■ Explain the procedure to the patient, and provide privacy. Wash your hands and put on gloves.

■ Unless the practitioner orders otherwise, schedule fundal assessments every 15 minutes for the first hour after delivery, every 30 minutes for the next 2 to 3 hours, every hour for the next 4 hours, every 4 hours for the rest of the first postpartum day, and every 8 hours until the patient's discharge.

■ Give prescribed analgesics before fundal checks, if indicated. Teach the patient relaxation techniques (such as deep breathing) *to help her cope with discomfort.*

■ Encourage the patient's efforts to urinate *because bladder distention impairs uterine contraction by pushing the uterus up and aside.* You may need to catheterize the patient if she can't urinate or if the uterus becomes displaced with increased bleeding.

■ Lower the head of the bed until the patient lies in a supine position. If this position causes discomfort — especially if she has had cesarean surgery — keep the head of the bed slightly elevated.

■ Expose the abdomen for palpation and the perineum for observation. Watch for bleeding, clots, and tissue expulsion while massaging the fundus.

■ Gently compress the uterus between both hands *to evaluate uterine firmness.* (See *Hand placement for fundal palpation and massage,* page 878.) Note the level of the fundus above or below the umbilicus in fingerbreadths or centimeters.

■ If the uterus seems soft and boggy, gently massage the fundus with a circular motion until it becomes firm. Simply cupping the uterus between your hands may also stimulate contraction. Alternatively, massage the fundus with the side of the hand above the fundus. Without digging into the abdomen, gently compress and release, always supporting the lower uterine segment with the other hand. Observe for lochia flow during massage.

Hand placement for fundal palpation and massage

A full-term pregnancy stretches the ligaments supporting the uterus, placing the uterus at risk for inversion during palpation and massage. To guard against this, use your hands to support and fix the uterus in a safe position. Here's how.

Place one hand against the patient's abdomen at the symphysis pubis level. This steadies the fundus and prevents downward displacement. Place the other hand at the top of the fundus, cupping it (as shown below).

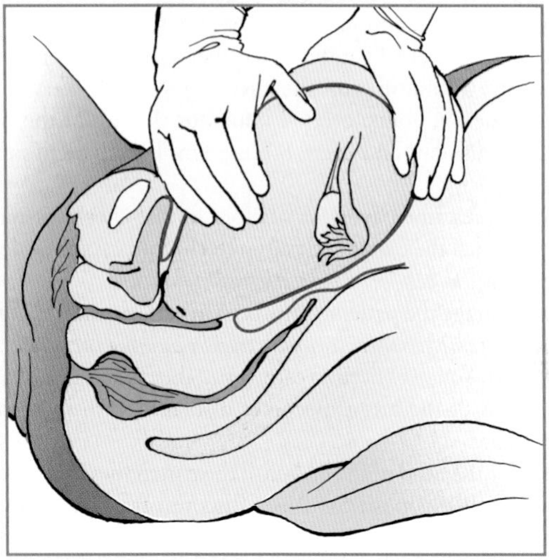

■ Massage long enough to produce firmness. The sensitive fundus needs only gentle pressure. *This should produce the desired results without causing excessive discomfort.*
■ Notify the practitioner immediately if the uterus fails to contract and if heavy bleeding occurs. If the fundus becomes firm after massage, keep one hand on the lower uterus and press gently toward the pubis *to expel clots.*
■ Clean the perineum and apply a clean perineal pad. Help the patient into a comfortable position. (See *Postpartum perineal care.*)

Special considerations

■ *Because incisional pain makes fundal palpation uncomfortable for the patient who has had a cesarean delivery,* provide pain medication beforehand as ordered. If the lochia flow diminishes after 4 hours, the practitioner may permit fewer fundal checks than usual, especially if the patient is receiving oxytocin.
■ If the patient has had a vertical abdominal incision for a cesarean delivery, palpate the uterus from the sides *to determine tone.*

NURSING ALERT *Absence of lochia may signal a clot blocking the cervical os. Subsequent heavy bleeding may result if a change in position dislodges the clot. Take vital signs to assess for hypovolemic shock.*

Complications

Because the uterus and its supporting ligaments are usually tender after delivery, pain is the most common complication of fundal palpation and massage. Excessive massage can stimulate premature uterine contractions, causing undue muscle fatigue and leading to uterine atony or inversion.

Documentation

Record vital signs, fundal height in centimeters or fingerbreadths, and position (midline or off-center) and tone (firm, or soft and boggy). Document massage and note the passage of any clots. Record excessive bleeding and your notification of the practitioner.

SELECTED REFERENCES

American Academy of Pediatrics and American College of Obstetricians and Gynecologists. *Guidelines for Perinatal Care,* 5th ed. Elk Grove Village, Ill.: AAP, 2002; Washington, D.C.:ACOG, 2002.

American College of Obstetricians and Gynecologists. "ACOG Practice Bulletin: Clinical Management Guidelines for Obstetricians-Gynecologists Number 76, October 2006: Postpartum Hemorrhage," *Obstetrics and Gynecology* 108(4):1039-47, October 2006.

Anderson, J.M., and Etches, D. "Prevention and Management of Postpartum Hemorrhage," *American Family Physician* 75(6):875-82, March 2007.

Pillitteri, A. *Maternal and Child Health Nursing: Care of the Childbearing and Childrearing Family*, 5th ed. Philadelphia: Lippincott Williams & Wilkins, 2007.

NEONATAL MONITORING

APGAR SCORING

Named after its developer, Virginia Apgar, the Apgar score quantifies the neonatal heart rate, respiratory effort, muscle tone, reflexes, and color. Each category is assessed 1 minute

Postpartum perineal care

Vaginal birth (which stretches and sometimes tears the perineal tissues) and episiotomy (which may minimize tissue injury) usually leave the patient with perineal edema and tenderness. Postpartum perineal care aims to relieve this discomfort, promote healing, and prevent infection.

Performed after the patient eliminates, perineal hygiene involves cleaning and drying the perineum and assessing the wound area and the lochia (blood and debris sloughed from the placental site and the decidua). Red immediately after delivery, the lochia turns pinkish brown in 4 to 7 days and appears white during the second and third weeks after delivery. This discharge decreases gradually but may continue for up to 6 weeks.

Cleaning the perineum

- Typically, you'll use a water-jet irrigation system or a peribottle to clean the perineum. Assist the patient to the bathroom, wash your hands, and put on gloves.
- If you're using a water-jet irrigation system, insert the prefilled cartridge containing antiseptic or medicated solution into the handle, and push the disposable nozzle into the handle until you hear it click into place. Instruct the patient to sit on the commode. Next, place the nozzle parallel to the perineum and turn on the unit. Rinse the perineum for at least 2 minutes from front to back. Then turn off the unit, remove the nozzle, and discard the cartridge. Dry the nozzle, and store it appropriately for later use.
- If you're using a peribottle, fill it with cleaning solution and instruct the patient to pour it over the perineal area.
- Help the patient to stand up before you flush the commode *to avoid spraying the perineum with contaminated water.*
- Assist her in applying a new perineal pad before returning to bed. Instruct her to apply the pad front to back *to avoid infection.*
- Before discharge, teach the patient how to perform perineal care.

Assessing healing progress

- Inspect the perineum regularly. To do so, first put on gloves.
- Ensure adequate lighting, and place the patient in lateral Sims' position *to best expose the perineum and anal area* (as shown below).

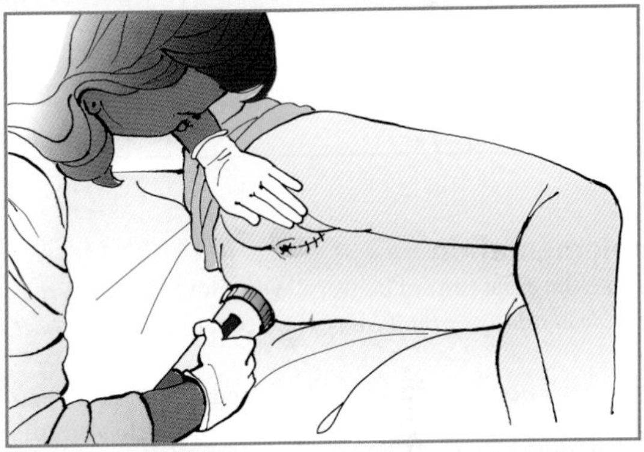

- When inspecting the wound area, be alert for such signs of infection as unusual swelling, redness, and foul-smelling drainage.

after birth and again 5 minutes later. Scores in each category range from 0 to 2. The highest score is 10—the greatest possible sum of the five categories.

The Apgar score should be assigned by health care providers who haven't provided direct nursing or medical care to the mother or fetus during labor. These individuals have direct involvement with birth outcomes, which may bias the scoring.

The evaluation at 1 minute indicates the neonate's initial adaptation to extrauterine life. The evaluation at 5 minutes gives a clearer picture of overall status.

If the neonate doesn't breathe or his heart rate is less than 100 beats/minute immediately after delivery, call for help and begin resuscitation at once. Don't wait for a 1-minute Apgar test score.

Equipment

Apgar score sheet or neonatal assessment sheet ▪ stethoscope ▪ clock with second hand or Apgar timers ▪ gloves. (See *Recording the Apgar score,* page 880.)

Preparation of equipment

If you use Apgar timers, make sure both timers are on at the instant of birth.

Recording the Apgar score

Use this chart to record the neonatal Apgar score at 1 minute and 5 minutes after birth. For each category, assign a score of 0 to 2 as shown. A total score of 7 to 10 indicates good condition; 4 to 6, fair condition (the neonate may have moderate central nervous system depression, muscle flaccidity, cyanosis, and poor respirations); 0 to 3, danger (the infant needs immediate resuscitation, as ordered).

SIGN	APGAR SCORE		
	0	1	2
Heart rate	Absent	Less than 100 beats/minute (slow)	More than 100 beats/minute
Respiratory effort	Absent	Slow, irregular	Vigorous cry
Muscle tone	Flaccid	Some flexion and resistance to extension of extremities	Active motion
Reflex irritability	No response	Grimace or weak cry	Vigorous cry
Color	Pallor, cyanosis	Pink body, blue extremities	Completely pink

Implementation

■ Note the exact time of delivery. Wear gloves *for protection from blood and body fluids*. Dry the neonate *to prevent heat loss*.

■ Place the neonate in a 15-degree Trendelenburg position *to promote mucus drainage*. Then position his head with the nose slightly tilted upward *to straighten the airway*.

■ Assess the neonate's respiratory efforts. If necessary, supply stimulation by rubbing his back or gently flicking his foot.

■ If the neonate exhibits abnormal respiratory responses, begin neonatal resuscitation according to the guidelines of the American Heart Association (AHA) and the American Academy of Pediatrics. Then use the Apgar score and the normal resuscitation AHA guidelines to judge the progress and success of resuscitation efforts. If resuscitation efforts prove futile, you'll need to implement measures for dealing with stillbirth. (See *Dealing with a stillbirth*.)

■ If the neonate exhibits normal responses, assign the Apgar score at 1 minute after birth.

■ Repeat the evaluation at 5 minutes after birth, and record the score.

Assessing neonatal heart rate

■ Using a stethoscope, listen to the heartbeat for 30 seconds, and record the rate. To obtain beats per minute, double the rate. Alternatively, palpate the umbilical cord where it joins the abdomen, monitor pulsations for 6 seconds, and multiply by 10 to obtain beats per minute. Assign a 0 for no heart rate, a 1 for a rate under 100 beats/minute, and a 2 for a rate greater than 100 beats/minute.

Assessing respiratory effort

■ Count unassisted respirations for 60 seconds, noting quality and regularity (a normal rate is 30 to 50 respirations/minute). Assign a 0 for no respirations; a 1 for slow, irregular, shallow, or gasping respirations; and a 2 for regular respirations and vigorous crying.

Assessing muscle tone

■ Observe the extremities for flexion and resistance to extension. This can be done by extending the limbs and observing their rapid return to flexion — the neonate's normal state. Assign a 0 for flaccid muscle tone; a 1 for some flexion and resistance to extension; and a 2 for normal flexion of elbows, knees, and hips, with good resistance to extension.

Assessing reflex irritability

■ Observe the neonate's response to nasal suctioning or to flicking the sole of his foot. Assign a 0 for no response, a 1 for a grimace or weak cry, and a 2 for a vigorous cry.

Dealing with a stillbirth

If a fetus that's mature enough to survive extrauterine life dies before or during delivery, the event is called a stillbirth and the fetus, a stillborn. Features of maturity include a gestational age of 16 weeks or more and a length of $6^1/4''$ (15.8 cm) or more. Delivery of a less-mature fetus is called a spontaneous abortion.

Nursing interventions

Besides measuring, weighing, identifying, and preparing the stillborn for the morgue, you'll need to provide emotional support to the parents. They'll need comfort and care whether or not they expected the stillbirth.

If the parents expected the stillbirth, help them continue working through their grief—especially if they've delayed grieving while waiting for delivery. If the parents didn't expect the stillbirth, help them express their anger and relieve their grief in positive ways. Refer them to appropriate support groups.

Offer bereaved parents the opportunity to hold the stillborn. If possible, provide a photograph, identification bracelet, or another memento. If they refuse these mementos, file them with the chart so that the parents can obtain them later, if desired.

Assessing color

- Observe skin color, especially at the extremities. Assign a 0 for complete pallor and cyanosis, a 1 for a pink body with blue extremities (acrocyanosis), and a 2 for a completely pink body.
- *To assess color in a dark-skinned neonate,* inspect the oral mucous membranes and conjunctiva, the lips, the palms, and the soles.

Special considerations

- If the patient and her support person don't know about the Apgar score, discuss it with them during early labor, when they'll be more receptive to new knowledge. *To prevent confusion or misunderstanding at delivery,* explain to them what will occur and why. Add that this is a routine procedure.
- If the neonate requires emergency care, make sure a member of the delivery team offers appropriate support.
- Closely observe the neonate whose mother receives heavy sedation just before delivery. Even if he has a high Apgar score at birth, he may exhibit secondary effects of sedation in the nursery. Be alert for respiratory depression or unresponsiveness.

Documentation

Record the Apgar score on the Apgar score sheet or the neonatal assessment sheet required by your facility. Be sure to indicate the total score and the signs for which points were deducted to guide postnatal care.

SELECTED REFERENCES

American Academy of Pediatrics and American College of Obstetricians and Gynecologists. *Guidelines for Perinatal Care,* 5th ed. Elk Grove Village, Ill.: AAP, 2002; Washington, D.C.:ACOG, 2002.

Mattson, S., and Smith, J., eds. *Core Curriculum for Maternal-Newborn Nursing,* 3rd ed. Philadelphia: W.B. Saunders Co., 2004.

VITAL SIGNS

Measuring vital signs establishes the baseline of any neonatal assessment. Typically, you'll visually assess the respiratory rate by watching and counting the neonate's breaths, although you may auscultate the lungs with a pediatric stethoscope and watch for labored or abnormal breathing. You'll measure the heart rate apically, also with a pediatric stethoscope, and take the first neonatal temperature rectally to verify rectal patency. Subsequent temperature readings are axillary to avoid injuring the rectal mucosa. Blood pressure readings may be assessed by sphygmomanometer or by palpation or auscultation. An electronic vital signs monitor may also be used. (See "Temperature," page 12; "Pulse," page 14; "Blood pressure," page 18; and "Respiration," page 24.)

When the neonate arrives in the nursery, additional procedures may be required to ensure his safety and progress. Depending on your facility's protocol, these procedures may include an identification and weight check, placement in radiant warming equipment, rectal temperature measurement, a vitamin K injection to stimulate neonatal clotting mechanisms, and eye treatments with an antibiotic to guard against infections.

Equipment

Pediatric stethoscope ▪ watch with second hand ▪ gloves ▪ thermometer (electronic with rectal probe and cover) ▪ water-

Normal vital signs in full-term neonates

Use these ranges (or those established by your facility) to guide assessment of neonatal status.

Respiratory rate
30 to 50 breaths/minute

Heart rate (apical)
110 to 160 beats/minute

Temperature
Axillary: 97.5° to 99° F (36.4° to 37.2° C)
Rectal: one degree higher

Blood pressure
Systolic: 60 to 80 mm Hg
Diastolic: 40 to 50 mm Hg

soluble lubricant ▪ sphygmomanometer with 1″ (2.5-cm) cuff.

Preparation of equipment

Assemble the equipment beside the patient. Apply the cover to the rectal probe. Using water-soluble lubricant, coat the thermometer or probe cover before taking a rectal temperature.

Implementation

- Confirm the neonate's identity using two patient identifiers according to your facility's policy.
- Wash your hands.

Determining respiratory rate

- Observe respirations first, before the neonate becomes active or agitated. Watch and count respiratory movements for 1 minute. Then record the result. (See *Normal vital signs in full-term neonates.*)
- Expect to see mostly diaphragmatic respirations. Also expect an irregular respiratory rate and pattern, varying from slow and shallow to rapid and deep. Abnormally fast breathing (tachypnea) may signal a problem. A lapse of 15 seconds or more after a complete respiratory cycle (one expiration and one inspiration) indicates apnea.
- Check for labored breathing (sometimes from blocked nasal passages). Observe for uneven chest expansion, nasal flaring, visible chest retractions, expiratory grunts, and inspiratory stridor (a high-pitched sound audible without a stethoscope).
- *To evaluate breath sounds,* auscultate the anterior and posterior lung fields, placing the stethoscope over each lung lobe for at least 5 seconds for a total of 1 minute. Normal breath sounds are clear and the same bilaterally. Immediately after birth, you may hear a few crackles resulting from retained fetal lung fluid.
- Observe the chest for symmetrical movement as it rises and falls. Also, determine any difference between the anterior and posterior diameters of the chest, which normally are equal. *Unequal diameters suggest hyperinflated lungs or respiratory distress.*

Assessing heart rate

- Place the stethoscope over the apical impulse on the fourth or fifth intercostal space at the left midclavicular line over the cardiac apex. Listen to and count the heartbeats for 1 minute *to learn the heart rate and to detect any abnormalities in quality or rhythm.*
- If you hear an unorthodox rhythm, assess whether the irregularity follows a definite or random pattern. *This evaluation helps to identify the type of abnormality.* For example, atrial fibrillation is an irregular rhythm with an irregular pattern.
- Auscultate for variations from the normal "lub-dub" systole-diastole sounds. Determine whether the first and second heart sounds are separate and distinct or split into two sounds. Assess for extra heartbeats and sounds that stretch into the next sound. *Such abnormal sounds may indicate a heart murmur, for example, from a patent ductus arteriosus, as blood rushes through the abnormal opening.*

Taking a rectal temperature

- Wash your hands and put on gloves.
- With the neonate lying in a supine position, firmly grasp his ankles with your index finger between them *to prevent skin trauma.* Place a diaper over the penis of a male neonate *to absorb urine if he urinates.*
- Still holding the neonate's ankles, insert the lubricated thermometer no more than ½″ (1.3 cm) — *inserting it any farther could cause rectal injury.* Place the palm of your hand on his buttocks, and hold the thermometer between your index and middle fingers. *This stabilizes the thermometer if the neonate moves suddenly. To inhibit the defecation response induced by inserting a rectal thermometer,* press the buttocks together. If you meet resistance during insertion, withdraw the thermometer and notify the practitioner.
- Hold an electronic thermometer until the temperature registers. (See "Temperature," page 12.) Remove the ther-

mometer, and read the number on the digital display. Record the result.

Taking an axillary temperature

- Dry the axillary skin. Then place the thermometer in the axilla, and hold it along the outer aspect of the neonate's chest between the axillary line and the arm for at least 3 minutes; *axillary temperature takes this long to register.* Hold an electronic thermometer in place until the temperature registers.
- Reassess axillary temperature in 15 to 30 minutes if it registers outside the normal range. If the temperature remains abnormal, notify the practitioner. *A subnormal temperature may result from infection, and an elevated temperature may result from dehydration or may reflect the environment, such as a malfunctioning overhead warmer.*
- Document the temperature.

Determining blood pressure

- Measure blood pressure in a quiet neonate.
- Make sure the blood pressure cuff is small enough for the patient (cuff width should be about one-half of the circumference of the neonate's arm) *because the cuff size affects accurate readings.*
- Wrap the cuff one or two fingerbreadths above the antecubital or popliteal area. With the stethoscope held directly over the chosen artery, hold the cuffed extremity firmly *to keep it extended* and inflate the cuff no faster than 5 mm Hg/second. (See *Alternative methods for assessing neonatal blood pressure.*)
- *To determine whether subsequent blood pressure assessments measure within the neonate's normal range,* compare subsequent blood pressure readings with baseline values. Report any significant deviation.

Special considerations

- If desired, count respirations while auscultating the heart rate.
- When listening to neonatal heart tones immediately after birth, you may hear murmurs resulting from a delayed closing of fetal blood shunts.
- Excessive neonatal activity — such as restlessness and crying during a vital signs assessment — may elevate the heart rate above normal. Therefore, describe the neonate's activity along with measured findings.

Documentation

Record vital signs and related measurements in your notes, a neonatal appraisal form, or a flowchart. Include any observations about the neonate's condition such as abnormal breath sounds.

Alternative methods for assessing neonatal blood pressure

Besides using a standard sphygmomanometer for assessing neonatal blood pressure, you may use palpation or auscultation.

Palpation

Feel for the neonate's radial or brachial pulse, which is the systolic blood pressure.

Auscultation

If you're using a pediatric stethoscope with amplification, listen for diastolic and systolic sounds at the brachial artery.

If you're using a Doppler blood pressure monitor, place the cuff directly over the brachial or popliteal artery *to ensure an accurate reading.* The device automatically inflates the cuff. *For greatest accuracy,* keep the cuffed arm or leg extended during cuff inflation. (Observe the extremity's color *because duskiness signifies reduced blood flow.*)

SELECTED REFERENCES

American Academy of Pediatrics and American College of Obstetricians and Gynecologists. *Guidelines for Perinatal Care,* 5th ed. Elk Grove Village, Ill.: AAP, 2002; Washington, D.C.:ACOG, 2002.

Darnall, R.A., et al. "The Late Preterm Infant and the Control of Breathing, Sleep, and Brainstem Development: A Review," *Clinics in Perinatology* 33(4):883-914, December 2006.

Devrim, I., et al. "Measurement Accuracy of Fever by Tympanic and Axillary Thermometry," *Pediatric Emergency Care* 23(1):16-19, January 2007.

Laptook, A.R., et al. "Admission Temperature of Low Birth Weight Infants: Predictors and Associated Mortalities," *Pediatrics* 119(3):e643-49, March 2007.

Mattson, S., and Smith, J., eds. *Core Curriculum for Maternal-Newborn Nursing,* 3rd ed. Philadelphia: W.B. Saunders Co., 2004.

Pillitteri, A. *Maternal and Child Health Nursing: Care of the Childbearing and Childrearing Family,* 5th ed. Philadelphia: Lippincott Williams & Wilkins, 2007.

Podoll, A., et al. "Inaccuracy in Pediatric Outpatient Blood Pressure Measurement," *Pediatrics* 119(3):e538-43, March 2007.

SIZE AND WEIGHT

A beginning point for many neonatal assessments, size and weight measurements establish the baseline for accurately monitoring normal growth. Anthropometric dimensions and weight help detect such disorders as small size for gestational age, hydrocephalus, and intracranial bleeding. You'll take these measurements in the nursery during routine checkups and sometimes at the neonate's home. Then you'll compare the results with previous measurements and with normal values.

Normally the neonate's head circumference measures the same as or more than his chest circumference. An exception occurs during the first 24 hours after birth, when head molding leaves the head circumference slightly smaller than the chest circumference. The head's contour usually returns to normal in 2 to 3 days. (See *Average neonatal size and weight.*)

The neonate's weight varies with gender, gestational age, heredity, and other factors. A firstborn usually weighs less at birth than later siblings. The neonate of a diabetic mother tends to be large. Because of an erratic feeding pattern and passage of urine and meconium, the normal neonate loses between 5% and 10% of his birth weight during the first few days. However, he usually regains this weight in 10 days. Normal weight gain for the neonate is 5 to 7 oz (141.7 to 198.4 g) weekly.

Equipment

Crib or examination table with a firm surface ▪ scale with tray ▪ scale paper, if necessary ▪ tape measure ▪ length board ▪ gloves, if the neonate hasn't been bathed yet.

Disposable paper tape measures are available. Cloth tape measures aren't recommended *because they can stretch, leading to inaccurate measurements.*

Preparation of equipment

Put clean paper on the scale *to promote warmth and prevent cold stress.* Balance the scale at zero as directed by the manufacturer.

Implementation

- Confirm the neonate's identity using two patient identifiers according to your facility's policy.
- Explain the procedure to the parents if they're present. Wash your hands, and put on gloves if you haven't bathed the neonate yet.
- To begin, position the neonate in a supine position in the crib or on the examination table. Remove all clothing but his diaper (if he has one). Be sure to record all measurements.

Measuring head circumference

- Slide the tape measure over the neonate's head (as shown below). *To arrive at the greatest circumference,* draw the tape snugly across the center of the forehead and the most prominent portion of the posterior head (the occiput).

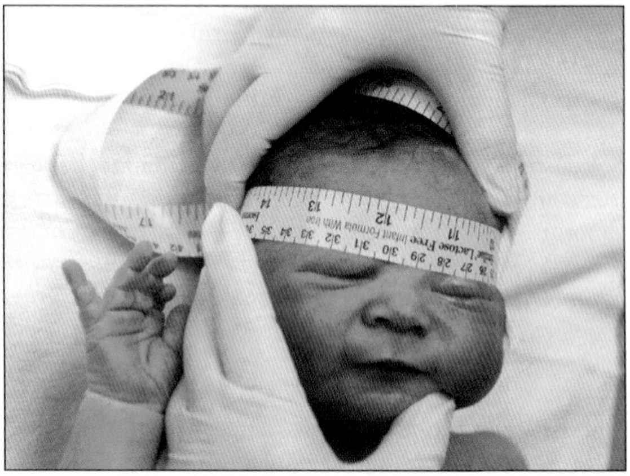

Measuring chest circumference

- Place the tape under the back, and wrap it snugly around the chest at the nipple line (as shown below). *To ensure accuracy,* keep the back and front of the tape level.

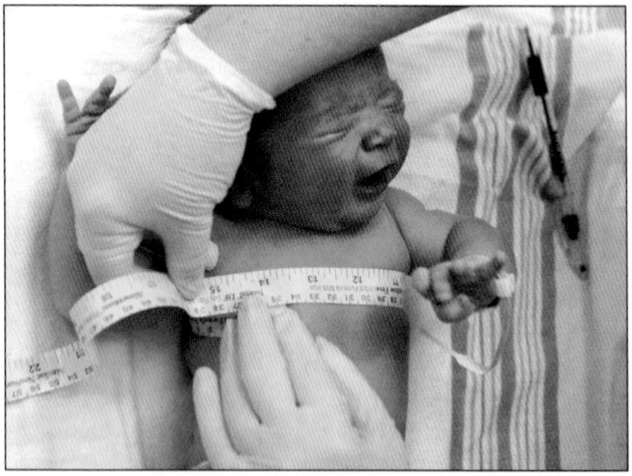

- Take the measurement after the neonate inspires and before he begins to exhale.

Measuring head-to-heel length

- Fully extend the neonate's legs with the toes pointing up. Measure the distance from the heel to the top of the head (as shown top of next page). If possible, have someone extend the legs by pressing down gently on the knees, or use a length board if available.

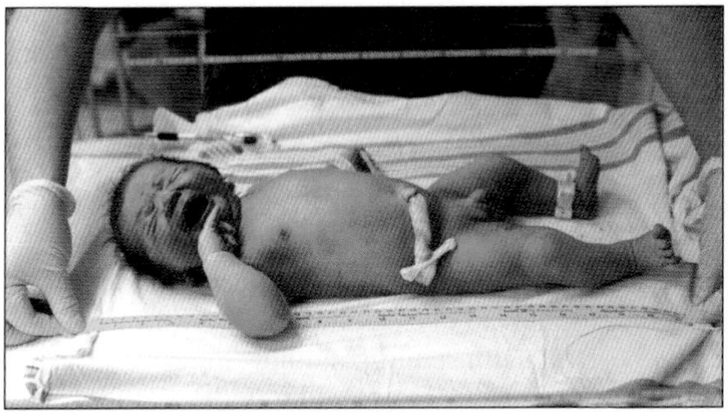

Weighing the neonate

■ Take this measurement before, not after, a feeding. Remove the neonate's diaper before placing him in the middle of the scale tray.

■ Note the neonate's weight. Keep one hand poised over him at all times *to prevent accidents.* Work quickly *to avoid having the scale become soiled or wet and to prevent neonatal heat loss.*

■ Return the neonate to the crib or examination table.

■ If the neonate has clothing or equipment on him (such as an I.V. armband), be sure to record this information.

■ Clean the scale tray *to prevent cross-contamination among neonates.*

Measuring abdominal girth

■ Place the neonate in a supine position, and measure his girth just above the umbilicus. Although not an anthropometric measurement, *the size of this expanse may suggest an abnormality such as an obstruction.*

■ When you finish, diaper and dress the neonate. Return him to his crib, if necessary, or give him to a parent who can hold and comfort him.

Special considerations

■ Keep in mind that head swelling or molding after delivery may skew initial head circumference measurements.

■ Another way to measure length is to place the neonate on paper, such as that used on examination tables. Mark the paper at the heel, with the toes pointing straight up, and at the head; measure the distance between the marks.

■ Various scale models are available. Be sure to learn how to read and operate the one available to you. If you use a model that measures metrically, supply the parents with a table of metric equivalents for use at home.

Documentation

Record each weight and dimension measurement in your notes or neonatal assessment sheet. During routine checkups, remember to share information with the parents, who may also be documenting their child's weight and dimensions.

Average neonatal size and weight

Besides weight, anthropometric measurements include head and chest circumferences and head-to-heel length. These measurements serve as a baseline and show whether the neonate's size is within normal ranges. Anthropometric measurements also reveal the presence of a significant problem or anomaly — especially if values stray far from the mean.

Average initial anthropometric ranges are:

■ Head circumference: 13″ to 14″ (33 to 35.5 cm)

■ Chest circumference: 12″ to 13″ (30.5 to 33 cm)

■ Head to heel length: 18″ to 21″ (46 to 53 cm)

■ Weight: 5 lb 8 oz to 8 lb 13 oz (2,495 to 3,998 g).

SELECTED REFERENCES

American Academy of Pediatrics and American College of Obstetricians and Gynecologists. *Guidelines for Perinatal Care,* 5th ed. Elk Grove Village, Ill.: AAP, 2002; Washington, D.C.:ACOG, 2002.

Bowden, V., and Greenberg, C.S. *Pediatric Nursing Procedures,* 2nd ed. Philadelphia: Lippincott Williams & Wilkins, 2007.

Mattson, S., and Smith, J., eds. *Core Curriculum for Maternal-Newborn Nursing,* 3rd ed. Philadelphia: W.B. Saunders Co., 2004.

Pillitteri, A. *Maternal and Child Health Nursing: Care of the Childbearing and Childrearing Family,* 5th ed. Philadelphia: Lippincott Williams & Wilkins, 2007.

APNEA MONITORING

Apnea in the neonate is defined as cessation of breathing for 20 seconds or longer, or for a shorter period if accompanied by cyanosis or bradycardia. (See *Categories of apnea,* page 886.) Apnea monitors provide an early alert to the caregiver when the breathing rate ceases, allowing for immediate life-saving interventions.

These monitors may be used for vulnerable neonates, such as those born prematurely, those who have survived a life-threatening medical emergency, and those with neurologic disorders, neonatal respiratory distress syndrome, bronchopulmonary dysplasia, congenital heart disease with heart

Categories of apnea

Apnea has long been recognized as a clinical problem in neonates. Considerable investigative and clinical attention has been directed toward this condition. Although progress has been made and certain categories of apnea have been delineated, the cause remains unclear in many situations. Below are listed six categories of apnea.

- Apnea is the cessation of respiratory airflow. This pause in respiration can be the result from central or diaphragmatic (no respiratory effort), obstructive (usually due to upper airway obstruction), or mixed causes. Short (15 seconds), central apnea can be normal at all ages.
- Pathologic apnea is characterized by cyanosis; abrupt, marked pallor or hypotonia; or bradycardia and a prolonged respiratory pause.
- Periodic breathing is a breathing pattern in which there are three or more respiratory pauses of greater than 3 seconds' duration with less than 20 seconds of respiration between pauses. Periodic breathing can be a normal event.
- Apnea of prematurity is periodic breathing with pathologic apnea in a premature neonate. Apnea of prematurity usually ceases by 37 weeks' gestation but occasionally persists to several weeks past term.
- Apparent life-threatening event is an episode characterized by some combination of apnea (central or occasionally obstructive), color change (usually cyanotic or pallid but occasionally erythematous or plethoric), marked change in muscle tone (usually marked limpness), choking, or gagging.
- Apnea of infancy is an unexplained episode of cessation of breathing for 20 seconds or longer, or a shorter respiratory pause associated with bradycardia, cyanosis, pallor, and marked hypotonia.

failure, a tracheostomy, a personal history of sleep-induced apnea, a family history of sudden infant death syndrome, or acute drug withdrawal.

According to the American Academy of Pediatrics, cardiorespiratory monitoring shouldn't be done at home for neonates to prevent sudden infant death syndrome (SIDS) because research hasn't shown a definitive link between apnea monitoring and prevention of SIDS.

Two types of monitors are used most commonly. The thoracic impedance monitor uses chest electrodes to detect conduction changes caused by respirations. The newest models have alarm systems and memories that record cardiorespiratory patterns. The apnea mattress, or underpad monitor, relies on a transducer connected to a pressure-sensitive pad, which detects pressure changes resulting from altered chest movements.

To guard against potentially life-threatening apneic episodes in vulnerable neonates, monitoring begins in the hospital (or birthing center) and continues at home. Parents need to learn how to operate the monitor, what actions to take when the alarm sounds, and how to revive an infant with cardiopulmonary resuscitation (CPR). Crucial steps for correctly using a monitor include testing the alarm system, positioning the sensor properly, and setting the controls correctly. (See *Using a home apnea monitor.*)

According to the National Institutes of Health, the criteria for discontinuing monitoring should be based on the neonate's clinical condition. Clinical experience and the literature support discontinuation when neonates with apparent life-threatening events have been free from significant alarms or apnea (vigorous stimulation or resuscitation wasn't needed) for 2 to 3 months. Additionally, assessing the neonate's ability to tolerate stress (immunizations, illnesses) during this time is advisable.

Equipment

Monitor unit ▪ electrodes ▪ leadwires ▪ electrode belt ▪ electrode gel, if needed ▪ pressure transducer pad, if using apnea mattress ▪ stable surface for monitor placement.

Prepackaged and pretreated disposable electrodes are available.

Implementation

- Confirm the neonate's identity using two patient identifiers according to your facility's policy.
- Explain the procedure to the parents, as appropriate, and wash your hands.
- Plug the monitor's power cord into a grounded wall outlet. Attach the leadwires to the electrodes, and attach the electrodes to the belt. If appropriate, apply conduction gel to the electrodes. (Alternatively, apply gel to the neonate's chest, place the electrodes over the gel, and attach the electrodes to the leadwires. Then secure the belt.)
- *To hold the electrodes securely in position,* wrap the belt snugly but not restrictively around the neonate's chest at the point of greatest movement — optimally at the right and left midaxillary line about ¾″ (2 cm) below the axilla. Be sure to position the leadwires according to the manufacturer's instructions.
- Follow the color code to connect the leadwires to the patient cable. Then connect the cable to the proper jack at the rear of the monitoring unit.

■ Turn the sensitivity controls to maximum *to facilitate tuning when adjusting the system.*
■ Set the alarms according to recommendations so that an apneic period lasting for a specified time activates the signal.
■ Turn on the monitor. If the monitor has two alarms—one to signal apnea, one to signal bradycardia—both will sound as part of the initial self-test of the monitor.
■ Adjust the sensitivity controls until the indicator lights blink with each breath and heartbeat.
■ If you use an apnea mattress, assemble the monitor and pressure transducer pad according to the manufacturer's directions.
■ Plug the monitor into a grounded wall outlet. Then plug the cable of the transducer pad into the monitor.
■ Touch the pad *to make sure it works.* Watch for the monitor's respiration light to blink.
■ Follow the manufacturer's instructions for pad placement.
■ If you have difficulty obtaining a signal, place a foam rubber pad under the mattress, and sandwich the transducer pad between the foam pad and the mattress.
■ If you hear the apnea or bradycardia alarm during monitoring, immediately check the neonate's respirations and color, but don't touch or disturb him until you confirm apnea.
■ If he's still breathing and his color is good, readjust the sensitivity controls or reposition the electrodes, if necessary.
■ If he isn't breathing, but his color looks normal, wait 10 seconds *to see if he starts breathing spontaneously.* If he isn't breathing and he appears pale, dusky, or blue, immediately try to stimulate breathing in these ways: Sequentially, place your hand on the neonate's back, rub him gently, or flick his soles gently. If he doesn't begin to breathe at once, start CPR. (For detailed instructions, see "Cardiopulmonary resuscitation, infant," page 924.)

Special considerations

■ *To ensure accurate operation,* don't put the monitor on top of any other electrical device. Make sure it's on a level surface and can't be bumped easily.
■ Avoid applying lotions, oils, or powders to the neonate's chest, *where they could cause the electrode belt to slip.* Periodically check the alarm by disconnecting the sensor plug. Then listen for the alarm to sound after the preset time delay.
■ In addition to apnea monitoring, the neonate will frequently receive a respiratory stimulant, such a theophylline or caffeine.

Complications

An apneic episode resulting from upper airway obstruction may not trigger the alarm if the neonate continues to make respiratory efforts without gas exchange. However, the monitor's bradycardia alarm may be triggered by the decreased

HOME CARE

Using a home apnea monitor

If a neonate in your care will require the use of a home apnea monitor, you'll need to prepare his parents to operate the equipment safely, correctly, and confidently. First, review the neonate's breathing problem with his parents. Explain that the monitor will warn them of breathing or heart rate changes.

Then offer the following guidelines:

■ Advise the parents to prepare their home and family for the equipment, for example, by providing a sturdy, flat surface for the monitor and by posting emergency telephone numbers (practitioner, nurse, equipment supplier, and ambulance) that are readily accessible.
■ Teach other responsible family members how to use the monitor safely. Suggest that older siblings, grandparents, babysitters, and other caregivers learn cardiopulmonary resuscitation (CPR).
■ Instruct the parents to notify local service authorities—police, ambulance service, telephone company, and electric company—if their neonate uses an apnea monitor *so that alternative power can be supplied if a failure occurs.*
■ Explain to the parents how a monitor with electrodes works. Advise them to make sure the respirator indicator goes on each time the neonate breathes. If it doesn't, describe troubleshooting techniques such as moving the electrodes slightly. Tell them to try this technique several times.
■ Show the parents how to respond to the apnea and bradycardia alarms. Direct them to check the color of the neonate's oral tissues. If the tissues appear bluish and the neonate isn't breathing, tell them to call loudly and touch him—gently at first, then more urgently, as needed. Tell them to stop short of shaking him. If he doesn't respond, urge them to begin CPR.
■ Advise the parents to keep the operator's manual attached to or beside the monitor and to consult it as needed. Explain that an activated loose-lead alarm, for example, may indicate a dirty electrode, a loose electrode patch, a loose belt, or a disconnected or malfunctioning wire or monitor.

How to instill medication for neonatal eye prophylaxis

Using your nondominant hand, gently raise the neonate's upper eyelid with your index finger and pull down the lower eyelid with your thumb. Using your dominant hand, apply the ordered ophthalmic antibiotic ointment in a line along the lower conjunctival sac (as shown below). Then close the eyes *to allow ointment to spread across the conjunctiva.* Repeat the procedure for the other eye.

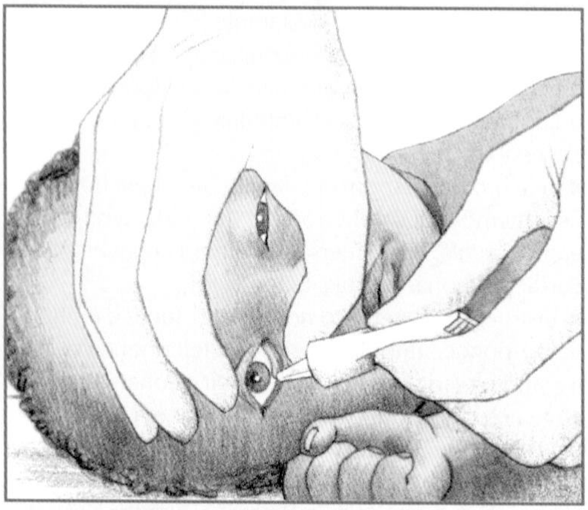

heart rate resulting from the vagal stimulation (which accompanies obstruction).

If you're using a thoracic impedance monitor without a bradycardia alarm, you may interpret bradycardia during apnea as shallow breathing *because this type of monitor fails to distinguish between respiratory movement and the large cardiac stroke volume associated with bradycardia.* In this case, the alarm won't sound until the heart rate drops below the apnea limit.

Documentation

Record all alarm incidents. Document the time and duration of apnea. Describe the neonate's color, the stimulation measures implemented, and any other pertinent information. Document any medications given.

SELECTED REFERENCES

American Academy of Pediatrics. "Policy Statement: Apnea, Sudden Infant Death Syndrome, and Home Monitoring," *Pediatrics* 111(4):914-17, April 2003.

Bowden, V., and Greenberg, C.S. *Pediatric Nursing Procedures,* 2nd ed. Philadelphia: Lippincott Williams & Wilkins, 2008.

Hall, K.L., and Zalman, B. "Evaluation and Management of Apparent Life-Threatening Events in Children," *American Family Physicians* 71(12):2301-308, June 2005.

Silvestri, J.M., et al. "Factors that Influence Use of a Home Cardiorespiratory Monitor for Infants: The Collaborative Home Infant Monitoring Evaluation," *Archives of Pediatric and Adolescent Medicine* 159(1):18-24, January 2005.

NEONATAL TREATMENTS

EYE PROPHYLAXIS

The instillation of antibiotic ointment into the neonate's eyes prevents blindness and eye damage from conjunctivitis due to *Neisseria gonorrhoeae* and *Chlamydia,* which the neonate may have acquired from the mother as he passed through the birth canal. This treatment is legally required in most states. It's recommended to prevent gonococcal ophthalmia but efficacy against Chlamydia eye infections isn't clear.

The Centers for Disease Control and Prevention (CDC) recommends a single application of Erythromycin (0.5%) ointment or Tetracycline ophthalmic ointment (1%).

Equipment

Ophthalmic antibiotic ointment, as ordered.

Preparation of equipment

Remove the cap from the ointment container. A single-dose ointment tube should be used *to prevent contamination and spread of infection.*

Implementation

- Confirm the patient's identity using two patient identifiers according to your facility's policy.
- If the parents are present for the procedure, explain that state law mandates neonatal eye prophylaxis. Forewarn them that the neonate may cry and that the treatment may irritate his eyes. Reassure them that these are temporary effects.
- Wash your hands and put on gloves.
- *To ensure comfort and effectiveness,* shield the neonate's eyes from direct light, tilt his head slightly to the side of the intended treatment, and instill the medication. (See *How to instill medication for neonatal eye prophylaxis.*)
- Close and manipulate the eyelids to spread the medication over the eye.

Special considerations

■ Treatment should be administered immediately upon admission if the neonate is born outside of the facility.

Documentation

If you perform neonatal eye prophylaxis in the delivery room, record the treatment on the delivery room form. If you perform it in the nursery, document it in your notes.

SELECTED REFERENCES

American Academy of Pediatrics and American College of Obstetricians and Gynecologists. *Guidelines for Perinatal Care,* 5th ed. Elk Grove Village, Ill.: AAP, 2002; Washington, D.C.: ACOG, 2002.

Department of Health and Human Services, Centers for Disease Control and Prevention (CDC). "Sexually Transmitted Diseases Treatment Guidelines 2002." Available at *http://www.cdc.gov/STD/treatment/4-2002TG.htm.*

Pillitteri, A. *Maternal and Child Health Nursing: Care of the Childbearing and Childrearing Family,* 5th ed. Philadelphia: Lippincott Williams & Wilkins, 2007.

THERMOREGULATION

A large body surface-to-mass ratio, reduced metabolism per unit area, limited amounts of insulating subcutaneous fat, vasomotor instability, and limited metabolic capacity make all neonates susceptible to hypothermia. To stay warm when he's cold-stressed, the neonate metabolizes brown fat. Unique to neonates, brown fat has energy-producing mitochondria in its cells, which enhance its capacity for heat production.

Brown fat metabolism effectively warms the body but only within a narrow temperature range. Without careful external thermoregulation, the neonate may become chilled. Hypoxia, acidosis, hypoglycemia, pulmonary vasoconstriction, and even death may result.

Thermoregulation provides a neutral thermal environment that helps the neonate maintain a normal core temperature with minimal oxygen consumption and caloric expenditure. Although it varies with the neonate, the average core temperature is 97.7° F (36.5° C).

Two kinds of thermoregulators are common in a hospital nursery: radiant warmers and incubators. The radiant warmer controls environmental temperature while the nurse gives initial care in the delivery room. Then, when the neonate arrives in the nursery, another radiant warmer may be used until his temperature stabilizes and he can occupy a bassinet. If the temperature doesn't stabilize or if the neonate has a condition that affects thermoregulation, a temperature-controlled incubator will house him. (See *Understanding thermoregulators,* page 890.)

Equipment

Radiant warmer or incubator (if necessary) ■ blankets ■ washcloths or towels ■ skin probe ■ adhesive pad ■ water-soluble lubricant ■ thermometer ■ clothing (including a cap) ■ optional: stockinette gauze.

Preparation of equipment

Turn on the radiant warmer in the delivery room, and set the desired temperature. Warm the blankets, washcloths, or towels under a heat source.

Implementation

Continue nursing measures to conserve neonatal body warmth until the patient's discharge.

In the delivery room

■ Place the neonate under the radiant warmer, and dry him with the warm washcloths or towels *to prevent heat loss by evaporation.*

■ Pay special attention to drying his scalp and hair. Then, if you take him off the warmer, make sure you cover his head (which makes up about 25% of neonatal body surface) with a ready-made cap *to prevent heat loss.*

■ Perform required procedures quickly *to reduce the neonate's exposure to cool delivery room air.*

■ Wrap him in the warmed blankets. If his condition permits, give him to his parents *to promote bonding.*

■ Transport the neonate to the nursery in the warmed blankets. Use a transport incubator when the nursery is far from the delivery room.

In the nursery

■ Remove the blankets and cap, and place the neonate under the radiant warmer.

■ Use the adhesive pad to attach the temperature control probe to his skin in the right upper abdominal quadrant. *This lets the servo control maintain neonatal axillary skin temperature between 97.5° and 99.5° F (36.4° and 37.5° C) or rectal temperature of 97.8° to 99° F (36.5° to 37.2° C).* If the neonate will lie prone, put the skin probe on his back *to ensure accurate temperature control and avoid false-high readings from the neonate lying on the probe.* Don't cover the device with anything *because this could interfere with the servo control.* Be sure to raise the warmer's side panels *to prevent accidents.*

■ Lubricate the thermometer, and take the neonate's rectal temperature on admission *to assess for rectal patency and to determine core temperature.* Take axillary temperatures thereafter *to avoid injuring delicate rectal mucosa.* Usually, axillary temperature readings are lower than the core temperature.

EQUIPMENT

Understanding thermoregulators

Thermoregulators preserve neonatal body warmth in various ways. A radiant warmer maintains the neonate's temperature by *radiation*. An incubator maintains the neonate's temperature by *conduction* and *convection*.

Temperature settings

Radiant warmers and incubators have two operating modes: *nonservo* and *servo*. The nurse manually sets temperature controls on nonservo equipment; a probe on the neonate's skin controls temperature settings on servo models.

Other features

Most thermoregulators come with alarms. Incubators have the added advantage of providing a stable, enclosed environment, which protects the neonate from evaporative cooling.

Radiant warmer

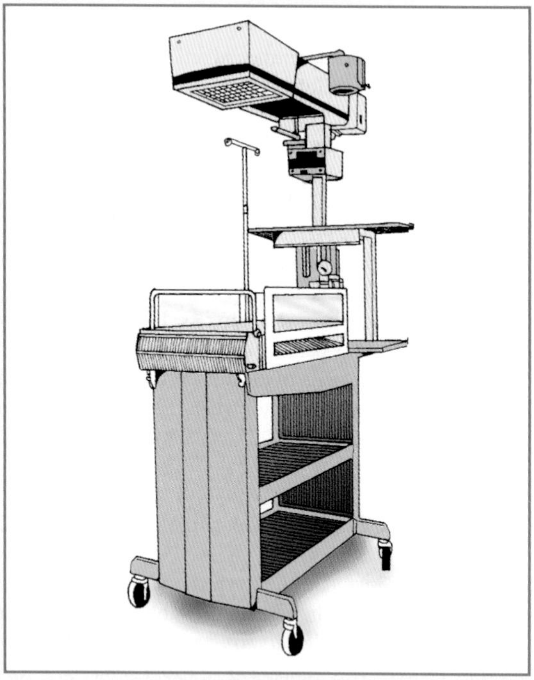

Incubator

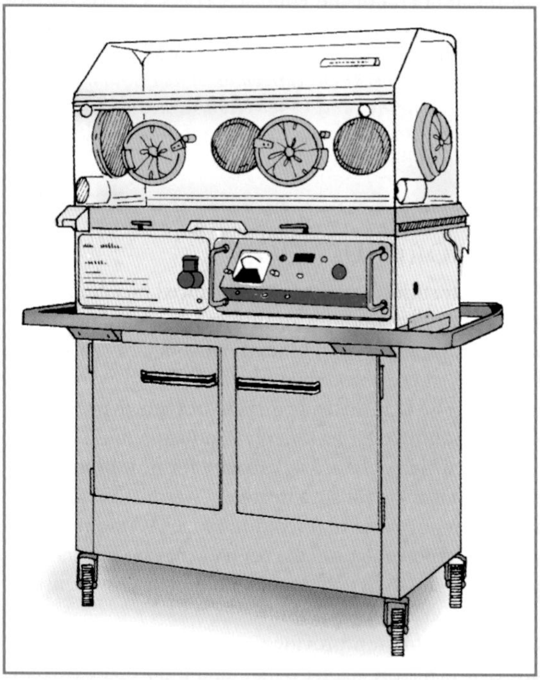

Take axillary temperatures every 15 to 30 minutes until the temperature stabilizes, then every 4 hours *to ensure stability.*

- Sponge-bathe the neonate under the warmer only after his temperature stabilizes and his glucose level is normal, and leave him under the warmer until his temperature remains stable.
- Take appropriate action if the temperature doesn't stabilize. The neonate should be warmed slowly, *as rapid warming may cause heat-induced apnea, hypotension, and shock.* If the neonate is in a double-walled incubator, begin by setting the air temperature at 96.8° F (36° C). Increase humidity *to decrease heat loss.* Retake the neonate's temperature in 15 to 30 minutes. If the temperature continues to fall, increase the incubator air temperature to 98.6° F (37° C) and evaluate the environment for missed sources of heat loss. If the neonate's temperature continues to fall after 15 minutes, increase the air temperature to 99.5° F (37.5° C) and consider adding a radiant warmer over the incubator *to increase external wall temperatures.* Check for signs of infection, which can cause hypothermia.

■ Apply a skin probe to the neonate in an incubator as you would for a neonate in a radiant warmer. Move the incubator away from cold walls or objects.

■ Perform all required procedures quickly *to maintain a neutral thermal environment and to minimize heat loss.* Close portholes in the hood immediately after completing any procedure, *also to reduce heat loss.* If procedures must be performed outside the incubator, do them under a radiant warmer.

■ To leave the hospital or to move to a bassinet, a neonate must be weaned from the incubator. Slowly reduce the incubator's temperature to that of the nursery. Check periodically for hypothermia. *To ensure temperature stability,* never discharge the neonate to home directly from an incubator.

■ When the neonate's temperature stabilizes, dress him, put him in a bassinet, and cover him with a blanket.

Special considerations

■ Always warm oxygen before administering it to a neonate *to avoid initiating heat loss from his head and face.*

■ *To prevent conductive heat loss,* preheat the radiant warmer bed and linen; warm stethoscopes and other instruments before use; and pad the scale with paper or a preweighed, warmed sheet before weighing the neonate.

■ *To avoid convective heat loss,* place the neonate's bed out of direct line of an open window, fan, or an air-conditioning vent.

■ *To control evaporative heat loss,* dry the neonate immediately after delivery. When bathing the neonate, expose only one body part at a time; wash each part thoroughly, and then dry it immediately.

■ Review the reasons for regulating body temperature with the neonate's family. Instruct them to keep him wrapped in a blanket and out of drafts when he isn't in the bassinet, both in the facility and at home. In a warm place, guard against overheating the neonate.

Complications

Hypothermia from ineffective natural or external thermoregulation can inhibit weight gain *because the neonate must use caloric energy to maintain his temperature.* Hyperthermia can cause increased oxygen consumption and apnea. Both conditions can result from equipment failures or insufficient monitoring.

Documentation

Name the heat source, and record its temperature and the neonate's temperature, whenever taken. Document any complications that result from using thermoregulatory equipment.

SELECTED REFERENCES

Bowden, V., and Greenberg, C.S. *Pediatric Nursing Procedures,* 2nd ed. Philadelphia: Lippincott Williams & Wilkins, 2007.

Mattson, S., and Smith, J., eds. *Core Curriculum for Maternal-Newborn Nursing,* 3rd ed. Philadelphia: W.B. Saunders Co., 2004.

Pillitteri, A. *Maternal and Child Health Nursing: Care of the Childbearing and Childrearing Family,* 5th ed. Philadelphia: Lippincott Williams & Wilkins, 2007.

Sherman, T.I. "Optimizing the Neonatal Thermal Environment," *Neonatal Network* 25(4):251-60, July-August 2006.

Watkinson, M. "Temperature Control of Premature Infants in the Delivery Room," *Clinics in Perinatology* 33(1):43-53, March 2006.

OXYGEN ADMINISTRATION

The neonate with signs and symptoms of respiratory distress — such as cyanosis, pallor, tachypnea, nasal flaring, bradycardia, hypothermia, retractions, hypotonia, hyporeflexia, expiratory grunting, and arterial blood gas (ABG) levels indicating hypoxia — will probably need oxygen. Also, because of his small size and special respiratory requirements, he'll need special equipment and administration techniques.

In an emergency, for instance, a handheld resuscitation bag and a small oxygen mask may be sufficient until more permanent measures can be initiated. When the neonate requires additional oxygen above the ambient concentration, the oxygen can be delivered by means of an oxygen hood or nasal prongs. If he needs continuous positive airway pressure (CPAP) to prevent alveolar collapse at the end of a breath (as in respiratory distress syndrome), he may receive oxygen through a nasopharyngeal or an endotracheal (ET) tube. (Oxygenation typically improves with CPAP and any pulmonary shunting tends to decrease.) If the neonate can't breathe on his own or needs to conserve his energy, he may receive oxygen through a ventilator.

No matter which system delivers the oxygen, the therapy is potentially hazardous to the neonate. The gas must be warmed and humidified to prevent hypothermia and dehydration. In high concentrations over prolonged periods, oxygen can cause retrolental fibroplasia (which results in blindness). If the concentration is too low, hypoxia and central nervous system damage may occur. Also, depending on how it's delivered, oxygen can contribute to bronchopulmonary dysplasia.

In some cases, extracorporeal membrane oxygenation, an alternative to oxygen administration, may help neonates who have severe hypoxia. This technique also relies on a supplemental oxygen source. (See *Extracorporeal membrane oxygenation,* page 892.)

Extracorporeal membrane oxygenation

Available in designated centers throughout the United States, extracorporeal membrane oxygenation (ECMO) was developed from cardiopulmonary bypass methods used during heart surgery. In this procedure, a machine circulates the patient's venous blood outside his body, passes the blood through a membrane oxygenator, and returns the newly oxygenated blood to the circulation. ECMO circuitry works by venoarterial bypass or venovenous bypass methods.

For neonates who meet stringent criteria, indications for ECMO include hyaline membrane disease, meconium aspiration, and congenital heart defects. Typically, the procedure is used as a last resort after maximum ventilatory support measures fail and when survival chances drop below 10%.

For neonates who require long-term oxygen therapy at home, special delivery systems are available. (See *Comparing home oxygen delivery systems.*)

Equipment

Oxygen source (wall, cylinder, or liquid unit) ▪ compressed air source ▪ flowmeters ▪ nasal prongs ▪ blender or Y connector ▪ large- and small-bore oxygen tubing (sterile) ▪ warming-humidifying device ▪ blood gas analyzer ▪ thermometer ▪ stethoscope ▪ nasogastric (NG) tube.

For handheld resuscitation bag and mask delivery: Specially sized mask with handheld resuscitation bag ▪ manometer with connectors. (The resuscitation bag must have a pressure-release valve.)

For oxygen hood delivery: Appropriate-sized oxygen hood.

For nasal prong delivery: Nasal prongs.

For CPAP delivery: Manometer with connectors ▪ nasopharyngeal or ET tube ▪ water-soluble lubricant ▪ hypoallergenic tape.

For delivery with a ventilator: Ventilator unit with manometer and in-line thermometer ▪ specimen tubes for ABG analyses ▪ ET tube ▪ optional: pulse oximeter.

Preparation of equipment

Wash your hands. Gather the necessary equipment, and assemble it according to manufacturer's recommendations.

To calibrate the oxygen analyzer: Turn the analyzer on and read the results. Room air should be about 21% oxygen. Check the analyzer power or battery level. Expose the analyzer probe to 100% oxygen and adjust sensitivity as necessary. Then recheck the amount of oxygen in room air.

To set up a handheld resuscitation bag and mask: Place the resuscitation bag and mask in the crib. Connect the large-bore oxygen tubing to the mask outlet. Then use connectors and small-bore tubing to connect a manometer to the bag. Next, connect the free end of the oxygen tubing to the warming-humidifying device, and fill the device with sterile water. Turn on the device when you're ready to use it, or prepare it according to the manufacturer's instructions.

Connect another piece of small-bore tubing to the inlet of the warming-humidifying device. Attach a Y connector to the opposite end of this tubing. Place a piece of small-bore tubing on each end of the Y connector, and connect the pieces of tubing to the flowmeters. Place an in-line thermometer as close as possible to the delivery end of the apparatus.

To set up an oxygen hood: Bring a clean oxygen hood and tubing if needed to the neonate's bedside. If the neonate was receiving oxygen via bag and mask, remove them from the connecting tubing. Attach the oxygen hood to this tubing. Place an in-line thermometer as close to the neonate as possible whenever using warmed oxygen.

Implementation

- Always wash your hands before working with a neonate *to prevent cross-contamination after handling other neonates.*

Using a handheld resuscitation bag and mask

- Turn on the oxygen and compressed air flowmeters to the prescribed flow rates.
- Place the mask on the neonate's face. Don't cover the neonate's eyes. Check pressure settings and mask size *to ensure that air doesn't leak from the mask's edges.*
- As you work to stabilize the neonate, have another staff member notify the practitioner immediately.
- Provide 40 to 60 breaths/minute. Use enough pressure to cause a visible rise and fall of the neonate's chest. Provide enough oxygen to maintain pink nail beds and mucous membranes. If you can't reach the practitioner during the emergency, deliver the oxygen percentage defined by your hospital's emergency policy.
- Continuously watch the neonate's chest movements and listen to breath sounds. Avoid overventilation, *which will blow off too much carbon dioxide and cause apnea.* If the neonate's heart rate falls below 100 beats/minute and fails to rise, continue to use the handheld resuscitation bag until the heart rate rises to 100 beats/minute or higher.
- Insert an NG tube *to vent air from the neonate's stomach.*

HOME CARE

Comparing home oxygen delivery systems

If a neonate in your care is discharged on oxygen, the delivery system prescribed may depend on such factors as equipment availability and parental skill levels. Other factors to consider include the liter flow (or oxygen concentration) required and appropriate administration equipment, for example, nasal cannula or catheter, oxygen hood, tent, high-flow mask, or nebulizer.

The nasal cannula, which provides a direct flow of oxygen to the nostrils, is the most common oxygen delivery device for home use. It imposes the fewest restrictions on a child attempting to interact with the environment. For instance, attaching extension tubing (up to 50′ [15.2 m]) to the cannula allows the child to move freely from room to room. However, the cannula can become dislodged from the nostrils with extensive manipulation. Velcro straps or adhesive dressings can reduce this risk by securing the cannula in the proper position. Common oxygen sources include the oxygen concentrator, cylinder oxygen, and liquid oxygen. When selecting the appropriate system for home care, the health care team looks at advantages and disadvantages, such as those that follow.

SYSTEM	ADVANTAGES	DISADVANTAGES
OXYGEN CONCENTRATOR		
Separates oxygen from ambient air and provides low-flow oxygen	■ Cost-effective for the neonate who needs continuous low-flow oxygen	■ Can't be used with a high-flow mask or nebulizer ■ Requires electricity ■ Requires an oxygen cylinder as a backup in case of malfunction or power failure ■ Bulky and noisy ■ Emits heat
CYLINDER OXYGEN		
Uses oxygen stored as a gas in a cylinder with a valve	■ Cost-effective for the neonate who requires high-flow oxygen or intermittent oxygen for up to 12 hours daily ■ Can be used with a high-flow oxygen mask, a nasal cannula, a nasal catheter, or a nebulizer ■ Portable when a small cylinder is used	■ Requires a humidification source if the flow must exceed 0.75 L ■ Must be used with caution and kept in a stand or cart; safety cap must be fastened securely in case the neonate falls
LIQUID OXYGEN		
Uses oxygen stored in a liquid state under high pressure in a cylinder with a valve	■ Cost-effective for the neonate who needs continuous low- to moderate-flow oxygen ■ Usually can be used with any oxygen delivery method ■ Smaller and more lightweight than other oxygen systems ■ Refillable, portable units available for when the neonate travels	■ Humidification source required if flow must exceed 0.75 L ■ May cause burns if oxygen comes into contact with skin during transfer from a stationary to a portable unit ■ Upright position required for cylinder

Using an oxygen hood

- Remove the connecting tubing from the face mask and connect it to the oxygen hood. Activate oxygen and a compressed air source, if needed, at ordered flow rates.
- Place the oxygen hood over the neonate's head.
- Measure the amount of oxygen the neonate is receiving with the oxygen analyzer. Be sure to place the analyzer probe close to the neonate's nose. Adjust the oxygen to the prescribed amount.

Using nasal prongs

- Match the prong size to the neonate's nose. Apply a small amount of water-soluble lubricant to the outside of the prongs. Turn on the oxygen and compressed air, if necessary. Connect the prongs to the oxygen tubing. Insert the prongs into the nose and steady them.
- Be sure to clean the prongs each shift *to ensure patency.*

Using CPAP

- Position the neonate on his back with a rolled towel under his neck *to keep the airway open without hyperextending the neck.*
- If you're administering oxygen through a nasopharyngeal or an ET tube, obtain the correct size tube. Turn on the oxygen and compressed air source. Then assist the practitioner with inserting the ET tube, attaching the oxygen delivery system (as set up for mask and bag delivery), and taping the tube in place. Next, insert an NG or orogastric tube, and leave it in place *to keep the stomach decompressed,* if ordered. Leave it open unless the neonate is receiving gavage feedings. Suction the nasal passages and oropharynx every 2 hours or as needed *to maintain an open airway.* Apply suction only while removing the suction catheter.

Using a ventilator

- Turn on the ventilator and set the controls, as ordered.
- Help the practitioner insert the ET tube, if appropriate.
- Connect the ET tube to the ventilator, and tape the tube securely.
- As with any delivery system, carefully watch the manometer *to maintain pressure at the prescribed level.* Also monitor the in-line thermometer *for correct temperature.*
- Monitor ABG levels every 15 to 20 minutes (or other reasonable interval) after any changes in oxygen concentration or pressure. Draw blood samples for ABG analysis from an umbilical artery catheter, radial artery catheter, or radial artery puncture. If desired, obtain capillary blood by warmed heel stick — this provides accurate levels of pH and carbon dioxide, but not oxygen. If ordered, monitor oxygen perfusion with pulse oximetry or mixed venous oxygen saturation monitoring.
- Keep the practitioner aware of ABG levels *so he can order appropriate changes in oxygen concentration.* Usually, partial pressure of oxygen is maintained at 60 to 90 mm Hg for an arterial sample and at 40 to 60 mm Hg for a capillary sample.
- Auscultate the lungs for crackles, rhonchi, and bilateral breath sounds.

Special considerations

- When administering oxygen, always take safety precautions *to avoid fire or explosion.* As soon as possible, explain the situation and the procedures to the parents. Take measures to keep the neonate warm *because hypothermia impedes respiration.*
- Check ABG levels at least every hour whenever the unstable neonate receives high oxygen concentrations or experiences a clinical change. If he doesn't respond to oxygen administration, check for congenital anomalies.
- Perform neonatal chest auscultation carefully *to hear subtle respiratory changes.* Also be alert for respiratory distress signs, and be prepared to perform emergency procedures. If required, perform chest physiotherapy and percussion, as ordered. Follow with suctioning *to remove secretions.* As ordered, discontinue oxygen when the neonate's fraction of inspired oxygen (FIO_2) reaches room air level and his arterial oxygen stabilizes at 60 to 90 mm Hg. Repeat ABG analysis 20 to 30 minutes after discontinuing oxygen and thereafter as ordered by the practitioner or by your facility's policy.
- If the neonate will receive oxygen over a lengthy time span, prepare his parents or other caregivers to administer oxygen at home.

Complications

Infection or "drowning" can result from overhumidification, which allows water to collect in tubing and then provides a growth medium for bacteria or suffocates the neonate. Hypothermia and increased oxygen consumption can result from administering cool oxygen. Metabolic and respiratory acidosis may follow inadequate ventilation.

Pressure ulcers may develop on the neonate's head, face, and around the nose during prolonged oxygen therapy. A pulmonary air leak (pneumothorax, pneumomediastinum, pneumopericardium, interstitial emphysema) may develop spontaneously with respiratory distress or result from forced ventilation. Decreased cardiac output may come from excessive CPAP.

Documentation

Note any respiratory distress that requires oxygen administration, the oxygen concentration given, and the delivery method. Record each change in oxygen concentration and the neonate's FIO_2 as measured by the oxygen analyzer. Note all routine checks of oxygen concentration. Document all ABG values, the times that samples were obtained, the neonate's condition during therapy, times suctioned, the amount and consistency of mucus, the type of continuous oxygen monitoring (if any), and any complications. Note respiratory rate, and describe breath sounds and any signs of additional respiratory distress.

SELECTED REFERENCES

American Heart Association. "2005 American Heart Association Guidelines for Cardiopulmonary Resuscitation and Emergency Cardiovascular Care," *Circulation* 112:iv-1-iv-203, December 2005.

Bowden, V., and Greenberg, C.S. *Pediatric Nursing Procedures*, 2nd ed. Philadelphia: Lippincott Williams & Wilkins, 2008.

Finer, N.N., et al. "Delivery Room Continuous Positive Airway Pressure/Positive End Expiratory Pressure in Extremely Low Birth Weight Infants: A Feasibility Trial," *Pediatrics* 114(3):651-57, September 2004.

Higgins, R.D., et al. "Executive Summary of the Workshop on Oxygen in Neonatal Therapies: Controversies and Opportunities for Research," *Pediatrics* 119(4):790-96, April 2007.

Jackson, J.K., et al. "Standardizing Nasal Cannula Oxygen Administration in the Neonatal Intensive Care Unit," *Pediatrics* 118(suppl 2):S187-96, November 2006.

Mattson, S., and Smith, J., eds. *Core Curriculum for Maternal-Newborn Nursing,* 3rd ed. Philadelphia: W.B. Saunders Co., 2004.

Shoemaker, M.T., et al. "High Flow Nasal Cannula Versus Nasal CPAP for Neonatal Respiratory Disease: A Retrospective Study," *Journal of Perinatology* 27(2):85-91, February 2007.

PHOTOTHERAPY

Phototherapy involves exposing the neonate to high-intensity fluorescent light that breaks down bilirubin (a pigment of red blood cells [RBCs]) for transport to the GI system and excretion. The treatment is commonly given to neonates with hyperbilirubinemia — a symptom of physiologic jaundice, breast-milk jaundice, or hemolytic disease. Phototherapy continues until bilirubin drops to normal levels because unchecked hyperbilirubinemia can lead to kernicterus (deposits of unconjugated bilirubin in the brain cells), permanent brain damage, and even death.

Physiologic jaundice — resulting from the neonate's high RBC count and short RBC life span — develops 2 to 3 days after delivery in about 50% of full-term neonates and 3 to 5 days in about 80% of premature neonates.

Breast-feeding jaundice typically develops several days after birth. It's thought to be related to decreased caloric intake and hydration due to ineffective breast-feeding. The American Association of Pediatrics (AAP) recommends early and frequent breast-feeding for the neonate; this helps stimulate peristalsis, which increases bilirubin excretion.

Treatment for hemolytic disease, a much more serious condition, includes phototherapy and exchange transfusions. In pathologic jaundice, which occurs within 12 hours of birth and raises serum bilirubin levels above 13 mg/dl, phototherapy may be used with appropriate treatment of the underlying cause.

There's continuing controversy regarding the management of jaundice in the healthy neonate. Several key issues include determining when to initiate phototherapy using total serum bilirubin level as an indicator, adverse effects of phototherapy versus adverse effects of hyperbilirubinemia, and whether phototherapy should be continuous or intermittent. The AAP has guidelines regarding initiating phototherapy treatment in the neonate. (See *AAP phototherapy guidelines,* page 896.)

Equipment

Phototherapy unit ▪ photometer ▪ opaque eye mask ▪ thermometer ▪ urometer ▪ surgical face mask or small diaper ▪ optional: thermistor (if the phototherapy unit is combined with a temperature-controlled radiant heat warmer) or incubator (if the neonate is small for his gestational age); bilimeter.

Prepackaged eye coverings are available.

Preparation of equipment

Set up the phototherapy unit about 18″ (46 cm) above the neonate's crib. Verify placement of the light-bulb shield *because this device filters ultraviolet rays and protects the neonate from broken bulbs.* If the neonate is in an incubator, place the phototherapy unit at least 3″ (7.6 cm) above the incubator *to promote sufficient airflow and prevent overheating.* Turn on the lights. Place a photometer probe in the middle of the crib *to measure the energy emitted by the lights.* The AAP recommends an energy range of 8 to 10 $\mu w/cm^2$/nanometer for low-intensity phototherapy and 30 $\mu w/cm^2$/nanometer or higher for high-intensity therapy.

Implementation

- Confirm the neonate's identity using two patient identifiers according to your facility's policy.
- Verify the practitioner's order to initiate therapy.
- Explain the procedure to the parents *to reduce their anxiety and guilt and to ensure cooperation.*
- Record the neonate's initial bilirubin level and his axillary temperature *to establish baseline measurements.*
- Place the opaque eye mask over the neonate's closed eyes. Fasten the mask securely enough to stay in place and to prevent the neonate from opening his eyes, but loosely enough to ensure circulation and avoid pressure on the eyeballs. *This*

AAP phototherapy guidelines

The American Academy of Pediatrics (AAP) has recommendations on when to initiate phototherapy for treating hyperbilirubinemia in neonates. Term neonates who are clinically jaundiced before 24 hours aren't considered healthy and require further evaluation.

AGE (HOURS)	TOTAL SERUM (TSB) LEVEL CONSIDER BILIRUBIN BASED ON CLINICAL JUDGEMENT	TSB LEVEL TREAT WITH PHOTOTHERAPY
25 to 48	≥ 12	≥15
49 to 72	≥15	≥18
> 72	≥17	≥20

Reproduced with permission from American Academy of Pediatrics. "Practice Parameter: Management of Hyperbilirubinemia in the Healthy Term Newborn," *Pediatrics* 94:558-65, October 1994.

protects the eyes and prevents reflex bradycardia and head molding.

■ Clean the eyes periodically *to remove drainage and check circulation.*

■ Remove eye patches for 5 to 10 minutes every 4 hours *to observe for irritation or drainage,* and also remove them for short periods during parental visits *to encourage bonding.*

■ Undress the neonate *to expose the most skin to the most light.* Remember to place a diaper under him and to cover male genitalia with a surgical mask or a small diaper *to catch urine and to prevent possible testicular damage from the heat and light waves.*

■ Take the neonate's axillary temperature 30 minutes after phototherapy is started and then every 2 hours *to make sure the neonate maintains a normal and stable body temperature.*

■ If the neonate is in a servo-controlled incubator or a radiant warmer, place the thermistor on the neonate's side and cover it with opaque or reflective tape. *This prevents frequent sensor changes and protects the sensor from direct energy.*

■ Provide additional warmth, if necessary, by adjusting the warming unit's thermostat.

■ Monitor elimination. Note urine and stool amounts and frequency. Weigh the neonate twice daily, and watch for dehydration signs (dry skin, poor turgor, depressed fontanels) *because phototherapy increases fluid loss through stools and evaporation.*

■ Clean the neonate carefully after each bowel movement *because the loose green stools that result from phototherapy can excoriate the skin.* Don't apply ointment *because this can cause burns under phototherapy lights.*

■ Check urine specific gravity with a urometer *to gauge the neonate's hydration status.*

■ Feed the neonate every 3 to 4 hours and offer water between feedings *to ensure adequate hydration and to boost gastric motility.* Make sure water intake doesn't replace breast milk or formula. The breast-fed neonate should be encouraged to eat every 2 to 3 hours (8 to 10 times in 24 hours). Don't give the breast-feeding neonate supplements with water or dextrose.

■ Reposition the neonate every 2 hours *to expose all body surfaces to the light and to prevent head molding and skin breakdown from pressure.*

■ Assess jaundice by blanching the skin with digital pressure over a bony prominence and determine the underlying color of the skin in the blanched area.

■ Check the bilirubin level at least once every 24 hours—more often if levels rise significantly. If you don't use a bilimeter, turn off the phototherapy unit before drawing venous blood for testing *because the lights may degrade bilirubin in the blood sample, resulting in inaccurate test results.*

■ Notify the practitioner if the bilirubin level nears 20 mg/dl in full-term neonates, or 15 mg/dl in premature neonates, *because these levels may lead to kernicterus.*

■ Review the neonatal and maternal histories for clues to possible hyperbilirubinemia causes. Also watch for signs of infection and metabolic disorders, and check the neonate's hematocrit for polycythemia. Inspect the neonate for hematoma, bruising, petechiae, and cyanosis. If the phototherapy unit has blue lights, turn them off for the examination *because these lights can mask cyanosis.*

Special considerations

■ If the neonate cries excessively during phototherapy, place a blanket roll on each side of him *to give him a feeling of security.*

■ If the practitioner diagnoses breast-feeding jaundice (suspending breast-feeding temporarily), teach the mother to express milk manually or with a pump. Encourage continued breast-feeding when indicated. Reassure the parents by explaining that jaundice is transitory. If possible, give phototherapy treatment in the mother's room *to facilitate bonding and to decrease parental anxiety and guilt feelings.*

Home care

Home phototherapy programs are safe and effective alternatives for treating uncomplicated neonatal jaundice. Teach the parents how to perform the procedure, and encourage their compliance. Explain that testing will continue until results show serum bilirubin at acceptable levels. Provide written instructions at discharge.

Complications

Phototherapy may cause complications, such as dehydration due to increases in insensible water loss, hypothermia or hyperthermia as a result of total skin surface exposure, diarrhea, and bronze baby syndrome (an idiopathic darkening of the skin, serum, and urine). Changes in feeding and activity patterns and hormonal secretions may follow prolonged therapy.

Documentation

At least once every 2 hours, note the progress of phototherapy and that the neonate's eyes remain protected. Record the time of all bilirubin testing, and plot results. Document eye covering changes and eye care given. Keep records of measured radiant energy — initially and then every 8 hours. Document neonatal time away from lights, for example, for feeding or other procedures. Note fluid intake and the amount of urine and feces eliminated. Describe any changes in skin appearance and character, in feeding patterns, and in activity level.

SELECTED REFERENCES

American Academy of Pediatrics. Subcommittee on Hyperbilirubinemia. "Management of Hyperbilirubinemia in the Newborn Infant 35 or More Weeks of Gestation: Practice Guideline," *Pediatrics* 114(1):297-316, July 2004.

Bowden, V., and Greenberg, C.S. *Pediatric Nursing Procedures*, 2nd ed. Philadelphia: Lippincott Williams & Wilkins, 2008.

National Association of Neonatal Nurses. Position Statement 3040: Prevention of Bilirubin Encephalopathy and Kernicterus in Newborns, August 2003.

Pillitteri, A. *Maternal and Child Health Nursing: Care of the Childbearing and Childrearing Family*, 5th ed. Philadelphia: Lippincott Williams & Wilkins, 2007.

Schwoebel, A., and Gebbaro, S. "Neonatal Hyperbilirubinemia," *Journal of Perinatal and Neonatal Nursing* 20(1):103-107, January-March 2007.

NEONATAL FEEDING

BREAST-FEEDING ASSISTANCE

Breast-feeding is the safest, simplest, and least-expensive way to provide complete infant nourishment. Components of successful and satisfying breast-feeding include proper breast care, normal milk flow, and a comfortably positioned mother and infant.

Breast-feeding is contraindicated for a mother with a severe chronic condition, such as active untreated tuberculosis, human immunodeficiency virus infection, some forms of hepatitis, severe heart disease, or drug or alcohol addiction.

Equipment

Nursing or support bra ■ pillow ■ protective cover, such as cloth diaper or small towel ■ optional: commercially available breast pads without plastic liners, or pads made from sanitary napkins, gauze, cloth diapers, or cotton handkerchiefs; instructional materials.

Implementation

■ Explain the procedure to the mother and provide privacy.
■ Encourage the mother to drink a beverage before and during or after breast-feeding. *This ensures adequate fluid intake, which helps to maintain milk production.*
■ Encourage the mother to attend to personal needs and to change the infant's wet or soiled diaper before breast-feeding begins *to avoid interruptions during feeding time.*
■ Wash your hands and instruct the mother to wash hers.
■ Help the mother find a comfortable position, for example, the cradle or side-lying position, *to promote the letdown reflex.* (See *Breast-feeding positions,* page 898.) Have her expose one breast and rest the nape of the infant's neck in the crook of her arm, supporting his back with her forearm. Use pillows to support the infant, as needed.
■ Urge the mother to relax during breast-feeding *because relaxation also promotes the letdown reflex.* Inform her that she may feel a tingling sensation when letdown occurs and that milk may drip or spray from her breasts. Tell her the reflex may also be initiated by hearing the infant's cry.
■ Guiding the mother's free hand, have her place her thumb on top of the exposed breast's areola and her first two fin-

Breast-feeding positions

Ordinarily, a maternity patient chooses a breast-feeding position that's comfortable and efficient. If the patient experiences discomfort in one position, she can choose another. By changing positions periodically, she can alter the infant's grasp on the nipple and thereby avoid contact friction on the same area. As appropriate, suggest the following typical breast-feeding positions.

Cradle position

The cradle position is the most common position for breast-feeding. The mother sits in a comfortable chair and cradles the infant's head in the crook of her arm. If desired, she can support her elbow with pillows *to minimize tension and fatigue.* She can also tuck the infant's lower arm alongside her body *so it stays out of the way.* The infant's mouth should remain even with the nipple, and his stomach should face and touch the mother's stomach (as shown below).

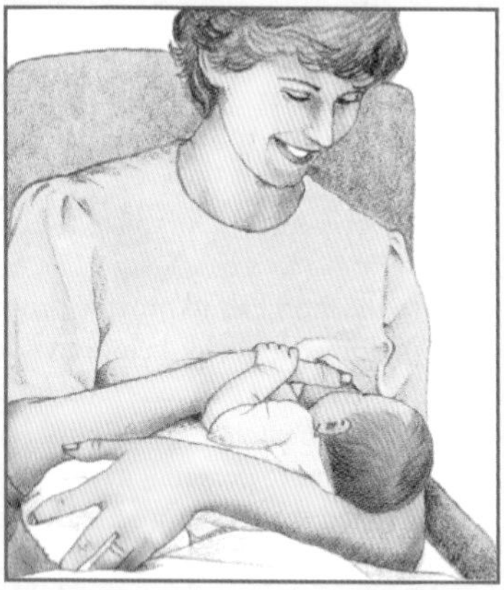

Side-lying position

The mother may choose the side-lying position for breast-feeding at night or during recovery from a cesarean delivery. She lies on her side with her stomach facing the infant's and the infant's head near her breast, and as the infant's mouth opens, she pulls him toward the nipple (as shown below).

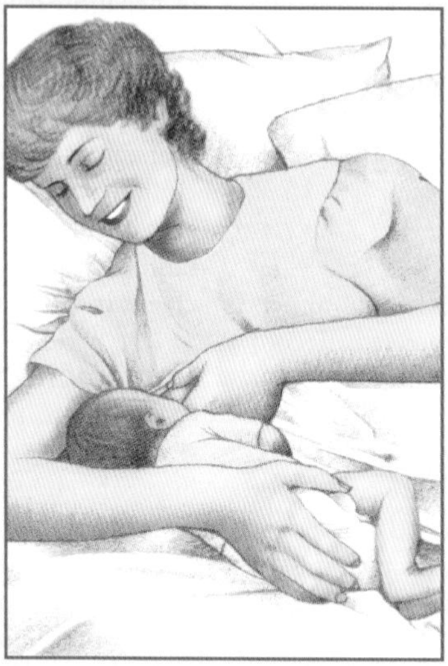

Football position

Commonly selected by a mother with large breasts or one who has had a cesarean delivery, the football position is also useful for feeding twins or infants who are small or premature. The mother sits in a comfortable chair with a pillow under her arm on the nursing side with the infant's body under her arm. She places her hand under the infant's head and brings it close to the breast while placing the fingers of her other hand above and below the nipple. As the infant's mouth opens, she pulls his head close to her breast (as shown below).

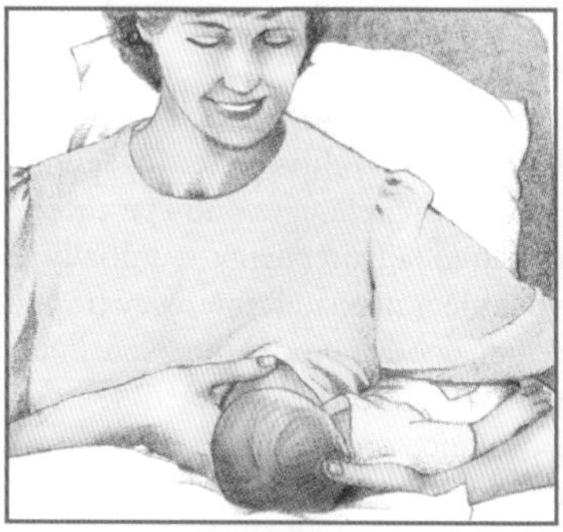

gers beneath it, forming a "C" with her hand. Turn the infant so that he faces the breast.

■ Tell the mother to stroke the infant's cheek located nearest her exposed breast or the infant's upper lip with the nipple. *This stimulates the rooting instinct, causing the infant to open his mouth wide.* Emphasize that she shouldn't touch the infant's other cheek *because he may turn his head toward the touch and away from the breast.*

■ When the infant opens his mouth and roots for the nipple, instruct the mother to insert the nipple and as much of the areola as possible into his mouth. *This helps him to exert sufficient pressure with his lips, gums, and cheek muscles on the milk sinuses below the areola.*

■ Check for occlusion of the infant's nostrils by the mother's breast. If this happens, reposition the infant to give him room to breathe.

■ Suggest that the mother begin nursing the infant for at least 15 minutes on each breast — even longer if the infant seems to want to continue to feed on that breast.

■ To alternate breasts, instruct the mother to slip a finger into the side of the infant's mouth *to break the seal* and move him to the other breast.

■ *To burp the infant,* show the mother how to hold the infant in an upright forward-tilting position with one hand supporting his chest and chin. Tell her to gently pat or rub the infant's back *to expel any ingested air.* Help her place a protective cover, such as a cloth diaper, under the infant's chin.

■ Instruct the mother to feed the infant at the other breast. If she wishes, and if the infant remains awake, she may nurse him longer. *A demand-feeding routine, in which the infant feeds according to his hunger and desire, establishes an abundant, steady milk supply appropriate for the infant's requirements (the more the infant needs, the more milk the mother produces). What's more, frequent nursing satisfies the infant's need to suck. It also promotes bonding.*

■ When the mother finishes breast-feeding, have her place the infant on his back. However, if the mother wishes to hold the infant longer, encourage her to do so. *Touching enhances bonding.*

■ Instruct the mother to air-dry her nipples for 15 minutes after she finishes feeding, and give her additional breast-care instructions as necessary. (See *Breast care for new mothers.*)

■ Encourage the mother's breast-feeding efforts. To boost these efforts, urge her to eat balanced meals, to drink at least eight 8-oz glasses of fluid daily (preferably water), and to nap daily for at least the first 2 weeks after giving birth. Answer her questions about breast-feeding and provide instructional materials, if available. Before she goes home, inform her about local breast-feeding and parenting support groups such as La Leche League International.

■ Teach the mother to observe for breast engorgement, which occurs 48 to 72 hours after delivery. If traditional relief measures fail to trigger the letdown reflex, warm packs may be applied to the breast immediately up to 15 minutes before breast-feeding. Cool or ice packs may be applied between feedings for comfort. Notify the practitioner if engorgement occurs.

■ Instruct the patient to report signs of mastitis—a red, tender, or warm breast and fever—which may occur after discharge.

Special considerations

■ Instruct the mother to use the side-lying position for breast-feeding on the delivery table. *This reduces discomfort from pressure on the episiotomy (if she had one).* Alternatively, you can adjust the table so that she can sit up. *Because the mother will probably be exhausted from delivery or drowsy from medication,* stay with her during this time.

■ Inform the mother that infants routinely lose weight (several ounces) during the first days of life. Advise her that colostrum, her first milk, is yellow, rich in protein and antibodies, and secreted in small amounts. Her true milk, which is thin and bluish, won't appear for several days.

■ Advise a mother who's breast-feeding twins that using the football position allows her to feed both infants at once. Instruct her to alternate breasts and infants at each feeding. If the mother prefers to nurse one infant at a time, make sure

HOME CARE

Breast care for new mothers

A mother who plans to breast-feed her infant should prepare her breasts as directed by her practitioner. After the infant's birth, she'll need to maintain breast tissue integrity. Although postpartum care varies for breast-feeding and non-breast-feeding mothers, both may benefit from the following guidelines.

For the breast-feeding mother

■ Instruct the mother to wash her areolae and nipples with water, without soap or a washcloth, *to avoid washing away the natural oils and keratin.*

■ Advise the mother with sore or irritated nipples to apply ice compresses just before breast-feeding. *This numbs and firms the nipples, making them less sensitive and easier for the infant to grasp.*

■ Suggest that lubricating the nipple with a few drops of expressed breast milk before feeding may help prevent tenderness.

■ Recommend placing breast pads over the nipples to collect colostrum or milk, which commonly leaks during the first few breast-feeding weeks. Advise replacing pads often *to guard against infection.*

■ Inform the mother that breast milk comes in 2 to 5 days after delivery and is accompanied by a slight temperature elevation and breast changes—increased size, warmth, and firmness.

■ Tell the mother that a well-fitting support bra may help control engorgement.

■ Advise the mother with engorged breasts to apply warm compresses, massage the breasts, take a warm shower, or express some milk before feeding. *This dilates the milk ducts, promotes letdown, and makes the nipples more pliable.*

For the non–breast-feeding mother

■ Instruct the mother to clean her breasts using the same technique as the breast-feeding mother. Add that she may use soap, however.

■ Advise her to wear a support bra *to help minimize engorgement and to decrease nipple stimulation.*

■ Advise her to avoid stimulating the nipples or manually expressing her milk to *minimize further milk production.* Instead, provide pain medication, as ordered, ice packs, or a breast binder.

the nursery and the mother both keep track of which infant came first during each feeding.

- Reassure her that there's no standard schedule for breast-feeding and that developing a comfortable breast-feeding routine takes time. Assure her that the infant is getting enough to eat if he seems content after feeding, voids 6 to 8 times per day, and gains weight.
- Tell her to expect uterine cramping during breast-feeding until her uterus returns to its original size. These contractions result from released oxytocin, a natural hormone that prompts the uterus to return to a nonpregnant state. Oxytocin also initiates the letdown reflex, thereby allowing the milk to flow from the alveoli into the ducts.
- If the infant shows little interest in breast-feeding, reassure the mother that he may need several days to learn and to adjust. If the infant is sleepy, encourage the mother to offer the breast frequently but to refrain from forcing him to nurse. Instead, advise her to try rubbing the infant's feet, unwrapping his blanket, changing his diaper, changing her position or the infant's position, and manually expressing milk and then allowing the infant to suckle. *A balky infant may suck eagerly if milk is flowing.*
- If the infant fails to nurse sufficiently and dehydration seems likely, have the mother give him expressed milk through a medicine dropper or small syringe. Instruct her to avoid frequent feeding with a bottle *because the infant may develop nipple confusion due to the artificial nipple and reject the mother's nipple.*
- Advise the mother to start breast-feeding with the breast she used last at the previous feeding *to help avoid breast engorgement.* Suggest attaching a safety pin to the bra strap supporting the breast she last used to serve as a reminder.
- Advise the mother not to take any drugs (including over-the-counter and herbal remedies) unless prescribed or approved by her practitioner *because some drugs pass through the breast milk to the infant.*

Complications

Breast engorgement may result from venous and lymphatic stasis and alveolar milk accumulation. Mastitis occurs postpartum in about 1% of mothers. It usually results from a pathogen that passes from the infant's nose or pharynx into breast tissue through a cracked or fissured nipple.

Documentation

After helping the mother breast-feed, note the areas in which she needs further instruction and help. Document patient teaching. Also document the time of feeding on each breast, the infant's suckling ability, difficulty in arousing the infant, positions of feeding, and assessment of the mother's nipples.

Selected references

Bowden, V., and Greenberg, C.S. *Pediatric Nursing Procedures*, 2nd ed. Philadelphia: Lippincott Williams & Wilkins, 2008.

Komara, C., et al. "Intervening to Promote Early Initiation of Breast-Feeding in the LDR," *American Journal of Maternal Child Nursing* 32(2):117-21, March-April 2007.

Mattson, S., and Smith, J., eds. *Core Curriculum for Maternal-Newborn Nursing,* 3rd ed. Philadelphia: W.B. Saunders Co., 2004.

Moore, E., et al. "Randomized Control Trial of Very Early Mother-Infant Skin-to-Skin Contact and Breast-Feeding Status," *Journal of Midwifery and Women's Health* 52(2):116-25, March-April 2007.

Swanson, V., et al. "Initiation and Continuation of Breast-Feeding: Theory of Planned Behavior," *Journal of Advanced Nursing* 50(3):272-82, May 2005.

Breast pumps

By creating suction, manual and electric breast pumps stimulate lactation. Indicated for a mother who wants to maintain milk production while she and her infant are separated or while illness temporarily incapacitates one or the other, or both, a breast pump can also relieve engorgement or collect milk for a premature infant with a weak sucking reflex.

The mother can also use a pump to reduce pressure on sore or cracked nipples or to reestablish her milk supply if a weaned infant becomes allergic to formula. She can also use it to collect milk from inverted nipples or to express milk mechanically when she can't express milk by hand or with a manual pump. Electric pumps are more effective and efficient than manual pumps. (See *Comparing breast pumps.*)

Equipment

Manual or electric breast pump ■ sterile collection bag or bottle (to store milk if desired) ■ optional: warm compresses and pillows.

An electric breast pump should come with a sterile, single-use accessory kit, which many pump manufacturers supply. The kit contains shields, milk cups, an overflow bottle, and tubing. These parts can be washed with soap and water and then sterilized for repeated use.

Preparation of equipment

Assemble the breast pump according to the manufacturer's instructions. If milk will be stored or frozen, thoroughly clean any removable parts that the milk will touch.

Implementation

- Explain the procedure to the patient.

■ Give her time to attend to personal needs first *so she won't have to interrupt the procedure for this purpose.* Also, advise her to wash her hands.
■ Instruct the patient to drink a beverage before and after breast pumping. *This ensures sufficient fluid intake to maintain adequate milk production.*
■ Help the patient to assume a comfortable position and to relax. Offer pillows for support. Provide privacy, and instruct her to uncover her breast completely *to prevent lint and dirt from entering the milk-collection container.*
■ If the patient's breasts are engorged, have her apply warm compresses for 5 minutes or take a warm shower *to dilate the milk ducts and stimulate the letdown reflex.*
■ *To help trigger the release of milk-producing hormones,* instruct the patient to use her thumb and forefinger to stimulate the nipple and areola for 1 to 2 minutes.

Using a manual pump

■ Instruct the patient to place the flange or shield against her breast with the nipple in the center of the device. Then tell her to use her other hand to operate the piston portion of the pump *to draw the milk from the breast.* Have her pump each breast in this manner until the milk stops flowing.
■ If the milk will be stored or frozen, direct the patient to fill a sterile plastic bottle with the milk from the collection container.

Using a battery-powered or electric breast pump

■ Unless the pump is battery-powered, make sure the pump has a three-pronged plug to ground it *to prevent electric shock.*
■ Instruct the patient to set the suction regulator on low. Tell her to hold the collection unit upright *to prevent milk from being sucked into the machine.* Have her center her nipple in the shield, which she'll place against the breast.
■ Direct her to activate the machine and adjust the suction regulator *to achieve a comfortable pressure.* Have her check the operator's manual *to determine the pressure setting at which the pump functions most efficiently.*
■ Instruct her to pump each breast for 5 to 8 minutes or until the spray grows scant. Then pump each breast again for 3 to 5 minutes and then again for 2 to 3 minutes.
■ If the patient is pumping both breasts simultaneously, tell her to pump for 15 to 20 minutes until the spray goes scant.
■ Tell the patient to remove the shield from the breast by inserting a finger between the breast and the shield *to break the vacuum seal.* Then she should return the suction regulator to the low setting and turn off the machine.
■ If the milk will be stored or frozen, pour it from the collection unit into a sterile plastic container. (If it's to be frozen, place it in the freezer immediately.)

EQUIPMENT

Comparing breast pumps

Breast pumps are available in battery-operated and electric models. The pump that's best for your patient depends on such factors as the pump's purpose and the patient's situation. A description of common pumps and their features follows.

Battery-powered pump

Having a battery-powered motor, this pump can be operated with one hand. Easy to clean, it's a good choice for mothers who work outside the home or who need a breast pump only for short-term use.

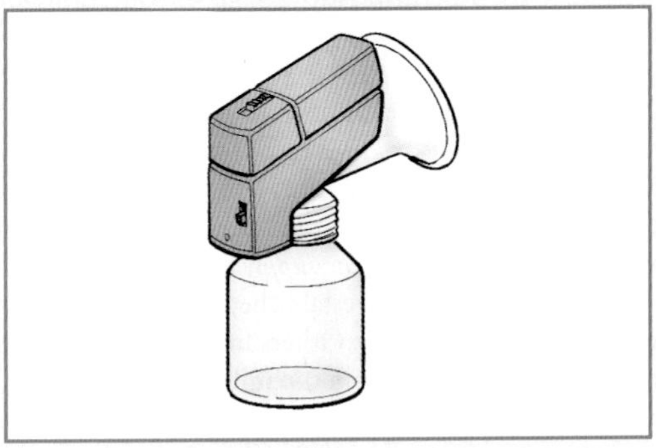

Electric pump

Usually used in hospitals, this gentle, efficient pump plugs into an electrical outlet and can be operated with one hand. It's available as a small 2-lb model or as a larger model about the size of a small sewing machine. Inform your patient that the larger model can be rented from a pharmacy or medical supply company.

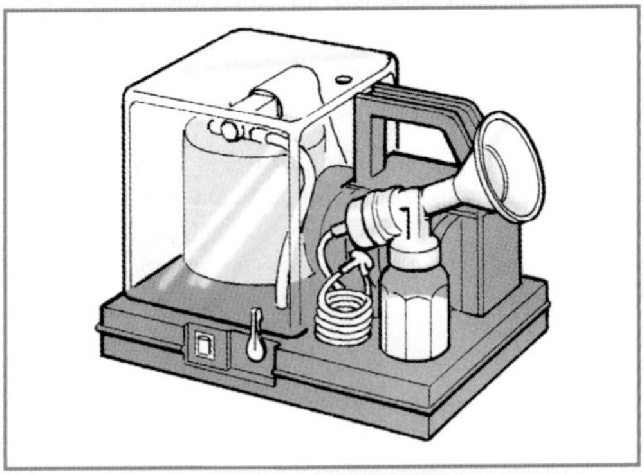

■ If the infant will drink the milk directly, pour it into a sterile bottle.
■ Label the collected milk with the date, the time of collection, and the amount. Also, make sure the label contains the infant's name if applicable.

Concluding the procedure

■ Instruct the patient to air-dry her nipples for about 15 minutes.
■ Instruct her to disassemble the removable parts of the pump and wash them according to the manufacturer's directions.

Special considerations

■ Provide emotional support *to alleviate the mother's distress related to the infant's absence at feeding time.*
■ Be sure to use a sterile plastic (not glass) collection bottle for the milk *because antibodies in the breast milk will adhere to a glass bottle.*
■ If the patient will use a breast pump for some time, have her pump her breasts every 2 to 3 hours *because neonates nurse 8 to 12 times every 24 hours.* Remind her to pump her breasts at night *because the breasts need round-the-clock stimulation to produce an adequate supply of milk.*
■ After the milk supply is established, some mothers may need to pump once nightly. Others find that they can sleep for 6 hours and still maintain the milk supply.
■ Breast milk can be stored in the refrigerator for 48 hours and in the freezer at 0° F (–17.8° C) for up to 6 months.

Complications

Common complications include nipple injury from suction and contaminated milk from improperly cleaned equipment or incorrect storage.

Documentation

Record the duration that the patient pumped each breast, the amount of milk collected, and the patient's tolerance of the procedure.

SELECTED REFERENCES

Brown, S.L., et al. "Breast Pump Adverse Events: Reports to the Food and Drug Administration," *Journal of Human Lactation* 21(2):169-74, May 2005.

Mattson, S., and Smith, J., eds. *Core Curriculum for Maternal-Newborn Nursing,* 3rd ed. Philadelphia: W.B. Saunders Co., 2004.

Pillitteri, A. *Maternal and Child Health Nursing: Care of the Childbearing and Childrearing Family,* 5th ed. Philadelphia: Lippincott Williams & Wilkins, 2007.

Swanson, V., et al. "Initiation and Continuation of Breast-Feeding: Theory of Planned Behavior," *Journal of Advanced Nursing* 50(3):272-82, May 2005.

Ueker, A.E. "Answering Questions About Breast Pumps," *LEAVEN* 37(1):12-13, February-March 2007.

BOTTLE-FEEDING

When a neonate requires a special diet or when a mother can't or chooses not to breast-feed, formula is the next-best food source. Formula preparations supply all needed vitamins and nutrients and can be administered by anyone. Most formulas used in hospitals come ready-to-feed in disposable containers. Some formulas and equipment, however, may require advance preparation, such as mixing and sterilization. The American Academy of Pediatrics (AAP) recommends the use of commercially prepared formula over animal milks or homemade preparations for the infant's first year.

Because formulas must be sterile, they're prepared either by the sterile method (in which all articles used in formula preparation are sterilized before mixing) or by the terminal heat method (in which the formula is prepared with clean technique and then sterilized using a home sterilizer). In the United States, some pediatricians recommend clean technique and tap water for formulas because water supplies are clean and safe in most areas.

A normal neonate takes 15 to 20 minutes to consume a 1- to 1½-oz portion of formula and usually feeds every 3 to 4 hours.

Equipment

Commercially prepared formula or ingredients ■ bottle, nipple, and cap ■ tissue or cloth ■ gown.

Hospitals commonly use disposable bottle and nipple units for neonatal feeding.

Preparation of equipment

If you're using commercially prepared formula, uncap the formula bottle and make sure the seal wasn't previously broken *to ensure sterility and freshness.* Then screw on the nipple and cap. Keep the protective sterile cap over the nipple until the neonate is ready to feed. If you're preparing formula, follow the manufacturer's instructions or the practitioner's prescription. Administer the formula at room temperature or slightly warmer.

NURSING ALERT *Don't heat formula in a microwave.*

Implementation

■ Confirm the neonate's identity using two patient identifiers according to your facility's policy.

- Wash your hands.
- Invert the bottle and shake some formula on your wrist *to test the patency of the nipple hole and the formula's temperature.* The nipple should be firm — not soft — *to prevent collapse from sucking.* The nipple hole should allow formula to drip freely but not to stream out. *If the hole is too large, the neonate may aspirate formula; if it's too small, the extra sucking effort he expends may tire him before he can empty the bottle.*
- Sit comfortably in a semireclining position, and cradle the neonate in one arm to support his head and back. *This position allows swallowed air to rise to the top of the stomach where it's more easily expelled.* If he can't be held, sit by him and elevate his head and shoulders slightly.
- Place the nipple in the neonate's mouth while making sure the tongue is down, but don't insert it so far that it stimulates the gag reflex. He should begin to suck, pulling in as much nipple as is comfortable. If he doesn't start to suck, stroke him under the chin or on his cheek, or touch his lips with the nipple *to stimulate his sucking reflex.*
- As the neonate feeds, tilt the bottle upward *to keep the nipple filled with formula and to prevent him from swallowing air.* Watch for a steady stream of bubbles in the bottle. This indicates proper venting and flow of formula. If the neonate pushes out the nipple with his tongue, reinsert the nipple. *Expelling the nipple is a normal reflex. It doesn't necessarily mean that the neonate is full.*
- Always hold the bottle for a neonate. If left to feed himself, he may aspirate formula or swallow air if the bottle tilts or empties. *Experts link bottle propping with an increased incidence of otitis media and dental caries in older infants.*

NURSING ALERT *Never put a neonate to bed with a bottle.*

- Burp the neonate after each ½ oz of formula *because he'll typically swallow some air even when fed correctly.* Hold the neonate upright in a slightly forward position, supporting his head and chest with one hand. Alternatively, position a clean cloth *to protect your clothing,* and hold the neonate upright over your shoulder, or place him facedown across your lap. *The change in position helps the gas to rise or "bring up the bubble."* In either case, rub or gently pat his back until he expels the air.
- After you finish feeding and burping the neonate, place him on his back as recommended by the AAP. Neonates are prone to regurgitation because of an immature cardiac sphincter. *Positioning on the back has been demonstrated to reduce the incidence of sudden infant death syndrome.*
- Discard any remaining formula, and properly dispose of all equipment.

Special considerations

- Change feeding duration by changing the size of the nipple or the nipple hole; *the neonate tires if he feeds too long, and his sucking needs aren't met if he doesn't feed long enough.*
- Be sure to note how much formula is in the bottle before and after the feeding. Use the calibrations along the side of the container *to calculate the amount of formula consumed.*
- Be alert for aspiration in the neonate who has a diminished sucking or swallowing reflex and who may have difficulty feeding. Also take appropriate measures according to hospital policy to feed the neonate with cleft lip and palate.
- Teach parents how to properly prepare and (if required) sterilize formula, bottles, and nipples, and how to feed and burp the neonate. Although most hospitals have a feeding schedule, advise the mother that she may switch to a more flexible demand-feeding schedule when at home. Forewarn her that the neonate may not feed well on his first day home *because of the new activity and environment.* Inform parents about the forms of formula available (ready-to-feed, concentrate, powders) *so that they can choose the most convenient form.*
- Prepare parents to expect the neonate to regurgitate formula. Explain that regurgitation (merely an overflow that typically follows feeding) shouldn't be confused with vomiting (a more complete emptying of the stomach accompanied by symptoms not associated with feeding).

Complications

Bottle-propping may allow the nipple to block the airway, causing suffocation; it may also lead to otitis media, aspiration, or dental caries. Lung infection or death may follow aspiration of regurgitated formula.

Documentation

Record the time and type of feeding, the amount of formula consumed, how well the neonate fed, and whether he appeared satisfied. Note any regurgitation or vomiting. If the mother feeds him, observe and describe their interactions. Document any patient teaching provided.

SELECTED REFERENCES

Bowden, V., and Greenberg, C.S. *Pediatric Nursing Procedures,* 2nd ed. Philadelphia: Lippincott Williams & Wilkins, 2008.

Flint, A., et al. "Cup Feeding Versus Other Forms of Supplemental Enteral Feeding for Newborn Infants Unable to Fully Breast-Feed," *Cochrane Database of Systematic Reviews* (2):CD005092, April 2007.

Goldfield, E.C., et al. "Coordination of Sucking, Swallowing, and Breathing and Oxygen Saturation During Early Infant Breast-Feeding and Bottle-Feeding," *Pediatric Research* 60(4):450-55, October 2006.

Mattson, S., and Smith, J., eds. *Core Curriculum for Maternal-Newborn Nursing,* 3rd ed. Philadelphia: W.B. Saunders Co., 2004.

GAVAGE FEEDING

Gavage feeding involves passing nutrients directly to the neonate's stomach by a tube advanced nasally or orally. If a neonate can't suck (because of prematurity, illness, or congenital deformity) or is at risk for aspiration (because of gastroesophageal reflux, ineffective gag reflex, or easy tiring), gavage feeding may supply nutrients until he can take food by mouth.

Unless the neonate has problems with the feeding tube, the nurse usually inserts it orally before each feeding and withdraws it after the feeding. This intermittent method stimulates the sucking reflex. If the neonate can't tolerate this, the nurse advances the tube nasally and leaves it in place for 24 to 72 hours. Gavage feeding is contraindicated for neonates without bowel sounds or with suspected intestinal obstruction, severe respiratory distress, or massive gastroesophageal reflux.

Equipment

Feeding tube (#5 French for nasogastric [NG] feeding of premature neonate; #8 French for others) ▪ feeding reservoir or large (20- to 50-ml) syringe ▪ prescribed formula or breast milk ▪ sterile water ▪ tape measure ▪ tape ▪ stethoscope ▪ gloves ▪ two 3-ml syringes ▪ optional: bowl and pacifier. A commercial feeding reservoir is available.

Preparation of equipment

Allow the formula or breast milk to warm to room temperature, if necessary. Wash your hands, and open the sterile water if it comes in a small-sized disposable container. Remove the syringe or reservoir and the feeding tube from the packaging.

Implementation

- Identify the neonate and verify the practitioner's orders.
- Using a tape measure, determine the length of tubing needed to ensure placement in the stomach. You'll usually measure from the tip of the nose to the tip of the earlobe to the xiphoid process. Mark the tube at the appropriate distance with a piece of tape. Measure from the bottom. Alternatively, you may also measure using the feeding tube itself.
- Place the neonate in a supine position. Elevate the head of his mattress one notch. Otherwise, place him in a supine position or tilted slightly to his right with head and chest slightly elevated.
- Put on gloves. Stabilize the neonate's head with one hand, and lubricate the feeding tube with sterile water with the other hand.
- Insert the tube smoothly and quickly up to the premeasured tape mark. For oral insertion, pass the tube toward the back of the throat. For nasal insertion, pass the tube toward the occiput in a horizontal plane.
- Synchronize tube insertion with throat movement if the neonate swallows *to facilitate tube passage into the stomach.* During insertion, watch for choking and cyanosis—signs that a tube has entered the trachea. If these occur, remove the tube and reinsert it. Also watch for bradycardia and apnea resulting from vagal stimulation.
- If the tube will remain in place, tape it flat to the neonate's cheek. *To prevent possible nasal skin breakdown,* don't tape the tube to the bridge of his nose.
- Make sure the tube is in the stomach (and not the lungs) by aspirating residual stomach contents with the syringe. Check the content's pH *because gastric contents are highly acidic. This helps confirm tube placement.* Note the volume obtained, and then reinject it *to avoid altering the neonate's buffer system and electrolyte balance.* Alternatively, as ordered, reduce the feeding volume by the residual amount, or prolong the interval between feedings.
- If you suspect that the tube is displaced, advance it several centimeters farther and test again. *Don't* begin feeding until you're certain the tube is in the stomach.
- When the tube is in place, connect the feeding reservoir or syringe to the top of the tube, fill the feeding reservoir or syringe with formula or breast milk, and start the feeding.
- If the neonate is on your lap, hold the container about 4″ (10 cm) above his abdomen. If he's lying down, hold it between 6″ and 8″ (15 and 20 cm) above his head. When using a commercial feeding reservoir, look for air bubbles in the container, *an indicator of formula passage.*
- Regulate flow by raising and lowering the container so that the feeding takes 15 to 20 minutes, the average time for a bottle-feeding. *To prevent stomach distention, reflux, and vomiting,* don't let the feeding proceed too rapidly.
- When the feeding is finished, pinch off the tubing before air enters the neonate's stomach. *This helps prevent distention and fluid leakage into the pharynx during tube removal, and consequent aspiration.*
- Withdraw the tube smoothly and quickly. If the tube will remain in place, flush it with several milliliters of sterile water, if ordered.
- Burp the neonate *to decrease abdominal distention.* Hold him upright or in a sitting position. Use one hand to support his head and chest and your other hand to gently rub or pat his back until he expels the air.

■ Place him on his stomach (only if he's being monitored with a cardiac-respiratory monitor) or right side for 1 hour after feeding *to facilitate gastric emptying and to prevent aspiration if he regurgitates.*
■ Don't perform postural drainage and percussion until 1 hour or more after feeding.

Special considerations

■ Use the NG approach for the neonate who must keep the feeding tube in place *because this approach holds the tube more securely than the orogastric approach.* Alternate the nostril used at each insertion *to prevent skin and mucosal irritation.*

Note: When possible, the oral route should be used for gavage feedings rather than the nasal route *because the neonate is an obligatory nose breather.*
■ Observe the premature neonate for indications that he's ready to begin bottle- or breast-feeding: strong sucking reflex, coordinated sucking and swallowing, alertness before feeding, and sleep after feeding.
■ Provide the neonate with a pacifier during feeding *to soothe him, to help prevent gagging, and to promote an association between sucking and the full feeling that follows feeding.*

Complications

Gagging with regurgitation causes loss of nutrients. An indwelling NG tube can irritate mucous membranes and cause nasal airway obstruction, epistaxis, and stomach perforation. A feeding tube may kink, coil, or knot and become obstructed, preventing feeding.

Documentation

Record the amount of residual fluid and the amount currently taken. Note the type and amount of any vomitus as well as any adverse reactions to tube insertion or feeding.

SELECTED REFERENCES

Bowden, V., and Greenberg, C.S. *Pediatric Nursing Procedures,* 2nd ed. Philadelphia: Lippincott Williams & Wilkins, 2008.

Mattson, S., and Smith, J., eds. *Core Curriculum for Maternal-Newborn Nursing,* 3rd ed. Philadelphia: W.B. Saunders Co., 2004.

Pinelli, J., and Symington, A. "Nonnutritive Sucking for Promoting Physiologic Stability and Nutrition in Preterm Infants," *Cochrane Database of Systematic Reviews* (4):CD001071, October 2005.

Premji, S.S. "Enteral Feeding for High-Risk Neonates: A Digest for Nurses into Putative Risk and Benefits to Ensure Safe and Comfortable Care," *Journal of Perinatal & Neonatal Nursing* 19(1):59-71, January-March 2005.

Street, J., et al. "Implementing Feeding Guidelines for NICE Patient <2000g Results in Less Variability in Nutrition Outcomes," *Journal of Parenteral and Enteral Nutrition* 30(6):515-18, November-December 2006.

SPECIAL PROCEDURES

CIRCUMCISION

Steeped in controversy and history, circumcision (the removal of the penile foreskin) is thought to promote a clean glans and to minimize the risk of phimosis (tightening of the foreskin) in later life.

Current scientific evidence indicates potential medical benefits for the circumcised male neonate. Indeed, studies have shown that circumcision may reduce the risk of penile cancer, decrease the risk of contracting a urinary tract infection, and lessen the risk of contracting a sexually transmitted disease. After reviewing available research, however, the American Academy of Pediatrics (AAP) concluded that there are no absolute medical indications for routine circumcision. They recommend that the parents should be provided with information about the potential benefits and risks and counseled to make a decision that's in the best interest of the child. The AAP also states that if the decision is made for circumcision, procedural analgesia should be provided.

In Judaism, circumcision is a religious rite (known as a *bris*) performed by a mohel (a specialist trained in both the medical procedure and Jewish law) on the 8th day after birth, when the neonate officially receives his name. Because most neonates are discharged before this time, the bris rarely occurs in the hospital.

There are two methods currently used in practice for performing circumcision. These include use of the Gomco clamp, Plastibell, or Mogen clamp.

Circumcision using a Gomco or Mogen clamp involves using the clamp to stabilize the penis while removing the foreskin. With this device, a cone that fits over the glans provides a cutting surface and protects the glans penis. The other technique uses a plastic circumcision bell (Plastibell) over the glans and a suture tied tightly around the base of the foreskin. This method prevents bleeding. The resultant ischemia causes the foreskin to slough off within 5 to 8 days. This method is thought to be painless because it stretches the foreskin, which inhibits sensory conduction.

Circumcision is contraindicated in neonates who are ill or who have bleeding disorders, ambiguous genitalia, or congenital anomalies of the penis, such as hypospadias or epispadias, because the foreskin may be needed for later reconstructive surgery.

Equipment

Circumcision tray (contents vary but usually include circumcision clamps, various-sized cones, scalpel, probe, scissors, forceps, sterile basin, sterile towel, and sterile drapes) ▪ antiseptic solution ▪ restraining board with arm and leg restraints ▪ sterile gloves ▪ petroleum gauze ▪ sterile 4″ × 4″ gauze pads ▪ optional: sutures, plastic circumcision bell, antimicrobial ointment, topical or local anesthetic, sterile marker, sterile labels, overhead warmer.

Preparation of equipment

Using a Gomco clamp: Assemble the sterile tray and other equipment in the procedure area. Open the sterile tray and pour antiseptic solution into the sterile basin. Using sterile technique, place sterile 4″ × 4″ gauze pads and petroleum gauze on the sterile tray. Arrange the restraining board and direct adequate light on the area.

Using a plastic circumcision bell: Assemble sterile gloves, sutures, restraining board, petroleum gauze and, if ordered, antibiotic ointment. A mohel usually brings his own equipment.

Preparing for analgesia administration

Currently there are several methods to provide analgesia to the neonate during a circumcision.

▪ Eutectic mixture of local anesthetics (EMLA cream) consists of the application of a cream containing 2.5% lidocaine and 2.5% prilocaine, administered 60 to 90 minutes before the procedure along with the application of an occlusive dressing. Research supports that the neonate who receives EMLA cream cries less and experiences less of an increase in heart rate during the procedure.

▪ Dorsal penile nerve block (DPNB) is administered using a 27G needle to inject 0.4 ml of 1% lidocaine at both the 10 and 2 o'clock positions at the base of the penis. Bruising at the injection site is the most reported complication.

▪ Subcutaneous ring block (SRB) involves administration of 0.8 ml of 1% lidocaine at the midshaft of the penis. The SRB appears to prevent crying and increases in heart rate more consistently than DPNB or EMLA cream. No complications have been reported to date.

▪ Neonates should also be given acetaminophen immediately after the procedure for pain relief.

Implementation

▪ Confirm the neonate's identity using two patient identifiers according to your facility's policy.

▪ Make sure the parents understand the procedure and have signed the proper consent form.

▪ Withhold feeding for at least 1 hour before the procedure *to reduce the possibility of emesis and aspiration.*

▪ Place the neonate on the restraining board. Restrain his arms and legs only during the procedure *to decrease distress.* Remain with the neonate *to offer comfort and produce a safe environment.*

▪ Assist the physician, as necessary, throughout the procedure, and comfort the neonate, as needed.

Using a Gomco clamp

▪ After putting on sterile gloves, the physician will clean the penis and scrotum with antiseptic solution and drape the neonate.

▪ He'll apply a Gomco clamp to the penis, loosen the foreskin, insert the cone under it *to provide a cutting surface and to protect the penis,* and remove the foreskin.

▪ Then he'll cover the wound with sterile petroleum gauze *to prevent infection and control bleeding.*

Using a plastic bell

▪ The physician will slide the plastic bell device between the foreskin and the glans penis.

▪ Then he'll tie a suture tightly around the foreskin at the coronal edge of the glans. The foreskin distal to the suture will become ischemic, and then atrophic. After 5 to 8 days, the foreskin will drop off with the plastic bell attached, leaving a clean, well-healed excision. No special care is required, but watch for swelling, *which may indicate infection or interfere with urination.*

Providing aftercare

▪ Remove the neonate from the restraining board, and assess for bleeding.

▪ If povidone-iodine was used before the procedure, wash it off with sterile water.

▪ Place the neonate on his back *to minimize pressure on the excisional area.* Leave him diaperless for 1 to 2 hours *to observe for bleeding and to reduce possible chafing and irritation.*

▪ Show the neonate to his parents to reassure them that he's all right.

▪ After you rediaper the neonate, change his diaper as soon as he voids. If the dressing falls off, clean the wound with warm water *to minimize pain from urine on the circumcised area.* Don't remove the original dressing until it falls off (usually after the first or second voiding).

▪ Check for bleeding every 15 minutes for the 1st hour and then every hour for the next 24 hours. If bleeding occurs, apply pressure with sterile gauze pads. Notify the physician if bleeding continues.

▪ Loosely diaper the neonate *to prevent irritation.* At each diaper change, apply ordered antimicrobial ointment, petroleum jelly, or petroleum gauze until the wound appears healed. Avoid leaving the neonate under the radiant warmer after placing petroleum gauze on the penis *because the area might burn.*

■ Teach the parents to watch for drainage, redness, or swelling. Don't remove the thin, yellow-white exudate that forms over the healing area within 1 to 2 days. *This normal incrustation protects the wound until it heals in 3 to 4 days.*

■ Don't discharge the neonate until he has voided.

Special considerations

■ Always be sure to show parents the circumcision before discharge *so they can ask any questions and so you can teach them how to care for the area.*

■ If the neonate's mother has human immunodeficiency virus (HIV) infection, circumcision will be delayed until the physician knows the neonate's HIV status. *The neonate whose mother has HIV infection has a higher-than-normal risk of infection.*

Home care

■ Inform the mother that the circumcision site may appear yellow in light-skinned neonates and lighter than the surrounding skin in dark-skinned neonates. Tell her that this signifies healing and isn't a cause for concern.

■ Instruct the mother to observe the circumcision site regularly for pus or bloody discharge, *which may indicate delayed healing or infection.* If these signs occur, she should notify the practitioner.

■ Tell the mother that the rim of the device used for circumcision may remain in place after discharge from the hospital. Reassure her that the rim will fall off harmlessly in 3 or 4 days. If it doesn't fall off after 1 week, tell her to notify the practitioner *because a retained rim may lead to infection.*

Complications

After a Gomco clamp procedure, infection and bleeding may occur. The skin of the penile shaft can adhere to the glans, resulting in scarring or fibrous bands. The most severe complications are urethral fistulae and edema. Incomplete amputation of the foreskin can follow application of the plastic circumcision bell.

Documentation

Note the time and date of the circumcision, any parent teaching, any excessive bleeding, and that voiding occurred before discharge.

Selected references

"Circumcision Policy Statement. American Academy of Pediatrics. Task Force on Circumcision," *Pediatrics* 103(3):686-93, March 1999.

Association of Women's Health, Obstetric, and Neonatal Nurses (AWHONN). "Neonatal Skin Care. Evidence-Based Clinical Practice Guideline." Washington D.C.: AWHONN, January 2001.

National Association of Neonatal Nurses. "Position Statement on Pain Management in Infants. #3019." Glenview, Ill.: NANN, April 1999. Available at *www.nann.org/public/articles/3019.doc.*

Weiss, H. "Male Circumcision as a Preventative Measure against HIV and Other Sexually Transmitted Diseases," *Current Opinions in Infectious Disease* 29(1):66-72, February 2007.

RhoGAM administration

RhoGAM is a concentrated solution of immune globulin containing Rh_o(D) antibodies. I.M. injection of RhoGAM keeps the Rh-negative mother from producing active antibody responses and forming anti-Rh_o(D) to Rh-positive fetal blood cells and endangering future Rh-positive infants. Maternal immunization to the Rh antigen commonly results from transplacental hemorrhage during gestation or delivery. If unchecked during gestation, incompatible fetal and maternal blood can lead to hemolytic disease in the neonate.

RhoGAM is indicated for the Rh-negative mother after abortion, ectopic pregnancy, or delivery of a neonate having Rh_o(D)-positive or Du-positive blood and Coombs'-negative cord blood, accidental transfusion of Rh-positive blood, amniocentesis, abruptio placentae, or abdominal trauma. A RhoGAM injection should be given within 72 hours to prevent future maternal sensitization.

Subsequent pregnancies of the Rh-negative mother require screening to detect previous inadequate RhoGAM administration or low Rh-positive antibody titers.

Administration of RhoGAM at approximately 28 weeks' gestation can also protect the fetus of the Rh-negative mother. The dose is determined according to the fetal packed red blood cell (RBC) volume that enters the mother's blood. A volume under 15 ml usually calls for one vial of RhoGAM; a significant fetomaternal hemorrhage calls for more than one vial if the fetal packed RBC volume exceeds 15 ml.

Equipment

3-ml syringe ■ 22G 1½" needle ■ RhoGAM vial ■ alcohol pads ■ gloves ■ triplicate form and patient identification (from the blood bank or laboratory).

Implementation

■ Confirm the patient's identity using two patient identifiers according to your facility's policy.

- Explain RhoGAM administration to the patient, and answer her questions. If the patient refuses the injection, notify the practitioner.
- Obtain a history of allergies and reaction to immunizations.
- Two nurses must check the vial's identification numbers and sign the triplicate form that comes with the RhoGAM. Complete the form, as indicated. Attach the top copy to the patient's chart. Send the remaining two copies, along with the empty RhoGAM vial, to the laboratory or blood bank.
- Provide privacy, wash your hands, and put on gloves.
- Withdraw the RhoGAM from the vial with the needle and syringe.
- Check landmarks for gluteal position, clean the gluteal injection site, and administer the RhoGAM I.M.
- Give the patient a card that identifies her Rh-negative status, and instruct her to carry it with her or keep it in a convenient location.

Special considerations

- After the procedure, watch for redness and soreness at the injection site.
- Provide an opportunity for the patient to voice any guilt or anxiety she may feel if she perceives her body as acting against the fetus.

Complications

Complications rarely occur after a single RhoGAM injection; when they do, they tend to be mild and confined to the injection site. After multiple injections (given after Rh mismatch), complications may include fever, myalgia, lethargy, discomfort, splenomegaly, or hyperbilirubinemia.

Documentation

Record the date, the time, and the site of the RhoGAM injection. If applicable, note the patient's refusal to accept a RhoGAM injection. Document patient teaching about RhoGAM. Also note whether the patient received a card identifying her Rh-negative status.

SELECTED REFERENCES

American Academy of Pediatrics and American College of Obstetricians and Gynecologists. *Guidelines for Perinatal Care,* 5th ed. Elk Grove Village, Ill.: AAP, 2002; Washington, D.C.: ACOG, 2002.

Mattson, S., and Smith, J., eds. *Core Curriculum for Maternal-Newborn Nursing,* 3rd ed. Philadelphia: W.B. Saunders Co., 2004.

Pillitteri, A. *Maternal and Child Health Nursing: Care of the Childbearing and Childrearing Family,* 5th ed. Philadelphia: Lippincott Williams & Wilkins, 2007.

17 ■ Pediatric care

INTRODUCTION

Caring for pediatric patients demands specialized knowledge and skills. A child's physiologic immaturity heightens his response to illness and to treatment regimens, and his small size narrows the margin for error in treatment. In addition, although children tend to recover more rapidly from an illness than adults do, they have a higher risk of serious complications.

When you care for a child, you need to consider his level of growth and development. For example, young children have only rudimentary motor skills and limited comprehension, making them especially prone to injury. Therefore, you need to remain alert to possibly dangerous situations and take steps to ensure the child's safety.

Keep in mind, too, that even though a child is ill, he still needs sensory and social stimulation. Therefore, you need to include play in your pediatric care plans. Besides promoting development and fostering a sense of security and well-being, play allows children to release the stress and tension that result from the unfamiliar surroundings and activities they encounter in the hospital.

Remember to include the parents in all aspects of their child's care. Encourage them to maintain their roles as caregivers and to continue including the child as a member of the family—especially during long-term hospitalization. Doing so will help to achieve the overall goal of pediatric care: to create a positive environment that promotes the physical and emotional health of the child and his family.

SPECIMEN COLLECTION

URINE COLLECTION

Collecting a urine specimen for laboratory analysis allows screening for urinary tract infection and renal disorders, evaluation of treatment, and detection of systemic and metabolic disorders.

Although a child without bladder control can't provide a clean-catch midstream urine specimen, the pediatric urine collection bag provides a simple, effective alternative. It offers minimal risk of specimen contamination without resorting to catheterization or suprapubic aspiration. Because the collection bag is secured with adhesive flaps, its use is contraindicated in a patient with extremely sensitive or excoriated perineal skin. Alternative methods of collecting urine from small children include the use of an inside-out disposable diaper or a test tube.

Equipment

For a random specimen: Pediatric urine collection bag (individually packaged) ▪ urine specimen container ▪ label ▪ laboratory request form ▪ two disposable diapers of appropriate size ▪ scissors ▪ gloves ▪ washcloth ▪ soap ▪ water ▪ towel ▪ bowl ▪ linen-saver pad.

For a culture and sensitivity specimen: Sterile pediatric urine collection bag ▪ sterile urine specimen container ▪ label ▪ laboratory request form ▪ two disposable diapers of appropriate size ▪ scissors ▪ gloves ▪ sterile bowl ▪ sterile or distilled water ▪ sterile 4″ × 4″ gauze pads ▪ antiseptic skin cleaner ▪ alcohol pad ▪ 3-ml syringe with needle ▪ linen-saver pad.

For a timed specimen: 24-hour pediatric urine collection bag (individually packaged) with evacuation tubing ▪ 24-hour urine specimen container ▪ label ▪ laboratory request form ▪ scissors ▪ two disposable diapers of appropriate size ▪ gloves ▪ washcloth ▪ soap ▪ water ▪ bowl ▪ towel ▪ sterile 4″ × 4″ gauze pads ▪ compound benzoin tincture ▪ small medicine cup ▪ 35-ml luer-lock syringe or urometer ▪ tubing stopper ▪ specimen preservative such as formaldehyde solution ▪ linen-saver pad.

Kits containing sterile supplies for clean-catch collections are commercially available and may be used to obtain a culture and sensitivity specimen.

Preparation of equipment

Check the practitioner's order for the type of specimen needed, and assemble the appropriate equipment. Check the patient's chart for allergies (for example, to iodine). Complete the laboratory request form *to avoid delay in sending the specimen to the laboratory.* Wash your hands.

With scissors, make a 2″ (5.1-cm) slit in one diaper, cutting from the center point toward one of the shorter edges. Later, you'll pull the urine collection bag through this slit when you position the bag and diaper on the patient. Pour water into the bowl; use sterile water and a sterile bowl if you need to collect a specimen for culture and sensitivity.

If you need a culture and sensitivity specimen, check the expiration date on each sterile package, and inspect for tears. Put on new gloves and open several packages of sterile 4″ × 4″ gauze pads.

If you need a timed specimen and will use benzoin in liquid form, pour it into the medicine cup. Cut the tubing on the urine collection bag so that only 6″ (15.2 cm) remain attached. Discard the excess. Place the stopper in the severed end of the tubing. If you're going to use a urometer for the patient who voids large amounts, don't cut the tubing; simply attach the device.

Implementation

- Confirm the child's identity using two patient identifiers according to your facility's policy.
- Explain the procedure to the patient, if he's old enough, and to his parents. Provide privacy, especially if the patient is beyond infancy.

Collecting a random specimen

- Wash your hands.
- Place the patient on a linen-saver pad.
- Clean the perineal area with soap, water, and a washcloth, working from the urinary meatus outward *to prevent contamination of the urine specimen.* Wipe gently *to prevent tissue trauma and stimulation of urination.* Separate the labia of the female patient and retract the foreskin of the uncircumcised male patient *to expose the urinary meatus.* Thoroughly rinse the area with clear water and dry with a towel. Don't use powders, lotions, or cream *because these counteract the adhesive.*
- Place the patient in the frog position, with his legs separated and knees flexed. If necessary, have the patient's parent hold him while you apply the collection bag.
- Remove the protective coverings from the collection bag's adhesive flaps. For the female patient, first separate the labia and gently press the bag's lower rim to the perineum. Then, working upward toward the pubis, attach the rest of the adhesive rim inside the labia majora. For the male patient, place the bag over the penis and scrotum, and press the adhesive rim to the skin.
- After the bag is attached, gently pull it through the slit in the diaper to prevent compression of the bag by the diaper and to allow observation of the specimen immediately after the patient voids. Then fasten the diaper on the patient.
- When urine appears in the bag, put on gloves and gently remove the diaper and the bag. Hold the bag's bottom port over the collection container, remove the tab from the port, and let the urine flow into the container.
- Measure the output, if necessary.
- Label the specimen and attach the laboratory request form to the container. Send it directly to the laboratory. Remove and discard gloves.
- Put the second diaper on the patient, and make sure he's comfortable.

Collecting a culture and sensitivity specimen

Follow the procedure for collecting a random specimen, with these modifications.

- Use sterile or distilled water, an antiseptic skin cleaner, and sterile 4″ × 4″ gauze pads to clean the perineal area.
- After putting on gloves, clean the urinary meatus; then work outward. Wipe only once with each gauze pad; then discard it.
- After the patient urinates, remove the bag and use an alcohol pad to clean a small area of the bag's surface. Puncture the clean area with the needle, and aspirate urine into the syringe.
- Inject the urine into the sterile specimen container. Be careful to keep the needle from touching the container's sides *to maintain sterility.* Remember, a large volume of urine is unnecessary *because only about 1 ml of urine is needed to perform this test.* Then remove and discard your gloves.

Collecting a timed specimen

- Check the practitioner's order for the duration of the collection and the indication for the procedure. Prepare the patient, put on gloves, and clean the perineum as for random specimen collection.
- If getting the bag to adhere is difficult, apply compound benzoin tincture to the perineal area, if ordered, *so that the collection bag will adhere better and you won't have to reapply it during the collection period.* If using liquid benzoin, dip a gauze pad into the medicine cup containing it. If using benzoin spray, cover the genitalia with a gauze pad before spraying *to prevent tissue trauma.*
- Allow the benzoin to dry. Then apply the collection bag, pull the bottom of the bag and the tubing through the slit in the diaper, and fasten the diaper. Remove and discard your gloves.
- Check the collection bag and tubing every 30 minutes to ensure a proper seal *because any leakage prevents collection of a complete specimen.*
- When urine appears in the bag, put on gloves and remove the stopper in the bag's tubing. Then attach the syringe to the end of the tubing, and aspirate the urine. Remove the syringe and insert the stopper into the tubing.
- Discard the specimen and begin timing the collection.
- When the next urine specimen is obtained, add the preservative to the 24-hour specimen container along with the specimen and refrigerate it or keep it on ice, as per your facility's protocol, *to keep the sample stable.*
- Periodically empty the collection bag *to prevent dislodgment of the collection bag.* Each time you remove urine, add it to the specimen container; then use the syringe to inject a small amount of air into the collection bag *to prevent a vacuum, which can block urine drainage.*
- When the prescribed collection period has elapsed (or as nearly as possible), stop the collection and send the total accumulated specimen to the laboratory.

■ Put on gloves and wash the perineal area thoroughly with soap and water *to remove the benzoin;* then put the second diaper on the patient.

Special considerations

■ Whatever the collection method used, avoid forcing fluids *to prevent dilution of the specimen, which can alter test results.* For a random collection or a culture and sensitivity collection, obtain a first-voided morning specimen, if possible.

■ If the collection bag becomes dislodged during timed collection, immediately reapply benzoin and attach another collection bag *to prevent loss of the specimen and the need to restart the collection.*

■ To collect a urine specimen from an infant or a young child with extremely sensitive or excoriated perineal skin, use the inside-out disposable diaper method. Place cotton balls in the perineal area of the diaper to absorb urine. After he has voided, remove the diaper and squeeze urine from the cotton balls into a specimen cup. Alternatively, tape a test tube to a male patient's penis to collect urine.

Complications

Adhesive from the rim of the collection bag can cause skin excoriation.

Documentation

Record the date, time, and method of collection. Also record the name of the test, the amount of urine collected (if necessary), and the time of specimen transport to the laboratory. Document any use of restraints, any complications, and the patient's tolerance of the procedure. Note the patient's and family's responses to any teaching.

SELECTED REFERENCES

Bowden, V., and Greenberg, C.S. *Pediatric Nursing Procedures,* 2nd ed. Philadelphia: Lippincott Williams & Wilkins, 2008.

Pillitteri, A. *Maternal & Child Health Nursing: Care of the Childbearing and Childrearing Family,* 5th ed. Philadelphia: Lippincott Williams & Wilkins, 2007.

TREATMENTS

DRUG ADMINISTRATION

Because a child responds to drugs more rapidly and unpredictably than an adult does, pediatric drug administration requires special care. Such factors as age, weight, body surface area, and drug form and route may dramatically affect a child's response to a drug. For example, because of his thin epithelium, a neonate or an infant absorbs topical medications much faster than an older child does.

Certain disorders also affect a child's response to medication. For example, gastroenteritis increases gastric motility, which in turn impairs absorption of certain oral medications. Liver or kidney disorders can hinder the metabolism of some medications.

Usual drug administration techniques may need adjustment to account for the child's age, size, and developmental level. A tablet for a young child, for example, may be crushed and mixed with a liquid for oral administration. In addition, the injection site and needle size will vary depending on the child's age and physical development.

Equipment

For oral medications: Prescribed medication ■ plastic disposable syringe, plastic medicine dropper, or spoon ■ medication cup ■ water, syrup, or jelly (for tablets) ■ optional: fruit juice.

For injectable medications: Prescribed medication ■ appropriately sized syringe and needle ■ alcohol pads ■ gloves ■ gauze pads ■ cold compresses ■ adhesive bandage.

Preparation of equipment

Check the practitioner's order for the prescribed drug, dosage, and route. Compare the order with the drug label, check the drug expiration date, and review the patient's chart for drug allergies.

Carefully calculate the dosage, if necessary, and have another nurse verify it. Typically, you'll double-check dosages for potentially hazardous or lethal drugs, such as insulin, heparin, digoxin, epinephrine, and opioids. Check your hospital's policy *to learn which drugs must be calculated and checked by two nurses.*

For giving an injection, select the appropriate needle. Typically, for I.M. injections in infants, you'll use a 25G 1″ needle, and in older children, a 23G 1″ needle. For subcutaneous injections, select a ¾″ or ½″ needle and, for intradermal medications, a 27G ½″ needle. To administer viscous medications, select a larger-gauge needle.

Implementation

■ Confirm the child's identity using two patient identifiers according to your facility's policy.

■ Assess the child's condition to determine the need for the medication and the effectiveness of previous therapy.

■ Carefully observe the child for a rash, pruritus, cough, or other signs of an adverse reaction to a previously administered drug.

- Explain the procedure to the child and his parents. Use terms the child can understand.
- Provide privacy, especially for an older child.

Giving oral medication to an infant

- Use a plastic syringe without a needle or a drug-specific medicine dropper to measure the dose. If the medication comes in tablet form, first crush the tablet (if appropriate) and mix it with water or syrup. Then draw the mixture into the syringe or dropper.
- Pick up the infant, raising his head and shoulders or turning his head to one side *to prevent aspiration.* Hold the infant close to your body *to help restrain him.*
- Using your thumb, press down on the infant's chin *to open his mouth.*
- Slide the syringe or medicine dropper into the infant's mouth alongside his tongue. Release the medication slowly *to let the infant swallow and to prevent choking.* If appropriate, allow him to suck on the syringe as you expel the medication.
- If not contraindicated, give fruit juice after giving medication.
- Then place a particularly small or inactive infant on his back *to decrease the risk of sudden infant death syndrome,* as recommended by the American Academy of Pediatrics. Allow an active infant to assume a position that's comfortable for him; avoid forcing him into a side-lying position *to prevent agitation.*

Giving oral medication to a toddler

- Use a plastic, disposable syringe or dropper to measure liquid medication. Then transfer the fluid to a medication cup.
- Elevate the toddler's head and shoulders *to prevent aspiration.*
- If possible, ask him to help hold the cup *to enlist his cooperation.* Otherwise, hold the cup to the toddler's lips, or use a syringe or a spoon to administer the liquid. Make sure the toddler ingests all of the medication.
- If the medication is in tablet form, first crush the tablet, if appropriate, and mix it with water, syrup, or jelly. Use a spoon, syringe, or dropper to administer the medication. (See *Drugs that shouldn't be crushed,* page 914.)

Giving oral medication to an older child

- If possible, let the child choose the liquid medication mixer and a beverage to drink after taking the medication.
- If appropriate, allow him to choose where he'll take the medication, for example, sitting in bed or sitting on a parent's lap.
- If the medication comes in tablet or capsule form, and if the child is old enough (between ages 4 and 6), teach him how to swallow solid medication. (If he knows how to do this, review the procedure with him *for safety's sake.*) Tell him to place the pill on the back of his tongue and to swallow it immediately by drinking water or juice. Focus most of your explanation on the water or juice *to draw the child's attention away from the pill.* Make sure the child drinks enough water or juice *to keep the pill from lodging in his esophagus.* Afterward, look inside the child's mouth *to confirm that he swallowed the pill.*
- If the child can't swallow the pill whole, crush it (if appropriate) and mix it with water, syrup, or jelly. Alternatively, after checking with the child's practitioner, order the medication in liquid form.

Giving an I.M. injection

- Choose an injection site that's appropriate for the child's age and muscle mass. (See *I.M. injection sites in children,* page 915.)
- Position the patient appropriately for the site chosen, and locate key landmarks, for example, the posterior superior iliac spine and the greater trochanter. Have someone help you restrain an infant; seek an older child's cooperation before enlisting assistance.
- Put on gloves. Clean the injection site with an alcohol pad. Wipe outward from the center with a spiral motion *to avoid contaminating the clean area.*
- Grasp the tissue surrounding the site between your index finger and thumb *to immobilize the site and to create a muscle mass for the injection.*
- Insert the needle quickly, using a darting motion. If you're using the ventrogluteal site, insert the needle at a 45-degree angle toward the knee.
- Aspirate the plunger to ensure that the needle isn't in a blood vessel. If no blood appears, inject the medication slowly so that the muscle can distend to accommodate the volume.
- Withdraw the needle and gently massage the area with a gauze pad *to stimulate circulation and enhance absorption.*
- Provide comfort and praise.

Giving a subcutaneous injection

- Select from these possible sites: the middle third of the upper outer arm, the middle third of the upper outer thigh, or the abdomen. You may apply a cold compress to the injection site *to minimize pain.*
- Put on gloves, and prepare the injection site with alcohol.
- Pinch the tissue surrounding the site between your index finger and thumb *to ensure injection into the subcutaneous tissue.* Holding the needle at a 45- to 90-degree angle, quick-

Drugs that shouldn't be crushed

When administering medication to infants and children, remember that not all pills can be crushed for easier administration. The list below shows common drugs that shouldn't be crushed; the reason the drug shouldn't be crushed is shown in parentheses beside the drug name.

Accutane, Amnesteem, Sotret (irritant)
Allegra-D (extended release)
Augmentin XR (extended release)
Avinza (extended release)
Azulfidine EN-Tabs (enteric coated)
Bisacodyl (enteric coated)
Bromfed (slow release)
Bromfed-PD (slow release)
Cardizem CD, LA (slow release)
Ceftin (taste)
Chloral Hydrate (liquid within a capsule, taste)
Chlor-Trimeton Allergy 12 Hour (slow release)
Chromagen (taste, irritant)
Cipro (taste)
Claritin-D 12 Hour (slow release)
Claritin-D 24-hour (slow release)
Colace (liquid within a capsule, taste)
Compazine Spansule (slow release)
Concerta (extended release)
Creon (enteric coated)
Dallergy (slow release)
Dallergy Jr. (slow release)
Deconamine SR (slow release)
Depakene (slow release, mucous membrane irritant)
Depakote (enteric coated)
Dexedrine Spansule (slow release)
Diamox Sequels (slow release)
Dimetapp Extentabs (slow release)
Drisdol (liquid filled)
Dristan (protective coating)
Drixoral (slow release)
Dulcolax (enteric coated)
Easprin (enteric coated)
Ecotrin (enteric coated)
Ecotrin Maximum Strength (enteric coated)
E.E.S. 400 Filmtab (enteric coated)
Entex LA (slow release)
ERYC (delayed release, enteric coated)
Ery-Tab (enteric coated)
Erythrocin Stearate (enteric coated)
Erythromycin Base (enteric coated)
Extendryl SR, JR (slow release)
Feldene (mucous membrane irritant)
Feosol (enteric coated)
Feratab (enteric coated)
Fero-Folic 500 (slow release)
Fergon (slow release)
Fero-Grad-500 (slow release)
Ferro-Sequel (slow release)
Fumatinic (slow release)
Geocillin (taste)
Guaifed (slow release)
Guaifed-PD (slow release)
Guaifenex PSE (slow release)
Humibid DM, LA (slow release)
Iberet (slow release)
ICAPS Plus (slow release)
ICAPS Time Release (slow release)
Kaon-Cl (slow release)
K-Dur (slow release)
Klor-Con (slow release)
Klotrix (slow release)
K-Tab (slow release)
Levbid (slow release)
Levsinex Timecaps (slow release)
Macrobid (slow release)
Metadate CD, ER (extended release)
Methylin ER (extended release)
Micro-K (slow release)
Motrin (taste)
Mucinex (extended release)
M S Contin (slow release)
Norpace CR (slow release)
Oramorph SR (slow release)
Pancrease MT (enteric coated)
PCE (slow release)
Phenergan (taste)
Phenytek (extended release)
Prelu-2 (slow release)
Prevacid (delayed release)
Pro-Banthine (taste)
Procanbid (slow release)
Respaire SR (slow release)
Ritalin-SR, Ritalin LA (slow release)
Rondec-TR (slow release)
Slo-bid Gyrocaps (slow release)
Slo-Niacin (slow release)
Slow Fe (slow release)
Slow-Mag (slow release)
Tegretol-XR (extended release)
Ten-K (slow release)
Tessalon Perles (slow release)
Theochron (slow release)
Theoclear L.A. (slow release)
Theolair-SR (slow release)
Theo-24 (slow release)
Topamax (taste)
T-Phyl (slow release)
Tylenol Extended Relief (slow release)
Uniphyl (slow release)
Vantin (taste)
Verelan (slow release)
Zyrtec-D 12-hour (extended release)

ly insert it into the tissue. Release your grasp on the tissue, and slowly inject the medication. Remove the needle quickly *to decrease discomfort.* Unless contraindicated, gently massage the area *to facilitate the drug's absorption.*

Giving an intradermal injection

- Put on gloves and pull the patient's skin taut (the site of choice is the inner aspect of the forearm).
- Insert the needle, bevel up, at a 10- to 15-degree angle just beneath the outer skin layer.

I.M. injection sites in children

When selecting the best site for a child's I.M. injection, consider:

- the child's age, weight, and muscular development
- the type of drug you're administering
- the amount of subcutaneous fat over the injection site
- the drug's absorption rate.

Vastus lateralis and rectus femoris

For a child under age 3, you'll typically use the vastus lateralis or rectus femoris muscle for an I.M. injection. Constituting the largest muscle mass in this age-group, the vastus lateralis and rectus femoris have fewer major blood vessels and nerves.

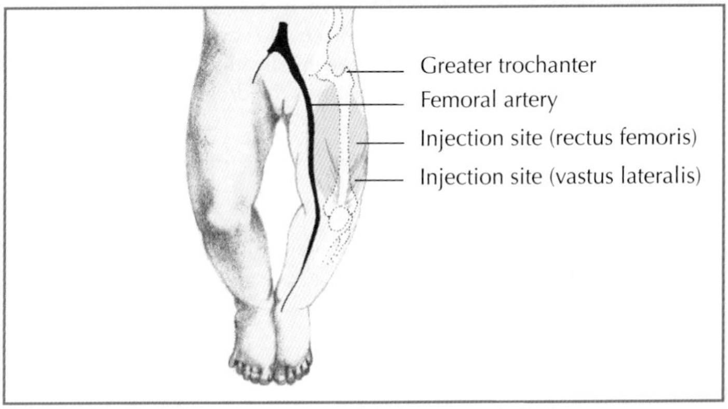

Ventrogluteal and dorsogluteal

For a child who can walk and is over age 3, use the ventrogluteal and dorsogluteal muscles. Like the vastus lateralis, the ventrogluteal site is relatively free from major blood vessels and nerves. Before you select either site, make sure that the child has been walking for at least 1 year *to ensure sufficient muscle development.*

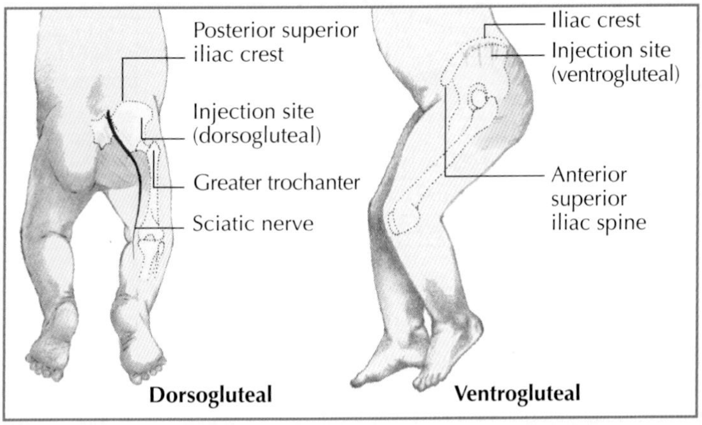

Deltoid

For a child older than 18 months who needs rapid medication results, consider using the deltoid muscle for the injection. Because blood flows faster in the deltoid muscle than in other muscles, drug absorption should be faster. However, be careful when using this site *because the deltoid doesn't develop fully until adolescence.* In a younger child, it's small and close to the radial nerve, which may be injured during needle insertion.

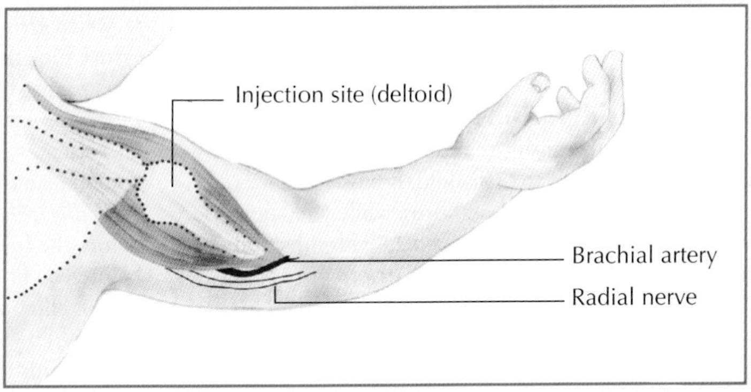

HOME CARE

Using subcutaneous injectors

Available for use by patients at home, subcutaneous injectors feature disposable needles or pressure jets to deliver doses of prescribed medications such as short-acting insulin. Appropriate for use in children, these devices deliver medication safely and accurately. Some brands have disposable needles and replaceable cartridges. Others require the patient to draw medications from standard bottles. A pressure jet deposits the drug in subcutaneous tissue.

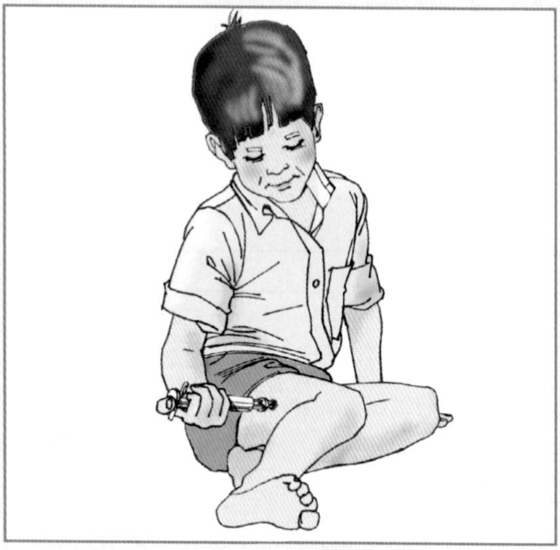

Although still relatively expensive, these devices are easy to use. For example, studies indicate that jet-injected insulin disperses faster and is absorbed more rapidly *because it avoids the puddling effect common with needle delivery.*

Needle injection

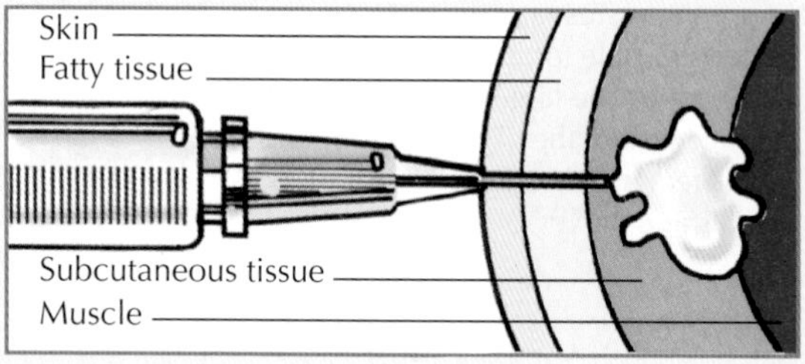

Pressure-jet injection

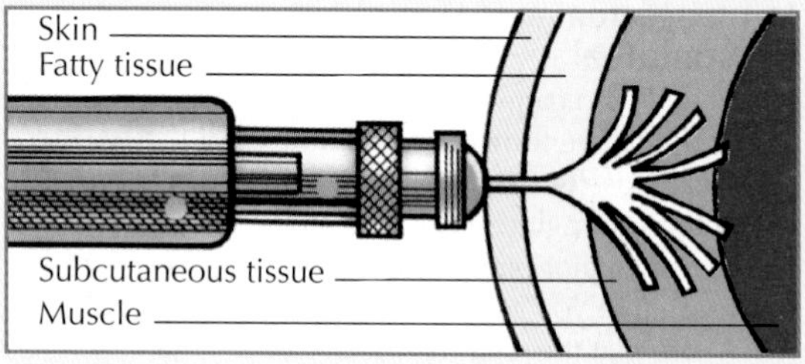

■ Slowly inject the medication, and watch for a bleb to appear. Quickly remove the needle, being careful to maintain the injection angle. If appropriate—for example, if the injection is related to allergy testing—draw a circle around the bleb, and avoid massaging the area *to avoid interfering with test results.*

Special considerations

■ Don't hesitate to consult the parents for tips on successfully giving medication to their child. If possible, have a parent administer a prescribed oral drug while you supervise. However, avoid asking a parent to help with injections *because the child may perceive the parent as a cause of pain.*

■ Aim for a trusting relationship with the child and his parents *so that you can offer support and promote cooperation even when a medication causes discomfort.* If the child will receive one injection, allow him to choose from the appropriate sites. However, if he'll receive numerous injections, remember that site rotation must follow a set pattern. Allow the child to play with a medication cup or syringe and to pretend to give medication to a doll.

■ When giving medication to an older child, be honest. Reassure him that distaste or discomfort will be brief. Emphasize that he must remain still *to promote safety and minimize discomfort.* Explain to the child and his parents that an assistant will help the child remain still, if necessary. Keep your explanations brief and simple.

■ *To divert the child's attention,* have him start counting just before the injection, and challenge him to try to reach 10 before you finish the injection. If the child cries, don't scold him or allow the parents to scold him. Have one of the parents hold a younger child and praise him for allowing you to give him the injection. You can also apply an adhesive bandage to the injection site *as a form of reward or badge.*

■ If the prescribed medication comes only in tablet form, consult the pharmacist (or an appropriate drug reference book) *to make sure crushing the tablet won't invalidate its effectiveness.* Avoid adding medication to a large amount of liquid such as the child's milk or formula *because the child may not drink the entire amount, resulting in an inaccurate dose of medication.*

■ Because infants and toddlers can't tell you what effects they're experiencing from a medication, you must be alert for signs of an adverse reaction. Compile a list of appropriate emergency drugs, calculating the dosages to the patient's weight. Post the list near the patient's bed *for reference in an emergency.*

■ If you have any doubt about proper medication dosage, always consult the practitioner who ordered the drug. Double-check information in a reliable drug reference.

Home care

Teach the parents about the proper dosage and administration of all prescribed medications. If the parents will administer a liquid medication, advise them to use a commercially available, disposable oral syringe to measure the dose. *To ensure an accurate dose,* advise them to avoid using a teaspoon. Teach them how to use the oral syringe. Use written materials — a medication instruction sheet, for example — *to reinforce your teaching.* If appropriate, teach the child and his parents about subcutaneous injectors. (See *Using subcutaneous injectors.*)

Documentation

Record the medication, form, dosage, date, time, route, and site of administration. Document the effect of the medication, the patient's tolerance of the procedure, complications, and nursing interventions. Note instructional activities related to medications.

Selected references

Bowden, V., and Greenberg, C.S. *Pediatric Nursing Procedures,* 2nd ed. Philadelphia: Lippincott Williams & Wilkins, 2008.

Ellis, J.A., et al. "Selling Comfort: A Survey of Interventions for Needle Procedures in a Pediatric Hospital," *Pain Management Nursing* 5(4):144-52, December 2004.

Garcia-Garcia, E., et al. "Long-term Use of Continuous Subcutaneous Insulin Infusion Compared with Multiple Daily Injections of Glargine in Pediatric Patients," *Journal of Pediatric Endocrinology & Metabolism* 20(1):37-40, January 2007.

Hohenhaus, S.M. "Giving Liquid Medications to Pediatric Patients," *Journal of Emergency Nursing* 32(1):69-70, February 2006.

The Joint Commission. *Comprehensive Accreditation Manual for Hospitals: The Official Handbook.* Standard MM 1.10 to MM 7.10.2007.

King, L. "Subcutaneous Insulin Injection Technique," *Nursing Standard* 17(34):45-52, May 2003.

Pillitteri, A. *Maternal & Child Health Nursing: Care of the Childbearing and Childrearing Family,* 5th ed. Philadelphia: Lippincott Williams & Wilkins, 2007.

I.V. THERAPY

In children, I.V. therapy may be prescribed to administer medications or to correct a fluid deficit, improve serum electrolyte balance, or provide nourishment. Primary nursing concerns related to pediatric I.V. therapy include correlating the I.V. site and equipment with the reason for therapy and the patient's age, size, and activity level. For example, a foot or scalp vein I.V. site may be used for infants, whereas a peripheral hand or wrist vein may be more suitable for ambulatory older children.

During I.V. therapy, the nurse must continually assess the patient and the infusion to prevent fluid overload and other complications.

Equipment

Prescribed I.V. fluid ■ volume-control set with microdrip tubing ■ infusion pump ■ I.V. pole ■ normal saline solution or sterile dextrose 5% in water (D5W) for injection ■ antiseptic solution ■ alcohol pads ■ 3-ml syringe ■ child-size butterfly I.V. catheter ■ tourniquet ■ ½″ or 1″ sterile tape ■ catheter securement device ■ gloves ■ optional: air eliminator I.V. filter.

To promote compliance and reduce the discomfort associated with catheter insertion, consider using a transdermal anesthetic cream. (See *Easing the pain of venipuncture,* page 918.)

Preparation of equipment

Gather the I.V equipment and take it to the patient's bedside. Check the expiration date on the I.V. fluid and inspect the I.V. container (an I.V. bag for leakage, a bottle for cracks). Examine the I.V. tubing for defects or cracks. Make sure the packaging surrounding the I.V. catheter remains intact.

Open the wrappings on the I.V. solution and the volume-control tubing set. Close all clamps on the tubing set; then insert the tip of the tubing set into the entry port of the I.V. bag or bottle. (If you're using an I.V. bag, be sure to hold the bag upright when attaching the tubing. *This will keep the sterile air inside the bag from escaping and making the fluid level difficult to read.*)

Easing the pain of venipuncture

For some children, receiving a needle stick—especially during venipuncture—can be a traumatic experience. You can lessen your pediatric patient's anxiety, reduce his pain, and improve compliance during the procedure by applying a transdermal anesthesia cream before the venipuncture. Here are a few guidelines for the use of this cream:

- Transdermal anesthesia cream (commonly known by the brand name EMLA cream) is supplied in a eutectic mixture of lidocaine 2.5% and prilocaine 2.5%. A eutectic mixture has a melting point below room temperature, allowing it to penetrate intact skin as far as the fat layer. The onset, depth, and duration of the anesthesia depend on how long the cream is allowed to stay on the skin. The minimum duration of application is 60 minutes; the maximum is 180 minutes.
- Apply the cream in a thick layer to clean, dry, intact skin at the intended venipuncture site. Then cover it with a transparent occlusive dressing, being careful not to spread the cream.
- Note the time of application on the dressing with a marking pen. When you're ready to perform the venipuncture, carefully remove the dressing. Wipe off the cream, clean the site with an antiseptic solution, and perform the venipuncture as usual.
- EMLA cream is also indicated for pain relief for various other procedures, including lumbar puncture, port access, bone marrow aspiration, insertion of a peripherally inserted central venous catheter, withdrawal of blood samples for arterial blood gas analysis and other laboratory tests, I.M. injection, and superficial skin surgery. It can be used on adults and on children who are at least 1 month old. Local reactions may include erythema and edema. Avoid administering EMLA cream to individuals with a known sensitivity to lidocaine or prilocaine.

Hang the bottle or bag from the I.V. pole. Open the clamp between the bag and the volume-control set and allow 30 to 50 ml of solution to flow into the calibrated chamber. Close the clamp.

Squeeze the drip chamber located below the calibrated chamber or volume-control set *to create a vacuum.* Release the drip chamber and allow it to fill halfway with solution. Then release the clamp below the drip chamber *so that fluid flows into the remaining tubing, removing any air.* After the tubing fills, close the clamp.

If you're using an infusion pump, attach the I.V. tubing to the infusion cassette, and insert the cassette into the infusion pump. Prime the cassette tubing according to the manufacturer's instructions. If you're using an air eliminator I.V. filter, attach the filter to the end of the cassette tubing. *To prevent air bubbles from entering the patient's circulatory system,* place the filter as close to the patient as possible. *To minimize the risk of infection,* maintain sterility at the tip of the I.V. tubing until you connect it to the I.V. catheter.

Cut as many strips of ½″ or 1″ tape as you'll need to secure the I.V. line. Prepare a syringe with 3 ml of flush solution—either the normal saline solution or D_5W.

Implementation

- Confirm the child's identity using two patient identifiers according to your facility's policy.
- Ask the patient (or his parents) whether he's allergic to any type of tape.
- Explain the reason for the I.V. therapy. Reassure the parents, and enlist their assistance in explaining the procedure to the patient in terms he can understand.
- Be sure to have a staff member available to assist you. Inform the parents that the staff member will help the patient remain still, if necessary, during the procedure.
- Wash your hands and put on gloves.
- Select the insertion site for the butterfly catheter. (See *Common pediatric I.V. sites.*) Aim the needle for the most distal site possible, and avoid placing the I.V. line in the patient's dominant arm or in areas of flexion, if possible. Avoid previously used or sclerotic veins.
- *To locate an appropriate scalp vein,* carefully palpate the site for arterial pulsations. If you feel these pulsations, select another site. Then, before inserting the I.V. line, prepare the selected site, as ordered.
- *To find an appropriate peripheral site,* apply a tourniquet to the patient's arm or leg and palpate a suitable vein.
- If you're inserting a butterfly catheter, flush the tubing connected to the butterfly with D_5W or normal saline solution.
- Clean the insertion site with the alcohol pad and antiseptic solution.
- Insert the I.V. needle into the vein. Watch for blood to flow backward through the catheter or butterfly tubing, *which confirms that the needle is in the vein.*
- Loosen the tourniquet, and attach the I.V. tubing to the hub of the catheter. Begin the infusion.
- Secure the device by applying a piece of ½″ tape over the hub. Next, place a piece of tape, adhesive side up, under-

neath and perpendicular to the device. Lift the ends of the tape and crisscross them over the device. (For more information, see *Methods of taping a venous access site,* page 354.) Alternately, you may secure the catheter using a catheter securement device. Further secure and protect the I.V. line, as needed. (See *Protecting an I.V. site,* page 920.)

NURSING ALERT *Remember to use only sterile tape under the transparent dressing.*

- Adjust the infusional flow, as ordered, by using the clamp on the I.V. volume-control tubing or by setting the infusion rate on the infusion pump.
- Add solution hourly (or as needed) from the I.V. bag to the volume-control set.
- Assess the I.V. site frequently for signs of infiltration, and check the I.V. bottle or bag for the amount of solution infused.
- Change the I.V. dressing every 24 hours, according to your facility's policy, or as needed *to prevent infection.* Change the I.V. tubing every 96 hours and the I.V. solution bottle or bag every 24 hours. Label the I.V. bottle or bag, tubing, and volume control set with the time and date of change.
- Change the I.V. insertion site every 72 hours, if possible, *to minimize the risk of infection.* If you inserted the I.V. line without proper skin preparation (during an emergency, for example), change the site sooner.

Common pediatric I.V. sites

Below are the most common sites for I.V. therapy in infants and children. Peripheral hand, wrist, or foot veins are typically used with older children, whereas scalp veins are used with an infant.

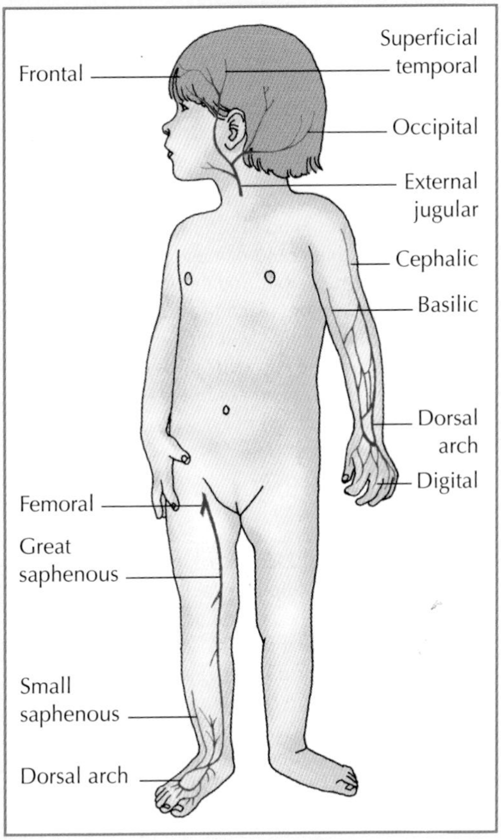

Special considerations

- When selecting an I.V. site, try not to use a site that impairs the child's ability to seek comfort. For example, if an infant typically sucks his right thumb, avoid placing the I.V. catheter in his right arm.
- Forewarn parents if you'll start the I.V. infusion in a scalp vein. Also tell them that you may have to shave hair from a small section of the infant's head.
- Ask an older child to participate in selecting the I.V. site, if possible, *to give him a sense of control.* If the child is mobile, aim for an I.V. site on the upper extremity *so that he can still get out of bed.* Avoid starting the I.V. infusion in the same arm as the patient's identification band, unless you first remove the band and replace it on the other arm, *to prevent potential circulatory impairment.*
- Evaluate the need for restraints after inserting the I.V. line. Apply them only if I.V. displacement seems imminent and other methods (distraction techniques, wrapping gauze around the site) have failed. If you must use restraints, assess the patient's skin integrity and provide hourly skin care *to prevent skin breakdown.* Remove the restraints at frequent intervals *to let the patient move freely.* Encourage the parents to hold and comfort the patient when he's unrestrained.
- *For precise regulation of the I.V. infusion,* use a volumetric infusion pump. These pumps infuse fluids at a predetermined rate regardless of temperature fluctuations, vessel variations, or fluid volume changes. Before using an infusion pump, review the operator's manual.
- After inserting the I.V. catheter, reward preschool and school-age patients. Popular rewards are colorful stickers to wear on clothes or on the I.V. dressing.
- You may apply an antimicrobial ointment over the I.V. site *to prevent infection.*

Home care

- Children who require long-term I.V. medications or nourishment may continue receiving I.V. therapy at home. Assess for conditions that promote successful home I.V. therapy — first and foremost, a patient and a parent (or other

Protecting an I.V. site

Protecting a child's I.V. site can be a challenge. An active child can easily dislodge an I.V. line, which will necessitate your reinserting it—thus causing him further discomfort. A child may also injure himself by dislodging the I.V. line.

To prevent a child from dislodging an I.V. line, first secure the needle or catheter carefully. Tape the I.V. site as you would for an adult, so that the skin over the tip of the venipuncture device is easily visible. However, avoid overtaping the site *because doing so makes it harder to inspect the site and the surrounding tissue.*

If the child is old enough to understand, warn him not to play with or jostle the equipment, and teach him how to walk with an I.V. pole to minimize tension on the line. If necessary, you can restrain the extremity.

You should also create a protective barrier between the I.V. site and the environment using one of the following methods.

Paper cup

Consider using a small paper cup to protect a scalp site. First, cut off the cup's bottom. (Make sure there are no sharp edges that could damage the child's skin.)

Next, cut a small slot through the top rim to accommodate the I.V. tubing. Place the cup upside down over the insertion site, so the I.V. tubing extends through the slot. Then, secure the cup with strips of tape (as shown at right). *The opening you cut in the cup allows you to examine the site.*

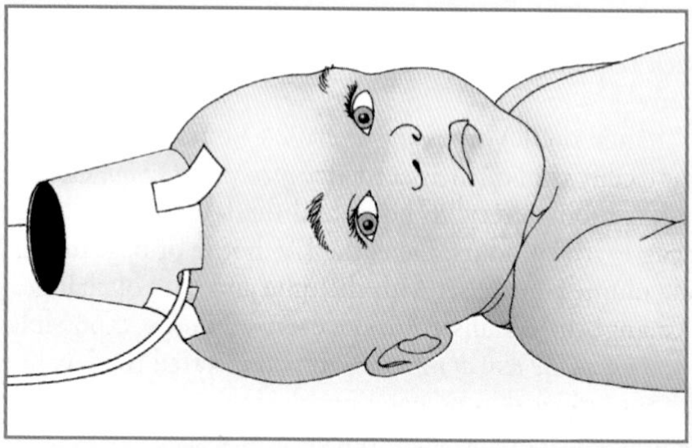

Stockinette

Cut a piece of 4″ (10.2-cm) stockinette the same length as the patient's arm. Slip the stockinette over the patient's arm, and lay the arm on an arm board. Then grasp the stockinette at both sides of the arm, and stretch it under the arm board. Securely tape the stockinette beneath the arm board (as shown at right).

Note: You may also protect a scalp site by placing a stockinette on the patient's head, leaving a hole to allow access to the site.

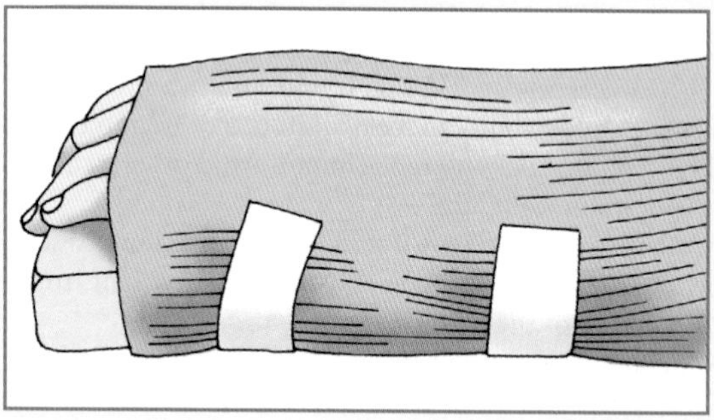

I.V. shield

Peel off the strips covering the adhesive backing on the bottom of the shield. Position the shield over the site so that the I.V. tubing runs through one of the shield's two slots. Then firmly press the shield's adhesive backing against the patient's skin (as shown at right). The shield's clear plastic composition allows you to see the I.V. site clearly.

If the shield is too large to fit securely over the site, just cut off the shield's narrow end below the two air holes. Now you can easily shape the device to the patient's arm.

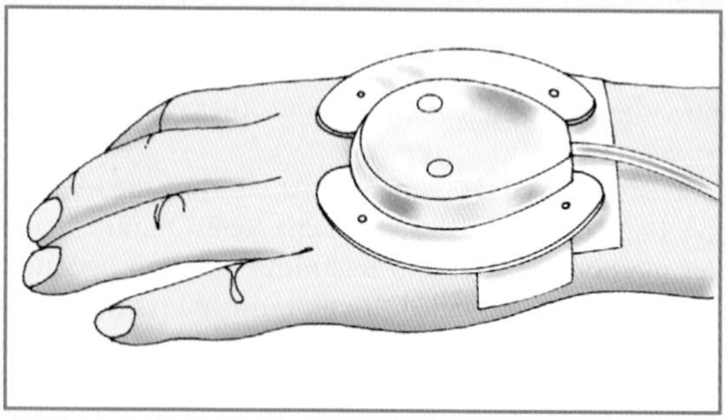

caregiver) who can and want to participate in home I.V. therapy. Other factors include availability of relief caregivers to provide occasional assistance (especially in an emergency); a conducive home environment with electricity, running water, a telephone, refrigeration, and storage space for supplies; an area set up for solution and tubing changes and I.V. site care; and an accessible hospital in case the patient needs emergency assistance or routine reinsertion of an I.V. line.

- Teach the parents (and the patient, if appropriate) how to identify and manage complications, such as site infiltration and clotting in the I.V. catheter. Show them how to operate equipment such as the infusion pump. Supplement verbal instructions with written patient-teaching materials for later reference. Before discharge, watch the parents operate the infusion pump for 24 hours so that you can identify areas in which they need further instruction and skills that require refinement.
- At discharge, arrange for a home health nurse to visit the patient daily for 2 or 3 days to support and guide initial home therapy. Inform the parents that after her daily visits, the home health nurse will probably visit every 2 to 3 days to assess the I.V. site, provide care, and answer questions.

Complications

Complications of I.V. therapy include infection, fluid overload, electrolyte imbalance, infiltration, and circulatory impairment.

Documentation

Record the date and time of the I.V. infusion, the insertion site, and the type and size of I.V. catheter. Note the patient's tolerance of the procedure. Describe patient- and parent-teaching activities. Document the condition of the I.V. site according to hospital policy. If infiltration affects the I.V. site, document the condition of the site at every shift change until the condition resolves.

SELECTED REFERENCES

Centers for Disease Control and Prevention. "Guidelines for the Prevention of Intravascular Catheter-Related Infections," *MMWR* 51(RR-10):1-26, August 2002.

Rosenthal, K. "Tailor Your I.V. Insertion Techniques for Special Populations," *Nursing* (5):36-41, May 2005.

"Standard 14. Documentation. Infusion Nursing Standards of Practice," *Journal of Infusion Nursing* 29(1S):S22-23, January-February 2006.

"Standard 16. Product Labeling. Infusion Nursing Standards of Practice," *Journal of Infusion Nursing* 29(1S):S23-24, January-February 2006.

"Standard 23. Expiration and Beyond-Use Dates. Infusion Nursing Standards of Practice," *Journal of Infusion Nursing* 29(1S):S29, January-February 2006.

"Standard 48. Administration Set Change. Infusion Nursing Standards of Practice," *Journal of Infusion Nursing* 29(1S):S48-49, January-February 2006.

"Standard 51. Catheter Site Care. Infusion Nursing Standards of Practice," *Journal of Infusion Nursing* 29(1S):S57-66, January-February 2006.

"Standard 53. Phlebitis. Infusion Nursing Standards of Practice," *Journal of Infusion Nursing* 29(1S):S58-59, January-February 2006.

"Standard 54. Infiltration. Infusion Nursing Standards of Practice," *Journal of Infusion Nursing* 29(1S):S59-60, January-February 2006.

"Standard 55. Extravasation. Infusion Nursing Standards of Practice," *Journal of Infusion Nursing* 29(1S):S61-62, January-February 2006.

"Standard 56. Infection. Infusion Nursing Standards of Practice," *Journal of Infusion Nursing* 29(1S):S62-63, January-February 2006.

CARDIOPULMONARY RESUSCITATION, CHILD

An adult who needs cardiopulmonary resuscitation (CPR) typically suffers from a primary cardiac disorder or an arrhythmia that has stopped the heart. An infant or a child who needs CPR typically suffers from hypoxia caused by respiratory difficulty or respiratory arrest.

Most pediatric crises requiring CPR are preventable. They include:

- motor vehicle accidents
- drowning
- burns
- smoke inhalation
- falls
- poisoning
- suffocation
- choking (usually from inhaling a plastic bag or small foreign bodies, such as toys and food).

Other causes of cardiopulmonary arrest in children include laryngospasm and edema from upper respiratory infections and sudden infant death syndrome.

Based on the same principle as CPR in adults, the procedure, when performed on children and infants, aims to restore cardiopulmonary function by pumping the victim's heart and ventilating the lungs until natural function resumes. However, CPR techniques differ depending on whether the patient is an adult, a child, or an infant.

For CPR purposes, the American Heart Association defines a patient by age. An infant is under age 1; a child is age

1 to puberty. Survival chances improve the sooner CPR begins and the faster advanced life-support systems are implemented. However speedily you undertake CPR for a child, though, first determine whether the patient's respiratory distress results from a mechanical obstruction or an infection, such as epiglottitis or croup. Epiglottitis or croup requires immediate medical attention, not CPR. CPR is appropriate only when the child isn't breathing.

Equipment

CPR requires no special equipment except a hard surface on which to place the patient and a child-size bag-valve mask, if available.

Implementation

- Gently shake the apparently unconscious child's shoulder and shout at her *to elicit a response.* If the child is conscious but has difficulty breathing, help her into a position that best eases her breathing—if she hasn't naturally assumed this position.
- Call for help to alert others and to enlist emergency assistance. If you're alone and the child isn't breathing, perform CPR for five cycles (2 minutes) before calling for help. One cycle for a lone rescuer is 30 chest compressions and two breaths.
- Position the child in a supine position on a firm, flat surface (usually the ground). The surface should provide the resistance needed for adequate chest compressions. If you must turn the child from a prone position, support her head and neck and turn her as a unit *to avoid injuring her spine* (as shown below).

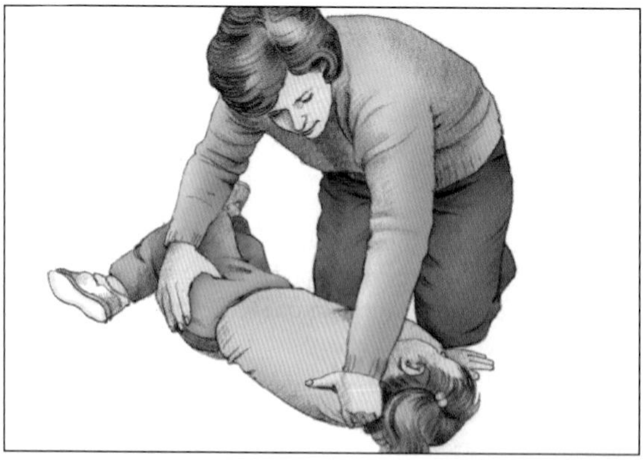

Establishing a patent airway

- Kneel beside the child's shoulder. Place one hand on the child's forehead and gently lift her chin with your other hand to open her airway (as shown top of next column). Avoid fingering the soft neck tissue *to avoid obstructing the airway.* Never let the child's mouth close completely.

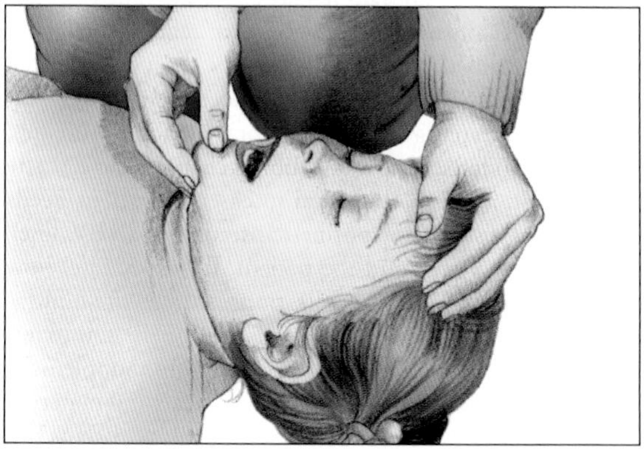

- If you suspect a neck injury, use the jaw-thrust maneuver *to open the child's airway to keep from moving the child's neck.* To do this, kneel beside the child's head. With your elbows on the ground, rest your thumbs at the corners of the child's mouth, and place two or three fingers of each hand under the lower jaw. Lift the jaw upward.
- While maintaining an open airway, place your ear near the child's mouth and nose to evaluate her breathing status (as shown below). Look for chest movement, listen for exhaled air, and feel for exhaled air on your cheek.

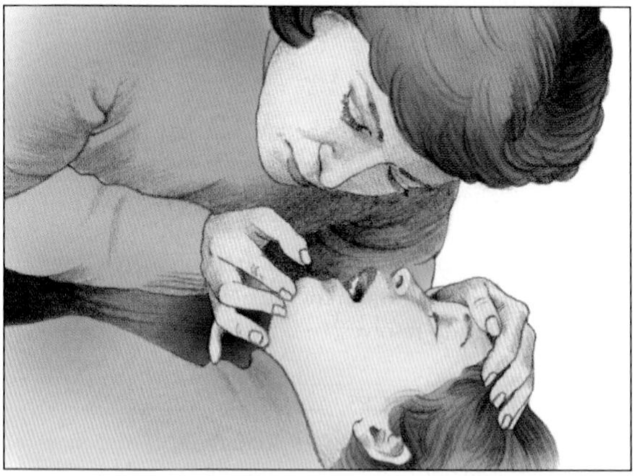

- If the child is breathing, maintain an open airway and monitor respirations.

Restoring ventilation

- If the child isn't breathing, maintain the open airway position, and take a breath. Then pinch the child's nostrils shut, and cover the child's mouth with your mouth (as shown top of next page). Give two slow breaths (1 to 1½ seconds/breath), and pause between each.

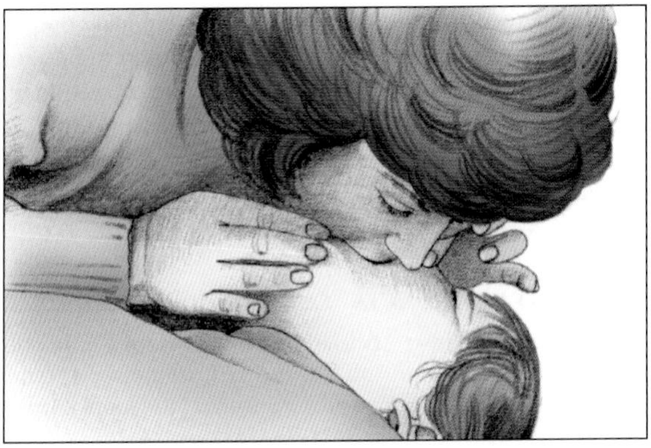

■ If your first attempt at ventilation fails to restore the child's breathing, reposition the child's head to open the airway and try again. If you're still unsuccessful, the airway may be obstructed by a foreign body. (See "Obstructed airway management, child, page 926.")
■ After you free the obstruction, check for breathing and pulse. If absent, proceed with chest compressions.

Restoring heartbeat and circulation
■ Assess circulation by palpating the carotid artery for a pulse.
■ Locate the carotid artery with two or three fingers of one hand. (You'll need the other hand to maintain the head-tilt position that keeps the airway open.) Place your fingers in the center of the child's neck on the side closest to you, and slide your fingers into the groove formed by the trachea and the sternocleidomastoid muscles (as shown below). Palpate the artery for 5 to 10 seconds *to confirm the child's pulse status.*

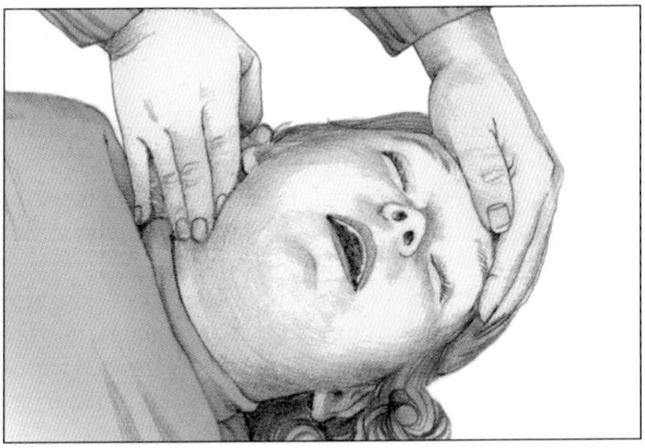

■ If you feel the child's pulse, continue rescue breathing, giving one breath every 3 seconds (20 breaths/minute).
■ If you can't feel a pulse or the pulse is less than 60 beats/minute with signs of poor perfusion, begin chest compressions.

■ Kneel next to the child's chest. Using the hand closest to her feet, locate the lower border of the rib cage on the side nearest you (as shown below).

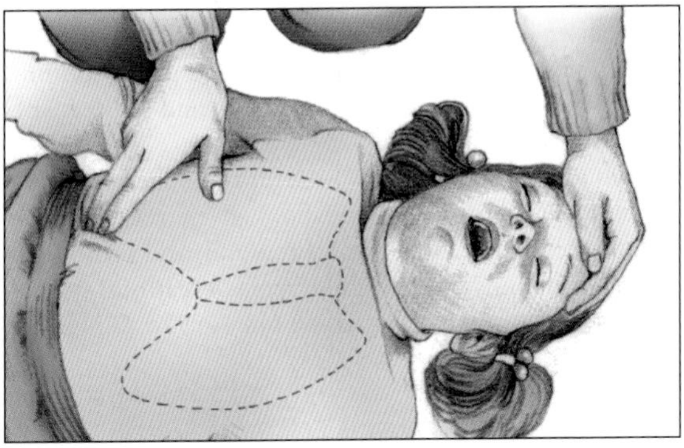

■ Hold your middle and index fingers together, and move them up the rib cage to the notch where the ribs and sternum join. Put your middle finger on the notch and your index finger next to it (as shown below).

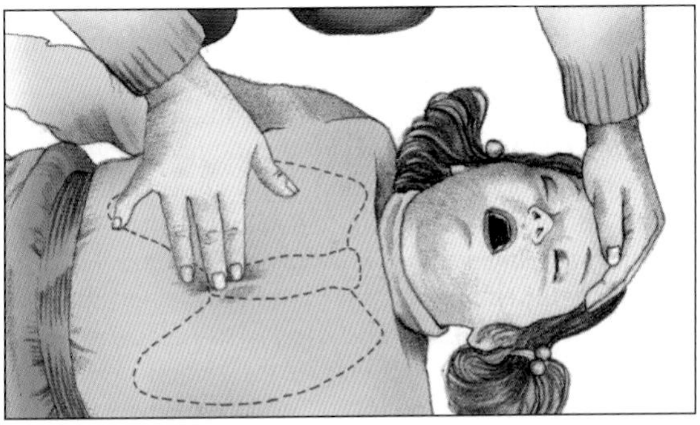

■ Lift your hand and place the heel just above the spot where the index finger was. The heel of your hand should be aligned with the long axis of the sternum (as shown below).

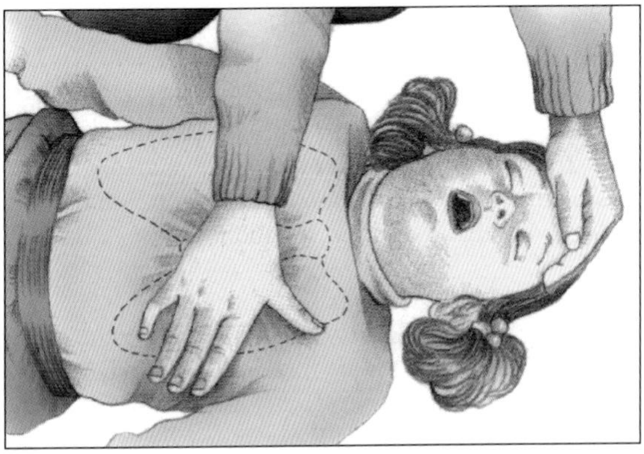

- Using the heel of one hand only, apply enough pressure to compress the child's chest downward ⅓ to ½ depth of the chest. Deliver cycles of 30 compressions and two breaths.
- After five cycles (2 minutes) of CPR, call the emergency medical service and get an automatic external defibrillator (AED), if appropriate. If you can't detect a pulse, continue chest compressions and rescue breathing and use the AED after five cycles.
- If you can detect a pulse, check for spontaneous respirations. If you fail to detect respirations, give one breath every 3 to 5 seconds (12 to 20 breaths/minute), and continue to monitor the pulse. If the child begins breathing spontaneously, keep the airway open and monitor the respirations and pulse.

Special considerations

- A child's tongue can easily block her small airway. If this occurs, simply opening the airway may eliminate the obstruction.
- When performing chest compressions, take care to ensure smooth motions. Keep your fingers off, and the heel of your hand on, the child's chest at all times. Also, time your motions so that the compression and relaxation phases are equal *to promote effective compressions.*
- If the child has breathing difficulty and a parent is present, find out whether the child recently had a fever or an upper respiratory tract infection. If so, suspect epiglottitis. In this instance, don't attempt to manipulate the airway *because laryngospasm may occur and completely obstruct the airway.* Allow the child to assume a comfortable position, and monitor her breathing until additional assistance arrives.
- Persist in attempts to remove an obstruction. As hypoxia develops, the child's muscles will relax, allowing you to remove the foreign object.
- During resuscitation efforts, make sure someone communicates support and information to the parents.
- If available, use a bag-valve mask over the child's nose and mouth when performing ventilations.

Complications

CPR can cause complications if the compressor doesn't place his hands properly on the sternum. These complications include fractured ribs, a lacerated liver, and punctured lungs. Gastric distention, a common complication, results from giving too much air during ventilation.

Documentation

Document all of the events of resuscitation and the names of the individuals who were present. Record whether the child suffered cardiac or respiratory arrest. Note where the arrest occurred, the time CPR began, how long the procedure continued, and the outcome. Document any complications — for example, a fractured rib, a bruised mouth, or gastric distention — as well as actions taken to correct them.

If the child received advanced cardiac life support, document which interventions were performed, who performed them, when they were performed, and what equipment was used.

Selected references

"2005 American Heart Association Guidelines for Cardiopulmonary Resuscitation and Emergency Cardiovascular Care: Pediatric Basic Life Support," *Circulation* 112(Suppl 24):IV-156-IV-166, December 2005.

Mutchner, L. "ABC's of CPR — Again," *AJN* 107(1):60-69, January 2007.

Samson, R.A., et al. "Outcomes of In-Hospital Ventricular Fibrillation in Children," *New England Journal of Medicine* 354(22):2328-39, June 2006.

Cardiopulmonary resuscitation, infant

An adult who needs cardiopulmonary resuscitation (CPR) typically suffers from a primary cardiac disorder or an arrhythmia that has stopped the heart. An infant or a child who needs CPR typically suffers from hypoxia caused by respiratory difficulty or respiratory arrest.

Most pediatric crises requiring CPR are preventable. They include:

- motor vehicle accidents
- drowning
- burns
- smoke inhalation
- falls
- poisoning
- suffocation
- choking (usually from inhaling a plastic bag or small foreign bodies, such as toys and food).

Other causes of cardiopulmonary arrest in infants include laryngospasm and edema from upper respiratory infections and sudden infant death syndrome.

Based on the same principle as CPR in adults, the procedure, when performed on children and infants, aims to restore cardiopulmonary function by pumping the victim's heart and ventilating the lungs until natural function resumes. However, CPR techniques differ depending on whether the patient is an adult, a child, or an infant.

For CPR purposes, the American Heart Association defines a patient by age. An infant is under age 1; a child is age 1 to puberty. Survival chances improve the sooner CPR begins and the faster advanced life-support systems are implemented. However speedily you undertake CPR for an infant, though, first determine whether the patient's respiratory distress results from a mechanical obstruction or an infection, such as epiglottitis or croup. Epiglottitis or croup requires immediate medical attention, not CPR. CPR is appropriate only when the infant isn't breathing.

Equipment

CPR requires no special equipment except a hard surface on which to place the patient and an infant-size bag-valve mask, if available.

Implementation

- Gently tap the foot of the apparently unconscious infant and call out his name.
- For a sudden, witnessed collapse, call for help or call emergency medical services. If you did not witness the collapse, perform resuscitation measures for 2 minutes; then call for help. You may move an uninjured infant close to a telephone, if necessary.
- Place the infant supine on a hard surface.
- Open the airway using the head-tilt, chin-lift maneuver, unless contraindicated by trauma. Don't hyperextend the infant's neck.
- Place your ear near the infant's mouth and nose *to evaluate his breathing status.* Look for chest movement, listen for exhaled air, and feel for exhale air on your cheek.
- If the infant is breathing, maintain an open airway and monitor respirations.

Restoring ventilation

- If the infant isn't breathing, take a breath and tightly seal your mouth over the infant's nose and mouth (as shown below).

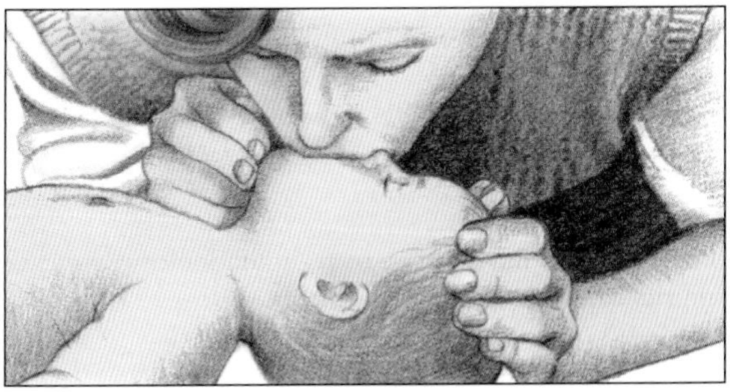

- Deliver two *gentle* puffs of air *because an infant's lungs hold less air than an adult's.* If the infant's chest rises and falls, then the amount of air is probably adequate.
- Continue rescue breathing with one breath every 3 to 5 seconds (12 to 20 breaths/minute) if you can detect a pulse and the pulse rate is greater than or equal to 60 beats/minute.
- Assess the infant's pulse by palpating the brachial artery located inside the infant's upper arm between the elbow and the shoulder (as shown below). If you find a pulse and the pulse is greater than or equal to 60 beats/minute, continue rescue breathing but don't initiate chest compressions.

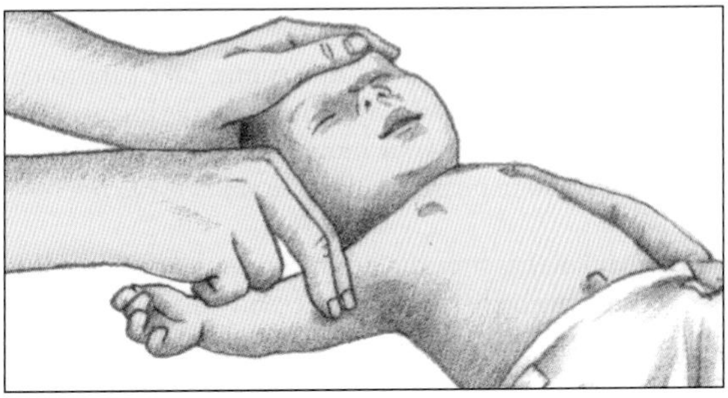

- Begin chest compressions if you find no pulse or the pulse rate is less than 60 beats/minute with signs of poor perfusion. *To locate the correct position on an infant's sternum for chest compressions,* draw an imaginary horizontal line between the infant's nipples. Place three fingers on the sternum, directly below—and perpendicular to—the nipple line. Then lift up your index finger so that the middle and ring finger lie one finger's width below the nipple line (as shown below). Use these two fingers to depress the sternum here ⅓ to ½ the depth of the chest at 100 compressions/minute.

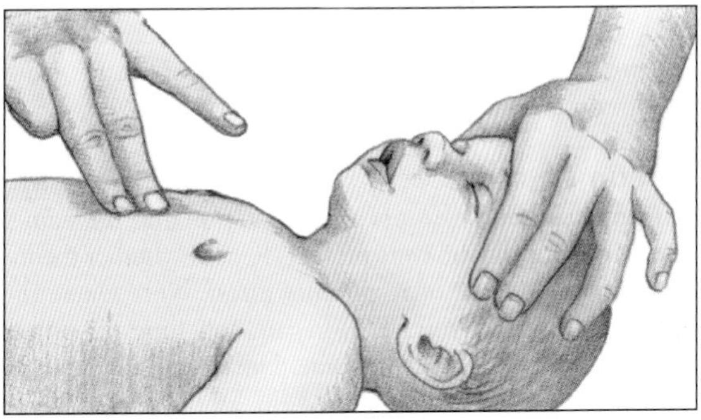

- Supply two breaths after every 30 compressions if you are the only rescuer. If two rescuers are involved, deliver two breaths for every 15 compressions.
- Be aware that, if available, you should use a bag-valve mask over the infant's nose and mouth when performing ventilations.

Special considerations

■ If two rescuers are available, the two thumb-encircling hands technique is preferred for chest compressions. Place your hands around the infant's chest with your fingers around the thorax and place your thumbs together on the lower half of the sternum. Compress the sternum with your thumbs and squeeze your fingers for counterpressure.

■ An infant's tongue can easily block her small airway. If this occurs, simply opening the airway may eliminate the obstruction.

■ When performing chest compressions, take care to ensure smooth motions. Keep your fingers on the infant's chest at all times. Also, time your motions so that the compression and relaxation phases are equal *to promote effective compressions.*

■ If the infant has breathing difficulty and a parent is present, find out whether the infant recently had a fever or an upper respiratory tract infection. If so, suspect epiglottitis. In this instance, don't attempt to manipulate the airway because laryngospasm may occur and completely obstruct the airway. Allow the infant to assume a comfortable position, and monitor her breathing until additional assistance arrives.

■ During resuscitation efforts, make sure someone communicates support and information to the parents.

■ If available, use a bag-valve mask over the infant's nose and mouth when performing ventilations.

Complications

CPR can cause complications if the compressor doesn't place his hands properly on the sternum. These complications include fractured ribs, a lacerated liver, and punctured lungs. Gastric distention, a common complication, results from giving too much air during ventilation.

Documentation

Document all of the events of resuscitation and the names of the individuals who were present. Record whether the infant suffered cardiac or respiratory arrest. Note where the arrest occurred, the time CPR began, how long the procedure continued, and the outcome. Document any complications — or example, a fractured rib, a bruised mouth, or gastric distention — as well as actions taken to correct them.

If the infant received advanced cardiac life support, document which interventions were performed, who performed them, when they were performed, and what equipment was used.

SELECTED REFERENCES

"2005 American Heart Association Guidelines for Cardiopulmonary Resuscitation and Emergency Cardiovascular Care: Pediatric Basic Life Support," *Circulation* 112(Suppl 24):IV-156-IV-166, December 2005.

OBSTRUCTED AIRWAY MANAGEMENT, CHILD

Obstructed airway can occur when a foreign body lodges in the throat or bronchus; when the patient aspirates blood, mucus, or vomitus; when the tongue blocks the pharynx; and when the patient experiences traumatic injury, bronchoconstriction, or bronchospasm. Obstruction causes anoxia, which leads to brain damage and death in 4 to 6 minutes.

If the child or infant is able to cough or make sounds, the airway obstruction is mild, and you shouldn't interfere. If the child or infant can't cough or make a sound, the airway obstruction is severe, and you should intervene by performing abdominal thrusts on a child and back blows and chest thrusts on an infant. Abdominal thrusts aren't recommended for infants because they may damage his liver.

Implementation

■ If the child is conscious and can stand, perform subdiaphragmatic abdominal thrusts (Heimlich maneuver) until the object is expelled.

■ If you see the object, remove it. Never perform a blind finger-sweep on a child because it may push the foreign body farther back into the pharynx and damage the oropharynx.

■ If the victim becomes unresponsive, call for help, and perform cardiopulmonary resuscitation.

■ Before giving rescue breaths, look into the mouth and if you can see the foreign body, remove it.

■ If you don't see the object, attempt ventilations and follow with chest compressions.

Special considerations

■ If the patient vomits, wipe out his mouth *to prevent additional obstruction.*

■ Even if efforts to clear the airway don't seem to be effective, keep trying.

Complications

The child may have nausea or regurgitation or experience injuries caused by abdominal thrusts.

Documentation

Record date and time of procedure and note patient's actions before the obstruction.

Document approximate length of time it took to clear the airway and record type and size of object removed. Note vital signs after procedure and document complications and nursing actions taken.

SELECTED REFERENCES

"2005 American Heart Association Guidelines for Cardiopulmonary Resuscitation and Emergency Cardiovascular Care: Pediatric Advanced Life Support," *Circulation* 112(Suppl 24):IV-167-IV-187, December 2005.

OBSTRUCTED AIRWAY MANAGEMENT, INFANT

Obstructed airway can occur when a foreign body lodges in the throat or bronchus; when patient aspirates blood, mucus, or vomitus; when the tongue blocks the pharynx; and when the patient experiences traumatic injury, bronchoconstriction, or bronchospasm. Obstruction causes anoxia, which leads to brain damage and death in 4 to 6 minutes.

If the infant or child is able to cough or make sounds, the airway obstruction is mild, and you shouldn't interfere. If the infant or child can't cough or make a sound, the airway obstruction is severe, and you should intervene by performing back blows and chest thrusts on an infant and abdominal thrusts on a child. Abdominal thrusts aren't recommended for infants because they may damage his liver.

Implementation

- Regardless of whether the infant is conscious, place him face down so that he's straddling your arm with his head lower than his trunk.
- Rest your forearm on your thigh and deliver five back blows with the heel of your hand between the infant's shoulder blades.
- If you haven't removed the obstruction, place your free hand on the infant's back.
- Supporting his neck, jaw, and chest with your other hand, turn him over onto your thigh.
- Keep his head lower than his trunk.
- Imagine a line between the infant's nipples and place the index finger of your free hand on his sternum, just below this imaginary line. Then place your middle and ring fingers next to your index finger and lift the index finger off his chest.
- Deliver five chest thrusts as you would for chest compression, but at a slower rate. *Don't perform abdominal thrust on an infant because it may damage the infant's liver.*
- Repeat the above steps until you've relieved the obstruction or the infant becomes unconscious.
- If the infant becomes unconscious, call for help, and start to perform cardiopulmonary resuscitation. (See "Cardiopulmonary resuscitation, infant," page 924.)
- Before performing rescue breaths, you should look in the infant's mouth for the foreign body. If you see the object, remove it. *Never perform a blind finger-sweep on an infant because it may push the foreign body farther back into the pharynx and damage the oropharynx.*
- Attempt ventilation and follow with chest compressions until the object is removed.

Special considerations

- If the patient vomits, wipe out his mouth to prevent additional obstruction.
- Persist in attempts to remove an obstruction. As hypoxia develops, the infant's muscles will relax, allowing you to remove the foreign object.

Complications

Complications may include nausea, regurgitation, or injuries caused by chest thrusts.

Documentation

Record date and time of procedure and note patient's actions before the obstruction.

Document approximate length of time it took to clear the airway and record type and size of object removed. Note vital signs after procedure and document complications and nursing actions taken.

SELECTED REFERENCES

"2005 American Heart Association Guidelines for Cardiopulmonary Resuscitation and Emergency Cardiovascular Care: Pediatric Advanced Life Support," *Circulation* 112(Suppl 24): IV-167-IV-187, December 2005.

BRYANT'S TRACTION

Also called *vertical suspension,* Bryant's traction is used primarily to reduce developmental hip dislocations in children. With the patient lying in a supine position in a bed or crib, the traction extends the legs vertically at a 90-degree angle to the body. Even if the disorder affects only one leg, the patient will have traction applied to both legs to prevent hip rotation and to ensure equal stress on the legs and even, bilateral bone growth.

Bryant's traction continues for 2 to 4 weeks. Afterward, the patient may be immobilized in a hip-spica cast. (See "Hip-spica cast care," page 929.) Usually chosen for children under age 2 who weigh 25 to 30 lb (11.3 to 13.6 kg),

Maintaining body alignment and traction

Keeping the child's body in the correct position with Bryant's traction requires precision as well as continual supervision and adjustment.

At the same time that the traction apparatus holds the patient's legs perpendicular to the mattress, you'll need to ensure that his buttocks stay slightly elevated *to provide countertraction* and that his shoulders stay flat and in the same position on the mattress *to maintain body alignment.* The use of weights help maintain the elevation of the buttocks and proper alignment (as shown at right).

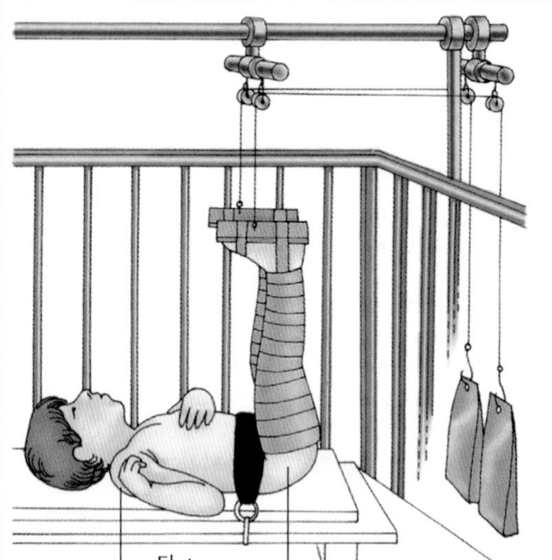

Bryant's traction is contraindicated for heavier children because the risk of positional hypertension rises with increased weight.

Equipment

Traction setup (supplied by the orthopedic department) ▪ moleskin traction straps ▪ elastic bandages ▪ foam rubber padding ▪ cotton balls ▪ compound benzoin tincture ▪ adhesive tape ▪ jacket restraint ▪ optional: clippers, cotton batting, convoluted foam mattress, sheepskin pad.

Preparation of equipment

Assist the physician and orthopedic technician with measuring and cutting the moleskin straps and with assembling the traction equipment.

Implementation

- Thoroughly explain the purpose and function of the traction *to enhance learning and alleviate patient and family anxiety*. If possible, use visual aids to illustrate your teaching. Keep a diagram handy for parents and a doll in traction for the patient.
- Ask the parents whether their child is sensitive or allergic to rubber or to adhesive tape.
- If the patient has hairy legs, clip the hair to ensure good contact between the moleskin traction straps and the skin.
- Apply the compound benzoin tincture, if ordered, to the patient's legs *to protect the skin.*
- Assist the physician or orthopedic technician with placing foam rubber padding and moleskin traction straps against the patient's legs and securing the straps with elastic bandages from foot to thigh. If the patient is allergic to rubber or to adhesive tape, wrap the legs in cotton batting before applying the straps.
- If necessary to keep the patient positioned properly, apply a jacket restraint to keep the weights from pulling the patient forward and altering the tractional force.
- Carefully monitor the circulatory status of the patient's legs 15 minutes and 30 minutes after applying initial traction. Then check circulatory status every 2 hours *to detect any impairment caused by traction.* Assess capillary refill, skin color, sensation, movement, temperature, peripheral pulses, and bandage tightness. If you detect circulatory compromise, loosen the elastic bandages and notify the patient's practitioner.
- Take care to position the elastic bandages precisely. Unless contraindicated, periodically remove the bandages from the unaffected leg *to assess circulation and provide skin care.*

When doing so, have another person hold the traction straps in place *to prevent slipping.* Don't unwrap the affected leg unless ordered to do so by the patient's practitioner.

- Check the patient's position regularly *to ensure optimum traction.* Be sure to raise the patient's buttocks high enough off the mattress *to allow one hand to slide between the skin and the mattress.* Avoid raising the buttocks too high, though, *because this may reduce the effectiveness of traction.*
- Try marking the bed sheet with an "X" at the correct shoulder position *as a guide to correct body alignment.* Near the patient's bed, post an illustration of the correct alignment to guide other nurses and caregivers. (See *Maintaining body alignment and traction.*)
- Provide skin care every 4 hours, focusing especially on the back, buttocks, and elbows — *the areas most prone to breakdown.* Place a convoluted foam mattress or a sheepskin pad — or both — beneath the patient *to help prevent or alleviate skin problems.*
- Inspect the traction apparatus at least every 2 hours *to ensure the correct weight.* Make sure the weights hang freely, the pulleys glide easily, the ropes aren't frayed, and the knots remain snugly tied and taped.
- Encourage the patient to take deep breaths at least every 2 hours *to minimize his risk of developing hypostatic pneumonia.*
- Review the patient's diet *to ensure that he consumes enough fiber and fluid to prevent constipation and urinary stasis.* (Infants should consume about 130 ml of fluid for each kilogram of body weight every 24 hours; toddlers should consume about 115 ml/kg.)
- Promote safety by keeping the side rails raised on the patient's bed whenever you aren't at the bedside.

Special considerations

- To promote regular deep breathing and guard against pneumonia, allow the patient to blow a horn, whistle, pinwheel, or bubbles heartily or encourage him to sing. This promotes lung expansion and enjoyment at the same time.
- *Because a child can't always tell you that he's in pain,* carefully observe his behavior, facial expression, and cry to judge discomfort levels. Besides needing an analgesic or sedative, the patient may need an antispasmodic medication *to relieve irritable muscles and prevent muscle spasms.*
- *To foster development, diversion, and mobility,* provide age-appropriate games and activities as permitted within the confines of traction. For infants, this can include mobiles, music boxes, and rattles. Toddlers may enjoy puppets, large-pieced puzzles, and dolls. Involve the family in their child's care and recreational activities *to increase the patient's sense of security and to minimize the family's anxiety.* If hospital policy permits, consider moving the infant's crib to the playroom *so that he can be around other children.*
- Eating and drinking are difficult and inconvenient for the patient in Bryant's traction because of the head-down position. *To facilitate digestion and encourage eating* — especially if the patient refuses food — place a small pillow under his head at mealtime. If possible, allow him to choose his own foods, and encourage his family to bring food from home.
- *To minimize patient movement,* change bed linens every other day unless the linens get wet or soiled. Keep sheets taut and wrinkle-free *to help prevent skin breakdown.*

Complications

Although generally safe, Bryant's traction may lead to pneumonia from restricted lung expansion resulting from the head-down position. Skin necrosis may result from bandages wrapped too tightly. Other complications include urinary stasis and constipation.

Documentation

Record the date and time that traction was applied, the amount of weight applied, and the patient's circulatory status, skin condition, and position. Note whether weights hang freely. Document changes in the patient's status, and describe the patient's and family's responses to the traction. Also note the patient's and family's responses to any patient teaching.

SELECTED REFERENCES

Bowden, V., and Greenberg, C.S. *Pediatric Nursing Procedures,* 2nd ed. Philadelphia: Lippincott Williams & Wilkins, 2008.

Flynn, J.M., and Schwend, R.M. "Management of Pediatric Femoral Shaft Fractures," *Journal of the American Academy of Orthopedic Surgeons* 12(5):347-59, September-October 2004.

Pillitteri, A. *Maternal & Child Health Nursing: Care of the Childbearing and Childrearing Family,* 5th ed. Philadelphia: Lippincott Williams & Wilkins, 2007.

HIP-SPICA CAST CARE

After orthopedic surgery to correct a fracture or deformity, a patient may need a hip-spica cast to immobilize both legs. Occasionally, the physician may apply a hip-spica cast to treat an orthopedic deformity that doesn't require surgery.

Caring for a patient in a hip-spica cast poses several challenges, including protecting the cast from urine and feces, keeping the cast dry, ensuring proper blood supply to the legs, and teaching the patient and his parents how to care for the cast at home.

Understanding the hip-spica cast

As you talk with parents about their child's hip-spica cast, describe how it will extend from the child's lower rib margin (or sometimes from the nipple line) down to the tips of the toes on the affected side and to the knee on the opposite, unaffected side. Mention that it expands at the waist to allow the child to eat comfortably. A stabilizer bar positioned between the legs keeps the hips in slight abduction and separates the legs.

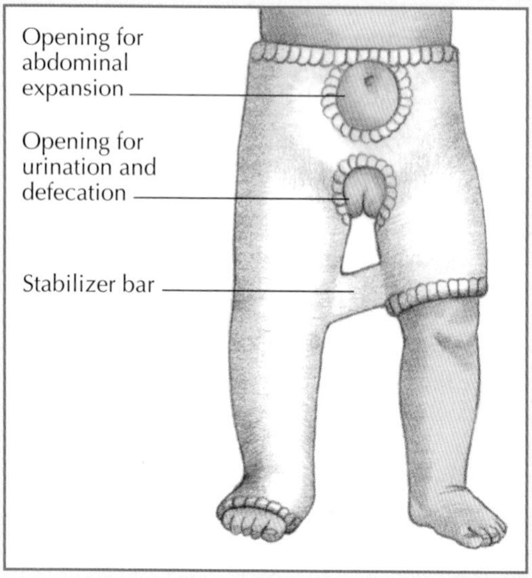

Infants usually adapt more easily to the cast than older children, but both need encouragement, support, and diversionary activity during their prolonged immobilization.

Equipment

Waterproof adhesive tape ■ moleskin or plastic petals ■ cast cutter or saw ■ scissors ■ nonabrasive cleaner ■ hair dryer ■ optional: disposable diaper or perineal pad.

Implementation

■ Before the physician applies the cast, describe the procedure to the patient and his parents. For patients ages 3 to 12, illustrate your explanation. Draw a picture, present a diagram, or use a doll with a cast or an elastic gauze dressing wrapped around its trunk and limbs. (See *Understanding the hip-spica cast.*)

■ After the physician constructs the cast, keep all but the perineal area uncovered. Provide privacy by draping a small cover over this opening. Turn the patient every 1 to 2 hours *to speed drying time.* Be sure to turn the patient to his unaffected side *to prevent adding pressure to the affected side.* If the patient is an infant, you can turn him by yourself. If the patient is an older child or an adolescent, seek assistance before attempting to turn him. When turning the patient, don't use the stabilizer bar between his legs for leverage. *Excessive pressure on this bar may disrupt the cast.* Handle a damp cast only with your palms *to avoid misshaping the cast material.*

■ After the cast dries, inspect the inside edges of the cast for stray pieces of casting material *that can irritate the skin.* (A traditional hip-spica cast requires 24 to 48 hours to dry. However, a hip-spica cast made from newer, quick-drying substances takes only 8 to 10 hours to dry. If made of fiberglass, it will dry in less than 1 hour.)

■ Cut several petal-shaped pieces of moleskin and place them, overlapping, around the open edges of the cast *to protect the patient's skin.* Use waterproof adhesive tape around the perineal area.

■ Give the patient a sponge bath to remove any cast fragments from his skin.

■ Assess the patient's legs for coldness, swelling, cyanosis, or mottling. Also assess pulse strength, toe movement, sensation (numbness, tingling, or burning), and capillary refill. Perform these circulatory assessments every 1 to 2 hours while the cast is wet and every 2 to 4 hours after the cast dries.

■ If the cast is applied after surgery, remember that the most accurate way to assess for bleeding is to monitor vital signs. A visible blood spot on the cast can be misleading: One drop of blood can produce a circle 3″ (7.6 cm) in diameter.

■ Check the patient's exposed skin for redness or irritation, and observe the patient for pain or discomfort caused by hot spots (pressure-sensitive areas under the cast). Also be alert for a foul odor. *These signs and symptoms suggest a pressure ulcer or infection.*

■ *To relieve itching,* set a handheld hair dryer on "cool." Then blow air under the cast. Warn the patient and his parents not to insert any object (such as a ruler, coat hanger, or knitting needle) into the cast to relieve itching by scratching *because these objects could disrupt the suture line, break adjacent skin, and introduce infection.* Also, be vigilant in ensuring that small objects or food particles don't become lodged under the cast and cause skin breakdown and infection.

■ Encourage the patient's family to visit and participate in his care and recreation. This increases the patient's sense of security and enhances the parents' sense of participation and control.

Special considerations

- If the patient is incontinent (or isn't toilet trained), *protect the cast from soiling.* Tuck a folded disposable diaper or perineal pad around the perineal edges of the cast. Then apply a second diaper to the patient, over the top of the cast, to hold the first diaper in place. Also, tuck plastic petals into the cast *to channel urine and feces into a bedpan.* If the cast still becomes soiled, wipe it with a nonabrasive cleaner and a damp sponge or cloth. Then air-dry it with a hair dryer set on "cool."
- Keep a cast cutter or saw available at all times *to remove the cast quickly in case of an emergency.*
- During mealtimes, position older children on their abdomens *to promote safer eating and swallowing.*
- Before removing the cast, reassure the parents and the patient that the noisy sawing process is painless. Explain how the saw works and that it will stop automatically after it cuts the cast.

Home care

- Before discharge, teach the parents how to care for the cast, and give them an opportunity to demonstrate their understanding. Include instructions for checking circulatory status, recognizing signs of circulatory impairment, and notifying the practitioner. Also demonstrate how to turn the child, apply moleskin, clean the cast, and ensure adequate nourishment.
- Teach the parents to treat dry, scaly skin around the cast by washing the child's skin frequently. After the cast is removed, they may apply baby oil or other lotion to soothe the skin. Urge them to schedule and keep all follow-up medical appointments.

Complications

Complications associated with a hip-spica cast come from immobility. They include constipation, urinary stasis, renal calculi, skin breakdown, respiratory compromise, and contractures. Frequent turnings, range-of-motion exercises, incentive spirometry, and adequate hydration and nutrition can minimize complications.

Documentation

Record the date and time of cast care. Describe circulatory status in the patient's legs, and record measurements of any bleeding or drainage. Note the condition of the cast and the patient's skin. Describe all skin care given.

Record findings of bowel and bladder assessments. Note patient and family tolerance of the cast. Document patient- and family-teaching topics discussed as well.

SELECTED REFERENCES

Cassinelli, E.H., et al. "Spica Cast Application in the Emergency Room for Select Pediatric Femur Fractures," *Journal of Orthopedic Trauma* 19(10):709-16, November-December 2005.

Flynn, J.M., and Schwend, R.M. "Management of Pediatric Femoral Shaft Fractures," *Journal of the American Academy of Orthopedic Surgeons* 12(5):347-59, September-October 2004.

Pillitteri, A. *Maternal & Child Health Nursing: Care of the Childbearing and Childrearing Family,* 5th ed. Philadelphia: Lippincott Williams & Wilkins, 2007.

Index

A

i refers to an illustration; t refers to a table.

B

i refers to an illustration; t refers to a table.

C

i refers to an illustration; t refers to a table.

D

i refers to an illustration; t refers to a table

E

i refers to an illustration; t refers to a table.

i refers to an illustration; t refers to a table.

J

K

L

i refers to an illustration; t refers to a table.

O

P

i refers to an illustration; t refers to a table

i refers to an illustration; t refers to a table.

Q

R

S

i refers to an illustration; t refers to a table.

i refers to an illustration; t refers to a table

U

i refers to an illustration; t refers to a table.

V

W

XY

Z